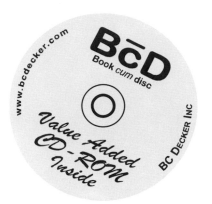
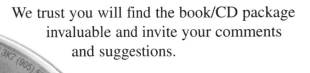

Advanced Therapy in

CARDIAC SURGERY

SECOND EDITION

Advanced Therapy in CARDIAC SURGERY

SECOND EDITION

Kenneth L. Franco, MD

Associate Professor of Surgery
Division of Cardiothoracic Surgery
University of Nebraska College of Medicine
Omaha, Nebraska

Edward D. Verrier, MD

Professor and Vice Chair of Surgery
Chief, Division of Cardiothoracic Surgery
University of Washington School of Medicine
Seattle, Washington

2003
BC Decker Inc
Hamilton • London

BC Decker Inc.

P.O. Box 620, LCD 1
Hamilton, Ontario L8N 3K7
Tel: 905-522-7017; 800-568-7281
Fax: 905-522-7839; 888-311-4987
E-mail: info@bcdecker.com
Website: www.bcdecker.com

ISBN 1-55009-061-5
Printed in Spain

Sales and Distribution

United States
BC Decker Inc.
P.O. Box 785
Lewiston, NY 14092-0785
Tel: 905-522-7017; 800-568-7281
Fax: 905-522-7839; 888-311-4987
E-mail: info@bcdecker.com
Website: www.bcdecker.com

Canada
BC Decker Inc.
20 Hughson Street South
P.O. Box 620, LCD 1
Hamilton, ON L8N 3K7
Tel: 905-522-7017; 800-568-7281
Fax: 905-522-7839; 888-311-4987
E-mail: info@bcdecker.com
Website: www.bcdecker.com

Foreign Rights
John Scott & Company
International Publishers' Agency
P.O. Box 878
Kimberton, PA 19442
Tel: 610-827-1640
Fax: 610-827-1671
E-mail: jsco@voicenet.com

Japan
Igaku-Shoin Ltd.
Foreign Publications Department
3-24-17 Hongo, Bunkyo-ku
Tokyo, Japan 113-8719
Tel: 3 3817 5680
Fax: 3 3815 6776
E-mail: fd@igaku-shoin.co.jp

U.K., Europe, Scandinavia, Middle East
Elsevier Science
Customer Service Department
Foots Cray High Street
Sidcup, Kent
DA14 5HP, UK
Tel: 44 (0) 208 308 5760
Fax: 44 (0) 181 308 5702
E-mail: cservice@harcourt.com

Singapore, Malaysia, Thailand, Philippines, Indonesia, Vietnam, Pacific Rim, Korea
Elsevier Science Asia
583 Orchard Road
#09/01, Forum
Singapore 238884
Tel: 65-737-3593
Fax: 65-753-2145

Australia, New Zealand
Elsevier Science Australia
Customer Service Department
STM Division
Locked Bag 16
St. Peters, New South Wales, 2044
Australia
Tel: 61 02 9517-8999
Fax: 61 02 9517-2249
E-mail: stmp@harcourt.com.au
Website: www.harcourt.com.au

Mexico and Central America
ETM SA de CV
Calle de Tula 59
Colonia Condesa
06140 Mexico DF, Mexico
Tel: 52-5-5553-6657
Fax: 52-5-5211-8468
E-mail: editoresdetextosmex@prodigy.net.mx

Argentina
CLM (Cuspide Libros Medicos)
Av. Córdoba 2067 - (1120)
Buenos Aires, Argentina
Tel: (5411) 4961-0042/(5411) 4964-0848
Fax: (5411) 4963-7988
E-mail: clm@cuspide.com

Brazil
Tecmedd
Av. Maurílio Biagi, 2850
City Ribeirão Preto – SP – CEP: 14021-000
Tel: 0800 992236
Fax: (16) 3993-9000
E-mail: tecmedd@tecmedd.com.br

To our wives and families;
To our teachers, residents, and colleagues; and
To our patients

CONTENTS

PREFACE

Four years have passed since the publication of the first edition of *Advanced Therapy in Cardiac Surgery*. Advances in technology have brought about changes in minimally invasive coronary artery surgery, minimally invasive mitral valve surgery, surgery for atrial fibrillation, and mechanical support for the failing heart. We have gained a better understanding of stem cells and growth factors and of the future role they may play in angiogenesis and cardiac repair. Progress continues in the field of xenotransplantation with the development of alphaGal knockout pigs and new methods to treat acute vascular rejection. We believe it was important to publish the second edition of this textbook now to reflect these advances and also to summarize other changes that have occurred in the field of cardiac surgery. Many new topics have been added and most of the chapters have been written by new authors. We hope readers will enjoy the second edition as much as they did the first.

We wish to express our sincere gratitude to all of our colleagues who took time from their busy practices to help make this textbook possible. The support and dedication of the staff at BC Decker Inc made our lives easier, and for that we are very thankful.

Kenneth L. Franco, MD
Edward D. Verrier, MD
December 2002

CONTRIBUTORS

KEITH D. AARONSON, MD, MS
Assistant Professor of Medicine
Department of Internal Medicine
University of Michigan Medical Center
Ann Arbor, Michigan

GABRIEL S. ALDEA, MD
Professor of Surgery
Division of Cardiothoracic Surgery
University of Washington School of Medicine
Seattle, Washington

ABDULAZIZ A. AL-KHALDI, MD, PHD
Senior Resident
Division of Cardiac Surgery
McGill University
Montreal, Quebec, Canada

KIT V. AROM, MD, PHD
Cardiovascular Surgeon
Cardiac Surgical Associates, PA
Minneapolis, Minnesota

John H. Artrip, MD
Clinical Fellow
Department of Surgery
New York Presbyterian Hospital
New York, New York

DAVID A. ASHBURN JR, MD
Research Fellow
Division of Cardiovascular Surgery
Hospital for Sick Children
Toronto, Ontario, Canada

F. GREGORY BAUMANN, PHD
Research Professor
Department of Surgery
New York University School of Medicine
New York, New York

WILLIAM E. BESCHORNER, MD
Adjunct Professor of Surgery
Department of Surgery
University of Nebraska Medical Center
Omaha, Nebraska

SANDRA G. BURKS, BSN
Department of Surgery
University of Virginia
Charlottesville, Virginia

ANTONIO MARIA CALAFIORE, MD
Chief of Cardiac Surgery
Department of Cardiology and
    Cardiac Surgery
S. Camillo de Lellis Hospital
Chieti, Italy

DUKE E. CAMERON, MD
Professor of Surgery
Division of Cardiac Surgery
Johns Hopkins Hospital
Baltimore, Maryland

ALAIN CARPENTIER, MD, PHD
Professor of Cardiovascular Surgery
Department of Cardiovascular Surgery
Broussais Hospital
Paris, France

BARBARA CATTADORI, MD, MS
Department of Cardiovascular Surgery
Broussais Hospital
Paris, France

JUAN CARLOS CHACHQUES, MD, PHD
Professor of Cardiovascular Surgery
Department of Cardiovascular Surgery
Broussais Hospital
Paris, France

W. RANDOLPH CHITWOOD JR, MD
Professor and Chair
Department of Surgery
East Carolina University School of Medicine
Greenville, North Carolina

RAY CHU-JENG CHIU, MD, PHD
Professor of Surgery
Division of Cardiac Surgery
McGill University
Montreal, Quebec, Canada

ALBERT J. CHONG, MD
Senior Research Fellow
Department of Surgery
University of Washington School of Medicine
Seattle, Washington

JOSEPH C. CLEVELAND JR, MD
Assistant Professor of Surgery
Division of Cardiothoracic Surgery
University of Colorado Health
    Sciences Center
Denver, Colorado

RICHARD P. COCHRON, MD
Surgical Director
Central Maine Heart and Valve Institute
Central Maine Medical Center
Lewiston, Maine

ROBBIN G. COHEN, MD
Associate Professor of Surgery
Department of Cardiothoracic Surgery
Keck School of Medicine
University of Southern California
Los Angeles, California

STEPHEN B. COLVIN, MD
Chief of Cardiothoracic Surgery
Department of Surgery
New York University School of Medicine
New York, New York

JOHN V. CONTE, MD
Associate Professor of Surgery
Division of Cardiac Surgery
Johns Hopkins Hospital
Baltimore, Maryland

MARCO CONTINI, MD
Department of Cardiology and
    Cardiac Surgery
S. Camillo de Lellis Hospital
Chieti, Italy

DENTON A. COOLEY, MD
President and Surgeon-in-Chief
Texas Heart Institute
Houston, Texas

JAMES L. COX, MD
Chair and CEO
The World Heart Foundation
Washington, DC

MICHAEL D. DAKE, MD
Associate Professor of Radiology
Chief, Division of Cardiovascular and
    Interventional Radiology
Stanford University School of Medicine
Stanford, California

RALPH J. DAMIANO JR, MD
John M. Shoenberg Professor of Surgery
Chief, Division of Cardiac Surgery
Washington University School of Medicine
St. Louis, Missouri

MICHELE DI MAURO, MD
Department of Cardiology and
    Cardiac Surgery
S. Camillo de Lellis Hospital
Chieti, Italy

MICHAEL D. DIODATO JR, MD
Research Fellow
Department of Surgery
Washington University School of Medicine
St. Louis, Missouri

JOHN R. DOTY, MD
Division of Cardiac Surgery
Johns Hopkins Hospital
Baltimore, Maryland

ROBERT D. DOWLING, MD
Associate Professor of Surgery
Division of Cardiothoracic Surgery
University of Louisville School of Medicine
Louisville, Kentucky

BRIAN W. DUNCAN, MD
Surgical Director of Mechanical
  Circulatory Support
Department of Pediatric and Congenital
  Heart Surgery
The Cleveland Clinic Children's Hospital
Cleveland, Ohio

NILOO M. EDWARDS, MD
Assistant Professor of Surgery
Director of Heart Transplantation
Division of Cardiothoracic Surgery
Columbia College of Physicians
  and Surgeons
New York, New York

RONALD C. ELKINS, MD
Professor of Surgery
Division of Thoracic and Cardiovascular
  Surgery
University of Oklahoma Health
  Sciences Center
Oklahoma City, Oklahoma

ROBERT W. EMERY, MD
Surgeon-in-Chief
Division of Cardiothoracic Surgery
Minneapolis Heart Institute
Minneapolis, Minnesota

M. ARISAN ERGIN, MD, PHD
Professor of Surgery
Department of Cardiothoracic Surgery
Mount Sinai School of Medicine
New York, New York

ANTHONY L. ESTRERA, MD
Assistant Professor of Surgery
Department of Cardiothoracic and
  Vascular Surgery
University of Texas Medical School
Houston, Texas

VOLKMAR FALK, MD, PHD
Department of Cardiac Surgery
University of Leipzig
Leipzig, Germany

KENNETH L. FRANCO, MD
Associate Professor of Surgery
Division of Cardiothoracic Surgery
University of Nebraska College of Medicine
Omaha, Nebraska

DAVID A. FULLERTON, MD
Professor of Surgery
Chief, Division of Cardiothoracic Surgery
Northwestern University Medical School
Chicago, Illinois

JAN D. GALLA, MD, PHD
Assistant Professor of Surgery
Department of Cardiothoracic Surgery
Mount Sinai Medical Center
New York, New York

AUBREY C. GALLOWAY, MD
Professor of Surgery
Division of Cardiothoracic Surgery
New York University School of Medicine
New York, New York

SANJIV K. GANDHI, MD
Assistant Professor of Surgery
Department of Surgery
University of Pittsburgh
Pittsburgh, Pennsylvania

JOSE P. GARCIA, MD
Assistant Professor of Surgery
Department of Cardiothoracic Surgery
Albert Einstein College of Medicine
Bronx, New York

MAURICIO GARRIDO, MD
Research Fellow
Department of Surgery
Columbia University
New York, New York

JEFFREY P. GOLD, MD
Professor and Chair
Department of Cardiovascular and
  Thoracic Surgery
Albert Einstein College of Medicine
Bronx, New York

BERNARD S. GOLDMAN, MD, FRCSC
Professor of Surgery
Division of Cardiothoracic Surgery
University of Toronto
Toronto, Ontario, Canada

STEVEN M. GORDON, MD
Associate Clinical Professor of Surgery
Ohio State University School of Medicine
Columbus, Ohio

LAMAN A. GRAY JR, MD
Professor of Surgery
Chief, Division of Cardiothoracic Surgery
University of Louisville School of Medicine
Louisville, Kentucky

G. RANDALL GREEN, MD
Surgery Fellow
Department of Surgery
University of Virginia Health Sciences Center
Charlottesville, Virginia

EUGENE A. GROSSI, MD
Professor of Surgery
Division of Cardiothoracic Surgery
New York University School of Medicine
New York, New York

FREDERICK L. GROVER, MD
Professor and Chair
Department of Surgery
University of Colorado Health
  Sciences Center
Denver, Colorado

CHAD E. HAMNER, MD
Surgery Fellow
Department of Surgery
Mayo Clinic Foundation
Rochester, Minnesota

CRAIG R. HAMPTON, MD
Senior Research Fellow
Department of Surgery
University of Washington School of Medicine
Seattle, Washington

DAVID N. HELMAN, MD
Surgery Fellow
Division of Cardiac Surgery
Massachusetts General Hospital
Boston, Massachusetts

ARLEN R. HOLTER, MD
Cardiovascular Surgeon
Cardiac Surgical Associates, PA
Minneapolis, Minnesota

KEITH A. HORVATH, MD
Associate Professor of Surgery
Division of Cardiothoracic Surgery
Northwestern University Medical School
Chicago, Illinois

TAM T. HUYNH, MD
Assistant Professor of Surgery
Department of Cardiothoracic and
  Vascular Surgery
University of Texas Medical School
Houston, Texas

STEPHAN JACOBS, MD
Department of Cardiac Surgery
University of Leipzig
Leipzig, Germany

W. R. ERIC JAMIESON, MD, FRCS (C),
FACS, FACC, CCFP (C)
Professor of Surgery
Department of Surgery
University of British Columbia
Vancouver, British Columbia, Canada

DAVID JAYAKAR, MD
Assistant Professor of Surgery
Division of Cardiac Surgery
University of Chicago Hospital
Chicago, Illinois

VALLUVAN JEEVANANDAM, MD
Professor of Surgery
Chief, Division of Cardiac Surgery
University of Chicago Hospital
Chicago, Illinois

JACOB JOSEPH, MD
Assistant Professor of Medicine
Department of Internal Medicine
University of Arkansas School for
  Medical Sciences
Little Rock, Arkansas

AFTAB R. KHERANI, MD
Research Fellow
Department of Surgery
Columbia University College of
  Physicians and Surgeons
New York, New York

ROBERT C. KING, MD
Assistant Professor of Surgery
Division of Cardiothoracic Surgery
University of Washington School of Medicine
Seattle, Washington

JAMES K. KIRKLIN, MD
Professor of Surgery
Director of Cardiothoracic Transplantation
Division of Cardiothoracic Surgery
University of Alabama at Birmingham
Birmingham, Alabama

JAMES J. KLEIN, MD
Assistant Clinical Professor of Surgery
Department of Cardiothoracic Surgery
Mount Sinai School of Medicine
New York, New York

JON A. KOBASHIGAWA, MD
Clinical Professor of Medicine
Department of Medicine
David Geffen School of Medicine at UCLA
Los Angeles, California

RALF KRAKOR, MD, PhD
Department of Cardiac Surgery
University of Leipzig
Leipzig, Germany

DAVID C. KRESS, MD
Department of Cardiothoracic Surgery
St. Luke's Medical Center
Milwaukee, Wisconsin

IRVING L. KRON, MD
William H. Muller Jr Professor and Chair
Department of Surgery
University of Virginia Health Sciences Center
Charlottesville, Virginia

TIMOTHY J. KROSHUS, MD, PhD
Cardiovascular Surgeon
Cardiac Surgical Associates, PA
Minneapolis, Minnesota

KARYN S. KUNZELMAN, PhD
Director of Surgical Research
Central Maine Heart and Valve Institute
Central Maine Medical Center
Lewiston, Maine

BRUCE W. LYTLE, MD
Department of Cardiothoracic Surgery
Cleveland Clinic Foundation
Cleveland, Ohio

HARI MALLIDI, MD
Surgical Resident
Department of Surgery
University of Toronto
Toronto, Ontario, Canada

HERSH S. MANIAR, MD
Surgical Resident
Department of Surgery
Cornell Medical Center
New York, New York

DAVID W. MARKHAM, MD
Fellow in Cardiology
Department of Internal Medicine
Duke University Medical Center
Durham, North Carolina

PATRICK M. MCCARTHY, MD
Surgical Director, Kaufman Center for
  Heart Failure
Program Director, Heart Transplantation
Department of Thoracic and Cardiovascular
  Surgery
Cleveland Clinic Foundation
Cleveland, Ohio

DAVID C. MCGIFFIN, MD
Professor of Surgery
Division of Cardiothoracic Surgery
University of Alabama at Birmingham
Birmingham, Alabama

PHILIPPE MENASCHÉ, MD, PhD
Department of Thoracic and Cardiovascular
  Surgery
Hospital Bichat
Paris, France

CHARLES C. MILLER III, PhD
Associate Professor of Surgery
Department of Cardiothoracic and
  Vascular Surgery
University of Texas Medical School
Houston, Texas

FRIEDRICH W. MOHR, MD, PhD
Department of Cardiac Surgery
University of Leipzig
Leipzig, Germany

TADASHI MOTOMURA, MD, PhD
Assistant Professor of Surgery
Michael E. DeBakey Department of Surgery
Baylor College of Medicine
Houston, Texas

MICHAEL S. MULLIGAN, MD
Assistant Professor of Surgery
Division of Cardiothoracic Surgery
University of Washington School of Medicine
Seattle, Washington

NORIYUKI MURAI, MD, PhD
Adjunct Instructor of Surgery
Michael E. DeBakey Department of Surgery
Baylor College of Medicine
Houston, Texas

YUKIHIKO NOSÉ, MD, PhD
Professor of Surgery
Michael E. DeBakey Department of Surgery
Baylor College of Medicine
Houston, Texas

MEHMET C. OZ, MD
Associate Professor of Surgery
Director of Cardiovascular Institute
Columbia University College of Physicians
  and Surgeons
New York, New York

FRANCIS D. PAGANI, MD, MS
Associate Professor of Surgery
Division of Cardiac Surgery
University of Michigan Medical Center
Ann Arbor, Michigan

SOON J. PARK, MD
Associate Professor of Surgery
Division of Cardiothoracic Surgery
University of Minnesota School of Medicine
Minneapolis, Minnesota

JIGNESH K. PATEL, MD, PhD
Assistant Clinical Professor of Medicine
Department of Medicne
David Geffen School of Medicine at UCLA
Los Angeles, California

PIERO PELINI, MD
Department of Cardiology and
  Cardiac Surgery
S. Camillo de Lellis Hospital
Chieti, Italy

FRANK A. PIGULA, MD
Assistant Professor of Surgery
Division of Pediatrics Cardiac Surgery
University of Pittsburgh School of Medicine
Pittsburgh, Pennsylvania

TIMOTHY H. POHLMAN, MD
Professor of Surgery
Division of Cardiothoracic Surgery
University of Washington School of Medicine
Seattle, Washington

EYAL E. PORAT, MD
Assistant Professor of Surgery
Department of Cardiothoracic and
  Vascular Surgery
University of Texas Medical School
Houston, Texas

SUNIL M. PRASAD, MD
Surgical Resident
Department of Surgery
Washington University School of Medicine
St. Louis, Missouri

GREG H. RIBAKOVE, MD
Associate Professor of Surgery
Division of Cardiothoracic Surgery
New York University School of Medicine
New York, New York

TODD K. ROSENGART, MD, FACS
Chief of Cardiothoracic Surgery
Evanston Hospital
Evanston, Illinois

HAZIM J. SAFI, MD
Professor and Chair
Department of Cardiothoracic and
  Vascular Surgery
University of Texas Medical School
Houston, Texas

HARTZELL V. SCHAFF, MD
Stuart W. Harrington Professor of Surgery
Chief, Department of Cardiothoracic
  Surgery
Mayo Medical School
Rochester, Minnesota

ZULFIKAR A. SHARIF, MD
Surgical Research Resident
Department of Surgery
Wayne State University School of Medicine
Detroit, Michigan

RAM SHARONY, MD
Research Fellow
Department of Surgery
New York University School of Medicine
New York, New York

WILLIAM D. SPOTNITZ, MD
Professor and Chief
Division of Cardiothoracic Surgery
University of Florida at Gainsville
Gainsville, Florida

LARRY W. STEPHENSON, MD
Professor and Chief
Division of Cardiothoracic Surgery
Wayne State University School of Medicine
Detroit, Michigan

LARS G. SVENSSON, MD, PhD
Director, Center for Aortic Surgery and
    Marfan Syndrome Clinic
Department of Cardiovascular Surgery
Cleveland Clinic Foundation
Cleveland, Ohio

DAVID O. TAYLOR, MD
Director, Heart Failure Special Care Unit
Department of Cardiology
Cleveland Clinic Foundation
Cleveland, Ohio

DORIS A. TAYLOR, PhD
Associate Professor of Medicine
Department of Internal Medicine
Duke University Medical Center
Durham, North Carolina

SANJEEV TREHAN, MD
Staff Cardiologist
Division of Cardiology
St. Francis Hospital
Tulsa, Oklahoma

PATRICIA URSOMANNO, MA
Clinical Research Coordinator
Department of Surgery
New York University School of Medicine
New York, New York

EDWARD D. VERRIER, MD
William K. Edmark Professor of Surgery
Chief, Division of Cardiothoracic Surgery
Vice Chair of Surgery
University of Washington School of Medicine
Seattle, Washington

VENKATARAMANA VIJAY, MD
Assistant Professor of Surgery
Department of Cardiovascular and
    Thoracic Surgery
Albert Einstein College of Medicine
Bronx, New York

GIUSEPPE VITOLLA, MD
Department of Cardiology and
    Cardiac Surgery
S. Camillo de Lellis Hospital
Chieti, Italy

GUS J. VLAHAKES, MD
Associate Professor of Surgery
Division of Cardiac Surgery
Massachusetts General Hospital
Boston, Massachusetts

THOMAS WALTHER, MD, PhD
Department of Cardiac Surgery
University of Leipzig
Leipzig, Germany

GARY D. WEBB, MD, FRCPC
The Bitove Family Professor of Adult
    Congenital Heart Disease
Department of Medicine/Cardiology
University of Toronto
Toronto, Ontario, Canada

STEPHEN WESTABY, MS, PhD, FETCS
Department of Cardiac Surgery
Oxford Heart Center
John Radcliffe Hospital
Oxford, United Kingdom

WILLIAM G. WILLIAMS, MD, FRCSC
Professor of Surgery
Department of Surgery
University of Toronto
Toronto, Ontario, Canada

ANDREW I. YEE, BS
Medical Student
Vanderbilt University School of Medicine
Nashville, Tennessee

CHAPTER 1

USE OF TISSUE SEALANTS IN CARDIAC SURGERY

WILLIAM D. SPOTNITZ, MD, SANDRA G. BURKS, BSN

The field of cardiac surgery remains one characterized by a wonderful blend of challenging pathology, intricate physiology, and significant technical challenge. Present trends toward minimally invasive surgery and procedures on older patients with more advanced stages of illness are creating new challenges for the cardiac surgeon. The already established coagulopathic substrate caused by heparin anticoagulation with or without fibrinolysis from the cardiopulmonary bypass pump establishes an environment in which improvements in methods to achieve hemostasis are clearly beneficial. The evolving and rapidly developing field of hemostats and tissue sealants provides an extremely useful new technology that will be of great value. This chapter discusses the currently approved and available tissue sealants that are effective in cardiac surgery. Both on- and off-label indications, as well as newer uses of these agents, are described.

As the craft of surgery has evolved over many centuries, the use of suture to approximate tissue layers and to close bleeding blood vessels has become a widely established standard form of treatment. Sutures have been available for this purpose since the second century BC.[1] In contrast, however, the use of surgical glue is a recent phenomenon that has gained the attention of clinicians only in the latter portion of the twentieth century. One factor stimulating the development of new surgical techniques has been the explosive growth in the methods of treating coronary artery disease in the twentieth century. Dr. John Gibbons performed the first cardiac operation using cardiopulmonary bypass in 1954. By 1977, more than 300,000 coronary artery bypass graft (CABG) operations were being performed each year.

The prototype of modern surgical glue, fibrin sealant, was first available in Europe in 1972. Although widely used outside of the United States for 25 years, this agent did not initially receive approval from the United States Food and Drug Administration (FDA). The FDA was concerned about the risk of viral disease transmission with this two-component pooled-plasma tissue-adhesive product and thus withheld approval. More recently,

clinical trials demonstrating efficacy of these products have been subject to concerns over clinical relevance beyond statistical significance. However, as consensus is building over the value of these agents, the ability to obtain market approval appears to be increasing. The FDA approved fibrin sealant in May 1998, with indications including hemostasis in cardiac and splenic surgery, as well as colonic sealing. Since 1998, multiple new agents have received approval for use, and new generations of agents are undergoing laboratory evaluation as well as clinical testing. Thus, the field of tissue sealants is a new and growing field that should provide multiple valuable materials for use by the cardiac surgeon.

A simple analogy gives insight into the value of these new surgical sealants. To best facilitate the manipulation of surgical tissue, a skilled surgeon, much as an accomplished cabinetmaker, must have the appropriate tools. The master cabinetmaker has a wide variety of saws to choose from, as does a skilled surgeon in choosing the appropriate scalpel or scissors. Similarly, the cabinetmaker has different screws and nails with which to join materials, and the surgeon has a variety of different suture materials, which are best suited for particular situations requiring tissue apposition. The cabinetmaker also uses glue as an important element in the creation of fine furniture. Until recently, however, the surgeon has not had the ability to use surgical glues or sealants. Thus, these new agents are an extremely important and valuable new addition to the surgical armamentarium. These materials are particularly useful for the cardiac surgeon whose specialty requires the utmost precision and technical expertise. The cardiac surgeon, much as the master artisan of fine furniture, now has a useful new class of adhesives that can be extremely helpful in facilitating successful clinical outcomes.

It can be useful to consider additional elements of the artisan analogy. The skills of a fine cabinetmaker are acquired over a number of years in a process that may require mentoring by a capable, competent, and caring mentor. A similar training period has been the mainstay of clinical cardiac surgery. During this period of training, the surgeon develops clinical skill in manipulating tissues as well as clinical judgment in the care of patients. The use of surgical adhesives, being a new technology, has not been an integral part of the educational process of young surgeons in training. Thus, their experience with these agents is relatively recent and underdeveloped. The new surgical hemostats and tissue adhesives are associated with a learning curve. Each agent requires its own appropriate indication, specific method of preparation, and application technique. Thus, it is important to get both cognitive and hands-on knowledge of the appropriate uses of these agents. Inappropriate use of these materials can limit their success and minimize their value to the surgeon.

In addition to the agents discussed in this chapter, new agents are presently under development and are being introduced rapidly into the marketplace. Each of these agents can be judged against the standard of an ideal tissue adhesive. The characteristics of an ideal tissue adhesive (Table 1-1) include efficacy, safety, usability, affordability, and approvability.[2] For these agents to be licensed by the FDA, they must be safe and effective. If an agent is considered safe, there must be no adverse effects in either the long- or short-term as a result of the agent or its metabolites. There must be no risk of infection, tissue injury or destruction, or carcinogenicity as a result of using the material. In terms of efficacy, the material should be capable of performing in an objectively measured and clinically appreciated manner. In other words, the agent must provide a statistically significant and, most importantly, clinically relevant benefit in patients. The issue of efficacy can be a particularly challenging one. Efficacy of these agents for each surgical specialty may be different, and even within a surgical specialty, efficacy varies from one specific application to another. For example, a cardiac surgeon who desires to seal a vascular anastomosis and to prevent bleeding needs an agent that can prevent needle-hole bleeding and that can seal weakened tissues. It may be desirable to have the agent exhibit these activities prior to removing vascular clamps and pressurizing an anastomosis. On the other hand, after the vascular clamps are removed and bleeding is evident at an anastomosis, it may be desirable to have an agent that can effectively stop active bleeding at a specific site. Thus, efficacy, even in a limited application such as anastomotic hemostasis, may require different capabilities. A liquid agent can be very effective at providing hemostasis and sealing an anastomosis prior to active hemorrhage after the removal of vascular clamps. However, a more substantial material may be required to stop active bleeding, as a liquid agent could be easily washed away by the flow of blood. Thus, efficacy can be different depending upon the specific surgical application.

Usability is also a critical element in allowing surgical sealants to be used in the operating room. To use these agents, the material frequently has to be reconstituted and prepared by the operating room staff. A complex and time-consuming reconstitution procedure for the tissue adhesive makes the agent harder to use and reduces surgeon and nurse enthusiasm for the material. An agent requiring a prolonged period of preparation also requires significant anticipation on behalf of the staff in order for it to be ready. This anticipation can result in a costly wasting of an agent if it is later determined that the agent is no longer required. Thus, the most useful agent is rapidly reconstitutable and does not require specialized storage facilities; instead, it can be kept on the operating room shelf. Also inherent in the concept of usability is the degree to which specialized applicators are available for delivering the tissue sealant to the appropriate surgical site. For example, a linear suture line may require a specific applicator capable of providing tissue sealant to a limited area with specific precise control of the flow of sealant. On the other hand, application to a large diffuse bleeding area may require a spray device capable of delivering efficiently and effectively the material over a broad surface. Additional examples include comparison of the applicators required for efficient use during a cardiac surgical operation requiring a median sternotomy versus a procedure performed through a smaller incision that may require a thoracoscope. The design and choice of specific applicators are critical elements in the successful use of tissue sealants.

Affordability is an important element because cost-effectiveness is under continuous review and health care dollars are limited and carefully monitored. The cost of an ideal tissue adhesive may be the most significant element in its success in the marketplace. The cost-effectiveness of surgical tissue sealants can be increased by achieving a reduction in operating room time, hospital length of stay, and outpatient recovery time. However, additional supporting data with respect to cost issues are still required as the present number of studies proving cost-effectiveness is extremely limited. Finally, approvability or the ability of the tissue adhesive to obtain licensure by the FDA, and hence market access, is an essential element. It took fibrin sealant 25 years to gain approval for use in the United States. It is hoped that newer agents entering the marketplace can be designed and tested so that the approval process is facilitated while maintaining excellent standards of safety and efficacy.

TABLE 1-1. Characteristics of an Ideal Tissue Adhesive

1. Safety	The product and its metabolites must produce no short- or long-term negative effects.
2. Efficacy	The agent must be proven scientifically and clinically effective.
3. Usability	The material must be easily reconstitutable in the operating room and applicable in an efficient manner.
4. Cost	The use of the adhesive should reduce the overall cost of the procedure.
5. Approvability	The licensure of the product should be obtainable within a reasonable period of time.

The following sections discuss the currently available tissue adhesives that may be useful for the cardiac surgeon in detail. These agents represent the first generation of materials of this type, but they are already proving very useful to the surgeon experienced in their capabilities. In addition to the obvious on-label clinical benefits of the agents, off-label additional advantages of these agents, including the ability to provide the capacity for drug delivery and tissue engineering, are illustrated.

Available Agents

Each of the available agents is reviewed below. All are FDA approved and discussed in the order of market approval since May 1998 (Table 1-2).

Fibrin Sealant

Fibrin sealant received approval by the FDA in May 1998. On-label indications include use as a hemostatic agent in cardiac surgical operations and in splenic trauma repair.[3] It is also approved for sealing colonic anastomoses at the time of colostomy closure. The commercial form of fibrin sealant comes as a two-component liquid with hemostatic and adhesive properties. It consists of concentrated human thrombin and fibrinogen containing trace amounts of calcium and factor XIII. The materials are derived from pooled human plasma. The fibrinogen in the presence of thrombin is cleaved and cross-linked to produce the final form of the fibrin sealant. The mixture contains bovine aprotinin, which functions as a stabilizer of fibrin and retards fibrinolysis. Polymerization of the fibrin sealant from the liquid components to a gel form

takes approximately 15 s, and reaches its final stage within approximately 2 min. The strength of fibrin sealant is influenced by the concentration of fibrinogen, and the speed of the polymerization process is regulated by the concentration of thrombin. The FDA has approved distribution of fibrin sealant by two different companies, which both market the identical product (Tisseel VH, Baxter Healthcare, Glendale, California, and Hemaseel APR, Haemacure Corporation, Sarasota, Florida).

Because both the fibrinogen and thrombin components of fibrin sealant are derived from human plasma, there is a potential risk of viral or other blood-borne disease transmission. To minimize this risk, donors are screened to eliminate those at highest risk for blood-borne diseases, and the product undergoes heat pasteurization and ultrafiltration. These methods are designed to enhance viral inactivation. To date, there are no documented cases of hepatitis or human immunodeficiency virus transmission from this product in more than 5 million cases worldwide. Because the product contains bovine aprotinin used as an antifibrinolytic in order to modify the rate of fibrin sealant degradation, there is a small risk of allergic reaction. Reports of complications with fibrin sealant in its present commercial form are rare.

Fibrin sealant components must be stored in a refrigerator at 2 to 6°C. The components are supplied as lyophilized powders, which must be reconstituted in a mixing and thawing process that includes saline containing calcium chloride and bovine aprotinin. The entire reconstitution process takes approximately 20 min and requires a special device supplied by the manufacturers to

TABLE 1-2. The Uses of Currently Approved Tissue Adhesives

Brand Names	Components	FDA Approval	Indications
Tisseel VH; Hemaseel APR	Fibrin sealant (pooled human plasma)	May 1998	Biologic hemostatic agent used in cardiopulmonary bypass procedures and splenic trauma, and for sealing of anastomoses in the closure of temporary colostomies.
Dermabond	2-Octyl-cyanoacrylate	August 1998	Device for topical closure of external lacerations and simple incisions.
FloSeal	Bovine collagen and bovine thrombin	December 1999	Device approved for surgical procedures (other than ophthalmic and urologic) as an adjunct to hemostasis when control of bleeding by ligature or conventional procedures is ineffective or impractical.
CoStasis	Bovine collagen and bovine thrombin + autologous human plasma	June 2000	Sprayable liquid hemostatic device for cardiovascular, general, hepatic, and orthopedic surgery.
FocalSeal-L	PEG polymer/hydrogel	May 2000	Light-activated synthetic device approved as an adjunct to standard closure of visceral pleural air leaks incurred during elective pulmonary resection.
BioGlue	Bovine albumin cross-linked with glutaraldehyde	Human Device Exemption: December 1999; full approval: December 2001	Device approved as an adjunct to standard methods of achieving hemostasis in adult patients with open surgical repair of large vessels (such as aorta, femoral, and carotid arteries).
CoSeal	PEG polymer/hydrogel	December 2001	Totally synthetic device approved for use in sealing arterial and/or venous reconstruction.

facilitate the mixing and thawing process. The reconstituted components are mixed during the application and begin to set up within 15 s of application to the clinical site. The commercial manufacturer provides fibrinogen as a concentration of 75 to 115 mg/mL to enhance the strength of the product, and thrombin at a concentration of 500 IU/mL in order to facilitate the rate of reaction. The sealant is distributed in a 1 mL kit that contains 1 mL of fibrinogen and 1 mL of thrombin and costs $75 to $100 (US) per milliliter. The 1 mL kit produces 2 mL of the final fibrin sealant. Larger volume kits, specifically 2 mL and 5 mL, are available.

The advantages of the commercial product include high concentrations of fibrinogen and thrombin, which enhance the strength and rapidity of polymerization, thus increasing the usefulness of the agent in the operating room. Also, the addition of aprotinin as a stabilizer enhances the stability of the sealant, making it resistant to fibrinolysis. Because the components of the adhesive are virally inactivated, the risk of blood-borne disease transmission appears to be significantly reduced. This commercial form of fibrin sealant also avoids the use of topical bovine thrombin.

Additional methods of producing fibrin sealant were developed prior to the FDA's May 1998 approval of the commercial product. Specifically, surgeons used concentrated solutions of fibrinogen combined with topical bovine thrombin to produce fibrin sealant. Blood bank cryoprecipitate can be used as a source of concentrated fibrinogen, or a concentrated fibrinogen can be obtained from the patient's own blood or from outdated units of plasma devoid of unstable clotting factors.[4,5] Methods of obtaining fibrinogen from the patient's own blood have the advantage of reducing the likelihood of blood-borne disease transmission. The use of outdated acutely frozen plasma avoids the waste of unstable clotting factors that are present in routine cryoprecipitate and is a valuable means of reversing coagulopathies in patients requiring the intravenous administration of clotting factors. The fibrinogen concentrations that can be obtained using cold or chemical precipitation techniques are less than those in the commercial product. Specifically, they vary between 15 and 35 mg/mL. Thus, this material may be weaker than that which is obtainable commercially. An additional limitation of the noncommercial form of fibrin sealant produced in the blood bank is that there is no stand-alone human thrombin product presently available in the United States. Thus, in order to produce fibrin sealant, it is necessary to combine concentrated human fibrinogen with the commercially available topical bovine thrombin. Reports of coagulopathy as a result of the use of topical bovine thrombin exist.[6,7] This is believed to occur when the body produces an antibody response to impurities in the bovine thrombin which can cross-react with the body's own clotting factors producing a coagulopathic state.

There is literature supporting fibrin sealant use in a wide variety of on- and off-label applications. Reports exist using both the commercial and blood bank–derived products.[8,9] In fact, the use of fibrin sealant in cardiac surgical procedures appears to account for the majority of fibrin sealant presently employed. This occurs predominantly in reoperation CABG procedures, valve replacements or repairs, complex congenital heart operations, and surgery on the aorta. It can be used to seal suture lines (Figures 1-1 and 1-2), vascular conduits, cannulation sites, vascular anastomoses, patches, dissections, catheterization sites, and diffusely bleeding surfaces. Particularly in reoperative cardiac surgery (Figures 1-3 and 1-4), fibrin sealant can be used to stop diffuse bleeding from the mediastinum secondary to scarring and adhesion. It may reduce the perioperative need for blood products.

There are two types of primary application devices for fibrin sealant available through the commercial manufacturers. One device is capable of providing for linear application of the sealant by using a dual syringe holder that allows for mixing of the components and delivery

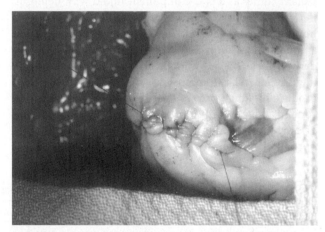

FIGURE 1-1. Closure of the apex of the left ventricle at the site of an aneurysm repair.

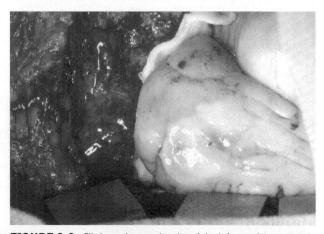

FIGURE 1-2. Fibrin sealant at the site of the left ventricle aneurysm repair after application by using a gas-driven spray applicator.

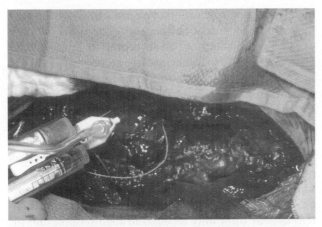

FIGURE 1-3. Spray application of fibrin sealant to stop capillary bleeding following reoperation CABG with mitral valve repair.

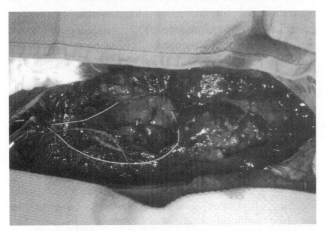

FIGURE 1-4. Operative field after completed spray application of fibrin sealant.

through a 19-gauge needle tip. This precise applicator tip is well suited for applying the sealant to localized suture lines but may clog if repeated applications are required. The manufacturers provide multiple tips to remedy this problem. The second major application method is a gas-driven spray application device. This device provides for the broad application of small aerosolized droplets of the adhesive components. Excellent mixing is produced over a wide surface area. This may result in a more efficient use of fibrin sealant and may reduce the volume of agent required for a specific application, resulting in improved cost-effectiveness. A variety of other catheter tips and handheld spray tips are also available for the discerning clinician.

There is a learning curve for the appropriate use of any of these new agents; it consists of hands-on use of the material and related device applicators. To most effectively apply fibrin sealant as a hemostat, the site of intended application must be as dry as possible. Because the agent is applied in a liquid form it is desirable to minimize active bleeding at the application site prior to appli-

cation of the sealant. Otherwise, during the period of polymerization, active bleeding washes away the liquid fibrin sealant before it can harden and produce hemostasis. One example of a method to reduce active bleeding to facilitate the application of fibrin sealant is the application of fibrin sealant to cardiovascular anastomoses prior to the release of cross-clamps. In this setting, the blood vessel is not pressurized and the fibrin sealant can be applied and polymerized prior to pressurization of the vessel and the development of active bleeding. If 2 to 3 min can be permitted for the formation of the fibrin sealant prior to release of vascular clamps, the fibrin sealant is very effective at reducing hemorrhage. Because fibrin sealant has polymerized in a relatively bloodless field in this setting, it is maximally effective at achieving hemostasis. Such an application of fibrin sealant, however, requires anticipation on the part of the surgeon. Specifically, the 20-min preparation time makes it necessary for the operating surgeon to request this material in advance of its use so that the circulating staff in the operating room can have it prepared before it is required. After reconstitution, fibrin sealant remains usable for approximately 4 h.

Although the application of fibrin sealant to a relatively bloodless field is desirable, this is not always practical. In such a case, the use of a carrier sponge of cellulose or collagen can be extremely helpful.[9] The sponge can be soaked in fibrinogen and then activated with thrombin just prior to application. The sponge is then applied to the active bleeding site. Thus, the sponge serves as a method of carrying the fibrin sealant to the bleeding site and achieves hemostasis through the manual pressure of the surgeon's hand on the sponge against the bleeding site. If bleeding is controlled for the 2 to 3 min required for the polymerization of the fibrin sealant by using this technique, effective hemostasis will be achieved. Obviously, if bleeding continues, in spite of the pressure on the sponge, effective hemostasis will likely not be achieved after 2 to 3 min of pressure. This carrier sponge method of fibrin sealant delivery is the most effective means of using this agent to control active bleeding and can be a very valuable adjunct to cardiac surgical procedures. It must be remembered that the best treatment for an actively bleeding blood vessel is the placement of an appropriate suture by using excellent surgical technique. However, if the bleeding is not suturable, fibrin sealant may be an excellent adjunctive method for achieving hemostasis.

A particular note of caution should be provided to the cardiac surgeon using fibrin sealant or any other thrombin-containing tissue hemostat or sealant. The use of heparin during cardiopulmonary bypass and vascular surgical procedures to avoid thrombosis is a mainstay of modern surgery. The last step in the clotting cascade, where heparin has its effect, is at the level of thrombin. Thus, a competitive interaction of exogenous thrombin and heparin can occur that may result in a reversal of the heparin effect, causing thrombosis. This can be particularly significant for a patient on cardiopulmonary bypass and could potentially result in thrombosis of the cardiopulmonary bypass pump. Patients in whom fibrin sealant is being used while on cardiopulmonary bypass should have the residual fibrin sealant components removed from the operative field by using the discard sucker. Do not use the pump sucker to clear these components; in fact, pump suckers should be removed from the operative field when fibrin sealant is being used. A second note of caution regards the thrombotic effect of thrombin in fibrin sealant on microvascular anastomoses. This was recently studied and it was suggested that thrombin concentrations $\leq$ 500 IU/mL as are currently available in the FDA-licensed product do not have significant deleterious effects on microvascular anastomoses.[10] Thrombin concentrations of > 500 IU/mL may have a negative impact on these anastomoses.

Additional newer uses of fibrin sealant include its use in minimally invasive procedures, atrial and ventricular septal defect closure, free wall rupture, and adhesion prevention. Fibrin sealant has been used to assist with newly developed microvascular anastomoses that can be performed by using intraluminal stents, for bioengineering of vascular grafts, and for the slow-release distribution of medications and other therapeutic factors.[11]

With respect to future capabilities, fibrin sealant is a versatile system capable of delivery of drugs and biologics.[12] Fibrin sealant can be used as a slow-release mechanism for a drug delivery of antibiotics, growth factors, and chemotherapeutic agents. Recent evidence suggests that fibrin sealant containing appropriate antibiotics may be effective at treating bacterial endocarditis and for sterilizing infected graft sites. A final note with respect to the capabilities of fibrin sealant beyond hemostasis and sealing of tissues includes its ability to provide lymphostasis. This is particularly remarkable in sites where extensive dissection is performed and seroma formation is likely. The literature also includes references to using fibrin sealant as a means of dealing with thoracic duct injuries occurring at the time of cardiac surgery in order to achieve lymphostasis.

Cyanoacrylate

2-Octyl-cyanoacrylate (Dermabond, Ethicon Inc., Somerville, NJ) was approved in 1998 as a new mechanism of closing skin incisions. Approved for topical skin application only and not indicated for internal use, this agent can be used for the closure of skin wounds that are not under extreme tension. It is the only commercially available tissue adhesive approved by the FDA for skin closure. The agent is helpful in closing traumatic skin lacerations, as well as for closure of skin incisions at the time of elective surgical procedures.[13–15] The skin edges are held in apposition while the cyanoacrylate is applied in layers along the entire length of the wound for a width of approximately 1 to 2 cm. The manufacturer recom-

mends repeated applications, separated by 30 s each, for a total of three layers of the material. The tissue adhesive works by polymerizing as it comes in contact with hydroxyl ions. A spontaneous release of heat occurs as the 2-octyl-cyanoacrylate forms, causing a sensation of warmth in the patient. The cyanoacrylate itself is extremely strong with internal bonding strength that exceeds the strength of the skin itself. The agent remains adherent to the skin for approximately 7 to 10 days during the period of wound healing, and is then spontaneously shed from the wound as the superficial layers of skin exfoliate. Thus, the adhesive is removed as the superficial layers of the skin are sloughed. The recommendation against using this material in high tension areas is not because of weakness in the adhesive itself, but rather because of the weakness of the superficial layers of the skin to which the adhesive bonds. Consequently, it is not recommended for use across joint surfaces or other extremely high-tension areas. The cyanoacrylate can be removed if necessary by application of petroleum-based products, which reduces the adherence strength of the agent and results in its easier removal.

Cyanoacrylate is marketed by the manufacturer in crushable 0.5 mL ampules (Figure 1-5) that cost approximately $25 (US). Depending on the length of the incision, it may take multiple ampules to cover a wound sufficiently. The ampules can be stored at room temperature. Application of the material to the skin surface is facilitated by the single-dose delivery system, which, after crushing, allows the liquid cyanoacrylate to be effectively delivered to the skin surface.

Because of its high strength characteristics, easy storage, and inexpensive costs, the internal use of cyanoacrylate is extremely desirable. However, cyanoacrylate is presently approved for external use only. Significant carcinogenicity in animals and humans treated internally with cyanoacrylates has been reported.[16] Until a safer form of this agent is developed, its use in internal settings is not recommended.

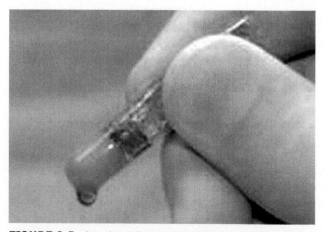

FIGURE 1-5. Ampule applicator of cyanoacrylate used for delivery of tissue adhesive.

With respect to the specific use of this agent, as with any wound closure technique, meticulous technique and thorough cleansing of the wound prior to closure is important. Accurate approximation of the skin edges by using forceps or fingers with eversion of the skin edges is recommended. For the ideal cosmetic result, a subcutaneous layer of sutures should be placed prior to closing the skin with cyanoacrylate. This minimizes contraction of the subcutaneous tissues that may cause wound dimpling and accentuate the negative appearance of a scar.

This agent can be an effective adjunct to routine methods of skin closure. For example, after closure of saphenous vein harvest-site incisions by using subcutaneous and subcuticular sutures, cyanoacrylate can be an adjunctive technique for sealing the skin. It functions as an effective barrier against the leakage of serous or lymphatic drainage from the leg wound sites and may reduce the risk of infection associated with these weeping incisions. Particularly in obese patients who require extensive dissection to harvest saphenous veins, this adjunctive technique may be effective in reducing wound drainage and potentially eliminating saphenous vein harvest-site infections.

With respect to new developments in the future of cyanoacrylate tissue adhesives, it is possible that less carcinogenic forms of this agent with minimal inflammatory responses in tissues can be developed. Efforts to develop cyanoacrylates with enhanced biodegradability may result in materials that can be characterized by great strength and can be used internally with a satisfactory safety profile.

Collagens and Thrombins

Active bleeding can be controlled effectively by using bovine thrombin and collagen because it is delivered as a gel rather than a liquid.[17,18] This product (FloSeal, Fusion Medical Technologies, Mountain View, California) is approved by the FDA as a hemostatic device that is effective at controlling bleeding during a wide variety of surgical procedures, including cardiac and vascular surgery.[17,18] The thicker consistency of this material, which simulates toothpaste (Figure 1-6), enhances its ability to remain at a site of active bleeding without being washed away. The manufacturer recommends the use of manual pressure for a period of 2 to 3 min following application of the agent in order to achieve hemostasis. A moist sponge will not stick to the device as the material sticks only to objects covered with blood. Thus, this agent maximizes effectiveness by remaining at the active bleeding site, allowing manual pressure application, and combining the commercial product's bovine collagen and thrombin with the patient's own blood fibrinogen to form a gel patch that can swell by as much as 20%. Repetitive applications of the bovine collagen and thrombin gel, if bleeding persists, are possible and are highly effective at controlling active bleeding. The swelling of the agent itself adds to the tamponade effect of the materials, but at present it is not

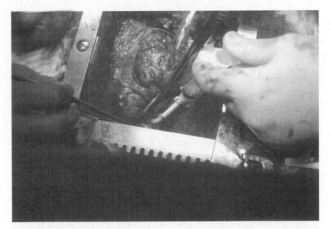

FIGURE 1-6. Application of bovine collagen and thrombin to site of bleeding at aortic suture line.

recommended for use in urologic or ophthalmologic procedures. This device costs approximately $140 (US) for a 5 mL kit that can be stored at room temperature. To prepare for application of the gel, bovine collagen and thrombin are mixed in a process that requires less than 5 min of preparation time in the operating room suite. With widespread approval for a variety of hemostatic indications, the agent is widely used in cardiac, vascular, spinal, and head and neck surgery to achieve rapid hemostasis at a site of active bleeding.

As mentioned earlier, the major risk factor associated with products containing bovine thrombin is related to antibody formation.[6,7] Impurities in bovine thrombin can potentially stimulate an immune response in human beings, resulting in the formation of antibodies that may cross-react with the body's own clotting factors. This antibody formation may cause inactivation of necessary human clotting proteins, causing a coagulopathy in the patient. Previous exposure may increase the likelihood of antibody responses and may lead to adverse outcomes.[7] Efforts have and are being made by the manufacturers of bovine thrombin to enhance the purification of this material in order to reduce the risk of antibody formation. Coagulopathy, which is reported rarely with the use of bovine thrombin, appears to occur when the patient develops antibodies against bovine thrombin and factor V, which may cross-react with human clotting factors. Surgeons should consider this potential complication when using this agent, particularly in a reexposure setting. The gelatin matrix is biodegraded at the site of application over a period of approximately 6 to 8 weeks.

The unique value of this agent is its ability to be particularly effective at the site of active bleeding. Designed as a thicker material capable of being combined with pressure and with inherent swelling capacity, this agent is highly effective for active bleeding. However, as a sealant for use prior to the development of active bleeding, this agent is ineffective. The material requires the interaction with blood containing fibrinogen in order to provide hemostatic effectiveness; thus it should be used in settings where active bleeding is occurring and not used as a sealant prior to the development of bleeding. It would not be effective at sealing a vascular anastomosis that was not pressurized and still under the application of vascular clamps. In this setting, without blood, the agent would not be activated. However, after removal of the vascular clamps, with the development of active bleeding from the anastomosis, this agent would be indicated and is useful. The manufacturer recommends a period of 2 min of pressure to maximize the hemostatic effect.

Thrombin, Collagen, and Plasma

This system consists of topical bovine thrombin and collagen, which can be combined with plasma obtained from the patient to form a hemostatic agent. The patient's own blood is fractionated into plasma and red cells by using a small tabletop centrifuge. The plasma can then be combined with topical bovine thrombin and collagen to form a fibrin sealant plus collagen (CoStasis, Cohesion Technologies, Palo Alto, California). The patient's own plasma is employed in this system and is combined with thrombin and collagen to produce a form of fibrin sealant based on the patient's own plasma fibrinogen enhanced with collagen. This material is prepared in the operating room at the time of the surgical procedure and was approved by the FDA in June 2000 as a device to stop active bleeding at the time of general, hepatic, and cardiovascular surgical operations.[19,20] A small tabletop centrifuge permits the patient's plasma to be separated from red cells. This plasma fraction is obtained in a syringe as a source of the patient's own fibrinogen and platelets. It can be prepared in advance of the patient's surgery, saving valuable operating room time. A second prefilled syringe containing thrombin and collagen is then used in the operating room at the time of surgical need. A dual syringe applicator is used for mixing of the thrombin and collagen component with the fibrinogen component. The system produces a sprayable collagen-based material to enhance delivery options. The resultant fibrin mixed with collagen is an effective hemostatic agent, which is biodegraded in the body in a period of 8 weeks. The concentration of fibrinogen in this material does not equal that of commercial fibrin sealant, but the effectiveness of this resultant fibrin is augmented by its combination with collagen. A variety of kit sizes are available for this product, and prefilled collagen and thrombin syringes can be kept in a refrigerator for periods of up to 24 months. Because this product contains topical bovine thrombin, the caution suggested in earlier sections of this chapter with respect to the development of coagulopathy applies to this agent as well.

Platelet Gels

The perfusionist familiar with rapid transfusion, hemoconcentrates, or other blood cell saving devices is capable of preparing platelet gels at the time of cardiac surgical operations.[21,22] The disposables required are frequently provided by the manufacturers of cell washing equipment or cardiopulmonary bypass circuits (Sorin, Haemonetics, Medtronic, Cobe). A platelet gel consisting of fibrinogen, platelets, and white cells can be prepared from the patient's own blood by using technology (Harvest Technologies Corporation, Plymouth, Massachusetts) to maximize the yields of platelets. This gel may enhance bone and tissue healing. When the concentrated platelets, white cells, and fibrinogen-rich plasma are mixed with commercially available bovine thrombin, a platelet gel clot is formed. The fibrin that is formed is enhanced by platelets and white cells. It has been suggested that the additional growth factors and other substances in this environment may contribute to improved wound healing and reparative processes. Although not as highly concentrated as commercial fibrin sealant, it has been suggested that platelet gels may be more cost-effective. No randomized controlled study presently exists to support this contention. This product is not approved by the FDA for use in cardiac surgery.

Polyethylene Glycol Polymers

Polyethylene glycol (PEG) polymers represent a new hydrogel family of tissue adhesives that are capable of bonding effectively to human tissues. The first such agent approved in the United States by the FDA is a PEG polymer capable of achieving pneumatosis at the time of lung resection. This agent (FocalSeal-L, Focal Incorporated, Lexington, Massachusetts) was approved in May 2000 for closure of fissural pleural air leak incurred in elective pulmonary resection. This PEG polymer is a light-activated synthetic device that is capable of reducing air leaks following pulmonary operations. This strong adhesive is commercially distributed by the manufacturer in the form of a two-component material. Tissues are first treated with a primer which prepares the tissue for the application of the PEG polymer. The application process consists of the initial brush application of the primer to the surface of the lung. This is followed by the application of the PEG polymer to the lung parenchyma. The PEG polymer is carefully worked into the lung tissues by using a second brush applicator separate from that used to apply the primer. After application of the PEG polymer, a light source (470 to 520 nm), consisting of a resterilizable wand connected to a light source box, is used to activate the PEG polymer and to form the final tissue adhesive. The entire process takes approximately 10 to 15 min and does require careful technique.

The primer and polymer require storage at −20° and 4°C, respectively. Application of the PEG polymer costs approximately $55 (US) per milliliter. The light source and wand needed for this system must be purchased separately.

The adhesive itself is very strong and has excellent adherence characteristics on the surface of the lung parenchyma.[23] In the multicenter trial used to obtain approval for this agent in patients undergoing lung resection, the polymer-treated patients were three times less likely to develop postoperative air leaks than were those patients who were treated with standard therapy alone.[24] This material remains present for as long as 6 months after application because it is biodegraded slowly. Approximately 36% is thought to remain at 6 months. Because this agent is relatively new, no long-term safety data are available. Physicians who are using this agent are encouraged to continue to exercise vigilance with respect to infection rates and potential long-term effects. The use of this agent in cardiac surgical applications has not been thoroughly explored or approved.

A second PEG polymer device (CoSeal, Cohesion Technologies, Palo Alto, California) was approved by the FDA in December 2001. This agent consists of two distinct PEG polymers that are combined to form a hydrogel sealant. This material is approved for use in sealing arterial and/or venous anastomoses during vascular reconstruction procedures. The synthetic device does not require light activation but cross-links to itself and to the underlying tissues on application. The agent is applied as a sprayable liquid through a dual syringe delivery system, and polymerizes within seconds of application. The agent is fully matured within approximately 60 s.

This PEG polymer is available in 2 and 4 mL single-patient use kits. The material is stored refrigerated at 2° to 8°C, and can be prepared within minutes in the operating room by using the delivery system kit, which is supplied with the product. Preparation involves mixing the two PEG polymers (which are supplied as a powder) with a liquid buffer solution, using a transferring syringe. The two then-ready PEG polymers are combined in the hand-held device for application to the tissues. The material is resorbed within weeks of application.

Albumin Glutaraldehyde

Albumin cross-linked with glutaraldehyde received approval as a sealing agent in vascular operations on large vessels in December 2001. Prior to FDA approval, it had been used under a human device exemption for the treatment of patients with aortic dissection. The products consist of bovine albumin, which is cross-linked by glutaraldehyde to form a strong adhesive bond. The manufacturer supplies the material (BioGlue, CryoLife, Inc., Kennesawa, Georgia) as a gun (Figure 1-7) containing both albumin and glutaraldehyde, which are effectively mixed at the time of application. The adhesive solidifies within a period of 20 to 30 s. Maximum strength is achieved within a period of 2 to 3 min. In its initial use as a method of enhancing the strength of the aorta at the time of aortic dissection, albumin cross-linked with glutaraldehyde was extremely effective at sealing vascular

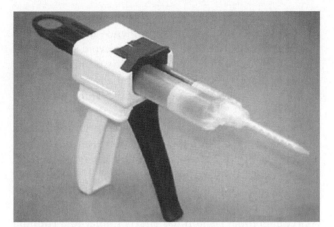

FIGURE 1-7. Applicator gun used to apply albumin cross-linked with glutaraldehyde to vascular tissues.

anastomoses and achieving hemostasis.[25,26] The agent was carefully applied between the dissected layers of the aorta in order to reapproximate the intima and adventitia. In the process of aortic dissection, the media is destroyed and the thin adventitia and intima layers become very fragile and difficult to suture. The treatment of type A aortic dissection requires replacement of the ascending aorta with a tube graft in order to avoid hemorrhage, cardiac tamponade, and death. The ability to suture the tube graft to dissected aortic tissue can be significantly improved by the use of albumin cross-linked with glutaraldehyde. In addition to using the adhesive to help obliterate the false lumen space between the adventitia and intima, the glue can be used to seal the anastomoses themselves. Not only does the material result in a strengthening of the friable layers of the aorta, but it also can be used to prevent leakage of blood from the anastomotic suture line. Thus, this material is capable of strengthening the fragile aortic tissues and of sealing the anastomosis. Initial studies of perioperative morbidity and mortality suggested significant benefit from the use of albumin cross-linked with glutaraldehyde.

This material comes in kits containing albumin and glutaraldehyde. The cost of the kit is approximately $450 (US). The material is stored at room temperature. Preparation requires assembly of the applicator gun, which can be completed in a period of several minutes by the scrub nurse in the operating room.

Cautions with respect to this agent include concerns over the long-term effects of this material on aortic tissues and the healing of vascular anastomoses. The literature cites some difficulties with an earlier glutaraldehyde, resorcinol, and formaldehyde (GRF) adhesive otherwise known as "French glue." It has been suggested that this agent could be associated with long-term complications, including tissue degradation, which may lead to recurrent aortic root dissection, aortic insufficiency, and false aneurysm formation.[27] Long-term studies with respect to this newer form of albumin and glutaraldehyde, which does not use formaldehyde in this setting, are pending, but concerns about similar problems exist.[28] For the present, caution needs to be used to avoid overdose of glutaraldehyde, which can result in tissue necrosis. The effects of glutaraldehyde could potentially reduce healing at the site of a vascular anastomosis. Thus, this agent should be used sparingly and with care. It is best to use an extremely thin layer and to guard against the application or dislodgement of the adhesive into a critical area such as a nerve or the ostium of a coronary artery. Potentially fatal myocardial infarction or later stenosis of the coronary artery due to inadvertent placement of this agent should be avoided. In addition, the use of this material in a circumferential fashion has effects similar to a running suture on vascular anastomoses that may be subject to later growth. Thus, the use of albumin cross-linked with glutaraldehyde in a pediatric population may result in a lack of growth of the anastomosis. Just as interrupted or absorbable sutures are more appropriate in the pediatric population in order to allow for later tissue growth, avoidance of the circumferential application of albumin cross-linked with glutaraldehyde can also help to facilitate later vascular anastomotic growth and enlargement.

Personal Experience

This section reviews the best uses of surgical tissue hemostats and sealants in cardiac surgery with respect to the author's personal experience. An attempt is made to differentiate between the agents to suggest the clinical situation in which each is best deployed. In the current cost-cutting environment, many operating rooms attempt to choose between the available agents, as opposed to stocking all of the materials, in order to save shelf space and to reduce expenses. In the author's experience, multiple agents are required for the effective care of cardiac surgical patients. Limiting the armamentarium to one or two agents may not allow for effective patient care. Multiple agents with different capabilities, just as multiple types of sutures, may be required for the best management of the patient.

Fibrin sealant is best used as a hemostatic sealant that is applied prior to significant active bleeding. Thus, it can be effectively used to control slow capillary bleeding from pericardial and epicardial adhesions at the time of reoperative cardiac surgery. This is particularly true when the agent is sprayed onto the operative field, allowing for a thoroughly mixed and thin layer of the hemostatic agent to be applied to the appropriate surfaces. Similarly, the agent can be applied to vascular anastomoses prior to removal of vascular clamps or prior to removal of the aortic cross-clamp. This allows the adhesive to polymerize and reach maximum strength prior to resumption of full intra-arterial pressure. If fibrin sealant is required at an active bleeding site, it is best to deliver it with a carrier sponge of cellulose or collagen. The carrier sponge allows the liquid fibrin sealant to be delivered to the active bleed-ing site without washing away and also allows pressure to be applied to facilitate hemostasis.

The use of plasma and collagen with bovine thrombin or platelet gels with bovine thrombin is similar to that of fibrin sealant. These agents each have their own specific advantages and disadvantages with respect to strength, cost, and additional levels of effectiveness. These agents, however, remain members of the fibrin sealant family because they depend on the interaction of fibrinogen and thrombin to form fibrin as a means of achieving hemostasis and sealing. At present each requires the use of bovine thrombin.

Cyanoacrylate is an extremely strong tissue adhesive that can be used to close the skin. Its strength is limited only by the strength of the superficial layers of epithelium as the glue strength exceeds that of the superficial layers of the dermis. This extremely strong and relatively inexpensive material is not approved for internal use because of the risks of carcinogenicity. In the hands of the cardiovascular surgeon, this agent may be valuable for use as an adjunctive means of sealing the skin after routine suture closure of the skin has been achieved. In this setting, the adhesive can be used to prevent the leakage of serous lymphatic fluids from a wound. This use may be able to reduce incidence of wound infection and prolonged hospitalization that is sometimes associated with wound drainage at the site of a saphenous vein harvest.

Bovine collagen and thrombin gel matrix is a potent hemostatic agent for the treatment of active bleeding. Because it is applied as a toothpaste-like material rather than a liquid, it is not easily washed away from the site of active bleeding. In addition, direct pressure with a moist sponge can be applied to the gel without the danger of the gel sticking to the sponge. Rather, the gel will only stick to the bleeding site and not to the moist sponge. Thus, there are two advantages to this agent at the site of active bleeding. It is less likely to be washed away and it can be easily combined with manual pressure. In addition, the material can be reapplied repeatedly if necessary in order to completely achieve hemostasis. This agent obviously would not be effective at sealing anastomosis prior to active bleeding. It would not be indicated in this setting as it requires combination with fibrinogen found in blood for effectiveness.

PEG polymers can be used effectively to seal lung air leaks. There are situations in cardiac surgery, particularly in reoperative procedures, where air leaks in the surface of the lung develop. Elimination of these air leaks may be important to minimize the risk of wound infection and later complications. In this setting, the cardiac surgeon could employ these PEG polymers to control pulmonary parenchymal air leaks. The process of applying these agents is somewhat time-consuming at present. The new PEG polymer system recently approved for vascular anastomoses has not yet been used clinically in sufficient numbers of the author's patients to allow the author to provide additional comments.

Albumin cross-linked with glutaraldehyde is an extremely powerful and strong tissue adhesive. It is capable of strengthening tissues as well as achieving strong tissue opposition. In addition, it can seal anastomoses. Although extremely strong, this agent needs to be used sparingly in order to avoid potentially toxic effects of glutaraldehyde on human tissue. In addition, its use at vascular anastomoses should be carefully considered because glutaraldehyde may reduce healing by retarding bridging of endothelial cells at the anastomotic site. The agent should be used carefully in anastomoses subject to further growth as circumferential application may, like running suture, restrict anastomotic growth and enlargement.

Future

The agents reviewed in this chapter represent the initial phases of development of new hemostatic tissue sealants and adhesives. Clinical trials and development work continue with a variety of agents. These materials, as well as those currently on the market, are valuable new additions to the surgical armamentarium.

A variety of additional off-label capabilities may be combined with those currently described, including drug delivery and tissue engineering. Cardiac surgeons have traditionally been on the forefront of new technology and development. At best, these new materials will be employed successfully by cardiac surgeons. Further new uses and capabilities may be developed. As with all new interventions, careful clinical observation and follow-up will be required to determine the best, safest, and most cost-effective uses of these modalities.

References

1. Spotnitz WD, Falstrom JK, Rodeheaver GT. The role of sutures and fibrin sealant in wound healing. Surg Clin North Am 1997;77:1–19.
2. Spotnitz WD. History of tissue adhesives. In: Sierra D, Saltz R, editors. Surgical adhesives and sealants, current technology and applications. Lancaster, PA: Technomic; 1996. p. 3–11.
3. Rousou J, Gonzalez-Lavin L, Cosgrove D, et al. Randomized clinical trial of fibrin sealant in patients undergoing resternotomy or reoperation after cardiac operations. J Thorac Cardiovasc Surg 1989;97:194–203.
4. Siedentop K, Harris D, Ham K, et al. Extended experimental and preliminary surgical findings with autologous fibrin tissue adhesive made from patient's own blood. Laryngoscope 1986;96:1062–4.
5. Spotnitz WD, Mintz PD, Avery N, et al. Fibrin glue from stored human plasma: an inexpensive and efficient method for local blood bank preparation. Am Surg 1987;53:460–4.
6. WL Daniels TM, Fisher PK, et al. Antibodies to bovine thrombin and coagulation factor V associated with the

7. use of topical bovine thrombin or fibrin glue: a frequent finding. Blood 1993;82:59a.
7. Ortel TL, Mercer MC, Thames EH, et al. Immunologic impact and clinical outcomes after surgical exposure to bovine thrombin. Ann Surg 2001;233:88–96.
8. Schlag G. Fibrin sealing in surgical and nonsurgical fields. Vols. 1–8. Berlin: Springer-Verlag; 1994.
9. Spotnitz WD. Fibrin sealant in the United States: clinical use at the University of Virginia. Thromb Haemost 1995;74:482–5.
10. Frost-Arner L, Spotnitz WD, Rodeheaver GT, et al. Comparison of the thrombogenicity of internationally available fibrin sealants in an established microsurgical model. J Plastic Reconstruct Surg 2001;108:1655–60.
11. Spotnitz WD. New developments in the use of fibrin sealant: a surgeon's perspective. J Long-Term Eff Med Implants 1997;7:243–53.
12. MacPhee M, Singh M, Brady R, et al. Fibrin sealant: a versatile delivery vehicle for drugs and biologics. In: Sierra D, Saltz R, editors. Surgical adhesives and sealants, current technology and applications. Lancaster, PA: Technomic; 1996. p. 109–20.
13. Quinn J, Drzewiecki A, Li M, et al. A randomized, controlled trial comparing a tissue adhesive with suturing in the repair of pediatric facial lacerations. Ann Emerg Med 1993;22:1130–5.
14. Quinn J, Wells G, Sutcliffe T, et al. A randomized trial comparing octyl-cyanoacrylate tissue adhesive and sutures in the management of lacerations. JAMA 1997;277(19):1527–30.
15. Toriumi DM, O'Grady K, Devang D, Bagal A. Use of octyl-2-cyanoacrylate for skin closure in facial plastic surgery. Plast Reconstr Surg 1998;102:2209–19.
16. Samson D, Marshall D. Carcinogenic potential of isobutyl-2-cyanoacrylate. J Neurosurg 1986;65:571–2.
17. Oz MC, Cosgrove DM, Badduke BR, et al. Topic N and The Fusion Matrix Study Group. Controlled clinical trial of a novel hemostatic agent in cardiac surgery. Ann Thorac Surg 2000;69:1376–82.
18. Reuthebuch O, Lachat ML, Vogt O, et al. FloSeal: a new hemostyptic agent in peripheral vascular surgery. Clin Cardiovasc Surg 2000;204–6.
19. Chapman W, Sherman R, Boyce S, et al. A novel collagen-based composite offers effective hemostasis for multiple surgical indications: results of a randomized controlled trial. Surgery 2001;129:445–50.
20. Chapman W, Clavien P, Fung J, et al. Effective control of hepatic bleeding using a novel collagen-based composite combined with autologous plasma: results of a randomized controlled trial. Arch Surg 2000;13:1200–4.
21. Hill AG, Hood AG, Reeder GD, et al. Perioperative autologous sequestration II: a differential centrifugation technique for autologous component therapy: methods and results. Am Acad Cardiovasc Perfusion 1993;14:122–5.
22. Hood AG, Hill AG, Reeder GD, et al. Perioperative autologous sequestration III: a new physiologic glue with wound healing properties. Am Acad Cardiovasc Perfusion 1993;14:126–9.
23. Ranger WR, Halpin D, Sawhney AS, et al. Pneumostasis of experimental air leaks with a new photopolymerized synthetic tissue sealant. Am Surg 1997;63:788–95.

24. Wain JC, Kaiser LR, Johnstone DW, et al. Trial of a novel synthetic sealant in preventing air leaks after lung resection. Ann Thorac Surg 2001;71:1623–9.

25. Hewitt CW, Marra SW, Kann BR, et al. BioGlue surgical adhesive for thoracic aortic repair during coagulopathy: efficacy and histopathology. Ann Thorac Surg 2001;71: 1609–12.

26. Raanani E, Latter DA, Errett LE, et al. Use of "BioGlue" in aortic surgical repair. Ann Thorac Surg 2001;72:638–40.

27. Bingley JA, Gardner MAH, Stafford EG, et al. Late complications of tissue glues in aortic surgery. Ann Thorac Surg 2000;69:1764–8.

28. Kazui T, Washiyama N, Bashar AHM, et al. Role of biologic glue repair of proximal aortic dissection in the development of early and midterm redissection of the aortic root. Ann Thorac Surg 2001;72:509–14.

CHAPTER 2

ANTICOAGULATION FOR MEDICAL DEVICES

DAVID N. HELMAN, MD, GUS J. VLAHAKES, MD

Anticoagulation, which has always been an important issue in the postoperative management of patients undergoing prosthetic heart valve replacement, has become increasingly important in the field of cardiac surgery over the last decade as the frequency of use of mechanical circulatory support devices has increased. Adding to the continued evolution of the field of post–cardiotomy anticoagulation is the recent addition of new anticoagulant and antiplatelet drugs targeted at different steps in the thrombotic process. Even as design strategies aimed at improving device resistance to thrombus formation evolve, it is likely that pharmacologic approaches to minimizing thrombus formation on prosthetic surfaces in contact with blood will continue to be necessary for the foreseeable future. Always underlying decisions regarding anticoagulant regimens is the balance that must be achieved between risk of thromboembolic complications versus risk of bleeding complications.

Blood–Device Interface and Clotting Cascade

The underlying problem that must be solved if a prosthetic device is to coexist in contact with the blood is that of thrombus formation at the blood–device interface. There are two aspects of this interface that are potentially amenable to modification to reduce thrombogenicity: (1) prosthetic material properties and device design, and (2) coagulability of blood. Both of these elements are important in achieving reduced thrombus formation. A prosthetic device in contact with blood initiates coagulation via the intrinsic pathway of the clotting system. This process is effected through the interaction of factor XII, high-molecular-weight kininogen (HMWK), and prekallikrein.[1] Experimental evidence exists that the main component adsorbed onto a foreign surface from plasma is fibrinogen at first, but that this fibrinogen layer is converted to HMWK over time.[2] Platelets do not adhere to HMWK like they do to fibrinogen, and this is part of the explanation for prosthetic surfaces becoming less thrombogenic over time.[2] Contact of factor XII with a foreign surface results in an activated protease form of factor XII, known as factor XIIa, which stimulates the remainder of the intrinsic coagulation cascade.[1] The end result of this clotting process is the conversion of fibrinogen to fibrin, which is mediated by the production of thrombin, the final protease to be generated in the clotting cascade.[3] All of the steps in the coagulation cascade are potential sites for pharmacologic intervention to minimize clotting in the presence of prosthetic medical devices.

Platelet Activation and Aggregation

In addition to the clotting cascade, platelets play a vital role in the formation of thrombus, particularly on the surface of a prosthetic device. Platelets are deposited on an artificial surface when it comes in contact with blood.[1] As platelets adhere to the surface, they are activated in terms of their expression of glycoprotein (GP) IIb/IIIa receptors.[4] The GPIIb/IIIa receptor is the most abundant receptor on the platelet cell membrane.[5] The importance of these GPIIb/IIIa receptors lies in their capacity to aggregate platelets by making use of fibrinogen as a connector to link platelets to one another. It is interesting that the GPIIb/IIIa receptors in inactivated platelets do not have a high affinity for fibrinogen, whereas these same receptors in activated platelets avidly bind fibrinogen.[6] The central role of the GPIIb/IIIa receptor in platelet aggregation has made it an attractive target for pharmacologic intervention.

Approaches to Prosthetic Device Surface Design

In addition to pharmacologic manipulation of the blood and its components, design of prosthetic device surfaces is the other variable in the interaction at the blood–device interface that can be addressed to minimize the potential for thrombosis. A number of strategies have been conceived to engineer prosthetic surfaces of both heart valves and mechanical circulatory support devices to reduce thrombogenicity.

Surface reactive groups on implanted prosthetic materials are thought to be one of the factors that promote the ultimate activation of the complement system leading to the hypothesis that the elimination of these surface reactive groups might minimize complement activation.[7] Another potential surface modification involves the binding of inert biomaterials, such as albumin, to the surface to interfere with the detection of the surface as foreign.[8] Prosthetic surfaces exposed to blood rapidly adsorb proteins, which is followed by deposition of fibrinogen.[2] It is attractive to think of facilitating the adsorption of proteins onto the surface that would block the adsorption of fibrinogen and thus reduce device thrombogenicity.

Attempts have been made to coat prosthetic device surfaces with living cells to minimize thrombogenicity. In a series of in vivo studies, Bernhard and associates inoculated the surface of a polyurethane circulatory support pump with cultured bovine fetal fibroblasts and found that this reduced thromboembolic complications.[9]

As an alternative to coating devices with living cells, designers of prosthetic heart valves and mechanical circulatory support devices have employed various tactics in an effort to promote the overgrowth of a biologic surface that would coat the newly implanted device and minimize thrombosis. Bjork and associates coated the surface of prosthetic heart valves with 40 μm diameter microspheres to increase the porosity of the valve surface and promote the growth of a nonthrombogenic endothelial surface.[10]

The design of the HeartMate I left ventricular assist device (VAD) (Thoratec Corp., Pleasanton, California) incorporates a textured surface coated with sintered titanium microspheres with the goal of reducing thromboembolism.[11,12] This approach results in a blood-contacting surface that is rapidly coated with an adherent "neo-intima" with a resultant need for acetylsalicylic acid (ASA) as the only antithrombotic treatment required for patients with this VAD.[13] Subsequent studies of this device demonstrate that although this biologic lining does exist on the surface of the VAD, an overall procoagulant state does exist with sustained thrombin generation because of deposition and activation of hematopoietic precursor and monocytic cells from the blood.[14,15]

Another method of decreasing prosthetic surface thrombogenicity was realized by bonding of anticoagulant drugs to the prosthetic surface. This was successfully accomplished with heparin-bonded circuits for use in cardiopulmonary bypass (CPB) and is covered in detail in another chapter in this text.[16] Heparin-bonding has also been used in the Berlin Heart VAD, which uses a coating of heparin on the inner surface of its polyurethane pump and silicone cannulae (Mediport, Berlin, Germany).[17] There are other molecules, including those that promote fibrinolysis, that might be bound to prosthetic device surfaces to improve biocompatibility.[18–20] It is possible that this strategy may be employed in implantable devices in the future.

Anticoagulant Drugs

Parenteral Anticoagulants

The cardiac surgical patient often first encounters parenteral anticoagulant drugs just prior to being supported with CPB. The standard anticoagulant for this purpose is unfractionated heparin (UH). Although UH is useful for CPB and for short-term intravenous anticoagulation, it is not without its limitations and adverse effects. There now exists a number of options for parenteral anticoagulation with less-complicated administration and monitoring requirements than UH, as well as for patients who have a history of heparin-induced thrombocytopenia (HIT). Whether or not any of these drugs will supplant UH as the standard anticoagulant for CPB remains to be seen.

Patients with a history of HIT pose a challenge in terms of anticoagulation, both in the operating room in preparation for CPB, as well as in the short-term inpatient setting. A number of parenteral anticoagulants are available that can be used in this setting. Although a detailed summary of these parenteral anticoagulants is beyond the scope of this chapter, recent comprehensive reviews are available in the literature.[21,22]

To date, there are not many reported uses of the GPIIb/IIIa inhibitors in the setting of CPB. One exception to this is a strategy that Koster and associates have used to anticoagulate a patient with HIT for CPB.[23] Their approach involved using UH and tirofiban, a GPIIb/IIIa inhibitor, in combination. Their rationale was that the tirofiban would act to inhibit platelet aggregation and thus prevent the potential complications of HIT and thrombosis.[23]

Oral Anticoagulants

Warfarin is the drug of choice for long-term anticoagulation for patients with prosthetic heart valves in the outpatient setting. Warfarin acts via antagonism of vitamin K, which is needed to synthesize clotting factors II, VII, IX, and X. Therapeutic levels of warfarin reduce the liver's production of clotting factors II, VII, IX, and X by 30 to 50% and lessen the activity of those factors that are produced to 10 to 40% of normal.[3] It should be noted that the plasma half-lives of the vitamin K–dependent factors (II, VII, IX, and X) vary significantly, with times up to 50 h; thus, it may take several days for the full anticoagulant effect of warfarin to be realized even though the international normalized ratio (INR) may be in the target range.[3]

Warfarin is the major component of the antithrombotic strategy in the United States for patients with prosthetic heart valves and some long-term mechanical circulatory support devices. Warfarin is often combined with an antiplatelet agent in the setting of prosthetic devices. There is experimental evidence that the benefit of warfarin in the setting of a foreign surface does not stem from a reduction in thrombus formation; rather, it stems from a reduction in the size of emboli.[24] This may be one reason why combining ASA with warfarin may be beneficial.

There are many studies in the literature on the subject of warfarin with or without additional antithrombotic drugs in the setting of patients with prosthetic heart valves. However, many of these studies are difficult to interpret because it is not always clear how closely patients' actual INRs matched the target range over time.

While proven to be an effective anticoagulant, chronic warfarin therapy does put the patient at increased risk of complications from hemorrhage, and the INR must be carefully monitored. The reported risk of serious bleeding complications with chronic warfarin therapy is between 0.2 and 2.2 occurrences per 100 patient years.[25] The trade-off between risk of thromboembolism and bleeding complications, as well as individual patient characteristics, such as propensity to fall, must be weighed when determining the target INR for a patient with a prosthetic cardiac device.

Antiplatelet Drugs (Parenteral and Oral)

The selection of available antiplatelet agents approved by the Food and Drug Administration (FDA) recently expanded with the addition of the GPIIb/IIIa inhibitors. Historically, antithrombotic therapy for patients with mechanical heart valves was based upon the use of warfarin in combination with an antiplatelet agent. The most commonly used antiplatelet agent in this setting is ASA. ASA, which interferes with thromboxane A_2–mediated platelet aggregation, is a relatively weak antiplatelet drug when compared to the GPIIb/IIIa inhibitors, which inhibit platelet aggregation without regard to the initial stimulus of platelet aggregation.[5]

Although the majority of the new antiplatelet agents are available only in intravenous form and are meant for short-term use, one of the new GPIIb/IIIa inhibitors, clopidogrel, is also available in an oral form. Much of the current information regarding the newer antiplatelet drugs comes from the literature reporting on percutaneous coronary interventions during which these agents are increasingly used. A review by Al Suwaidi and associates of studies employing GPIIb/IIIa inhibitors during percutaneous coronary stenting procedures showed a decrease in the frequency of myocardial enzyme elevation by 40 to 50% when compared to procedures performed without the use of GPIIb/IIIa inhibitors.[26]

Although there is presently no literature on the subject of the oral GPIIb/IIIa inhibitors used in the setting of prosthetic valves, it is possible that these drugs may be used in this setting in the future. Clopidogrel, an oral GPIIb/IIIa inhibitor, has been reported as a component of the antithrombotic regimens for patients with VADs.[27,28]

Dipyridamole and ticlopidine are antiplatelet drugs that have been used as well in the setting of prosthetic heart valves and mechanical circulatory support systems. Dipyridamole, which interferes with platelet function by increasing the cellular concentration of adenosine 3',5'-monophosphate, has been combined with warfarin in patients with mechanical heart valves.[3,29] Ticlopidine works to inhibit platelet aggregation via an effect on the GPIIb/IIIa receptor on platelets.[3] The use of ticlopidine has been limited as an antiplatelet agent as a result of an incidence of severe neutropenia of approximately 1%, as well as because of reported cases of thrombotic thrombocytopenic purpura.[26]

Oral antithrombotic regimens for patients with prosthetic heart valves and long-term mechanical circulatory support devices will undoubtedly continue to evolve, likely continuing to make use of warfarin as an anticoagulant component with the addition of an antiplatelet drug. The new antiplatelet drugs will have to be evaluated in terms of their potential to provide improved protection from thromboembolic complications while potentially allowing for a lower INR with a lower risk of bleeding complications.

One issue that the cardiac surgeon is increasingly faced with is the necessity of operating on patients that have been receiving continuous intravenous infusions of the new GPIIb/IIIa inhibitors. There is certainly a concern for increased hemorrhagic complications in performing an operative procedure in this setting. Concern about taking patients on intravenous abciximab, a GPIIb/IIIa inhibitor, to the operating room stems from the fact that after discontinuing abciximab, platelet aggregation and bleeding time remain altered for 12 to 48 h.[30] Abciximab is bound to circulating platelets for as long as 21 days, but the half-life of abciximab is only 25 min, so its effects can be reversed via platelet transfusion.[31] Lincoff and associates conducted a randomized, placebo-controlled trial of patients undergoing coronary artery bypass grafting after percutaneous coronary interventions used either abciximab or a placebo.[31] They found that postoperative mediastinal chest tube drainage was virtually identical and that the difference in the rates of re-exploration for bleeding for the two groups were statistically insignificant. It remains to be seen whether these findings will hold true for the other novel antiplatelet drugs. It does appear that the cardiac surgeon will be faced with an increasing number of patients with unstable angina who are referred for surgery while on intravenous antiplatelet agents.

Summarized in Figure 2-1 are the mechanisms of thrombus formation as a result of blood contact with a prosthetic surface, as well as the sites of actions of the antithrombotic drugs discussed above.

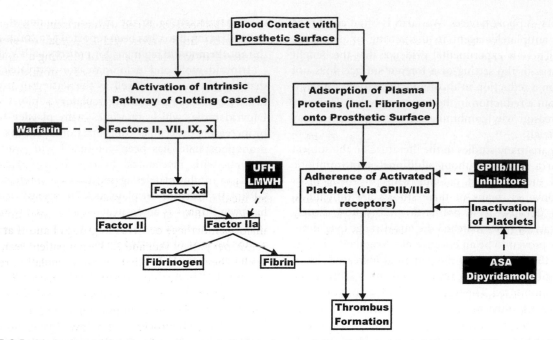

FIGURE 2-1. Mechanisms of thrombus formation on prosthetic surfaces and sites of pharmacologic intervention. ASA = acetylsalicylic acid; LMWH = low-molecular-weight heparin; UFH = unfractionated heparin.

Antithrombotic Strategies for Prosthetic Heart Valves

Anticoagulation for heart valve replacement and repair has evolved since the inception of surgical correction of valvular heart disease. Historically, higher levels of anticoagulation were used than are recommended by most today. With more anticoagulation comes the increased risk of hemorrhagic complications, a factor that has been the impetus to maintain patients on lower levels of anticoagulation while still achieving acceptably low frequencies of thrombotic complications. The overall incidence of thromboembolic complications in patients with mechanical heart valves on warfarin therapy is approximately 1% per patient year.[32] On the other hand, bleeding complications have been reported to occur in patients taking warfarin at the rate of 0.7 to 6.6% per patient year.[33] Minimization of thromboembolic complications and bleeding complications requires a balance in terms of level of antithrombotic therapy. Individual patient characteristics, making a patient more prone to clot or bleed, necessitate customization of antithrombotic regimens to achieve an optimal outcome. A number of factors, specific to patients with prosthetic heart valves, can be identified that impact the desired level of anticoagulation. Table 2-1 shows these factors and the direction in which they influence anticoagulation levels.

Bioprosthetic Valves

Bioprosthetic heart valves are inherently less thrombogenic than mechanical heart valves, and for this reason patients with bioprosthetic valves have historically been

TABLE 2-1. Patient Characteristics Modifying Level of Antithrombotic Treatment

Characteristic	Effect on Desired Level of Antithrombotic Treatment
Decreased ejection fraction	↑
Atrial fibrillation	↑
Enlarged left atrium	↑
Left atrial thrombus	↑
History of embolic stroke	↑
Hypercoagulable state	↑
History of previous bleeding	↓
Gait instability	↓

treated with lower levels of anticoagulation than those with mechanical valves. One additional factor that is generally agreed upon is that bioprosthetic valves in the aortic position are less likely to form a thrombus than those in the mitral position. For this reason, the need for anticoagulation for bioprosthetic valves in the aortic position is a topic that has generated some controversy. There are those who argue that all bioprosthetic valves, regardless of position, require anticoagulation for the first 3 postoperative months. On the side of no need for warfarin in the early (< 3 months) postoperative period are Moinuddeen and associates, who retrospectively analyzed 195 patients undergoing bioprosthetic aortic valve replacement.[34] They found no statistically significant difference in cerebral ischemic events nor bleeding complications between patients treated with warfarin for the first 3 postoperative months and patients not treated with warfarin.

Blair and associates retrospectively reviewed 370 patients who underwent Carpentier-Edwards bioprosthetic valve replacement in the aortic and mitral positions and who were treated postoperatively with ASA only, warfarin only, or no antithrombotic therapy.[35] They concluded that for porcine valves in the aortic position, ASA was the only antithrombotic therapy necessary. For porcine valves in the mitral position, they recommended that the patient's antithrombotic regimen should be determined by the patient's individual characteristics, and if the patient was in sinus rhythm, ASA alone might be adequate. Others have recommended that patients in sinus rhythm with mitral or aortic bioprosthetic valves only need anticoagulation during the first 3 postoperative months.[36]

Mechanical Valves

There is less controversy with regard to mechanical heart valves in that it is nearly uniformly agreed that patients with mechanical valves in place require anticoagulation. The rate of major thromboembolism in patients with mechanical heart valves has been reported at approximately 4% per patient year with no antithrombotic treatment, 2% per patient year with antiplatelet treatment, and 1% per patient year with warfarin treatment.[32] A number of factors, other than specific patient characteristics, have been implicated in an increased risk of thromboembolism, including (1) caged-ball valves, (2) mitral valve prostheses, and (3) multiple prosthetic valves.[36]

Recommendations for anticoagulation for mechanical heart valves have evolved over the years. In 1989, the American College of Chest Physicians and the National Heart, Lung, and Blood Institute (ACCP-NHLBI) issued a consensus guideline that recommended an INR of 3.0 to 4.5 for mechanical heart valves.[37] A subsequent revision by these organizations was made in 1992 to lower the goal INR for mechanical heart valves to 2.5 to 3.5 to minimize the risk of bleeding complications.[37]

Efforts have been made to standardize the reporting of complications related to prosthetic valves and level of anticoagulation. Akins has developed a "composite thromboembolism and bleeding index" in an effort to accurately combine reported data on thromboembolic and hemorrhagic complications in anticoagulated patients with mechanical valves in order to make comparisons between valves and anticoagulation regimens.[38] This rate of complications is calculated by summing all thromboembolic and bleeding events and dividing by the cumulative patient years of follow-up.

Cannegieter and associates used retrospective data to determine an "optimal" INR for mechanical valves.[39] They concluded that the optimal INR to minimize the risk of both thromboembolic complications and bleeding complications is 2.5 to 4.9 and recommended a target INR of 3.0 to 4.0 to achieve the optimal level of anticoagulation. In addition, they concluded that ASA in addition to warfarin was most useful in the setting where control of the INR was not good.

ASA has been combined with warfarin in patients with mechanical heart valves with the goal of allowing a reduced INR to reduce the risk of bleeding complications while maintaining a low risk of thromboembolism. Meschengieser and associates have investigated this in a prospective randomized trial comparing two groups of patients with mechanical heart valves: group I included patients with an INR goal of 2.5 to 3.5 and who were given 100 mg of ASA per day; group II included patients with an INR goal of 3.5 to 4.5 with no ASA.[40] Meschengieser and associates found that patients in group I and group II had an incidence of embolic episodes of 1.32% per patient year and 1.48% per patient year, respectively. Episodes of major hemorrhage occurred in groups I and II at rates of 1.13% per patient year and 2.33% per patient year, respectively. They concluded that the anticoagulation regimens offered similar protection from thromboembolic complications and that there was not an increased occurrence of gastrointestinal bleeding with the addition of ASA.

Altman and associates also investigated antithrombotic regimens in patients with mechanical heart valves.[41] They compared patients taking ASA (330 mg per day), dipyridamole (75 mg twice daily), and acenocoumarol. They separated their patients into two groups: those with an INR of 2.0 to 3.0 and those with an INR of 3.0 to 4.5. They found that the risk of thromboembolism was not statistically different between the two groups but that the risk of bleeding complications was significantly lower in the group with an INR of 2.0 to 3.0, leading them to conclude that an INR of 2.0 to 3.0 is safer.

Turpie and associates evaluated the addition of 100 mg of ASA per day to warfarin treatment with a goal INR of 3.0 to 4.5 in patients with mechanical heart valves or with bioprosthetic heart valves plus atrial fibrillation or a history of thromboembolism with a randomized, placebo-controlled trial.[42] They found that the addition of ASA had these effects: (1) the rate of thromboembolism decreased from 4.6% per patient year to 1.6% per patient year, and (2) the rate of bleeding increased from 6.6% per patient year to 8.5% per patient year. The authors concluded that the added risks of warfarin plus ASA were outweighed by the benefits.

In addition to ASA, dipyridamole has been used in combination with warfarin in an effort to safely reduce the target INR in patients with mechanical valves. Kontozis and associates followed 200 patients with St. Jude valves with a mean follow-up of 52 ± 24 months.[29] The anticoagulation regimen used in this group of patients was warfarin to achieve a target INR of 2.0 to 2.5 with 300 mg of dipyridamole per day. The median INR was 1.88 ± 0.54. The results of this study showed a thromboembolic rate of 1.5% per patient year with a rate of major bleeding of 1.3% per patient year, leading the authors to conclude that low-level warfarin therapy with the addition of dipyridamole was reasonable for St. Jude mechanical valves.

Massel and associates undertook a meta-analysis of reports on patients with prosthetic heart valves treated with warfarin and ASA or dipyridamole.[43] They concluded that antiplatelet therapy, particularly low-dose ASA, with warfarin reduces the risk for systemic thromboembolism and death in these patients while increasing the risk of major bleeding only slightly.

A relatively new concept in anticoagulation for mechanical heart valves is the use of low-molecular-weight heparin (LMWH); however, there is not yet an abundance of reported data on this topic. Lev-Ran and associates described two treatment failures with this approach.[44] Their two patients had mechanical bileaflet valves, one in the mitral position and one in the aortic position. Both patients were treated with enoxaparin, a LMWH, after warfarin treatment had to be discontinued, and both went on to have thrombosis of their mechanical valves after 32 weeks and 37 weeks of enoxaparin treatment. Anti–factor Xa levels were apparently not followed in these patients. Two other small case series of successful use of long-term LMWH in patients with mechanical heart valves have been reported.[45,46]

LMWH treatment has been used successfully in the immediate postoperative period following mechanical heart valve implantation. Montalescot and associates treated patients immediately after valve implantation with LMWH instead of UH while waiting for oral anticoagulant therapy to become therapeutic.[47] They monitored anti–factor Xa levels and found the LMWH treatment to be effective as an alternative to UH. The use of LMWH, if shown to be reliable, might allow for earlier hospital discharge following valve replacement while waiting for therapeutic warfarin levels to be achieved.

Consensus Recommendations for Antithrombotic Therapy for Prosthetic Heart Valves

In an effort to synthesize clinical data on the subject of antithrombotic therapy for prosthetic heart valves, consensus guidelines have been drafted. Table 2-2 summa-rizes recommendations from a recent ACCP consensus conference.[33] General recommendations for patients with mechanical valves include the following: (1) all patients with mechanical valves require oral anticoagulation, and (2) UH or LMWH should be used until a therapeutic INR has been achieved for 2 days. General recommendations for patients with bioprosthetic valves include (1) oral anticoagulation for 3 months for mitral or aortic valve replacement, (2) UH or LMWH until a therapeutic INR has been achieved for 2 days, and (3) long-term ASA (80 mg daily) for patients in sinus rhythm.

Another set of recommendations for antithrombotic therapy comes from a recent American College of Cardiology/American Heart Association task force on practice guidelines for valvular heart disease, as shown in Table 2-3.[48] General recommendations include (1) addition of ASA (80 to 100 mg daily) if not on ASA, and (2) warfarin (INR 3.5 to 4.5) in high-risk patients when ASA cannot be used.[48]

In addition to heart valve replacements, many patients undergo repairs, particularly of the mitral valve, often incorporating prosthetic annuloplasty rings. There is not much data in the literature with regard to antithrombotic strategies for these patients. One recommendation from the Mayo Clinic, extrapolated from their experience with valve replacement, is that patients undergoing valve repair who are in sinus rhythm should be treated with warfarin with a goal INR of 2.5 for 6 weeks to 3 months followed by 325 mg of ASA per day indefinitely.[37]

Antithrombotic Strategies for Ventricular Assist Devices

Mechanical circulatory support systems have evolved rapidly over the last decade to the point now where there are feasible alternatives available for patients with end-stage heart failure as a bridge to heart transplantation, as well as for those patients in need of shorter-term

TABLE 2-2. American College of Chest Physicians Consensus Recommendations on Antithrombotic Therapy for Prosthetic Heart Valves

Valve Type	Modifying Factor	Antithrombotic Regimen
St. Jude, Carbomedics, Medtronic-Hall	AVR	Warfarin (INR 2–3)
Mechanical: bileaflet	AVR, AF	Warfarin (INR 2.5–3.5) or INR 2–3 and ASA 80 mg daily
Mechanical: tilting disk or bileaflet	MVR	Warfarin (INR 2.5–3.5) or INR 2–3 and ASA 80 mg daily
Mechanical: caged-ball	None	Warfarin (INR 2.5–3.5) and ASA 80–100 mg daily
Mechanical: any type	Additional risk factors	Warfarin (INR 2.5–3.5) and ASA 80–100 mg daily
Bioprosthetic	None	Warfarin (INR 2–3) for 3 months, then ASA 80 mg daily
Bioprosthetic	AF	Warfarin (INR 2–3)
Bioprosthetic	LA thrombus	Warfarin (INR 2–3)
Bioprosthetic	History of systemic TE	Warfarin (INR 2–3) for 3 to 12 months

AF = atrial fibrillation; ASA = acetylsalicylic acid; AVR = aortic valve replacement; INR = international normalized ratio; LA = left atrial; MVR = mitral valve replacement; TE = thromboembolism.
Reproduced with permission from Stein PD et al.[33]

TABLE 2-3. American College of Cardiology/American Heart Association Consensus Recommendations on Antithrombotic Therapy for Prosthetic Heart Valves

Indication	Antithrombotic Regimen
First 3 months after valve replacement	Warfarin (INR 2.5–3.5)
More than 3 months after valve replacement	
Mechanical valve	
AVR and no risk factor*	
Bileaflet valve or Medtronic-Hall valve	Warfarin (INR 2–3)
Other disk valves or Starr-Edwards valve	Warfarin (INR 2.5–3.5)
AVR plus risk factor*	Warfarin (INR 2.5–3.5)
MVR	Warfarin (INR 2.5–3.5)
Bioprosthesis	
AVR and no risk factor*	ASA 80–100 mg daily
AVR and risk factor*	Warfarin (INR 2–3)
MVR and no risk factor*	ASA 80–100 mg daily
MVR and risk factor*	Warfarin (INR 2.5–3.5)

ASA = acetylsalicylic acid; AVR = aortic valve replacement; INR = international normalized ratio; MVR = mitral valve replacement.
*Risk factors: atrial fibrillation, left ventricular dysfunction, previous thromboembolism, hypercoagulable conditions.
Reproduced with permission from Bonow RO et al.[48]

circulatory support for reversible conditions such as myocarditis. Device design has evolved to the point where there are several FDA-approved pulsatile devices designed for long-term support, as well as a number of new axial flow and pulsatile devices undergoing human trials now. For VADs in particular, the thromboembolic rate historically has been approximately 20%.[49] This rate has decreased with modifications to the designs of pumps and cannulae as well as improvements in pharmacologic regimens. Antithrombotic strategies vary for mechanical circulatory support devices as a function of their design in terms of the properties of the blood-contacting surfaces, as well as the type of pumping action. Both the device itself and individual patient characteristics dictate the antithrombotic strategy that must be followed.

Table 2-4 illustrates representative antithrombotic regimens that are used at various centers for a number of the available mechanical circulatory support devices. As with prosthetic heart valves, antithrombotic treatment plans for patients with support devices must be tailored to patients' individual medical characteristics. It should be noted that not all of these devices are approved for use by the FDA.

Special Situations

When patients with a prosthetic heart valve or mechanical circulatory support device in place experience bleeding problems (eg, from gastrointestinal hemorrhage or intracranial hemorrhage), a decision has to be made regarding modification of the existing antithrombotic regimen. Any reduction in level of antithrombotic therapy has the potential for the generation of thromboembolism, while the bleeding complication often demands a change in therapy. There is insufficient literature addressing this situation. One recent retrospective study of 52 patients undergoing anticoagulation with warfarin for mechanical heart valves analyzed the discontinuation of anticoagulation in the setting of intracranial hemorrhage.[57] The goal of the study was to assess the risk of ischemic stroke following the discontinuation of anticoagulation in this group of patients, 27% of which had a history of previous ischemic stroke. This study found that the cumulative risk for ischemic stroke at 30 days in patients with mechanical heart valves who have had warfarin anticoagulation discontinued is 3%, although it did not specify the mean duration of anticoagulation discontinuation, and concluded that 1- to 2-week discontinuation of anticoagulation therapy in these patients is safe.[57]

Life-threatening bleeding complications may require complete cessation of anticoagulation, with the attendant

TABLE 2-4. Representative Antithrombotic Strategies for VADs

Device	Device Type	Support Duration	Antithrombotic Regimen	Reference
Abiomed BVS-5000	Pulsatile, EC	Short-term	IV heparin with ACT 200 seconds	50
Cardiac Assist Technologies AB-180	Centrifugal, EC	Short-term	No systemic drugs, heparin into pump	51
Thoratec HeartMate LVAD	Pulsatile, IC	Long-term	ASA 325 mg daily	13
Baxter Novacor LVAS	Pulsatile, IC	Long-term	Warfarin with INR 2.0–2.5, clopidogrel	27
Thoratec VAD	Pulsatile, EC	Long-term	Warfarin with INR 3.0–3.5	52
Berlin Heart LVAD	Pulsatile, EC	Long-term	Warfarin with INR 2.5–3.5, ASA 50 mg daily, clopidogrel 375 mg daily	28
Thoratec HeartMate II LVAD	Axial, IC	Long-term	Planned warfarin with INR 1.5–2.5, ASA, dipyridamole	53
Jarvik 2000 LVAD	Axial, IC	Long-term	Warfarin with INR 2.0	54
MicroMed DeBakey LVAD	Axial, IC	Long-term	Warfarin with INR 2.0–2.5, ASA, clopidogrel	55
CardioWest TAH	Pulsatile, IC	Long-term	Warfarin with INR 2.5–3.5, ASA, dipyridamole, pentoxifylline, clopidogrel	56

ACT = activated clotting time; ASA = acetylsalicylic acid; EC = extracorporeal; IC = intracorporeal; INR = international normalized ratio; IV = intravenous; LVAD = left ventricular assist device; LVAS = left ventricular assist system; TAH = total artificial heart; VAD = ventricular assist device.

risk of thrombosis, while less-severe bleeding episodes may simply necessitate a decrease in the level of anticoagulation.

Summary

Patients with valvular heart disease or heart failure will continue to benefit from the development of prosthetic valves and mechanical circulatory support devices with decreased thrombogenicity, as well as anticoagulant and antiplatelet drugs with increased efficacy and safety profiles. The relevance to the cardiac surgeon of these antithrombotic strategies will likely become increasingly important as it now appears that the number of long-term mechanical circulatory support devices implanted annually is likely to continue to grow.[58] As in the past, the goal will be to design optimal antithrombotic regimens, making use of anticoagulants as well as antiplatelet agents, to provide freedom from both thromboembolic and bleeding complications in patients with prosthetic heart valves and implanted circulatory support systems.

References

1. Edmunds LH. Extracorporeal perfusion. In: Edmunds LH, editor. Cardiac surgery in the adult. New York: McGraw-Hill; 1997. p. 255–94.
2. Vroman L, Adams AL, Fischer GC, et al. Interaction of high-molecular-weight kininogen, factor XII, and fibrinogen in plasma at interfaces. Blood 1980;55:156–9.
3. Majerus PW, Broze GJ, Miletich JP, et al. Anticoagulant, thrombolytic, and antiplatelet drugs. In: Hardman JG, Limbird LE, editors. Goodman and Gilman's the pharmacological basis of therapeutics. 9th ed. New York: McGraw-Hill; 1996. p. 1341–60.
4. Sheppeck RA, Bentz M, Dickson C, et al. Examination of the roles of glycoprotein Ib and glycoprotein IIb/IIIa in platelet deposition on an artificial surface using clinical antiplatelet agents and monoclonal antibody blockade. Blood 1991;78:673–80.
5. Lefkovits J, Plow EF, Topol EJ. Platelet glycoprotein IIb/IIIa receptors in cardiovascular medicine. N Engl J Med 1995;332:1553–9.
6. Jen CJ, Lin JS. Direct observation of platelet adhesion to fibrinogen- and fibrin-coated surfaces. Am J Physiol 1991;261:H1457–63.
7. Schoen FJ, Claggett GP, Hill JD, et al. The biocompatibility of artificial organs. ASAIO Trans 1987;33:824–33.
8. Bamford CH, Al-Lamee KG. Chemical methods for improving haemocompatibility of synthetic polymers. Clinical Materials 1992;10:243–61.
9. Bernhard WF, Colo NA, Szycher M, et al. Development of a nonthrombogenic collagenous blood-prosthetic interface. Ann Surg 1980;192:369–81.
10. Bjork VO, Sternlieb JJ, Kaminsky DB. Optimal microporous surface for endothelialization of metal heart valves in the blood stream. Scand J Cardiovasc Surg 1990;24:97–100.
11. Rose EA, Levin HR, Oz MC, et al. Artificial circulatory support with textured interior surfaces: a counterintuitive approach to minimizing thromboembolism. Circulation 1994;90:87–91.
12. Dasse KA, Chipman SD, Sherman CW, et al. Clinical experience with textured blood contacting surfaces in ventricular assist devices. ASAIO Transactions 1987;33:418–25.
13. Slater JP, Rose EA, Levin HR, et al. Low thromboembolic risk without anticoagulation using advanced-design left ventricular assist devices. Ann Thorac Surg 1996;62:1321–7.
14. Spanier T, Oz M, Levin H, et al. Activation of coagulation and fibrinolytic pathways in patients with left ventricular assist devices. J Thorac Cardiovasc Surg 1996;112:1090–7.
15. Spanier TB, Chen JM, Oz MC, et al. Time-dependent cellular population of textured-surface left ventricular assist devices contribute to the development of a biphasic systemic procoagulant response. J Thorac Cardiovasc Surg 1999;118:404–13.
16. Aldea GS, Doursounian M, O'Gara P, et al. Heparin-bonded circuits with a reduced anticoagulation protocol in primary CABG: a prospective, randomized study. Ann Thorac Surg 1996;62:410–8.
17. Koster A, Loebe M, Sodian R, et al. Heparin antibodies and thromboembolism in heparin-coated and noncoated ventricular assist devices. J Thorac Cardiovasc Surg 2001;121:331–5.
18. Janvier G, Baquey C, Roth C, et al. Extracorporeal circulation, hemocompatibility, and biomaterials. Ann Thorac Surg 1996;62:1926–34.
19. Wendel HP, Ziemer G. Coating-techniques to improve the hemocompatibility of artificial devices used for extracorporeal circulation. Eur J Cardiothorac Surg 1999;16:342–50.
20. De Somer F, Francois K, van Oeveren W, et al. Phosphorylcholine coating of extracorporeal circuits provide natural protection against blood activation by the material surface. Eur J Cardiothorac Surg 2000;18:602–6.
21. Follis F, Schmidt CA. Cardiopulmonary bypass in patients with heparin-induced thrombocytopenia and thrombosis. Ann Thorac Surg 2000;70:2173–81.
22. Frederiksen JW. Cardiopulmonary bypass in humans: bypassing unfractionated heparin. Ann Thorac Surg 2000:70:1434–43.
23. Koster A, Loebe M, Hansen R, et al. Alterations in coagulation after implantation of a pulsatile Novacor LVAD and the axial flow MicoMed DeBakey LVAD. Ann Thorac Surg 2000;70:533–7.
24. Madras PN, Thomson CL, Johnson WR. The effect of Coumadin upon thrombus forming on foreign surfaces. Artif Organs 1980;4:192–8.
25. Braunwald E. Valvular heart disease. In: Brauwald E, Zipes DP, Libby P, editors. Heart disease. 6th ed. Philadelphia: WB Saunders; 2001. p. 1643–713.
26. Al Suwaidi J, Berger PB, Holmes DR. Coronary artery stents. JAMA 2000;284:1828–36.
27. Robbins RC, Kown MH, Portner PM, et al. The totally implantable Novacor left ventricular assist system. Ann Thorac Surg 2001;71:S162–5.
28. Loebe M, Kaufman F, Hetzer R. The Berlin heart. In: Goldstein DJ, Oz MC, editors. Cardiac assist devices. Armonk, NY: Futura Publishing Company, 2000. p. 275–87.

29. Kontozis L, Skudicky D, Hopley MJ, et al. Long-term follow-up of St. Jude medical prosthesis in a young rheumatic population using low-level warfarin anticoagulation: an analysis of the temporal distribution of causes of death. Am J Cardiol 1998;81:736–9.

30. Tcheng JE, Ellis SG, George BS. Pharmacodynamics of chimeric glycoprotein IIb/IIIa integrin antiplatelet antibody Fab 7E3 in high-risk coronary angioplasty. Circulation 1994;90:1757–64.

31. Lincoff AM, LeRoy AL, Despotis GJ, et al. Abciximab and bleeding during coronary surgery: results from the EPI-LOG and EPISTENT trials. Ann Thorac Surg 2000;70:516–26.

32. Cannegieter SC, Rosendaal FR, Briet E. Platelets/thromboembolism: thromboembolic and bleeding complications in patients with mechanical heart valve prostheses. Circulation 1994;89:635–41.

33. Stein PD, Alpert JS, Bussey HI, et al. Antithrombotic therapy in patients with mechanical and biological prosthetic heart valves. Chest 2001;119:220S–7S.

34. Moinuddeen K, Quin J, Shaw R, et al. Anticoagulation is unnecessary after biological aortic valve replacment. Circulation 1998;98 Suppl II:95II–8II.

35. Blair KL, Hatton AC, White WD, et al. Comparison of anticoagulation regimens after Carpentier-Edwards aortic or mitral valve replacement. Circulation 1994;90:214–9.

36. Vongpatanasin W, Hillis LD, Lange RA. Prosthetic heart valves. N Engl J Med 1996;335:407–16.

37. Tiede DJ, Nishimura RA, Gastineau DA, et al. Modern management of prosthetic valve anticoagulation. Mayo Clin Proc 1998;73:665–80.

38. Akins CW. Results with mechanical cardiac valvular prostheses. Ann Thorac Surg 1995;60:1836–44.

39. Cannegieter SC, Rosendaal FR, Wintzen AR, et al. Optimal oral anticoagulant therapy in patients with mechanical heart valves. N Engl J Med 1995;333:11–7.

40. Meschengieser SS, Fondevila CG, Frontroth J, et al. Low-intensity oral anticoagulation plus low-dose aspirin versus high-intensity oral anticoagulation alone: a randomized trial in patients with mechanical prosthetic heart valves. J Thorac Cardiovasc Surg 1997;113:910–6.

41. Altman R, Rouvier J, Gurfinkel E, et al. Comparison of two levels of anticoagulant therapy in patients with substitute heart valves. J Thorac Cardiovasc Surg 1991;101:427–33.

42. Turpie A, Gent M, Laupacis A, et al. A comparison of aspirin with placebo in patients treated with warfarin after heart-valve replacement. N Engl J Med 1993;329:524–9.

43. Massel D, Little SH. Risks and benefits of adding antiplatelet therapy to warfarin among patients with prosthetic heart valves: a meta-analysis. J Am Coll Cardiol 2001;37:569–78.

44. Lev-Ran O, Kramer A, Gurevitch J, et al. Low-molecular-weight heparin for prosthetic heart valves: treatment failure. Ann Thorac Surg 2000;69:264–6.

45. Weitz JI. Low-molecular-weight heparins. N Engl J Med 1997;337:688–98.

46. Lee LH, Liauw PLY, Ng ASH. Low-molecular-weight heparin for thromboprophylaxis during pregnancy in 2 patients with mechanical mitral valve replacement. Thromb Haemost 1996;76:628–30.

47. Montalescot G, Polle V, Collet JP, et al. Low-molecular-weight heparin after mechanical heart valve replacement. Circulation 2000;101:1083–6.

48. Bonow RO, Carabello B, deLeon AC, et al. Guidelines for the management of patients with valvular heart disease: executive summary: a report of the American College of Cardiology/American Heart Association task force on practice guidelines (committee on management of patients with valvular heart disease). Circulation 1998;98:1949–84.

49. Goldstein DJ, Oz MC, Rose EA. Implantable left ventricular assist devices. N Engl J Med 1998;339:1522–33.

50. Samuels LE, Holmes EC, Thomas MP, et al. Management of acute cardiac failure with mechanical assist: experience with ABIOMED BVS 5000. Ann Thorac Surg 2001;71:S67–72.

51. Magovern JA, Sussman MJ, Goldstein AH, et al. Clinical results with the AB-180 left ventricular assist device. Ann Thorac Surg 2001;71:S121–4.

52. Pennington DG, Oaks TE, Lohmann DP. The Thoratec device. In: Goldstein DJ, Oz MC, editors. Cardiac assist devices. Armonk, NY: Futura Publishing Company; 2000. p. 251–62.

53. Griffith BP, Kormos RL, Borovetz HS, et al. HeartMate II left ventricular assist system: from concept to first clinical use. Ann Thorac Surg 2001;71:S116–20.

54. Westaby S, Banning AP, Jarvik R, et al. First permanent implant of the Jarvik 2000 heart. Lancet 2000;356:900–3.

55. Noon GP, Morley DL, Suellen I, et al. Clinical experience with the MicroMed DeBakey ventricular assist device. Ann Thorac Surg 2001;71:S133–8.

56. Copeland J, Arabia F, Smith R, et al. The CardioWest total artificial heart. In: Goldstein DJ, Oz MC, editors. Cardiac assist devices. Armonk, NY: Futura Publishing Company; 2000. p. 341–55.

57. Phan TG, Koh M, Wijdicks EFM. Safety of discontinuation of anticoagulation in patients with intracranial hemorrhage at high thromboembolic risk. Arch Neurol 2000;57:1710–3.

58. Rose EA, Gelijns AC, Moskowitz AJ, et al. Long-term use of a left ventricular assist device for end-state heart failure. N Engl J Med 2001;345:1435–43.

CHAPTER 3

PROPHYLAXIS AGAINST ATRIAL FIBRILLATION FOLLOWING OPEN HEART SURGERY

JOSEPH C. CLEVELAND JR, MD, FREDERICK L. GROVER, MD

Atrial fibrillation is the most common arrhythmia occurring after cardiac surgery, with an estimated incidence of 20 to 40% following cardiac surgery.[1,2] Although cardiac surgeons routinely dismiss postoperative supraventricular tachycardias as a mere nuisance, current data suggest that atrial fibrillation following cardiac surgery may result in significant morbidity.[1,3] Atrial fibrillation is associated with complications including thromboembolism, a need to institute further therapy with potential adverse effects (pharmacologic), and a prolonged hospital stay with a resultant increase in resources and cost.[1,4] This chapter reviews the risk factors, proposed pathogenesis of atrial fibrillation, and pharmacologic or electrical strategies to prevent or decrease the incidence of atrial fibrillation following cardiac surgery.

Risk Factors for Atrial Fibrillation Following Cardiac Surgery

Prior investigations have established several risk factors to identify patients at high risk for atrial fibrillation following cardiac surgery. The most robust clinical risk factor associated with postoperative atrial fibrillation is increasing age.[1–6] The risk for developing atrial fibrillation is less than 5% for patients who are younger than the fourth decade, roughly 25 to 30% for patients in the sixth decade of life, and nearly 60% for patients in the eighth decade of life.[7] Attempts to correlate metabolic and morphologic changes in atrial tissue with atrial fibrillation are attractive mechanistic hypotheses to explain this association. Changes in atrial tissue such as atrophy of myocytes, increased lipopigment deposition, and vacuolation of atrial tissue have yielded a variable correlation with the development of postoperative atrial fibrillation.[8] Clearly, these investigations are important, as they may shed

important insights into the mechanism whereby increasing age promotes postoperative atrial fibrillation.

A multitude of other risk factors (Table 3-1) have also been identified as predictive for the development of postoperative atrial fibrillation. These other risk factors have not been consistently observed across all studies, however. Creswell and colleagues identified increasing patient age, preoperative use of digoxin, a history of rheumatic disease, the presence of chronic obstructive pulmonary disease, and increasing aortic cross-clamp time as independent risk factors associated with the development of atrial fibrillation.[3] Mathew and colleagues identified these independent risk factors for the development of atrial fibrillation: advanced age, a history of atrial fibrillation or congestive heart failure, male sex, and a resting heart rate of greater than 100 beats per minute.[2] In addition, these investigators identified pulmonary vein venting, bicaval cannulation, postoperative atrial pacing, and prolonged aortic cross-clamp times as independent procedural related risk factors for the development of postoperative atrial fibrillation. Targeting a high-risk group with prophylaxis seems appealing. However, based upon

TABLE 3-1. Risk Factors for Developing Postoperative Atrial Fibrillation

- Age
- History of atrial fibrillation or congestive heart failure
- Male sex
- Preoperative use of digoxin
- Chronic obstructive pulmonary disease
- History of rheumatic heart disease
- Resting heart rate > 100 bpm
- Prolonged aortic cross-clamp time
- Bicaval cannulation
- Pulmonary vein venting

the broad clinical risk factors identified to date, it seems prudent to offer prophylaxis to all patients.

Adverse Outcomes Associated with Postoperative Atrial Fibrillation

The development of postoperative atrial fibrillation is clearly not predictive of an increased mortality. This fact has largely been responsible for the perception that this particular arrhythmia is somehow "benign." However, it is incontrovertible that patients who develop atrial fibrillation following cardiac surgery have a more complicated, prolonged postoperative recovery.[1,3] Indeed, Creswell and colleagues reported an increased incidence of postoperative stroke (3.3% vs 1.4%) in patients who developed postoperative atrial fibrillation.[3] Almassi and colleagues also reported a 5.3% incidence of cardiovascular accident (CVA) in postoperative atrial fibrillation versus 2.4% in patients without postoperative atrial fibrillation.[1] Patients who develop atrial fibrillation are further placed at risk for developing heart failure if they have marginal ventricular function postoperatively, or if they develop a very rapid ventricular response. Lastly, the treatment of atrial fibrillation with pharmacologic agents is associated with significant adverse effects. Many of the antiarrhythmic agents can produce hypotension, bradycardia, and potentially lethal proarrhythmic changes such as torsades de pointes. As mentioned earlier, the mere implementation of a new drug to treat this disorder obligates the patient to a more complicated postoperative course.

The management of postoperative atrial fibrillation consumes a substantial amount of health care resources, in addition to placing the patient at risk for increased perioperative morbidity.[4,9] Diagnostic studies, including electrocardiograms, serum chemistries, and arterial blood gas determinations, in patients who experience atrial fibrillation are often unrevealing of a serious metabolic or ischemic basis for this arrhythmia. However, these tests are routinely performed in many institutions, and they represent a significant cost in terms of health care resources. More importantly, as the peak incidence of atrial fibrillation is between the second and fourth postoperative day, patients must remain in a monitored bed status (step-down unit) until the arrhythmia resolves or until the ventricular rate is reliably controlled. Thus, the development of atrial fibrillation lengthens the overall hospital stay after cardiac surgery, and it increases the acuity level of the patient. In fact, atrial fibrillation after cardiac surgery is estimated to cost an additional $562 million (US) per year following coronary artery bypass graft (CABG) alone.[9] It is the summation of the patient-specific increases in morbidity, CVA, risks of additional medications, and the increased health care resource utilization that make this arrhythmia a serious and costly postoperative complication.

Pathogenesis of Atrial Fibrillation Following Cardiac Surgery

The mechanism(s) leading to atrial fibrillation following cardiac surgery is (are) multifactorial and incompletely understood. Elegant studies by Sato and colleagues have characterized the electrophysiologic abnormalities in the atria of animals subjected to cardiopulmonary bypass.[10] Simplistically, it appears that cardiopulmonary bypass (CPB) induces changes in the dispersion of refractoriness of the atrium. Dispersion of refractoriness describes the orderly progression of the normal short periods of refractoriness in the left atrium to the longer periods of refractoriness in the right atrium. Normally, areas of short refractoriness do not lie adjacent to longer periods of refractoriness. This change from relatively ordered, homogenous areas of refractory periods (preoperative state) to nonhomogenous (postoperative state) areas of short and long refractory periods lying adjacent to one another promotes fibrillation in the atria. It was proposed that relative atrial ischemia during aortic cross-clamping was a possible mechanism producing these changes. Plausible hypotheses to promote these changes in the dispersion of refractoriness with CPB include atrial ischemia, effects of cardioplegia and CPB, volume/fluid shifts occurring postoperatively, and direct injury to the right atrium with cannulation.[10,11]

These hypotheses appeared to explain the mechanisms of atrial fibrillation until the recent era of off-pump coronary artery bypass (CAB), which is also associated with a significant incidence of postoperative atrial fibrillation. Conflicting reports regarding the influence of off-pump CAB upon the postoperative incidence of atrial fibrillation exist. Siebert and colleagues found no difference in the rate of postoperative atrial fibrillation in patients undergoing off-pump CAB (10.2%) versus patients (9.2%) with conventional CAB procedures.[12] Conversely, Hernandez and colleagues found a significant reduction —from a 26% incidence of postoperative atrial fibrillation following conventional CAB to 21% in the off-pump group—in the Northern New England Cardiovascular Disease Study Group.[13] Thus, many of the proposed mechanisms invoking CPB or global atrial ischemia seem less plausible to explain these electrophysiologic changes. An attractive unifying hypothesis is a combination of pericarditis with a local inflammatory response, and the presence of a hyperadrenergic state postoperatively. Both of these mechanisms are present whether CAB is performed on or off pump, and could explain the predisposition of patients toward the development of atrial fibrillation after cardiac surgery. The hypothesis is supported by the observation that β-receptor antagonists play an important role in decreasing the incidence of postoperative atrial fibrillation. Lastly, histologic studies of atrial tissue may elucidate mechanisms favoring the development of atrial fibrillation. At the time of surgery, Ad and colleagues found myolysis and lipofuscin in the right atrium of patients undergoing CAB and correlated these changes with the occurrence of atrial fibrillation postoperatively.[8] Currently, it appears that several mechanisms may contribute to the development of atrial fibrillation and the characterized changes in the refractory period throughout the atrium following cardiac surgery.

Pharmacologic Prophylaxis against Atrial Fibrillation

Numerous pharmacologic strategies attempt to reduce the incidence of postoperative atrial fibrillation. Overall, most reported studies demonstrate a positive effect with a variety of pharmacologic agents; to date, however, no singular particular agent or combination of agents has completely eliminated atrial fibrillation following cardiac surgery.

Digitalis was one of the earliest antiarrhythmic agents employed. Johnson and colleagues found a reduction in postoperative atrial fibrillation, from 25 to 5%, with digitalis preparation.[14] Based upon this study, digitalis became widely employed to prevent atrial fibrillation. Its use today, however, is limited. Studies exist that suggest an increased risk of postoperative arrhythmias in patients treated with digoxin. More contemporary experience with digoxin alone as a preventive agent does not reduce the incidence of atrial fibrillation to less than 20%.

Magnesium infusions have also been examined in relation to preventing atrial fibrillation after cardiac surgery. Casthely and colleagues studied the effect of perioperative and postoperative magnesium infusions in 140 patients.[15] The group that received magnesium pre– and post–cardiopulmonary bypass had the lowest incidence of atrial fibrillation. We routinely administer magnesium postoperatively to our patients for 48 h to diminish the incidence of atrial fibrillation.

Procainamide (Vaughn Williams class Ia) has been used to treat and to prevent atrial fibrillation after cardiac surgery. When administered in a randomized blinded controlled trial to subjects for 5 days after cardiac surgery, procainamide reduced the incidence of atrial fibrillation compared to control subjects.[16] While this evidence supports the use of this agent, procainamide is not easily administered, it is associated with torsades de pointes, serum levels of its metabolites must be followed, and toxicity can develop. Therefore, we have not used this agent routinely for prophylaxis.

β-Receptor antagonists have been extensively studied as prophylactic agents to prevent atrial fibrillation post cardiac surgery. Several studies have individually confirmed the efficacy of these agents in reducing the incidence of postoperative atrial fibrillation. A meta-analysis of β-receptor antagonists revealed a significant decrease in the likelihood of patients developing atrial fibrilla-

tion.[17] Patients who received β-receptor antagonists had an odds ratio of 0.28 (95% confidence interval, 0.21–0.36) for developing atrial fibrillation. A subsequent meta-analysis corroborated these observations and noted a significant reduction in the incidence of atrial fibrillation in patients receiving either β-receptor antagonists alone or in combination with digoxin.[18] Clearly, β-receptor antagonists have several other salutary benefits, and they represent extremely attractive agents in the prevention of atrial fibrillation following cardiac surgery. In addition, β-receptor antagonists have the appeal of attenuating the hyperadrenergic state following cardiac surgery. Thus, a physiologic rationale also exists for their use. As the vast majority of our patients are already placed on β-receptor antagonists preoperatively, we reinstitute β-receptor antagonists as soon as possible after cardiac surgery (usually on postoperative day [POD] 1). We routinely use metoprolol, beginning at a dose of 25 mg po bid, and increasing the dose until the patient's preoperative dose is achieved.

Sotalol, a class III agent with β-receptor antagonist properties, is also widely used to prevent atrial fibrillation.[19] Sotalol has proven efficacious as an agent that decreases the incidence of atrial fibrillation in all but two studies.[20] Although sotalol has proven efficacy, two specific properties of this agent deserve mention. Sotalol's β-receptor antagonist properties are potent, and significant episodes of bradycardia are common during therapy. More importantly, sotalol prolongs the QT interval and can predispose patients to potentially lethal arrhythmias, including torsades de pointes.

Amiodarone is another pharmacologic agent that has enjoyed much popularity as a prophylactic agent against atrial fibrillation. Amiodarone is also a class III agent, with very weak adrenergic receptor–blocking properties. Most studies that used amiodarone for prevention against atrial fibrillation have noted a decreased incidence in patients receiving amiodarone. Daoud and colleagues administered amiodarone (200 mg po tid) for 7 days before cardiac surgery.[21] They subsequently noticed a reduction in the incidence of atrial fibrillation in those patients receiving amiodarone (23%), as compared to control patients (42%). Total hospital costs were lowered in the amiodarone group ($18,375 [US]) versus control patients ($23,387 [US]). Their study, however, relegated patients to a 1-week oral loading regimen preoperatively. As an increasing proportion of our patients are operated upon shortly after cardiac catheterization, the 1-week loading regimen used in this study is unavailable to a substantial number of patients.

The Amiodarone Reduction in Coronary Heart (ARCH) trial conducted by Guarnieri and colleagues attempted to remedy some of the criticisms of the prior Daoud study.[22] They administered 1 g of amiodarone IV immediately postoperatively to patients undergoing cardiac surgery. The vast majority of these patients underwent CAB only, and they demonstrated a decrease in the incidence of atrial fibrillation with postoperative amiodarone prophylaxis. Although demonstrating a decreased incidence of atrial fibrillation (35% treated vs 47% control), interestingly enough, there was no difference in the hospital length of stay between the amiodarone and placebo groups. Furthermore, this study reported that control subjects had an incidence of atrial fibrillation of 47%, whereas amiodarone-treated patients still had an incidence of atrial fibrillation that was 35%. Critics of this study note that the amiodarone-treated group had an incidence of atrial fibrillation which approaches that of placebo-treated patients in other studies. In addition, amiodarone did not decrease the length of hospital stay.

More recently, Giri and colleagues queried whether oral amiodarone in combination with β-receptor antagonists could decrease the likelihood of developing atrial fibrillation after cardiac surgery.[23] They evaluated both patients who could be loaded orally 5 days prior to surgery and patients who could only receive 1 day of preoperative oral loading. They noted a decrease in atrial fibrillation from 38% in controls to 23% in amiodarone-treated patients. Even more notably, there was a significant difference in favor of amiodarone in the prevention of postoperative CVA, and ventricular tachycardia. Others have noted favorable effects when amiodarone has been administered perioperatively to prevent atrial fibrillation following cardiac surgery.[24,25] Amiodarone is a safely administered drug, but it does have a long half-life, and pulmonary toxicity can occur, but this adverse effect is usually associated with prolonged use. It would appear that amiodarone is most efficacious when administered preoperatively to prevent atrial fibrillation following cardiac surgery.

Effects of Biatrial Pacing to Prevent Atrial Fibrillation

Although prophylactic administration of a variety of pharmacologic agents such as β-adrenergic–receptor antagonists, amiodarone, and sotalol reduce the incidence of atrial fibrillation following cardiac surgery, there is still an appreciable 15 to 25% occurrence of this arrhythmia. Observational studies in patients with atrial fibrillation show that chronic, simultaneous dual atrial pacing may reduce the rate of atrial fibrillation recurrence. Thus, it seems logical that biatrial pacing could reduce the incidence of atrial fibrillation following cardiac surgery.

Three randomized, controlled trials evaluating biatrial pacing in the prophylaxis of postoperative atrial fibrillation exist. Fan and colleagues evaluated 132 patients without a history of atrial fibrillation who underwent cardiac surgery (CAS).[26] Patients were randomized into four groups: control (no pacing), right atrial pacing, left atrial pacing, or biatrial pacing. The patients in the pacing groups were paced at either 90 beats per minute or 10 beats per minute greater than the intrinsic heart rate (maximum paced rate = 120 bpm). Overdrive pacing was continued for 5 days, and patients were continuously monitored with telemetry for this period. The incidence of atrial fibrillation was 42% in controls, 36% in left-atrial-only-paced, 33% in right-atrial-only-paced, and 13% in biatrial-paced patients. Furthermore, the length of stay was significantly reduced in the biatrial pacing group (7 days versus 9 days in the control group). Daoud and colleagues similarly randomized 118 patients to right atrial pacing (atrial inhibited [AAI] mode), right atrial triggered (AAT) pacing, or biatrial pacing (triggered mode).[27] Both patients and investigators were blinded to the pacing technique, and patients were followed on telemetry postoperatively. Patients were paced until 24 h prior to discharge, and atrial fibrillation was defined as any atrial fibrillation that lasted longer than 5 min. The incidence of atrial fibrillation in the right-atrium-only-paced patients was approximately 30%, whereas biatrial pacing reduced the incidence of postoperative atrial fibrillation to 10%. In contrast to Fan and colleagues, this study revealed no difference in postoperative length of stay (PLOS) between the groups—all groups had a PLOS of approximately 7 days.[26] Levy and colleagues randomized 130 patients to biatrial pacing for 4 days or no pacing.[28] They observed a decrease from 39% incidence of atrial fibrillation in control subjects to 14% in biatrial-paced patients. In summary, these three trials consistently show a positive effect for biatrial pacing in reducing the incidence of atrial fibrillation following cardiac surgery.

Conclusions

Despite multiple strategies to prevent atrial fibrillation following cardiac surgery, this problem is the most common arrhythmia encountered in the postoperative period. Although viewed as an inconvenience by many cardiac surgeons, this arrhythmia may have serious adverse long-term outcomes, such as an increased incidence of CVA. Even if patient-related morbidity were unaffected by this arrhythmia, the societal costs in terms of additional days of hospitalization are enormous. An ideal prophylactic strategy is one that is easily administered, is effective across a wide range of patient population, is inexpensive, and is associated with minimal risk or adverse side effects. A singular "ideal" strategy to prevent postoperative atrial fibrillation following cardiac surgery does not exist. However, it seems reasonable to offer the following approach based upon the available data. (1) β-Receptor antagonists should be reinstituted as soon as possible after cardiac surgery. (2) Amiodarone should be administered preoperatively in an elective setting at a dose of 200 mg po tid for 1 week prior to surgery. It is less clear that amiodarone is as efficacious in preventing postoperative atrial fibrillation. (3) Maintenance of normal electrolyte levels (particularly potassium and magnesium) and avoidance of large volume shifts in the postoperative period are warranted. (4) Biatrial pacing may prove efficacious in preventing atrial fibrillation, but this modality will probably be used in conjunction with pharmacologic therapy to prevent postoperative atrial fibrillation. Unfortunately, less-invasive surgical strategies, such as off-pump CAB, may not uniformly reduce the incidence of atrial fibrillation. The problem of postoperative atrial fibrillation remains as an important postoperative complication, and until postoperative atrial fibrillation is better mechanistically understood, the approach to its prevention will largely require some degree of empiric therapy.

References

1. Almassi GH, Schowalter T, Nicolosi AC, et al. Atrial fibrillation after cardiac surgery: a major morbid event? Ann Surg 1997;226:(4)501–11.

2. Mathew JP, Parks R, Savino JS, et al. Atrial fibrillation following coronary artery bypass graft surgery: predictors, outcomes, and resource utilization. Multi-Center Study of Perioperative Ischemia Research Group. JAMA 1996; 276(4):300–6.

3. Creswell LL, Schuessler RB, Rosenbloom M, Cox JL. Hazards of postoperative atrial arrhythmias. Ann Thorac Surg 1993;56(3):405–9.

4. Aranki SF, Shaw DP, Adams DH, et al. Predictors of atrial fibrillation after coronary artery surgery. Current trends and impact on hospital resources. Circulation 1997; 94(3):390–7.

5. Fuller JA, Adams GG, Buxton B. Atrial fibrillation after coronary artery bypass grafting. Is it a disorder of the elderly? J Thorac Cardiovasc Surg 1989;97(6):821–5.

6. Leitch JW, Thomson D, Baird DK, Harris PJ. The importance of age as a predictor of atrial fibrillation and flutter after coronary artery bypass grafting. J Thorac Cardiovasc Surg 1990;100(3):338–42.

7. Ommen SR, Odell JA, Stanton MS. Atrial arrhythmias after cardiothoracic surgery. N Engl J Med 1997;337(12):209.

8. Ad N, Snir E, Vidne BA, Golomb E. Histologic atrial myolysis is associated with atrial fibrillation after cardiac operation. Ann Thorac Surg 2001;72(3):688–93.

9. Tamis JE, Steinberg JS. Atrial fibrillation independently prolongs hospital stay after coronary artery bypass surgery. Clin Cardiol 2000;23(3):155–9.

10. Sato S, Yamauchi S, Schuessler RB, et al. The effect of augmented atrial hypothermia on atrial refractory period, conduction, and atrial flutter/fibrillation in the canine heart. J Thorac Cardiovasc Surg 1992;104(2):297–306.

11. Cox JL. A perspective on postoperative atrial fibrillation. Semin Thorac Cardiovasc Surg 1999;11(4):299–302.

12. Siebert J, Anisimowicz L, Lango R, et al. Atrial fibrillation after coronary artery bypass grafting: does the type of procedure influence the early postoperative incidence. Eur J Cardiothorac Surg 2001;19(4):455–9.

13. Hernandez F, Cohn WE, Baribeau YR, et al. In-hospital outcomes of off-pump versus on-pump coronary artery bypass procedures: a multicenter experience. Ann Thorac Surg 2001;72(5):1528–33.

14. Johnson LW, Dickstein RA, Fruehan CT, et al. Prophylactic digitalization for coronary artery bypass surgery. Circulation 1976;53(5):819–22.

15. Casthely PA, Yoganathan T, Komer C, Kelly M. Magnesium and arrhythmias after coronary artery bypass surgery. J Cardiothorac Vasc Anesth 1994;8(2):188–91.

16. Laub GW, Janeira L, Muralidharan S, et al. Prophylactic procainamide for prevention of atrial fibrillation after coronary artery bypass grafting: a prospective, double-blind, randomized, placebo-controlled pilot study. Crit Care Med 1993;21(10):1474–78.

17. Andrews TC, Reimold SC, Berlin JA, Antman EM. Prevention of supraventricular arrhythmias after coronary artery bypass surgery. A meta-analysis of randomized control trials. Circulation 1991;84(5):III236–44.

18. Kowey PR, Taylor JE, Rials SJ, Marinchak RA. Meta-analysis of the effectiveness of prophylactic drug therapy in preventing supraventricular arrhythmia early after coronary artery bypass grafting. Am J Cardiol 1992; 69(9):963–5.

19. Suttorp MJ, Kingma JH, Peels HO, et al. Effectiveness of sotalol in preventing supraventricular tachyarrhythmias shortly after coronary artery bypass grafting. Am J Cardiol 1991;68(11):1163–9.

20. Jacquet L, Evenepoel M, Mareene F, et al. Hemodynamic effects and safety of sotalol in the prevention of supraventricular arrhythmias after coronary artery bypass surgery. J Cardiothorac Vasc Anesth 1994;8(4):431–6.

21. Daoud EG, Strickberger SA, Man KC, et al. Preoperative amiodarone as prophylaxis against atrial fibrillation after heart surgery. N Engl J Med 1997;337(25):1785–91.

22. Guarnieri T, Nolan S, Gottlieb SO, et al. Intravenous amiodarone for the prevention of atrial fibrillation after open heart surgery: the Amiodarone Reduction in Coronary Heart (ARCH) trial. J Am Coll Cardiol 1999; 34(2):343–7.

23. Giri S, White CM, Dunn AB, et al. Oral amiodarone for prevention of atrial fibrillation after open heart surgery, the Atrial Fibrillation Suppression Trial (AFIST): a randomized placebo-controlled trial. Lancet 2001;357 (9259):830–6.

24. Katariya K, DeMarchena E, Bolooki H. Oral amiodarone reduces incidence of postoperative atrial fibrillation. Ann Thorac Surg 1999;68(5):1599–603.

25. Lee SH, Chang CM, Lu MJ, et al. Intravenous amiodarone for prevention of atrial fibrillation after coronary artery bypass grafting. Ann Thorac Surg 2000;79(1):157–61.

26. Fan K, Lee KL, Chiu CS, et al. Effects of biatrial pacing in prevention of postoperative atrial fibrillation after coronary artery bypass surgery. Circulation 2000; 102(7):755–60.

27. Daoud EG, Dabir R, Archambeau M, et al. Randomized, double-blind trial of simultaneous right and left atrial epicardial pacing for prevention of post-open heart surgery atrial fibrillation. Circulation 2000;102(7): 761–5.

28. Levy T, Fotopoulos G, Walker S, et al. Randomized controlled study investigating the effect of biatrial pacing in prevention of atrial fibrillation after coronary artery bypass grafting. Circulation 2000;102(12):1382–7.

CHAPTER 4

WHAT'S NEW IN MYOCARDIAL PROTECTION

PHILIPPE MENASCHÉ, MD, PhD

Over these past years, the development of off-pump surgery and the emergence of exciting new technologies have somewhat reduced the interest formerly paid to myocardial protection. This trend has been further reinforced by the belief that techniques of myocardial protection had reached such a level of efficacy that it would be difficult to improve them further. An additional reason for some investigators to have stepped back from studies of myocardial protection is the frustrating discrepancy between the successful use of some interventions in the laboratory setting and their inability to positively affect patient outcomes. The free radical story is just one example of this discrepancy, and, as discussed below, preconditioning might also fail to meet the hopes raised by a bunch of enthusiastic experimental studies.

Nevertheless, it would be unfair to consider that all the problems associated with myocardial protection have been fully solved. Thus, a recent survey of 8,641 patients who underwent coronary artery bypass grafting (CABG) operations in northern New England indicates an overall mortality of 4.48%, of which 65% could be directly attributed to postoperative cardiac failure.[1] In the PURSUIT trial, which assessed the effects of a glycoprotein (GP) IIb/IIIa inhibitor in CABG patients with unstable angina, the 7-day mortality or myocardial infarction rate was 22.3% in the 692 patients of the control arm of the study.[2] Likewise, a high perioperative mortality (21.2%) was reported by the Mayo Clinic group in its series of 52 patients undergoing aortic valve replacement with a low ejection fraction (< 35%) and a borderline transvalvular gradient.[3] The 12.2% in-hospital mortality published in a collective review of 279 dialysis-dependent CABG patients provides additional evidence that there is still room for improvement and that, even though poor surgical outcomes may have a wide variety of causes, intraoperative myocardial injury remains a predominant factor, which justifies relentless efforts to try to minimize it by improving current techniques.[4] This endeavor is further supported by the common observations that cardiac surgical patients are increasingly older and that the toler-

ance to ischemia (and hypoxia) is reduced in aged human myocardium.[5]

Although there has been no major breakthrough in the field, ongoing experimental and clinical research has either validated already known concepts and techniques or opened new perspectives. Consequently, the current review focuses on these most recent advances.

Novelties in Cardioplegia Vehicles

Although cold crystalloid cardioplegia still has its proponents who claim that this technique is associated with excellent clinical outcomes, blood cardioplegia has been increasingly used because of the compelling evidence that it decreased myocardial damage during the cross-clamping period. In the recent literature, two papers from the same group have brought additional biologic evidence for the presumed superiority of blood cardioplegia by showing that it reduced postreperfusion production of neutrophil-derived superoxide radicals and neutrophil integrin expression, as compared with crystalloid cardioplegia.[6,7] Three other studies, published in 1999 and 2000, are of still greater relevance because they have focused on clinically meaningful end points. In a cohort of patients undergoing emergency surgery for unstable angina, Tomasco and associates showed that the risk of early death sharply increased as ejection fraction decreased in patients receiving crystalloid cardioplegia, whereas this parameter was no longer a predictor of mortality with the use of a blood vehicle.[8] Ibrahim and coworkers focused on patients with an ejection fraction of < 40% and exposed to either the crystalloid St. Thomas' solution or a similar blood-based solution.[9] They found that the latter technique significantly improved the rate of recovery of left ventricular function. These results are further extended by those from the CABG Patch trial.[10] This study, primarily designed to assess the effects of implanting a cardioverter defibrillator at the time of bypass surgery in patients with an ejection fraction < 36%, has provided the opportunity to collect data on the relationship between cardioplegic type and perioperative events. With the caveat that cardioplegia was not randomized, the study shows that when compared with patients receiving blood cardioplegia ($n = 695$), those receiving crystalloid cardioplegia ($n = 190$) were found to have significantly more operative deaths (2% vs 0.3%, $p = 0.02$), postoperative Q-wave myocardial infarctions (10% vs 2%, $p < 0.001$), shock (13% vs 7%, $p = 0.013$), and postoperative conduction defects (21.6% vs 12.4%, $p = 0.001$). In spite of the lack of randomization for cardioplegia, these data are unlikely to have been skewed in favor of the blood cardioplegia group as these patients had significantly more risk factors (diabetes mellitus, hypertension, and long cross-clamping time). Despite these advantages, there was no significant difference between crystalloid and blood cardioplegia for either 30-day (6% vs 4%, respectively) or late mortality (24% vs 21%, respectively) at a mean follow-up of 32 months. These delayed deaths, however, can be due to a variety of causes and do not negate the conclusion that the early postoperative outcomes, which are most influenced by intraoperative myocardial protection, are improved by the use of blood cardioplegia in this high-risk population of patients with severe left ventricular dysfunction.

For those using crystalloid cardioplegia, recent data outline the benefits of reducing the chloride content of St. Thomas' solution for limiting edema in normal rabbit hearts, but not in those hearts taken from animals with volume-overload congestive failure.[11,12] These studies are important for better understanding the role of volume-sensitive chloride channels, but their clinical relevance may be hampered by the fact that they are based on isolated cell models and that changes in the ionic content of St. Thomas's solution for clinical use would require customized formulations, which may be more complicated than relying on commercially available preparations. Other studies have re-emphasized the salutary effects of magnesium supplementation for limiting calcium overload and for improving preservation of coronary vascular contractile function.[13,14]

Novelties in Cardioplegia Delivery Strategies

Temperature

During the past decade, the introduction of warm-blood cardioplegia has probably been the major conceptual breakthrough in the field of myocardial preservation. In spite of a huge number of experimental and clinical studies comparing cold- versus warm-blood cardioplegia, it remains difficult to conclusively establish the superiority of one technique above the other. However, some recent publications suggest the following trends: (1) The assumption that continuous oxygenated perfusion of the normothermically arrested heart enables the perfect matching of energy demand and supply so that ischemia is eliminated is probably an oversimplification. Animal data show that even under these "ideal" conditions, some metabolic and functional myocardial damage may occur, possibly enhanced by the cessation of rhythmic contractions, the subsequent interruption of lymphatic flow, and, ultimately, edema.[15] (2) However, the magnitude of this injury is likely to be limited or at least transient, as clinical experience with warm-blood cardioplegia has overall been satisfactory.[15] In 1994, the Warm Heart Investigators Trial, in which CABG patients were randomized to cold-blood ($n = 872$) or warm-blood ($n = 860$) cardioplegia, showed that the latter technique was associated with significantly fewer enzymatic myocardial infarctions and low-output syndromes.[16] In a subsequent subanalysis of the original trial, the benefit drawn from warm-blood cardioplegia was found to be evenly distributed across all risk groups.[17] This trend toward improved cardioprotection with increased blood cardioplegia temperatures was recently supported by another randomized trial that reported a smaller postoperative troponin-I release after intermittent lukewarm-blood (18° to 20°C) or warm-blood (35° to 37°C) cardio-plegia as compared with intermittent cold-blood (6° to 8°C) cardioplegic perfusion.[18] Consistent with these results, analysis of aggregated data from several trials published during these past years supports a protective effect of warm-blood cardioplegia, if one considers the crude estimate of perioperative mortality: 1.3% (27 of 2,095 patients in the warm-blood series) versus 1.9% (40 of 2,074 patients in the cold-blood series).[19] Of note, the benefits of warm-blood cardioplegia (given in a continuous fashion) also seem to extend to high-risk valve operations.[20] Furthermore, as nonfatal perioperative events have been recognized to adversely influence late survival, it is not completely unexpected that in a large nonrandomized series of 6,064 CABG patients, warm/tepid-blood cardioplegia was also associated with better event-free late survival than was cold-blood cardioplegia.[21] (3) The initially attractive concept of aerobic arrest inherent in continuous oxygenated blood perfusion has been somewhat diverted by the subsequent introduction of an intermittent pattern of cardioplegia delivery. Although clinical experience with this approach has yielded overall satisfactory results (reviewed by Caputo and co-workers), particularly in comparison with cold crystalloid cardioplegia, it should be remembered that it has been developed to meet the surgeon's comfort rather than the myocardium's needs.[22,23] Indeed, "intermittent warm-blood cardioplegia" is not an homogeneous entity; instead, it encompasses a wide variety of regimens that differ with respect to cardioplegia temperature, duration of the ischemic intervals, and modalities (duration, flow, hematocrit) of the "catch-up" reperfusion phases. In 2000, Minatoya and colleagues published a study in which they claim that 30-min ischemic intervals at 37°C provide "clinically acceptable myocardial protection for CABG."[24]

This conclusion, which is based on rather soft end points, is in total contradiction with the experimental data published that same year by Torchiana and associates showing that 30-min normothermic ischemia produces major metabolic alterations even with antecedent cardioplegia delivery.[25] In clinical practice, the safety margin is likely to vary among patients, and, as shown in a recent pig study, tolerance to intermittent perfusion is reduced in hearts that are already in a state of metabolic deprivation as they proceed to cardioplegia.[26] As a general rule, it is probably safe that interruption of warm cardioplegia does not exceed 10 min, a value consistent with the early report from the Warm Heart Investigators trial, in which interruptions of cardioplegic delivery longer than 13 min were a risk factor for adverse outcomes.[27] When more extended periods of ischemia are anticipated, hypothermia becomes a necessary adjunct because even a modest decrease in temperature can provide an effective buffer against ischemic injury.[28] For this reason, this author still favors the routine use of antegrade arrest followed by retrograde cardioplegia because the low-pressure, low-flow backbleeding through coronary arteriotomies can be easily handled, thereby allowing a near-continuous heart perfusion, which is technically more difficult to achieve by the antegrade route. A recent study by Elwatidy and colleagues supports the superiority of this antegrade/retrograde tepid delivery technique over cold-blood cardioplegia delivered in a similar way or antegrade cold-crystalloid cardioplegia.[29] (4) Although it is a common practice to apply to warm-blood cardioplegia the 1:4 crystalloid to blood dilution ratio initially developed for cold perfusion, we and others have shown that minimal blood dilution (coined "minicardioplegia") is an effective means of optimizing aerobic metabolism through an increased oxygen supply during arrest.[30,31] The availability of flexible cardioplegia delivery devices that feature accurate control over the dilution ratio has probably accelerated the trend toward reducing the cardioplegic crystalloid component of blood cardioplegia mixtures (our practice entails perfusion of pure blood supplemented with a concentrated arrest solution made of potassium and magnesium).

In the setting of continued efforts to simplify cardioplegic techniques, a recent randomized trial in low-risk CABG patients has questioned the real utility of warm substrate-enriched induction/reperfusion blood cardioplegia in addition to intermittent cold-blood cardioplegia.[32] In this study, bracketing cold-blood cardioplegia delivery with these additional blood shots only resulted in a transient unsustained improvement in left ventricular systolic function immediately after bypass, without any difference in patient outcomes. One could argue that the study was not powered to detect such differences and that the benefits of supplemental warm induction/reperfusion might become more evident in high-risk patients, but these assumptions still remain purely speculative. In line with these results, two recent randomized studies have also failed to document any benefit of the terminal "hot shot" over unmodified reperfusion following cold-blood cardioplegia in low-risk valve or CABG operations.[33,34]

Route

Retrograde delivery of cardioplegia, either alone or, more commonly, in combination with antegrade perfusion, is now a well-established method of myocardial protection, as evidenced by its use in 64% of cases recorded by a collective survey of practice patterns in 1995.[35] In 1991, this author and colleagues reported clinical data suggesting that retrograde cardioplegia was likely to be most beneficial in patients with complete coronary artery obstructions, which makes sense because cardioplegia maldistribution and resulting myocardial ischemia can be easily anticipated from this anatomic pattern of disease.[36] The most recently published studies in this area re-emphasize this conclusion. Franke and co-workers randomized 58 patients to antegrade or retrograde crystalloid cardioplegia.[37] Twenty-four hours after bypass surgery, cardiac troponin-I concentration was significantly higher in the antegrade group (8.2 μg/L vs 3.2 μg/L), but the difference was still more striking in the subset of patients with subtotal stenosis or occlusion of one or more main coronary arteries where peak troponin-I values were fourfold higher when cardioplegia was given anteriorly. In another study dealing with 744 patients undergoing reoperative CABGs, a situation where native vessels and previously placed grafts are commonly occluded or critically stenosed, multivariate logistic regression analysis identified failure to use retrograde cardioplegia as the strongest independent predictor of in-hospital mortality (odds ratio, 2.8).[38] The efficacy of the coronary sinus route in optimizing myocardial preservation through a homogeneous distribution of cardioplegia is further demonstrated by its beneficial effects on postoperative outcomes in patients with severe left ventricular dysfunction. In 1996, Kaul and colleagues had already identified the nonuse of coronary sinus cardioplegia as a significant predictor of increased early mortality in patients with an ejection fraction < 0.20.[39] This conclusion is reinforced by the recently reported data from the Patch trial showing, in this cohort of patients with an ejection fraction < 0.36, that mixed (antegrade/retrograde) cardioplegia results in less inotrope and intra-aortic balloon pump use and less new conduction defects than does antegrade cardioplegia alone.[10] Of note, patients of the combined group also demonstrated a reduced incidence of postoperative right ventricular dysfunction, thereby supporting this author and colleagues previous observation that the experimental data suggesting the inability of retrograde cardioplegia to adequately preserve the right ventricle are probably not relevant to the human atherosclerotic heart.[40] In our early studies of retrograde cardioplegia, we had stressed, however, that right ventricular preservation was likely dependent on a juxta-atrial positioning of the balloon catheter so as to avoid mechanical blockade of the most distal tributaries of the coronary sinus. Two recent studies provide additional support to this concept. First, in pig hearts, myocardial perfusion in the posterior part of the interventricular septum and the posterior wall of the left ventricle, as assessed by magnetic resonance imaging, was improved by proximal location of the deflated retrograde catheter close to the coronary sinus orifice, as opposed to distal insertion of the catheter far into the sinus with the balloon fully inflated.[41] Second, in cadaver human hearts retroperfused with a radiopaque dye of similar viscosity as that of blood, optimal right and left ventricular perfusion occurred when the catheter tip was placed in the orifice of the coronary sinus and decreased as it was advanced more distally.[42] Put together, these data confirm that retrograde cardioplegia is an important component of myocardial protection in high-risk patients and that proper positioning of retrograde balloon catheters remains critical for optimizing the efficacy of this approach.

Novelties in Cardioplegia Additives

Adenosine

The potential use of this compound during cardiac operations is discussed in the following section on preconditioning.

Insulin

A recent randomized trial, which included 56 low-risk CABG patients, showed that supplementation of blood cardioplegia with insulin accelerated resumption of aerobic metabolism and improved functional recovery, independent of the concentration of glucose.[43] Unfortunately, in a much larger cohort of patients undergoing CABG for unstable angina and randomized to insulin cardioplegia ($n = 557$) or placebo ($n = 570$), insulin failed to provide any clinically meaningful benefit.[44] The usefulness of this additive to cardioplegia thus remains uncertain. Along this line, Lazar and associates recently revived the old concept of glucose-insulin-potassium by showing that this treatment regimen improved postoperative outcomes in diabetic patients.[45] Larger trials are clearly warranted before the true benefits of this mode of substrate enhancement can be conclusively validated.

L-Arginine

Although nitric oxide (NO) might be both friend and foe, through enhanced vasodilation and generation of the toxic peroxynitrite free radical, respectively, the trend has usually been to highlight the cardioprotective effects of an increased bioavailability of NO for reversing the endothelial dysfunction associated with cardioplegia and reperfusion. In practice, this can achieved by loading the myocardium with the NO precursor L-arginine. Unfortunately, the encouraging results obtained with this compound in several experimental studies contrast with the failure of the only randomized clinical trial to document any benefit of L-arginine supplementation to the blood cardioplegic solution.[46] Whether this negative result is due to an unexpectedly wrong concept, an inappropriate protocol of drug delivery, or an insufficient power of the study to detect a difference in the primary outcome measure (enzymatic markers of myocardial necrosis) remains to be determined.

Free Radical Scavengers

The free radical story is illustrative of the distressing gap between a physiopathologically attractive concept based on sound experimental data and the inability to translate it into clinically meaningful therapeutic interventions. Namely, the huge number of laboratory studies, most of which date back to one decade ago, showing the cardioprotective effects of enzymatic scavengers and antioxidants related to postischemic limitation of free radical–mediated tissue damage sharply contrasts with the paucity of clinical data. Some isolated studies have assessed the effects of antioxidants (mannitol, allopurinol, and vitamins C and E) or iron chelators (deferoxamine). At best, they have brought additional "proof of concept" but have failed to demonstrate substantial improvement in patient outcomes. Indeed, we know that such a demonstration would require large trials powered enough to detect differences in clinically meaningful end points such as mortality, Q-wave myocardial infarction, or other robust indices of myocardial injury. The complexity and cost of such trials have made pharmaceutical companies reluctant to undertake them. Thus, there is nothing really new in the field except for a recent experimental confirmation of the cardioprotection afforded by transition metal chelation. Thus although some scavengers are available for clinical use (metal chelators, such as deferoxamine, or thiol compounds, such as N-acetylcysteine, might be among the most effective), the methodological issues outlined earlier, along with the increasing use of blood cardioplegia, which likely minimizes reperfusion injury, probably explain that interest in the concept seems to have fainted during these last years.[47]

Novelties in Cardioprotective Concepts

Preconditioning

Ischemic preconditioning is an adaptive phenomenon by which a brief period of reversible ischemia renders the heart more tolerant to a subsequent, more prolonged period of ischemia. It is currently considered as one of the most powerful means of reducing infarct size and, presumably through this mechanism, improving function.

From the onset, the concept has been attractive for cardiac surgeons because the timed planning of aortic cross-clamping offers the possibility of implementing preischemic interventions. However, in spite of a large number of experimental studies that have yielded overall positive results, preconditioning has failed to become part of our current methods of myocardial protection. There are at least three reasons for this. First, as previously mentioned, the primary effect of preconditioning is to reduce infarct size, whereas its benefits on stunning are less clear. This may limit the relevance of the concept to cardiac surgery, except when standard methods are expected to provide less-than-optimal protection (ie, poor left ventricular function, left ventricular hypertrophy, long ischemic times), in which case, limiting the irreversible necrosis-related component of myocardial injury should logically translate into improved patient outcomes. Second, the idea of subjecting cardiac surgical patients to an intentional pre–cross-clamp ischemic stimulus is rather counterappealing. It is acknowledged that two recent studies have reported improved protection in ischemically preconditioned patients undergoing valve or coronary operations.[48,49] Of note, however, in these two studies, the cross-clamping times were relatively long (in the range of 90 min) and there was a five- to tenfold increase in postoperative myocardial muscle creatine kinase isoenzyme (CK-MB) release when compared to baseline values. These data are consistent with the previous assumption that it is primarily in case of suboptimal protection that preconditioning is likely to be a useful adjunct to standard methods. Other studies, however, have failed to document any benefit of ischemic preconditioning, and these discrepant data have likely reinforced the reluctance of most clinical surgeons to adopt this technique.[50,51] Third, we still lack preconditioning pharmacologic mimetics that are usable in humans and that have proven to be safe and effective. A careful dissection of the different steps of the preconditioning-induced signaling pathway is, therefore, critical for identifying the key mediators that could be elective targets for therapeutic interventions.

According to the classic scheme, signaling is initiated by activation of various membrane receptors by their agonists, particularly adenosine, bradykinin, opioid, and α-agonists. Receptor activation then causes phosphorylation and translocation of protein kinase C (PKC) and other downstream kinases, particularly tyrosine kinase and p38 mitogen-activated protein kinase (MAPK), whose phosphorylation correlates with the protection afforded by preconditioning.[52] This would ultimately lead to opening of adenosine triphosphate (ATP)–dependent sarcolemmal/mitochondrial potassium channels whose role in mediating a preconditioning type of cardioprotection in various species has been extended to the human heart by experiments that use right atrial trabeculae harvested during cardiac operations.[53,54] This paradigm, however, was recently challenged by some studies suggesting that mitochondrial potassium channels could actually act as *triggers* rather than *end effectors* of the signaling pathway.[55] According to this hypothesis, receptor activa-tion opens mitochondrial potassium channels, causing the mitochondria to produce oxygen-derived free radicals, which would then set the heart in a preconditioned state by oxidative activation of the kinase cascade.[56–58] This hypothesis is further supported by a recent study showing, in a clinically relevant model of atherosclerotic mouse, that the protective effects of ischemic preconditioning can be duplicated by exposure to hyperoxia.[59] The end effector of the pathway is not yet precisely identified, but heat shock protein 27 (HSP 27) is a possible candidate. This low-molecular-weight compound plays an important role in maintaining the integrity of the actin cytoskeleton, and it is mechanistically linked to the kinase cascade because it can be phosphorylated by the p38 MAPK.[60,61]

The previous considerations provide a framework for pharmacologic interventions designed to mimic preconditioning. Among receptor agonists that act at the onset of the signaling pathway, the most attractive for clinical use is adenosine, which has been the subject of extensive investigations. A summary of the most recent clinical data leads to the conclusion that this drug has yielded mixed results. In a study of 45 patients who were given adenosine according to a strict preconditioning protocol (5-min infusion of 140 μ/kg/min followed by 10 min of washout before cardioplegic arrest), this author and colleagues failed to document any protective effect of the drug on postoperative troponin-I release or patient outcomes, although there was some evidence that the preconditioning pathway had been "turned on," as reflected by increased myocardial tissue activities of 5'-nucleotidase (a surrogate marker for PKC activation).[62] It is possible, however, that this "preconditioning-type" scenario is not the best suited for exploiting the cardioprotective effects of adenosine. A recent study reported improved recovery of function in CABG patients when adenosine was given as a short pretreatment (200 μ/kg), immediately before aortic cross-clamping (ie, without an intervening period of drug-free washout).[63] Likewise, in the large trial previously conducted by Mentzer and co-workers, the salutary effects of adenosine on a composite outcome (high-dose dopamine, epinephrine use, insertion of a balloon pump, myocardial infarction, and death) were demonstrated in a protocol involving protracted exposure to the drug (before, during, and after cardioplegic arrest).[64] Additional studies are clearly warranted to better the conditions under which adenosine-induced protection on cellular and microvascular function can be optimized.

Regardless of whether ATP-sensitive channels are located upstream or downstream the kinase pathway, they represent the second major target for pharmacologic preconditioning mimetics. Unfortunately, the clinical use of potassium-channel agonists is still plagued with the limited availability of suitable compounds. Diazoxide, a selective opener of mitochondrial potassium channels that preserves the functional and structural integrity of these organelles and experimentally mimics the cardio-protective effects of ischemic preconditioning, is a potent hypotensive drug, and its administration before cross-clamping may raise some safety concerns.[65,66] It is also a drug that is no longer protected by a patent, which accounts for the limited interest of pharmaceutical companies in promoting its development for this indication. Nicorandil, which acts at the level of mitochondrial and sarcolemmal potassium channels, is not available for intravenous use (except in Japan), and, although feasible, an oral intake is probably not the type of regimen best suited for the acute setting of intraoperative myocardial protection. Furthermore, the protection expected from the channel-opening properties of nicorandil might be overwhelmed by the peripheral vasodilatory effects mediated by its nitrate-like action. In this context, a growing interest is legitimately paid to inhalational anesthetics (particularly, isoflurane and sevoflurane) commonly used during cardiac operations, and which also duplicate the cardioprotective effects of ischemic preconditioning by the opening of potassium channels. So far, experimental and preliminary clinical data have been encouraging and certainly warrant further investigations to assess whether an appropriate use of these agents, with respect to dosing and timing of administration, would elicit improved cardioprotection, in addition to taking advantage of their anesthetic effects.[67–69]

Finally, studies were also conducted in an attempt to reproduce the delayed (~24 h) protection afforded by ischemic preconditioning ("second window of protection"), which is thought to result from an increased expression of stress proteins. Unfortunately, the usual trigger of the upregulation of these cytoprotective proteins is heat shock, which is clearly irrelevant to clinical practice, hence the interest for the drug monophosphoryl lipid A, which is reported to similarly induce delayed protection.[70] This compound should be clinically tested in the near future.

Sodium/Proton Exchange Inhibition

During postischemic reperfusion, accumulated protons are extruded outside the cells in exchange for an influx of sodium ions. Because the ischemia-impaired sodium/potassium pump cannot cope with this excess of intracellular sodium ions, their efflux occurs through the sodium/calcium exchange, which then operates in a "reverse" mode. The ultimate result is an intracellular calcium overload and the attendant tissue damage. These considerations have led to the development of inhibitors of the sodium/proton exchange, which have been consistently shown experimentally to markedly reduce infarct size and stunning in models of regional and global myocardial ischemia, respectively. It is noteworthy that in a canine infarct model, sodium/proton exchange inhibition and ischemic preconditioning provided comparable protection against 60 min of ischemia, but the former approach was more efficacious in reducing infarct size when the occlusion time was extended to 90 min.

The combination of these two strategies produces additive cardioprotection, suggesting that they may act via separate complementary mechanisms.[71]

In the surgically relevant setting of cardioplegic arrest, sodium/proton exchange inhibition has been strikingly effective in improving postischemic recovery of function under both normothermic and hypothermic conditions, the maximal therapeutic efficacy being achieved with the use of the drug before and during arrest rather than only at the time of reperfusion. Interest in this approach is now reinforced by the availability of one exchange inhibitor, cariporide, for human use. In isolated rat hearts, measurements of intracellular calcium and pH by a dye and nuclear magnetic resonance spectroscopy, respectively, relate the functional benefits of cariporide to a reduction of calcium overload during ischemia and early reperfusion and to a prolongation of postischemic acidosis.[72] Such an acidosis actually contributes to cytoprotection through limitation of calcium overload and should not be a concern because it is mild and transient as mechanisms other than the sodium/proton exchanger come into play to regulate intracellular pH. In cardiac surgery, the use of cariporide might actually extend to off-pump CABG, as suggested by a recent study showing, in a sheep model of local ischemia mimicking the situation of beating-heart operations, that post–reperfusion stunning is abrogated by this drug.[73]

These laboratory data tend to be corroborated by the results of the large GUARDIAN clinical trial in which a benefit of cariporide was only found in the subgroup of approximately 3,000 CABG patients. Another study (EXPEDITION) is currently underway to further confirm the salutary effects of this drug on postoperative outcomes. Should the results be positive, it is likely that this drug, or others of the same class, will find a place in our armamentarium of perioperative cardioprotective strategies.

Alternates to Potassium

One paradox of myocardial protection is that although calcium overload is widely recognized as a culprit event in the genesis of postoperative cardiac dysfunction, hearts are universally arrested with potassium, which, by causing membrane depolarization, can trigger a calcium influx through voltage-dependent channels. Assuming that calcium overload is involved in the pathophysiology of reperfusion injury, it is noteworthy that, based on pathologic data, the latter has been reported to account for one-fourth of all deaths occurring after cold crystalloid arrest.[74] This emphasizes the potential clinical relevance of the different strategies that have been developed in an attempt to address this issue.

HYPERPOLARIZED ARREST

The rationale of this approach is that more negative membrane potentials (hyperpolarization) are associated with minimal ionic shifts, resulting in a limitation of calcium overload and better preservation of energy stores.

In practice, such a hyperpolarization can be achieved with potassium channel openers. A large number of experimental studies, many of which came from Damiano's laboratory, show that these drugs, when used as cardioplegic vehicles, are as, or even more, cardioprotective than standard crystalloid- or blood-based potassium arrest. Unfortunately, the clinical relevance of these results still remains limited because, as outlined earlier, only one of these compounds (nicorandil) is available for human use. Although nicorandil provides equivalent protection to potassium cardioplegia through its potassium channel–opening properties, the use, in this study, of an isolated heart model precluded assessing the systemic vasodilatation potentially related to the nitrate-like effects of the drug.[75] This issue is of major clinical relevance because high drug concentrations are likely to be required to achieve electromechanical arrest. Furthermore, the use of nicorandil during cardiac operations is hampered by the lack of an injectable form.

On the other hand, recent data open some interesting perspectives in that they suggest that potassium-channel openers could be useful as *adjuncts* to standard potassium-based cardioplegia because of their ability to keep membrane potential at more negative values, with a resulting reduction in calcium influx.[76] However, although some studies support this hypothesis, other studies yield more mixed results.[77,78] Thus, in a rabbit model of global ischemia, addition of the mitochondrial potassium-channel opener diazoxide to a potassium/magnesium-based cardioplegic solution further reduced infarct size but failed to improve recovery of function when compared with cardioplegia alone.[79] Ducko and colleagues also have been unable to demonstrate any benefit of supplementing St. Thomas' solution with pinacidil.[80] Indeed, the putative efficacy of these drugs is likely to be influenced by several variables, particularly temperature, pharmacologic profile, and mode of delivery (eg, pinacidil cardioplegia was only superior to St. Thomas' solution when given in a continuous mode).[81] Further studies are clearly warranted to explore this possibility of blunting some of the untoward effects of potassium cardioplegia through the concomitant use of potassium channel openers.

Along this line, a recent original study has reported that estrogens (17β-estradiol) could prevent hyperkalemia-induced calcium overload by a mechanism that might involve activation of potassium channels.[82] These experiments, however, were conducted in isolated cardiomyocytes and clearly require further validation in more clinically relevant large-animal models before estrogen supplementation to standard potassium-based cardioplegic solutions can be reasonably considered.

β-BLOCKADE

This technique is a sort of trade-off between off-pump and conventional surgery. It shares in common with standard CABG the institution of cardiopulmonary bypass and aortic cross-clamping. However, the heart is not arrested; it is only slowed by continuous normokalemic blood perfusion supplemented with the short-acting β-blocker esmolol. The underlying rationale is that blood perfusion should avoid ischemia while maintenance of rhythmic contractions is expected to eliminate the edema-related component of postoperative dysfunction. Bleeding through the arteriotomies is managed by the same tricks as those used during beating-heart operations.

In spite of some encouraging reports, this technique has not yet gained large clinical acceptance, and its real benefits remain unclear.[83,84]

Novelties in Methods of Assessment

Among new end points that can be useful for assessing cardioprotective techniques, cardiac natriuretic hormones are raising a growing interest. A recent study by Chello and associates has reported a tight correlation between plasma levels of atrial and brain natriuretic factors and left ventricular function, as assessed by echocardiography, after CABG surgery.[85] Should these preliminary data be confirmed, these hormonal assays might provide a reliable means of noninvasively assessing the occurrence and extent of postoperative heart failure.

In conclusion, the major novelty in the field of myocardial protection has probably been the identification of new therapeutic targets such as ATP-sensitive potassium channels and/or the sodium/proton exchanger. Of utmost importance is the recognition that inflammatory mediators *systemically* released during cardiopulmonary bypass can also have a negative *myocardial* impact. The most recently reported example of this interplay is the improvement in postoperative outcome in patients with severe left ventricular dysfunction following leukocyte depletion from blood cardioplegia.[86] Because anti-inflammatory strategies are discussed in another chapter, they are not addressed here except to emphasize that any intervention that mitigates the inflammatory response to bypass can likely be also categorized as a cardioprotective intervention.

References

1. O'Connor GT, Birkmeyer JD, Dacey LJ, et al. Results of a regional study of modes of death associated with coronary artery bypass grafting. Ann Thorac Surg 1998;66:1323–8.
2. Marso SP, Bhatt DL, Roe MT, et al. Enhanced efficacy of eptifibatide administration in patients with acute coronary syndrome requiring in-hospital coronary artery bypass grafting. Circulation 2000;102:2952–8.
3. Connolly HM, Oh JK, Schaff HV, et al. Severe aortic stenosis with low transvalvular gradient and severe left ventricular dysfunction: result of aortic valve replacement in 52 patients. Circulation 2000;101:1892–4.
4. Liu JY, Birkmeyer NJO, Sanders JH, et al. Risks of morbidity and mortality in dialysis patients undergoing

coronary artery bypass surgery. Circulation 2000;102: 2973–7.

5. Mariani J, Ou R, Bailey M, et al. Tolerance to ischemia and hypoxia is reduced in aged human myocardium. J Thorac Cardiovasc Surg 2000;120:660–7.

6. Kalawski R, Balinski M, Bugajski P, et al. Stimulation of neutrophil activation during coronary artery bypass grafting: comparison of crystalloid and blood cardioplegia. Ann Thorac Surg 2001;71:827–31.

7. Kalawski R, Deskur E, Bugajski P, et al. Stimulation of neutrophil integrin expression during coronary artery bypass grafting: comparison of crystalloid and blood cardioplegic solutions. J Thorac Cardiovasc Surg 2000;119:1270–7.

8. Tomasco B, Cappiello A, Fiorilli R, et al. Surgical revascularization for acute coronary insufficiency: analysis of risk factors for hospital mortality. Ann Thorac Surg 1997;64: 678–83.

9. Ibrahim MF, Venn GE, Young CP, Chambers DJ. A clinical comparative study between crystalloid and blood-based St Thomas' hospital cardioplegic solution. Eur J Cardiothorac Surg 1999;15:75–83.

10. Flack JE, Cook JR, May SJ, et al. Does cardioplegia type affect outcome and survival in patients with advanced left ventricular dysfunction? Results from the CABG Patch trial. Circulation 2000;102 (19 Suppl 3):III84–9.

11. Sun X, Ducko CT, Hoenicke EM, et al. Mechanisms responsible for cell volume regulation during hyperkalemic cardioplegic arrest. Ann Thorac Surg 2000;70:633–8.

12. Danetz JS, Davies RD, Clemo HF, Baumgarten CM. Rabbit ventricular myocyte volume changes as a direct result of crystalloid cardioplegia in congestive heart failure induced by aortic regurgitation. J Thorac Cardivasc Surg 2000;119:826–33.

13. Matsuda N, Tofukuji M, Morgan KG, Sellke F. Coronary microvascular protection with Mg^{2+}: effects on intracellular calcium regulation and vascular function. Am J Physiol 1999;276:H1124–30.

14. Tofukuji M, Matsuda N, Dessy C, et al. Intracellular free calcium accumulation in ferret vascular smooth muscle during crystalloid and blood cardioplegic infusions. J Thorac Cardiovasc Surg 1999;118:163–72.

15. Elvenes OP, Korvald C, Ytrebo LM, et al. Myocardial metabolism and efficiency after warm continuous blood cardioplegia. Ann Thorac Surg 2000;69:1799–805.

16. The Warm Heart Investigators. Randomised trial of normothermic versus hypothermic coronary bypass surgery. Lancet 1994;343:559–63.

17. Christakis GT, Lichtenstein SV, Buth KJ, et al. The influence of risk on the results of warm heart surgery: a substudy of a randomized trial. Eur J Cardiothorac Surg 1997;11:515–20.

18. Chocron S, Kaili D, Yan Y, et al. Intermediate lukewarm (20°C) antegrade intermittent blood cardioplegia compared with cold and warm blood cardioplegia. J Thorac Cardiovasc Surg 2000;119:610–6.

19. Fremes SE, Tamariz MG, Abramov D, et al. Late results of the Warm Heart Trial. The influence of nonfatal cardiac events on late survival. Circulation 2000;102 (19 Suppl 3): III339–45.

20. Nagaoka H, Hirooka K, Ohnuki M, Fujiwara N. Effectiveness of continuous warm blood cardioplegia in cardiac valve re-replacement. J Heart Valve Dis 1999;8:124–30.

21. Mallidi H, Sever J, Tamariz M, et al. The short and long-term effects of warm/tepid cardioplegia [abstract]. Circulation 2000;102:II-829.

22. Caputo M, Ascione R, Angelini GD, et al. The end of the cold era: from intermittent cold to intermittent warm blood cardioplegia. Eur J Cardiothorac Surg 1998;14:467–75.

23. Jacquet LM, Noirhomme PH, Van Dyck MJ, et al. Randomized trial of intermittent antegrade warm blood versus cold crystalloid cardioplegia. Ann Thorac Surg 1999;67: 471–7.

24. Minatoya K, Okabayashi B, Shimada I, et al. Intermittent antegrade warm blood cardioplegia for CABG: extended interval of cardioplegia. Ann Thorac Surg 2000;69: 74–6.

25. Torchiana DF, Vine AJ, Shebani KO, et al. Cardioplegia and ischemia in the canine heart evaluated by ^{31}P magnetic resonance spectroscopy. Ann Thorac Surg 2000;70: 197–205.

26. Ericsson AB, Kawakami T, Vaage J. Intermittent warm blood cardioplegia does not provide adequate myocardial resuscitation after global ischaemia. Eur J Cardiothoracic Surg 1999;16:233–9.

27. Lichtenstein SV, Naylor CD, Feindel CM, et al. Intermittent warm blood cardioplegia. Circulation 1995;92 (19 Suppl 2):II341–6.

28. Fiore AC, Swartz MT, Nevett R, et al. Intermittent antegrade tepid versus cold blood cardioplegia in elective myocardial revascularization. Ann Thorac Surg 1998;65: 1559–65.

29. Elwatidy AMF, Fadalah MA, Bukhari EA, et al. Antegrade crystalloid cardioplegia vs antegrade/retrograde cold and tepid blood cardioplegia in CABG. Ann Thorac Surg 1999;68:447–53.

30. Menasché Ph, Touchot B, Pradier F, et al. Simplified method for delivering normothermic blood cardioplegia. Ann Thorac Surg 1993;55:177–8.

31. Hayashida N, Isomura T, Sato T, et al. Minimally diluted tepid blood cardioplegia. Ann Thorac Surg 1998;65: 615–21.

32. Wallace AW, Ratcliffe MB, Nosé PS, et al. Effect of induction and reperfusion with warm substrate-enriched cardioplegia on ventricular function. Ann Thorac Surg 2000;70:1301–7.

33. Edwards R, Treasure T, Hossein-Nia M, et al. A controlled trial of substrate-enhanced, warm reperfusion ("hot shot") versus simple reperfusion. Ann Thorac Surg 2000;69:551–5.

34. Chocron S, Alwan K, Yan Y, et al. Warm reperfusion and myocardial protection. Ann Thorac Surg 1998;66: 2003–7.

35. Robinson LA, Schwarz GD, Goddard DB, et al. Myocardial protection for acquired heart disease surgery: results of a national survey. Ann Thorac Surg 1995;59:361–72.

36. Menasché P, Subayi JB, Veyssié L, et al. Efficacy of coronary sinus cardioplegia in patients with complete coronary artery occlusions. Ann Thorac Surg 1991;51: 418–23.

37. Franke U, Wahlers T, Cohnert U, et al. Retrograde versus antegrade crystalloid cardioplegia in coronary surgery: value of troponin-I measurement. Ann Thorac Surg 2001;71:249–53.

38. Borger MA, Rao V, Weisel RD, et al. Reoperative coronary bypass surgery: effect of patent grafts and retrograde cardioplegia. J Thorac Cardiovasc Surg 2001;121:83–90.

39. Kaul TK, Agnihotri AK, Fields BL, et al. Coronary artery bypass grafting in patients with an ejection fraction of twenty percent or less. J Thorac Cardiovasc Surg 1996;111:1001–12.

40. Menasché P, Fleury JP, Droc L, et al. Metabolic and functional evidence that retrograde warm blood cardioplegia does not injure the right ventricle in human beings. Circulation 1994;90(5 Pt 2):II310–5.

41. Tian G, Xiang B, Dai G, et al. The effects of retrograde cardioplegia technique on myocardial perfusion and energy metabolism: a magnetic resonance imaging and localized phosphorus 31 spectroscopy study in isolated pig hearts. J Thorac Cardiovasc Surg 2000;120:544–51.

42. Tosson R, Kuschkowitz F, Dasbach G, Laczkovics A. Relationship between position of the coronary sinus catheter and distribution of cardioplegia. J Heart Valve Dis 1999;8:120–3.

43. Rao V, Borger MA, Weisel RD, et al. Insulin cardioplegia for elective coronary bypass surgery. J Thorac Cardiovasc Surg 2000;119:1176–84.

44. Rao V, Christakis GT, Weisel RD, et al. The insulin cardioplegia trial: reaching the limits of myocardial protection for CABG. Presented at the 81st Annual Meeting of the American Association for Thoracic Surgery, May 6–9, 2001, San Diego, CA.

45. Lazar HL, Chipkin S, Philippides G, et al. Glucose-insulin-potassium solutions improve outcomes in diabetics who have coronary artery operations. Ann Thorac Surg 2000;70:145–50.

46. Carrier M, Pellerin M, Pagé PL, et al. Can L-arginine improve myocardial protection during cardioplegic arrest? Results of a phase I pilot study. Ann Thorac Surg 1998;66:108–12.

47. Karck M, Tanaka S, Berenshtein E, et al. The push-and-pull mechanism to scavenge redox-active transition metals: a novel concept in myocardial protection. J Thorac Cardiovasc Surg 2001;121:1169–78.

48. Li G, Chen S, Lu E, Li Y. Ischemic preconditioning improves preservation with cold blood cardioplegia in valve replacement patients. Eur J Cardiothorac Surg 1999;15:653–7.

49. Wu Z-K, Tarkka MR, Pehkonen E, et al. Beneficial effects of ischemic preconditioning on right ventricular function after coronary artery bypass grafting. Ann Thorac Surg 2000;70:1551–7.

50. Perrault LP, Menasché P, Bel A, et al. Ischemic preconditioning in cardiac surgery: a word of caution. J Thorac Cardiovasc Surg 1996;112:1378–86.

51. Kaukoranta PK, Lepojärvi MPK, Ylitalo KV, et al. Normothermic retrograde blood cardioplegia with or without preceding ischemic preconditioning. Ann Thorac Surg 1997;63:1268–74.

52. Weinbrenner C, Liu GS, Cohen MV, Downey JM. Phosphorylation of tyrosine 182 of p38 mitogen-activated protein kinase correlates with the protection of preconditioning in the rabbit heart. J Mol Cell Cardiol 1997;29:2383–91.

53. Gross GJ, Fryer RM. Sarcolemmal versus mitochondrial ATP-sensitive K+ channels and myocardial preconditioning. Circ Res 1999;84:973–9.

54. Pomerantz BJ, Robinson TN, Morrell TD, et al. Selective mitochondrial adenosine triphosphate-sensitive potassium channel activation is sufficient to precondition human myocardium. J Thorac Cardiovasc Surg 2000;120:387–92.

55. Pain T, Yang X-M, Critz SD, et al. Opening of mitochondrial K_{ATP} channels triggers the preconditioned state by generating free radicals. Circ Res 2000;87:460–6.

56. Baines CP, Goto M, Downey J. Oxygen radicals released during ischemic preconditioning contribute to cardioprotection in the rabbit myocardium. J Mol Cell Cardiol 1997;29:207–16.

57. O'Rourke B. Myocardial K_{ATP} channels in preconditioning. Circ Res 2000;87:845–55.

58. Forbes RA, Steenbergen C, Murphy E. Diazoxide-induced cardioprotection requires signaling through a redox-sensitive mechanism. Circ Res 2001;88:802–9.

59. Li G, Tokuno S, Tähepôld P, et al. Preconditioning protects the severely atherosclerotic mouse heart. Ann Thorac Surg 2001;71:1296–304.

60. Baines CP, Liu GS, Birincioglu M, et al. Ischemic preconditioning depends on interaction between mitochondrial K_{ATP} channels and actin cytoskeleton. Am J Physiol 1999;276:H1361–8.

61. Sugden PH, Clerk A. "Stress-responsive" mitogen-activated protein kinases (c-Jun N-terminal kinases and p38 mitogen activated protein kinases) in the myocardium. Circ Res 1998;83:345–52.

62. Belhomme D, Peynet J, Florens E, et al. Is adenosine preconditioning truly cardioprotective in coronary artery bypass surgery? Ann Thorac Surg 2001;70:590–4.

63. Wasir H, Bhan A, Choudhary SK, et al. Pretreatment of human myocardium with adenosine. Eur J Cardiothoracic Surg 2001;19:41–6.

64. Mentzer RM, Rahko PS, Molina-Viamonte V, et al. Safety, tolerance, and efficacy of adenosine as an additive to blood cardioplegia in humans during coronary artery bypass surgery. Am J Cardiol 1997;79(12A):38–43.

65. Ozcan C, Holmuhamedov EL, Jahangir A, Terzic A. Diazoxide protects mitochondria from anoxic injury: implications for myopreservation. J Thorac Cardiovasc Surg 2001;121:298–306.

66. Ghosh S, Standen NB, Galiñanes M. Evidence for mitochondrial K_{ATP} channels as effectors of human myocardial preconditioning. Cardiovasc Research 2000;45:934–40.

67. Kersten JR, Schmeling TJ, Hettrick DA, et al. Mechanism of myocardial protection by isoflurane: role of adenosine triphosphate-regulated potassium (K_{ATP}) channels. Anesthesiology 1996;85:794–807.

68. Toller WG, Kersten JR, Pagel PS, et al. Sevoflurane reduces myocardial infarct size and decreases the time threshold for ischemic preconditioning in dogs. Anesthesiology 1999;91:1437–46.

69. Belhomme D, Peynet J, Louzy M, et al. Evidence for preconditioning by isoflurane in coronary artery bypass graft surgery. Circulation 1999;100 (19 Suppl):II-340–4.

70. Yoshida T, Engelman RM, Engelman DT, et al. Preconditioning of swine heart with monophosphoryl lipid A improves myocardial preservation. Ann Thorac Surg 2000;70:895–900.

71. Gumina RJ, Buerger E, Eickmeier C, et al. Inhibition of the Na$^+$/H$^+$ exchanger confers greater cardioprotection against 90 min of myocardial ischemia than ischemic preconditioning in dogs. Circulation 1999;100:2519–26.

72. Strömer H, de Groot MCH, Horn M, et al. Na$^+$/H$^+$ exchange inhibition with HOE642 improves postischemic recovery due to attenuation of Ca^{2+} overload and prolonged acidosis on reperfusion. Circulation 2000;101:2749–55.

73. Hendrikx M, Rega F, Jamaer L, et al. Na$^+$/H$^+$-exchange inhibition and aprotinin administration: promising tools for myocardial protection during minimally invasive CABG. Eur J Cardiothorac Surg 2001;19:633–9.

74. Weman SM, Karhunen PJ, Penttilä A, et al. Reperfusion injury associated with one-fourth of deaths after coronary artery bypass grafting. Ann Thorac Surg 2000;70:807–12.

75. Jayawant AM, Lawton JS, Hsia P-W, Damiano RJ. Hyperpolarized cardioplegic arrest with nicorandil. Advantages over other potassium channel openers. Circulation 1997;96 (19 Suppl):II-240–6.

76. Lopez JR, Jahangir R, Jahangir A, et al. Potassium channel openers prevent potassium-induced calcium loading of cardiac cells: possible implications in cardioplegia. J Thorac Cardiovasc Surg 1996;112:820–31.

77. Dorman BH, Hebbar L, Clair MJ, et al. Potassium channel opener-augmented cardioplegia. Protection of myocyte contractility with chronic left ventricular dysfunction. Circulation 1997;96 (19 Suppl):II-253–9.

78. Monti F, Iwashiro K, Picard S, et al. Adenosine triphosphate-dependent potassium channel modulation and cardioplegia-induced protection of human atrial muscle in an in vitro model of myocardial stunning. J Thorac Cardiovasc Surg 2000;119:842–8.

79. Toyoda Y, Levitsky S, McCully JD. Opening of mitochondrial ATP-sensitive potassium channels enhances cardioplegic protection. Ann Thorac Surg 2001;71:1281–9.

80. Ducko CT, Stephenson ER, Jayawant AM, et al. Potassium channel openers; are they effective as pretreatment or additives to cardioplegia? Ann Thorac Surg 2000;69:1363–8.

81. Jayawant M, Stephenson ER, Damiano RJ. Advantages of continuous hyperpolarized arrest with pinacidil over St. Thomas' hospital solution during prolonged ischemia. J Thorac Cardiovasc Surg 1998;116:131–8.

82. Jovanovic S, Jovanovic A, Shen WK, Terzic A. Protective action of 17β-estradiol in cardiac cells: implications for hyperkalemic cardioplegia. Ann Thorac Surg 1998;66:1658–61.

83. Kuhn-Régnier F, Natour E, Dhein S, et al. Beta-blockade versus Buckberg blood-cardioplegia in coronary bypass operation. Eur J Cardiothorac Surg 1999;15:67–74.

84. Yasuda T, Kamiya H, Tanaka Y, Watanabe G. Ultra–short-acting cardioselective beta-blockade attenuates postischemic cardiac dysfunction in the isolated rat heart. Eur J Cardiothorac Surg 2001;19:647–52.

85. Chello M, Mastroroberto P, Perticone F, et al. Plasma levels of atrial and brain natriuretic peptides as indicators of recovery of left ventricular systolic function after coronary artery bypass. Eur J Cardiothorac Surg 2001;20:140–6.

86. Roth M, Kraus B, Scheffold T, et al. The effect of leukocyte-depleted blood cardioplegia in patients with severe left ventricular dysfunction: a randomized, double-blind study. J Thorac Cardiovasc Surg 2000;120:642–50.

CHAPTER 5

BLOOD CONSERVATION FOR OPEN HEART SURGERY

TODD K. ROSENGART, MD, FACS

Efforts at reducing the use of homologous blood in cardiac surgery date back nearly to the advent of cardiopulmonary bypass (CPB) itself, but the goal of performing "bloodless" open heart surgery—without homologous blood transfusions—remains elusive even today. Even in the most recent series, homologous blood transfusions have been required in 30 to 70% of open heart surgery patients, with two to four donor exposures required per patient.[1–3] In fact, it has been estimated that at least 10% of the nation's blood supply is used for patients undergoing open heart surgery.[4]

The impetus for blood conservation in open heart surgery has several origins, including (1) national blood shortages that surface periodically and refocus attention on blood conservation; (2) new and/or undetectable infectious sequelae of transfusion (most recently, for example, concerns over West Nile virus) that threaten both the quality and quantity of the blood supply; and (3) incompatibility and other immunologic reactions that persist as problems associated with any allogeneic blood transfusion.[5,6] Currently, cost and resource efficiency considerations also play a prominent role in mandating a reduction in blood transfusions. Equally important to all these considerations is a prevalent and overwhelming patient concern for avoiding blood transfusions.

Several studies have found that the risk factors for transfusion in open heart surgery include both essentially fixed parameters—such as age, gender, and body mass—and other parameters that may be subject to modification by appropriate therapeutic interventions.[7–9] The latter group includes two independent predictors: the preoperative red cell mass and the postoperative chest tube output, which have been the subject, in one way or another, of most recent attempts at blood conservation. Because the preoperative red cell mass and perioperative bleeding represent independent risk factors for transfusion,[7–9] only a blood conservation strategy that addresses both these parameters will allow for a truly effective *bloodless* surgical outcome.

Although many new technical and pharmacologic modalities have been used separately to avoid homologous transfusion, the isolated, nonprogrammatic, and often sporadic application of these measures to a patient population at increasing risk for transfusion has limited progress toward "bloodless" open heart surgery. The results of numerous previous trials of single-component therapies in which homologous transfusions were successfully reduced but not eliminated are consistent with our hypothesis that comprehensively addressing the independent risk factors for transfusion is a prerequisite to the total avoidance of homologous transfusion. For example, obligatory intraoperative red cell transfusion can become necessary in the patient with a low hematocrit level on bypass, owing to a low preoperative red cell mass and hematocrit, even if an effective hemostatic regimen resulted in minimal postoperative bleeding. Conversely, the transfusion of coagulation factors or red cells may be required in the patient with a coagulopathy and excessive bleeding postoperatively, even if the preoperative red cell mass and hematocrit have been optimized. Furthermore, efforts directed at avoiding coagulopathy or anemia, but not both of these transfusion predictors, ignore the fact that it is the total number of red cell and coagulation factor donor exposures that determines the risk of infectious transmittal. It is thus critical to consider all homologous transfusions in developing a strategy for bloodless surgery.

An Algorithmic Multimodality Blood Conservation Strategy

A series of technical and pharmacologic modalities can be combined into a multimodality blood conservation strategy in order to address the risk factors for blood transfusion following open heart surgery in a comprehensive manner. This strategy was initially used in the performance of cardiac surgery in Jehovah's Witnesses patients,[10] a group of patients who refuse all transfusions on religious grounds. The algorithmic application of a stratified blood conservation program, which represents a refinement of the compulsory multimodality strategy used for the high-risk Jehovah's Witnesses patients, has also been reported.[11] Both these strategies are designed to reduce bleeding and the need for allogeneic transfusion by comprehensively addressing the risk factors for bleeding and transfusion, as discussed above, and optimally incorporating appropriate blood conservation measures into an integrated program. The algorithmic approach takes into account the relative risk/benefit of each intervention, a consideration that is important in terms of patient safety as well as in light of the mounting pressure of medical economics.

The described series of technical and pharmacologic interventions was blood conserving, directed toward minimizing both the hemodilution and the coagulopathy associated with CPB in order to mitigate preoperative red cell mass and postoperative chest tube output as transfusion risk factors, respectively. Technical interventions include modifications in the performance of cardiopulmonary bypass, intraoperative autologous blood donation, normovolemic hemodilution, and perioperative blood salvage; these interventions represent simple, generally inexpensive measures that are safe and effective in decreasing transfusion requirements. Recent pharmacologic advances allowing enhancement of the hematopoietic and coagulation systems have provided additional useful means of blood conservation, and these have also been included in the protocol. These interventions can be grouped together as five specific strategies, which are discussed below: (1) maximize autologous blood generation/regeneration; (2) minimize unnecessary hemodilution; (3) minimize autologous blood loss/maximize autologous blood salvage; (4) optimize coagulation status/minimize coagulopathic insult; and (5) transfuse allogeneic blood only when physiologically necessary (Table 5-1).

Strategy 1: Maximize Autologous Blood Generation/Regeneration

A critical initial component of the conservation protocol is to ensure that the patient will have an adequate hematocrit while on bypass. This can be accurately predicted from a nomogram based upon the patient's gender, height, and weight, to determine the total blood volume, multiplied by their baseline hematocrit to determine preoperative red cell mass,[12] which, in turn, is entered into an equation that incorporates the anticipated pump prime volume and thereby allows calculation of the hemodilution effects of the crystalloid pump prime.[12] The end point for these calculations is the minimum safely tolerable hematocrit on bypass. While such a value cannot be determined absolutely for all patients, a large retrospective study by Fang and colleagues determined that a minimum on-bypass hematocrit of less than 16% in low-risk patients and 18% in high-risk patients predicted a significantly greater incidence of adverse events when compared to patients with correspondingly higher hematocrit values.[13] Consequently, if the patient is a Jehovah's Witness or if blood transfusion is otherwise contraindicated, and if the estimated on-bypass

TABLE 5-1. Strategies and Specific Interventions Constituting the New York Hospital-Cornell Medical Center Blood Conservation Program

Strategy	Intervention

1. Maximize autologous blood generation	Erythropoietin
	    Iron
	    Vitamin C
	    Folate
	    Vitamin B$_{12}$

2. Minimize hemodilution	Minimize crystalloid administration Retrograde autologous priming (RAP) Small-volume oxygenator/circuitry
3. Minimize autologous losses	Meticulous technique Cell saver—exclusive use Intraoperative autologous donation Shed mediastinal blood autotransfusion Positive end-expiratory pressure Minimize use of pads/sponges

4. Optimize coagulation status	Full and sustained rewarming
	Antifibrinolytics
	    Aprotinin (full or half dose)
	    Amicar®

5. Minimize unnecessary transfusions	Adhere to strict transfusion guidelines Early return to operating room for excessive bleeding

hematocrit is inadequate (less than 18%), surgery is delayed until adequate erythropoietin therapy can be administered. If the hematocrit is adequate or transfusion is not otherwise contraindicated, surgery is not delayed.

Red cell mass is enhanced using a high-dosage erythropoietin regimen of 300 U/kg intravenous load, followed by maintenance therapy of 500 U/kg subcutaneously every other day.[14] This regimen is supplemented by oral or intravenous iron, folate, and vitamin C. This "high-dose" erythropoietin therapy results in a dramatic early rise in hematocrit and sustained increases in erythropoiesis above that obtained with a standard dosage regimen with this protocol.[8,10] Hematocrit increases of 2 to 3% per day can be anticipated within approximately 5 to 7 days after initiating this erythropoietin regimen. This treatment regimen is effective even in patients with anemia secondary to hemolysis from perivalvular prosthetic leaks, in whom endogenous erythropoietin levels and erythropoiesis would be expected to be maximized.

Erythropoietin therapy is continued postoperatively until a hematocrit of 30% is obtained. The initial postoperative hematocrit often approximates the preoperative hematocrit, which is normally greater than 30%, so that postoperative erythropoietin therapy usually is not required.

Erythropoietin therapy is expensive, with a hospital cost for the high-dose regimen described in our Jehovah's Witnesses series of approximately $4,000 (US), exclusive of daily hospital charges. Erythropoietin therapy has consequently been shifted to an outpatient regimen that uses a visiting nurse service to administer the therapy. The use of alternative means of maintaining the preoperative hematocrit, thereby avoiding obligatory transfusions associated with excessively low hematocrit values, is also emphasized. Minimizing the hemodilution associated with cardiopulmonary bypass is one such critical strategy.

Strategy 2: Minimize Unnecessary Hemodilution

Hemodilution, the direct result of the mixing of the patient's blood volume with the crystalloid CPB circuit prime, is a unique and obligatory feature of open heart surgery as currently practiced, and it imposes a significant risk for red blood cell transfusions.[15–17] Decreases in hematocrit with the institution of bypass are directly proportional to the dilution of the red cell mass caused by the asanguinous pump prime volume. This decrease in hematocrit may lead directly to obligatory red cell transfusions during or after open heart surgery, as a result of unacceptably lowered hematocrits. The hematocrit resulting from the hemodilution associated with CPB can be directly calculated as the product of the patient's hematocrit and the patient's red cell mass (volume) as a fraction of the crystalloid CPB prime volume plus the red cell volume, as previously described.[17] Red cell mass, the product of blood volume times hematocrit, can be determined by using a nomogram based on the initial hematocrit, height, weight, and gender. Thus, the patients in whom specific interventions to minimize hemodilution could play a critical role in avoiding transfusion may also be predicted preoperatively.

Incremental improvements have been made in decreasing the hemodilution associated with CPB through such methods as the use of "low-prime" oxygenators.[16] In this technique, the crystalloid prime volume can be decreased to 1,200 to 1,400 mL from 2,000 mL by using a small-volume oxygenator and small-diameter tubing in patients with a body mass of less than 65 kg. This decrease in hemodilution results in a significant reduction in homologous red blood cell transfusions.[16] Nevertheless, a significant margin for minimizing hemodilution, thereby decreasing homologous red cell transfusions, can be achieved by using a technique called *retrograde autologous priming* (RAP).[17,18] During the RAP procedure, the crystalloid CPB prime is evacuated from the pump circuit at the initiation of bypass in advance of the patient's blood column (Figure 5-1). RAP significantly decreases the hemodilution associated with bypass and, accordingly, minimizes red blood cell transfusions during and after open heart surgery.[17] In a study of primary coronary bypass patients (*n* = 30), the lowest hematocrit during CPB was 22 ± 3% versus 20 ± 3% in RAP and control patients, respectively (*p* = .002). One (3%) of 30 RAP patients received transfusion intraoperatively whereas 7 (23%) of 30 control patients required transfusion during surgery (*p* = .03). The number of patients receiving any

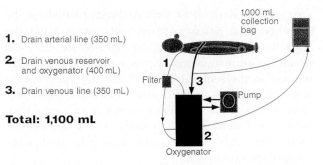

1. Drain arterial line (350 mL)

2. Drain venous reservoir and oxygenator (400 mL)

3. Drain venous line (350 mL)

Total: 1,100 mL

FIGURE 5-1. Schematic of the retrograde autologous prime (RAP) technique. *1. Arterial line drainage.* Blood is allowed to drain through the pump arterial line from the aorta through the filter, into the recirculation line and up into a 1000-mL transfer bag. *2. Venous reservoir and oxygenator drainage.* The arterial pump is slowly advanced until pump prime is cleared from the oxygenator into the recirculation bag. *3. Venous line drainage.* As bypass is commenced, the venous line prime is drained into the recirculation bag. The recirculation bag is rehung to allow for crystalloid transfusion as necessary. Reproduced with permission from Rosengart TK et al.[10]

homologous red cell transfusions in the two groups during the entire hospitalization was 8 of 30 (27%) versus 16 of 30 (53%), respectively (*p* = .03).

Both low-prime circuitry and RAP are essentially cost-free techniques that are easily applied and well tolerated, and they can significantly reduce transfusion requirements in coronary artery bypass graft (CABG) patients. The direct result of these techniques is higher hematocrits during CPB, providing an increased margin of safety in patients with low preoperative red cell mass and/or hematocrit, and decreasing allogeneic red cell requirements. Because of the reduced hemodilution associated with these techniques, the demands for preoperative erythropoietin therapy to boost the preoperative red cell mass are accordingly limited.

Strategy 3: Minimize Autologous Blood Loss/ Maximize Autologous Blood Salvage

The potential to generate higher hematocrits during CPB, as described above, in turn acts synergistically and improves the opportunity to apply other blood conservation strategies. Intraoperative autologous blood donation (IAD), whereby the patient's own blood is removed at the start of surgery, stored, and then transfused back to the patient following CPB, is one such strategy. The use of IAD alone significantly decreases red blood cell transfusion requirements.[12] Although the mechanism underlying this reduction in transfusion requirement remains unresolved, the removal of large blood volumes, as opposed to the more conventional smaller-volume IAD, is advocated because of evidence in the literature and in preliminary studies that large-volume IAD more favorably affects postoperative hematocrit and blood loss with incremental minimal risk. Large-volume IAD was designed to achieve a targeted hematocrit of 18% on bypass, based on the hypothesis that unless a critical mass was donated, the impact of this blood in terms of the total red cell mass would be inconsequential. Application of this protocol resulted in the removal of approximately 1,200 mL of blood, or almost one-third of the estimated blood volume, in patients in whom this technique was employed. As discussed above, this magnitude of IAD is significantly greater than that removed in most previous studies but was well tolerated.

The other technical components designed to minimize autologous loss during surgery include meticulous hemostatic technique, avoidance of the use of lap pads, which can absorb a significant amount of unrecoverable blood, and exclusive use of the cell saver intraoperatively. It should be noted that the cell saver blood, and all autologous blood, is reinfused via a continuous circuit to accede to the religious specifications of Jehovah's Witnesses patients.[8,10] Unlike the IAD blood, the cell saver blood is usually exposed to heparin and to the bypass circuit prior to collection. The cell saver blood, lacking the potential benefit of being unexposed to these coagulopathic sources, is reinfused as needed to maintain an acceptable minimum hematocrit and is not held in reserve until after CPB, as is the case with IAD blood.

The reinfusion of shed mediastinal blood, collected via specialized pleural and mediastinal drains, is a potentially lifesaving technical innovation.[10] This shed mediastinal blood can be administered back to the patient in a continuous circuit, as described above. In reality, intraoperative use of aprotinin and attention to hemostasis have minimized postoperative blood loss to the point that shed blood autotransfusion has rarely been required, serving mainly as a safeguard against unanticipated postoperative bleeding. Additional technical measures to minimize postoperative blood loss include full rewarming during CPB, appropriate use of positive end-expiratory pressure for tamponade, and the use of topical and intravenous fluid-warming devices.

Perhaps the most important postoperative conservation strategy is the simple technical intervention of minimizing blood draws for laboratory determinations, which can account for up to 250 mL of blood loss over the course of a hospitalization. By using pediatric blood tubes and by eliminating unnecessary testing, hospital staff can significantly reduce this kind of blood loss.

Strategy 4: Optimize Coagulation Status/ Minimize Coagulopathic Insult

Use of the serine protease inhibitor aprotinin to minimize the coagulopathic insult associated with cardiopulmonary bypass is a major strategy of blood conservation. Aprotinin was first introduced into clinical use in 1953 for the treatment of acute pancreatitis. Use of aprotinin in cardiac surgery dates back to the observations reported by Tice and colleagues in 1963.

The current era of aprotinin therapy dates to the serendipitous discovery by the Hammersmith group that a high-dose regimen (5 to 6 million units average total dose) significantly reduced bleeding in an experimental model of lung inflammation and, subsequently, in cardiac surgical patients.[19,20] Since that time, aprotinin use has repeatedly been demonstrated to produce about a 30 to 50% decrease in bleeding and blood transfusion in patients undergoing open heart surgery, as demonstrated primarily in trials of primary and reoperation coronary bypass surgery.[20–24]

The mechanism of action of aprotinin is multifactorial and highly complex, acting at multiple loci in the coagulation cascade (Figure 5-2). Aprotinin blocks the activation of kallikrein at the start of the cascade and blocks plasmin activation at the terminus of the cascade, but also affects the activity of all the intermediary products normally affected by these two key mediators.[25,26]

Aprotinin also appears to be specifically capable of blocking the transendothelial migration capability of leukocytes. The complex effects of aprotinin activity are highlighted by its effects on platelet function. Specifically, aprotinin appears to interact with platelets by blocking thrombin-mediated proteolysis and consequent activation of protease-activated receptor (PAR)-1 on the surface of platelets, thereby both inhibiting platelet aggregation (antithrombotic effect) and, as a consequence of this antiaggregation mechanism, preserving platelet function (hemostatic effect).[26]

Presumably on the basis of these antiinflammatory properties, it was recently suggested that aprotinin decreases the incidence of stroke and other adverse sequelae of cardiopulmonary bypass.[27] In an aggregate analysis of 1,800 patients enrolled in placebo-controlled trials, aprotinin use was associated with approximately a 50% reduction in the incidence of stroke after CABG surgery (2.6% vs 1.0%: placebo vs "full-dose" aprotinin, $p < .009$).[27]

The "full Hammersmith" regimen, based upon the initial Hammersmith experience mentioned above, represents the current standard dose of reference for all aprotinin treatment strategies. This regimen is used in the high-risk Jehovah's Witnesses patients and reoperative populations. The high-dose aprotinin regimen is administered as follows: a small (10,000 kallikrein-inhibiting units [KIU]) intravenous test dose is given at the initiation of the surgery, to assess for anaphylaxis. This is followed approximately 10 min later by an intravenous loading dose of 2 million KIU (280 mg) of aprotinin and a CPB pump prime load of 2 million units. An intravenous maintenance infusion of 0.5 million units (70 mg) per hour is then continued until the end of the operation. Because of the interaction of aprotinin with the celite reagent used in performing activated clotting times (ACTs), ACT is maintained at a level of 750 s with interval re-administration of heparin, as previously described.[20] While "half-dose" and "pump-prime" doses are

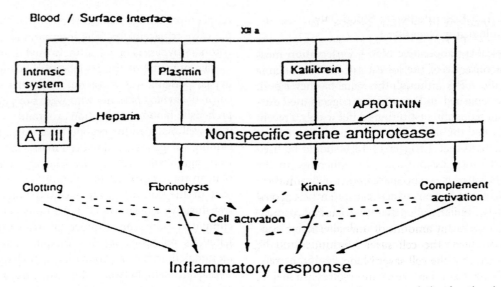

FIGURE 5-2. Schematic depicting multiple sites at which aprotinin is likely to act to enhance coagulation function during and after cardiopulmonary bypass. AT III = antithrombin. Reproduced with permission from Pifarre R. Anticoagulation hemostasis and blood preservation in cardiovascular surgery. Philadelphia: Hanley and Belfus; 1990.

also advocated as being efficacious, safety and efficacy data with these dose regimens are conflicting.[28]

The potential side effects of aprotinin use include a reported increase in the risk of graft thrombosis and/or myocardial infarction, as well as renal dysfunction.[20–23] The international post-CABG angiography study reported by Alderman and colleagues contains perhaps the most definitive data in regard to graft patency.[24] In this study, aprotinin did not adversely affect graft patency in patients at low risk for graft occlusion (US sites), but at sites with a greater prevalence of risk factors for graft occlusion (Danish and Israeli sites), aprotinin use was associated with an incidence of graft occlusion of 23% as compared to 12.4% in placebo controls. Despite criticism that randomization should have neutralized such differences, the authors claim an overall risk ratio of aprotinin-induced graft closure of 1.05 after adjustment for these risk factors. Pooled analyses of randomized trials have similarly failed to show an increased incidence of mortality, myocardial infarction, or renal dysfunction associated with aprotinin use.[28]

It would seem intuitive that prohemostatic therapy following coronary bypass surgery, as with the use of aprotinin, might be undesirable in terms of graft patency, given data generated over the past two decades suggesting that perioperative antiplatelet therapy induces a degree of coagulopathy that enhances graft patency. On the other hand, given the complexity of pro- and antithrombotic as well as antiinflammatory effects of aprotinin, the actual risk of side effects of this agent must be determined by actual, rather than postulated, outcomes data. Although lingering concerns remain regarding toxicities associated with aprotinin use, exhaustive trial data have failed to clearly demonstrate such risks and may have yielded evidence of additional benefit,

such as in the amelioration of stroke. A full-dose aprotinin regimen is advocated in high-risk patients such as Jehovah's Witnesses, reoperations, or patients with a preexisting coagulopathy, in whom major coagulopathic bleeding may be expected.

Other antifibrinolytic agents, including ε-aminocaproic acid (EACA, or Amicar) and the related agent tranexamic acid (TA), also reduce bleeding and blood transfusions in open heart surgery.[29] These compounds act by blocking plasminogen binding to fibrin, therefore effectively blocking plasminogen activation and, consequently, fibrinolysis. Both EACA and TA differ from aprotinin in their inability to inhibit kallikrein activity and in that they are without the general antiproteolytic activity of aprotinin. The only significant difference between TA and EACA is that TA is approximately 10 times more potent than EACA.

A meta-analysis performed by Fremes and colleagues that includes clinical trials completed since 1980 concluded that both EACA/TA and aprotinin significantly decreased transfusion requirements when compared to placebo (32% and 53%, respectively, $p < .0001$).[30] Although the effects of aprotinin and those of the antifibrinolytics were not statistically different in this analysis, only aprotinin decreased the absolute frequency of postoperative transfusion requirements in terms of the percentage of patients transfused compared with a placebo ($p < .0001$, 23% reduction). EACA is an effective agent for treating postbypass coagulopathies and is used prophylactically for most lower-risk patients in whom aprotinin is not administered. Aprotinin and EACA should not be used in the same patient because of the potential risk of pathologic coagulative complications with the combined use of these agents.

Strategy 5: Transfuse Allogeneic Blood Only When Physiologically Necessary

Another critical intraoperative blood conservation measure is the acceptance of the lowest safe level of anemia during and after CPB. Although this value has never been definitively established and transfusion triggers used during CPB by surgeons and institutions differ widely, a recent analysis suggested the safety of a 15% transfusion trigger but also suggested that a trigger of 18% should be used when comorbidities are present.[13] By adherence to the stated triggers, patients can be spared potentially unnecessary allogeneic transfusion, which can often be ordered inappropriately. Similarly, allogeneic platelets and coagulation factors are not transfused unless all alternative non-transfusion measures were appropriately instituted and the patient continues to bleed at a clinically significant rate. The coagulopathy associated with CPB resolves in a majority of patients, and adherence to these transfusion protocols eliminated patients' requiring return to the operating room for control of a mechanical source of bleeding.

Clinical Trials

Aside from the studies reported above of specific components of the multimodality blood conservation program, the application of the complete program in 50 Jehovah's Witnesses patients and 100 consecutive other patients has also been reported.[10,11] Figures 5-3 and 5-4 outline the specific protocols employed in these studies. The experience in the cases of Jehovah's Witnesses patients includes the successful performance of complex procedures in both the adult and the pediatric populations,[31] including reoperations, congenital heart reconstruction, and multiple valve replacements. The internal mammary artery in coronary bypass is now routinely used in these patients.

The outcome of the 30 Jehovah's Witnesses coronary bypass patients was compared with that of 30 primary coronary bypass patients who were not part of the comprehensive blood conservation program.[10] The two groups were well matched for preoperative transfusion risks, including age, gender, and red cell mass. Chest tube outputs were significantly less in the Jehovah's Witnesses group than in the control group (Figure 5-5). Fifty-seven percent of the control group received homologous blood transfusions, a mean of 3.0 ± 4.8 units per patient, when compared with the absence of transfusions for the Jehovah's Witnesses patients. In spite of this transfusion requirement in the control patients, discharge hematocrits were equivalent between the two groups (Figure 5-6). There was no difference in operative mortality between groups, and the diagnosis-related group (DRG)–matched lengths of stay and ancillary costs were similar, and in many cases decreased, in the Jehovah's Witnesses patients when compared to the control population.

In the clinical trial examining the algorithmic application of the blood conservation strategy, 100 consecutive patients underwent coronary bypass surgery without any homologous transfusion, in comparison with the transfusion of a mean of 2.2 ± 6.7 units of allogeneic blood per patient (34 patients [38%] transfused) in a well-matched group of 90 patients undergoing CABG, in whom the multimodality blood conservation program was not applied but in whom an identical set of transfusion guidelines was enforced (control group).[11] The control patients

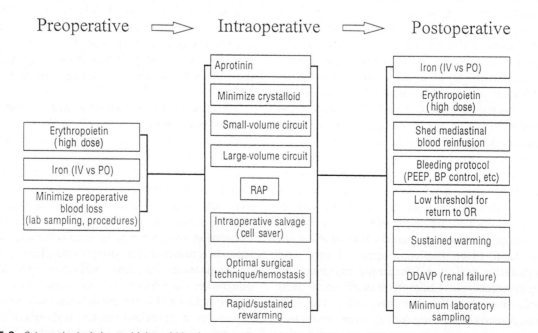

FIGURE 5-3. Schematic depicting multiphased blood conservation strategy as applied for Jehovah's Witnesses patients. Reproduced with permission from Rosengart TK et al.[10] (BP = blood pressure; DDAVP = desmopressin acetate; OR = operating room; PEEP = positive end-expiratory pressure.)

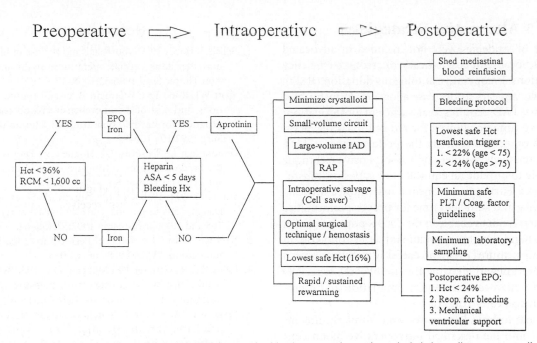

Preoperative ⟹ Intraoperative ⟹ Postoperative

FIGURE 5-4. Multimodality algorithm applied to the 100 consecutive blood conservation patients. Included are all measures applied during the preoperative, intraoperative, and postoperative periods. Reproduced with permission from Helm RE et al.[11] (ASA = acetylsalicylic acid; EDO = erythropoietin; Hct = hematocrit; Hx = history; PLT = platelet; RCM = red cell mass.)

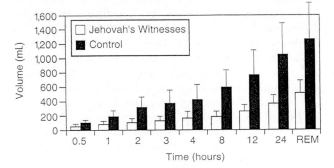

FIGURE 5-5. Chest tube output at various time points following operation for first-time coronary bypass control and Jehovah's Witnesses patients (*n* = 30). Significant differences (p < .05) were noted at all time points. REM = chest tube removal. Reproduced with permission from Rosengart TK et al.[10]

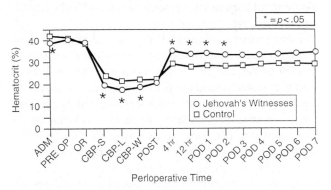

FIGURE 5-6. Serial hematocrits at specified time points for Jehovah's Witnesses and control patients (*n* = 30). Significant differences in hematocrit were noted at specified time points. Reproduced with permission from Rosengart TK et al.[10] ADM = admittance; OR = operating room; CBP = cardiopulmonary bypass; L = low; POD = postoperative day; S = start; W = wean from bypass.)

experienced almost twice the volume of postoperative blood loss at 12 h, when compared to the multimodality (MMD) group (660 ± 270 mL vs 370 ± 180 mL, *p* < .001). Total costs in each of the three major DRGs were equivalent or significantly less in the MMD group, when compared with the matched control patients.

Eight MMD patients experienced hematocrits of less than the stated 16% transfusion trigger during CPB (and no patient reached the 22% postoperative trigger). These eight patients, in whom no neurologic or other complication was noted, were successfully transfused to a hematocrit of 16% or above with available autologous blood (IAD or cell saver). This observation supports the hypothesis that patients can be spared potentially unnecessary allogeneic transfusion simply by adhering to predeter-

mined transfusion triggers, in addition to using the other blood conservation measures described in this chapter.

Performing transfusion-less pediatric open heart surgery still remains problematic because of the large relative volume of pump prime as compared to red cell mass and the profound consequent hemodilution that occurs in the neonate and young child. Nevertheless, the use of hemoconcentration in the operating room has significantly enhanced the postbypass hematocrits that can be achieved in these patients,[31] and selected pediatric patients can undergo open heart surgery without transfusion and with discharge hematocrits that are comparable to admission hematocrits.

Alternative Strategies

A number of strategies were not included in advocated algorithms because of cost, efficacy, or resource efficiency considerations. Preoperative autologous donation (PAD), for example, appears to decrease allogeneic transfusions, but effective PAD requires that sufficient postdonation/preoperative time be allowed for red cell mass regeneration; PAD otherwise restricts the performance of IAD, which is a relatively simpler and less-expensive technique that is likely to provide an equivalent or superior transfusion product. Furthermore, anemia may induce myocardial ischemia, and sufficient time for proper performance of PAD often is not available in the CABG population. On the other hand, use of recombinant erythropoietin in conjunction with PAD may be useful in accelerating red cell regeneration and allowing the use of PAD, especially in the non-CABG cardiac surgery population and if erythropoietin costs are reduced.

Additional technical measures were similarly not incorporated into the described intraoperative blood conservation program because their utility was uncertain or their cost-benefit ratios were unclear. These measures include platelet plasmapheresis, heparin-coated and other biocompatible circuitry, hemofiltration, and leukocyte filtration devices.

Desmopressin acetate (DDAVP) is a synthetic analog of the hormone vasopressin but is devoid of the vasoconstrictor effects of the native hormone. Desmopressin acetate appears to enhance platelet adhesion by augmenting the release from endogenous stores in endothelial cells and increasing the circulating levels of von Willebrand's factor and factor VIII coagulant protein. Although initial reports on the effects of DDAVP in CPB surgery were encouraging, multiple subsequent studies have generally failed to demonstrate similar benefits. Desmopressin acetate is consequently not used, except in patients with specific platelet defects.

It should be noted that significant blood conservation has been demonstrated with off-pump coronary bypass surgery.[32] This outcome is not surprising, given the absence of the hemodilution and coagulopathy obtained in avoiding the use of cardiopulmonary bypass, and given the opportunity to use less heparin in off-pump procedures. Because of the potential of a relatively hypercoagulable state in off-pump versus standard CABG patients, antifibrinolytic agents are not used in these patients.

Finally, although holding much promise, artificial blood substitutes have not advanced into standard critical practice.

Conclusion

Comprehensive risk factor–based application of multiple blood conservation measures in an optimized, integrated, and algorithmic manner can safely and significantly decrease bleeding and the need for allogeneic transfusion in CABG surgery in a cost-effective manner.

References

1. Belisle S, Hardy JF. Hemorrhage and the use of blood products after adult cardiac operations: myths and realities. Ann Thorac Surg 1996;62:1908–17.
2. Scott WJ, Rode R, Castlemain B, et al. Efficacy, complications, and cost of a comprehensive blood conservation program for cardiac operations. J Thorac Cardiovasc Surg 1992;103:1001–7.
3. Goodnough LT, Despotis GJ, Hogue CW, Ferguson TB. On the need for improved transfusion indicators in cardiac surgery. Ann Thorac Surg 1995;60:473–80.
4. Surgenor DM, Wallace EL, Churchill WH, et al. Red cell transfusions in coronary artery bypass surgery (DRGs 106 and 107). Transfusion 1992;32:458–64.
5. NIH Consensus Conference. Perioperative red blood cell transfusion. JAMA 1988;260:2700–3.
6. Jones JW, Rawitscher RE, McLean TR, et al. Benefit from combining blood conservation measures in cardiac operations. Ann Thorac Surg 1991;51:541–6.
7. Magovern JA, Sakert T, Benckart DH, et al. A model for predicting transfusion after coronary artery bypass grafting. Ann Thorac Surg 1996;61:27–32.
8. Rosengart TK, Helm RE, Klemperer J, et al. Combined aprotinin and erythropoietin use: results with Jehovah's Witnesses. Ann Thorac Surg 1994;58:1397–403.
9. Ferraris VA, Gildengorin V. Predictors of excessive blood use after coronary artery bypass grafting: a multivariate analysis. J Thorac Cardiovasc Surg 1989;98:492–7.
10. Rosengart TK, Helm RE, DeBois WJ, et al. Open heart operations without transfusion using a multimodality blood conservation strategy in Jehovah's Witness patients: implications for a "bloodless" surgical technique. J Am Coll Surg 1997;184:432–40.
11. Helm RE, Rosengart TK, Klemperer JD, et al. Comprehensive multimodality blood conservation: 100 consecutive CABG operations without transfusion. Ann Thorac Surg 1998;65:125–36.
12. Helm RE, Klemperer J, Rosengart TK, et al. Intraoperative autologous blood donation preserves red cell mass but does not decrease postoperative bleeding. Ann Thorac Surg 1996;62:1431–41.
13. Fang WC, Helm RE, Krieger KH, et al. Impact of minimum hematocrit during cardiopulmonary bypass on mortality in patients undergoing coronary artery surgery. Circulation 1997;96 Suppl 9:194–9.
14. Helm RE, Gold JP, Rosengart TK, et al. Erythropoietin in cardiac surgery. J Card Surg 1993;8(5):579–606.
15. Jansen PG, Te Velthuis H, Bulder ER, et al. Reduction in prime volume attenuates the hyperdynamic response after cardiopulmonary bypass. Ann Thorac Surg 1995;60:544–50.
16. DeBois WJ, Sukhram Y, McVey J, et al. Reduction in homologous blood transfusions using a low prime circuit. J Extracorp Technol 1996;28(2):58–62.
17. Rosengart TK, DeBois W, O'Hara M, et al. Retrograde autologous priming (RAP) for cardiopulmonary bypass: a safe and effective means of decreasing hemodilution and transfusion requirements. J Thorac Cardiovasc Surg 1998;115:426–39.
18. Balachandran S, Cross MH, Karthikeyan S, et al. Retrograde autologous priming of the cardiopulmonary bypass cir-

cuit reduces blood transfusion after coronary artery surgery. Ann Thorac Surg 2002;73:1912–8.

19. Van Oeveren W, Jansen NJG, Bidstrup BP, et al. Effect of aprotinin on hemostatic mechanisms during cardiopulmonary bypass. Ann Thorac Surg 1987;44;640–5.

20. Royston D, Bidstrup BP, Taylor KM, Sapsford RN. Effect of aprotinin on need for blood transfusions after repeat open heart surgery. Lancet 1987;2:1289–91.

21. Cosgrove DM III, Heric B, Lytle BW, et al. Aprotinin therapy for reoperative myocardial revascularization: a placebo-controlled trial. Ann Thorac Surg 1992;54:1031–8.

22. Lemmer JH Jr, Stanford W, Bonney SL, et al. Aprotinin for coronary bypass operations: efficacy, safety, and influence on early saphenous vein graft patency. J Thorac Cardiovasc Surg 1994;107:543–53.

23. Levy JH, Pifarre R, Schaff HV, et al. A multicenter, double-blind, placebo-controlled trial of aprotinin for reducing blood loss and the requirement for donor-blood transfusion in patients undergoing repeat coronary artery bypass grafting. Circulation 1995;92:2236–44.

24. Alderman EL, Levy JH, Rich JB, et al. Analyses of coronary graft patency after aprotinin use: results from the international multicenter aprotinin graft patency experience (IMAGE) trial. J Thorac Cardiovasc Surg 1998;116:716–30.

25. Landis RC, Asimakopoulous G, Poullis M, et al. The antithrombotic and antiinflammatory mechanisms of action of aprotinin. Ann Thorac Surg 2001;72:2169–75.

26. Mojcik CF, Levy JH. Aprotinin and the systemic inflammatory response after cardiopulmonary bypass. Ann Thorac Surg 2001;71:745–54.

27. Murkin JM. Attenuation of neurologic injury during cardiac surgery. Ann Thorac Surg 2001;72:S1838–44.

28. Smith PK, Muhlbaier LH. Aprotinin: safe and effective only with the full-dose regimen. Ann Thorac Surg 1996;62:1575–7.

29. Blauhut B, Harringer W, Bettelheim P, et al. Comparison of the effects of aprotinin and tranexamic acid on blood loss and related variables after cardiopulmonary bypass. J Thorac Cardiovasc Surg 1994;108:1083–91.

30. Fremes SE, Wong BI, Lee E, et al. Meta-analysis of prophylactic drug treatment in the prevention of postoperative bleeding. Ann Thorac Surg 1994;58:1580–8.

31. Rosengart TK, Lang S, Helm RE, Friedman D. Open heart surgery in the pediatric Jehovah's Witness population: no longer "Russian roulette." Pediatr Cardiol 1996;17:430–3.

32. Ascione R, Willimas S, Lloyd DT, et al. Reduced postoperative bloodless and transfusion requirement after beating heart coronary operation: a prospective randomized study. J Thorac Cardiovasc Surg 2001;121:689–96.

CHAPTER 6

USE OF HEPARIN-BONDED CARDIOPULMONARY BYPASS CIRCUITS WITH ALTERNATIVES TO STANDARD ANTICOAGULATION

GABRIEL S. ALDEA, MD

Systemic anticoagulation to prevent the activation of the coagulation system has been the standard practice during cardiopulmonary bypass. Young's work in a primate model has shown suppression of fibrin monomer production when the activated clotting time (ACT) exceeds 400 s, establishing an industry "gold standard."[1] With these anticoagulation parameters, despite the application of many blood conservation strategies, as many as 30 to 70% of all patients undergoing coronary artery bypass graft (CABG) require homologous transfusions. Recent investigators question this standard and suggest that an ACT of 300 s is equally safe.[2–5] Heparin itself (independent of cardiopulmonary bypass) can cause fibrinolysis and platelet degranulation, and heparin–protamine complexes may further activate inflammation.[6,7] If extracorporeal perfusion can be performed safely with lower levels of anticoagulation and without increased thrombogenic risk, it is possible to achieve improved hemostasis and a decrease in the need for homologous transfusion with its associated morbidity and cost. The contact of blood with the large, artificial, nonendothelialized surfaces of the cardiopulmonary bypass circuit results in an intense surface interaction initiated by formed and unformed blood elements. Accentuated by the shear stresses, turbulence, cavitation, and osmotic forces of artificial flow, an intense stimulation of many biologic reactions occur, including the coagulation, fibrinolytic, complement, kallikrein, and kinin systems. This cross-stimulation is further amplified and results in activation and consumption of platelets, activation and degranulation of leukocytes, destruction of red blood cells, and the release of anaphylaxins, oxygen free radicals, and endotoxins. The biologic effects of these reactions are clinically described as the "postperfusion syndrome." These responses can be characterized as

changes in two principle categories: (1) coagulation and thrombosis, and (2) generalized inflammation. The role of novel "biocompatible" extracorporeal surfaces and perfusion techniques is to attenuate these responses.

Heparin-bonded circuits (HBCs) were developed in an attempt to limit the activation of the coagulation system. The binding of heparin to artificial surfaces was first reported by Gott.[8] Recently, the heparin-binding process was extended to the entire extracorporeal circuit ("tip-to-tip"). Heparin is bound to artificial surfaces by one of several processes: ionic binding, grafting, multiple point covalent binding, and end point covalent attachment.

Within minutes of bypass, an adsorbed plasma protein layer covers these surfaces. The composition and characteristics of this protein layer are thought to confer the properties of HBC.[9] The use of heparin-bonded circuits attenuates the activation of neutrophils, platelets, and complement during cardiopulmonary bypass by altering the blood–surface interface.[10–17] Although improved biocompatibility and thromboresistance of HBCs have been inferred from these findings, the safety and clinical relevance of these findings are still debated.[18,19] The thromboresistant properties of HBCs have also led to a resurgence of interest to assess and redefine optimal anticoagulation during cardiopulmonary bypass.[4] Despite their potential theoretic benefits, several areas have to be better defined and understood prior to wide application of HBCs to cardiac surgery, including (1) defining the optimal technical and perfusion environment to use HBCs and accentuate any possible potential clinical benefits; (2) determining the safety of using HBCs, with emphasis on thrombogenic potential and occurrence of any clinical complications; (3) determining clinical benefit over the use of conventional circuits; (4) determining the effect of anticoagulation protocol (full versus lower) on clinical outcome and thrombogenic potential; (5) defining whether the clinical benefits derived from the use of HBCs can be imparted to all patients undergoing cardiac surgery or are limited to a high-risk patient population or procedures; (6) exploring possible mechanisms by which HBCs may influence clinical outcomes and determine areas for future advance; and, finally, (7) evaluating the contribution of cardiotomy suction to the deleterious effects previously attributed to cardiopulmonary bypass (CPB) itself. Our initial experience with these techniques was limited to a high-risk patient population (Jehovah's Witnesses patients and catheterization laboratory emergencies requiring CABG), with outstanding clinical results.[20] Following this initial successful experience, a series of studies was undertaken to define the possible benefits and limitations of HBCs.

Methods

An integrated blood conservation strategy was developed and uniformly applied to all patients undergoing CABG.[21] It involves the routine use of many clinically proven "best practice" strategies. The precise techniques and composition of the "tip-to-tip" heparin-bonded cardiopulmonary bypass circuits were previously described in detail. These techniques include the use of maximal cell saving; large-bore directional arterial cannulas to minimize shear rates; centrifugal pumps; hollow-fiber membrane oxygenators; closed venous reservoirs; elimination of routine use of cardiotomy suckers to minimize blood–air interface (except in open cardiac procedures); low prime volume (< 600 mL) to minimize dilution; near-normothermic bypass (core temperature of > 34°C [93.2°F] to avoid active cooling); precise heparin and protamine titration dose-response assays; routine use of ε-aminocaproic acid (Amicar); strict protocols delineating thresholds for transfusion; meticulous attention to technical detail; and, finally, a concerted effort by the surgeons, perfusionists, anesthesiologists, and nurses to minimize homologous transfusion.

Outcomes

A prospective study of 234 patients undergoing primary, non-emergent CABG was continued to more definitively demonstrate the efficacy and safety of these techniques.[21] Four hundred and four patients undergoing primary CABG were randomized and treated with HBCs and lower anticoagulation protocol (LAP; activated clotting time [ACT] > 280 s) or conventional non-HBCs (NHBCs) with full anticoagulation protocol (FAP) (ACT > 480 s).[22] Only reoperations and catheterization laboratory emergencies were excluded (which were treated exclusively with HBCs and LAP). Techniques of cardiopulmonary bypass, clinical pathways leading to transfusion, extubation, intensive care unit (ICU), and hospital discharge were standardized and uniformly applied. Preoperative risk profiles were similar in both treatment groups. The

patients' acuity was higher than average, with 72% of patients undergoing CABG within 24 h of angiography because of urgent clinical presentation. Patients had a mean age of 65 ± 10 years, ejection factor (EF) 46 ± 12%, 33% incidence of diabetes mellitus, 79% incidence of hypertension, 48% incidence of prior myocardial infarction (MI), and 11% incidence of prior cerebrovascular accident/transient ischemic attack (CVA/TIA) with an Society of Thoracic Surgeons predicted mortality of 3.8 ± 2.1% (nearly twice the reported expected STS national database average for the same time period [ie, 1.9%]). Preoperative and discharge hematologic parameters were similar in the HBC and NHBC treatment groups, demonstrating strict adherence to transfusion protocol (Table 6-1). By design, patients treated with HBCs received lower heparin doses, had lower activated clotting times during cardiopulmonary bypass, and required lower protamine reversal doses (Table 6-2). Mediastinal tube drainage in the first 24 h following surgery was reduced in the HBC group. Both the incidence and magnitude of homologous transfusion were reduced with HBCs and LAP (43% reduction). Patients treated with HBCs had a shorter duration of ventilator support as well as shorter ICU and hospital stays (Table 6-3). In addition, when compared with patients treated with NHBCs, patients treated with HBCs had a reduced incidence of postoperative MI, inotropic requirement, pulmonary complications, thromboembolic complications, atrial fibrillation, and the occurrence of any other postoperative complication (see Table 6-3). Although the incidence of clinical thromboembolic complications was lower in patients treated with HBCs, the magnitude of intravascular particulate emboli generated during CPB was further quantified by subjecting arterial filters to scanning electron micrographic analyses. The percentage of the arterial filter covered by microscopic debris was carefully quantified and was 83% lower in patients treated with HBCs and LAP (6.1 ± 5.6% vs 35.1 ± 18.2%, $p = 2.1E-6$). Representative sets of arterial filters from patients treated with

TABLE 6-1. Discharge Hematologic Profile

Variable	NHBC (n = 202)	HBC (n = 202)	p Value
Hgb (g/dL)	9.1 ± 1.4	9 0 ± 1.3	.55
Hematocrit	26.7 ± 4.0%	26.5 ± 3.7%	.66
Platelets (10³)	129 ± 45%	133 ± 48%	.32

Hgb = hemoglobin; HBC = heparin-bonded circuit; NHBC = non-HBC.

TABLE 6-2. Anticoagulation Protocol

Variable	NHBC (n = 202)	HBC (n = 202)	p Value
Heparin dose (USP/kg)	410 ± 292	176 ± 62	2.8E-70
ACT high (s)	534 ± 95	378 ± 79	1. 1E-54
ACT low (s)	401 ± 292	291 ± 56	5.9E-66
Protamine reversal (mg)	208 ± 78	112 ± 50	6.0E-39

ACT = activated clotting time; HBC = heparin-bonded circuit; NHBC = non-HBC; USP = U.S. Pharmacopeia.

TABLE 6-3. Comparison of Morbidity and Mortality in Patients Treated with NHBCs and HBCs

Variable	NHBC (n = 202)	HBC (n = 202)	p Value	Odds Ratio (95% CI)
Homologous transfusion				
Incidence	46.5%	36.6%*	0.04	—
Magnitude (units)	3.47 ± 8.37	1.98 ± 4.40*	0.03	—
Mediastinal drainage (mL/24 h)	660 ± 412	581 ± 254*	0.02	—
Ventilator support (h)	18.8 ± 39.1	12.8 ± 13.9*	0.04	—
ICU stay (h)	29.9 ± 28.8	20.3 ± 14.3*	0.007	—
Hospital stay (days)	6.8 ± 4.3	5.9 ± 2.2*	0.02	—
Mortality	1.98%	0.50%	0.18	—
Return to OR for postoperative bleeding	2.48%	1.49%	0.48	—
Perioperative MI	3.96%	0.99%*	0.05	0.24 (0.05–1.16)
Postoperative inotropes	7.4%	1.5%*	0.003	0.19 (0.05–0.66)*
Postoperative CVA/TIA	1.49%	0.50%	0.31	—
Ventilator > 3 days	4.46%	0.50%*	0.01	0.11 (0.01–0.85)*
Pneumonia	2.98%	0.48%	0.76	—
Tracheostomy	2.48%	0.50%	0.10	—
Atrial fibrillation	36.1%	26.4%*	0.03	0.63(0.41–0.96)*
Renal failure	2.97%	1.49%	0.31	—
Vascular	1.49%	0.50%	0.31	—
MI + CVA/TIA + vascular	6.44%	1.98%*	0.025	0.29 (0.09–0.91)*
Any postoperative complication	41.1%	28.7%*	0.009	0.58 (0.38–0.87)*

CVA/TIA = cerebrovascular accident/transient ischemic attack; HBC = heparin-bonded circuit; ICU = intensive care unit; MI = myocardial infarction; NHBC = nonheparin-bonded circuit; OR = operating room.
* $p < 0.05$.

HBCs and NHBCs are compared in Figures 6-1 and 6-2. The incidence and magnitude of homologous transfusion were significantly lower in patients treated with HBCs and could result from several confounding factors. The direct influence of the use of HBCs on homologous transfusion was confirmed with the use of multivariate logistic regression analysis. In addition to the use of HBCs, only preoperative hematocrit, age, total pump time, gender, and body surface area (BSA) were demonstrated to be factors that were significantly and independently correlated with the administration of homologous transfusion (Table 6-4). Compared to men, women were 5.8 times more likely to receive homologous transfusion ($p < .0001$, 95% CI 3.6 to 9.3).Women treated with HBCs had a 65% reduction in the magnitude of transfusion (2.6 ± 3.8 vs 6.0 ± 11.3 units, $p = .03$). An important relation-ship was noted between the magnitude of homologous transfusion, time to extubation, incidence of postoperative complications, and length of hospital stay (and therefore cost) (Table 6-5). This relationship was further confirmed by using multivariate analysis of pre-, intra-, and postoperative variables. Homologous transfusion was confirmed to be a significant predictor of time to extubation, incidence of postoperative complications, and length of hospital stay.

Factors that were significantly correlated with time to extubation (listed in their order of relative importance) were the occurrence of homologous transfusion, postoperative inotropic requirement, and age. Factors that were significantly correlated with occurrence of postoperative complications were age, time of extubation, and homologous transfusion. Finally, the factors that were signifi-

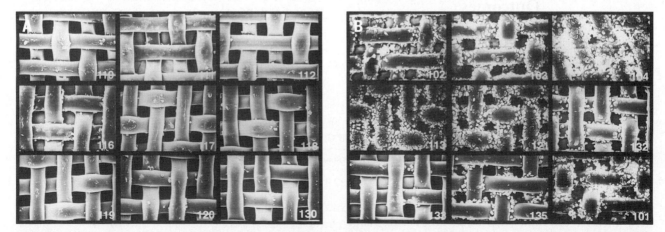

FIGURE 6-1. Scanning electron micrographs (× 200 original magnification) of nine representative arterial filters at the conclusion of CPB. *A,* Patients treated with HBCs with LAP. *B,* Patients treated with NHBCs and FAP.

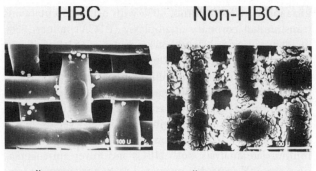

HBC   Non-HBC

- ⇓ACT 223 sec   ⇓ACT 460 sec

FIGURE 6-2. Close-up scanning electron micrographs of two representative patients (× 200 original magnification). The filter on the left is from a patient treated with HBCs, with the lowest ACT on CPB of 223 s. The filter on the right is from a patient treated with conventional NHBCs, with a lowest ACT on bypass of 460 s.

TABLE 6-4. Independent Determinants of the Occurrence of Homologous Transfusion

Variable	Coefficient	SE of Coefficient	Probability
Preoperative hematocrit	−0.310	0.044	< .000001
Age	0.056	0.016	.0005
Total pump time	0.024	0.007	.0004
Use of HBC	−0.785	0.302	.009
Gender	0.820	0.380	.03
BSA	−1.741	0.863	.04
Preoperative renal failure (Cr > 2.5)	0.488	0.676	.53
Prior CVA/TIA	1.45	1.47	.33

BSA = body surface area; Cr = creatinine; CVA/TIA = cerebrovascular accident/transient ischemic attack; HBC = heparin-bonded circuit.

cantly and independently correlated with length of hospital stay (and therefore cost) were postoperative pulmonary complications, atrial fibrillation, postoperative renal dysfunction, occurrence of homologous transfusion, total pump time, and postoperative MI. It is possible that clinical improvements noted with the use of HBCs are based on their isolated effect on a small group of patients receiving large amounts of homologous transfusion. To exclude this possibility, a group of patients who received massive homologous transfusions, defined as patients receiving more than 8 homologous units, was identified. This small group of 41 patients (22 NHBC patients and 19 HBC patients) represented 10.1% of the total study population of 404 patients and was responsible for 69% of all the homologous units transfused

(769 of 1,100 units). After exclusion of this group, clinical outcomes were analyzed, reconfirming the significant improvements noted with the use of HBCs and LAP (see Table 6-3). HBCs may improve clinical outcomes primarily by reducing homologous transfusion.

Alternatively, the blunted "inflammatory response" to cardiopulmonary bypass may also affect clinical outcomes. To evaluate this second mechanism, an analysis of the subset of patients not receiving any transfusion was performed, and these patients had uniformly outstanding clinical outcomes. The overall incidence of any postoperative complication was reduced in patients treated with HBCs and LAP, when compared to those patients treated with NHBCs and FAP (21.9% versus 33.3%, $p < .05$, odds ratio 0.56, 95% CI 0.32 to 0.98).

Ionic versus Covalent HBCs

The specific method of heparin bonding (ionic versus covalent) may influence clinical outcomes. Possible differences were assessed in a prospective randomized study of 404 patients. The relative efficacy of ionic and covalent HBCs were compared to their identical NHBCs.

Ionic and covalent HBCs were also compared to each other. When compared to an equivalent NHBC, patients treated with an ionic HBC required fewer homologous transfusions (2.0 ± 4.2 versus 3.4 ± 8.2 units, $p < .05$), had fewer postoperative complications (29% versus 41%, $p < .05$), and had a shorter hospital stay (6.2 ± 2.6 versus 7.1 ± 5.2 days, $p < .05$). Similarly, when compared to identical NHBCs, patients with covalent-bound HBCs required fewer homologous transfusions (2.0 ± 4.7 versus 3.5 ± 7.6 units, $p < .05$), had fewer postoperative complications (27.7% versus 42.1%, $p < .05$), and had a shorter hospital stay (5.7 ± 1.6 versus 6.4 ± 3.2 days, $p < .05$). When compared to each other, ionic- and covalent-bound HBCs resulted in a similar magnitude of improvement in clinical outcomes (no statistical differences by analysis of variance).

Effect of Anticoagulation Protocol on Clinical Outcomes in Patients Treated with HBCs

It was unclear whether it was the HBCs or the lower anticoagulation protocol which was most responsible for the improved clinical outcomes. To determine the effect of anticoagulation protocol on clinical outcomes and thrombin

TABLE 6-5. Effect of Homologous Transfusion on Clinical Outcomes

Homologous Units (%)	Number	Hospital Stay (d)	Time to Extubation (h)	Postoperative Complications (%)
0	236 (58.4%)	5.4 ± 1.6	10.3 ± 4.1	27.1
1–2	84 (20.8%)	6.6 ± 3.0*	14.5 ± 14.1*	35.7
3–4	34 (8.4%)	7.9 ± 4.3**	17.6 ± 53.9	44.1**
5–8	15 (3.7%)	8.6 ± 61	32.3 ± 59.9	53.3
>8	41 (10.1%)	10.7 ± 6.8***	64.7 ± 5.7***	63.4***

* $p < .05$ vs 0 homologous units; ** $p < .05$ vs 1 to 2 homologous units; *** $p < .05$ vs 3 to 4 homologous units

generation in patients treated exclusively with HBCs, 244 consecutive patients undergoing primary CABG were randomized to either an LAP (ACT > 250 s) or an FAP (ACT > 450 s).[23] When compared to patients who were treated with FAP, patients treated with LAP had a lower incidence (24.2% versus 35.8%, $p < .05$) and magnitude (0.50 ± 0.92 versus 1.08 ± 2.10 units, $p = .005$) of homologous transfusion. Clinical outcomes were uniformly outstanding in patients treated with HBCs in both anticoagulation treatment groups. However, patients treated with LAP had a lower incidence of thromboembolic complications, defined as the combined incidence of MI, CVA/TIA, and vascular events (0.8 versus 5.0%, $p < .05$, odds ratio 0.12 with 95% CI of 0.01 to .95), and a modest reduction in hospital stay (5.3 ± 1.2 versus 5.7 ± 1.7 days, $p = .05$).

Effect of Anticoagulation Protocol Thrombin Generation in Patients Treated with HBCs

Thrombin generation during CPB was assessed in a subset of 58 patients by measuring thrombin–antithrombin complexes and fragment F1.2. Thrombin generation increased during CPB in both treatment groups but correlated poorly to the anticoagulation protocol and ACT (r2 = 0.03). No differences in the number of microemboli detected by transcranial Doppler (TCD) analysis during CPB were noted between anticoagulation protocols. Most detected microemboli (> 70%) were associated with direct aortic manipulation during insertion and removal of cannulae, partial or complete clamping, and unclamping. A detailed neurologic and neuropsychological cognitive evaluation demonstrated similar outcomes in the LAP and FAP treatment groups. Patients treated with HBCs had a low incidence of neurologic events as compared to other reports.[23] In addition, these patients had a more rapid and complete recuperation of neuropsychological function. Although 87% of patients had demonstrable neuropsychological deficits immediately after CABG (postoperative day 4), less than 11% of patients exhibited any deficit 4 weeks following operative procedure.

Effect of HBCs and Anticoagulation Protocol in Patients Undergoing Emergency CABG

The morbidity related to emergency CABG might be of such magnitude as to obscure any potential benefits related to the use of HBCs. A retrospective study of 206 patients undergoing emergency CABG (defined as surgical procedure immediately following catheterization, mandated by clinical circumstances) was undertaken to assess the effects of HBCs on clinical outcomes in this high-risk patient subset.[24] Risk profiles of patients treated with HBCs and NHBCs were similar, with 47% incidence of preoperative

intraaortic balloon pump, 40% with acute percutaneous transluminal coronary angioplasty (PTCA) failure, 73% incidence of prior MI, and 38% incidence of left ventricular ejection fraction of < 40%. More than 90% of patients were on aspirin and intravenous heparin preoperatively. Compared to patients treated with NHBCs, in patients treated with HBCs, there was similar incidence (80% versus 85%) but a lower magnitude (5.5 ± 9.3 versus 23.6 ± 29.2 units, $p = .008$) of homologous transfusion. Using multivariate analysis, both HBCs and lower anticoagulation protocol were demonstrated to be independent predictors of homologous transfusion. Patients undergoing CABG with HBCs had a lower incidence of perioperative MI (2.6% versus 12.3%, $p = .03$) and inotropic requirement (18% versus 38%, $p = .005$). The incidence of any thromboembolic complications was reduced with HBCs (6% versus 16%, $p = .02$), as was the incidence of serious complications (13% versus 29%, $p = .01$; odds ratio 0.37, 95% CI 0.18 to 0.75). This resulted in shorter ICU (31 versus 92 h, $p = .009$) and hospital stays (7.8 ± 5.7 versus 11.1 ± 8.9 days, $p = .03$).

Use of HBCs in Valve Surgery

The outcomes of 120 patients undergoing valve surgery with HBCs and LAP were compared to the outcomes of 232 patients treated with NHBCs and FAP in a retrospective study of 352 patients.[25] When compared to patients who were treated with NHBCs, patients who were treated with LAP had a lower incidence (64.2% versus 85.8%, $p = .0001$) and magnitude (6.9 ± 13.0 versus 18.6 ± 26.2 units, $p < .00001$) of homologous transfusion. Postoperative chest-tube drainage (558 ± 466 versus 1054 ± 911 mL, $p < .00001$), incidence of reoperation for bleeding (2.5% versus 8.2%, $p = .04$), and the overall incidence of any postoperative complication (42% versus 56%, $p = .02$) were also significantly reduced. Multivariate analysis identified use of HBCs as an independent predictor of decreased transfusion and postoperative complications. Two patients in the HBC with LAP group and none in the NHBC with FAP group required early reintervention valve thrombosis when small mechanical prostheses (annular size < 29 mm) were implanted in the mitral position. Although this incidence was not statistically significant ($p = .22$), because of the potential for early valve thrombosis, higher levels of anticoagulation were recommended for mechanical valve implantation when an LAP is used. In the past 2 years, with an anticoagulation protocol maintaining an ACT > 350 s during CPB, no early valve thrombosis was noted in a consecutive series of over 400 patients.

Effect of Cardiotomy Suction

A prospective randomized study was performed to evaluate the independent effects of HBC and disassociate them from those of cardiotomy suction in patients undergoing non-emergency CABG performed with ACT > 450 s.[26]

HBCs preserved platelet function regardless of use of cardiotomy suction. However, this study conclusively demonstrated that the use of cardiotomy suction, especially with non-HBCs, resulted in a dramatic progressive increase in markers of thrombin generation, and granulocyte activation (polymorphonuclear [PMN] elastase), as well as of neuronal injury (neuron-specific enolase and S-100 beta) previously attributed to artificial perfusion and CPB itself. The use of HBCs with elimination of cardiotomy section (exclusive use of cell saver) in patients undergoing CABG resulted in a modest (200 mL) increase in cell-saver volume and resulted in near-complete blunting of thrombin generation, platelet activation, granulocyte activation, and markers of neuronal injury (Figures 6-3 to 6-8).

Learning Curve

The improved outcomes described above represent a progressive experience and familiarity of cardiothoracic surgeons, perfusionists, and anesthesiologists, who have used these techniques in more than 3,000 patients. The anticoagulation protocol was gradually lowered to the current levels and thresholds after safety and efficacy were confirmed. Over the past 4 years (1994 to 1997), we noted progressive reduction in the incidence of homologous transfusion (52% versus 36%, versus 25% versus 15%), magnitude of transfusion (4.1 versus 1.9 units versus 0.5 versus 0.3 units), and hospital stays (6.5 versus 5.9 days versus 5.2 versus 4.5 days). A gradual adjustment of the anticoagulation protocol is recommended to reflect the team's experience and familiarity with these techniques.

Discussion

Enhanced biocompatibility with HBCs was introduced to decrease the 30 to 70% incidence of homologous transfusion noted despite the broad application of many blood conservation strategies and in an attempt to blunt the "inflammatory response" to artificial perfusion which is responsible for much of the morbidity associated with

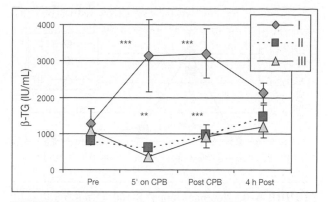

FIGURE 6-4. Platelet activation: β-TG. (** $p \leq .01$ I vs II; *** $p \leq .001$ I vs III.) β-TG = beta thromboglobulin.

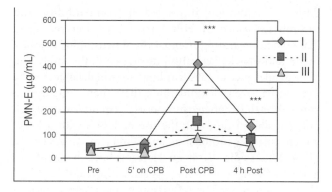

FIGURE 6-5. Inflammation: polymorphonuclear elastase (PMN-E). (* $p \leq .05$ I vs II; *** $p \leq .001$ I vs III.)

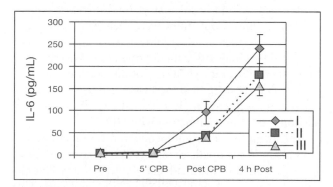

FIGURE 6-6. Inflammation: interleukin (IL)-6.

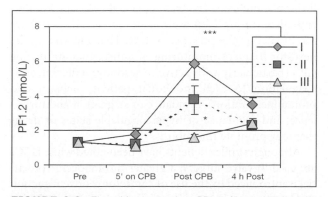

FIGURE 6-3. Thrombin generation: PF1.2. (* $p \leq .05$ II vs III; *** $p \leq .001$ I vs III.)

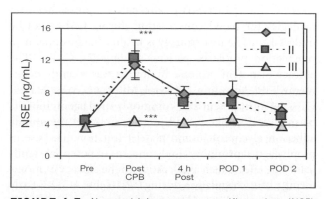

FIGURE 6-7. Neuronal injury: neuron-specific enolase (NSE). (*** $p \leq .001$ I and II vs III.) (POD = postoperative day.)

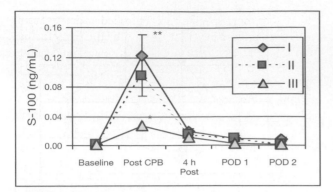

FIGURE 6-8. Neuronal injury: S-100. (* $p \le .05$ II vs III; ** $p \le .01$ I vs III.) (POD = postoperative day.)

CPB.[27–29] Although improved biocompatibility and thromboresistance of HBCs have been inferred from studies demonstrating attenuation of neutrophil, complement, and platelet activation during CPB, the safety and clinical relevance of these findings are still debated.[4–21] We have conclusively demonstrated that when compared to conventional (nonheparin-bonded) circuits with a full anticoagulation protocol, the use of HBCs with a lower anticoagulation protocol as an adjunct to an integrated blood conservation strategy decreases both the incidence and magnitude of homologous transfusion and improves clinical outcomes. The reduction in parameters, such as time to extubation, pulmonary complications, incidence of postoperative MI, and inotropic requirement, resulted in shorter ICU and hospital stays (and therefore cost).[21] Improved clinical outcomes were seen with HBCs and LAP in all patients undergoing CABG and were not restricted to a high-risk patient population. We especially noted these outcomes when cardiotomy suction was eliminated and an integrated perfusion strategy was used. These improvements are less dramatic when cardiotomy suction is used in conjunction with HBCs.[26]

The magnitude of homologous transfusion appears to be an important predictor of clinical outcomes such as time to extubation and incidence of postoperative complication, as well as length of hospital stay and cost. This underscores the importance of maximizing all blood conservation efforts. Two alternative approaches and strategies for blood conservation during CABG can be undertaken. The first strategy is to alter the postoperative coagulation profile of patients undergoing CABG. The efficacy of potent protease inhibitors was recently documented.[30,31] Aprotinin (Trasylol, Miles Inc., West Haven, CT), the most potent and commonly used agent, inhibits plasmin and kallikrein and preserves platelet membrane adhesion glycoprotein and platelet function. The use of prophylactic aprotinin raised concerns of potential significant side effects such as alteration in the efficacy of monitoring of anticoagulation during CPB (celite ACT).[32] Early experience noted a trend toward a higher incidence of perioperative Q-wave MI and graft occlusion on postmortem

examination, which was thought to be related to a potential hypercoagulable state.[33] These concerns have raised the issue of inadequate anticoagulation in earlier series, perhaps related to the direct effect of aprotinin on celite ACT, resulting in suboptimal anticoagulation. More recently, a low incidence of adverse events, such as graft thrombosis and renal failure, was reported and dispelled many earlier concerns despite the presence of a hypercoagulable state.[34–36] Sensitization and allergic reactions with repeated use have also been reported. Finally, aprotinin is expensive, imposing an additional cost of nearly $1,000 (US) per patient when used as recommended, with a full (Hammersmith) loading dose.[30,32] Although we use aprotinin selectively in aortic surgery or other complex cardiac surgery, we do not use it for routine CABG (primary or reoperative). We suggest an alternative strategy to enhance blood conservation during on-pump CABG surgery. Instead of altering the perioperative coagulation balance with hemostasis-promoting drugs, we use more thromboresistant circuits (heparin bonded) with lower systemic anticoagulation. It is unclear whether homologous transfusion directly causes deleterious clinical effects or is a sensitive but indirect marker of patient acuity. The main mechanism by which HBCs with LAP improve outcomes appears to be improved hemostasis (better preservation of platelet function and number) and a decrease in homologous transfusion along with a blunted inflammatory response to artificial perfusion. The hemostatic effect is underestimated by measurement of postoperative mediastinal tube output, which does not take into account differences in intraoperative blood losses or possible effects on intravascular volume. In addition to a reduction in homologous transfusion, the use of HBCs also results in a significant reduction in the incidence of postoperative complications, which is also noted in patients not receiving any homologous transfusions. This suggests that in addition to their hemostatic benefits, HBCs may exert a salutary beneficial effect by attenuating postcardiopulmonary bypass "inflammation" and its associated complications.

We also have conclusively demonstrated that HBCs with LAP, when used appropriately in CABG, do not increase the risk of clinical, microscopic, or hematologic thromboembolism. The technique and risks of thromboembolism during CPB are not unique to HBCs but are accentuated in the presence of LAP. This underscores the need for frequent monitoring of anticoagulation during CPB (particularly with active rewarming), tailoring anticoagulation to each individual patient (heparin and protamine titration), avoidance of stagnation and turbulence, and avoidance of hypercoagulable states or drugs that may promote thrombosis.

Although similar benefits have been noted when HBCs are used in valve surgery, a greater thrombogenic potential is introduced by the use of cardiotomy or vent suction and by extensive blood–air interface, which occurs during open cardiac procedures. Based on our earlier clinical experience, we have modified our anticoagulation protocol to reflect these concerns (to ACT > 350 s), with improved clinical outcomes.

Our work challenges several commonly accepted precepts in cardiac surgery, especially on-pump CABG. One such notion is that cardiotomy suction and open systems (which are used ubiquitously) are safe. Another is that CPB results in obligatory and unalterable hemostatic, inflammatory, and systemic insults. Our data and those of others suggest that the use of an HBC with a closed system (strict avoidance of cardiotomy suction when used with an integrated perfusion strategy described above) blunts and nearly eliminates all these perturbations. These perturbations were the main impetus to pursue off-pump CABG surgery. Further studies comparing a new gold standard of using biocompatible HBC with appropriate integrated techniques (either empty beating or cardioplegic arrested heart) to off-pump CABG are necessary prior to abandoning excellent established long-term results (durability) with on-pump "best practice" techniques for the yet-to-be-documented long-term outcomes of off-pump CABG.

We suggest that applying HBCs to cardiac surgery in general and to CABG in particular is both safe and effective and that it results in significant improvement in clinical outcomes. These improved outcomes with dramatic reductions in morbidity compare very favorably with the incidence of MI reported in previous studies comparing CABG and PTCA (less than 1% versus 6 to 8%) and CVA (less than 1% versus 6%) and has profound implications on the choice of optimal therapy.[36,37] The added cost of this technology has to be weighed against its potential benefits and ease of use. Currently, the cost of these circuits is less than the cost administration of a single homologous blood transfusion, and the circuits require only minor modification in surgical and perfusion techniques.

Future Advances

In addition to active research to develop even more effective biocompatible cardiopulmonary bypass surfaces, alternatives to heparin anticoagulation and protamine reversal are being explored. The search for alternatives to heparin are mainly prompted by better recognition of the syndrome of heparin-induced thrombocytopenia. These include use of porcine versus bovine heparin, low-molecular-weight heparinoids (such as Fragmin), urokinase, r-hirudin, ancrod, iloprost or prostacyclin alone or in addition to heparin, Orgaran, and specific active-site blockade of factor IXa, among many.[38–43] Alternatives to heparin reversal (protamine) include recombinant platelet factor and heparinase I (Neutralase), as well as heparin removal devices.[44,45] Results are, at best, preliminary, and unfortunately, many of these alternatives to heparin anticoagulation are more difficult to reverse. We

believe that more specific and controlled anticoagulation (and reversal) used in conjunction with HBCs may further improve clinical outcomes. Currently, many innovations and alternative approaches to standard multivessel surgical revascularization are being explored. Such approaches attempt to limit the morbidity related to standard surgical incisions (median sternotomy) or to cardiopulmonary bypass. These include percutaneous approaches with multivessel PTCA or stent placement (chemically eluting), minimal-access surgical approaches with beating-heart surgery (avoiding CPB), and minimal-access approaches that use femoral bypass, perhaps enhanced by robotic techniques. These new approaches have to be practical, economical, and have short- and long-term outcomes comparable to a new "gold standard" of CABG, with more complete arterial revascularization performed with biocompatible cardiopulmonary bypass surfaces.

References

1. Young JA, Kisher CT, Doty DB. Adequate anticoagulation during cardiopulmonary bypass determined by activated clotting time and appearance of fibrin monomer. Ann Thorac Surg 1978;26:231–40.
2. Gravlee GP, Haddon WS, Rothberger HK, et al. Heparin dosing and monitoring during cardiopulmonary bypass. J Thorac Cardiovasc Surg 1990;99:518–27.
3. Cardoso PFG, Yamazaki F, Keshavjee S, et al. A reevaluation of heparin requirement during cardiopulmonary bypass. J Thorac Cardiovasc Surg 1991;101:153–60.
4. von Segesser LK, Weiss BK, Pasic M, et al. Risks and benefits of low systemic heparinization during open heart operations. Ann Thorac Surg 1994;58:391–8.
5. Ovrum E, Holen EA, Tangen G, et al. Completely heparinized cardiopulmonary bypass and reduced systemic anticoagulation: clinical and hemostatic effects. Ann Thorac Surg 1995;60:365–71.
6. Khuri SF, Valeri R, Losclazo J, et al. Heparin causes platelet dysfunction and indices of fibrinolysis before cardiopulmonary bypass. Ann Thorac Surg 1995;60:1008–14.
7. Cavarocchi NC, Schaff HV, Orszulak TA, et al. Evidence for complement activation by protamine-heparin interaction after cardiopulmonary bypass. Surgery 1985;98:525–31.
8. Gott VL, Whiffen JD, Datton RC. Heparin bonding on colloidal graphite surfaces. Science 1963;142:1297–8.
9. Edmunds LH Jr. Breaking the blood-biomaterial barrier. ASAIO J 1995;41:824–30.
10. Fosse E, Oddvar M, Johnson E, et al. Reduced complement and granulocyte activation with heparin-coated cardiopulmonary bypass. Ann Thorac Surg 1994;58:472–7.
11. Wendel HP, Heller W, Hoffmeister HE. Pathway of platelet protection in heparin-coated devices and its significance for cardiac surgery. Trans Soc Biomater 1995;21:281.
12. Gu YJ, van Oeveren W, Akkerman C, et al. Heparin-coated circuits reduce the inflammatory response to cardiopulmonary bypass. Ann Thorac Surg 1993;55:917–22.
13. Pekna M, Hagman L, Halden E, et al. Complement activation during cardiopulmonary bypass: effects of immobilized heparin. Ann Thorac Surg 1994;58:421–4.

14. Ovrum E, Mollnes TE, Fosse E, et al. High and low heparin dose with heparin-coated cardiopulmonary bypass circuits: activation of complement and granulocytes. Ann Thorac Surg 1995;60:1755–61.

15. Jansen PGM, Velthuis H, Huybregts RAJM, et al. Reduced complement activation and improved post-operative performance after cardiopulmonary bypass with heparin-coated circuits. J Thorac Cardiovasc Surg 1995;110:829–34.

16. Gu YJ, van Oeveren W, van der Kamp KWHJ, et al. Heparin coating of extracorporeal circuits reduces thrombin formation in patients undergoing cardiopulmonary bypass. Perfusion 1991;6:221–5.

17. Ovrum E, Holen EA, Tangen G, et al. Completely heparinized cardiopulmonary bypass and reduced systemic heparin: clinical and hemostatic effects. Ann Thorac Surg 1995;60:365–71.

18. Gorman RC, Ziats NP, Gikakis N, et al. Surface-bound heparin fails to reduce thrombin formation during clinical cardiopulmonary bypass. J Thorac Cardiovasc Surg 1996;111:1–12.

19. Edmunds LH Jr. Surface-bound heparin—panacea or peril? Ann Thorac Surg 1994;58:285–6.

20. Aldea GS, Shapira OM, Treanor P, et al. Effective use of heparin-bonded circuits and lower anticoagulation for coronary artery grafting in Jehovah's Witnesses. J Cardiac Surg 1996;11:12–17.

21. Aldea GS, Doursounian M, O'Gara P, et al. Heparin-bonded circuits with a reduced anticoagulation protocol in primary CABG: a prospective, randomized study. Ann Thorac Surg 1996;62:410–8.

22. Aldea GS, Doursounian M, O'Gara P, et al. Heparin-bonded circuits with a reduced anticoagulation protocol improve clinical outcomes in patients undergoing primary CABG. A prospective randomized trial [abstract]. 22nd Annual Meeting of the Western Thoracic Surgical Association, Maui, Hawaii, 1996;7:30.

23. Aldea GS, O'Gara P, Shapira OM, et al. Effect of anticoagulation protocol on clinical outcomes in patients undergoing CABG with heparin-bonded circuits. Ann Thorac Surg 1998;65:425–33.

24. Aldea GS, Lilly K, Guadiani JM, et al. Heparin-bonded circuits improve clinical outcomes in emergency CABG. J Card Surg 1997;12:389–97.

25. Shapira OM, Aldea GS, Zelingher J, et al. Enhanced blood conservation and improved clinical outcome after valve surgery using heparin-bonded cardiopulmonary bypass circuits. J Card Surg 1996;11:307–17.

26. Aldea GS, Soltow LO, Chandler WL, et al. Elimination of cardiotomy suction limits: thrombin generation, platelet activation and inflammation in patients undergoing CABG treated with heparin-bonded circuits . J Thorac Cardiovasc Surg 2002;123(4):742–55

27. LoCicero J III, Massad M, Gandy K, et al. Aggressive blood conservation in coronary artery surgery: impact on patient care. J Cardiovasc Surg 1990;31:559–63.

28. Jones JW, Rawitscher RE, Mclean TR, et al. Benefits from combining blood conservation measures in cardiac operations. Ann Thorac Surg 1991;51:541–6.

29. Scott WJ, Rode R, Castelmain B, et al. Efficacy, complication, and cost of a comprehensive blood conservation program for cardiac operations. J Thorac Cardiovasc Surg 1992;103:1001–7.

30. Fremes SE, Wong BI, Lee E, et al. Meta-analysis of prophylactic drug treatment in the prevention of postoperative bleeding. Ann Thorac Surg 1994;58:1580–8.

31. Rosengart TK, Helm RE, Klempere J, et al. Combined aprotinin and erythropoietin use for blood conservation: result with Jehovah's Witnesses. Ann Thorac Surg 1994;58:1397–1403.

32. Tabuchi N, Njo TL, Tigchelaar I, et al. Monitoring of anticoagulation in aprotinin-treated patients during heart operations. Ann Thorac Surg 1994;58:774–7.

33. Cosgrove DM III, Heric B, Lytle BW, et al. Aprotinin therapy for re-operative myocardial revascularization: a placebo-controlled study. Ann Thorac Surg 1992;54:1031–8.

34. Feindt PR, Walcher S, Volkmer I, et al. Effect of high dose aprotinin in aortocoronary bypass grafting. Ann Thorac Surg 1995;60:1076–80.

35. Feindt P, Sefert U, Volkmer I, et al. Is there a phase of "hypercoagulability" when aprotinin is used in cardiac surgery? Eur J Cardiothorac Surg 1994:8(6):308–13.

36. Okita Y, Takamoto S, Ando M, et al. Is the use of aprotinin safe with deep hypothermic circulatory arrest in aortic surgery? Investigation on blood coagulation. Circulation 1996;94 Suppl 9:II-177–81.

37. Pocock SJ, Henderson RA, Rickards AF, et al. Meta-analysis of randomized trials comparing angioplasty with bypass surgery. Lancet 1995;346:1184–9.

38. Roach GW, Kanchuger M, Mangano CM, et al. Adverse cerebral outcomes after coronary artery surgery. N Engl J Med 1996;335:1857–63.

39. Henny CP, Ten Cate H, Ten Cate JW, et al. A randomized blind study comparing standard heparin and a new low molecular weight heparinoid in cardiopulmonary bypass in dogs. J Lab Clin Med 1985;106:187–96.

40. Potzsch B, Madlener K, Seelig C, et al. Monitoring r-hirudin anticoagulation during cardiopulmonary bypass—assessment of whole blood ecarin clotting time. Thromb Haemost 1997;77:920–5.

41. Zulys VJ, Teasdale SJ, Michel ER, et al. Ancrod (Arvin) as an alternative to heparin anticoagulation for cardiopulmonary bypass. Anesthesiology 1989;71:870–87.

42. Addonizio VP, Fisher CA, Bowen JC, et al. Prostacyclin in lieu of anticoagulation with heparin for extracorporeal circulation. Trans ASAIO 1981;27:304–7.

43. Wilhelm MJ, Schmid C, Kececioglu D, et al. Cardiopulmonary bypass in patients with heparin-induced thrombocytopenia using Org 10172. Ann Thorac Surg 1996;61:920–4.

44. Dehmer GJ, Lange RA, Tate DA, et al. Randomized trial of recombinant platelet factor 4 versus protamine for reversal of anticoagulation in humans. Circulation 1996;94 Suppl 9:II-347–52.

45. Michelsen LG, Kikura M, Levy JH, et al. Heparinase I (Neutralase) reversal of systemic anticoagulation. Anesthesiology 1996;85:339–46.

CHAPTER 7

ANTI-INFLAMMATORY STRATEGIES IN CARDIAC SURGERY

ALBERT J. CHONG, MD, CRAIG R. HAMPTON, MD,
TIMOTHY H. POHLMAN, MD, EDWARD D. VERRIER, MD

"Inflammation in itself is not to be considered as a disease ... and in disease, where it can alter the diseased mode of action, it likewise leads to a cure; but where it cannot accomplish that salutary purpose, ... it does mischief."

John Hunter, *Treatise on the Blood, Inflammation, and Gunshot Wounds*, London, 1794

Cardiovascular disease is the leading cause of death in the United States today.[1] Open heart surgery remains one of the mainstay treatments for both acquired and congenital heart disease. The evolution of the field of cardiac surgery was made possible by the development of the heart–lung machine. John Gibbon Jr, after beginning his work on a pump oxygenator in the 1930s, successfully repaired an atrial septal defect using a cardiopulmonary bypass (CPB) device in 1953.[2] With this landmark event, the era of open heart surgery was born. Most cardiac surgical procedures today use the heart–lung machine, providing a bloodless field and a still heart, so that repair can take place in a controlled and precise environment.

The trauma of cardiac surgical procedures and the nonphysiologic environment created by the cardiopulmonary machine elicit an undesired, extravagant systemic inflammatory state in the patient (Figure 7-1). The clinical spectrum of this inflammatory response ranges from patients exhibiting a few minor clinical sequelae to those with a severe form consisting of bleeding, thromboembolism, and multiple organ dysfunction, and, ultimately, failure. The clinical result of this detrimental response is termed the *postpump syndrome*, or the *systemic inflammatory response syndrome (SIRS)*, similar to that seen in septic shock or trauma. The widespread damaging effects associated with SIRS may include every major organ system, including the lung, brain, kidney, gut, and heart.[3–5]

Up to 10% of patients undergoing cardiac surgical procedures with CPB become affected with a clinically apparent form of SIRS.[6] That most patients successfully recover without complications from this disseminated inflamma-

tory state attests to the variability of individual response, as well as to the tremendous physiologic reserve and ability to prevent widespread organ damage. Although the degree of systemic inflammatory response and the subsequent clinical sequelae have significant interindividual variability, the patients who are at increased risk include those patients with advanced age, severely impaired left ventricular function, or multiple comorbidities.[7] Because of the increasing high-risk demographics of patients requiring cardiac surgical procedures, research efforts have focused on the mechanism of SIRS and possible therapeutic strategies to reduce the systemic inflammation and the resultant clinical consequences.

SIRS is complex and involves the activation of multiple interdependent and redundant inflammatory systems at both the humoral and cellular levels (see Figure 7-1). The activators of these inflammatory cascades during cardiac operations include the trauma of the surgical procedure and the components of CPB, such as the membrane oxygenators and roller pumps; bioincompatible artificial surfaces; and the oxidative stress of ischemia and reperfusion. In addition to the initiation of the coagulation cascade, humoral inflammatory systems that become activated include kallikrein, fibrinolysis, and complement (see Figure 7-1).[3,8] Furthermore, virtually every cell type becomes activated directly by the surgical procedure and CPB, as well as through the products of the humoral inflammatory cascades. These activated cells subsequently release pro-inflammatory cytokines such as interleukin (IL)-1β, IL-6, IL-8, and tumor necrosis factor (TNF)-α, which further potentiate the systemic inflammatory reaction by further activating inflammatory cascades and cells. This process leads to a highly redundant and interdependent systemic inflammatory reaction, which, when unfettered, will ultimately result in multiple organ failure.

This chapter initially discusses the mechanism of activation of humoral inflammatory systems and the resultant systemic inflammatory response. The latter portion of this chapter focuses on the therapeutic strategies to

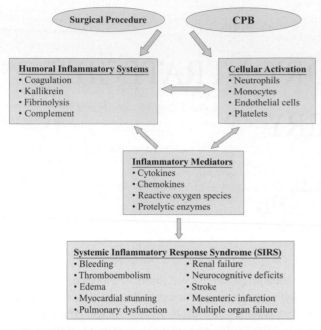

FIGURE 7-1. Mechanism of systemic inflammatory response. Activation of humoral inflammatory cascades and multiple cell types leads to elaboration of inflammatory mediators, resulting in systemic inflammatory response syndrome (SIRS). This schematic highlights the interdependence and redundancy of these systems, providing opportunity for amplification at multiple steps.

minimize the systemic inflammatory response, thereby possibly reducing the morbidity and mortality of cardiac operations.

Inflammatory Systems

Coagulation and Kallikrein Systems

The coagulation and kallikrein systems contribute to the SIRS by the production of numerous inflammatory mediators, which activate other humoral inflammatory cascades and multiple inflammatory cell types. The intrinsic coagulation and kallikrein systems are intimately associated with the plasma protein factor XII (Hageman factor), which undergoes autoactivation upon contact with negatively charged surfaces (eg, CPB circuit and exposed subendothelial extracellular matrix), producing factor XIIa and factor XIIf (Figure 7-2). Factor XIIa then initiates two inflammatory systems: intrinsic coagulation and kallikrein cascades. Factor XIIa activates factor XI, thereby initiating the intrinsic coagulation pathway. The extrinsic coagulation cascade is activated by tissue factor, an integral membrane protein produced by endothelial cells and monocytes. The ultimate products of both the intrinsic and extrinsic coagulation pathways are thrombin and fibrin clot. Thrombin can also induce the production of tissue factor by the endothelium and monocytes, thereby creating a positive feedback loop on the activation of the extrinsic coagulation pathway.[9,10]

The products of the coagulation cascade, in addition to providing hemostasis, are intimately involved in the pro-inflammatory response. Thrombin contributes to the formation of diffuse microemboli, resulting in a microcirculatory "no reflow" phenomenon, which may potentiate the ischemia/reperfusion injury.[11,12] Moreover, thrombin, through the protease-activated receptor (PAR), activates platelets and endothelial cells and promotes chemotaxis of monocytes and neutrophils (see Figure 7-2).[9,13] Fibrinogen and fibrin also contribute to the inflammatory response by stimulating the production of cytokines and chemokines in monocytes, neutrophils, fibroblasts, and endothelial cells.[14]

Factor XIIa in the presence of high-molecular-weight kininogen (HMWK) converts prekallikrein to kallikrein, a protease with serine at its active site (see Figure 7-2). Kallikrein and factor XIIa in a positive feedback loop further activate factor XII. Kallikrein activates multiple inflammatory pathways. First, kallikrein principally stimulates neutrophils to release superoxide and hydrogen peroxide as well as proteolytic enzymes such as elastase and cathepsin.[15,16] Second, kallikrein promotes the release of bradykinin from surface-bound HMWK.[17] Bradykinin is a potent inducer of smooth-muscle contraction and increased capillary permeability.[18] This promotes further injury by causing edema and facilitating the movement of polymorphonuclear cells (PMNs) into tissues, resulting in elaboration of destructive proteolytic enzymes.[17,19] Third, kallikrein and bradykinin directly activate the fibrinolytic system (see Figure 7-2) by activating prourokinase, while bradykinin stimulates the release of tissue plasminogen activator (t-PA) from endothelial cells. Fourth, kallikrein also augments the activation of the complement system by cleaving C5 to produce C5a, a potent anaphylatoxin with numerous inflammatory properties (see "Complement System" for further details).

Activation of the factor XII/kallikrein system during cardiac operations has been confirmed in numerous experimental and clinical studies. Multiple studies demonstrate a rise in kallikrein–C1-inhibitor complex, a measure of kallikrein activation, and a decrease in prekallikrein levels with onset of CPB.[18,20,21] More importantly, activation of the kallikrein–kinin system is related to the development of postoperative organ dysfunction.[20] Seghaye and colleagues found that multisystem organ failure may be related to increased kallikrein activation.[22] Patients with low prekallikrein levels that failed to return to baseline after cardiac surgery exhibited a tendency toward developing multisystem organ failure.

The activation of the kallikrein system during cardiac operations with CPB significantly contributes to the systemic inflammatory response by further activating multiple inflammatory cell types and other humoral inflammatory systems. This process highlights the redundancy and the interdependence of the systemic inflammatory response. Furthermore, as described above, patients

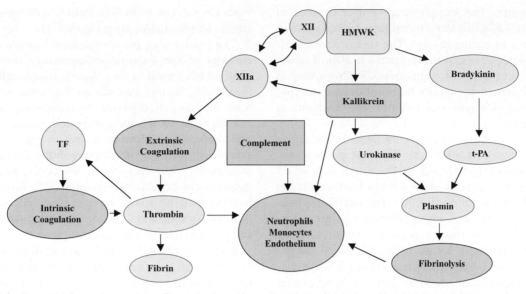

FIGURE 7-2. Humoral inflammatory systems. The activation of humoral cascades (intrinsic and extrinsic coagulation, complement, kallikrein, and fibrinolysis) is interdependent. Multiple interactions between the cascades and the redundancy of the systems allow for amplification at numerous steps. HMWK = high-molecular-weight kininogen; TF = tissue factor; t-PA = tissue plasminogen activator.

with increased activation of the kallikrein system tended toward development of increased morbidity. Therefore, strategies to minimize the activation of the kallikrein system may have profound influences in blunting the systemic inflammatory response and reducing postoperative morbidity and mortality after cardiac surgical procedures.

Fibrinolytic System

The fibrinolytic system can be activated by multiple pathways and potentiates the SIRS by generation of numerous inflammatory mediators. First, factor XII, upon activation via contact with negatively charged surfaces, initiates the extrinsic coagulation cascade, producing thrombin and releasing kallikrein and bradykinin from HMWK (see Figure 7-2). Thrombin is a potent stimulus for the release of t-PA from endothelial cells.[23] t-PA cleaves plasminogen to plasmin that digests fibrin, thereby degrading fibrin clot. Thrombin also induces the release of tissue factor from endothelial cells and monocytes, thereby leading to further production of thrombin and amplifying the fibrinolytic response.[9,24] Second, kallikrein potentiates fibrinolysis indirectly by activating prourokinase and directly by cleaving plasminogen to plasmin. Plasmin also directly activates factor XII, forming another positive feedback cycle.

In addition to disrupting hemostasis, fibrinolysis produces fibrin split products, which promote inflammation. Fibrin stimulates TNF-α and IL-1β expression by monocytes and chemokine secretion by endothelial cells, fibroblasts, and neutrophils.[14,24,25] Furthermore, fibrin stimulates the production of chemokines from monocytes.[25] Fibrin-degradation products (FDPs) have also been implicated in platelet dysfunction, endothelial injury, and impaired fibrin production.[24]

Multiple experimental and clinical studies demonstrate activation of the fibrinolytic system during cardiac surgical procedures.[26–30] Although the activation of fibrinolysis is inevitable in cardiac operations (and all surgical procedures in general), excessive activation of this system is associated with poorer clinical outcome. Cvachovec and colleagues showed that among patients undergoing cardiac operations, those with evidence of excessive fibrinolysis by thromboelastography required more fluid resuscitation and inotropic support postoperatively.[31] Moreover, the only deaths from this study were of patients exhibiting excessive fibrinolysis; all these patients succumbed to multiorgan failure and sepsis. These findings suggest that those patients with excessive fibrinolysis had poorer clinical outcomes.

The interdependence of the kallikrein and fibrinolytic systems underscores the potentially dangerous mechanism of uncontrolled activation and amplification of the systemic inflammatory response. Because of this redundancy in the inflammatory systems, potential therapies need to target the inhibition of multiple inflammatory cascades.

Complement System

Complement activation has been the subject of intense investigation to find potential therapeutic targets to minimize the morbidity and mortality seen after cardiac operations from the systemic inflammatory response. There are several causes for activation of complement: contact of blood elements with the foreign surfaces of the CPB circuit; surgical procedure; ischemia/reperfusion injury; endotoxin; products of the fibrinolytic and kallikrein–kinin cascades; and drugs administered, such as heparin and protamine. The complement system consists of approximately 30 plasma and membrane-bound proteins activated in a cascading fashion. The significance of this system is demonstrated by the fact that 5 to 10% of serum proteins are complement components.[32] This system is an integral part of the body's humoral defense mechanism, as well as a powerful initiator and mediator of inflammation.

Complement activation can be initiated through three different pathways (Figure 7-3). The first pathway, the classical pathway, is activated by the interaction of C1 with clustered Fc regions of antibodies bound to target antigens of invading foreign cells.[33] The alternative (second) pathway is an antibody-independent pathway activated by numerous triggers such as foreign surfaces, damaged tissue, shear forces, hypoxia-induced oxygen free radicals, and t-PA.[33] These triggers amplify the continuous low-level basal activation of C3. During cardiac surgical procedures, this pathway represents the major route of activation of the complement system. The third pathway is initiated by the binding of mannose-binding lectin, also known as mannan/mannose-binding protein, to carbohydrate moieties on the surfaces of bacteria, yeast, parasites, and viruses.[34] The complement system can also be directly activated by components of other inflammatory pathways such as kallikrein, plasmin, thrombin, and factor XIIf. All these pathways ultimately converge to form C3 convertase, an enzyme that cleaves C3 to its activated forms, C3a and C3b. C3b subsequently cleaves C5 to generate C5a, a potent anaphylatoxin, and C5b, which

binds C6, C7, C8, and C9 to form C5b-9, the membrane attack complex (MAC) (see Figure 7-3).

The products of the complement cascade are potent effectors of the systemic inflammatory response. The MAC attaches itself to the cell surface and forms a transmembrane channel that allows the influx of ions and water into the cell, disabling the maintenance of osmotic and chemical equilibrium, ultimately leading to cell lysis and death.[35] Furthermore, C5b-9 increases endothelial expression of leukocyte adhesion molecules, upregulates interleukin and chemokine secretion, and inhibits endothelium-dependent relaxation.[36–39] C4b and C3b bind to their respective receptors on cell surfaces and facilitate opsonization of complement-coated particles and the clearance of immune complexes.[40]

C3a, C4a, and C5a cause degranulation of basophils and mast cells, releasing numerous inflammatory mediators such as histamine, leukotrienes, and thromboxane.[41] These complement products also directly contract smooth muscle and endothelium, causing an increase in vascular permeability. C5a as well as its cleaved product C5a desArg are the most potent anaphylatoxins produced by the complement cascade.[42] They elicit numerous biologic activities that potentiate the systemic inflammatory response. Nanomolar concentrations of C5a and C5a desArg cause chemotaxis and activation of neutrophils, resulting in the production of oxygen free radicals and release of histotoxic enzymes such as myeloperoxidase, elastase, and cathepsin.[42–45] C5a and C5a desArg also activate monocytes and endothelial cells, resulting in the

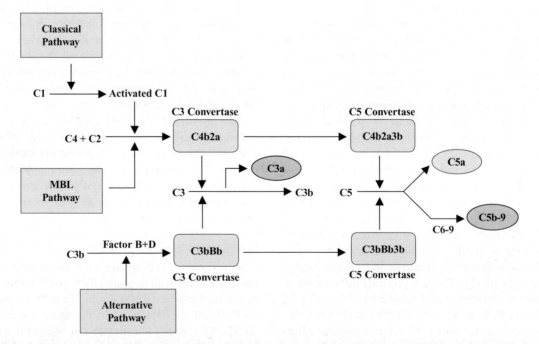

FIGURE 7-3. Complement cascade. The complement cascade can be activated by three different pathways (classical, alternative, and mannose-binding lectin). The three major products of this system are C3a, C5a, and C5b-9 (membrane attack complex), which are potent inflammatory mediators. The sequential cascading fashion of activation allows for multiple amplification steps and possible therapeutic targets for inhibition. MBL = mannose binding lectin.

expression of leukocyte adhesion molecules and the production of interleukins, chemokines, TNF-α, and tissue factor.

Numerous studies demonstrate the activation of the complement system and correlate the degree of activation with postoperative morbidity. Chenoweth and colleagues, in a landmark study, studied the levels of complement products in patients undergoing coronary artery bypass graft (CABG) with CPB in the early 1980s.[46] The investigators discovered that C3a levels became elevated within 10 min of the onset of bypass and continued to increase, peaking at approximately five times the preoperative levels by the end of the operation. Subsequent studies found a similar rise in activated complement product levels, including C3a, C4a, and C5b-9.[47,48] More importantly, C3a levels were prognostic for the probability of postoperative pulmonary, renal, and cardiac dysfunction.[47] Studies also demonstrate that the administration of protamine to reverse the anticoagulant effects of heparin caused a 2- to 11-fold increase in C4a levels through the activation of C1, thereby initiating the classical pathway.[49,50]

The complement system represents a significant defense against foreign pathogens; however, uncontrolled activation following cardiac operations with CPB is associated with increased postoperative end-organ dysfunction involving every organ system. Although numerous endogenous inhibitors exist to control the activation of the complement cascade, studies demonstrate significant elevations of activated complement products during and after cardiac operations. Furthermore, complement products induce the activation of multiple inflammatory systems and cell types, creating a potentially dangerous positive feedback loop. Therefore, therapies aimed at inhibiting the activation of the complement system or its potent inflammatory end products may reduce the morbidity and mortality of cardiac operations.

Anti-inflammatory Strategies

Pharmacologic Strategies

SERINE PROTEASE INHIBITORS

Numerous clinical and experimental studies establish that serine protease inhibitors effectively inhibit the systemic inflammatory response. However, although a decrease in blood loss occurs with the use of serine protease inhibitors, studies fail to show improvements in other clinical end points or an association between the use of serine protease inhibitors and improved clinical course.

Serine proteases, molecules with the amino acid serine at their active site, are enzymes that are central to the processes of coagulation and inflammation. Examples of serine proteases include thrombin, coagulation factors, complement products, kallikrein, trypsin, elastase, and cathepsin. Inhibitors of serine proteases regulate and prevent uncontrolled activation of these potent enzymes. Of the serine protease inhibitors, the broad-spectrum agent isolated from bovine lung tissue, aprotinin, and the synthetic compounds, nafamostat (FUT-175) and gabexalate (FOY), are the most widely studied in both experimental and clinical settings. By inhibiting key enzymes in coagulation and inflammation, serine protease inhibitors were initially employed to minimize the inflammatory response of acute pancreatitis, then later to treat septic shock syndromes.[51,52] However, shortly thereafter, the ability of these agents to decrease blood loss and transfusion requirements after cardiac operations was recognized. Royston and his colleagues first reported the use of high-dose aprotinin in a randomized study of high-risk patients undergoing repeat open heart surgery.[53] They demonstrated a reduction in blood loss and transfusion requirements in those who received aprotinin. Multiple subsequent randomized placebo-controlled studies confirm this finding; high-dose aprotinin therapy reduces mediastinal drainage (by 31% to 81%), transfusion requirements (by 35% to 97%), and the number of patients requiring transfusions of blood products (by 40% to 88%).[54–57]

While the benefits of serine protease inhibitors in reducing blood loss and transfusion requirements are well established, it is becoming increasingly clear that serine protease inhibitors also blunt the systemic inflammatory response in patients undergoing cardiac surgical procedures. The vast majority of the mediators in these inflammatory cascades are serine proteases; hence, the goal would be to administer an appropriate dose of antiprotease and inhibit these inflammatory cascades, minimizing the morbidity and mortality seen after cardiac surgical procedures. However, although experimental and clinical studies of serine protease inhibitors show biochemical evidence for inhibition of SIRS, most studies fail to demonstrate any clinical benefit, except for blood loss.

Numerous studies demonstrate that serine protease inhibitors prevent the activation of humoral inflammatory cascades including kallikrein, fibrinolytic, and complement systems.[18,21,58–63] Serine protease inhibitors also exert further anti-inflammatory effects through inhibition of cellular activation, which occurs during cardiac surgical procedures. Studies suggest that serine protease inhibitors exhibit significant anti-inflammatory properties through their actions on neutrophils: first, neutrophil activation is limited in the bypass circuit; second, neutrophil extravasation is reduced; and third, neutrophil release of toxic enzymes and free radicals is inhibited.[60,64–69] Furthermore, serine protease inhibitors decreased the expression of adhesion molecules and cytokines by endothelial cells.[70]

Cardiac surgical procedures with CPB result in both quantitative and qualitative platelet disorder, including decrease in platelet number, derangement of platelet function, and activation of platelets. Some of the hemostatic effects of aprotinin are attributed to prevention of the aforementioned effects of cardiac surgical procedures and CPB on platelets.[65,71–74] Aprotinin inhibits platelet activation by evaluating activation markers, platelet microparticle formation, and shape change.[73–75] Furthermore, these serine protease inhibitors block thrombin-induced platelet activation.[76–78]

Numerous clinical studies have evaluated aprotinin's anti-inflammatory effects by examining cytokine levels in patients undergoing cardiac operations. Aprotinin decreases levels of TNF-α, IL-1β, IL-8, and IL-6 in plasma of patients undergoing CPB, as well as in human serum circulated through a simulated extracorporeal circuit.[30,68,79]

Despite the abundance of experimental and clinical studies demonstrating aprotinin's ability to decrease cytokine release, reduce cellular activation, and inhibit activation of inflammatory cascades such as complement, fibrinolysis, and kallikrein, no studies to date have conclusively shown improvements in clinical end points, except for blood loss, in patients undergoing cardiac operations. The plasma protease pathways that contribute to the systemic inflammatory response are interrelated and at times redundant; hence, pharmacologic attenuation of SIRS with protease inhibitors will be a challenge. Therefore, studies involving the combination of serine protease inhibitors with other modalities of anti-inflammatory therapies are needed to evaluate the role of antiprotease treatment in improving clinical outcome.

COMPLEMENT INHIBITORS

Activation of the complement system during cardiac operations elicits a potent inflammatory response through cellular activation and elaboration of chemokines and cytokines, with subsequent tissue damage and organ dysfunction. The complement system is involved in numerous disease states, including vasculitis, glomerulonephritis, hemolytic anemia, allergic neuritis, and burn injury.[80–84] Hence, inhibition of complement at various points in the cascade is a potential therapeutic target to minimize the systemic inflammatory response of cardiac surgical procedures, thereby reducing postoperative morbidity and mortality. To inhibit the activation of the complement cascade, numerous complement inhibitors have been developed (Table 7-1). Although multiple studies demonstrate effective blockade of complement activation by complement inhibitors, unfortunately, results from studies evaluating clinical outcomes are disappointing. The following section describes the results of studies evaluating the complement inhibitors listed in Table 7-1.

Rinder and associates employed a simulated extracorporeal circulation model to examine the effects of complement activation blocker-2 (CAB-2) on monocytes, neutrophils, and platelets.[85] CAB-2 is the product of a chimeric gene constructed from the genes encoding membrane cofactor protein (MCP) and decay accelerating factor (DAF), combining the inhibitory properties of these regulatory proteins through inhibition of both C3 and C5 convertases. The addition of CAB-2 to the simulated circuit blocked the generation of C3a, C5a, and C5b-9.

Furthermore, CAB-2 inhibited the activation of monocytes, neutrophils, and platelets. Therefore, inhibition of both classical and alternative pathways of complement activation by CAB-2 blunts the cellular activation that occurs during CPB.

Among the naturally occurring complement regulatory proteins, complement receptor-1 (CR1) is best characterized as a potential therapeutic tool to minimize the deleterious effects of complement activation in cardiac operations. CR1 binds both C3b and C4b, thereby inhibiting C3 and C5 convertases, and serves as a cofactor for factor I–mediated degradation of C3b and C4b.[86,87] Weisman and colleagues developed a soluble complement receptor-1 (sCR1) lacking the transmembrane and cytoplasmic domains, thereby overcoming its limitation as an effective regulator of complement activation.[88] In vitro, sCR1 blocked activation of complement by both alternative and classical pathways. Furthermore, Weisman and colleagues demonstrated a decrease in myocardial infarct size and a reduction in C5b-9 deposition in a rat model of ischemia/reperfusion injury.[88] In a neonatal pig CPB model, Chai and colleagues showed that sCR1 attenuated the deleterious effects of CPB on pulmonary and cardiac function.[89] Lazar and associates confirmed this finding by demonstrating decreased pulmonary and cardiac dysfunction in pigs undergoing coronary revascularization with sCR1 treatment.[90]

Although a generalized complement inhibition strategy would theoretically produce a more potent and widespread anti-inflammatory effect, inhibition of both classical and alternative pathways increase the susceptibility to infections.[91] Moreover, patients with early classical complement pathway product deficiencies exhibited lupus symptomology.[92] Therefore, research efforts have recently focused on more selective inhibition of the complement system.

Factor D is the rate-limiting enzyme involved in the activation of the alternative complement pathway.[93,94] Investigators have studied the effects of a monoclonal antibody to factor D in experimental settings. Addition of a monoclonal antibody specific for factor D protected

TABLE 7-1. Complement Inhibitors and the Mechanism of Action

Complement Inhibitor	Mechanism of Action
Complement activation blocker-2 (CAB-2)	Inhibits C3 and C5 convertase
Soluble complement receptor-1 (sCR-1)	Binds C3b and C4b, inhibiting C3 and C5 convertase
Factor D antibody	Binds factor D, inhibiting activation of alternative pathway
Properdin antibody	Inhibits properdin, inhibiting stabilization of C3 convertase
C5 antibody	Binds C5, inhibiting C5 activation to form C5a and C5b
Compstatin	Binds C3, inhibiting C3 activation to form C3a

isolated rabbit hearts from complement-mediated injury by preserving myocardial function.[95] Fung and colleagues, in a simulated CPB circuit model, found that monoclonal antibody to factor D effectively blocked the alternative complement pathway by inhibiting the production of Bb, C3a, C5b-9, and C5a.[96] Moreover, activation of platelets and neutrophils as well as production of IL-8 were suppressed by antifactor D monoclonal antibody.

A specific inhibitor of C3 convertase has also been studied as a therapeutic strategy to prevent the activation of the alternative complement pathway. C3 convertase, which is composed of C3bBb, is stabilized by properdin (factor P).[97] Monoclonal antibody to properdin, in a simulated extracorporeal circuit, completely inhibited the generation of C3a and C5b-9 and reduced activation of neutrophils and platelets.[98] Alternative complement pathway-specific inhibitor may have limited effectiveness because C3b generated from the classical pathway can activate the alternative pathway. However, the relative contribution of this phenomenon to the activation of the alternative complement pathway has not been studied. Interestingly, antiproperdin monoclonal antibody blocked the formation of C5b-9 after activation of the classical complement pathway by heparin–protamine complex.[98] Hence, the production of active complement species through the activation of the alternative complement pathway via the classical pathway plays a significant role. Antiproperdin monoclonal antibody shows promise as a potential therapeutic agent to decrease the systemic inflammatory response of cardiac surgery.

Recently, a C3-binding synthetic peptide (Compstatin) was developed.[99] This anticomplement agent, unlike others described here, is a small peptide consisting of 13 amino acid residues, making it simple and inexpensive to manufacture. Addition of Compstatin to the blood circulated in a simulated extracorporeal circuit resulted in effective inhibition of C3a and C5b-9 generation and suppression of leukocyte activation.[100]

Production of C3b is essential for clearance of circulating immune complexes and proper phagocytosis of bacteria and fungi.[101] Deficiency of C3 predisposes patients to recurrent life-threatening infections and increased risk of autoimmune diseases such as systemic lupus erythematosus and glomerulonephritis.[101] Inhibition of the complement system at the level of C5, however, would prevent the formation of C5a and C5b-9, while preserving the production of C3b. Patients with deficiency of C5 are more susceptible to *Neisseria* infections; however, the course of the infection is more benign when compared to patients without a C5 deficiency.[101] Humanized monoclonal antibodies against C5 have been developed to bind C5 and prevent its cleavage into C5a and C5b-9.[102,103] The addition of monoclonal antibody to C5 in a simulated extracorporeal circuit resulted in profound inhibition of C5a and C5b-9 production and suppressed the activation of neutrophils and platelets.[104] Fitch and colleagues performed a prospective randomized trial in patients undergoing CABG with CPB to evaluate the effects of anti-C5 monoclonal antibody.[105] Patients receiving anti-C5 monoclonal antibody treatment exhibited decrease in leukocyte activation, 40% attenuation of myocardial injury, 80% decrease in new cognitive deficits, and a 1 unit reduction in postoperative blood loss. These data suggest that C5 inhibition with anti-C5 monoclonal antibody may be a promising therapeutic target for reduction of the morbidity and mortality seen after cardiac surgery through prevention of complement-mediated inflammation and tissue damage, while preserving C3b-mediated immune competence. Currently, plans for a phase III trial are underway to further evaluate the effects of anti-C5 therapy.

Multiple complement inhibitors have been developed and studied in both experimental and clinical settings. Although studies have demonstrated effective reduction of complement activation, unfortunately, studies have not conclusively shown clinical benefit. The redundancy of the multiple inflammatory cascades would make it unlikely that inhibition of the complement system alone would produce clinical improvements. Therefore, clinical improvements will likely require combining complement inhibitors with other modalities of anti-inflammatory therapies.

CORTICOSTEROIDS

Corticosteroids have been used to treat patients with a variety of inflammatory disorders, even before the mechanism of this drug was discovered. Numerous investigators have demonstrated the effectiveness of steroids in decreasing the systemic inflammation in patients undergoing cardiac surgical procedures. However, most studies have failed to show the translation of these beneficial effects on the biochemical profile into improvements in clinical outcome.

The beneficial effects of corticosteroids were first demonstrated in animals and patients with shock and sepsis.[106] Because of the similar physiologic sequelae seen in the setting of sepsis and CPB, initial studies focused on the hemodynamic effects of corticosteroids to decrease vasoconstriction during CPB and to prevent postoperative low cardiac output syndrome.[107,108] The pathophysiologic rationale for the use of steroids during CPB, however, has evolved drastically since this time. Although the mechanism of corticosteroids remains incompletely defined, it is currently believed that possible benefits of corticosteroids during cardiac surgical procedures are derived from its inhibitory effects on the inflammatory cascades and cellular activation. Corticosteroids freely penetrate the plasma membrane of inflammatory cells and bind to the glucocorticoid receptor.[109] This complex interacts with the promoter regions of multiple pro- and anti-inflammatory genes, thereby ultimately preventing the initiation and amplification of systemic inflammation. Through this molecular mechanism, corticosteroids have been shown in vitro to prevent the elaboration of multiple pro-inflammatory chemokines and cytokines such as IL-1, IL-2, IL-3, IL-6, interferon-γ, granulocyte-macrophage colony-stimulating factor (GM-CSF), and TNF-α.[109–112] Furthermore, corticosteroids enhance the generation of macrophage inhibitory factor.[113] Consequently, steroids, directly and indirectly through these inflammatory mediators, prevent the activation of neutrophils and monocytes.[114] Corticosteroids, in addition, stimulate the synthesis of lipocortin-1, inhibiting phospholipase A_2, subsequently preventing the production of potent inflammatory agents such as prostaglandins, leukotrienes, and thromboxanes.[115]

These anti-inflammatory effects of corticosteroids have also been demonstrated in patients undergoing cardiac surgical procedures with CPB. Numerous studies show that methylprednisolone treatment significantly reduced the plasma levels of IL-1, IL-6, IL-8, and TNF-α in patients undergoing cardiac operations.[116–123] Moreover, corticosteroids augmented the production of anti-inflammatory mediators such as IL-4 and IL-10 associated with cardiac surgical procedures.[124–126] Neutrophil activation was also significantly blunted with corticosteroids.[127–129] Furthermore, although a few studies reveal an inhibition of complement production with methylprednisolone treatment, most studies fail to demonstrate a significant effect on complement activation with administration of corticosteroids.[116,118,130–134]

Unfortunately, while most studies show a beneficial effect of steroids on the balance of pro- and anti-inflammatory mediators, demonstration of improvements in clinical end points have been disappointing and less consistent. While some small prospective studies have found improved postoperative hemodynamics with steroid treatment, others demonstrated not only no significant impact on postoperative course with steroid treatment, but also increased morbidity, such as significantly elevated blood glucose levels.[119,122,135] Tassani and colleagues found benefits of methylprednisolone on cytokine levels in a prospective, randomized, double-blinded study of 52 patients undergoing elective CABG.[136] The patients receiving steroid treatment had improved postoperative hemodynamics and pulmonary function as well as a decreased duration of mechanical ventilation. All the patients also received aprotinin in addition to methylprednisolone. The combined anti-inflammatory effect of a protease inhibitor and a corticosteroid may have improved the clinical course in the patients in this study. More importantly, this finding suggests that improved clinical outcomes with reduced morbidity and mortality in patients undergoing cardiac surgical procedures may require the use of multiple anti-inflammatory modalities.

However, more recent clinical studies performed by Chaney and his colleagues demonstrate that methylprednisolone treatment of patients undergoing cardiac surgical procedures with CPB not only fail to provide clinical benefits, but may be detrimental to the postoperative course.[137,138] The first investigation was a prospective, randomized, placebo-controlled study of 60 patients undergoing elective CABG with CPB.[137] Corticosteroid treatment did not reduce complement activation. Furthermore, patients in the methylprednisolone group had significantly decreased pulmonary function and required more postoperative inotropic support and more prolonged mechanical ventilation. These findings suggested that corticosteroid treatment of cardiac surgical patients may induce detrimental hemodynamic and pulmonary effects, lengthening the duration of mechanical ventilation. In a subsequent larger study with varying dosing regimens, these same investigators corroborated these findings.[138] Hence, these results suggest that corticosteroid treatment does not offer any clinical benefit and may worsen clinical course by inducing hyperglycemia and prolonging mechanical ventilation.

In summary, despite improvements in biochemical profiles in patients receiving steroids, clinical improvements have not been consistently demonstrated. The results of multiple experimental and clinical studies demonstrate that corticosteroid pretreatment of patients undergoing cardiac surgical procedures with CPB decrease pro-inflammatory mediators while enhancing the production of anti-inflammatory mediators. However, whether these beneficial changes offer clinical benefit remains controversial. Furthermore, recent studies suggest a detrimental effect of corticosteroids on postoperative course. Larger prospective randomized studies are required to determine the optimal dose and timing of corticosteroids, as well as possible beneficial or detrimental effects on clinical outcome. Moreover, recognizing the redundancy of the inflammatory cascades, studies employing combinations of corticosteroids with other anti-inflammatory agents such as protease inhibitors or anticomplement therapies need to be conducted to investigate possible additive or synergistic effects, leading to reduced postoperative morbidity and mortality. In total, given the aforementioned data, the routine use of corticosteroids in cardiac surgical procedures is not warranted or cannot be substantiated.

ANTIOXIDANTS

Generation of reactive oxygen species during cardiac surgical procedures plays a major role in initiation and amplification of SIRS as well as the subsequent tissue destruction and end-organ damage.[139–142] Major sources of oxygen-derived free radicals include activated neutrophils and xanthine oxidase catalysis of the oxidation of hypoxanthine in reperfused tissues.[143,144] These reactive oxygen species induce damage to cellular components through peroxidation of membrane lipids, proteins, and other cellular structures.[145–148] Furthermore, oxidation of antiproteases such as α_1-antiprotease renders these protective enzymes dysfunctional.[147] Reactive oxygen species also promote amplification of the systemic inflammatory response by activating inflammatory cascades such as complement, and by inducing the release of cytokines from endothelial cells and neutrophils.[143,145]

Among the numerous theoretical approaches to limiting the toxic effects of oxygen-derived free radicals, investigators have focused on supplementing the patient's antioxidant defensive mechanisms. Studies demonstrate a depletion of endogenous antioxidants such as alpha-tocopherol (vitamin E) and ascorbic acid (vitamin C) in patients undergoing cardiac surgical procedures.[149,150] The depletion of antioxidants was prevented by exogenous supplementation before the onset of surgical procedures.[141,149] Moreover, exogenous supplementation also blunted the increase in levels of oxygen-derived free radicals such as hydrogen peroxide in patients undergoing CPB.[141] Multiple animal studies employing exogenous supplementation of alpha-tocopherol or ascorbic acid, used alone or in combination, demonstrate attenuation of the free radical–mediated amplification of the inflammatory response and tissue damage.[151,152]

The studies in patients undergoing cardiac surgical procedures, however, have not shown clear clinical benefit with exogenous administration of antioxidants. A prospective randomized study of 48 patients given intravenous or oral supplementation of alpha-tocopherol or ascorbic acid demonstrated that the exogenous supplementation of oxidants prevented the depletion of these vitamins.[149] The plasma levels of creatine phosphokinase MB, a marker for myocardial injury, and malondialdehyde, a product of lipid peroxidation, were decreased in patients receiving supplementation. However, the study failed to demonstrate an improvement in ventricular function or a reduction in the incidence of ventricular arrhythmias or amount of inotropic requirements. Butterworth and colleagues performed a prospective randomized clinical trial evaluating the effects of pegorgotein, a superoxide anion scavenger, in 67 patients undergoing CABG with CPB.[153] The administration of pegorgotein produced no improvements in neuropsychological deficits or myocardial function. Westhuyzen and colleagues, in a prospective randomized study of 76 patients undergoing elective CABG with or without CPB, alpha-tocopherol and ascorbic acid supplementation prevented the depletion of these antioxidants; however, the study failed to demonstrate a decrease in myocardial injury or improvements in myocardial function.[141]

Although the idea of exogenous supplementation of a patient's antioxidant defenses to reduce the free radical–mediated injury seems promising, no studies have consistently demonstrated a clinical benefit in patients undergoing cardiac surgical procedures. The negative results from clinical studies may be because antioxidant supplementation aims to minimize the injury induced by one of the end products of a highly redundant and already amplified systemic inflammation. Therefore, studies combining antioxidants with other modalities of therapy are needed to further explore the possible benefits of antioxidant supplementation.

PHOSPHODIESTERASE INHIBITORS

Phosphodiesterase inhibitors such as milrinone possess potent inotropic and vasodilatory effects and thus are beneficial in patients with congestive heart failure or myocardial instability after cardiac operations.[154–156] Phosphodiesterase inhibitors, by interfering with the breakdown of cyclic adenosine monophosphate (cAMP), increase cAMP levels, thereby increasing intracellular calcium.[157,158]

The increase in intracellular cAMP and resultant rise in intracellular calcium by administration of phosphodiesterase inhibitors may also have anti-inflammatory effects. Intracellular cAMP has been reported to inhibit the transcriptional process of TNF-α messenger ribonucleic acid (mRNA) production.[159] Furthermore, experimental studies demonstrate that phosphodiesterase inhibitors decreased the elaboration of inflammatory mediators by monocytes and inhibited the activation of neutrophils by cytokines.[157,159,160] Animal studies also show reduction of inflammatory cytokines such as IL-1β and TNF-α, and improved myocardial function.[157,160,161]

A limited number of clinical studies show a suppression of the inflammatory response with improvements in clinical parameters by treating patients undergoing cardiac surgical procedures with phosphodiesterase inhibitors. Prospective randomized studies of patients receiving milrinone during cardiac operations demonstrate a decrease in the production of IL-1β and IL-6, which are inversely correlated with cAMP levels.[162,163] Moreover, improvements in hemodynamics and a reduction in gastric mucosal acidosis, indicating increased end-organ perfusion, have been demonstrated. Similar results were found with another phosphodiesterase inhibitor, olprinone.[164] Patients receiving olprinone had increased levels of the anti-inflammatory cytokine IL-10.

Hayashida and colleagues evaluated the effects of colforsin dapropate hydrochloride, a derivative of forskolin, on patients undergoing CABG with CPB.[165] Similar to phosphodiesterase inhibitors, colforsin, an activator of adenylate cyclase, increases intracellular cAMP and calcium levels, as well as having potent inotropic and vasodilatory effects in vitro and in vivo.[158,166,167] The patients receiving colforsin had decreased plasma levels of IL-1β, IL-6, and IL-8, along with increased cAMP levels. Furthermore, these patients had improved pulmonary and myocardial function. Another phosphodiesterase inhibitor, pentoxifylline, was also shown to decrease levels of IL-6, IL-8, and TNF-α in patients undergoing cardiac operations.[168]

Phosphodiesterase inhibitors, by increasing the intracellular cAMP levels, seem to decrease the systemic inflammatory response by blunting the elaboration of cytokines by monocytes and neutrophils. Moreover, the results of these experimental and small clinical studies are encouraging and have suggested improvements in pulmonary and myocardial function with the use of phosphodiesterase inhibitors. However, these preliminary results need to be assessed in larger clinical trials to determine the true safety and efficacy of phosphodiesterase inhibitors when used in this context.

Modification of Surgical Technique

CPB with cardioplegic arrest is a standard part of most cardiac surgical procedures performed contemporaneously. The use of this extracorporeal device provides a still and bloodless surgical field so that the procedure can occur in a controlled environment. However, as detailed above, CPB is a well-recognized elicitor of a systemic inflammatory response in patients, ultimately resulting in tissue damage and end-organ dysfunction. Strategies to minimize the systemic inflammation from CPB, thereby reducing the attendant clinical sequelae, include modification of the bypass circuit or the complete elimination of the heart–lung machine from the surgical procedure. Strategies to modify the CPB circuit include heparin-bonded circuits, elimination of cardiotomy suction, leukocyte depletion, and modified ultrafiltration. Heparin-bonded circuits and elimination of cardiotomy suction are discussed in Chapter 6, "Use of Heparin-Bonded Cardiopulmonary Bypass Circuits with Alternatives to Standard Anticogulation." The first part of this section briefly discusses modifications of surgical techniques including off-pump CABG, minimally invasive CABG, and biventricular bypass, while the latter part of this section focuses on the remaining strategies of CPB circuit modification, with particular focus on leukocyte depletion and modified ultrafiltration.

OFF-PUMP AND MINIMALLY INVASIVE CABG

The widely held belief that avoidance of CPB may reduce morbidity has caused a resurgence of interest in performing open heart surgery without CPB.[169–172] Improvements in technology and the development of cardiac stabilizers have made off-pump coronary artery bypass (OPCAB) a reality for many patients. Moreover, attempts to further reduce the systemic inflammatory response have led to the minimally invasive coronary artery bypass grafting (MICAB) technique, where off-pump coronary revascularization is performed through a small anterolateral thoracotomy, thereby minimizing the contribution of the surgical procedure.[169] The effectiveness of these new and evolving surgical techniques continues to be evaluated in both experimental and clinical settings.

Multiple studies have been performed to evaluate the role of OPCAB and MICAB in decreasing the systemic inflammatory response, thereby improving the clinical outcomes. Although the majority of studies evaluating the biochemical markers of inflammation show an attenuation of the systemic inflammation in patients undergoing OPCAB or MICAB, the clinical studies evaluating the clinical course of these patients demonstrate conflicting results.[171,173–180] However, elimination of the CPB and a minimally invasive surgical approach may prove beneficial to certain patient subpopulations such as those with advanced age or multiple comorbidities. Prospective randomized trials with larger patient groups and selected subgroups (elderly, left ventricular dysfunction, renal insufficiency, or calcified ascending aorta) are needed to further evaluate the possible reduction of systemic inflammatory response and subsequent improvement in clinical course of patients undergoing OPCAB or MICAB. For further details on this topic, please see Chapter 10, "Off-Pump Coronary Artery Bypass Grafting."

BIVENTRICULAR BYPASS

As described above, elimination of the nonphysiologic environment created by the CPB may blunt the systemic inflammatory response, with subsequent reduction in postoperative morbidity. Recognizing that the lungs may be a significant source of systemic inflammatory mediators after standard cardiac surgical procedures, there has been a resurgence of interest in a bilateral bypass technique with deep hypothermic arrest, introduced by Drew and Anderson in 1959.[181,182] This technique involves the use of the patient's own lungs as an oxygenator in a bilateral cardiac bypass circuit during CABG. The process entails double arterial cannulation (aorta and pulmonary artery) and double atrial cannulation (left and right atria) while the patient's lungs are mechanically ventilated.

In addition to eliminating CPB as a source of activation of humoral and cellular inflammatory cascades, this technique may minimize the elaboration of cytokines by the lungs upon reperfusion after a period of ischemia that occurs with standard CPB. Glenville and colleagues alluded to this anti-inflammatory benefit by reporting the reduction of neutrophil sequestration in the lungs in a group of 20 patients undergoing CABG with biventricular bypass.[183] A more extensive investigation was performed by Richter and colleagues in a prospective randomized trial of 30 patients undergoing elective CABG.[184] The patients undergoing biventricular bypass, as opposed to the traditional CPB, had decreased levels of IL-6 and IL-8. These patients also had decreased postoperative blood loss with reduced transfusion requirements. Furthermore, these patients also had improved pulmonary function and required shorter duration of mechanical ventilator support. This study demonstrated that the Drew–Anderson technique, although requiring double arterial and atrial cannulation, is safe and may be effective in reducing the systemic inflammatory response and improving clinical outcome. Further studies are required to validate its efficacy.

Modification of CPB Circuit

CPB has been demonstrated to potentiate the systemic inflammatory reaction in patients undergoing cardiac operations through the contact of humoral and cellular components of the blood with foreign surfaces and the traumatic shear forces of roller pumps and suction devices. Therefore, investigators have focused on the possible benefits of modifying the CPB circuit to reduce the systemic inflammatory response. The role of heparin-bonded circuits and elimination of cardiotomy suction are discussed in Chapter 6 "Use of Heparin-Bonded Cardiopulmonary Bypass Circuits with Alternatives to Standard Anticoagulation". The following section will focus on leukocyte depletion and modified ultrafiltration.

LEUKOCYTE DEPLETION

Although neutrophils play a major role in the defense against foreign pathogens, uncontrolled recruitment and activation of these inflammatory cells have been implicated as the mediator of numerous inflammatory diseases such as rheumatoid arthritis, ulcerative colitis, and SIRS.[185,186] There are multiple inflammatory mediators that induce the chemotaxis, adherence, and activation of neutrophils, including contact with synthetic surfaces, C5a, kallikrein, leukotriene B$_4$, hypoxia, thrombin, fibrin-degradation products, and cytokines.[9,14,19,42] Neutrophils are activated by numerous inflammatory mediators elaborated during cardiac surgical procedures with CPB. With the onset of CPB, neutrophils decrease in number as a result of hemodilution and adsorption to the extracorporeal circuit, followed by widespread activation.[187] Activation of neutrophils during cardiac surgical procedures has been demonstrated in multiple experimental and clinical studies by showing upregulation of integrin expression and increases in levels of enzymes such as myeloperoxidase and elastase.[188–190] Leukocyte filters were first introduced to reduce the large number of leukocytes that contaminated standard red cell transfusions.[191] Technical improvements of these filters led to their introduction into the field of cardiac surgery in the early 1990s.[192] The concept of leukocyte filtration to minimize and reduce the effects of toxic enzymes and inflammatory mediators released by neutrophils has led to numerous studies with conflicting results.

Numerous studies demonstrate the mechanism of neutrophil activation by inflammatory mediators. Neutrophils respond to these mediators by rolling, adhering, and transmigrating across the endothelial layer to reach the extravascular interstitium.[147] The expression of selectins (E-selectin, P-selectin, and L-selectin) on endothelial cells and neutrophils accomplishes a low-affinity association between these two cells.[193,194] The upregulation of integrins such as leukocyte factor antigen (LFA)-1 (CD11a/CD18) and Mac-1 (CD11b/CD18) on neutrophils then bind to endothelial adhesion molecules of the immunoglobulin superfamily such as intercellular adhesion molecule-1 (ICAM-1), vascular cell adhesion molecule-1 (VCAM-1), and platelet-endothelial cell adhesion molecule (PECAM); this process results in a firm adherence of neutrophils to the endothelium, resulting in transmigration.[193] These

activated neutrophils then release histotoxic enzymes such as elastase, myeloperoxidase, collagenase, gelatinase, and other proteolytic enzymes. In addition, activated neutrophils also release multiple cytokines and oxygen free radicals such as hydrogen peroxide, oxygen halides, and hydroxyl anion.[147] These events may ultimately lead to pathologic tissue destruction, generation of pro-inflammatory mediators, and recruitment and activation of more inflammatory cells.

To minimize the pro-inflammatory and destructive processes of neutrophils, investigators have evaluated the possible benefits of leukocyte depletion during cardiac operations. Three different methods of leukocyte depletion have been employed during cardiac surgical procedures: (1) systemic leukocyte reduction with an arterial filter encompassing the entire duration of CPB; (2) strategic leukocyte filtration initiated during reperfusion with an arterial or a venous filter; and (3) leukocyte depletion of blood cardioplegia.

Multiple studies evaluating the effects of leukocyte depletion in patients undergoing cardiac surgical procedures have produced conflicting results. Although most studies have found decreased neutrophil activation and circulating cytokine levels with the use of leukocyte depletion, these studies fail to demonstrate improvements in hemodynamics, pulmonary function, and length of hospital stay.[195–209] Some studies indicate that although the filter prevents the recirculation of neutrophils into the systemic circulation by their adhesion to the filter, it may actually activate these "trapped" neutrophils and promote the release of soluble pro-inflammatory mediators that can enter the systemic circulation.[207] Larger prospective randomized studies with optimization of filtration techniques are needed to further evaluate the anti-inflammatory effects and subsequent clinical benefits of leukocyte depletion. Furthermore, the combination of leukocyte filters with other efficacious extracorporeal circuit modifications (eg, heparin-bonded circuit and elimination of cardiotomy suction) may hold even more promise in reducing the morbidity and mortality of cardiac surgical procedures.

MODIFIED ULTRAFILTRATION

Recognizing that elaboration of pro-inflammatory mediators correlates with postoperative morbidity, modified ultrafiltration has been used. In the pediatric population, the use of modified ultrafiltration during cardiac surgical procedures with CPB has produced favorable results.[210–212] The employment of modified ultrafiltration decreased the levels of pro-inflammatory cytokines and reduced postoperative morbidity by shortening length of hospital and ICU stay and by decreasing the duration of mechanical ventilator support. However, the benefits of modified ultrafiltration are less clear in the adult cardiac surgical population.

Ultrafiltration is a convective process in which the patient's blood is filtered across a porous membrane, allowing small molecules with a mass less than the pore size of the filter and water to be removed by a transmembrane pressure gradient.[213] Modified ultrafiltration refers to the conduction of ultrafiltration immediately after the termination of CPB, with the inlet of the filter positioned close to the arterial cannula and its outlet returning blood directly to the right atrium.[213] In addition to reducing extravascular water and increasing the hematocrit, modified ultrafiltration has been shown to lower plasma levels of activated complement products and cytokines in the pediatric population.[210,212] The studies in the adult population, however, are limited.

Multiple investigators have studied the impact of modified ultrafiltration in patients undergoing CABG with CPB. Tassani and colleagues studied the effects of modified ultrafiltration in 43 patients undergoing CABG with CPB.[214] Patients receiving ultrafiltration treatment had lower plasma levels of IL-8 and increased pulmonary function, resulting in shorter duration of mechanical ventilation. Boga and colleagues also performed a similar study in 40 patients undergoing CABG.[215] However, cytokine levels remained unaltered with modified ultrafiltration. Grunenfelder and associates investigated the role of modified ultrafiltration in a prospective randomized study of 47 patients undergoing CABG with CPB.[216] Although patients in the ultrafiltration group had reduced levels of cytokines (IL-6, IL-8, TNF-α) and adhesion molecules (E-selectin, ICAM), the investigators were unable to demonstrate any significant impact on clinical course. Luciani and colleagues recently performed a large prospective randomized study of modified ultrafiltration in 573 patients undergoing cardiac surgical procedures.[217] This study included a large proportion of high-risk patients with advanced age and multiple comorbidities. Although hospital mortality remained the same, postoperative cardiac, pulmonary, neurologic, and gastrointestinal complications were significantly reduced in patients receiving modified ultrafiltration. These results show promise in decreasing the systemic inflammatory response and reducing postoperative morbidity with the use of modified ultrafiltration, especially in high-risk patients. Further studies are needed to corroborate these encouraging results.

Conclusion

Cardiac operations elicit a systemic inflammatory response in patients, inducing the elaboration of multiple cytokines, chemokines, and destructive enzymes. This inflammatory reaction involves multiple cell types and humoral cascades which are interdependent and redundant, allowing for amplification at numerous steps. When this systemic inflammatory response is unfettered, a wide spectrum of clinical consequences may result, including thromboembolism, bleeding, fluid retention, and multiple organ dysfunction and failure. Therefore, investigative efforts have focused on understanding the mechanism of the SIRS to develop potential therapeutic targets to inhibit this inflammatory response, thereby possibly improving clinical outcome. Multiple therapeutic methods have been investigated, including pharmacologic inhibitors and modifications of surgical technique and CPB circuit. Although studies demonstrate an attenuation of the systemic inflammatory response through the use of these therapies in experimental and clinical settings, studies fail to conclusively show clinical benefit from these therapies. The specificity of each of these therapies may be unable to minimize the deleterious effects of a systemic inflammatory response resulting from the activation of multiple, interdependent, and redundant inflammatory cascades and cell types. Hence, further studies investigating the biochemical and clinical effects of a combination of anti-inflammatory therapies are needed. Moreover, further studies delineating the molecular mechanism of activation of cellular and humoral inflammatory cascades may lead to additional potential therapeutic targets such as mitogen-activated protein (MAP) kinases (p38, JNK, ERK) and transcription factors (NF-κB, AP-1, ATF-3, Egr-1). Discussion of the molecular mechanism of inflammation is beyond the scope of this chapter, and the reader is referred to excellent recent comprehensive reviews.[218–225]

References

1. American Heart Association. 2002 Heart and stroke statistical update. Dallas (TX): American Heart Association; 2001.
2. Gibbon JH Jr. Application of a mechanical heart and lung apparatus in cardiac surgery. Minn Med 1954;37:171–5.
3. Royston D. The inflammatory response and extracorporeal circulation. J Cardiothorac Vasc Anesth 1997;11:341–54.
4. Royston D. Preventing the inflammatory response to open-heart surgery: the role of aprotinin and other protease inhibitors. Int J Cardiol 1996;53 Suppl:S11–37.
5. Asimakopoulos G, Smith PL, Ratnatunga CP, Taylor KM. Lung injury and acute respiratory distress syndrome after cardiopulmonary bypass. Ann Thorac Surg 1999; 68:1107–15.
6. Cremer J, Martin M, Redl H, et al. Systemic inflammatory response syndrome after cardiac operations. Ann Thorac Surg 1996;61:1714–20.
7. Westaby S. Organ dysfunction after cardiopulmonary bypass. A systemic inflammatory reaction initiated by the extracorporeal circuit. Intensive Care Med 1987;13:89–95.
8. Edmunds LH Jr. Inflammatory response to cardiopulmonary bypass. Ann Thorac Surg 1998;66:S12–6; discussion S25–8.
9. Coughlin SR. Sol Sherry lecture in thrombosis: how thrombin "talks" to cells: molecular mechanisms and roles in vivo. Arterioscler Thromb Vasc Biol 1998;18:514–8.
10. Osterud B. Tissue factor expression by monocytes: regulation and pathophysiological roles. Blood Coagul Fibrinolysis 1998;9 Suppl 1:S9–14.
11. Carden DL, Granger DN. Pathophysiology of ischaemia-reperfusion injury. J Pathol 2000;190:255–66.

12. Reffelmann T, Kloner RA. The "no-reflow" phenomenon: basic science and clinical correlates. Heart 2002;87:162–8.

13. Coughlin SR. Thrombin signalling and protease-activated receptors. Nature 2000;407:258–64.

14. Szaba FM, Smiley ST. Roles for thrombin and fibrin(ogen) in cytokine/chemokine production and macrophage adhesion in vivo. Blood 2002;99:1053–9.

15. Schapira M, Despland E, Scott CF, et al. Purified human plasma kallikrein aggregates human blood neutrophils. J Clin Invest 1982;69:1199–202.

16. Wachtfogel YT, Pixley RA, Kucich U, et al. Purified plasma factor XIIa aggregates human neutrophils and causes degranulation. Blood 1986;67:1731–7.

17. Bhoola KD, Figueroa CD, Worthy K. Bioregulation of kinins: kallikreins, kininogens, and kininases. Pharmacol Rev 1992;44:1–80.

18. Fuhrer G, Gallimore MJ, Heller W, Hoffmeister HE. Aprotinin in cardiopulmonary bypass—effects on the Hageman factor (FXII)— kallikrein system and blood loss. Blood Coagul Fibrinolysis 1992;3:99–104.

19. Cugno M, Nussberger J, Biglioli P, et al. Increase of bradykinin in plasma of patients undergoing cardiopulmonary bypass: the importance of lung exclusion. Chest 2001;120:1776–82.

20. Kongsgaard UE, Smith-Erichsen N, Geiran O, et al. Different activation patterns in the plasma kallikrein-kinin and complement systems during coronary bypass surgery. Acta Anaesthesiol Scand 1989;33:343–7.

21. Wachtfogel YT, Harpel PC, Edmunds LH Jr, Colman RW. Formation of C1s-C1-inhibitor, kallikrein-C1-inhibitor, and plasmin-alpha 2-plasmin-inhibitor complexes during cardiopulmonary bypass. Blood 1989;73:468–71.

22. Seghaye MC, Duchateau J, Grabitz RG, et al. Complement activation during cardiopulmonary bypass in infants and children. Relation to postoperative multiple system organ failure. J Thorac Cardiovasc Surg 1993;106:978–87.

23. Miller BE, Levy JH. The inflammatory response to cardiopulmonary bypass. J Cardiothorac Vasc Anesth 1997;11: 355–66.

24. Kluft C, Dooijewaard G, Emeis JJ. Role of the contact system in fibrinolysis. Semin Thromb Hemost 1987;13:50–68.

25. Smiley ST, King JA, Hancock WW. Fibrinogen stimulates macrophage chemokine secretion through toll-like receptor 4. J Immunol 2001;167:2887–94.

26. Gelb AB, Roth RI, Levin J, et al. Changes in blood coagulation during and following cardiopulmonary bypass: lack of correlation with clinical bleeding. Am J Clin Pathol 1996;106:87–99.

27. Chan AK, Leaker M, Burrows FA, et al. Coagulation and fibrinolytic profile of paediatric patients undergoing cardiopulmonary bypass. Thromb Haemost 1997;77: 270–7.

28. Bick RL. The clinical significance of fibrinogen degradation products. Semin Thromb Hemost 1982;8:302–30.

29. Tabuchi N, de Haan J, Boonstra PW, van Oeveren W. Activation of fibrinolysis in the pericardial cavity during cardiopulmonary bypass. J Thorac Cardiovasc Surg 1993;106:828–33.

30. Whitten CW, Greilich PE, Ivy R, et al. D-Dimer formation during cardiac and noncardiac thoracic surgery. Anesth Analg 1999;88:1226–31.

31. Cvachovec K, Horacek M, Vislocky I. A retrospective survey of fibrinolysis as an indicator of poor outcome after cardiopulmonary bypass and a possible early sign of systemic inflammation syndrome. Eur J Anaesthesiol 2000;17:173–6.

32. Muller-Eberhard HJ. Molecular organization and function of the complement system. Annu Rev Biochem 1988;57: 321–47.

33. Volanakis JE, Frank MM. The human complement system in health and disease. New York: M. Dekker; 1998. p. 656.

34. Turner MW. Mannose-binding lectin: the pluripotent molecule of the innate immune system. Immunol Today 1996;17:532–40.

35. Morgan BP. Regulation of the complement membrane attack pathway. Crit Rev Immunol 1999;19:173–98.

36. Kilgore KS, Flory CM, Miller BF, et al. The membrane attack complex of complement induces interleukin-8 and monocyte chemoattractant protein-1 secretion from human umbilical vein endothelial cells. Am J Pathol 1996;149:953–61.

37. Tedesco F, Pausa M, Nardon E, et al. The cytolytically inactive terminal complement complex activates endothelial cells to express adhesion molecules and tissue factor procoagulant activity. J Exp Med 1997;185:1619–27.

38. Stahl GL, Reenstra WR, Frendl G. Complement-mediated loss of endothelium-dependent relaxation of porcine coronary arteries. Role of the terminal membrane attack complex. Circ Res 1995;76:575–83.

39. Collard CD, Agah A, Reenstra W, et al. Endothelial nuclear factor-kappaB translocation and vascular cell adhesion molecule-1 induction by complement: inhibition with anti-human C5 therapy or cGMP analogues. Arterioscler Thromb Vasc Biol 1999;19:2623–9.

40. Collard CD, Lekowski R, Jordan JE, et al. Complement activation following oxidative stress. Mol Immunol 1999; 36:941–8.

41. Kilgore KS, Friedrichs GS, Homeister JW, Lucchesi BR. The complement system in myocardial ischaemia/reperfusion injury. Cardiovasc Res 1994;28:437–44.

42. Hugli TE, Muller-Eberhard HJ. Anaphylatoxins: C3a and C5a. Adv Immunol 1978;26:1–53.

43. Foreman KE, Glovsky MM, Warner RL, et al. Comparative effect of C3a and C5a on adhesion molecule expression on neutrophils and endothelial cells. Inflammation 1996;20:1–9.

44. Czermak BJ, Sarma V, Bless NM, et al. In vitro and in vivo dependency of chemokine generation on C5a and TNF-alpha. J Immunol 1999;162:2321–5.

45. Pan ZK. Anaphylatoxins C5a and C3a induce nuclear factor kappaB activation in human peripheral blood monocytes. Biochim Biophys Acta 1998;1443:90–8.

46. Chenoweth DE, Cooper SW, Hugli TE, et al. Complement activation during cardiopulmonary bypass: evidence for generation of C3a and C5a anaphylatoxins. N Engl J Med 1981;304:497–503.

47. Kirklin JK, Westaby S, Blackstone EH, et al. Complement and the damaging effects of cardiopulmonary bypass. J Thorac Cardiovasc Surg 1983;86:845–57.

48. Steinberg JB, Kapelanski DP, Olson JD, Weiler JM. Cytokine and complement levels in patients undergoing cardiopulmonary bypass. J Thorac Cardiovasc Surg 1993;106:1008–16.

49. Cavarocchi NC, Schaff HV, Orszulak TA, et al. Evidence for complement activation by protamine-heparin interaction after cardiopulmonary bypass. Surgery 1985;98:525–31.

50. Moore FD Jr, Warner KG, Assousa S, et al. The effects of complement activation during cardiopulmonary bypass. Attenuation by hypothermia, heparin, and hemodilution. Ann Surg 1988;208:95–103.

51. Hansson K, Lenninger S. Proteinase inhibitors in acute pancreatitis. Acta Chir Scand Suppl 1967;378:103–14.

52. Sardesal VM, Rosenberg JC. Proteolysis and bradykinin turnover in endotoxin shock. J Trauma 1974;14:945–9.

53. Royston D, Bidstrup BP, Taylor KM, Sapsford RN. Effect of aprotinin on need for blood transfusion after repeat open-heart surgery. Lancet 1987;2:1289–91.

54. Alajmo F, Calamai G, Perna AM, et al. High-dose aprotinin: hemostatic effects in open heart operations. Ann Thorac Surg 1989;48:536–9.

55. Fraedrich G, Weber C, Bernard C, et al. Reduction of blood transfusion requirement in open heart surgery by administration of high doses of aprotinin—preliminary results. Thorac Cardiovasc Surg 1989;37:89–91.

56. Dietrich W, Barankay A, Dilthey G, et al. Reduction of homologous blood requirement in cardiac surgery by intraoperative aprotinin application—clinical experience in 152 cardiac surgical patients. Thorac Cardiovasc Surg 1989;37:92–8.

57. Dietrich W, Spannagl M, Jochum M, et al. Influence of high-dose aprotinin treatment on blood loss and coagulation patterns in patients undergoing myocardial revascularization. Anesthesiology 1990;73:1119–26.

58. Sundaram S, Gikakis N, Hack CE, et al. Nafamostat mesylate, a broad spectrum protease inhibitor, modulates platelet, neutrophil and contact activation in simulated extracorporeal circulation. Thromb Haemost 1996;75:76–82.

59. Gott JP, Cooper WA, Schmidt FE Jr, et al. Modifying risk for extracorporeal circulation: trial of four antiinflammatory strategies. Ann Thorac Surg 1998;66:747–53; discussion 753–4.

60. Stammers AH, Huffman S, Alonso A, et al. The antiinflammatory effects of aprotinin in patients undergoing cardiac surgery with cardiopulmonary bypass. J Extra Corpor Technol 1997;29:114–22.

61. Lu H, Du Buit C, Soria J, et al. Postoperative hemostasis and fibrinolysis in patients undergoing cardiopulmonary bypass with or without aprotinin therapy. Thromb Haemost 1994;72:438–43.

62. Blauhut B, Gross C, Necek S, et al. Effects of high-dose aprotinin on blood loss, platelet function, fibrinolysis, complement, and renal function after cardiopulmonary bypass. J Thorac Cardiovasc Surg 1991;101:958–67.

63. Miyamoto Y, Hirose H, Matsuda H, et al. Analysis of complement activation profile during cardiopulmonary bypass and its inhibition by FUT-175. Trans Am Soc Artif Intern Organs 1985;31:508–11.

64. Fritz H, Wunderer G. Biochemistry and applications of aprotinin, the kallikrein inhibitor from bovine organs. Arzneimittelforschung 1983;33:479–94.

65. Wachtfogel YT, Kucich U, Hack CE, et al. Aprotinin inhibits the contact, neutrophil, and platelet activation systems during simulated extracorporeal perfusion. J Thorac Cardiovasc Surg 1993;106:1–9; discussion 9–10.

66. Redl H, Schlag G, Paul E, Schiesser A. Cellular (thrombocytes, granulocytes) effects of proteinase inhibitors—gabexylate, gabexate mesylate (FOY) and aprotinin. Resuscitation 1986;14:81–90.

67. Wachtfogel YT, Kettner C, Hack CE, et al. Thrombin and human plasma kallikrein inhibition during simulated extracorporeal circulation block platelet and neutrophil activation. Thromb Haemost 1998;80:686–91.

68. Soeparwata R, Hartman AR, Frerichmann U, et al. Aprotinin diminishes inflammatory processes. Int J Cardiol 1996;53 Suppl:S55–63.

69. Asimakopoulos G, Thompson R, Nourshargh S, et al. An anti-inflammatory property of aprotinin detected at the level of leukocyte extravasation. J Thorac Cardiovasc Surg 2000;120:361–9.

70. Asimakopoulos G, Lidington EA, Mason J, et al. Effect of aprotinin on endothelial cell activation. J Thorac Cardiovasc Surg 2001;122:123–8.

71. Royston D. High-dose aprotinin therapy: a review of the first five years' experience. J Cardiothorac Vasc Anesth 1992;6:76–100.

72. Weerasinghe A, Taylor KM. The platelet in cardiopulmonary bypass. Ann Thorac Surg 1998;66:2145–52.

73. van Oeveren W, Harder MP, Roozendaal KJ, et al. Aprotinin protects platelets against the initial effect of cardiopulmonary bypass. J Thorac Cardiovasc Surg 1990;99:788–96; discussion 796–7.

74. Mohr R, Goor DA, Lusky A, Lavee J. Aprotinin prevents cardiopulmonary bypass-induced platelet dysfunction. A scanning electron microscope study. Circulation 1992;86:II405–9.

75. Shigeta O, Kojima H, Jikuya T, et al. Aprotinin inhibits plasmin-induced platelet activation during cardiopulmonary bypass. Circulation 1997;96:569–74.

76. Landis RC, Asimakopoulos G, Poullis M, et al. The antithrombotic and antiinflammatory mechanisms of action of aprotinin. Ann Thorac Surg 2001;72:2169–75.

77. Landis RC, Haskard DO, Taylor KM. New antiinflammatory and platelet-preserving effects of aprotinin. Ann Thorac Surg 2001;72:S1808–13.

78. Poullis M, Manning R, Laffan M, et al. The antithrombotic effect of aprotinin: actions mediated via the protease activated receptor 1. J Thorac Cardiovasc Surg 2000;120:370–8.

79. Isbir CS, Dogan R, Demircin M, et al. Aprotinin reduces the IL-8 after coronary artery bypass grafting. Cardiovasc Surg 2001;9:403–6.

80. Vriesendorp FJ, Flynn RE, Pappolla MA, Koski CL. Complement depletion affects demyelination and inflammation in experimental allergic neuritis. J Neuroimmunol 1995;58:157–65.

81. Mathieson PW, Qasim FJ, Thiru S, et al. Effects of decomplementation with cobra venom factor on experimental vasculitis. Clin Exp Immunol 1994;97:474–7.

82. Cochrane CG. The role of complement in experimental disease models. Springer Semin Immunopathol 1984;7:263–70.

83. Couser WG, Baker PJ, Adler S. Complement and the direct mediation of immune glomerular injury: a new perspective. Kidney Int 1985;28:879–90.

84. Gelfand JA, Donelan M, Hawiger A, Burke JF. Alternative complement pathway activation increases mortality in a model of burn injury in mice. J Clin Invest 1982;70:1170–6.

85. Rinder CS, Rinder HM, Johnson K, et al. Role of C3 cleavage in monocyte activation during extracorporeal circulation. Circulation 1999;100:553–8.

86. Fearon DT. Regulation of the amplification C3 convertase of human complement by an inhibitory protein isolated from human erythrocyte membrane. Proc Natl Acad Sci U S A 1979;76:5867–71.

87. Iida K, Nussenzweig V. Complement receptor is an inhibitor of the complement cascade. J Exp Med 1981;153:1138–50.

88. Weisman HF, Bartow T, Leppo MK, et al. Soluble human complement receptor type 1: in vivo inhibitor of complement suppressing post-ischemic myocardial inflammation and necrosis. Science 1990;249:146–51.

89. Chai PJ, Nassar R, Oakeley AE, et al. Soluble complement receptor-1 protects heart, lung, and cardiac myofilament function from cardiopulmonary bypass damage. Circulation 2000;101:541–6.

90. Lazar HL, Bao Y, Gaudiani J, et al. Total complement inhibition: an effective strategy to limit ischemic injury during coronary revascularization on cardiopulmonary bypass. Circulation 1999;100:1438–42.

91. Swift AJ, Collins TS, Bugelski P, Winkelstein JA. Soluble human complement receptor type 1 inhibits complement-mediated host defense. Clin Diagn Lab Immunol 1994;1:585–9.

92. Morgan BP, Walport MJ. Complement deficiency and disease. Immunol Today 1991;12:301–6.

93. Lesavre PH, Muller-Eberhard HJ. Mechanism of action of factor D of the alternative complement pathway. J Exp Med 1978;148:1498–509.

94. Volanakis JE, Narayana SV. Complement factor D, a novel serine protease. Protein Sci 1996;5:553–64.

95. Tanhehco EJ, Kilgore KS, Liff DA, et al. The anti-factor D antibody, MAb 166-32, inhibits the alternative pathway of the human complement system. Transplant Proc 1999;31:2168–71.

96. Fung M, Loubser PG, Undar A, et al. Inhibition of complement, neutrophil, and platelet activation by an anti-factor D monoclonal antibody in simulated cardiopulmonary bypass circuits. J Thorac Cardiovasc Surg 2001;122:113–22.

97. Fearon DT, Austen KF. Properdin: binding to C3b and stabilization of the C3b-dependent C3 convertase. J Exp Med 1975;142:856–63.

98. Gupta-Bansal R, Parent JB, Brunden KR. Inhibition of complement alternative pathway function with anti-properdin monoclonal antibodies. Mol Immunol 2000; 37:191–201.

99. Sahu A, Kay BK, Lambris JD. Inhibition of human complement by a C3-binding peptide isolated from a phage-displayed random peptide library. J Immunol 1996; 157:884–91.

100. Nilsson B, Larsson R, Hong J, et al. Compstatin inhibits complement and cellular activation in whole blood in two models of extracorporeal circulation. Blood 1998; 92:1661–7.

101. Ross SC, Densen P. Complement deficiency states and infection: epidemiology, pathogenesis and consequences of neisserial and other infections in an immune deficiency. Medicine (Baltimore) 1984;63:243–73.

102. Wurzner R, Schulze M, Happe L, et al. Inhibition of terminal complement complex formation and cell lysis by monoclonal antibodies. Complement Inflamm 1991;8: 328–40.

103. Thomas TC, Rollins SA, Rother RP, et al. Inhibition of complement activity by humanized anti-C5 antibody and single-chain Fv. Mol Immunol 1996;33:1389–401.

104. Rinder CS, Rinder HM, Smith BR, et al. Blockade of C5a and C5b-9 generation inhibits leukocyte and platelet activation during extracorporeal circulation. J Clin Invest 1995;96:1564–72.

105. Fitch JC, Rollins S, Matis L, et al. Pharmacology and biological efficacy of a recombinant, humanized, single-chain antibody C5 complement inhibitor in patients undergoing coronary artery bypass graft surgery with cardiopulmonary bypass. Circulation 1999;100:2499–506.

106. Weil MH, Whigham H. Corticosteroids for reversal of hemorrhagic shock in rats. Am J Physiol 1965;209: 815–8.

107. Dietzman RH, Ersek RA, Lillehei CW, et al. Low output syndrome. Recognition and treatment. J Thorac Cardiovasc Surg 1969;57:138–50.

108. Replogle RL, Gazzaniga AB, Gross RE. Use of corticosteroids during cardiopulmonary bypass: possible lysosome stabilization. Circulation 1966;33:I86–92.

109. Refojo D, Liberman AC, Holsboer F, Arzt E. Transcription factor-mediated molecular mechanisms involved in the functional cross-talk between cytokines and glucocorticoids. Immunol Cell Biol 2001;79:385–94.

110. Mukaida N, Zachariae CC, Gusella GL, Matsushima K. Dexamethasone inhibits the induction of monocyte chemotactic-activating factor production by IL-1 or tumor necrosis factor. J Immunol 1991;146:1212–5.

111. Joyce DA, Gimblett G, Steer JH. Targets of glucocorticoid action on TNF-alpha release by macrophages. Inflamm Res 2001;50:337–40.

112. Chrousos GP. The hypothalamic-pituitary-adrenal axis and immune-mediated inflammation. N Engl J Med 1995;332:1351–62.

113. Calandra T, Bernhagen J, Metz CN, et al. MIF as a glucocorticoid-induced modulator of cytokine production. Nature 1995;377:68–71.

114. Boumpas DT, Chrousos GP, Wilder RL, et al. Glucocorticoid therapy for immune-mediated diseases: basic and clinical correlates. Ann Intern Med 1993;119:1198–208.

115. Perretti M, Flower RJ. Modulation of IL-1-induced neutrophil migration by dexamethasone and lipocortin 1. J Immunol 1993;150:992–9.

116. Engelman RM, Rousou JA, Flack JE 3rd, et al. Influence of steroids on complement and cytokine generation after cardiopulmonary bypass. Ann Thorac Surg 1995;60: 801–4.

117. Kawamura T, Inada K, Nara N, et al. Influence of methylprednisolone on cytokine balance during cardiac surgery. Crit Care Med 1999;27:545–8.

118. Jorens PG, De Jongh R, De Backer W, et al. Interleukin-8 production in patients undergoing cardiopulmonary bypass. The influence of pretreatment with methylprednisolone. Am Rev Respir Dis 1993;148:890–5.

119. Teoh KH, Bradley CA, Gauldie J, Burrows H. Steroid inhibition of cytokine-mediated vasodilation after warm heart surgery. Circulation 1995;92:II347–53.

120. Volk T, Schmutzler M, Engelhardt L, et al. Influence of amino steroid and glucocorticoid treatment on inflammation and immune function during cardiopulmonary bypass. Crit Care Med 2001;29:2137–42.

121. Yilmaz M, Ener S, Akalin H, et al. Effect of low-dose methyl prednisolone on serum cytokine levels following extracorporeal circulation. Perfusion 1999;14:201–6.

122. Fillinger MP, Rassias AJ, Guyre PM, et al. Glucocorticoid effects on the inflammatory and clinical responses to cardiac surgery. J Cardiothorac Vasc Anesth 2002;16:163–9.

123. Dernek S, Tunerir B, Sevin B, et al. The effects of methylprednisolone on complement, immunoglobulins and pulmonary neutrophil sequestration during cardiopulmonary bypass. Cardiovasc Surg 1999;7:414–8.

124. Wan S, LeClerc JL, Schmartz D, et al. Hepatic release of interleukin-10 during cardiopulmonary bypass in steroid-pretreated patients. Am Heart J 1997;133:335–9.

125. Wan S, DeSmet JM, Antoine M, et al. Steroid administration in heart and heart-lung transplantation: is the timing adequate? Ann Thorac Surg 1996;61:674–8.

126. Tabardel Y, Duchateau J, Schmartz D, et al. Corticosteroids increase blood interleukin-10 levels during cardiopulmonary bypass in men. Surgery 1996;119:76–80.

127. Jansen NJ, van Oeveren W, van Vliet M, et al. The role of different types of corticosteroids on the inflammatory mediators in cardiopulmonary bypass. Eur J Cardiothorac Surg 1991;5:211–7.

128. Hill GE, Alonso A, Spurzem JR, et al. Aprotinin and methylprednisolone equally blunt cardiopulmonary bypass-induced inflammation in humans. J Thorac Cardiovasc Surg 1995;110:1658–62.

129. Hill GE, Whitten CW, Landers DF. The influence of cardiopulmonary bypass on cytokines and cell–cell communication. J Cardiothorac Vasc Anesth 1997;11:367–75.

130. Andersen LW, Baek L, Thomsen BS, Rasmussen JP. Effect of methylprednisolone on endotoxemia and complement activation during cardiac surgery. J Cardiothorac Anesth 1989;3:544–9.

131. Boscoe MJ, Yewdall VM, Thompson MA, Cameron JS. Complement activation during cardiopulmonary bypass: quantitative study of effects of methylprednisolone and pulsatile flow. Br Med J 1983;287:1747–50.

132. Fosse E, Mollnes TE, Osterud A, Aasen AO. Effects of methylprednisolone on complement activation and leukocyte counts during cardiopulmonary bypass. Scand J Thorac Cardiovasc Surg 1987;21:255–61.

133. Ferries LH, Marx JJ, Ray JF. The effect of methylprednisolone on complement activation during cardiopulmonary bypass. J Extra Corpor Technol 1984;16:83–8.

134. Tennenberg SD, Bailey WW, Cotta LA, et al. The effects of methylprednisolone on complement-mediated neutrophil activation during cardiopulmonary bypass. Surgery 1986;100:134–42.

135. Kawamura T, Inada K, Okada H, et al. Methylprednisolone inhibits increase of interleukin 8 and 6 during open heart surgery. Can J Anaesth 1995;42:399–403.

136. Tassani P, Richter JA, Barankay A, et al. Does high-dose methylprednisolone in aprotinin-treated patients attenuate the systemic inflammatory response during coronary artery bypass grafting procedures? J Cardiothorac Vasc Anesth 1999;13:165–72.

137. Chaney MA, Nikolov MP, Blakeman BP, et al. Hemodynamic effects of methylprednisolone in patients undergoing cardiac operation and early extubation. Ann Thorac Surg 1999;67:1006–11.

138. Chaney MA, Durazo-Arvizu RA, Nikolov MP, et al. Methylprednisolone does not benefit patients undergoing coronary artery bypass grafting and early tracheal extubation. J Thorac Cardiovasc Surg 2001;121:561–9.

139. Sussman MS, Bulkley GB. Oxygen-derived free radicals in reperfusion injury. Methods Enzymol 1990;186:711–23.

140. Starkopf J, Zilmer K, Vihalemm T, et al. Time course of oxidative stress during open-heart surgery. Scand J Thorac Cardiovasc Surg 1995;29:181–6.

141. Westhuyzen J, Cochrane AD, Tesar PJ, et al. Effect of preoperative supplementation with alpha-tocopherol and ascorbic acid on myocardial injury in patients undergoing cardiac operations. J Thorac Cardiovasc Surg 1997; 113:942–8.

142. Clermont G, Vergely C, Jazayeri S, et al. Systemic free radical activation is a major event involved in myocardial oxidative stress related to cardiopulmonary bypass. Anesthesiology 2002;96:80–7.

143. Fantone JC, Ward PA. Role of oxygen-derived free radicals and metabolites in leukocyte-dependent inflammatory reactions. Am J Pathol 1982;107:395–418.

144. Rao PS, Cohen MV, Mueller HS. Production of free radicals and lipid peroxides in early experimental myocardial ischemia. J Mol Cell Cardiol 1983;15:713–6.

145. Cavarocchi NC, England MD, Schaff HV, et al. Oxygen free radical generation during cardiopulmonary bypass: correlation with complement activation. Circulation 1986;74:III130–3.

146. Hochstein P, Jain SK. Association of lipid peroxidation and polymerization of membrane proteins with erythrocyte aging. Fed Proc 1981;40:183–8.

147. Weiss SJ. Tissue destruction by neutrophils. N Engl J Med 1989;320:365–76.

148. Kettle AJ, Winterbourn CC. Superoxide modulates the activity of myeloperoxidase and optimizes the production of hypochlorous acid. Biochem J 1988;252:529–36.

149. Oktar GL, Sinci V, Kalaycioglu S, et al. Biochemical and hemodynamic effects of ascorbic acid and alpha-tocopherol in coronary artery surgery. Scand J Clin Lab Invest 2001;61:621–9.

150. Tangney CC, Hankins JS, Murtaugh MA, Piccione W Jr. Plasma vitamins E and C concentrations of adult patients during cardiopulmonary bypass. J Am Coll Nutr 1998;17:162–70.

151. Klein HH, Pich S, Lindert S, et al. Combined treatment with vitamins E and C in experimental myocardial infarction in pigs. Am Heart J 1989;118:667–73.

152. Massey KD, Burton KP. Alpha-tocopherol attenuates myocardial membrane-related alterations resulting from ischemia and reperfusion. Am J Physiol 1989;256: H1192–9.

153. Butterworth J, Legault C, Stump DA, et al. A randomized, blinded trial of the antioxidant pegorgotein: no reduction in neuropsychological deficits, inotropic drug support, or

myocardial ischemia after coronary artery bypass surgery. J Cardiothorac Vasc Anesth 1999;13:690–4.

154. Jaski BE, Fifer MA, Wright RF, et al. Positive inotropic and vasodilator actions of milrinone in patients with severe congestive heart failure. Dose-response relationships and comparison to nitroprusside. J Clin Invest 1985;75: 643–9.

155. Konstam MA, Cody RJ. Short-term use of intravenous milrinone for heart failure. Am J Cardiol 1995;75:822–6.

156. Monrad ES, Baim DS, Smith HS, Lanoue AS. Milrinone, dobutamine, and nitroprusside: comparative effects on hemodynamics and myocardial energetics in patients with severe congestive heart failure. Circulation 1986; 73:III168–74.

157. Yoshimura T, Usami E, Kurita C, et al. Effect of theophylline on the production of interleukin-1 beta, tumor necrosis factor-alpha, and interleukin-8 by human peripheral blood mononuclear cells. Biol Pharm Bull 1995;18:1405–8.

158. Seamon KB, Padgett W, Daly JW. Forskolin: unique diterpene activator of adenylate cyclase in membranes and in intact cells. Proc Natl Acad Sci U S A 1981;78:3363–7.

159. Verghese MW, McConnell RT, Strickland AB, et al. Differential regulation of human monocyte-derived TNF alpha and IL-1 beta by type IV cAMP-phosphodiesterase (cAMP-PDE) inhibitors. J Pharmacol Exp Ther 1995;272:1313–20.

160. Bergman MR, Holycross BJ. Pharmacological modulation of myocardial tumor necrosis factor alpha production by phosphodiesterase inhibitors. J Pharmacol Exp Ther 1996;279:247–54.

161. Takeuchi K, del Nido PJ, Ibrahim AE, et al. Vesnarinone and amrinone reduce the systemic inflammatory response syndrome. J Thorac Cardiovasc Surg 1999; 117:375–82.

162. Hayashida N, Tomoeda H, Oda T, et al. Inhibitory effect of milrinone on cytokine production after cardiopulmonary bypass. Ann Thorac Surg 1999;68:1661–7.

163. Yamaura K, Okamoto H, Akiyoshi K, et al. Effect of low-dose milrinone on gastric intramucosal pH and systemic inflammation after hypothermic cardiopulmonary bypass. J Cardiothorac Vasc Anesth 2001;15:197–203.

164. Yamaura K, Akiyoshi K, Irita K, et al. Effects of Olprinone, a new phosphodiesterase inhibitor, on gastric intramucosal acidosis and systemic inflammatory responses following hypothermic cardiopulmonary bypass. Acta Anaesthesiol Scand 2001;45:427–34.

165. Hayashida N, Chihara S, Tayama E, et al. Antiinflammatory effects of colforsin dapropate hydrochloride, a novel water-soluble forskolin derivative. Ann Thorac Surg 2001;71:1931–8.

166. Hosono M, Takahira T, Fujita A, et al. Cardiovascular and adenylate cyclase stimulant properties of NKH477, a novel water-soluble forskolin derivative. J Cardiovasc Pharmacol 1992;19:625–34.

167. Mori M, Takeuchi M, Takaoka H, et al. Effect of NKH477, a new water-soluble forskolin derivative, on arterial-ventricular coupling and mechanical energy transduction in patients with left ventricular systolic dysfunction: comparison with dobutamine. J Cardiovasc Pharmacol 1994;24:310–6.

168. Ustunsoy H, Sivrikoz MC, Bakir K, et al. The inhibition of pro-inflammatory cytokines with pentoxifylline in the cardiopulmonary bypass lung. Respir Med 2002;96:275–9.

169. Cremer J, Struber M, Wittwer T, et al. Off-bypass coronary bypass grafting via minithoracotomy using mechanical epicardial stabilization. Ann Thorac Surg 1997;63:S79–83.

170. Ascione R, Lloyd CT, Gomes WJ, et al. Beating versus arrested heart revascularization: evaluation of myocardial function in a prospective randomized study. Eur J Cardiothorac Surg 1999;15:685–90.

171. Buffolo E, de Andrade CS, Branco JN, et al. Coronary artery bypass grafting without cardiopulmonary bypass. Ann Thorac Surg 1996;61:63–6.

172. Pfister AJ, Zaki MS, Garcia JM, et al. Coronary artery bypass without cardiopulmonary bypass. Ann Thorac Surg 1992;54:1085–91; discussion 1091–2.

173. Struber M, Cremer JT, Gohrbandt B, et al. Human cytokine responses to coronary artery bypass grafting with and without cardiopulmonary bypass. Ann Thorac Surg 1999;68:1330–5.

174. Gu YJ, Mariani MA, van Oeveren W, et al. Reduction of the inflammatory response in patients undergoing minimally invasive coronary artery bypass grafting. Ann Thorac Surg 1998;65:420–4.

175. Diegeler A, Doll N, Rauch T, et al. Humoral immune response during coronary artery bypass grafting: a comparison of limited approach, "off-pump" technique, and conventional cardiopulmonary bypass. Circulation 2000;102:III95–100.

176. Wildhirt SM, Schulze C, Schulz C, et al. Reduction of systemic and cardiac adhesion molecule expression after off-pump versus conventional coronary artery bypass grafting. Shock 2001;16 Suppl 1:55–9.

177. Schulze C, Conrad N, Schutz A, et al. Reduced expression of systemic proinflammatory cytokines after off-pump versus conventional coronary artery bypass grafting. Thorac Cardiovasc Surg 2000;48:364–9.

178. Hernandez F, Cohn WE, Baribeau YR, et al. In-hospital outcomes of off-pump versus on-pump coronary artery bypass procedures: a multicenter experience. Ann Thorac Surg 2001;72:1528–33; discussion 1533–4.

179. Ascione R, Lloyd CT, Underwood MJ, et al. Economic outcome of off-pump coronary artery bypass surgery: a prospective randomized study. Ann Thorac Surg 1999; 68:2237–42.

180. Al-Ruzzeh S, George S, Yacoub M, Amrani M. The clinical outcome of off-pump coronary artery bypass surgery in the elderly patients. Eur J Cardiothorac Surg 2001;20: 1152–6.

181. Berglin E, Sandin O, Winstedt P, William-Olsson G. Extracorporeal circulation without an oxygenator in coronary bypass grafting. J Thorac Cardiovasc Surg 1986; 92:306–8.

182. Drew CE, Anderson IM. Profound hypothermia in cardiac surgery. Report of three cases. Lancet 1959;1:748–50.

183. Glenville B, Ross D. Coronary artery surgery with patient's lungs as oxygenator. Lancet 1986;2:1005–6.

184. Richter JA, Meisner H, Tassani P, et al. Drew–Anderson technique attenuates systemic inflammatory response syndrome and improves respiratory function after coronary artery bypass grafting. Ann Thorac Surg 2000;69:77–83.

185. Henson PM, Johnston RB Jr. Tissue injury in inflammation. Oxidants, proteinases, and cationic proteins. J Clin Invest 1987;79:669–74.

186. Malech HL, Gallin JI. Current concepts: immunology. Neutrophils in human diseases. N Engl J Med 1987;317:687–94.

187. Zahler S, Massoudy P, Hartl H, et al. Acute cardiac inflammatory responses to postischemic reperfusion during cardiopulmonary bypass. Cardiovasc Res 1999;41:722–30.

188. Butler J, Parker D, Pillai R, et al. Effect of cardiopulmonary bypass on systemic release of neutrophil elastase and tumor necrosis factor. J Thorac Cardiovasc Surg 1993;105:25–30.

189. Borowiec JW, Hagman L, Totterman TH, et al. Circulating cytokines and granulocyte-derived enzymes during complex heart surgery. A clinical study with special reference to heparin-coating of cardiopulmonary bypass circuits. Scand J Thorac Cardiovasc Surg 1995;29:167–74.

190. Faymonville ME, Pincemail J, Duchateau J, et al. Myeloperoxidase and elastase as markers of leukocyte activation during cardiopulmonary bypass in humans. J Thorac Cardiovasc Surg 1991;102:309–17.

191. Diepenhorst P, Sprokholt R, Prins HK. Removal of leukocytes from whole blood and erythrocyte suspensions by filtration through cotton wool. I. Filtration technique. Vox Sang 1972;23:308–20.

192. Gourlay T, Fleming J, Taylor KM. Laboratory evaluation of the Pall LG6 leukocyte depleting arterial line filter. Perfusion 1992;7:131–40.

193. Ilton MK, Langton PE, Taylor ML, et al. Differential expression of neutrophil adhesion molecules during coronary artery surgery with cardiopulmonary bypass. J Thorac Cardiovasc Surg 1999;118:930–7.

194. Jordan JE, Zhao ZQ, Vinten-Johansen J. The role of neutrophils in myocardial ischemia-reperfusion injury. Cardiovasc Res 1999;43:860–78.

195. Ichihara T, Yasuura K, Maseki T, et al. The effects of using a leukocyte removal filter during cold blood cardioplegia. Surg Today 1994;24:966–72.

196. Hayashi Y, Sawa Y, Nishimura M, et al. Clinical evaluation of leukocyte-depleted blood cardioplegia for pediatric open heart operation. Ann Thorac Surg 2000;69:1914–9.

197. Sawa Y, Matsuda H, Shimazaki Y, et al. Evaluation of leukocyte-depleted terminal blood cardioplegic solution in patients undergoing elective and emergency coronary artery bypass grafting. J Thorac Cardiovasc Surg 1994;108:1125–31.

198. Roth M, Kraus B, Scheffold T, et al. The effect of leukocyte-depleted blood cardioplegia in patients with severe left ventricular dysfunction: a randomized, double-blind study. J Thorac Cardiovasc Surg 2000;120:642–50.

199. Chen YF, Tsai WC, Lin CC, et al. Leukocyte depletion attenuates expression of neutrophil adhesion molecules during cardiopulmonary bypass in human beings. J Thorac Cardiovasc Surg 2002;123:218–24.

200. Chiba Y, Morioka K, Muraoka R, et al. Effects of depletion of leukocytes and platelets on cardiac dysfunction after cardiopulmonary bypass. Ann Thorac Surg 1998;65:107–13; discussion 113–4.

201. Morioka K, Muraoka R, Chiba Y, et al. Leukocyte and platelet depletion with a blood cell separator: effects on lung injury after cardiac surgery with cardiopulmonary bypass. J Thorac Cardiovasc Surg 1996;111:45–54.

202. Hurst T, Johnson D, Cujec B, et al. Depletion of activated neutrophils by a filter during cardiac valve surgery. Can J Anaesth 1997;44:131–9.

203. Mihaljevic T, Tonz M, von Segesser LK, et al. The influence of leukocyte filtration during cardiopulmonary bypass on postoperative lung function. A clinical study. J Thorac Cardiovasc Surg 1995;109:1138–45.

204. Fabbri A, Manfredi J, Piccin C, et al. Systemic leukocyte filtration during cardiopulmonary bypass. Perfusion 2001;16 Suppl:11–8.

205. Johnson D, Thomson D, Mycyk T, et al. Depletion of neutrophils by filter during aortocoronary bypass surgery transiently improves postoperative cardiorespiratory status. Chest 1995;107:1253–9.

206. Baksaas ST, Videm V, Mollnes TE, et al. Leucocyte filtration during cardiopulmonary bypass hardly changed leucocyte counts and did not influence myeloperoxidase, complement, cytokines or platelets. Perfusion 1998;13:429–36.

207. Lust RM, Bode AP, Yang L, et al. In-line leukocyte filtration during bypass. Clinical results from a randomized prospective trial. ASAIO J 1996;42:M819–22.

208. Mair P, Hoermann C, Mair J, et al. Effects of a leucocyte depleting arterial line filter on perioperative proteolytic enzyme and oxygen free radical release in patients undergoing aortocoronary bypass surgery. Acta Anaesthesiol Scand 1999;43:452–7.

209. Gu YJ, de Vries AJ, Boonstra PW, van Oeveren W. Leukocyte depletion results in improved lung function and reduced inflammatory response after cardiac surgery. J Thorac Cardiovasc Surg 1996;112:494–500.

210. Keenan HT, Thiagarajan R, Stephens KE, et al. Pulmonary function after modified venovenous ultrafiltration in infants: a prospective, randomized trial. J Thorac Cardiovasc Surg 2000;119:501–5; discussion 506–7.

211. Pearl JM, Manning PB, McNamara JL, et al. Effect of modified ultrafiltration on plasma thromboxane B_2, leukotriene B_4, and endothelin-1 in infants undergoing cardiopulmonary bypass. Ann Thorac Surg 1999;68:1369–75.

212. Shimpo H, Shimamoto A, Sawamura Y, et al. Ultrafiltration of the priming blood before cardiopulmonary bypass attenuates inflammatory response and improves postoperative clinical course in pediatric patients. Shock 2001;16 Suppl 1:51–4.

213. Elliott MJ. Ultrafiltration and modified ultrafiltration in pediatric open heart operations. Ann Thorac Surg 1993;56:1518–22.

214. Tassani P, Richter JA, Eising GP, et al. Influence of combined zero-balanced and modified ultrafiltration on the systemic inflammatory response during coronary artery bypass grafting. J Cardiothorac Vasc Anesth 1999;13:285–91.

215. Boga M, Islamoglu, Badak I, et al. The effects of modified hemofiltration on inflammatory mediators and cardiac performance in coronary artery bypass grafting. Perfusion 2000;15:143–50.

216. Grunenfelder J, Zund G, Schoeberlein A, et al. Modified ultrafiltration lowers adhesion molecule and cytokine

levels after cardiopulmonary bypass without clinical relevance in adults. Eur J Cardiothorac Surg 2000;17:77–83.

217. Luciani GB, Menon T, Vecchi B, et al. Modified ultrafiltration reduces morbidity after adult cardiac operations: a prospective, randomized clinical trial. Circulation 2001;104:I253–9.

218. Karin M. The regulation of AP-1 activity by mitogen-activated protein kinases. J Biol Chem 1995;270:16483–6.

219. Michel MC, Li Y, Heusch G. Mitogen-activated protein kinases in the heart. Naunyn Schmiedebergs Arch Pharmacol 2001;363:245–66.

220. Hai T, Wolfgang CD, Marsee DK, et al. ATF3 and stress responses. Gene Expr 1999;7:321–35.

221. Silverman ES, Collins T. Pathways of Egr-1–mediated gene transcription in vascular biology. Am J Pathol 1999;154:665–70.

222. Parry JV, Perry KR, Harbour S, et al. False negativity by an anti-HIV assay kit (IMx 8B32) and evaluation of its replacement (IMx 8C98). J Med Virol 1998;56:138–44.

223. Ghosh S, Karin M. Missing pieces in the NF-kappaB puzzle. Cell 2002;109 Suppl:S81–96.

224. Boyle EM Jr, Pohlman TH, Johnson MC, Verrier ED. Endothelial cell injury in cardiovascular surgery: the systemic inflammatory response. Ann Thorac Surg 1997;63:277–84.

225. Verrier ED, Morgan EN. Endothelial response to cardiopulmonary bypass surgery. Ann Thorac Surg 1998;66:S17–9; discussion S25–8.

CHAPTER 8

PREVENTION OF NEUROLOGIC INJURY DURING CARDIAC AND GREAT VESSEL SURGERY

JOSE P. GARCIA, MD, VENKATARAMANA VIJAY, MD, JEFFREY P. GOLD, MD

Neurologic injury has long been associated with cardiac and major vascular surgery. As surgeons and neurologists have come to better understand the etiology and management of these complications, the surgical armamentarium to prevent these injuries has grown rapidly. This chapter reviews the nature and etiology of these perioperative events and also reviews what is currently accepted as meaningful preventive and therapeutic modalities. This review is best divided between those procedures that employ the technology known as *cardiopulmonary bypass* and those that may be done without this technology.

Minimally invasive procedures have been marketed and popularized across the country and around the world. In many instances, what is really meant is small incision or port access surgery, rather than the true concept of minimally invasive or less traumatic. If the verb *to invade* truly means to conquer or to plunder, less traumatic or minimally invasive procedures should be those associated with the least amount of time required for long-term recovery and with the development of the most functional status as time passes. Consequently, prevention and management of all neurologic sequelae of cardiac and major vascular procedures is integral to the concept of minimally invasive surgery.

Cardiopulmonary bypass (CPB) has become the mainstay of cardiac surgery since its introduction by Gibbon in 1953. Until recently, use of CPB was synonymous with all cardiac surgery and, in particular, coronary artery bypass grafting (CABG), a procedure performed more than 300,000 times per year in the United States and more than 700,000 times per year around the world.[1] In addition, CPB is used for valve surgery and other complex adult and pediatric cardiac procedures, increasing the total to more than 2,000,000 procedures per year. In addition to the cost, complexity, and high degree of technical support associated with CPB, there has been mounting evidence of some degree of end-organ damage associated with its use. While most patients demonstrate no detectable clinical sequelae, for a minority of patients the results can be devastating.[1–3] Neurologic injury associated with cardiac surgery is not an uncommon complication. Varying degrees of manifestation have been recognized since the early days of CPB-based cardiac procedures.[4,5] Changes in cerebral flow, cerebral reperfusion injury, embolic events, and CPB-induced whole-body inflammatory response are the most commonly recognized etiologies of these injuries.[6] Neurologic incidents suffered with cardiac surgery can be grouped into three categories: stroke, cognitive defects, and encephalopathy. These episodes are well documented. The development of these complications is not limited to the field of cardiac surgery, and much of what we know about the etiology, course, treatment, and prevention of these complications has been obtained from patients undergoing other types of surgery, including trauma, orthopedic, and vascular surgery.[7,8]

Elderly patients (more than 70 years of age) are more susceptible to neurologic complications than are other patients. With the escalation in the number of octogenarians undergoing coronary artery revascularization and valvular replacement/repair, several studies show an increase in neurologic complications in these patients.[9] The overall mortality associated with cardiac surgery has declined over the last 20 years. This can be attributed to several factors, including better techniques for anesthesia, CPB, and myocardial preservation. Similar advances allowing for enhanced cerebral protection have not been accomplished, even though improvements in the CPB circuit have been made. The recent use of off-pump technology for coronary revascularization shows promise in decreasing the neurologic complications accompanying the traditional CPB approach. Economic issues affecting health care are an impetus for research in the prevention of these complications, which can be a significant financial burden on the patient, family, and the health care institution. Current research is focused on determining the incidence and the clinical significance of varying degrees of neurologic injury.[10]

To better understand the neurologic complications associated with cardiac surgery, we first must define these sequelae.[3] A stroke is a focal motor, sensory, or visual deficit lasting more than 24 h. A stroke can be further characterized as clinical injury noted on examination or a structural injury noted only on radiologic studies such as computed tomography (CT), magnetic resonance imaging (MRI), or positron emission tomography (PET) scanning. A cognitive injury is an alteration in thought, behavior, or consciousness, with or without notable focal sensory or motor neurologic signs. Alterations in psychomotor, linguistic, or memory functions are all forms of the separate domains of perioperative cognitive injury. Finally, encephalopathy is a more global injury characterized by obtundation, drowsiness, lethargy, or delirium without focal sensory or motor findings on physical examination or classic structural changes on CT, MRI, or PET scans.

Stroke

The incidence of stroke is largely dependent on known risk factors and the procedure performed. Approximately 5% of patients undergoing isolated coronary revascularization suffer stroke, while incidents increase to an average of 8% for isolated valve surgery.[11–13] Patients undergoing combined CABG-valve surgery have an 18% average incidence of stroke. The mortality for patients suffering a stroke following cardiac surgery varies between 22 and 36%. The overall incidence for all cardiac procedures varies between 4.7 and 5.2%.[14,15] Stroke in patients undergoing open heart surgery is usually apparent immediately after the procedure, with > 90% documented within 24 h postoperatively.[3,16,17] In addition, > 65% of patients will have multiple new cerebral infarcts on radiographic scanning. Studies show that the average post–CABG stroke patient has infarcts within six separate vascular territories of the brain.[18,19]

During the last decade, more octogenarians than ever before have presented for open heart surgery. Several studies have documented a significantly higher incidence of stroke in this patient population.[20,21] Patients younger than 60 years old who are undergoing CABG with CPB have a < 1% chance of stroke, whereas patients who are older than 80 years of age have a 9% chance of stroke.[21–23] In addition to age, several other risk factors increase the incidence of stroke. Severe aortic atheroma, as seen on transesophageal echocardiography (TEE), predisposes patients to a much higher risk of stroke.[24–26] Patients who display limited or no atheroma have a < 2% incidence of stroke, whereas patients with a grade IV or V aorta have a stroke rate as high as 40%. Of patients with carotid lesions < 50% have an incidence of perioperative stroke of ≤ 1%. Patients with significant carotid lesions, > 90%, have a stroke incidence of 6.5%. Note, however, that perioperative strokes are rarely related to the carotid stenosis.[27,28] The majority of patients with carotid disease also have underlying aortic disease, which is the most common source of embolic strokes. Studies show that patients with poor collateral cerebral flow as documented by ocular plethysmography have a higher stroke incidence (7.2%) than do patients with normal collateral (< 2%). Lastly, patients with a previous hemispheric stroke or a large infarct are at a higher risk of having a new stroke or expansion of the previous stroke.[29]

Cognitive Deficits

The incidence of neurocognitive deficits following open heart surgery with CPB has been a recent topic of interest and research. In one landmark study, Shaw and associates prospectively examined 312 patients undergoing CABG with CPB, employing standardized cognitive tests administered preoperatively and at 1 week and 6 months postoperatively. The overall stroke rate was 1.1%; however, 79% of patients manifested significant decrease in cognitive performance postoperatively. Similar results have been documented in other studies.[9,30,31]

Elderly patients with multiple comorbidities can now undergo cardiac surgery with low mortality rates, although they remain at a high risk of experiencing neurocognitive deficits. Many physicians overlook the significance of cognitive decline in the postoperative period because the deficit is only transient in a substantial number of patients. When formally tested, linguistic, memory, and psychomotor function reveal alterations in a pattern characteristic of cardiac surgery.[19,31,32] Longitudinal studies show that the severity of significant cognitive deficits subsides over time, but patients may have long-term cognitive decline and reduced level of overall cognitive functioning. Newman found that cognitive deficits are evident in approximately 53% of patients at discharge; the incidence decreased to 36% at 6 weeks and to 24% at 6 months. Five years after surgery, the incidence of cognitive decline was 42%.[9,30] Psychomotor function appears to be more affected than memory functions, whereas linguistic function is the best preserved. The incidences of psychomotor and cognitive abnormalities depend to a large extent on the definitions within the parameters of psychometric testing.[33] The long-term significance of these subtle measured changes is unknown. What is clear to all is that patients coming to the operating room with significant degrees of cognitive dysfunction are at the highest risk of perioperative deterioration and of long-term progressive deterioration. This is best demonstrated by patients diagnosed with preoperative dementia states, which states are commonly exacerbated following surgery. Recent studies demonstrate a dramatic reduction in the incidence of neurocognitive deficit when patients undergo off-pump coronary revascularization. Although the stroke incidence may not be significantly different, off-pump patients have negligible cognitive impairment when compared to an incidence as high as 90% in patients subjected to CPB.[34]

Encephalopathy

Encephalopathy is seen in 30 to 35% of patients undergoing cardiac procedures.[3] The most common presentation is confusion without focal neurologic deficits. Radiographic imaging is usually negative, although cerebral edema may be seen on MRI. Most symptoms peak within 24 h of surgery, and only 10% of patients have symptoms by the fourth postoperative day. Encephalopathy is not associated with existing aortic atherosclerotic disease, but it is related to age, alcoholism, narcotics, sedatives, and metabolic disturbances.[19] Encephalopathy is also associated with various types of preoperative substance abuse syndromes, metabolic conditions, and advanced dementia states.

Cause and Impact of Neurologic Injury

The etiologies of neurologic injury have been well defined, and there is extensive literature in this area. The most common cause of injury following CPB is embolization of atherosclerotic debris from the ascending aorta or the aortic arch.[35,36] Other factors contributing to neurologic injury include cerebral hypoperfusion, focal vasomotor spasm, cerebral reperfusion injury, CPB-induced inflammatory response, and toxic and metabolic effects. Research efforts have focused on identifying markers in blood and cerebrospinal fluid (CSF) correlating with neurologic injury. Well-established markers include cerebral spinal fluid lactate, adenylate kinase, and neuron-specific enolase. Recently, serum levels of S-100β have been found to correlate with adverse neurologic outcomes after cardiac surgery.[37–40] Many researchers in the field consider CSF and serum S-100β to be the "serum myocardial band isomer of creatinine phosphokinase" (MB-CPK) of neurologic tissue death. The prevalence of neurocognitive and encephalopathic alterations vary according to the complexity of the testing and the individual technician. This indicates the necessity of a reliable and objective marker correlating with neurologic injury. Objective tests allow for implementation of new interventions, especially in prospective trials.[6]

Neurologic injury, whether it be stroke or cognitive deficits, is most commonly caused by embolization during or following cardiopulmonary bypass.[41–43] Although most embolic events are caused by atherosclerotic debris, other sources include air, clot, and foreign material (pledgets). Extensive data have been gathered in an effort to determine the source, frequency, and severity of embolic events.[44,45] TEE and transcranial Doppler imaging of the middle cerebral artery are extremely useful for identifying the true nature of this problem.[24,25,46] Advanced atherosclerotic disease of the ascending aorta and transverse aortic arch are independent predictors of perioperative stroke, with incidences as high as 60%.

Numerous studies confirm the presence of embolic signals in the aorta and cerebral circulation in almost all patients undergoing cardiac surgery. In a prospective study of patients undergoing cardiac surgery with CPB, the average number of unilateral middle cerebral artery emboli detected was 535; the range was from 8 to 1,855. These emboli were correlated with vascular manipulation and were most notable following placement and release of the aortic cross-clamp (66%). Approximately half of the 535 emboli were evident within 4 min after release of the cross-clamp, and an additional 140 emboli were liberated following the partial aortic cross-clamp release. The emboli released during manipulation of the aorta are much larger than those particles that are noted randomly during the procedure, and are thought to be associated with the most significant and long-standing neurologic complications.

Attempts have been made to characterize the embolic particles in the cerebral circulation. In one study, 1,500 of the particles liberated within the first 4 min of clamp manipulation were carefully analyzed on more than 720,000 frames of echo imaging. The average embolic particle diameter was 0.8 mm, with a range from 0.3 to 2.9 mm in diameter.[47] The particle volume that corresponded to these diameters ranged from 0.01 to 12.5 mm³. A full 28% of the embolic particles associated with aortic manipulation had a diameter larger than 1 mm. This facilitated the calculation of the average aortic embolic load of particulate material, which was approximately 3.7 cc. This aortic embolic load ranged from 0.6 to 11.2 cc. The percentage of the total aortic embolic load entering the cerebral circulation varied from case to case, ranging from 3.9 to 18%. Therefore, the mean cerebral embolic load was 276 mm³ per patient, with a range of 60 to 510 mm³.

Significantly, the number of cerebral emboli relates not only to neurologic events but also to length of hospital stay and to cardiac events. The increase in length of stay is independent of any cardiac or neurologic complications. In a cohort of 82 patients prospectively evaluated with transcranial Doppler, patients who experienced a perioperative stroke had an average of 449 intraoperative cerebral emboli. Patients who did not have a perioperative stroke averaged 169 emboli. Patients who suffered myocardial infarction, shock, or ventricular tachycardia had an average cerebral embolic load of 393 emboli as compared to an average load of 163 emboli in those patients without any similar cardiac complications.

The length of hospital stay in patients without any major cardiac or neurologic complication increases from

8.6 days in those having fewer than 100 total emboli to 13.5 days in those patients having 100 to 300 cerebral emboli. The hospital stay increases to more than 40 days in patients having more than 500 detected cerebral emboli. These emboli, as determined by echo Doppler of the dominant one of the middle cerebral arteries, are frequently related to neurologic injuries as well as to cardiac and other extracardiac manifestations, which prolongs hospitalization and slows recovery.

These and numerous other intraoperative and postmortem studies reinforce the notion that aortic atherosclerosis in the setting of cardiac surgery is a predictor for associated cerebral embolization.[48] These emboli are particularly related to clamp manipulation of the aorta, which releases the greatest number, highest volume, and largest sizes of emboli.[49] The emboli are associated with major neurologic and cardiac complications, with prolonged hospitalization and a slow and frequently incomplete recovery. Thus, it is important to better understand the mechanism of release and transmission of these atherosclerotic particles and to develop strategies to alter their devastating sequelae.

Prevention of Neurologic Injuries

Numerous strategies have been proposed in an effort to decrease the risk and incidence of perioperative stroke, neurocognitive deficits, and encephalopathic alterations associated with cardiac surgery using CPB or techniques involving manipulation of the aorta. There is extensive evidence-based literature in this area, and several important studies are discussed here.[50–52] In addition, many strategies have been proposed, which are based on anecdotal cases that remain unproven. The areas of intervention can be divided into the preoperative, intraoperative, and postoperative phases.

Careful evaluation of the preoperative patient is critical in decreasing perioperative stroke incidence. Two important factors of the evaluation are patient selection and procedure selection.[53,54] The presence of advanced age, long-standing diabetes mellitus (especially insulin-dependent), long-standing and poorly controlled hypertension, chronic renal insufficiency, and advanced peripheral vascular disease are independent predictors of a high incidence of perioperative stroke or neurocognitive injury.[30] Patients who possess the genetic marker for apolipoprotein E4, as well as patients who have significant low albumin due to chronic malnutrition or chronic debilitation, are at a higher risk of perioperative stroke. As previously mentioned, patients with advanced atherosclerosis of the aorta, especially those with mobile plaque components, are at extremely high risk of embolic stroke.[24,25,46,54–56] Severe aortic disease is commonly associated with the other risk factors discussed above. The degree of the cardiac disease, the patient's overall condition, and possible nonsurgical alternatives should all be carefully considered in the preoperative cardiac surgical patient evaluation process.[57,58]

The relationship between cerebrovascular disease (CVD) and postoperative neurologic dysfunction in the cardiac surgery patient is of major interest. The independent risk factor of high-grade carotid artery disease and/or prior stroke has been described as an important predictor.[27,59,60] Studies have reported on the relationship between the severity of angiographically defined carotid stenosis and the risk of perioperative stroke. In patients with unilateral carotid stenosis (50–90%) and without symptoms of cerebrovascular disease, there was no increase in the risk of perioperative troke asscoaietd with coronary revascularization procedures. A later study showed that cardiac patients with 90% or greater carotid stenosis had a greater risk of ipsilateral stroke (6.2%) than did patients with 50 to 90% occlusion of the internal carotid artery.[61] Symptomatic patients, or patients with signs suggestive of cerebrovascular disease, should be referred for laboratory assessment of the cerebral circulation. Because the risk of stroke in a patient with a history of a transient ischemic attack (TIA) who undergoes a carotid endarterectomy (CEA) is 3 to 7% and the absolute risk of perioperative stroke associated with coronary revascularization is 5 to 7%, a decision to perform a prophylactic or combined CABG/CEA must be carefully considered. The approach to the cardiac patient with significant carotid disease (occlusion greater than 80%) has been extensively debated. Some patients with symptomatic carotid disease and high-grade coronary artery disease or aortic stenosis have been shown to do better with a combined procedure. Other subsets of patients with combined carotid and coronary disease are approached differently according to institutional philosophy.

The selection of the procedure affords the surgeon the ability to markedly decrease the risk of neurologic injury. First, there is now evidence that patients undergoing off-pump procedures have a significantly decreased risk of neurocognitive deficits (especially the elderly).[23,34,62–65] Coronary revascularization patients who are at increased risk for neurologic injury should be considered off-pump candidates. The mere cannulation of the aorta along with CPB is a risk factor and should be avoided if possible. Furthermore, procedures that omit aortic clamping, either cross- or partial clamping, will decrease the risks of neurologic problems. Arguably, the safest operation for coronary revascularization in octogenarians may be left internal mammary artery (LIMA)–radial vein composites with sequential anastomosis, especially if the posterior descending artery need not be bypassed. This approach has the added benefits of no CPB and no manipulation of the aorta or great vessels.

Other intraoperative techniques that may help to decrease neurologic injury are patient positioning and monitoring. Transient periods of deep Trendelenburg's position and left/right side up are reported to impact on preventing neurologic injury. Intraoperative tools that are often used to determine aortic pathology prior to cannulation include TEE and/or epiaortic imaging. Both techniques are also useful in identifying other cardiac pathology, especially left/right shunt, which could prove to be a source of air embolus potentially leading to neurologic injury. Routine preoperative evaluations include biplane chest x-rays, which often can demonstrate a calcified aortic arch. CT and fluoroscopy are extremely useful in detecting the aortic calcification. Only TEE, epiaortic imaging, and intravascular ultrasonography (IVUS) can accurately reveal the severity and extent of the intravascular atherosclerosis.[66–72] The presence of atherosclerotic aortic wall disease exceeding 10 mm or any mobile component of the plaque disease are critical findings with regard to the planning and safe completion of any procedure employing cardiopulmonary bypass. Inspection and manual palpation of the aorta can be extremely unreliable because it does not provide detail regarding plaque thickness or luminal mobility of plaque components. This is especially true when there is diffuse, soft, intramural plaque material. Arterial pressure monitoring is critical to ensure ideal blood pressure management before, during, and after CPB. Transcranial carotid Doppler ultrasonography and mixed venous and cerebral oxygen saturation meters have been used predominantly as research tools.[31,54,55,73–75]

Cardiopulmonary Bypass and Neurologic Injury

Several factors associated with CPB are implicated in determining the incidence of neurologic injury following cardiac surgery. Aortic cannulation (including type of cannula), bypass apparatus, arterial line filters, temperature, pH, pump flows, and duration of CPB can have a direct effect on morbidity. In addition, techniques often employed, including hemodilution, deep hypothermia, and de-airing, can play a major role in determining the incidence of neurologic injury following cardiac surgery.

Aortic cannulation is the cause of many cerebral vascular emboli; this has been confirmed by Doppler studies. The type of cannula (on-end-hole, side-hole, or "lighthouse-tipped" cannulas) and the material of the cannula (which can be either rigid plastic, soft plastic, or metal) have been advocated in different ways to minimize the incidence of perioperative stroke. The site of arterial cannulation, whether aortic or femoral, is not protective of stroke. Femoral cannulation can create a "sandblast" effect in atherosclerotic regions of the abdominal and thoracic aorta, which can be as diseased as the ascending aorta. Some investigators advocate the cannulation of the innominate or subclavian artery, either directly or with an intervening graft, in patients with severe aortic atherosclerosis. The cannula tip can be advanced into the thoracic aorta where any embolic "sandblasting" can be directed away from the cerebral circulation. It is impor-

tant to note that the subclavian artery can be rather fragile and that approximately 30% of subclavian arteries will have atherosclerotic disease if the proximal aorta is diseased. Judicious selection of target vessels for cardiopulmonary bypass inflow cannulation has been successful and reliable in otherwise high-risk patients.

In addition to emboli generated during aortic instrumentation, the type of CPB equipment can also affect the embolic load delivered to the brain. Centrifugal pumps seem to be favored over roller and other pumps. Using membrane instead of bubble oxygenators produces lower volumes of microparticulate air as measured by placing ultrasonic transducers over the arterial inflow cannula. The delivery of emboli into the cerebral microcirculation, documented by transcranial Doppler, is much greater with the bubble than with the membrane oxygenator. Arterial line filters have been advocated to minimize embolic events. These filters are effective in decreasing the embolic load, with the 20 mm type being more effective than a 40 mm filter (Padayachee). Arterial line filters can remove emboli material from the CPB circuit as well as from the cardiotomy suction reservoirs and venous drainage systems. The use of cardiotomy suction, even with arterial line filtration, is associated with a reported incidence of neurologic injury caused by the blood-air interface that is associated with characteristic postmortem histopathologic changes in the microvasculature of the brain in clinical and laboratory research environments. The lipid and debris-laden material that is suctioned from the pericardial well is not completely filtered and forms microscopic particulate emboli that cause diffuse and irreversible neurologic injury. Therefore, the minimization of cardiotomy suction and the use of quality filters appear to be very important. Arterial line leukocyte filtration that is used to reduce the overall perioperative leukocyte count is associated with a blunted inflammatory response to CPB. These types of leukoreduction filters appear to reduce the inflammatory neurologic components of bypass and embolization. Consequently, they have been anecdotally advocated to reduce the incidence and severity of stroke and other perioperative neurologic events.

There are no studies defining the optimal pump flow during CPB for patients undergoing either closed or open cardiac procedures. Some studies advocate high mean flow rates and a mean arterial pressure (MAP) between 70 and 90 mm Hg. The ideal pump flow provides adequate oxygen delivery without excess cerebral perfusion and the associated embolic load. It has been shown that with CPB at moderate hypothermia, normocapnia, nonpulsatile blood flow, and a MAP between 45 and 70 mm Hg, variation of pump flow between 1.0 and 2.0 L/min/m^2 did not alter cerebral blood flow.[76] Although not universally accepted, hypertensive patients appear to be better with higher MAPs on CPB.[77,78] Some investigators advocate the use of heparin-bonded tubing and pulsatile flow to reduce stroke, but this has not been widely accepted. In addition, there is some evidence that prolonged CPB duration may be a greater risk factor for neurologic dysfunction.[79]

Metabolic parameters controlled during CPB and postoperatively are extremely important. pH management (alpha stat vs pH stat) during periods of moderate and profound hypothermic circulation, as well as during circulatory arrest, is extremely important. Neurologic deficits are more commonly detected in patients who are managed with pH stat techniques than in patients who are managed with alpha stat techniques. Temperature-uncorrected blood-gas management techniques are preferable in adult patients undergoing hypothermic CPB.

Deep hypothermic circulatory arrest and low-flow CPB have been investigated intensively and are recognized as associated with all three major types of neurologic injury. Optimal temperatures, duration of arrest, cooling/rewarming rates, and use of neuroprotective medications (steroids and barbiturates and serum protease inhibitors) have been debated. Meticulous attention to warming and cooling rates and the avoidance of hypothermic CPB may prevent abnormal cerebral perfusion and the intense vasomotor spasm that can be associated with rapid changes in temperature.[80,81] The role of retrograde cerebral perfusion in cooling the central nervous system, providing a degree of neuroprotective benefit during the circulatory arrest period, and washing debris from extensively diseased aortas during complex reconstruction has been well debated.[82–85] The avoidance of hyperglycemic and hypoglycemic states, especially in long-standing diabetic patients and in neonates and infants, is believed to be very important. Rapid flux of glucose and other osmotically active materials are considered deleterious and are to be avoided during CPB.[86]

De-airing procedures are routine prior to weaning cardiac patients from cardiopulmonary bypass. Incomplete de-airing procedures have been implicated in perioperative stroke and encephalopathic changes. Multiple positioning maneuvers, cardiac manipulations, left-heart venting techniques, and CPB-assisted maneuvers are used by surgeons. These maneuvers are performed with the patient in the Trendelenburg position. TEE can be extremely useful as an aid in performing and for confirming complete de-airing. Many surgeons use high-flow CO_2, blowing it into the cardiac field, especially with valve surgery, using mini-incisions where manual manipulations are not possible. Although there is widespread use of this technique, there is no conclusive evidence that it decreases air embolism.[87] It does, however, frequently change the appearance of the intracavitary microbubbles imaged with TEE during de-airing and anecdotally increases the speed and completeness of de-airing while TEE monitoring is ongoing. It is important to recall that the CO_2 gas is frequently suctioned into the cardiotomy and vent lines, requiring an alteration in oxygenator gas-flow mixtures and rates.

Another area of recent research is in the development of specialized cannulas and instruments. The use of soft-padded aortic clamps or endovascular clamps offers ways to minimize or prevent aortic manipulation, which is the major cause of neurologic morbidity. Some surgeons advocate the use of single aortic cross-clamp for CABG or LIMA–radial vein grafts to prevent stroke in patients with advanced ascending aortic atherosclerosis. These approaches are superior to replacing heavily calcified aortas or performing extensive endarterectomies, which are associated with a high incidence of neurologic events and the associated mortalities.

A generation of endoaortic filtration devices (Embol-X, Mountain View, California) has been developed and widely deployed in Europe and to some extent in North America during the completion of a multicenter trial. These are either freestanding devices deployed into the aorta during off-pump coronary artery bypass (OPCAB) proximal anastomosis creation or are integrated into the aortic cannula for on-pump coronary and valvular procedures. The preliminary studies all demonstrate safety of deployment and removal of the filtration device and removal of atherosclerotic debris easily visible with the human eye in virtually all of the patients in whom it has been employed. Emboli retrieval devices for angioplasty and for cerebrovascular and peripheral vascular surgery are also in various stages of development and clinical use.

Specific pharmacologic agents used during the preoperative period, during CPB, and postoperatively have been studied in an effort to minimize the intense vasospasm associated with embolic and/or hypoperfusion stroke. Anti-inflammatory and calcium-channel blocking agents have been studied as possible means to decrease neurovascular spasm.[88–90] Data suggest that the anti-inflammatory effects of the widely used hemostatic agent aprotinin (Bayer Labs), when used in high-dose (full Hammersmith) regimen, will blunt some of the neurologic sequelae of CPB.[19] The relationship of these agents to the embolic phenomena is poorly understood. Various pharmacologic strategies have been employed in an attempt to decrease the neurologic and neurocognitive impairment associated with cardiac surgery and CPB. Protective anesthetics either maintain coupling of concomitant cerebral metabolic rate for oxygen ($CMRO_2$) and cerebral blood flow (CBF), or increase CBF while markedly decreasing $CMRO_2$.

Conclusion

Stroke, neurocognitive deficits, and encephalopathic changes are common complications associated with cardiac surgery.[91,92] Various strategies and monitoring technologies have been used to better understand the nature and extent of this problem. Surgeons have developed various techniques and tools to guide prevention and therapy. Great emphasis is placed on evaluation of the ascending and transverse aorta for the extent of athero-sclerotic disease because emboli from this source is the most common etiology for stroke. Cerebral hypoperfusion, cerebral reperfusion injury, focal vasospasm, metabolic derangement, and the inflammatory response seen with CPB are implicated in neurologic injury.

Preoperative evaluation and a well-planned operation are key if neurologic injury is to be prevented. Several risk factors are associated with a high incidence of neurologic events following cardiac surgery. Once these factors are identified, the operation should be tailored to reduce the risk. The patients with the highest incidence of neurologic injury are octogenarians with hypertension, diabetes, prior stroke, and diffuse peripheral vascular disease. Beating-heart revascularization and the use of T-grafts markedly decrease the incidence of neurologic defects in these and other patients. Despite innovative medical treatment regimens, definitive treatment of refractory heart disease still necessitates surgical revascularization and cardiopulmonary bypass. Percutaneous catheter interventions are themselves commonly associated with cerebral atheroemboli and to some extent with stroke, peripheral embolization, and cognitive changes. Therefore, we should continue to examine all possible strategies that can be used to decrease neurologic injury associated with this procedure. Even though the neurocognitive deficits seen postoperatively are subtle, they should not be discounted. The large number of cardiac procedures performed highlights the socioeconomic impact of even minor neurocognitive dysfunction, and further underscores the need for continued research and procedure development.

References

1. Roach G. Kanchuger M, Mora Mangano C, et al. Adverse cerebral outcomes after coronary bypass surgery. N Engl J Med 1996;335:1857–63.
2. Adkins ER. Quality of life after stroke: exposing a gap in nursing literature. Rehabil Nurs 1993:18:144–7.
3. Barbut D, Caplan LR. Brain complications of cardiac surgery. Curr Probl Cardiol 1997;22:449–80.
4. Johnson P. Markers of cerebral ischemia after cardiac surgery. J Cardiothorac Vasc Anesth 1996;1:120–6.
5. Kirkham FJ. Recognition and prevention of neurological complications in pediatric cardiac surgery. Pediatr Cardiol 1998;19:331–45.
6. Blauth CI, Schulenberg WE, Taylor KM. Cerebral micro-embolism during cardiopulmonary bypass: retinal microvascular studies in-vivo with fluorescein angiography. J Thorac Cardiovasc Surg 1988;95:668–76.
7. Moody DM, Bell MA, Challa VR, et al. Brain microemboli during cardiac surgery or aortography. Ann Neurol 1990;4:477–86.
8. Plestis KA, Navi DG, Russo M, Gold JP. Left atrial femoral bypass and CSF drainage decreases neurologic complications in repair of descending and thoracoabdominal aortic aneurysms. Ann Vasc Surg 2001;15(1):49–52.
9. Tuman KJ, McCarthy RJ, Najafi H, Ivankovich AD. Differential effects of advanced age on neurologic and cardiac risks of coronary artery operations. J Thorac Cardiovasc Surg 1992;104:1510–7.
10. Newman MF, Wolman R, Kanchuger M, et al. Multicenter preoperative stroke risk index for patients undergoing coronary artery bypass graft surgery. Multicenter Study of Perioperative Ischemia (McSPI) Research Group. Circulation 1996;94 Suppl 9:1174–80.
11. Cernaianu AC, Vassilidze TV, Flum DR, et al. Predictors of stroke after cardiac surgery. J Card Surg 1995;4(Pt 1):334–9.
12. Cheng RT. Neurological complications in heart disease. Baillieres Clin Neurol 1997;2:337–55.
13. Kuroda Y, Uchimoto R, Kaieda R, et al. Central nervous system complications after cardiac surgery; a comparison between coronary artery bypass grafting and valve surgery. Anesth Analg 1993;76:222–7.
14. Albes JM, Schistek R, Baier R, et al. Early and late results following coronary bypass surgery beyond the age of 75 years. Thorac Cardiovasc Surg 1991;39:289–93.
15. Libman RB, Wirkowski E, Neystat M, et al. Stroke associated with cardiac surgery. Determinants, timing, and stroke subtype. Arch Neurol 1997;54:83–7.
16. Ricotta JJ, Faggioli GL, Castilone A, Hassett JM. Risk factors for stroke after cardiac surgery: Buffalo Cardiac-Cerebral Study Group. J Vasc Surg 1995;2:359–64.
17. Mravinac CM. Neurologic dysfunctions following cardiac surgery. Crit Care Nurse Clin North Am 1991;4:691–8.
18. DuPlessis AJ, Treves ST, Hickey PR, et al. Regional cerebral perfusion abnormalities after cardiac operations. Single photon emission computed tomography (SPECT) findings in children with postoperative movement disorders. J Thorac Cardiovasc Surg 1994;107:1036–43.
19. Taylor KM. Brain damage during cardiopulmonary bypass. Ann Thorac Surg 1994;42:212–7.
20. Klima U, Wimmer-Greinecker G, Mair R, et al. The octogenarians—a new challenge in cardiac surgery? Thorac Cardiovasc Surg 1994;42:212–7.
21. Mills SA. Risk factor for cerebral injury and cardiac surgery. Ann Thorac Surg 1995;59:1296–9.
22. Rady MY, Ryan T, Starr NJ. Perioperative determinants of morbidity and mortality in elderly patients undergoing cardiac surgery. Crit Care Med 1998;2:225–35.
23. Rao V. Christakis GT, Weisel RD et al. Risk factors for stroke following coronary bypass surgery. J Card Surg 1995;4:468–74.
24. Barbut D, Lo YW, Hartman GS, et al. Aortic atheroma is related to outcome but not numbers of emboli during coronary bypass. Ann Thorac Surg 1997;64:454–9.
25. Barbut D, Yao FS, Lo YW, et al. Determination of size of aortic emboli and embolic load during coronary artery bypass grafting. Ann Thorac Surg. 1997;63:1262–7.
26. Amarenco P. Atherosclerotic disease of the aortic arch as a risk factor for recurrent ischemic stroke. N Engl J Med 1996;334:1216–21.
27. Babu SC, Shah PM, Singh BM, et al. Coexisting carotid stenosis in patients undergoing cardiac surgery: indications and guidelines for simultaneous operations. Am J Surg 1985;150:207–11.

28. Brener BJ, Brief DK, Alpert J, et al. A four-year experience with preoperative noninvasive carotid evaluation of two thousand twenty-six patients undergoing cardiac surgery. J Vasc Surg 1984:1:386–9.

29. Rorick MB, Furan AJ. Risk of cardiac surgery in patients with prior stroke. Neurology 1990;40:835–7.

30. Newman MF, Reves JG. Toward a new frontier in cardiac surgery. Ann Thorac Surg 1997;632:322–3.

31. Nollert G, Mohnle P, Tassani-Prell P, et al. Postoperative neuropsychological dysfunction and cerebral oxygenation during cardiac surgery. Thorac Cardiovasc Surg 1995;43:260–4.

32. Toner I, Taylor KM, Newman S, Smith PL. Cerebral functional changes following cardiac surgery: neuropsychological and EEG assessment. Eur J Cardiothorac Surg 1998;1:13–20.

33. Savageau JA, Stanton BA, Jenkins CD, Frater WM. Neuropsychological function following elective cardiac operations. A six-month reassessment. J Thorac Cardiovasc Surg 1982;84:595–600.

34. Diegeler A, Hirsch R, Schneider F, et al. Neuromonitoring and neurocognitive outcome in off-pump versus conventional coronary bypass operation. Ann Thorac Surg 2000;69(4):1162–6.

35. Stump DA, Rogers AT, Hammon JW, Newman SP. Cerebral emboli and cognitive outcome after cardiac surgery. J Cardiothorac Vasc Anesth 1996;1:113–8.

36. DiPasquale G, Pinelli G, Manini GL, et al. Cardiopathy and acute cerebrovascular insufficiency: prospective study with two dimensional echocardiography. G Ital Cardiol 1985;15:407–13.

37. Gao F, Harris DN, Sapsed-Byrne S, Sharp S. Neurone-specific enolase and Sangtec 100 assays during cardiac surgery: Part III—Does haemolysis affect their accuracy? Perfusion 1997;12:171–7.

38. Gao F, Harris DN, Sapsed-Byrne S, Sharp S. Neurone specific enolase and Sangtec 100 assays during cardiac surgery: Part I — The effects of heparin, protamine and propofol. Perfusion 1997;12:163–5.

39. Taggart DP, Bhattacharya K, Meston N, et al. Serum S-100 protein concentration after cardiac surgery: a randomized trial of arterial line filtration. Eur J Cardiothorac Surg 1997;4:465–9.

40. Westaby S, Johnson P, Parry AJ, et al. Serum S100 protein: a potential marker for cerebral events during cardiopulmonary bypass. Ann Thorac Surg 1996;61:88–92.

41. Clark RE, Brillman J, Davis DA, et al. Microemboli during coronary artery bypass grafting: genesis and effect on outcome. J Thorac Cardiovasc Surg 1995;109:249–58.

42. O'Brien JJ, Butterworth J, Hammon JW, et al. Cerebral emboli during cardiac surgery in children. Anesthesiology 1997;87:1063–9.

43. Wong DH. Perioperative stroke. Part II: cardiac surgeon and cardiogenic embolic stroke. Can J Anaesth 1991;38 (Pt 1):471–88.

44. Gill R, Murkin JM. Neuropsychological dysfunction after cardiac surgery: what is the problem? J Cardiothorac Vasc Anesth 1997;10:91–8.

45. William IM, Stephens JF, Richardson EP Jr, et al. Brain and retinal microemboli during cardiac surgery. Ann Neurol 1991;5:736–7.

46. Barbut D, Yao FS, Hager DN, et al. Comparison of transcranial Doppler ultrasonography and transesophageal echocardiography to monitor emboli during coronary artery bypass surgery. Stroke 1996;27:87–90.

47. Dexter F, Hindman BJ, Marshall JS. Estimate of the maximum absorption rate of microscopic arterial air emboli after entry into the arterial circulation during cardiac surgery. Perfusion 1996;6:445–50.

48. Diewick M, Tandler R, Mollhoff T, et al. Heart surgery in patients aged eighty years and above: determinants of morbidity and mortality. Thorac Cardiovasc Surg 1997:45:119–26.

49. Barbut D, Hinton RB, Szatrowski TP, et al. Cerebral emboli detected during bypass surgery are associated with clamp removal. Stroke 1994;25:2398–402.

50. Fessatidis I, Prapas S, Hevas A, et al. Prevention of perioperative neurologic dysfunction. A six-year perspective of cardiac surgery. J Cardiovasc Surg 1991;32(5):570–4.

51. Fisher M, Jonas S, Sacco RI. Prophylactic neuroprotection for cerebral ischemia. Stroke 1994;25:1075–80.

52. Utley JR. Techniques for avoiding neurologic injury during adult cardiac surgery. J Cardiothorac Vasc Anesth 1996: 1:38–43.

53. Amarenco P. Atherosclerotic disease of the aortic arch as a risk factor for recurrent ischemic stroke. N Engl J Med 1996;334:1216–21.

54. Barbut D, Lo YW, Gold JP, et al. Impact of embolization during coronary artery bypass grafting on outcome and length of stay. Ann Thorac Surg 1997;63:998–1002.

55. Barbut D, Gold JP. Aortic atheromatosis and risks of cerebral embolization. J Cardiothorac Vasc Anesth 1996; 10(1):24–9.

56. Konstadt SN, Reich DL, Kahn R, Viggiani RF. Transesophageal echocardiography can be used to screen for ascending aortic atherosclerosis. Anesth Analg 1995:81:225–8.

57. Roth BJ, Meyer CA. Coronary artery calcification at CT as a predictor for cardiac complications of thoracic surgery. J Comput Assist Tomogr 1997;4:619–22.

58. Sahar G, Raanani E, Brauner R, Vidne BA. Cardiac surgery in octogenarians. J Cardiovasc Surg (Torino) 1994;35 (6 Suppl 1):201–5.

59. Vingerhoets G, Van Notten G, Jannes C. Effect of asymptomatic carotid artery disease on cognitive carotid artery disease on cognitive outcomes after cardiopulmonary bypass. J Int Neuropsychol Soc 1996;3:236–9.

60. Walker WA, Harvey WR, Gaschen JR, et al. Is routine carotid screening for coronary surgery needed? Am Surg 1996;62:308–10.

61. Bettman MA, Katzen BT, Furlan AJ, et al. Carotid stenting and angioplasty: a statement for healthcare professionals from the Councils on Cardiovascular Radiology, Stroke, Cardiothoracic and Vascular Surgery, Epidemiology and Prevention. Stroke 1998;29(1):336–8.

62. Rao V, Christakis GT, Weisel RD, et al. Risk factors for stroke following coronary bypass surgery. J Card Surg 1995;4:468–74.

63. Murkin JM. The role of CPB management in neurobehavioral outcomes after cardiac surgery. Ann Thorac Surg 1995;59:1308–11.

64. Murkin JM, Newman SP, Stump DA, Blumenthal JA. Statement of consensus on assessment of neurobehavioral outcomes after cardiac surgery. Ann Thorac Surg 1995;59:1289–95.

65. Murkin JM, Baird DL, Martrzke JS, et al. Long-term neurological outcomes after cardiac surgery. Ann Thorac Surg 1995;59:1308–11.

66. Hartman GS, Peterson J, Konstadt SN, et al. High reproducibility in the interpretation of intraoperative transesophageal echocardiographic evaluation of aortic atheromatous disease. Anesth Analg 1996;82:539–43.

67. Murphy PM. Pro: intraoperative transesophageal echocardiography is a cost effective strategy for cardiac surgical procedures. J Cardiothorac Vasc Anesth 1997;2:246–9.

68. Nicolosi AC, Aggarwal A, Almassi GH, Olinger GN. Intraoperative epiaortic ultrasound during cardiac surgery. 1996;11(1):49–55.

69. Trehan N, Mishra M, Dhole S, et al. Significantly reduced incidence of stroke during coronary artery bypass grafting using transesophageal echocardiography. Eur J Cardiothorac Surg 1997;2:234–42.

70. Davila-Roman VG, Barzilai B, Wareing TH, et al. Intraoperative ultrasonographic evaluation of the ascending aorta in 100 consecutive patients undergoing cardiac surgery. Circulation 1991;84 Suppl 5:III47–53.

71. Davila-Roman VG, Phillips KJ, Daily NN, et al. Intraoperative transesophageal echocardiography and epiaortic ultrasound for assessment for atherosclerosis of the thoracic aorta. J Am Coll Cardiol 1996;28:942–7.

72. Marschall K, Kanchuger M, Kessler K, et al. Superiority of transesophageal echocardiography in detecting aortic arch atheromatous disease: identification of patients at increased risk of stroke during cardiac surgery. J Cardiothorac Vasc Anesth 1994;1:5–13.

73. Austin EH III, Edmonds HL Jr, Auden SM, et al. Benefit of neurophysiologic monitoring for pediatric cardiac surgery. J Thorac Cardiovasc Surg 1997;114:707–15, 717; discussion 715–6.

74. Nuwer MR. Intraoperative electroencephalography. J Clin Neurophysiol 1993;4:437–44.

75. Sebel PS. Central nervous system monitoring during open heart surgery: an update. J Cardiothorac Vasc Anesth 1998:12(2 Suppl 1):3–8.

76. Craver J, Bufkin BL, Weintraub WS, Guyton RA. Neurologic events after coronary bypass grafting: further observations with warm cardioplegia. Ann Thorac Surg 1995;59:1429–33.

77. Gold JP, Carlson ME, Hartman GS. Invited commentary. Ann Thorac Surg 200;69:1075–76.

78. Plestis KA, Gold JP. Importance of blood pressure regulation in maintaining adequate tissue perfusion during cardiopulmonary bypass. Semin Thorac Cardiovasc Surg 200;13(2):170–5.

79. Murkin JM, Martzke JS, Buchan AM, et al. A randomized study of the influence of perfusion techniques and pH management strategy in 316 patients undergoing coronary artery bypass surgery. II: neurologic and cognitive outcomes. J Thorac Cardiovasc Surg 1995;110:349–62.

80. McLean RF, Wong BI, Naylor CD, et al. Cardiopulmonary bypass, temperature and central nervous system dysfunction. Circulation 1994;90(5 Pt 2):II250–5.

81. Nathan HJ, Lavalle G. The management of temperature during hypothermic cardiopulmonary bypass: I—Canadian survey. Can J Anaesth 1995;42:669–71.

82. Coselli JS. Retrograde cerebral perfusion is an effective means of neutral support during deep hypothermic circulatory arrest. Ann Thorac Surg 1997;64:908–12.

83. Phoon CK. Deep hypothermic circulatory arrest during cardiac surgery: effects on cerebral blood flow and cerebral oxygenation in children. Am Heart J 1993;125:1739–48.

84. Rooney SJ, Pagano D, Bognolo G, et al. Aprotinin in aortic surgery requiring profound hypothermia and circulatory arrest. Eur J Cardiothorac Surg 1997;2:373–8.

85. Yerlioglou ME, Wolfe D, Mezrow CK, et al. The effect of retrograde cerebral perfusion after particulate embolization to the brain. J Thorac Cardiovasc Surg 1995;110:1470–85.

86. Jacobs A, Neveling M, Horst M, et al. Alterations of neuropsychological function and cerebral glucose metabolism after cardiac surgery are not related only to intraoperative microembolic events. Stroke 1998;29:660–7.

87. Hoka S, Okamoto H, Takahashi S, Yasui H. Adequate de-airing during cardiac surgery. J Cardiovasc Surg (Torino) 1995;36:201–2.

88. Murkin JM Cardiopulmonary bypass and the inflammatory response: a role for serine protease inhibitors? J Cardiothorac Vasc Anesth 1997;2 Suppl 1:19–23; discussion 24–5.

89. Forsman M, Olsnes BT, Semb G, Steen PA. Effects of nimodipine on cerebral blood flow and neuropsychological outcome after cardiac surgery. Br J Anaesth 1990;65:514–20.

90. Legault C, Furberg CD, Wagenknecht LE, et al. Nimodipine neuroprotection in cardiac valve replacement: report of an early terminated trial. Stroke 1996;27:593–8.

91. Galea J, Manche A. Cardiac surgery and the brain. N Engl J Med 1994;330(10):717.

92. Isgro F, Schmidt C, Pohl P, Saggau W. A predictive parameter in patients with brain related complications after cardiac surgery? Eur J Cardiothorac Surg 1997;4:640–4.

CHAPTER 9

POSTINFARCTION VENTRICULAR SEPTAL DEFECT REPAIR

ROBERT C. KING, MD, EDWARD D. VERRIER, MD

In the early 1950s, as the "Golden Era" of cardiac surgery began, postinfarction ventricular septal defect (VSD) was felt to be a uniformly fatal complication of acute myocardial infarction (AMI). Compilations of original reports demonstrated an associated mortality of 50% 1-week postseptal rupture. Few patients survived longer than 2 months, and those that did were reportable.[1,2] These odds were, of course, very attractive to the pioneers of cardiac surgery. The first reported successful repair of a postinfarction VSD is credited to Cooley in 1957.[3] Since that initial success, technical advances in the repair of these defects have not mirrored the rapid advances in many of the other disciplines of cardiac surgery. Advances in cardiac imaging and cardiopulmonary support have improved our ability to quickly diagnose and support those patients who develop a postinfarction murmur associated with hemodynamic deterioration caused by septal rupture. Unfortunately, surgeons are still left with the technical challenges of exposing the defect, determining the extent of infarction, resecting, and repairing only as much injured myocardium as is necessary, while deciding whether or not to correct ongoing coronary ischemia.

Only an estimated 1 to 2% of patients suffering AMI will go on to develop septal perforation. Of those patients, fewer still will make it to the operating room for attempted repair. Combine this with an increasing aggressiveness in the diagnosis and percutaneous treatment of coronary artery disease, and the incidence of postinfarction VSD may continue to decline.[4] Having said this, myocardial infarction resulting in septal perforation may be the sentinel event in as many as 80% of the patients who develop postinfarction VSD.[5] Combine this statistic with an increasing awareness of coronary artery disease in regions of the world with limited access to high-technology interventions, and the problem of postinfarction VSD remains. With an associated mortality of 10 to 40%, postinfarction VSD repair remains a high-risk procedure. Advances in applied therapies and surgical techniques continue to be limited by relatively small patient populations.

Studies in necropsy patients provide valuable insight into the anatomic and pathologic considerations that contribute to the development of postinfarction VSD. Despite the association with the occlusion of a single vessel supplying either the anterior or posterior septum, significant triple-vessel coronary artery disease ($\geq$ 75% diameter reduction) was demonstrated in 50 to 90% of autopsied patients.[6,7] The development of a postinfarction VSD was associated with an inferior wall infarction in approximately 55 to 75% of the cases. Approximately 70% of inferior VSDs were found to be more complex in nature because of serpiginous necrotic myocardial dissection planes. Most anterior wall defects were found to be simple through-and-through–type perforations.[7] Most surgical series have not reflected this preponderance of inferior wall defects or severity of associated coronary atherosclerosis as both of these characteristics probably contribute significantly to preoperative mortality.

Most postinfarction VSDs occur 2 to 7 days post myocardial infarction. The mean duration from infarction to septal perforation is 3 to 4 days. Appearance of a VSD prior to 2 days post infarction can be an ominous sign and is associated with a higher mortality.[8] Early postinfarction VSD most likely occurs following a large myocardial infarction. The size of the associated infarction is probably the reason for a higher operative mortality in this subgroup of patients. Patients developing a murmur post myocardial infarction should undergo immediate echocardiography. Confirmation of VSD can be achieved by the measurement of increased oxygen saturation in the right heart in combination with a 1.5:1 or greater shunt. The importance of right-heart catheterization in the setting of postinfarction VSD is decreasing as the combination of two-dimensional transthoracic Doppler echocardiography and transesophageal echocardiography approaches a diagnostic sensitivity and specificity of 100%.[9]

Intraaortic balloon pump (IABP) or intraaortic balloon counterpulsation should be considered early in the course for all patients who develop a postinfarction VSD. Early IABP placement can allow for resuscitation of stunned or ischemic myocardium while improving cardiovascular hemodynamics and enhancing end-organ perfusion. IABP placement in patients with signs of low cardiac output or ongoing cardiogenic shock should be mandatory. Improved survival has been observed in those patients who have received IABP support prior to postinfarction VSD repair.[10–12] Additionally, IABP support can be essential in patient stabilization, allowing for left-heart catheterization and coronary angiography prior to surgery.

Mandatory coronary angiography prior to postinfarction VSD repair cannot be supported in the setting of severe refractory cardiogenic shock. Immediate operative repair is indicated unless the patient's comorbidities preclude surgical candidacy. In most other patients, attempts should be made to stabilize the patient prior to performance of left-heart catheterization. Coronary artery bypass grafting (CABG) at the time of VSD repair neither decreases nor increases operative mortality.[13–15] However, North American literature demonstrates improved long-term survival in those patients receiving coronary revascularization at the time of postinfarction VSD repair.[13,16] In contrast, European reports show no long-term survival advantage for routine CABG at the time of VSD repair.[14,15] Whether or not this difference in long-term outcome reflects differences in access to single-vessel disease intervention remains to be determined. Evidence recommends coronary angiography in all stabilized patients, followed by an attempt at complete operative revascularization at the time of VSD repair. If single-vessel disease is encountered at the time of angiography, then revascularization becomes unnecessary.

Initial operative strategies for managing postinfarction VSD developed during the 1970s. Daggett painstakingly outlined the principles for successful VSD repair. Operative delay (6 weeks if possible), infarctectomy, patch closure of the VSD, and patch closure of the infarctectomy (two-patch technique) were felt to be essential components for ensuring good surgical outcomes.[11] The exact application of these philosophies varied with the anatomic site of the infarction. Apical infarcts could be managed by simple apical amputation with a "sandwiched" felt-buttressed closure of the resultant defect (Figure 9-1). Anterior and posterior defects were addressed through the infarcted myocardium. The infarcted myocardium was generously resected, and the resultant septal and free wall defects were then closed with two separate patches. Very small VSDs associated with small amounts of infarcted myocardium could be repaired primarily with felt-buttressed sutures. Most VSDs, however, required patch closure of the defect. Following successful septation of the heart, the free wall defect could be closed with a slightly redundant Dacron

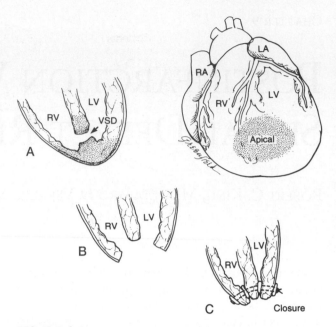

FIGURE 9-1. Repair of apical VSD (*A*) by débridement (*B*) and primary repair buttressed with pledgets or felt (*C*). LA = left atrium; LV = left ventricle; RA = right atrium; RV = right ventricle.

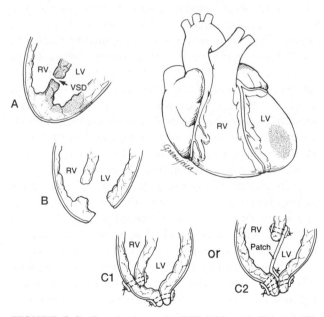

FIGURE 9-2. Repair of anterior VSD (*A*) by débridement (*B*), primary repair buttressed with pledgets or felt (*C1*), or patch repair buttressed with pledgets or felt (*C2*). LV = left ventricle; RV = right ventricle.

patch buttressed with felt strips or pledgets (Figures 9-2 and 9-3). In a posterior defect, the patch closing the VSD could be anchored to the mitral valve annulus. If frank papillary necrosis and/or rupture were present, mitral valve replacement was performed through the left atrium following septal repair and ventricular closure.

With time, the original Daggett principles underwent significant change. Operative delay was felt to deny surgi-

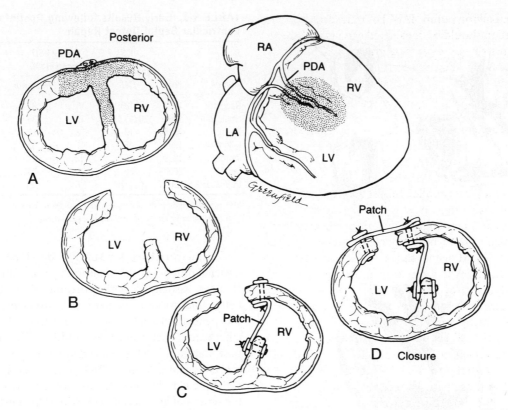

FIGURE 9-3. Repair of posterior VSD (*A*) by débridement (*B*), patch repair of VSD (*C*), and patch repair of infarctectomy (*D*). LA = left atrium; LV = left ventricle; PDA = posterior decending (coronary) artery; RA = right atrium; RV = right ventricle.

cal intervention to a subset of patients who were at risk for increased operative morbidity and mortality. As familiarity with postinfarction VSD repair increased, it became apparent that a significant percentage of patients in this high-risk subset could be salvaged by an operation and experience good long-term outcomes. Earlier repair (< 3 weeks) met with encouraging results.[17,18]

David, in an interest to decrease troublesome suture-line bleeding, switched patch materials from woven Dacron to bovine pericardium. In an effort to maximize right ventricular preservation, he developed the endocar-dial-patch (single-patch) exclusion technique (Figures 9-4 and 9-5). He approached the defect via a left ventriculo-tomy with very little, if any, infarctectomy. He then sewed a patch to what was felt to be the border of the septal infarction, well beyond the defect, in an attempt to "right ventricularize" the VSD. The left ventriculotomy was then closed with felt-buttressed Prolene sutures to include the infarcted free wall. The approach was similar for either anterior or posterior defects.[19]

Residual septal defect or recurrence following repair was not uncommon with wide infarctectomy. Out of an interest to decrease the rate of recurrence, two strategies, very similar to the endocardial patch exclusion technique, developed in Brazil and Japan in the late 1980s. Either synthetic or bioprosthetic patches were "tacked" around

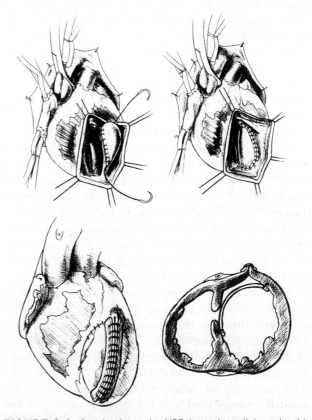

FIGURE 9-4. Repair of anterior VSD by endocardial patch with infarct exclusion. Pericardial patch is sutured to septum first, then to lateral wall.

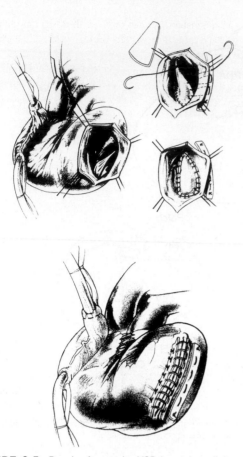

FIGURE 9-5. Repair of posterior VSD by endocardial patch with infarct exclusion. Pericardial patch is sutured to mitral annulus, septum, and posterior wall.

TABLE 9-1. Early Results following Postinfarction Ventricular Septal Defect Repair

Author	Year	Overall OM (%)	OM by VSD Location (%)		Recurrence (%)
			Anterior	Posterior	
Daggett[12]	1982	46 (25)*	15	37	NR
Skillington[18]	1990	20 (11.1)*	12	33	NR
David[19]	1995	13	13	13	NR
Killen[24]	1997	45	41	52	NR
Pretre[28]	1999	26	NR	NR	18
Deja[8]	2000	35	35	34	40
Labrousse[15]	2002	42 (27)*	NR	NR	8

OM = operative mortality; NR = not reported; VSD = ventricular septal defect.

* Percentage in parentheses represents most recent experience.

the zone of infarction to viable myocardium on both the septum and the involved free wall. This was done through a left ventricular approach without infarctectomy.[20,21] The septal patch was brought out through the infarctectomy and secured to a midline split of the exterior patch with buttressed sutures. The addition of a biologic glue to the "right ventricularized" repair was first carried out in Europe with encouraging results.[15,22] Although not necessarily representing a breakthrough in surgical technique, the addition of a biologic glue appeared to strengthen the infarct border, reinforce the septal repair, and improve hemostasis by sealing suture lines.

Outcomes following postinfarction VSD repair have improved during the past four decades despite a relatively small operative experience (Table 9-1). Early operation (prior to shock), avoidance of infarctectomy, improved surgical techniques, better myocardial protection strategies, and improved perioperative support technologies have contributed to improved outcomes. More importantly, most series have reported improving outcomes and decreasing recurrence rates as their own institutional experience has grown.[12]

Several correlates for survival developed as a better understanding of the anatomic and pathophysiologic changes associated with postinfarction VSD became better understood. Preoperative cardiogenic shock is an independent predictor for poor outcome when forcing an emergency operation.[8,23–25] Additionally, inferior wall postinfarction VSD is associated with a higher operative mortality and morbidity. Right ventricular infarction and subsequent right-heart failure occur more frequently in the setting of an inferior wall infarct. As stated previously, postmortem studies also demonstrate the complex serpiginous nature of inferior wall VSDs. This complexity may contribute to miscalculations in estimating the actual size and extent of septal infarction at the time of operation. Combine these findings with the difficult anatomic exposure of the inferior wall, and the challenges associated with repairing and managing inferior wall VSDs can be significant. Several factors also associated with poor outcome include a short interval from infarction to VSD appearance, proximal location of infarction, rapid onset of cardiogenic shock, and recurrence or residual VSD following repair. Most of these characteristics are likely secondary to a large myocardial infarction. Therefore, the size and location of the infarct associated with the development of a septal defect are the two most important factors in determining operative outcome. The degree of ongoing coronary artery ischemia and/or its correction at the time of operation has demonstrated little correlation to operative outcome.

Long-term benefits following postinfarction VSD repair have been demonstrated.[13,15,17–19] Most patients who undergo successful repair remain in class I or II New York Heart Association (NYHA) heart failure following recovery. The mean actuarial survival following postinfarction VSD repair approximates 65% at 5 years and 40% at 10 years.[26–28] Table 9-2 summarizes published long-term results. Operative mortality and long-term outcome were not significantly affected by age. Long-term benefit has been demonstrated in patients older than 70 years of age.[29,30] An aggressive operative strategy in patients older

TABLE 9-2. Long-Term Outcomes following Postinfarction Ventricle Septal Defect Repair

Author	Year	Actuarial Survival (%)			Class I or II NYHA (%)
		1 Year	5 Years	10 Years	
Daggett[12]	1982	NR	NR	NR	88.5
Skillington[18]	1990	78	71	40	80
David[19]	1995	80	66	NR	97
Killen[24]	1997	49.7	41.5	25.6	NR
Pretre[28]	1999	78	65	40	84
Deja[8]	2000	NR	46	NR	83
Labrousse[15]	2002	85*	63*	23*	NR

NR = not reported; NYHA = New York Heart Association symptoms of heart failure.

* Excluding operative mortality.

than 70 years of age should be encouraged prior to the occurrence of hemodynamic instability.

Postinfarction VSD remains a challenging problem for the cardiac surgeon today. It is a relatively uncommon complication following acute myocardial infarction. Several institutions have reported increasing success in managing these patients as their experience with repairing postinfarction VSDs has increased. Diagnosis and repair prior to hemodynamic compromise is advisable. Preservation of ventricular geometry and viable myocardium favors infarctotomy with minimal infarctectomy prior to patch closure of the VSD and free-wall repair. Stabilization and left-heart catheterization prior to surgical revascularization and VSD repair may improve long-term outcomes.

References

1. Sanders RJ, Kerr WH, Blount SG. Perforation of the interventricular septum complicating myocardial infarction. Am Heart J 1956;51:736.
2. Schlappi JC, Landale DG. Perforation of the infarcted interventricular septum. Am Heart J 1954;47:432.
3. Cooley DA, Belmonte BA, Zeis LB, et al. Surgical repair of ruptured interventricular septum following acute myocardial infarction. Surgery 1957;41:930–7.
4. Kinn JW, O'Neill WW, Benzuly KH, et al. Primary angioplasty reduces the risk of myocardial rupture compared to thrombolysis for acute myocardial infarction. Catheter Cardiovasc Diagn 1997;42:151–7.
5. Mann JM, Roberts WC. Cardiac morphologic observations after operative closure of acquired ventricular septal defect during acute myocardial infarction: analysis of 16 necropsy patients. Am J Cardiol 1987;60:981–7.
6. Mann JM, Roberts WC. Acquired ventricular septal defect during acute myocardial infarction: analysis of 38 unoperated necropsy patients and comparison with 50 unoperated necropsy patients without rupture. Am J Cardiol 1988;62:8–19.
7. Edwards BS, Edwards WD, Edwards JE. Ventricular septal rupture complicating acute myocardial infarction: identification of simple and complex types in 53 autopsied hearts. Am J Cardiol 1984;54:1201–5.
8. Deja MA, Szostek J, Widenka K, et al. Post infarction ventricular septal defect—can we do better? Eur J Cardiothorac Surg 2000;18:194–201.
9. Kishon Y, Igbal A, Oh JK, et al. Evolution of echocardiographic modalities in detection of postmyocardial infarction ventricular septal defect and papillary muscle rupture: study of 62 patients. Am Heart J 1993;126:667–75.
10. Blanche C, Khan SS, Matloff JM, et al. Results of early repair of ventricular septal defect after an acute myocardial infarction. J Thorac Cardiovasc Surg 1992;104:961–5.
11. Daggett WM, Guyton RA, Mundth ED, et al. Surgery for post-myocardial infarct ventricular septal defect. Ann Surg 1977;186:260–71.
12. Daggett WM, Buckley MJ, Akins CW, et al. Improved results of surgical management of postinfarction ventricular septal rupture. Ann Surg 1982;196:269–77.
13. Muehrcke DD, Daggett WM, Buckley MJ, et al. Postinfarct ventricular septal defect repair: effect of coronary artery bypass grafting. Ann Thorac Surg 1992;54:876–83.
14. Dalrymple-Hay MJR, Langley SM, Sami SA, et al. Should coronary artery bypass be performed at the same time as repair of a post-infarct septal defect? Eur J Cardiothorac Surg 1998;13:286–92.
15. Labrousse L, Choukroun JM, Chevalier F, et al. Surgery for post-infarction ventricular septal defect (VSD): risk factors for hospital death and long-term results. Eur J Cardiothorac Surg 2002;21:725–32.
16. Komeda M, Fremes SE, David TE. Surgical repair of postinfarction ventricular septal defect. Circulation 1990;82 Suppl IV:IV243–7.
17. Piwnica A, Menasche P, Beaufils P, et al. Long-term results of emergency surgery for postinfarction ventricular septal defect. Ann Thorac Surg 1987;44:274–6.
18. Skillington PD, Davies RH, Luff AJ, et al. Surgical treatment for infarct-related ventricular septal defects. J Thorac Cardiovasc Surg 1990;99:798–808.
19. David TE, Dale L, Zhao S. Postinfarction ventricular septal rupture: repair by endocardial patch with infarct exclusion. J Thorac Cardiovasc Surg 1995;110:1315–22.
20. da Silva JP, Cascudo MM, Baumgratz JF, et al. Postinfarction ventricular septal defect. J Thorac Cardiovasc Surg 1989;97:86–9.
21. Usui A, Murase M, Maeda M, et al. Sandwich repair with two sheets of equine pericardial patch for acute posterior post-infarction ventricular septal defect. Eur J Cardiothorac Surg 1993;7:47–9.
22. Musumeci F, Shukla V, Mignosa C, et al. Early repair of postinfarction ventricular septal defect with gelatin-resorcin-formol biological glue. Ann Thorac Surg 1996;62:486–8.
23. Cummings RG, Califf R, Jones RN, et al. Correlates of survival in patients with postinfarction ventricular septal defect. Ann Thorac Surg 1989;47:824–30.
24. Killen DA, Piehler JM, Borkon M, et al. Early repair of postinfarction ventricular septal rupture. Ann Thorac Surg 1997;63:138–42.
25. Anderson DR, Adams S, Bhat A, et al. Post-infarction ventricular septal defect: the importance of site of

infarction and cardiogenic shock on outcome. Eur J Cardiothorac Surg 1989;3:554–7.

26. Ellis CJ, Parkinson GF, Jaffe WM, et al. Good long-term outcome following surgical repair of post-infarction ventricular septal defect. Aust N Z J Med 1995;25: 330–6.

27. Deville C, Fontan F, Chevalier JM, et al. Surgery of post-infarction ventricular septal defect: risk factors for hospital death and long-term results. Eur Cardiothorac Surg 1991;5:167–75.

28. Pretre R, Ye Q, Grunenfelder J, et al. Operative results of "repair" of ventricular septal rupture after acute myocardial infarction. Am J Cardiol 1999;84:785–8.

29. Blanche C, Khan SS, Chaux A, et al. Postinfarction ventricular septal defect in the elderly: analysis and results. Ann Thorac Surg 1994;57:1244–7.

30. Muehrcke DD, Blank S, Daggett WM. Survival after repair of postinfarction ventricular septal defects in patients over the age of 70. J Card Surg 1992;7:290–300.

CHAPTER 10

OFF-PUMP CORONARY ARTERY BYPASS GRAFTING

ROBBIN G. COHEN, MD

For the last 40 years, cardiopulmonary bypass (CPB) has provided the platform that has enabled cardiac surgeons to perform coronary artery bypass grafting (CABG) on progressively older and sicker patients, with continually improving results. Despite this, few would argue that CPB accounts for a significant portion of the morbidity and mortality associated with CABG. The untoward effects of CPB are the result of both physiologic and mechanical factors. Exposing blood and its components to the non-physiologic surfaces of tubing, oxygenators, and filters, combined with the sheer stress associated with pumping and suction, leads to destruction of red cells, white blood cells, and platelets. This, coupled with the incorporation of abnormal substances from cardiac vents and pericardial suction devices, results in an inflammatory reaction associated with the release of cytokines, increased capillary permeability, and the potential for dysfunction of every major organ system in the body (Figure 10-1). In addition, the use of CPB usually requires manipulation of the aorta during cannulation and cross-clamping, which can result in atheromatous and air emboli to the brain and other major organs. Although advances in CPB technology and surgical technique have resulted in progressively safer cardiac surgical procedures over the years, the consequences of CPB can be severe. This is especially true in high-risk patients currently undergoing CABG.

Advances in surgical technique and instrumentation have led many cardiac surgeons throughout the world to adapt an off-pump beating-heart model with which to perform coronary artery bypass grafting. The introduction of coronary stabilizers, cardiac positioning devices, and mechanical anastomotic devices has served to facilitate these procedures in hopes of maintaining the momentum toward improved results with CABG. Although information is accumulating that suggests promising early results, it is not clear whether our goals of

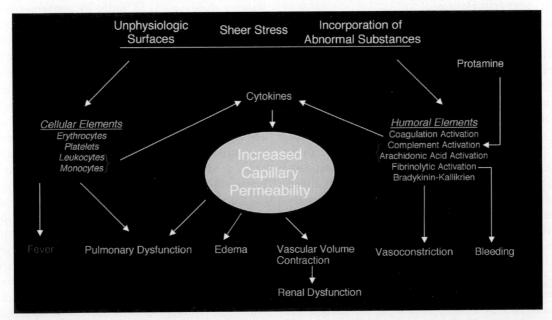

FIGURE 10-1. Toxicity of cardiopulmonary bypass.

safer CABG without compromising the long-term quality of the operation will be met. This chapter discusses the development, indications, operative technique, and results of off-pump CABG.

History

The earliest attempts at surgical myocardial revascularization occurred long before CPB became available to cardiac surgeons. In 1952, Vineburg reported his technique of implanting the internal mammary artery directly into the myocardium.[1] In 1958, Longmire and the University of California, Los Angeles group reported their experience with open coronary artery endarterectomy without CPB.[2] The early 1960s saw the successful integration of CPB into virtually every cardiac surgery operating room. This, combined with the introduction of coronary angiography by Sones and Shirey,[3] resulted in an explosion in the number of coronary bypass operations performed throughout the world. Although the use of CPB for CABG became the standard in most cardiac surgical centers, the deleterious effects of CPB, as well as limited resources in some countries, led some surgeons to continue to pursue CABG without CPB. In the early 1990s, both Buffolo and Benetti reported low mortality rates in patients undergoing off-pump CABG.[4,5] However, these operations tended to be associated with fewer grafts per patient when compared with on-pump groups. Furthermore, the long-term patency rate of coronary bypass grafts performed without CPB was uncertain. At the time, Gundry commented that he had observed both a high incidence of late mortality and poor long-term graft patency in patients undergoing CABG without CPB. He also warned that temporarily occluding the coronary arteries with sutures could result in injury to the coronary artery distal to the anastomosis, with subsequent graft closure.

As video-assisted technology became available to surgeons in other fields, many cardiac surgeons became interested in less invasive ways to perform CABG. In 1995, Benetti reported two cases of single-vessel CABG procedures using video-assisted techniques for taking down the left internal mammary artery (LIMA). This was followed by anastomosis of the LIMA to the left anterior descending artery via a small left anterior thoracotomy incision without the use of CPB.[6] Experience with this procedure grew worldwide as surgeons realized that they could perform limited CABG procedures with decreased hospital stays, less blood loss, and earlier return to normal activities (Figure 10-2). At the same time, devices designed to stabilize the target coronary arteries without causing hemodynamic compromise became available. These devices allowed for easier off-pump anastomoses, which translated into improved patency rates. Regardless, these operations were limited to single- and two-vessel CABG, which make up only a small portion of the number of CABG procedures performed worldwide each year.

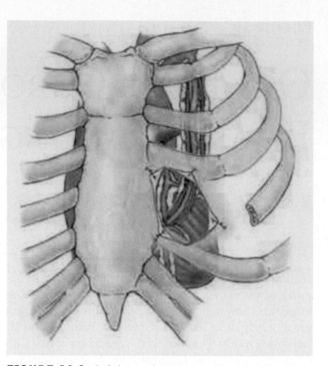

FIGURE 10-2. Left internal mammary artery to left anterior descending coronary artery via a limited anterior thoracotomy incision. Reproduced with permission from Fann J, Pompil M, Burdon T, et al. Port access coronary artery bypass grafting. In: Cohen R, Mack M, Fonger J, Landreneau R, editors. Minimally invasive cardiac surgery. St. Louis (MO): Quality Medical Publishing; 1999. p. 18–7.

To extend the proposed benefits of off-pump CABG to patients with multivessel coronary disease, two obstacles had to be overcome. The first was the ability to gain surgical exposure to coronary arteries on all surfaces of the heart, including the lateral and inferior walls, without significant hemodynamic compromise. The second was to be able to stabilize these vessels in order to perform anastomoses whose patency rates would be comparable to anastomoses performed on a quiet heart. Most surgeons abandoned attempts at performing off-pump CABG via small thoracotomy incisions or partial sternotomies and have returned to the standard sternotomy incision for off-pump CABG. Several methods and instruments were developed for elevating the heart in order to gain surgical exposure to the lateral and inferior surfaces. Probably the simplest was to place pericardial stay sutures deep on the lateral pericardium in order to rotate the heart on its axis. This maneuver, combined with clockwise rotation of the patient and relaxation on the right-sided pericardial stay sutures, was a reliable method of getting to the obtuse marginal and posterior descending coronary arteries without causing hemodynamic collapse (Figure 10-3). Suction devices have since been developed that attach to the apex of the heart, allowing it to be safely elevated on a flexible arm (Figure 10-4).

Several types of devices have been developed to stabilize the coronary arteries for off-pump CABG. The original devices consisted of prongs designed to isolate

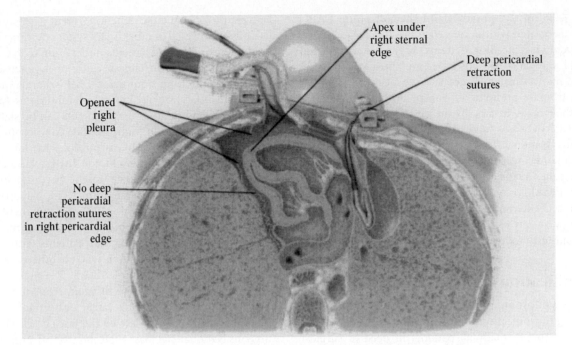

FIGURE 10-3. Use of deep pericardial stay sutures to rotate heart for exposure of coronary arteries on lateral aspect of the heart. Courtesy of Medtronic, Inc., Minneapolis, MN.

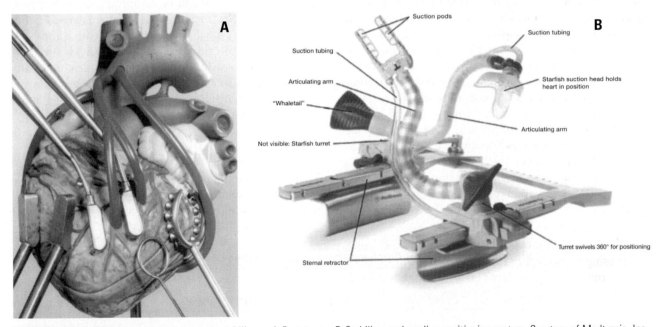

FIGURE 10-4. Evolution of coronary artery stabilizers. *A*, Prototypes. *B*, Stabilizer and cardiac positioning system. Courtesy of Medtronic, Inc., Minneapolis, MN.

the coronary artery between them either by pressure or by suction (see Figure 10-4). Early attempts at these devices were difficult to use and often led to suboptimal stabilization, resulting in difficult coronary anastomoses. Improvements in coronary stabilizers now allow them to be connected to the sternal retractor with flexible arms that allow better positioning of the heart as well as improved stabilization (see Figure 10-4). Other develop-

ments in instrumentation aimed at better off-pump coronary anastomoses include CO_2/H_2O misters, silastic tapes designed to occlude coronary arteries without injuring the vessel, and intracoronary shunts designed to limit ischemia during the coronary anastomoses.

As experience with off-pump CABG has grown, the surgical literature has been inundated with reports demonstrating improvements in results when compared with CABG on CPB. Many claim that off-pump CABG can be associated with decreased mortality, fewer neurologic events, less bleeding, better renal function, decreased hospital stay, and less cost. Despite these encouraging results, many cardiac surgeons have been reluctant to change from on-pump to off-pump CABG for the majority of their cases. In fact, by the end of 2001, fewer than 13% of CABG cases reported to the Society of Thoracic Surgeons National Database were performed without CPB. Potential reasons for this slow rate of acceptance include general satisfaction with the results obtained with on-pump CABG, concerns over the technical difficulty of off-pump CABG, and reluctance to adapt new techniques until they are proven in prospective randomized studies with long-term follow-up.

Indications for Off-Pump CABG

Varying philosophies exist among cardiac surgeons regarding the indications for off-pump CABG. Some surgeons feel that virtually all patients in need of surgical myocardial revascularization should undergo off-pump CABG, and they have set out to demonstrate that the operation is technically possible in everyone. Others feel that there is a selective role for off-pump CABG and that its use should be confined to those who are at high risk of developing complications with the use of CPB. For example, a young, otherwise healthy patient undergoing CABG has less than a 1% risk of cardiovascular accident (CVA) and may have little to gain by undergoing off-pump CABG. By contrast, a patient older than age 80 years with a history of prior CVA, calcified aorta, renal failure, diabetes, peripheral vascular disease, and smoking has almost a 40% chance of perioperative CVA when undergoing CABG and stands the most to gain by avoiding CPB with cannulation and cross-clamping of the aorta (Table 10-1).[7] Other examples of patients who might benefit from off-pump CABG include those with severely depressed left ventricular function, recent acute myocardial infarction, renal or other organ system dysfunction, or bleeding disorders, and patients undergoing redo CABG.

Patients who are unstable because of hypotension or arrhythmias resulting from myocardial ischemia or acute myocardial infarction are not good candidates for off-pump CABG. Sometimes these patients can be stabilized with intraaortic balloon pump (IABP) counterpulsation, after which off-pump CABG is possible. At our institution, we have a low threshold for IABP placement in patients whom we anticipate might become unstable because of ischemia or arrhythmias, in patients with recent large acute myocardial infarctions, in patients with severe left main disease, or in patients with significantly decreased left ventricular function. Patients with critical left main coronary artery lesions who are otherwise stable can safely undergo off-pump CABG.[8]

Although technically more difficult, reoperative coronary bypass surgery can be safely performed without CPB.[9] In fact, Mack's review of the Society of Thoracic Surgeons National Database indicates that off-pump techniques may offer a survival advantage in this subgroup of patients requiring myocardial revascularization.[10]

Off-pump CABG should not be performed in patients in whom the result might be compromised for technical reasons. Examples include young patients or diabetics who tend to have small coronary targets with diffuse calcific atherosclerotic disease. Off-pump CABG is also difficult in patients with extremely large hearts or hearts where the coronary arteries are located deep within the myocardium. CABG in these patients is usually more safely performed on CPB.

Operative Technique

There are a number of important differences in operative technique between on- and off-pump CABG, beginning with the operating room environment. The importance of

TABLE 10-1. Risk of Stroke after Traditional Coronary Artery Bypass Grafting

Calcified Aorta	Prior Stroke	Carotid Disease	Renal Failure	PVD	Smoking	DM	Predicted Risk		
							60 y	70 y	80 y
−	−	−	−	−	−	−	0.4	0.6	0.9
−	−	−	−	+	−	−	0.6	1.0	1.5
−	+	−	−	−	−	−	0.7	1.1	1.8
+	−	−	−	−	−	−	1.2	1.8	2.8
−	+	+	−	−	−	−	1.2	1.9	2.9
−	+	+	−	−	+	+	2.7	4.1	6.1
+	−	−	+	−	−	+	3.4	5.1	7.5
−	+	−	−	−	+	+	3.5	5.2	7.7
+	+	+	−	−	−	−	3.7	5.5	8.1
−	+	+	+	−	+	+	5.4	8.0	11.6
+	−	+	−	+	+	+	6.6	9.7	14.1
+	+	+	+	+	+	+	21.6	29.5	38.9

Reproduced with permission from John R, et al.[7]
DM = diabetes mellitus; PVD = peripheral vascular disease; y = years of age.

avoiding hypothermia cannot be overemphasized. As a result, the operating room is kept warm, and the patient is placed on a warming blanket. The cardiopulmonary bypass machine is usually not primed, but the perfusionist remains in the operating room and frequently assists with setting up the CO_2 blower/mister, suction for stabilizers, and performing activated clotting times at 20-min intervals. Off-pump CABG can be particularly challenging for the anesthesiologist, who has to deal with hemodynamic changes resulting from manipulation of the heart during anastomoses to the posterior and lateral coronary circulation. At times, the anesthesiologist will be required to administer vasopressors or inotropes to elevate the blood pressure during distal anastomoses on the lateral and posterior aspects of the heart. Other parts of the surgical procedure, such as placement of a side-biting clamp for proximal anastomoses or the use of the mechanical aortic connectors, require pharmacologic lowering of the blood pressure. Changes of position of the operating table are also frequent. Communication between the surgeon and anesthesiologist during off-pump CABG is key in order to be able to anticipate each other's moves, ensuring a smooth and orderly operation.

The patient is placed in the supine position with a roll under the shoulders. A radial arterial line and Swan-Ganz catheter are placed by the anesthesiologist. The patient is prepped and draped for a sternotomy incision. An intra-aortic balloon pump is placed in patients with severely depressed left ventricular function (ejection fraction [EF] < 25%) or recent myocardial infarction.

After making a standard sternotomy incision, the internal mammary arteries are dissected in the traditional manner. Greater and lesser saphenous vein grafts are harvested endoscopically. The pericardium is opened in the inverted-T fashion and its edges hung to the sternal retractor with stay sutures. The transverse pericardial incision at the diaphragm is extended farther posterior than usual on the right side, taking care not to injure the phrenic nerve. The heart is examined for the location, size, and quality of the target coronary arteries. Heparin (30 U/kg) is administered by the anesthesiologist. This is the same heparin dose normally used for CPB cases.

The order of coronary arteries bypassed depends on the patient's coronary anatomy and the pattern of coronary artery disease. Some surgeons believe that it is important to bypass collateralized vessels, followed by collateralizing vessels. If the left anterior descending (LAD) artery is significantly diseased, most prefer to begin by performing the left internal mammary artery to LAD artery anastomosis. We then routinely follow with diagonal arteries, ramus intermedius, and obtuse marginals, followed by the vessels of the right coronary circulation. The technical details of performing distal coronary anastomoses are described later in this section.

Once the internal mammary artery grafts are completed, we prefer to perform the proximal aortosaphenous vein graft anastomoses. This allows immediate revascularization of the myocardium supplied by each target vessel with the completion of each distal anastomosis. Previously, proximal anastomoses were performed by placing a side-biting clamp on the aorta after pharmacologically lowering the systolic blood pressure to approximately 90 mm Hg. We currently use proximal aortic connectors (St. Jude Medical Inc., St. Paul, MN) to perform most aortosaphenous vein graft anastomoses (Figure 10-5). Although long-term patency data with the use of these devices are not yet available, there are a number of advantages associated with their use. First, and most importantly, the need for manipulation of the aorta is significantly reduced. This is especially important during redo coronary bypass procedures where placement of proximal anastomoses is complicated by old graft and cannulation sites, and in patients with localized areas of atherosclerotic disease in the ascending aorta. The use of aortic connectors also has the potential to significantly reduce operating time. However, extra care must be taken to assure that graft length and position are correct in order to prevent kinking and early graft closure.

The performance of safe and reliable distal coronary anastomoses depends on adequate surgical exposure and stabilization of the target coronary artery, as well as creating a relatively bloodless field in which to sew. Whereas exposure of the coronary arteries on the anterior and anterolateral aspect of the heart is easily obtained, distal anastomoses on the lateral and posterior aspects of the beating heart can be technically challenging. Several maneuvers can be used that position the heart to expose the coronary arteries for off-pump CABG while maintaining hemodynamic stability. Many surgeons place two or three stay sutures under tension deep in the pericardium on the left side. At the same time, the pericardial traction sutures on the right pericardium are released. This rolls the apex of the heart toward the surgeon,

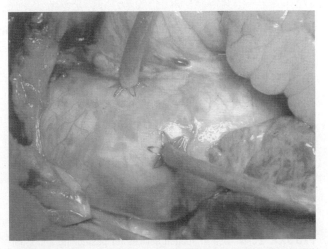

FIGURE 10-5. Proximal aortosaphenous vein graft anastomoses using a mechanical connector (St. Jude Medical Inc.).

exposing the lateral aspect of the heart (see Figure 10-3). This maneuver is facilitated by partially rotating the operating table clockwise. Although some surgeons routinely open the right pleural space to allow the heart to fall toward it during distal anastomoses on the lateral aspect of the heart, we have not found this to be necessary. Recently, suction devices were developed that adhere to the apex of the heart so that it can be retracted anteriorly on a flexible locking arm. The use of these devices facilitate exposure of the lateral and inferior aspects of the heart without the need for deep pericardial traction sutures (Figure 10-6).

Once the heart is positioned so that the target coronary artery is adequately exposed, the coronary stabilizer is placed to minimize movement in the area of the anastomosis. The epicardium over the target area on the coronary artery is dissected to ensure that the vessel is soft and as disease-free as possible in this area. The heart is then allowed to resume its normal position so that the graft length can be determined. This step is important as miscalculations in graft length can lead to undue tension and kinking of the graft at the proximal anastomosis if the graft is too short, and to kinking and occlusion of the graft if it is too long. Once the graft is oriented and cut to size, the heart is repositioned for the distal anastomosis and the stabilizer replaced. Soft silastic tapes are placed proximal and distal to the area of the planned arteriotomy and gently snared to occlude the vessel (Figure 10-7). Whereas some surgeons prefer only proximal occlusion of the coronary artery in order to assure that the artery distal to the anastomosis is uninjured, we have found this technique to be associated with excessive blood loss.

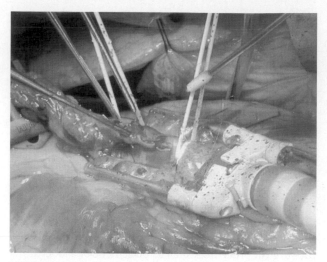

FIGURE 10-7. Off-pump anastomosis of LIMA to LAD artery, using proximal and distal silastic tapes (for temporary occlusion) and a suction stabilizer.

After the target coronary artery is positioned, stabilized, and occluded, we briefly pause to see that the patient is hemodynamically stable and that it is safe to proceed with the arteriotomy and distal coronary anastomosis. We have not found it necessary to perform ischemic preconditioning, nor do we routinely use intracoronary shunts. With this technique, we have found that the distal anastomoses are usually well tolerated. One exception is when the distal anastomosis is performed to the proximal right coronary artery, especially if the proximal lesion in the right coronary artery is not too severe. Temporary occlusion of the proximal to mid-right coronary artery can result in bradycardia and hemodynamic instability. Intracoronary shunts reduce the risk of problems in this situation. Visualization during distal coronary anastomoses is enhanced with the use of a CO_2 blower-mister, which is held by the surgical assistant. The velocity of the CO_2 should be kept at a minimum to avoid injury to the coronary endothelium.

Once a distal anastomosis is completed, it is important to release both silastic tapes, as well as the occluder on the graft, so that any air can be flushed out prior to tying down the suture. We routinely use a Doppler probe to evaluate the patency and flow characteristics of each graft, particularly the internal mammary artery graft to the LAD artery. A clearly discernible low-pitched sound during diastole assures a patent distal anastomosis.

After all coronary grafts are completed and checked for length, orientation, and hemostasis, a full dose of protamine is administered so that the activated clotting time is back to baseline. We do not routinely place atrial or ventricular pacing wires unless the patient has a history of arrhythmias or arrhythmias have occurred during the operation. Chest tubes are placed, and the sternotomy incision closed in the usual fashion, again

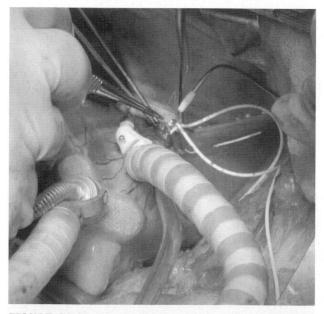

FIGURE 10-6. Use of suction devices for positioning and stabilization of an obtuse marginal coronary artery for a distal coronary anastomosis.

checking to see that the grafts lie comfortably without tension or kinking.

Postoperative Care

After the operation, patients remain sedated and on mechanical ventilation as they are transported to the intensive care unit, where they are closely monitored for hemodynamic instability, arrhythmias, and bleeding. In our experience, this allows for a smoother recovery than does extubating patients in the operating room. After 1 to 2 h of stability, short-acting anesthetics are discontinued and the patients weaned to extubation as they awaken from anesthesia. Most patients spend one night in the intensive care unit. Amiodarone is used prophylactically against arrhythmias. Aspirin and clopidogrel (Plavix) are administered on the first postoperative day. Whereas aspirin is continued indefinitely, clopidogrel is discontinued after 6 weeks. When postoperative atrial fibrillation occurs, it is treated with intravenous diltiazem.

Aggressive postoperative pain management is important after off-pump CABG. Intravenous and oral narcotics supplemented with ketorolac are most frequently used. In general, patients tend to be more awake earlier after off-pump CABG than when CPB is used. This makes early aggressive pain management important. Although we have tried other pain management modalities such as local anesthetic blocks, patient self-administered intravenous narcotic pumps, and oral cyclooxygenase (COX)-2 inhibitors, we have not seen significant improvements in post-operative analgesia with these methods.

Our experience suggests that postoperative deep venous thrombosis and pulmonary embolism may be more common after off-pump CABG when compared with CABG on CPB. Prophylaxis against deep venous thrombosis consists of compression boots and subcutaneous heparin, along with a policy of early and regular ambulation while hospitalized.

Results of Off-Pump CABG

Given the morbidity and physiologic consequences that can be associated with CPB, it seems intuitive that there should be an improvement in the results of off-pump CABG when compared with on-pump CABG. This has been more difficult to prove than one might expect. One of the problems lies in the fact that there continues to be a lack of prospective randomized studies comparing the two types of coronary surgery. In fact, over the past several years, most studies regarding the results of off-pump CABG are retrospective reviews of clinical series of off-pump operations compared with computer-matched groups of patients who had CABG performed on-pump. These studies, some of which have shown conflicting results, have led to confusion regarding which patients are likely to gain the most when their coronary bypass operations are performed without CPB. Furthermore, long-term results, especially those pertaining to graft patency and freedom from re-intervention, are scarce.

Cardiac Function and Arrhythmia

An important physiologic advantage of off-pump CABG is that it eliminates the necessity for a global cardiac ischemic period. Animal studies show that time of ischemic cardioplegic arrest is directly correlated with the degree of early cardiac dysfunction.[11] In his review article, Heames summarizes the effects of global ischemia on the heart and discusses the benefits of off-pump CABG.[12] Postoperative levels of troponin I and myocardial muscle creatine kinase isoenzyme (CK-MB) are lower after off-pump CABG when compared with CABG on CPB. Furthermore, myocardial lipid peroxidation is reduced, and oxidative metabolism recovers more rapidly after beating-heart surgery than with CPB.[13–15] This is not to say that temporary occlusion of major coronary arteries does not result in regional ischemia and the potential for myocardial stunning.[16] In fact, some surgeons advocate ischemic preconditioning and routine use of intracoronary shunts in order to prevent regional myocardial damage during off-pump CABG.[17–19] Others have shown that temporary local occlusion of major coronary arteries results in a transient decrease in myocardial function during occlusion, with complete recovery during reperfusion. This change was less significant with increasing degrees of coronary stenosis.[20]

Given the advances in cardiac protection during cardioplegic arrest, differences in postoperative ventricular function between off-pump CABG and CABG with CPB are difficult to document and are probably not significant in patients with normal or near-normal cardiac function. Experience with off-pump surgery in patients with left ventricular dysfunction is growing. Although mortality rates and postoperative improvement in ventricular function are comparable between off-pump CABG and CABG with CPB in this group, requirements for postoperative inotropic support, prolonged ventilation, and intensive care unit stay are all increased in the CPB group.[21] These results appear to justify an aggressive approach toward performing off-pump CABG in patients with severely depressed left ventricular dysfunction. Even when crossover to CPB becomes necessary, it has been shown that on-pump beating-heart CABG in this group can be associated with excellent results and improved long-term left ventricular function when compared to similar patients undergoing CABG with ischemic cardioplegic arrest.[22]

Atrial fibrillation is the most common complication after CABG. Although we have not been able to show an improvement in the rate of postoperative atrial fibrillation with off-pump CABG, this has not been the case in other reports. Stamou showed a significant rate of drop of the odds ratio for new-onset atrial fibrillation in a large series of off- versus on-pump CABG patients.[23] In this series, patients with persistent postoperative atrial fibrillation went on to have a higher postoperative in-hospital stroke rate and higher in-hospital mortality. In a prospective randomized trial comparing off- with on-pump CABG patients, Ascione and colleagues reported that CPB inclusive of cardioplegic arrest was an independent predictor of postoperative atrial fibrillation by stepwise multivariate regression analysis.[24]

Graft Patency

The question of whether short- and long-term patency rates after off-pump CABG are comparable to those obtained with CPB is perhaps the most hotly contested issue currently facing coronary surgeons. At present, little information exists regarding long-term patency and clinical results of off-pump CABG. Gundry followed 107 patients who underwent off-pump CABG between 1989 and 1990 for 7 years, and compared them with 112 patients who underwent CABG with CPB. Although survival and cardiac death rates were similar for the two groups, twice as many patients in the off-pump group required recatheterization (30% vs 16%), and 20% required a second revascularization procedure. Only 7% of patients who had CABG with CPB required re-intervention during the same time frame.[25] It should be noted that these operations were performed prior to the widespread use of coronary stabilizers and positioning devices for off-pump CABG. Since then, improvements in such instrumentation have led to generally reliable and reproducible coronary anastomoses. Puskas performed early angiographic follow-up of 125 consecutive off-pump CABG patients and found 100% patency of all internal mammary artery grafts and a total patency rate of 97.8%.[26] Lund determined that early angiographic patency of grafts after off-pump CABG was 95.3% to the LAD artery, 91.8% to the circumflex (CX), and 85.3% to the right coronary artery. Patency was inversely related to diameter of the grafted vessel in the LAD and CX areas.[27]

Many questions still have not been answered regarding the reliability of coronary anastomoses performed without CPB. Some surgeons believe that the coagulopathy generally associated with CPB may have a protective effect on graft patency and that a hypercoagulable state may accompany off-pump CABG. Kim and colleagues compared 1-year graft patency after off-pump CABG with that of conventional CABG and with on-pump beating CABG. In their study, the 1-year patency rate of saphenous vein grafts after off-pump CABG was significantly lower than either conventional CABG or on-pump beating CABG (67% vs 88% vs 86.8%). There was no difference in the patency rate of arterial grafts between the three groups.[28]

The issue of graft patency after off-pump CABG is further complicated by the addition of mechanical stapling devices currently used for proximal aortograft anastomoses and soon to be available for distal coronary anastomosis. Because these devices are based on a stent-like mechanism, concerns exist regarding their potential for early stenosis or graft occlusion. Furthermore, small deviations in graft angle or length when these devices are used can result in kinking and graft occlusion. Until more information is available regarding the long-term patency rate with mechanical anastomotic devices in clinical practice, their use in only selected patients may be warranted.

Perioperative Mortality

Numerous clinical reports in the surgical literature suggest that perioperative mortality was decreased in off-pump CABG when compared with similar groups of patients who underwent on-pump CABG. Mack's group in Dallas compared the results of 1,983 off-pump CABG patients with 6,466 patients undergoing CABG with CPB. In this study, early mortality was significantly decreased in the off-pump group (3.5% vs 1.8%), despite a lower predicted risk in the on-pump CABG group.[29] Cleveland and colleagues compared the results of on- and off-pump CABG using the Society of Thoracic Surgeons National Adult Cardiac Surgery Database for the years 1998 through 1999. During this period, 9.9% of CABG cases reported to the Society of Thoracic Surgeons National Database were performed without CPB. In this analysis of thousands of patients, the use of an off-pump procedure was associated with a statistically significant decrease in risk-adjusted operative mortality from 2.9% with conventional CABG to 2.3% in the off-pump group. Furthermore, the major complication rate was reduced from 14.1% in the CPB group to 10.6% in the off-pump group.[30] The Cleveland Clinic Group compared 441 consecutive off-pump patients with 502 CABG-with-CPB patients by using propensity-based matching. In this analysis, patients undergoing on-pump CABG had more three-vessel coronary artery disease, more left main disease, and higher New York Heart Association functional class. However, there was no difference in observed mortality between the two groups.[31]

Although a number of prospective randomized trials are currently underway, only a few that compare the results of off-pump CABG with CABG using CPB have been completed. In a report to the Twenty-third Congress of the European Society of Cardiology, Diegeler found no difference in mortality in a trial of 124 patients prospectively randomized to undergo either off- or on-pump CABG.[32] Puskas and colleagues reported similar hospital and 30-day mortality in a prospective randomized comparison of 200 unselected patients having off- versus on-pump CABG.[33] These results suggest that either off-pump CABG is not associated with the kind of improvement in results for which surgeons had hoped, or that surgeons have not yet identified which types of patients benefit the most. Akpinar showed no difference in perioperative mortality when comparing a large series of off- versus on-pump CABG patients. However, in patients who were deemed "high risk" by the Allegheny Clinic Risk Scoring Scale, the mortality rate was 3.9% in the off-pump group as compared with 7.9% in the on-pump group.[34] It makes sense that the higher the number of preoperative risk factors, the more a given patient stands to benefit from off-pump CABG. There is a need for more studies designed to identify which groups of patients will benefit the most from off-pump CABG. On a more discouraging note, Magee and colleagues recently published data to suggest that although morbidity is improved, mortality after off-pump CABG is not improved in diabetic patients when compared with the on-pump group.[35]

Neurologic Complications

Coronary artery bypass surgery has long been associated with both major and minor neurologic sequelae. Although most surgical reports estimate the rate of cerebrovascular accidents after CABG to be in the 2% range, the rate of postoperative neurologic abnormalities is probably much higher.[37] Roach and colleagues evaluated 2,108 patients from 24 US institutions for two categories of neurologic outcomes after conventional CABG.[36] They found the incidence of adverse cerebral outcomes after CABG to be 6.1%. Type I injuries (focal injury, or stupor or coma at discharge) accounted for 3.1%, while type II injuries (deterioration in intellectual function, memory deficit, or seizures) accounted for 3.0% of adverse cerebral outcomes. The consequences of perioperative adverse neurologic outcomes in this study emphasize their importance, and they are depicted in Table 10-2.

Most major neurologic sequelae after CABG are the result of thromboembolism, perioperative hypotension,

and hypoperfusion.[37,38] Thromboemboli and atheroemboli can be macroscopic and result from manipulation of the aorta during coronary surgery. Microemboli generated during CPB also contribute to poor neurologic outcomes after CABG, but their role is less clear. Off-pump CABG has the potential to decrease the incidence of adverse neurologic outcomes after CABG by two mechanisms. The first is by decreasing the amount of aortic manipulation by avoiding aortic cannulation and cross-clamping. Whereas many surgeons still prefer to use a side-biting clamp to perform proximal anastomoses, mechanical aortic anastomotic devices further decrease the potential for minimal aortic manipulation with off-pump CABG. The potential for microembolism is also decreased by avoiding CPB.

Although studies exist that show an overall decrease in stroke with off-pump CABG as compared to CABG with CPB, most show little or no difference.[39–41] This has been particularly true in prospective randomized trials that compare the two types of CABG operations.[33,42] The real question is whether off-pump CABG has the potential to reduce the rate of major adverse neurologic outcomes in patients who would normally be considered high risk for stroke. By using univariate analysis, Ricci and colleagues reported a significant decrease in the prevalence of stroke after off-pump CABG in patients over the age of 70 years.[43] However, CPB did not emerge as an independent predictor of stroke at multivariate analysis. The same group looked at the incidence of stroke after CABG in octogenarians and was able to perform 97 off-pump CABG operations without a perioperative stroke, compared to a stroke rate of 9.3% in an on-pump group of 172 patients.[44] This makes sense when one considers the risk factors for stroke with CABG. As previously mentioned in "Operative Techniques," John and colleagues showed that a patient older than age 80 years, with a history of calcified aorta, prior stroke, carotid disease, renal failure, peripheral vascular disease, smoking, and diabetes, has a stroke rate with conventional CABG that approaches 40% (see Table 10-1).[7] The potential for decreasing the risk of stoke when these risk factors exist lies in the ability to perform the operation with little or no manipulation of the ascending aorta.

Neurocognitive function can be significantly impacted in patients after on-pump CABG, particularly in the elderly.[45] In fact, Newman and colleagues showed an incidence of cognitive decline of 53% at discharge, 36% at 6 weeks, 24% at 6 months, and 42% at 5 years after traditional CABG.[46] Unfortunately, there was no control group in this study. However, the rates of cognitive decline were greater than would be expected from other studies observed in elderly patients.[47] Because neurocognitive function is usually considered to be an adverse reaction to CPB, one would expect to see improvement in the results of CABG in the off-pump groups. van Dijk, in a prospective randomized study in which psychologists who tested for cognitive function were blinded as to whether patients had undergone on or off-pump CABG, showed that patients

TABLE 10-2. Clinical Consequences of Adverse Cerebral Outcomes after Conventional Coronary Artery Bypass Grafting

Variable	Type 1 Outcome (N = 66)	Type II Outcome (N = 63)	No Adverse Cerebral Event (N = 1979)
Death during hospitalization – no. (%)	14 (21)	6 (10)	38 (2)
Duration of postoperative hospital stay – days			
Mean ± SD	25.3 ± 22.1	20.5 ± 25.2	9.5 ± 12.4
Median	17.6	10.9	7.7
Duration of ICU stay – days			
Mean ± SD	11.1 ± 15.4	6.6 ± 7.9	2.6 ± 3.5
Median	5.8	3.2	1.9
Discharged to home – no. (%)†	21 (32)	38 (60)	1773 (90)

Adapted from Roach GW et al.[36]

*$p < .001$ for all comparisons among the groups. ICU = intensive care unit.
†Patients not discharged to their homes either died or were discharged to intermediate- or long-term care facilities.

had improved cognitive outcomes at 3 months postoperation but that the effects were limited and became negligible at 12 months.[48] Diegeler, on the other hand, showed significant differences in postoperative S-100 serum levels as well as postoperative cognitive testing in 40 patients randomized to undergo off- versus on-pump CABG.[49] In his study, postoperative cognitive function using the Syndrom Kurtz Test Score was rated in a pathologic range in 18 of 20 patients undergoing on-pump CABG, compared to no impairments in the off-pump group.

It is becoming clearer that off-pump CABG has the potential to decrease adverse neurologic outcomes, especially in high-risk patients. These improvements are the result of avoidance of the physiologic consequences of CPB, as well as decreased manipulation of the aorta. Whereas improvements in low-risk patients, such as young patients without comorbidities, may be subtle or difficult to demonstrate, improvements in outcomes in elderly patients with multiple risk factors have the potential to be dramatic.

Postoperative Renal Function

The impact of cardiac surgery with CPB on renal function and its consequences is well known.[50,51] Although the nephrotoxicity of CPB has improved considerably over the years, the number of patients undergoing CABG who have preoperative renal dysfunction is growing as older and sicker patients are operated on. Off-pump CABG was associated with improved glomerular filtration as measured by creatinine clearance when compared with patients who underwent on-pump CABG. Furthermore, the urinary microalbumin/creatinine and fractional excretion of sodium are better in off-pump versus on-pump CABG patients.[52,53] Analyses of large groups of patients undergoing off-pump CABG show significantly decreased rates of renal failure. Mack reviewed the postoperative morbidity in 3,000 off-pump CABG patients and compared it with 14,609 patients who underwent CABG with CPB in the same multicenter database. He found the incidence of postoperative renal failure to be 0.97% in the CPB group, as compared with 0.5% in the off-pump group.[10] Cartier compared the effects of off- versus on-pump CABG on postoperative renal function in patients with preoperative renal insufficiency (creatinine level > 130 mmol/L). He found that although there seemed to be an overall benefit to off-pump CABG, deterioration in renal function was not necessarily prevented in that group.[54] We have seen similar results. Although dialysis can usually be prevented in off-pump CABG patients with preoperative renal dysfunction, creatinine levels frequently rise for 1 to 2 days before stabilizing or returning to preoperative levels. We attribute this to blood pressure fluctuations and pharmacologic manipulation, which occurs with the various cardiac positions during off-pump operations.

Respiratory Complications

Postoperative pulmonary complications after cardiac surgical procedures on CPB can be associated with atelectasis, pulmonary edema, inflammation, increased capillary permeability, and pleural effusions.[55] The possibility that these problems might be less prevalent by avoiding CPB has led off-pump CABG surgeons to strive for earlier postoperative extubation and shorter intensive care unit stays. In our early series of off-pump CABG operations, 40% of patients were extubated in the operating room. However, these patients tended to be more uncomfortable in the first few postoperative hours, frequently requiring large amounts of pain medication. We have returned to a policy of early but controlled extubation in the intensive care unit. In general, we have not seen an overall improvement in the incidence of respiratory complications in our off-pump CABG group. Similarly, Cox and colleagues showed that myocardial revascularization with or without cardiopulmonary bypass caused a similar degree of pulmonary dysfunction as assessed by alveolar-arterial oxygen gradient.[56] However, in our experience, the incidence of prolonged ventilation in patients with respiratory insufficiency does seem to have improved. Mack also showed a significantly decreased rate of prolonged ventilation in patients undergoing off-pump CABG when compared to CABG on CPB in a large series of patients.[57]

Postoperative Bleeding and Transfusions

The effects of cardiopulmonary bypass on homeostasis, platelet number and function, and in postoperative bleeding after cardiac surgery are well known.[58–60] As previously mentioned, the contact of blood and its components with nonphysiologic surfaces of the extracorporeal circuit, shear forces, activation of the complement system, and fibrinolysis contribute to platelet dysfunction that has the potential to result in postoperative bleeding.[61] Off-pump CABG has been consistently associated with decreased postoperative bleeding, decreased transfusion rate, and decreased return to the operating room for postoperative hemorrhage when compared to on-pump CABG.[62] In fact, these findings have been consistent throughout the surgical literature regarding off-pump bypass surgery. By avoiding the adverse effects of CPB, platelet function and number are preserved, clotting factor deficiencies and circulating anticoagulants are avoided, and postoperative chest tube output is less.[61]

Postoperative Stay and Hospital Cost

Postoperative hospital stay and hospital costs are difficult to assess because they are affected by so many variables. As a result, conflicting reports exist regarding cost benefits and hospital length of stay with off-pump CABG when compared to CABG on CPB. Retrospective analyses of large computer-matched groups demonstrate a significant improvement in hospital stay associated with off-pump CABG.[29] Puskas demonstrated a decrease in hospital stay from a mean of 5.7 days with on-pump CABG to 3.9 days with off-pump CABG.[63] Regarding cost, surgeons at the Bristol Heart Institute randomized patients to off- or on-pump CABG and found that off-pump CABG was significantly less costly than conventional CABG with respect to operating materials, bed occupancy, and transfusion requirements.[64] However, Bull and colleagues showed no significant difference between off-pump CABG and CABG with CPB with regard to cost, length of stay, or incidence of complications. Clearly, the potential for improvements in cost and length of stay depend on personal preferences and priorities of the individual surgeons. We found that eliminating CPB from operating room costs initially accounted for a 25% cost savings with off-pump CABG. This savings was quickly eliminated with the use of disposable coronary stabilizers, cardiac positioning devices, and mechanical stapling devices. Similarly, we have seen tremendous variation in hospital stays depending on the comfort levels of early discharge between different cardiologists, making standardized discharge policies difficult to implement. In our experience, overall length of hospital stay after CABG has depended more on these subjective factors than on whether or not CPB was used with CABG.

Conclusion

Off-pump CABG has the potential to further improve the results obtained with surgical myocardial revascularization. This is particularly important given the increased age and number of comorbidities seen in patients currently being referred for coronary surgery. Increased experience, along with well-designed prospective randomized trials, will enable surgeons to identify the most appropriate patient groups for off-pump CABG. At the same time, advances in instrumentation, including mechanical anastomotic devices, have the potential to increase the safety of these operations.

References

1. Vineburg AM. Treatment of coronary insufficiency by implantation of the internal mammary artery into the left ventricular myocardium. J Thorac Surg 1952;23:42–54.
2. Longmire WP, Cannon JA, Kattus A. Direct vision coronary endarterectomy for angina pectoris. N Engl J Med 1958; 259:993–9.
3. Sones FM Jr, Shirey EK. Cinecoronary arteriography. Mod Conc Cardiovasc Dis 1962;31:135.
4. Buffolo E, Andrade JC, Branco JN, et al. Myocardial revascularization without extracorporeal circulation. Seven-year experience in 593 cases. Eur J Cardiothorac Surg 1990;4:504–8.
5. Benetti FJ, Naselli G, Wood M, et al. Direct myocardial revascularization without extracorporeal circulation: experience in 700 patients. Chest 1991;100(2):312–6.
6. Benetti FJ, Ballester C. Use of thoracoscopy and a minimal thoracotomy in mammary-coronary bypass to the left anterior descending artery, without extracorporeal circulation: experience in 2 cases. J Cardiovasc Surg 1995; 36:159–61.
7. John R, Choudhri AF, Weinberg AD, et al. Multicenter review of preoperative risk factors for stroke after coronary artery bypass grafting. Ann Thorac Surg 2000;69(1):30–5.
8. Yeatman M, Caputo M, Ascione R, et al. Off-pump coronary artery bypass surgery for critical left main stem disease: safety, efficacy and outcome. Eur J Cardiothorac Surg 2001;19(3):239–44.
9. Stamou SC, Pfister AJ, Dullum MK, et al. Late outcome of reoperative coronary revascularization on the beating heart. Heart Surg Forum 2001;4(1):69–73.
10. Mack M. Off-pump CABG: what's proven, what's not. Presented at the Annual Meeting of the American College of Surgeons. New Orleans, October 2001.
11. Manchi A, Edmondson SJ, Hearse DJ. Dynamics of early postischemic myocardial functional recovery. Evidence of reperfusion induced injury? Circulation 1995;92: 526–34.
12. Heames RM, Gill RS, Ohri SK, Hett DA. Off-pump coronary artery surgery. Anaesthesia 2002;57(7):676–85.
13. Bouchard D, Cartier R. Off-pump revascularization of multivessel coronary artery disease has a decreased myocardial infarction rate. Eur J Cardiothorac Surg 1998;14:S20–4.
14. Wildhirt SM, Schulze C, Conrad N, et al. Reduced myocardial cellular damage and lipid peroxidation in off-pump versus conventional coronary artery bypass grafting. Eur J Med Res 2000;5(5):222–8.
15. Koh TW, Carr-White GS, DeSouza AC, et al. Intraoperative cardiac troponin T release and lactate metabolism during coronary artery surgery: comparison of beating heart with conventional coronary artery surgery with conventional bypass. Heart 1999;81:495–500.
16. Rubitzsch H, Ansorge K, Wollert HG, Eckel L. Stunned myocardium after off-pump coronary artery bypass grafting. Ann Thorac Surg 2001;71:352–5.
17. D'Ancona G, Donias HW, Bergsland J, Karamanoukian HL. Myocardial stunning after off-pump coronary artery bypass grafting: safeguards and pitfalls [letter]. Ann Thorac Surg 2001;72(6):2182–3.
18. Laurikka J, Wu ZK, Iisalo P, et al. Regional ischemic preconditioning enhances myocardial performance in off-pump coronary artery bypass grafting. Chest 2002; 121(4):1183–9.
19. Yeatman M, Caputo M, Narayan P, et al. Intracoronary shunts reduce transient intraoperative myocardial dysfunction during off-pump coronary operations. Ann Thorac Surg 2002;73(5):1411–7.
20. Brown PM, Kim VB, Boyer BJ, et al. Regional left ventricular systolic function in humans during off-pump coronary bypass surgery. Circulation 1999;100 Suppl 19:II125–7.
21. Kirali K, Rabus MB, Yakut N, et al. Early and long-term comparison of the on and off-pump bypass surgery in patients with left ventricular dysfunction. Heart Surg Forum 2002;5(2):177–81.

22. Prifti E, Bonacchi M, Giunti G, et al. Does on-pump beating-heart coronary artery bypass grafting offer better outcome in end-stage coronary artery disease patients? J Card Surg 2000;15(6):403–10.

23. Stamou SC, Dangas G, Hill PC, et al. Atrial fibrillation after beating heart surgery. Am J Cardiol 2000;86(1):64–7.

24. Ascione R, Caputo M, Calori G, et al. Predictors of atrial fibrillation after conventional and beating heart coronary surgery: a prospective, randomized study. Circulation 2000;102(13):1530–5.

25. Gundry SR, Romano MA, Shattuck OH, et al. Seven-year followup of coronary artery bypasses performed with and without cardiopulmonary bypass. J Thorac Cardiovasc Surg 1998;115(6):1273–7.

26. Puskas JD, Wright CE, Ronson RS, et al. Clinical outcomes and angiographic patency in 125 consecutive off-pump coronary bypass patients. Heart Surg Forum 1999; 2(3):216–21.

27. Lund O, Christensen J, Holme S, et al. On-pump versus off-pump coronary artery bypass: independent risk factors and off-pump graft patency. Eur J Cardiothorac Surg 2001;20(5):901–7.

28. Kim KB, Lim C, Lee C, et al. Off-pump coronary artery bypass may decrease the patency of saphenous vein grafts. Ann Thorac Surg 2001;72(3):S1033–7.

29. Magee MJ, Jablonski KA, Stamou SC, et al. Elimination of cardiopulmonary bypass improves early survival for multivessel coronary artery bypass patients. Ann Thorac Surg 2002;73(4):1196–202.

30. Cleveland JC Jr, Shroyer AL, Chen AY, et al. Off-pump coronary bypass grafting decreases risk-adjusted mortality and morbidity. Ann Thorac Surg 2001;72(4):1282–8.

31. Sabik JF, Gilliov AM, Blackstone EH, et al. Does off-pump coronary surgery reduce morbidity and mortality? J Thorac Cardiovasc Surg 2002;124:698–707.

32. Diegeler A et al. Presented at the XXIII Congress of the European Society of Cardiology. September 2001.

33. Puskas JD, Williams WH, Duke PG, et al. Off-pump coronary artery bypass provides complete revascularization while reducing myocardial injury, transfusion requirements and length of stay. Presented at the 82nd Annual Meeting of the American Association for Thoracic Surgery, 2002.

34. Akpinar B, Guden M, Sanisoglu I, et al. Does off-pump coronary artery bypass surgery reduce mortality in high risk patients? Heart Surg Forum 2001;4(3):231–6.

35. Magee MJ, Dewey TM, Acuff T, et al. Influence of diabetes on mortality and morbidity: off-pump coronary artery bypass grafting versus coronary artery bypass grafting with cardiopulmonary bypass. Ann Thorac Surg 2001; 72(3):776–80.

36. Roach GW, Kanchuger M, Mangano CM, et al. Adverse cerebral outcomes after coronary bypass surgery. N Engl J Med 1996;335(25):1857–63.

37. McKhann GM, Goldsborough MA, Borowicz LM, et al. Predictors of stroke risk in coronary artery bypass patients. Ann Thorac Surg 1997;63:516–21.

38. Mickleborough LL, Walker PM, Takagi Y, et al. Risk factors for stroke in patient undergoing coronary artery bypass grafting. J Thorac Cardiovasc Surg 1996;112:1250–8.

39. Karamanoukian HL, Donias HW, Bergsland J. Decreased incidence of postoperative stroke following off-pump coronary artery bypass. J Am Coll Cardiol 2002;39(5): 917–9.

40. Trehan N, Mishra M, Sharma OP, et al. Further reduction in stroke after off-pump coronary artery bypass grafting: a 10-year experience. Ann Thorac Surg 2001;72(3): S1026–32.

41. Hernandez F, Cohn WE, Baribeau YR, et al. In-hospital outcomes of off-pump coronary artery bypass procedures: a multicenter experience. Ann Thorac Surg 2001;72(5): 1528–33.

42. van Dijk D, Nierich AP, Jansen EW, et al. Early outcome after off-pump versus on-pump coronary bypass surgery: results from a randomized study. Circulation 2001;104(15):1761–6.

43. Ricci M, Karamanoukian HL, Dancona G, et al. On-pump and off-pump coronary artery bypass grafting in the elderly: predictors of adverse outcome. J Card Surg 2001; 16(6):458–66.

44. Ricci M, Karamanoukian HL, Abraham R, et al. Stroke in octogenarians undergoing coronary artery surgery with and without cardiopulmonary bypass. Ann Thorac Surg 2000;69(5):1471–5.

45. Newman MF, Croughwell ND, Blumenthal JA, et al. Effect of aging on cerebral autoregulation during cardiopulmonary bypass: association with postoperative cognitive dysfunction. Circulation 1994;90 Suppl II: II-243–9.

46. Newman MF, Kirchner JL, Phillips-Bute B, et al. Longitudinal assessment of neurocognitive function after coronary artery bypass surgery. N Engl J Med 2001;344(6): 396–402.

47. Haan MN, Shemanski L, Jagust WJ, et al. The role of APOE epsilon4 in modulating effects of other risk factors for cognitive decline in elderly persons. JAMA 1999;282: 40–6.

48. van Dijk D, Jansen EW, Hijman R, et al. Cognitive outcome after off-pump and on-pump coronary artery bypass graft surgery. JAMA 2002;287(11):1404–13.

49. Diegeler A, Hirsch R, Schneider F, et al. Neuromonitoring and neurocognitive outcome in off-pump versus conventional coronary bypass operations. Ann Thorac Surg 2000;69(4):1162–6.

50. Abel RM, Buckley MJ, Austen WG, et al. Etiology, incidence, and prognosis of renal failure following cardiac operations. J Thorac Cardiovasc Surg 1976;71:323–33.

51. Lema G, Meneses G, Urzua J, et al. Effects of extracorporeal circulation on renal function in coronary surgical patients. Anesth Analg 1995;81:446–51.

52. Ascione R, Lloyd CTG, Underwood MJ, et al. On-pump versus off-pump coronary revascularization: evaluation of renal function. Ann Thorac Surg 1999;68:493–8.

53. Loef BG, Epema AH, Navis G, et al. Off-pump coronary revascularization attenuates transient renal damage compared with on-pump coronary revascularization. Chest 2002;121(4):1190–4.

54. Cartier R. Off-pump surgery and chronic renal insufficiency [letter; comment]. Ann Thorac Surg 2000;69(6): 1995–6.

55. Barnas GM, Watson RJ, Green MD, et al. Lung and chest wall mechanical properties before and after cardiac surgery with cardiopulmonary bypass. J Appl Physiol 1992;73:1040–6.

56. Cox CM, Ascione R, Cohen AM, et al. Effect of cardiopulmonary bypass on pulmonary gas exchange: a prospective randomized study. Ann Thorac Surg 2000;69(1): 140–5.

57. Mack MJ, Magee MJ, Edgerton JR, et al. Beating heart techniques improved outcomes in coronary artery bypass grafting. Presented at the 81st Annual Meeting of the American Association for Thoracic Surgery. San Diego, CA, 2001.

58. Kawahito K, Kobayashi E, Iwasa H, et al. Platelet aggregation during cardiopulmonary bypass evaluated by a laser light scattering method. Ann Thorac Surg 1999;67: 79–84.

59. Holloway DS, Summaria L, Sandesara J, et al. Decreased platelet number and function and increased fibrinolysis contribute to postoperative bleeding in cardiopulmonary bypass patients. Thromb Haemost 1988;59: 62–7.

60. Liu B, Belboul A, Larsson S, Roberts D. Factors influencing haemostasis and blood transfusion in cardiac surgery. Perfusion 1996;11:131–43.

61. Ascione R, Williams FM, Lloyd CT, et al. Reduced postoperative blood loss and transfusion requirement after beating-heart coronary operations: a prospective randomized study. J Thorac Cardiovasc Surg 2001;121(4): 689–96.

62. Nader ND, Khadra WZ, Reich NT, et al. Blood product use in cardiac revascularization: comparison of on- and off-pump techniques. Ann Thorac Surg 1999;68(5):1640–3.

63. Puskas JD, Thourani VH, Marshall JJ, et al. Clinical outcomes, angiographic patency, and resource utilization in 200 consecutive off-pump coronary bypass patients. Ann Thorac Surg 2001;71(5):1477–83.

64. Ascione R, Lloyd CT, Underwood MJ, et al. Economic outcome of off-pump coronary artery bypass surgery: a prospective randomized study. Ann Thorac Surg 1999; 68(6):2237–42.

CHAPTER 11

ROBOTICS IN CARDIAC SURGERY

MICHAEL D. DIODATO JR, MD, HERSH S. MANIAR, MD,
SUNIL M. PRASAD, MD, RALPH J. DAMIANO JR, MD

Many surgical disciplines have been quick to adopt endoscopic technology because of the decreased morbidity and shorter recovery times.[1–3] These procedures are performed through small 5 to 10 mm ports with visualization using an endoscopic camera. Traditionally, most of these procedures have been excisional in nature rather than reconstructive and microsurgical. This is primarily a result of the limitations of conventional endoscopic instrumentation. For this reason, until recently, endoscopic approaches to cardiac surgery have not met with any success.

With the development of robotic surgical systems, or computer-assisted surgery, many of the limitations of conventional endoscopy have been overcome. While computers have long since transformed our office and hospital practice, they have had little direct impact upon the operating room. However, the introduction of computer-assisted surgery over the last several years has for the first time brought together the information technology revolution and the technical performance of surgery. In robotic surgery, there is a digital interface between the surgeon's hands and the instruments. This interface can be used to enhance surgical technical ability, thus enabling endoscopic microsurgery. Over the last few years, the use of robotic systems has allowed cardiac surgeons to perform minimally invasive endoscopic coronary artery bypass grafting (CABG) and valve procedures. This chapter summarizes the use of robotics in cardiac surgery and discusses their potential to transform our specialty.

History of Robotics

Aristotle is credited with the original concept of automation. In the fourth century B.C., he wrote, "If every instrument could accomplish its own work, obeying or anticipating the will of others...if the shuttle could weave, and the pick touch the lyre, without a hand to guide them, chief workmen would not need servants,..."[4]

The first generation of robots consisted of automatons. An automaton is a self-moving machine, constructed for the purpose of imitating animate motions.[5] Most of the earliest automatons were clock-controlled ornamentations. In the year 1350, an automated rooster was erected on top of the cathedral in Strasbourg, France. Within the same time period, an Arab named al-Jazari wrote a book on automatons. The book included an illustration of an automated Arab lady that filled and emptied a washbasin.[6] In 1774, Droz invented one of the most complicated automatons in history. The "automatic scribe" could write any message up to 40 characters long.[7] In 1801, Joseph Jacquard invented a textile machine operated by punch cards, which went into mass production as a programmable loom.[8] In 1805, Maillardet constructed a spring-activated automaton that could draw pictures and write in both French and English.[5] At the 1876 World's Fair, life-sized automatons, including brass instrument players, artists, and card magicians, entertained large audiences. A few years later, Thomas Edison used a condensed version of his phonograph invention in the design of the famous talking doll.[9]

Although this concept is centuries old, the term *robot* was first coined in 1920. It is a derivative of the Czech word for serf, "robota," and is attributed to the playwright Karel Capek and his play, *Rossum's Universal Robots* (Figure 11-1). The play was a parody on a utopian society where all menial labor was performed by machines thereby freeing man to enjoy a life of leisure. In 1940, Westinghouse created two of the first robots that used an electric motor for entire body motion in the rectangular coordinate plane.[9] Interestingly, the term *robotics* did not come into use until 1942, when Isaac Asimov published the story "Runaround" in the magazine *Astounding*. It was in this manuscript that Asimov's "Three Laws of Robotics" were expounded. These laws, which still hold validity for modern robotics, state that (1) robots may not injure a human being or, through inaction, allow a human to

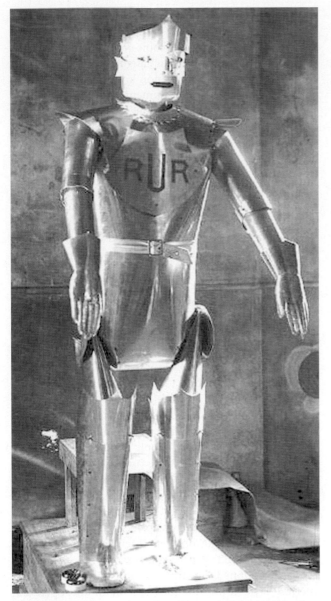

FIGURE 11-1. A representation of Rossum's Universal Robot from Karel Capek's play.

General Motors installed robots onto production lines in Trenton, NJ, in 1962. By 1964, artificial intelligence laboratories were opened at Massachusetts Institute of Technology, Stanford University, and the University of Edinburgh. In 1968, Shakey, a robot with visual capabilities, was developed at the Stanford Research Institute and was soon followed by a robotic arm that was electrically powered. Richard Hohn at Cincinnati Milacron Corporation developed the first commercially available minicomputer-controlled robot, T3 (the Tomorrow Tool) in 1973. Professor Scheinman, the developer of the Stanford arm, formed Vicarm Incorporated in 1974 to market an industrial-strength version of the arm, which was computer controlled. The National Aeronautics and Space Administration (NASA) used these arms on the Viking space probes.

By the beginning of the 1980s, with the computer industry just beginning to blossom, the robot industry experienced a time of rapid growth. Fujitsu Fanuc Company of Japan developed the first totally automated factory in 1980. New robotics companies were appearing nearly every month. However, by 1990, most of the small companies had been purchased by large conglomerates that now control what has become a $170 billion industry.[11] Throughout the 1990s, these robotics companies tried to deal with problems in the human-robot interface, and the first visual servo-controlled systems were developed. As computer technology evolved, effective feedback systems were developed, which spurred a second wave of start-up companies and research. Over the last decade, the field of robotics expanded from its early industrial origins and began to focus on new markets, including medicine.

Two main companies have produced surgical robotic systems for cardiac surgery: Computer Motion and Intuitive Surgical. Computer Motion, Inc. (Goleta, CA), was founded in 1989 by Yulun Wang, PhD, and introduced a voice-controlled arm, AESOP, to position and hold an endoscopic camera in 1993. In October 1994, AESOP became the first Food and Drug Administration (FDA)–cleared surgical robot. In November 1996, AESOP 2000 became the first voice-controlled robot cleared by the FDA. The ZEUS Robotic Microsurgical System was introduced into clinical use in September 1998.

Frederic Moll, MD, Robert Younge, and John Freund, MD, formed Intuitive Surgical in 1995 based on technology developed by Stanford Research Institute, now SRI International. The da Vinci Surgical System (Intuitive Surgical, Inc., Mountain View, CA) consisted of a surgeon console, a computer controller, and endoscopic instruments with articulated "endowrists" at the end of two surgical arms. The first robotically assisted cardiac surgeries in the world were performed using the da Vinci system. Dr. Carpentier, in Paris, performed a mitral valve procedure in April 1998. In the same month, Dr. Friedrich Mohr, in Leipzig, performed the first robotically assisted CABG.

come to harm; (2) a robot must obey the orders given to it by human beings except such orders that would conflict with the first law; and (3) a robot must protect its own existence as long as such protection does not conflict with the first or second laws.[10]

While there was progress in both computer development and robotics in the early twentieth century, it was the invention of the transistor in 1948 that accelerated the development of robots and computers. In 1951, Raymond Goetz developed a teleoperated articulated arm for the Atomic Energy Commission. George Devol designed the first programmable robot and coined the term *universal automaton* in 1954. He was the founder of the first robot company.

Overview and Advantages of Robotic Surgical Systems

Robotic systems have been developed to assist in endoscopic procedures. These systems consist of three main components: a surgeon interface device, a computer controller, and specially designed instrument tips attached to robotic arms. The surgeon controls the instrument handles from an interface device. His movements are subsequently relayed to and digitized by a computer controller. The information is then passed along to robotic arms, which are positioned on or near the operating table. Current surgical robotic arm systems are able to move with multiple degrees of freedom, simulating the movement of the human arm, elbow, and wrist.

A third robotic arm is capable of manipulating the endoscope and is controlled by the surgeon. The direct control of the robotic arm has eliminated the need for a human assistant. The robotic camera arm is more precise than a human assistant, and the number of times the camera needs cleaning has been reduced three- to fivefold.[12] With the AESOP arm, movements can be stored in the computer's memory and be returned to with a simple voice command. The endoscope allows for much greater magnification than traditional surgical loupes, enhancing the surgeon's visualization of the anatomic detail of small structures. Although the loss of depth perception because of two-dimensional video monitors has been a traditional drawback to endoscopic visualization,[13,14] both companies offer high-resolution three-dimensional monitors.[15]

The computer interface is the major difference between robotic and traditional surgery. It allows for digitization of the surgeon's movements. This "digital" information can then be manipulated by the computer to enhance surgical movement. The two principal manipulations include filtering and motion scaling. The filtration of high-frequency oscillating motion effectively eliminates the surgeon's natural tremor. This helps to overcome the disadvantages of traditional endoscopy, in which the long instruments significantly magnify even the smallest tremor. This elimination of tremor enhances precision and may even facilitate ambidexterity. The computer controller also permits a variable degree of motion scaling, anywhere from 1- to 10-fold, changing gross hand movements at the console to fine movements in the operative field. This phenomenon has been termed *scaled telepresence*[16] and aids the surgeon in operating on extremely small structures. Recent work in our laboratory shows that motion scaling is most responsible for the enhanced precision seen with robotic systems.

The instrumentation available with computer-assisted endoscopic surgery offers significant advantages over those instruments used for conventional handheld instruments. Conventional nonrobotic laparoscopic equipment is limited to four degrees of freedom (a degree of freedom is a direction in which an instrument can move). Furthermore, the operator's motions are reversed (ie, the tip and handle move in opposite directions), and shear forces on the laparoscopic instruments are high, leading to increased operator fatigue. These pitfalls are both caused by the phenomenon known as the "fulcrum effect."[17] Separating the instrument tip from the handle eliminates this problem. With the help of the computer controller, intuitive motion is restored such that when the surgeon moves the instrument handle one way, the instrument tip moves in the same direction. Robotic systems allow for more intuitive hand movements by maintaining both the natural eye–hand axis as well as the oculovestibular orientation. This is in sharp contrast to the mirror image movements required in conventional endoscopic surgery. Robotic systems also allow for more degrees of freedom in movement by including a "wrist" joint on the instrument, creating a more natural handlike articulation.

However, a drawback of these systems is the loss of direct human contact with the tissue. As a result of the design of the robotic system, there can be no true haptic or force feedback given to the surgeon. While computer software and laparoscopic surgical models are being developed to create accurate haptic sensation, these are not currently clinically available.

A final advantage of the robotic systems is improved ergonomics. Operator fatigue results from many factors during conventional laparoscopic procedures. The surgeon is required to stand at the operating table, in often awkward positions, depending on trocar placement. Furthermore, the video monitor may be situated in a way that does not allow for convenient unobstructed viewing. The resulting common complaints of neck and back stiffness may lead to less-than-optimal surgical performance. In robotically assisted surgery, the surgeon is seated at the console, positioned directly in front of the monitor. This interface style immerses the surgeon in the operating field, minimizes distractions, and increases operator comfort. This serves to increase the surgeon's concentration and focus on the task at hand. It has been hypothesized that these improved ergonomics should help the surgeon's performance remain optimal for longer periods of time.

In summary, with better visualization, improved dexterity, and reduced fatigue, robotically assisted cardiac surgery allows for a level of precision superior to that obtainable with conventional endoscopic and open surgical techniques. This has expanded the use of endoscopy into the clinical microsurgical and reconstructive specialties.

Current Robotic Systems

Computer Motion

The current version of AESOP was introduced in January 1998. This robotic arm controls the endoscope and is mounted on the operating table. AESOP responds to more than 20 simple voice commands (Figure 11-2).

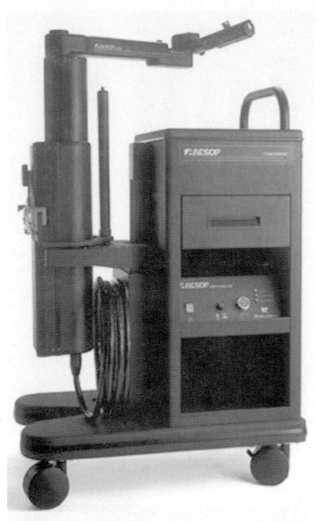

FIGURE 11-2. The AESOP robotic arm. It can be mounted to the operating table and accommodates most conventional endoscopes.

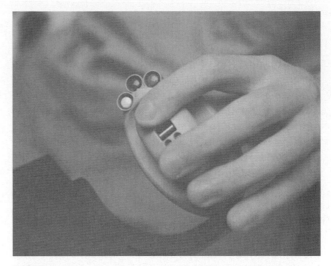

FIGURE 11-3. The Microwrist handle by Computer Motion.

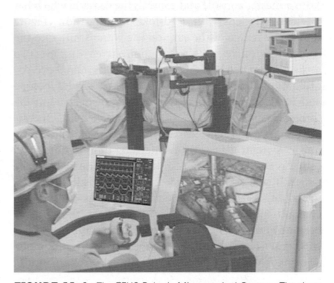

FIGURE 11-4. The ZEUS Robotic Microsurgical System. The three robotic arms are shown in the background, attached to the operating room table.

AESOP has eliminated the need for a dedicated camera holder and has an established track record of performance in more than 125,000 clinical procedures.[18]

The ZEUS Robotic Microsurgical System was introduced into clinical use in September 1998. Designed as a telemanipulator, the surgeon's movements are digitized and filtered by a signal processor, before being relayed to the robotic arms for the completion of a given movement. The surgeon is seated at an interface device or console. The surgeon holds form-fitted handles that provide an extremely sensitive natural robotic interface (Figure 11-3). The system mechanically relays the surgeon's hand movements to a computer controller.

Housed within the console is a 16-inch video monitor that displays the operative field (Figure 11-4). A three-dimensional flat-screen display is also available. The surgeon remains seated, with the endoscopic image displayed perfectly centered at eye level and close to the hands. Overall surgical performance has been shown to be improved by this surgeon-instrument orientation.[19] A second display

located immediately beneath the video monitor functions as a touch screen to provide control of instrument type, motion scaling, and performance characteristics of the instrument end-effectors.

The final components of the ZEUS system are the robotic arms, which are mounted on the operating table. These three arms are all lightweight (20 kilograms total) and independent, allowing for maximum flexibility in port placement. The surgical assistant and the remainder of the surgical team are positioned in close proximity to the robotic arms while the surgeon is seated away from the table at the ZEUS console. If necessary, the arms can be repositioned to accommodate the workspace requirements of the operative team.

The robotic arms hold the endoscopic instruments. Several of them have a designed "microwrist" near the instrument tip that provides for five degrees of freedom (Figure 11-5). The endoscopic instruments used in the ZEUS system are custom designed by Scanlan International (St. Paul, MN). More than 20 different end-effectors are offered, including needle drivers, ring forceps, tissue graspers, and microscissors. The instruments are between 3 and 5 mm in diameter and are easily inserted through 5 mm ports. These instruments are smaller than conventional endoscopic instruments, are reusable, and may be sterilized in the conventional manner. They are easily interchangeable during the operation, and the time to set up the ZEUS system has routinely been less than 20 min.[20]

Intuitive Surgical

The da Vinci Surgical System by Intuitive Surgical permits the intracavitary manipulation of various 2 to 4 mm instrument tips through six degrees of excursion, emulating the human wrist (Figure 11-6). The surgeon operates from a master console and controls the camera, which has a wide-angle lens with a 10-fold magnification (Figure 11-7). The image of the surgical site is transmitted to the surgeon through a high-resolution stereo display (two separate channels), which helps to restore hand–eye coordination. The Insite High-Resolution 3-D Endoscope and imaging processing equipment provide true-to-life three-dimensional images of the operative field. Operating images are enhanced, refined, and optimized by using image synchronizers, high-intensity illuminators, and camera control units. A robotic cart located at the patient's side positions and drives the wristlike devices, while an assistant adjusts and performs instrument changes (Figure 11-8). The operator at the console becomes immersed 1n the surgical landscape creating a "telepresence" with optimal access and dexterity. Robotic arms and "wrist" instruments are placed through 10 mm

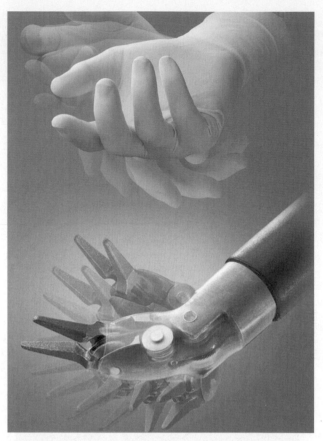

FIGURE 11-6. The da Vinci surgical EndoWrist provides articulation for surgical instruments.

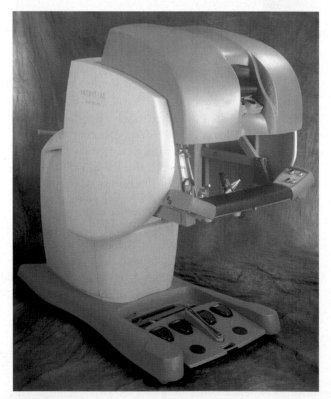

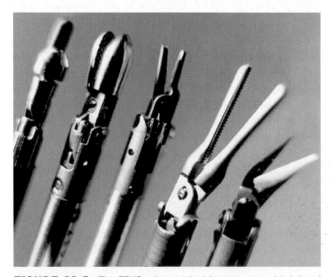

FIGURE 11-5. The ZEUS microsurgical instruments with jointed tips.

FIGURE 11-7. The da Vinci surgical console.

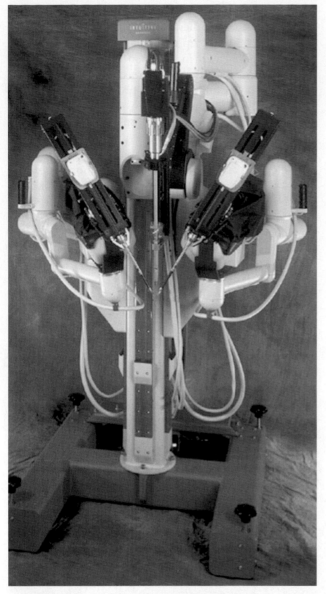

FIGURE 11-8. The da Vinci surgical robotic cart.

Robotics in Cardiac Surgery

Coronary Artery Bypass Grafting

There is extensive experience worldwide with robotically assisted CABG. While these operations are still performed on highly selected patients, spectacular progress has been made over the last several years. The worldwide experience for the ZEUS and the da Vinci systems is summarized below.

THE ZEUS EXPERIENCE

The European experience with the ZEUS system has principally been reported by Dr. Reichenspurner and his group in Munich.[21] They were the first in the world to use the ZEUS system, in September 1998. In August 2002, Dr. Reichenspurner reported that 41 patients had been operated upon using the ZEUS system between 1998 and 2001. These patients had single- or multivessel disease. The use of ZEUS occurred in a stepwise progression. In the initial 12 patients, the system was used for endoscopic internal thoracic artery (ITA) harvest. This was done to familiarize the surgeon with the device and the environment. The system was then used to perform 17 coronary anastomoses on arrested hearts in the next 13 patients. The anastomoses were performed endoscopically using robotic assistance and included left internal thoracic artery (LITA) to left anterior descending (LAD) ($n = 13$), right internal thoracic artery (RITA) to obtuse marginal (OM) ($n = 2$), and saphenous vein graft to diagonal targets ($n = 2$). The next 6 patients had the anastomoses (LITA to LAD) performed on a beating heart through a median sternotomy. Only one patient had to be converted to a manually performed anastomosis. The robotically assisted anastomoses took a median time of 21 min (range, 14 to 32 min) on the arrested and 25 min (range, 19 to 42 min) on the beating heart ($p =$ not significant). There was no significant difference in operating room (OR) time or date of discharge between these first two groups.

Two patients underwent endoscopic CABG with port-access cardiopulmonary bypass. LITA harvest took 83 and 110 min, and bleeding occurred in the first case, which required minithoracotomy to control. The anastomoses took 42 and 40 min to complete, and the surgeries took 4.5 and 5.3 h, respectively.

The last eight patients of this series underwent endoscopic CABG without cardiopulmonary bypass (CPB) on a beating heart. Median time for LITA harvest was 55 min (range, 43 to 74 min), and the median time for anastomotic completion was 32 min (range: 22 to 50 min). OR time was 5.5 h (range, 4.6 to 8.0 h), and median discharge day was 5.0 (range, 4 to 11 days). One patient was converted to an open procedure. The median times to perform the anastomoses were significantly longer in the endoscopic groups, but the median length of hospitalization was 5 days in the endoscopic groups and 8 days in the sternotomy groups. Postoperative angiography showed a

ports and converge in the surgical field. Six degrees of motion freedom are offered by this combination of trocar-positioned arms (insertion, pitch, and yaw) and articulated instrument wrists (roll, grip, pitch, and yaw). From the operating console, full x, y, and z-axis agility is effected by coordinating foot-pedal clutching and hand-motion sensors. Console surgeon hand activity is emulated precisely at the surgical field. Console foot pedals control the camera, its spatial orientation, and its focus. Moreover, if the surgeon's hands engage in a clumsy position, a foot-pedal clutching mechanism allows for easy and immediate repositioning. These eye–hand–foot interactions allow the surgeon to ratchet articulated wrists smoothly through every coordinate, configuring a myriad of complex instrument positions while providing maximum ergonomic comfort.

97% patency of all grafts, with only two anastomoses showing mild narrowing of less than 50%.

In the United States, Dr. Damiano and his group at Pennsylvania State University performed the first robotically assisted cardiac surgical procedure in North America, in December 1998.[22] The Food and Drug Administration approved a single-center clinical trial to evaluate the efficacy and safety of robotically assisted endoscopic CABG. Nineteen patients underwent a robotically assisted anastomosis of the LITA to the LAD. Primary outcome measurements were device-related complications and graft patency 6 to 8 weeks postoperatively.

All anastomoses were performed endoscopically through three-instrument ports (Figure 11-9). A modified subxiphoid approach was used for port placement. A zero-degree endoscope was attached to the AESOP voice-controlled robotic arm. A continuous end-to-side anastomosis was performed with a specially designed 7 cm double-armed 7–0 suture. Because this study was only approved for single-vessel bypass, all other grafts were completed manually prior to the robotic anastomosis.[23]

The system required an average set-up time of 16 ± 1 min. There were no intraoperative complications related to port placement or mechanical failures of the system. The time required to perform the LITA-to-LAD anastomosis was 22.5 ± 1.2 min, and the last five anastomoses were each performed in less than 20 min. Eighty-nine percent (17 of 19) of the grafts measured were patent and had excellent diastolic flow by ultrasound. Average graft flow was 38 ± 5 mL/min. Two of the grafts had inadequate flow and were manually reconstructed. The average intensive care unit (ICU) stay was 1.1 ± 1 days, and the average hospital stay was 4 ± 0.4 days. There was 100% late follow-up of these patients at 17 ± 4 months. At that time, there were no late complications and all patients were New York Heart Association (NYHA) class I. Eight weeks after surgery, graft patency was assessed by coronary angiography. This revealed all grafts to be patent and no graft stenosis of greater than 50%.[24]

In Canada, Dr. Boyd accumulated a significant experience with endoscopic ITA harvesting using the ZEUS system and has the largest series of totally closed endoscopic CABG. Initially, his group investigated the use of the AESOP robotic arm during ITA harvest.[25] In 55 consecutive patients, the ITA was harvested endoscopically using a 30° endoscope. Anastomoses were initially completed

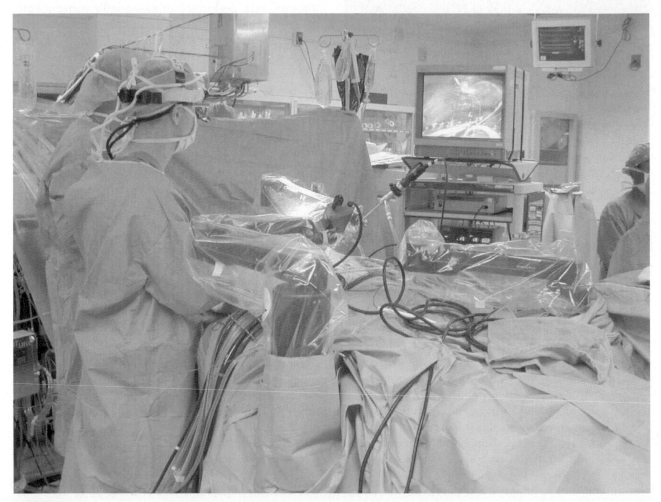

FIGURE 11-9. Intraoperative photograph of the ZEUS Robotic Microsurgical System in use for CABG.

manually through a limited thoracotomy. The average harvest time was 57 ± 23 min. Robotic camera assistance significantly reduced the number of endoscopic cleanings and was felt to facilitate the more difficult dissections. The AESOP arm reliably responded to more than 95% of verbal commands, and there was 100% patency in the 14 patients who underwent postoperative angiography.

Subsequently, the Harmonic Scalpel (Ethicon Endo-Surgery, Cincinnati, OH) was adapted to a ZEUS robotic arm, and 19 patients underwent LITA harvest using a robotically controlled Harmonic Scalpel with computer-assisted video control.[26] The investigators concluded that the ZEUS system could be used safely for ITA harvesting even when the anterior–posterior working space was limited. The advantages of the robotically controlled endoscope included greater exposure, superior image quality, and a consistent quality of assistance, which improved video dexterity and lessened surgeon fatigue.

Dr. Boyd's group has used the ZEUS system for beating-heart coronary anastomoses in 12 patients undergoing single-vessel CABG through a limited thoracotomy. The anastomotic times from ITA to LAD were 80 ± 27 min. No repair sutures were required, and average graft flows were 38 ± 24 mL/min. Postoperative angiography was performed on all patients, all anastomoses were patent, and 10 of 12 were Fitzgibbon's grade A.

Dr. Boyd has since performed a closed-chest totally endoscopic beating-heart CABG on six patients, using the ZEUS robotic system.[27] The first case was performed on September 24, 1999. Using a zero-degree endoscope,

the AESOP, and warm carbon dioxide gas insufflation, sufficient working space and visibility were established in the mediastinum. A specially designed sternal elevator also was employed to increase the anterior–posterior intrathoracic space. With the patients in a right lateral decubitus position, trocars were inserted in the third, fifth, and seventh interspaces along the mid to anterior axillary lines (Figure 11-10). In preparation for the beating-heart anastomosis, an articulating end stabilizer (Computer Motion, Goleta, CA) was inserted through a port in the second interspace at the axillary line for LAD stabilization.

In this clinical series, anastomotic times varied between 40 and 74 min (mean, 55.8 min). All anastomoses had acceptable flows with a mean of 28 mL/min (range, 12 to 46 mL/min), and no patient required conversion from the robotic technique. Median operative time was 6 h (range, 4.5 to 7.5 h). All patients underwent coronary angiography prior to discharge, and five of six grafts were found to be patent. One had a 50% stenosis in the region of the distal snare site. The average length of hospital stay was 4.0 ± 0.9 days. All patients were free from angina, had returned to work, and had normal exercise capacity at a mean follow up of 145.3 ± 29.6 days.[27]

THE DA VINCI EXPERIENCE

As of May 2001, the da Vinci telemanipulation system (Intuitive Surgical, Mountain View, CA) had been used in 1,250 endoscopic cardiac procedures ranging from the harvesting of arteries (1,137) to endoscopic CABG and

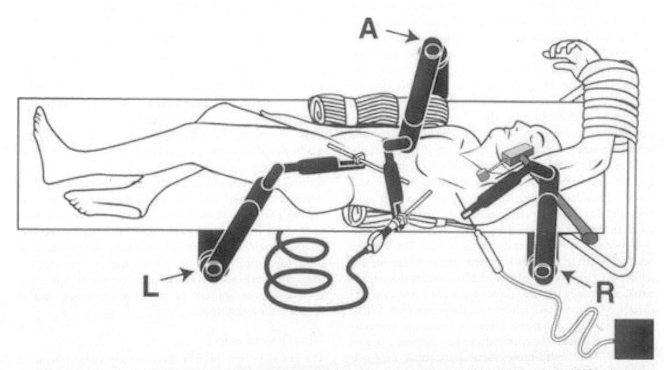

FIGURE 11-10. Port placement used by Dr. Boyd in London, Ontario, Canada, for endoscopic beating-heart CABG. *A* is the AESOP robotic arm. *R* is the right instrument arm. *L* is the left instrument arm. Note the left subclavicular placement of the endoscopic stabilizer.

mitral valve repair. This system was clinically introduced in 1998. Dr. Loulmet performed the first total endoscopic CABG using da Vinci in June 1998.[28]

Dr. Mohr and his group reported their experience in 131 patients undergoing coronary artery bypass grafting from December 1998 to April 2000.[29] This group also proceeded in a stepwise fashion, using the system initially to take down the ITA ($n = 81$), and then expanded its use to perform the ITA-to-LAD graft in a standard sternotomy ($n = 15$). The operation was then changed to a total endoscopic CABG on an arrested heart ($n = 27$) and then on a beating heart ($n = 8$). There were no technical problems reported, and 79 of 81 ITA takedowns were performed successfully. The average time for the ITA takedown was 48.3 ± 26.3 min, but in the last 20 patients, this improved to 35.4 ± 7.7 min. The anastomosis was performed manually in the initial ITA harvests, and there was a 96.3% patency on postoperative angiographic follow-up at 3 to 6 days. At 6 months' follow-up, all patients were free from angina. Through a sternotomy, the mean time to perform the anastomosis using the robotic system was 16 ± 11 min, and all anastomoses were patent postoperatively.

The group then progressed to the third stage of the trial, a total endoscopic CABG on an arrested heart. Twenty-two of 27 patients underwent the operation successfully. Four patients were converted to an open procedure during the operation, and one was converted postoperatively. There was no mortality, and at 3 months' follow-up, 95.4% of grafts were patent by angiography. The operation took 3.5 to 8 h to complete.

The final stage of this study had the surgeon performing a total endoscopic CABG on a beating heart. Eight patients were initially selected to undergo this procedure. Four patients achieved sufficient stabilization to undergo the procedure. Two patients completed the operation uneventfully; two needed revision of the anastomosis, one for occlusion of the graft and one for a low flow on angiography. In these four patients, the anastomosis was performed in 24 to 49 min. The other four patients were not able to undergo the procedure for several reasons, including small intracavitary space, calcification of the LAD, septal branch bleeding, and cardiac arrhythmia prior to LAD occlusion. This last patient had an anterior wall myocardial infarction and succumbed on the sixth postoperative day. All other patients had uneventful postoperative courses and were discharged between days 6 and 8.

Between May 1999 and January 2001, Dr. Stephan Schueler's group in Dresden used the da Vinci on 201 patients.[30] Group A consisted of 156 patients placed into either minimally invasive direct coronary bypass surgery (MIDCAB) ($n = 106$) without cardiopulmonary bypass or a robotically enhanced Dresden technique coronary artery bypass (REDT-CAB) with cardiopulmonary bypass ($n = 50$). All anastomoses were performed manually under direct visualization. The ITA was harvested endoscopically in these groups. In group B, eight patients had

endoscopic LITA takedown with robotically enhanced CABG via median sternotomy. In group C, 37 patients underwent totally endoscopic CABG, 8 on pump and 29 off pump.

The mortality rate was 0.6% (1 of 201) for all groups. Ten patients (4.9%) were converted intraoperatively to a conventional median sternotomy. Stress ECG was performed 4 weeks postoperatively in 97.5% of patients. Seven patients from group A (4.5%) had angina. Four of these patients had anastomotic stenosis. One patient in group B was found to have a previously undiagnosed lesion of the circumflex coronary artery by angiography and was treated with angioplasty. Of the 56 patients scheduled for total endoscopic CABG, 19 (33.9%) were converted to a MIDCAB procedure because of several factors, including calcification of the LAD, intramural LAD course, pleural adhesions, and difficulty with stabilization. There was no difference in the length of ICU stay, ventilation time, or hospital stay between any of the groups.

A third German group in Frankfurt, headed by Dr. Wimmer-Greinecker, has also been active using the da Vinci system for totally endoscopic CABG.[31] From June 1999 to February 2001, 45 patients had the procedure performed on an arrested heart. Thirty-seven patients had a single-vessel ITA-to-coronary artery bypass, and eight patients had double-vessel bypass. Initially, there was a 22% conversion rate, but this fell to 5% in the last 20 patients. All patients with angiographic follow-up had patent grafts. There was no mortality reported in this series. The anastomoses took an average of 18.4 ± 3.8 and 21.1 ± 6.3 min to complete in the single- and double-vessel groups, respectively. The cross-clamp time in these groups was 61 ± 16 min for single-vessel bypass and 99 ± 55 min for double-vessel bypass. The bypass time was 136 ± 32 min when only one bypass was performed and 197 ± 63 min when two bypasses were performed. When compared with a patient cohort receiving conventional CABG, there was no difference in ICU length of stay, ventilation requirement, or duration of hospital stay.

In summary, the experiences at centers around the world demonstrate the capabilities of robotic assistance for enabling endoscopic CABG. As surgeons become more experienced and computer components continue to develop, the safety and efficacy of these procedures will continue to improve. At present, totally endoscopic CABG is reserved for highly selected patients with limited disease. Widespread application awaits the development of more sophisticated robotic systems and the introduction of parallel technologies to aid in target site stabilization, to increase the amount of intrathoracic space, and to facilitate the anastomosis.

Mitral Valve Surgery

The first steps in minimally invasive valve surgery involved the use of smaller incisions than the traditional median sternotomy but were performed under direct vision.

Surgeons found that these incisions provided adequate exposure, and they reported encouraging results with low morbidity and mortality.[32,33] These initial experiences were often performed with HeartPort (Redwood City, CA) technology. This endovascular cardiopulmonary bypass system was usually inserted via the femoral vessels and, as a result, removed the perfusion tubing from the thoracic incision.[34] This made the operative field less cluttered and more accessible. Recently, several groups reported their experience with robotically assisted mitral valve surgeries through small thoracotomies.

In Europe, Dr. Mohr in Leipzig has one of the world's largest experiences with robotically assisted mitral valve surgery. A recent report included 449 patients over a 5-year period, June 1996 to July 2001.[35] Of these patients, 327 had a mitral valve repair and 122 had replacement. The procedure was changed during the middle of this study secondary to a high rate of complications, and the group adopted the procedure developed by Dr. Chitwood in 226 cases.[35] In 366 cases, the voice-controlled robotic-arm AESOP 3000 was used for videoscopic guidance. In only 23 cases was the procedure completely performed using the da Vinci telemanipulation system. The mean length of the surgical incision was 4.3 ± 0.5 cm, and the surgery was completed in 176 ± 56 min. These authors found a significant learning curve as the surgeons gained experience in the minimally invasive procedures. Only 9 patients had failed repairs, all in the first 80 patients. The addition of the da Vinci system "allows a precise controlled mitral valve repair, with the technical potential for a completely endoscopic procedure."[36] The authors concluded that patients were more satisfied with the minimally invasive procedure, had less pain, and were able to return to previous activities more quickly.

Working at the same time in Munich, Dr. Reichenspurner and his group reported similar results in 50 patients undergoing minimally invasive mitral valve procedures using HeartPort port-access technology and three-dimensional video assistance.[38] Twenty-four patients had replacements, and 20 patients had repairs, and there were multiple etiologies. The last 20 patients utilized the AESOP-controlled endoscope. These patients were compared to 49 patients undergoing the traditional procedure during the same time period. Using a right submammary incision, 4 to 7 cm in length, and a three-dimensional endoscopic camera (Vista Cardiothoracic Systems Inc., Westborough, MA), the surgeon was able to simultaneously see the operative site by looking into the incision and at the endoscopic picture inside of his helmet. The endoscopic picture was most useful in viewing the subvalvular apparatus and checking the position of sutures and knots. There was a trend toward longer duration of cardiopulmonary bypass and aortic cross-clamp time in the minimally invasive group. However, the length of stay in the ICU and hospital was less in the minimally invasive patients. In this series, there was no mortality and 85% of patients were in NYHA class I at 3 months' follow-up. These authors stressed the need for careful preoperative selection of patients for the minimally invasive repair.

In the United States, Dr. W. Randolph Chitwood and his team have progressively increased the role for computer assistance for both mitral valve repair and replacement.[38,39] In June 1998, this group performed the first video-directed mitral operation in the United States using an AESOP 3000–controlled endoscope. This initial series used a 5 to 6 cm submammary minithoracotomy for exposure. Dr. Chitwood compared 127 patients that underwent minimally invasive video-assisted mitral valve surgery with 100 sternotomy-based mitral valve procedures.[40] Of the 127 minimally invasive patients, 55 had a manually directed endoscope whereas 72 had a computer-directed endoscope (AESOP). The average cross-clamp times in the computer-directed minimally invasive and conventional groups were identical, but both were significantly lower than the manually directed minimally invasive group. Seven patients in the conventional group required reexploration for bleeding whereas none of the manually directed and only three of the robotically directed patients required reoperation. Moreover, 13% of the conventional sternotomy group had prolonged ventilatory requirements as compared to 0% and 1% in the manually and robotically directed groups, respectively. The 30-day operative mortality for the minimally invasive group was 2.3%, which was identical to their previously reported mortality rate for the conventional procedure. The length of hospital stay was significantly lower in the minimally invasive groups. The authors concluded that the minimally invasive approach was a safe and feasible approach to mitral valve surgery in the hands of an experienced surgeon. The surgeon-controlled camera tracking was more intuitive. Technically, the video assistance was particularly advantageous for providing stable lighting and vibration-free viewing of the subvalvular apparatus. These benefits have quickly helped transition this team and others from video-assisted surgery toward video-directed mitral procedures, where almost all of the procedure is performed under endoscopic vision.

Dr. Chitwood performed the first complete computer-enhanced robotic mitral valve repair in North America in May 2000.[41] The da Vinci system was used to perform this operation and seven subsequent operations. The procedure is still performed through a 5 to 6 cm incision, but all leaflet resections, chordal procedures, and defect closures are done with the da Vinci system. These procedures were undertaken in a highly select group.[42] His early results are promising and confirm the feasibility of robotically assisted valve surgery.

Investigators have now begun to use the ZEUS robotic system in mitral valve procedures. Using a "service entrance" incision and a right anterior 6 cm thoracotomy, Dr. Grossi was able to repair the mitral valve in a 50-year-old patient with posterior leaflet prolapse.[43] The valve repair required 3 h and 2 min of cardiopulmonary bypass, and the ZEUS robotic instrumentation was used for 69 min. Dr. Grossi has performed six minimally invasive mitral valve replacements in the laboratory, taking an average 69.3 ± 5.4 min to complete.[44]

In summary, the initial clinical trials of the robotic and telemanipulation systems show that they can be used to assist mitral valve surgery. There has been a significant learning curve with this technology, and its role and precise value in the surgical treatment of valvular heart disease remain to be determined.

Atrial Septal Surgery

Dr. Alfieri's group from Milan, Italy, has employed the da Vinci surgical system in the repair of atrial septal defects (ASDs) in seven patients.[45] Five patients had ASDs, while the other two had a patent foramen ovale with atrial septal aneurysms. All procedures were performed on an arrested heart. Four ports were placed into the right chest. An endoaortic balloon occluded the ascending aorta, and cardioplegia was delivered. Bypass was established using the HeartPort system. A right atriotomy was performed, and the defect was closed with interrupted (one patient) or continuous suture (six patients). All procedures were completed endoscopically, and there were no complications reported. At 1-month follow-up, all of the repairs were intact.

Dr. Michael Argenziano recently reported the use of the da Vinci robotic surgical system to close an ASD in a 33-year-old woman.[46] This procedure was performed on cardiopulmonary bypass using four thoracic ports. Cross-clamp time was 43 min. The patient was ambulatory within 15 h and was discharged on day 3. At 30-day follow-up, the patient was doing well.

Future Directions

Although there has been tremendous progress in the development of robotically assisted cardiac surgery over the last several years, there are still many challenges that must be overcome in order to widen the applicability of these techniques in the clinical arena. At present, these operations are often lengthy, technically difficult, and applicable to only carefully selected patients. However, as was seen after the introduction of laparoscopy in general surgery, the accumulation of surgical experience with this sophisticated instrumentation will, over time, improve operative choreography and shorten operative times. The development of parallel technologies to facilitate these procedures also will likely result in significant advances in the field.

One of the most significant challenges that face surgeons embarking on endoscopic procedures is the determination of optimal port placement. Both surgical experience and the use of computer guidance should facilitate this in the future. By using computerized tomography and magnetic resonance imaging, preliminary efforts toward the development of a three-dimensional virtual cardiac surgical planning platform have been initiated for use with totally endoscopic cardiac surgery.[47] Improved instrumentation will also aid the development of this field. Smaller and more precise instruments, perhaps with more flexibility in the shaft, may also simplify port placement in the future.

The real significance of robotically assisted cardiac surgery lies in the resultant integration of computers into the operating theater. Primarily, three areas will be impacted: surgeon control, intraoperative imaging, and information access. Future improvements in the digital–manual interface will continue to enhance a surgeon's technical ability with these systems. Endoscopic procedures will become more feasible as computers become more powerful, smaller, and less expensive. Continued technologic advancements in robotic systems should bring us closer to a more ideal surgical system over the next several years. This ideal system would include fully replicated master kinematics, a full range of end effectors, effective and simple site delivery, tactile feedback, superb three-dimensional optics, and data fusion capability to allow for computer- and image-guided surgery.

With further enhancements, simple surgical maneuvers may be able to be programmed in order to assist in suturing and in the performance of an anastomosis. Systems may eventually "learn" surgical techniques through the use of neural networks. This will allow present procedures to be performed less invasively, as well as enable surgeons to perform an ever-expanding repertoire of procedures previously thought impossible because of the inherent physical shortcomings of human beings.

Computer technology will also revolutionize intraoperative imaging. Undoubtedly, the future will see the introduction of image-guided cardiac surgery. Surgeons will be able to manipulate images intraoperatively and view digital echocardiograms, angiograms, and computed tomography and magnetic resonance imaging scans directly on the video monitor. Furthermore, these images could be superimposed on the operative field. Fusion of these images with endoscopic pictures will allow surgeons to precisely define the cardiac anatomy without direct visualization. Further manipulation of the digital visual interface may also make it possible to work on the beating heart in "virtual stillness." The movement of the robotic camera and instruments could be synchronized with each heartbeat, effectively canceling cardiac motion and increasing surgical precision.

Finally, there will be continued advances in information access. In the operating room, networked video monitors will provide access to the hospital information system and ancillary services. In addition, this system could be linked to local area networks, the global Internet, and the hospital library. This technology will allow surgeons to share their acumen with their colleagues around the globe via high-speed video links.

As cardiac surgeons, our challenge will be to not let ourselves be defined by the size of our incisions. We must become cardiac interventionists, performing percutaneous interventions on various intrathoracic structures. Our understanding of the anatomy of the chest and our training make us ideally suited to perform these procedures and handle the potential complications. The dawn of the era of computer-assisted surgery has commenced and promises to bring dramatic advances in our capabilities as cardiac surgeons in the treatment of all forms of cardiac pathology. The continued advance of robotic and computer technology has the potential to transform both the operating rooms and our specialty as we enter the new millennium. Computers and robots have allowed human beings to explore the reaches of the universe and the depths of the oceans. They have allowed us to delve into our past and see our future. Hopefully, with continued clinical research and developing technology, they will aid cardiac surgeons in performing our complex procedures with progressively less invasiveness and morbidity, adding yet another facet to their improvement of the human condition.

References

1. Rosen M, Ponsky J. Minimally invasive surgery. Endoscopy 2001;33(4):358–66.
2. Vilos GA, Alshimmiri MM. Cost-benefit analysis of laparoscopic versus laparotomy salpingo-oophorectomy for benign tubo-ovarian disease. J Am Assoc Gynecol Laparosc 1995;2(3):299–303.
3. Seifman BD, Wolf JS Jr. Technical advances in laparoscopy: hand assistance retractors, and the pneumodissector. J Endourol 2000;14(10):921–8.
4. Malone R. The robot book. New York: Push Pin Press; 1978. p. 26.
5. Asimov I, Frenkel K. Robots: machines in man's image. New York: Harmony Books; 1985.
6. Malone R. The robot book. New York: Push Pin Press; 1978. p. 31.
7. Malone R. The robot book. New York: Push Pin Press; 1978. p. 35.
8. Chauvry G. Joseph Jacquard and the weaving revolution. Available at: http://www.g7lyon.tm.fr/Lyon/hommes/jacq.g.htm (accessed October 12, 2002).
9. MicroMaster. The history of robotics. Available at http://members.tripod.com/MicroMaster/history.html (accessed October 7, 2002).
10. Asimov I. I, robot (a collection of short stories originally published between 1940 and 1950). London: Grafton Books; 1968.
11. History of robotics and robots. Available at http://www.geocities.com/Eureka/7331/hrorobot.htm (accessed September 15, 2002).
12. Kavoussi LR, Moore RG, Adams JB, et al. Comparison of robotic versus human laparoscopic camera control. J Urol 1995;6:2134–6.
13. Ballantyne GH. The pitfalls of laparoscopic surgery: challenges for robotics and telerobotic surgery. Surg Laparosc Endosc Percutan Tech 2002;12(1):1–5.
14. Falk V, Mintz D, Grunenfelder J, et al. Influence of three-dimensional vision on surgical telemanipulator performance. Surg Endosc 2001;15(11):1282–8.
15. Computer Motion Report. Santa Barbara, CA. Available at: http://www.computermotion.com/products.html; and Intuitive Surgical Systems, Mountain View, CA. Available at: http://www.intuitivesurgical.com/products/index.html (accessed October 4, 2002).
16. Dewey TM, Mack MJ. Lung cancer. Surgical approaches and incisions. Chest Surg Clin N Am 2000;10(4):803–20.
17. Porat O, Shoham M, Meyer J. Effect of control design on task performance in endoscopic tele-operation. Available at: http://robotics.technion.ac.il/projects/ori_project.html (accessed October 11, 2002).
18. Computer Motion Report. Santa Barbara (CA): June 2000.
19. Hanna GB, Shimi SM, Cuschieri A. Task performance in endoscopic surgery is influenced by location of the image display. Ann Surg 1998;227(4):481–4.
20. Damiano RJ Jr, Reichenspurner H, Ducko CT. Robotically assisted endoscopic coronary artery bypass grafting: current state of the art. Adv Card Surg 2000;12:37–57.
21. Detter C, Boehm DH, Reichenspurner H, et al. Robotically assisted coronary artery surgery with and without cardiopulmonary bypass—from first clinical use to endoscopic operation. Med Sci Monit 2002;8(7):MT118–23.
22. Damiano RJ Jr, Ehrman WJ, Ducko CT, et al. Initial United States clinical trial of robotically assisted endoscopic coronary artery bypass grafting. J Thorac Cardiovasc Surg 2000;119(1):77–82.
23. Damiano RJ Jr, Ducko CT, Stephenson ER Jr, et al. Robotically assisted coronary artery bypass grafting: a prospective single center clinical trial. J Card Surg 2000;15(4):256–65.
24. Prasad SM, Ducko CT, Stephenson ER, et al. Prospective clinical trial of robotically assisted endoscopic coronary grafting with 1-year follow-up. Ann Surg 2001;233(6):725–32.
25. Boyd WD, Kiaii B, Novick RJ, et al. RAVECAB: improving outcome in off-pump minimal access surgery with robotic assistance and video enhancement. Can J Surg 2001;44(1):45–50.
26. Kiaii B, Boyd WD, Rayman R, et al. Robot-assisted computer enhanced closed-chest coronary surgery: preliminary experience using a harmonic scalpel and ZEUS. Heart Surg Forum 2000;3(3):194–7.
27. Boyd WD, Rayman R, Desai ND, et al. Closed-chest coronary artery bypass grafting on the beating heart with the use of a computer-enhanced surgical robotic system. J Thorac Cardiovasc Surg 2000;120(4):807–9.
28. Loulmet D, Carpentier A, d'Attellis N, et al. Endoscopic coronary artery bypass grafting with the aid of robotic assisted instruments. J Thorac Cardiovasc Surg 1999;118(1):4–10.
29. Mohr FW, Falk V, Diegeler A, et al. Computer-enhanced "robotic" cardiac surgery: experience in 148 patients. J Thorac Cardiovasc Surg 2001;121:842–53.
30. Kappert U, Schneider J, Cichon R, et al. Development of robotic-enhanced endoscopic surgery for treatment of coronary artery disease. Circulation 2001;104 Suppl I; I-102–7.
31. Dogan S, Aybek T, Andresen E, et al. Totally endoscopic coronary artery bypass grafting on cardiopulmonary bypass with robotically enhanced telemanipulation:

report of forty-five cases. J Thorac Cardiovasc Surg 2002;123:1125–31.

32. Cosgrove DM, Sabik JF, Navia JL. Minimally invasive valve surgery. Ann Thorac Surg 1998;65:1535–8.

33. Navia JL, Cosgrove DM. Minimally invasive mitral valve operations. Ann Thorac Surg 1996;62:1542–4.

34. Grossi EA, La Pietra A, Galloway AC, et al. Videoscopic mitral valve repair and replacement using the port-access technique. Adv Card Surg 2001;13:77–88.

35. Onnasch JF, Schneider F, Falk V, et al. Five years of less invasive minimal surgery: from experimental to routine. Heart Surg Forum 2002;5(2):132–5.

36. Chitwood WR, Wixon CL, Elbeery JR, et al. Video-assisted minimally invasive mitral valve surgery. J Thorac Surg 1997;114:773–80.

37. Reichenspurner H, Boehm DH, Gulbins H, et al. Three-dimensional video and robot-assisted port-access mitral valve operation. Ann Thorac Surg 2000;69:1176–82.

38. Chitwood WR Jr, Nifong LW. Minimally invasive video-scopic mitral valve surgery: the current role of surgical robotics. J Card Surg 2000;15(1):61–75.

39. Chitwood WR Jr. Video-assisted and robotic mitral valve surgery: toward an endoscopic surgery. Semin Thorac Cardiovasc Surg 1999;11(3):194–205.

40. Felger JE, Chitwood WR Jr, Nifong LW, Holbert D. Evolution of mitral valve surgery: toward a totally endoscopic approach. Ann Thorac Surg 2001;72(4):1203–8; discussion 1208–9.

41. Chitwood WR Jr, Nifong LW, Elbeeery JE, et al. Robotic mitral valve repair: trapezoidal resection and prosthetic annuloplasty with the da Vinci Surgical System. J Thorac Cardiovasc Surg 2000;120;1171–2.

42. Felger JE, Nifong LW, Chitwood WR Jr. Robotic cardiac valve surgery: transcending the technologic crevasse! Curr Opin Cardiol 2001;16:146–51.

43. Grossi EA, LaPietra A, Applebaum RM, et al. Case report of robotic instrument-enhanced mitral valve surgery. J Thorac Cardiovasc Surg 2000;120;1169–71.

44. LaPietra A, Grossi EA, Derivaux CC, et al. Robotic-assisted instruments enhance minimally invasive mitral valve surgery. Ann Thorac Surg 2000;70:835–8.

45. Torraca L, Ismeno G, Quarti A, Alfieri O. Totally endoscopic atrial septal defect closure with a robotic system: experience with seven cases. Heart Surg Forum 2002; 5(2):125–7.

46. Argenziano M, Oz MC, DeRose JJ Jr, et al. Totally endoscopic atrial septal defect repair with robotic assistance. Heart Surg Forum 2002;5(3):194–297.

47. Friedl R, Preisack M, Schefer M, et al. CardioOp: an integrated approach to teleteaching in cardiac surgery. Stud Health Technol Inform 2000;70:76–82.

CHAPTER 12

BEATING-HEART BYPASS GRAFTING WITH TEMPORARY CARDIAC ASSIST

VOLKMAR FALK, MD, PhD, RALF KRAKOR, MD, PhD, THOMAS WALTHER, MD, PhD, FRIEDRICH W. MOHR, MD, PhD

Beating-heart surgery is widely accepted. However, some earlier studies indicate that because of difficulties with exposure of the posterior wall there is a tendency for incomplete revascularization. As a result, in several recent studies that compared on-pump and off-pump surgery, there were fewer grafts performed in the off-pump group.[1,2] Especially distal branches of the circumflex artery were less frequently revascularized. This was in part attributed to the hemodynamic changes that occur with tilting of the heart. Early experiments performed by Grundeman revealed that right ventricular outflow obstruction was the main cause for impaired hemodynamics with tilting of the heart.[3] While most of the hemodynamic impairment can be prevented by avoiding rapid tilting and by using a Trendelenburg position, some investigators advocate the use of temporary right-heart assist to overcome the problems associated with exposure of the posterior wall.[4] A number of devices for active right-heart support during beating-heart coronary artery bypass grafting have been developed and tested experimentally and clinically.

The Enabler

Technology

The Enabler (HemoDynamics, Yokneam, Israel) is an electrohydraulic electrocardiogram (ECG)-triggered right-heart bypass system to enhance right atrial to pulmonary artery flow while unloading the right ventricle. The system consists of a control console, a disposable pump-head, and a cannula. The control console is connected to the lower chamber of the pump-head by a water-filled tube. The pump-head contains two chambers that are separated by a flexible diaphragm. The cannula is filled with a sterile isotonic solution and connected to the pump-head's upper chamber. The valved cannula is placed within the right heart with its inlet portion in the right atrium and the outlet tip in the pulmonary artery (Figure 12-1). An ECG-triggered servocontroller controls the cyclical movement of water between the control console and the lower chamber

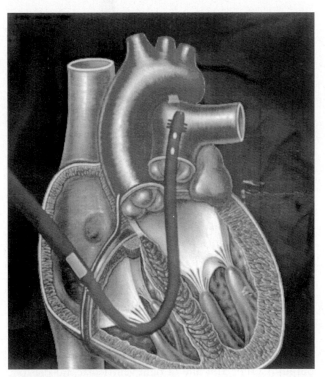

FIGURE 12-1. Enabler cannula.

of the pump-head. The diaphragm moves accordingly, sucking blood from the right atrium into the cannula and the upper chamber of the pump-head in diastole, which blood is expelled from the cannula into the pulmonary artery in systole (Figure 12-2). By means of valves in the cannula, blood flow is unidirectional during the two phases of the cardiac cycle. Insertion of the 24-French cannula is performed through the right jugular vein.

Experimental Results

Initially, the Enabler system was tested as a left-heart assist device in an animal model of acute heart failure. In heart failure, it effectively supported the circulation by increasing cardiac output and perfusion pressure.[5]

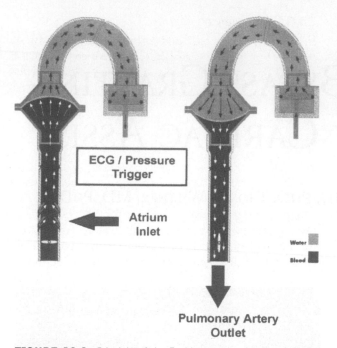

FIGURE 12-2. Principle of the Enabler system. An electrocardiogram (ECG)-triggered hydraulically driven membrane sucks the blood from the right atrium during diastole and expels it into the pulmonary artery during systole.

The experimental results with the use of the Enabler system for right ventricular support during beating-heart bypass grafting are conflicting. Dekker and colleagues reported their results with the Enabler system in an experimental study with eight sheep.[6] The cannula was introduced via the jugular vein and positioned with the inlet valve in the right atrium and outlet valve in the pulmonary artery. The Octopus was used to expose the inferior wall and the posterior wall of the left ventricle. The hemodynamic effects of this tilting with and without Enabler right ventricular support were recorded, including pressure volume (PV) loops as measured by conductance catheters in both ventricles. Accordingly, tilting caused a reduction in cardiac output (CO) of 31% and of right ventricular end-diastolic volume (RVEDV) of 44%, while right ventricular end-diastolic pressure (RVEDP) remained essentially unchanged. During right ventricular support with the Enabler system, CO remained 23% lower than pretilting values. The authors concluded that the Enabler cannot restore CO because of its limited output and because of a decrease in right ventricular output with activation of the system.[6] The authors also noted hemolysis, as expressed by an increase in free hemoglobin, with Enabler activation. No signs of damage to the endocardium or to the tricuspid and pulmonary valve were found. Similar experimental results were found by our group (Figure 12-3).

Clinical Experience

In 10 patients with triple-vessel disease, beating-heart bypass grafting using the Enabler for short-time right ven-

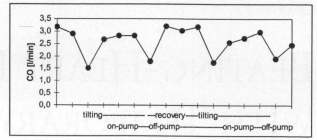

FIGURE 12-3. Hemodynamic data (sheep study). During tilting, cardiac output (CO) drops. With activation of the pump, CO is partially restored.

tricular support was performed. All patients underwent a median sternotomy. After heparinization, the cannula was inserted via the right atrium into the pulmonary artery under transesophageal echocardiography (TEE) control. Hemodynamics were assessed at rest, after insertion of the pump, and before, during, and after tilting maneuvers required to expose the obtuse marginal branches (with or without pump support). No technical mishaps occurred. All patients underwent successful bypass grafting. Mean arterial blood pressure (MAP) dropped during tilting from 65 ± 10 to 43 ± 15 mm Hg. The Enabler restored MAP to pretilting levels (65 ± 13 mm Hg). Similarly, CO recovered after an initial drop from baseline level to normal ranges. It was concluded that tilting of the heart is possible with less hemodynamic deterioration when using the Enabler for temporary right-heart support.[7]

Microaxial Flow Pumps

Technology

Microaxial flow pumps have also been used for temporary cardiac assist during off-pump coronary artery bypass (OPCAB) surgery in both experimental and clinical settings. Two pumps have been used: the Hemopump (Medtronic Inc., Minneapolis, Minnesota) and the Impella pump (Impella, Aachen, Germany).

Both pumps are high-speed rotary blood pumps that make use of the Archimedes' screw principle. A rotating impeller expels the blood through a small cannula.

While similar to the Hemopump, the Impella micropump is a sensorized axial flow pump with an integrated micromotor (Figure 12-4). This pump avoids the need for the long high-speed rotating wire that the Hemopump uses to connect to its external motor. The left-side Impella pump has an outer diameter of only 6.4 mm, allowing for a peripheral access. By measuring the difference between in- and outflow pressures, the pump can be precisely positioned. In combination with the rotary speed (up to 32,000 rotations per min), pump flow (up to 4.5 L/min) can be calculated. The right-side pump is mounted in a balloon cannula that is placed similarly to a pulmonary artery catheter (Figure 12-4).

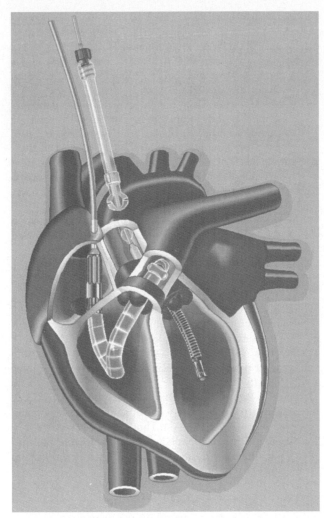

FIGURE 12-4. The Impella system for biventricular support.

Experimental Experience

The feasibility of using the Impella pump was shown by Meyns in an experimental study.[8] In 12 sheep, the left anterior descending (LAD), the intermediate branch, and the circumflex arteries were consecutively occluded for 10 min. One group of animals had no mechanical support, and the other group was treated with biventricular support by means of two intravascular micropumps that were inserted through the femoral artery and jugular vein, respectively. All of the pump-supported animals survived the procedure; one of the control animals died of ventricular fibrillation. At the end of the reperfusion period, the hemodynamic performance and myocardial contractility were significantly better in the pump-supported group. In addition, subendocardial blood flow measured by microspheres was significantly better in all areas of the left ventricle in the assisted group. The authors concluded that the supported heart is more resistant to repetitive local ischemia; consequently, support by microaxial pumps could increase the safety of beating-heart surgery, especially in more complex cases.

Clinical Experience

In a prospective, randomized multicenter study, 42 patients underwent assisted OPCAB in which two Impella pumps were used for biventricular intracorporeal circulation (group 1). The control group consisted of 38 patients who were operated on by using a conventional cardiopulmonary bypass set-up (group 2). Procedure time was 112 min ± 31.9 min (group 1) and 137.4 min ± 36.2 min (group 2). An average of 2.3 vessels were grafted in group 1, and an average of 2.2 vessels were grafted in group 2. During exposure of the back wall, mean pump flow was 3.7 (2.5 to 4.4) L/min in group 1 and 4.9 (3.6 to 6.2) L/min in group 2. Hemolysis defined by the level of free hemoglobin was lower than 20 mg/dL at all times, except for four patients (two in each group) with maximum levels of 100 mg/dL. There were no pump-related life-threatening or severe adverse events. The authors concluded that beating-heart procedures can be performed reliably and safely using biventricular microaxial flow pump assist.[9]

In another randomized trial, Hemopump-assisted beating-heart coronary artery bypass grafting was compared with conventional bypass grafting using cardiopulmonary bypass, aortic cross-clamping, and cardioplegic cardiac arrest. While similar procedure and assist times were reported, fewer grafts were performed in the Hemopump group (1.8 vs 2.5). The Hemopump group had less intraoperative blood loss and lower troponin-T levels.[10]

Discussion

The benefit of mechanical support during beating-heart coronary artery bypass grafting was demonstrated more than 10 years ago.[11] The Hemopump, as well as centrifugal pumps, has been successfully used for pump-assisted coronary revascularization on the beating heart. The Hemopump was not very practical because it did not allow for tilting of the heart.[12] At the same time, beating-heart coronary artery bypass grafting without mechanical support was introduced. Initially, hemodynamic problems with tilting of the heart were reported, and in trials that compared OPCAB with conventional surgery, fewer grafts were performed due to difficulties with exposure of the posterior and lateral walls. With the development of suction stabilizers, OPCAB has become a reliable technique that has found widespread application. Angiographic results are similar to those of conventional surgery. Better anesthesiologic management, as well as new devices such as the Expose device, have helped to overcome most of the hemodynamic problems associated with tilting of the heart. Thus, the clinical problem of impaired hemodynamics during tilting of the heart is rare.

Both the Enabler and the prior generation of rotary pumps have overcome some of the limitations of older pumps that were used for temporary cardiac assist during beating-heart bypass grafting. There is less hemolysis, the devices are smaller, and critical parts, such as the flexible shaft of the Hemopump, have been omitted. The devices restore cardiac output to some degree during tilting of the heart. Biventricular support preserves hemodynamics during tilting and ischemia (with coronary occlusion) and may lead to improved myocardial flow and contractility in the reperfusion phase.[13]

However, placing of the devices is time-consuming, and the device itself can interfere mechanically with tilting of the heart, requiring repositioning during the procedure. Although there are no reports describing complications as a result of using these devices, the potential of an injury exists. In addition, the use of these devices is associated with additional costs. Off-pump beating-heart bypass grafting is performed routinely in a number of centers and can be safely performed even in high-risk subgroups of patients with low ejection fraction or left-main stenosis. Thus, despite the technical evolution, there is rarely an indication to use these devices for temporary cardiac assist during beating-heart surgery.

References

1. Kshettry VR, Flavin TF, Emery RW, et al. Does multivessel, off-pump coronary artery bypass reduce postoperative morbidity? Ann Thorac Surg 2001;71:1751–2.
2. Bull DA, Neumayer LA, Stringham JC, et al. Coronary artery bypass grafting with cardiopulmonary bypass versus off-pump cardiopulmonary bypass grafting: does eliminating the pump reduce morbidity and cost? Ann Thorac Surg 2001;71:170–3.
3. Grundeman PF, Borst C, Verlaan CWJ, et al. Exposure of circumflex branches in the tilted, beating porcine heart: echocardiographic evidence of right ventricular deformation and the effect of right or left heart bypass. J Thorac Cardiovasc Surg 1999;118:316–23.
4. Suematsu Y, Ohtsuka T, Miyaji K, et al. Right heart mini-pump bypass for coronary artery bypass grafting: experimental study. Eur J Cardiothorac Surg 2000;18:276–81.
5. Nishimura Y, Meyns B, Ozaki S, et al. The Enabler cannula pump: a novel circulatory support system. Int J Artif Organs 1999;22:317–23.
6. Dekker AL, Geskes GC, Cramers AA, et al. Right ventricular support for off-pump coronary artery bypass grafting studied with bi-ventricular pressure-volume loops in sheep. Eur J Cardiothorac Surg 2001;19:179–84.
7. Autschbach R, Krakor R, Gummert J, et al. Intermittent mechanical right heart support for complete revascularisation of the heart in beating heart technique. Thorac Cardiovasc Surg 2000;48 Suppl I:82.
8. Meyns B, Sergeant P, Siess T, et al. Coronary artery bypass graft with biventricular microaxial pumps. Perfusion 1999;14:287–90.
9. Autschbach R, Rauch T, Engel M, et al. A new intracardiac microaxial pump: first results of a multicenter study. Artif Organs 2001;25:327–30.
10. Lonn U, Peterzen B, Carnstam B, Casimir-Ahn H. Beating heart coronary surgery supported by an axial blood flow pump. Ann Thorac Surg 1999;67:99–104.
11. Sweeney MS, Frazier OF. Device supported myocardial revascularization: safe help for sick hearts. Ann Thorac Surg 1992;54:1065–70.
12. Lonn U, Peterzen B, Granfeldt H, Casimir-Ahn H. Coronary artery operation with support of the Hemopump cardiac assist system. Ann Thorac Surg 1994;58:519–23.
13. Meyns B, Sergeant P, Nishida T, et al. Micropumps to support the heart during CABG. Eur J Cardiothorac Surg 2000;17:169–74.

CHAPTER 13

TOTAL ENDOSCOPIC BYPASS GRAFTING

VOLKMAR FALK, MD, PHD, STEPHAN JACOBS, MD, THOMAS WALTHER, MD, PHD, FRIEDRICH W. MOHR, MD, PHD

Rationale for Endoscopic Bypass Grafting

The goals of minimally invasive or less-invasive coronary artery bypass grafting are twofold: to reduce the surgical trauma by minimizing access and to obviate the need for extracorporeal circulation. Ideally, coronary artery bypass grafting would be performed endoscopically on the beating heart.

In the early 1990s, some groups developed techniques to perform coronary anastomoses on the beating heart.[1,2] With the development of mechanical stabilizers that provided sufficient local immobilization of the beating heart, patency rates became comparable to conventional on-pump surgery, and both the minimally invasive direct coronary artery bypass (MIDCAB) operation and off-pump coronary artery bypass (OPCAB) procedures have found widespread clinical application.[3–5]

Stimulated by the developments in other surgical specialties, endoscopic techniques were introduced in the field of cardiac surgery in the mid-1990s. Using conventional endoscopic instruments, some groups started with endoscopic harvesting of the internal thoracic artery.[6] At the same time, cardiopulmonary bypass systems, such as the Port-Access system, were introduced, which allowed for closed-chest cardiopulmonary bypass and cardiac arrest.[7] Closed-chest bypass grafting was, however, still not possible, primarily because of the limitations of conventional endoscopic instruments. The introduction of computer-enhanced instrumentation systems (robotics) has prepared the ground for true endoscopic bypass grafting. These telemanipulators enhance the dexterity, allow scaling of motions, and provide tremor filtering.[8] A number of groups have started to expand their minimally invasive programs with an endoscopic approach that uses the two currently available surgical telemanipulation systems. After extensive experimental trials, the first clinical studies have demonstrated the feasibility of total endoscopic coronary artery bypass (TECAB) grafting on the arrested and on the beating heart.[9,10]

Telemanipulation Technology

Two telemanipulation systems are currently commercially available, the Zeus (Computer Motion, Goleta, California) and the da Vinci (Intuitive Surgical, Mountain View, California) systems. The da Vinci system consists of two major components: a master console and a cart-mounted manipulator. The console houses the display system, the master handles, the user interface, and the electronic controller. The image of the surgical site is transmitted to the surgeon through a high-resolution stereo display. The system projects the image of the surgical site atop the surgeon's hands, while the controller transforms the spatial motion of the tools into the camera frame of reference. Hereby the system provides a natural hand-eye coordination. Motion scaling allows for various ratios for master and manipulator motions. By activating a foot switch, the operator is able to temporarily uncouple and reposition the masters in the working field, while the instrument tips remain stationary (indexing). A tremor filter is used to minimize involuntary motions. The patient-side cart consists of two instrument manipulators and a central camera manipulator. The instruments (end effectors) attach interchangeably to the two instrument manipulators that feature an automated instrument recognition system. By means of an endowrist, a total of 6° of freedom is provided, allowing for free motion and orientation of the tip in space. The system has been described in detail elsewhere.[8–12]

Technique of TECAB

In December 1998, the da Vinci system was introduced; its main focus was on endoscopic coronary surgery.[13] In the majority of cases, the system was used to harvest the internal thoracic artery (ITA) endoscopically. After an initial learning curve that was similar in most centers using this technology, harvest times for the left ITA are now in the range of 30 to 40 min, and the technique is routinely performed in a number of centers.[9,14,15]

For robotic-assisted ITA harvest, patients are placed in a supine position with the left chest slightly elevated and the left arm lowered. Single-lung ventilation of the right lung is performed. A 30° scope angled up is inserted at the fourth intercostal space (ICS). Continuous CO_2 insufflation is applied to enhance exposure by increasing the available space between the heart and the sternum. Although insufflation pressures up to 10 mm Hg are usually well tolerated, hemodynamic studies demonstrate an increase in right ventricular filling pressures, a decrease of intrathoracic blood volume index, and a decrease of right ventricular ejection fraction with increasing insufflation pressures. As a result, cardiac index and mean arterial pressure (MAP) may decrease despite a compensatory increase in heart rate.[16] The instrument ports are created in the third and sixth ICS. Depending on the individual's physiognomy, ports are created in a flat triangle (with the central camera port placed a little bit lower than the two instrument ports) or in an almost linear fashion following the anterior axillary line. The ideal position for the set-up joints of the instrument arms is 90° between the primary and secondary axis (shoulder) and 45° between the secondary and tertiary axis (elbow). For the camera arm, the net-sum of angles should be 0°, resulting in straight alignment of the scope and the central column. With this set-up there should be no necessity to move the set-up joints during the procedure. The remote centers should be placed correctly within the ports to provide the highest precision and lowest friction.

The ITA is usually dissected as a pedicle from the first rib to the sixth ICS by using low-energy cautery. Clips are rarely used. In cases of muscle or fat covering the ITA, initial dissection of the tissue, including the fascia, facilitate take-down. The precision of the instruments does also allow for a skeletonized take-down technique. Care must be taken to avoid injury of the subclavian vein and the phrenic nerve while dissecting the proximal part of the ITA. ITA harvesting is now routinely performed and permits the tailoring of the thoracotomy incision necessary for a MIDCAB procedure. Approximately 1,350 cases of robotic ITA take-downs have been reported for the da Vinci system alone. If the ITA is to be used for a TECAB procedure, the vessel is skeletonized distally, cut and trimmed for the anastomosis in situ by using the native tissue for countertraction. The pedicle is not detached from the chest wall until the anastomosis is finally performed so as to avoid torsion of the graft and any interference during pericardiotomy. For bilateral ITA take-down, the right pleural space is opened and the right ITA is dissected first, sometimes facilitated by the use of a 0° scope.

The first successful TECAB procedure on the arrested heart was reported by Loulmet.[17] Following ITA take-down, the pericardial fat is removed and a pericardial window is created. After the left anterior descending (LAD) artery is identified, femoro-femoral bypass is initiated by using the Port-Access system for closed-chest cardiopulmonary bypass and antegrade cardioplegic cardiac arrest. The anastomosis is then performed in a running fashion on the arrested heart through the same ports. More than 100 cases have been reported in the literature, mostly single-vessel revascularization of the ITA to the LAD. Cardiopulmonary bypass time and cross-clamp time are in the range of 80 to 120 and 40 to 60 min, respectively. The conversion rate to a sternotomy is now consistently less than 10%, and the reported patency rate for the TECAB procedure ranges from 95 to 100% prior to discharge and 96% at 3-month follow-up angiography.[18–20] In a few patients, the right ITA was used to graft the right coronary artery (RCA), and successful double-vessel TECAB to the LAD and RCA, as well as sequential grafting of the LAD and a diagonal branch, has been reported.[21–23] In addition, both ITAs may be harvested endoscopically, followed by a multivessel arterial revascularization on the arrested heart through a left parasternal minithoracotomy in the second interspace (Dresden technique).[24]

The development of endoscopic coronary artery bypass grafting on the beating heart required the development of endoscopic stabilizers and methods for temporary vascular occlusion. Complete endoscopic bypass grafting was first achieved in a canine model by using a nitinol-based self-expanding endoscopic stabilizer.[25,26] More advanced stabilizers have subsequently been developed, allowing articulation of the pads and thus providing easier placement. The last generation of endoscopic stabilizers also features vacuum assistance and an irrigation channel (Figure 13-1).

Vascular occlusion can be achieved by using vascular clamps or, more commonly, by using silastic bands that are either locked into the pads of the stabilizer or used in combination with a self-locking plate.

Complete TECAB procedures on the beating heart were first reported by groups in Leipzig and Dresden that used the da Vinci system and an endoscopic stabilizer that was inserted through a subxyphoidal port (Figure 13-2).[10,27] After the site for the anastomosis is identified, occlusion snares are placed around the vessel. Rather than pushing the needle through, the motion of the heart is used to passively move the needle through the tissue. Before insertion of the stabilizer, all suture material to be used should be placed into the chest to avoid CO_2 leaks later during the procedure. After the stabilizer is placed, the ITA is placed beneath the stabilizer. Alternatively, a first stitch can already be placed in the ITA while it is still attached to the chest wall. Before starting the anastomosis, instruments should be checked for the possible occurrence of singularities, and changes in set-up made accordingly. The irrigation is placed from behind, aiming at the site of the anastomosis. After occlusion (usually proximal and distal occlusion will be necessary because even a little bleeding from the anastomotic site is not well tolerated), the anastomosis is performed in the usual fashion. Approximately 80 closed-chest beating-heart procedures, including 3 double-vessel beating-heart TECABs using the da Vinci system, have been reported in the literature.[18,28] Based on an intention to treat, the conversion rate (elective conversion to a MIDCAB procedure) with this approach is currently in the range of 30 to 50%. LAD occlusion times are in the range of 25 to 40 min, and thus exceed those reported for MIDCAB procedures.

Others have used the Zeus system for closed-chest bypass grafting. Because of the lower level of dexterity of the Zeus telemanipulator, five to seven ports plus an additional working port (minithoracotomy) for assistance are needed. Because insufflation pressure cannot be maintained throughout the procedure, a sternal hook is used to provide additional space between the chest wall and the heart. Due to longer anastomotic times, a coronary shunt is used. A harmonic scalpel is usually used for ITA takedown, and the stabilizer is inserted parasternally in the second intercostal space.[29,30]

Discussion

Based on the experience presented here, it can be concluded that the use of telemanipulation systems is safe and allows for true endoscopic coronary artery bypass grafting. The use of the systems is currently restricted to a few indications (single-vessel bypass grafting of the LAD; occasionally, double-vessel grafting), but it is conceivable that they may be used for endoscopic multivessel procedures in the near future. Ergonomic human-machine interfaces and multilevel servo controlling allow for precise tissue handling despite the lack of fine tactile feedback.

However, operating times are still long and conversions to MIDCAB or open surgery are frequently necessary. A lot of steps that occur between ITA take-down and performing the anastomosis are hampered by the lack of assistance, limited space, the lack of fine tactile feedback, and a limited number of instruments. Among the difficulties are the handling of excessive epicardial fat, determination of the optimal site for an anastomosis, target vessel calcification, and backbleeding from septal branches. In addition, difficulties with positioning of the stabilizer or incomplete immobilization render beating-heart closed-chest bypass grafting difficult. Although removal of pericardial fat, identifying the target vessel, temporary vessel occlusion, delivering material inside the chest, and many more parts of the procedure are trivial in an open-chest scenario, they require a certain choreography to be mastered endoscopically. A low threshold for conversion is mandatory to avoid any risk for the patient. Elective conversion is safe and should not be considered a failure.

As with all new technologies, a learning curve has to be overcome and structured training is considered essential

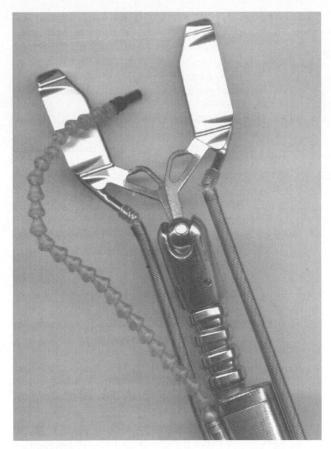

FIGURE 13-1. Latest generation of vacuum-assisted endoscopic stabilizer with irrigating channel.

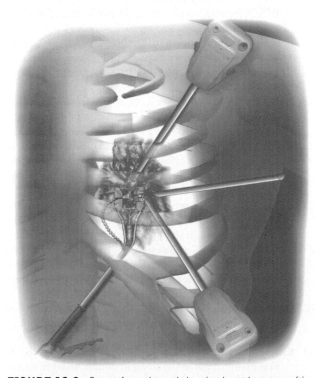

FIGURE 13-2. Set-up for endoscopic beating-heart bypass grafting of the left internal thoracic artery to the left anterior descending. The stabilizer is inserted through a subxyphoidal port.

for the procedural success. This includes a principal understanding of the system architecture of telemanipulation systems and the underlying human-machine interface technology. A team approach is crucial for success, and it is important that the table-side surgeon understands the basic mechanisms of joint motion of the manipulators in order to provide a set-up that allows an unrestricted range of motion. Take-down of the ITA should be routinely accomplished, before aiming at a complete TECAB procedure. For multivessel revascularization, endoscopic devices for exposure of the back wall of the heart need to be developed. Alternatively, different access routes (transabdominal, right chest) need to be explored. Endoscopic ultrasound probes may help to identify coronary pathology and to define the ideal location for an anastomosis in the absence of tactile feedback.[31]

With refinements in telemanipulator technology and the development of adjunct devices to enhance exposure, the technique of computer-enhanced endoscopic cardiac surgery will further evolve and may prove beneficial for selected patients. Smaller and more flexible modular robotic arms will be developed, and new control algorithms will eventually allow one operator to control multiple arms. Three-dimensional high-definition television (3D-HDTV) systems will provide even better optical resolution in the near future.[32] The application of multimodal 3D imaging and computational modeling of the range of motion of the robotic arms in an individual patient dataset may optimize preoperative planning of the procedure.[33] The use of preoperative imaging may also help to better identify suitable candidates for an endoscopic approach. Multidetector computed tomography (CT) scanning may help to preoperatively identify intramyocardial LADs, decreasing the risk of conversion or grafting to a diagonal branch.[34] New devices for facilitated anastomosis, such as the Ventrica magnetic coupling device, may facilitate endoscopic coronary artery bypass grafting in the future.

References

1. Califiore AM, Gianmarco GD, Teodori G, et al. Left anterior descending coronary artery grafting via left anterior small thoracotomy without cardiopulmonary bypass. Ann Thorac Surg 1996;61:1658–65.
2. Subramanian VA. Less invasive arterial CABG on a beating heart. Ann Thorac Surg 1997;63:68–71.
3. Diegeler A, Spyrantis N, Matin M, et al. The revival of surgical treatment for isolated proximal high-grade LAD lesions by minimally invasive coronary artery bypass grafting. Eur J Cardiothorac Surg 2000;17:501–4.
4. Ricci M, Karamanoukian HL, D'Ancona G, et al. Exposure and mechanical stabilization in off-pump coronary artery bypass grafting via a sternotomy. Ann Thorac Surg 2000;70:1736–40.
5. Arom KV, Flavin TF, Emery RW, et al. Safety and efficacy of off-pump coronary artery bypass grafting. Ann Thorac Surg 2000;69:704–10.
6. Duhaylongsod FG, Mayfield WR, Wolf RK. Thoracoscopic harvest of the internal thoracic artery: a multicenter experience in 218 cases. Ann Thorac Surg 1998;66:1012–7.
7. Mohr FW, Falk V, Diegeler A, et al. Minimally invasive Port-Access mitral valve surgery. J Thorac Cardiovasc Surg 1998;115:567–76.
8. Falk V, Diegeler A, Walther T, et al. Developments in robotic cardiac surgery. Curr Opin Cardiol 2000;15:378–87.
9. Falk V, Diegeler A, Walther T, et al. Total endoscopic coronary artery bypass grafting. Eur J Cardiothorac Surg 2000;17:38–45.
10. Falk V, Diegeler A, Walther T, et al. Total endoscopic off-pump coronary artery bypass grafting. Heart Surg Forum 2000;3:29–31.
11. Guthart GS, Salisbury JK. The Intuitive Telesurgery system: overview and application. Proc IEEE ICRA 2001. [In press]
12. Falk V. Robotic surgery. In: Yim AP, Hazelrigg SR, Izzat MB, et al, editors. Minimal access cardiothoracic surgery. Philadelphia: WB Saunders; 1999. p. 623–9.
13. Mohr FW, Falk V, Diegeler A, Autschbach R. Computer-enhanced coronary artery bypass surgery. J Thorac Cardiovasc Surg 1999;117:1212–3.
14. Kappert U, Cichon R, Schneider J, et al. Robotic coronary artery surgery—the evolution of a new minimally invasive approach in coronary artery surgery. Thorac Cardiovasc Surg 2000;48:193–7.
15. Cichon R, Kappert U, Schneider J, et al. Robotically enhanced "Dresden technique" with bilateral internal mammary artery grafting. Thorac Cardiovasc Surg 2000;48:189–92.
16. Raumanns J, Diegeler A, Falk V, et al. Hemodynamic effects of CO_2 insufflation under one-lung ventilation for robot-guided surgery. Anesth Analg 2000;90:SCA55.
17. Loulmet D, Carpentier A, d'Attellis N, et al. First endoscopic coronary artery bypass grafting using computer-assisted instruments. J Thorac Cardiovasc Surg 1999;118:4–10.
18. Mohr FW, Falk V, Diegeler A, et al. Computer-enhanced robotic cardiac surgery—experience in 148 patients. J Thorac Cardiovasc Surg 2001;121:842–53.
19. Kappert U, Schneider J, Cichon R, et al. Development of robotic enhanced endoscopic surgery for the treatment of coronary artery disease. Circulation 2001;104 Suppl I:I-102–7.
20. Dogan S, Aybek T, Andressen E, et al. Totally endoscopic coronary artery bypass can be performed with a low conversion rate. Heart Surg Forum 2001;4 Suppl II:84.
21. Aybeck T, Dogan S, Andressen E, et al. Robotically enhanced totally endoscopic right internal thoracic coronary artery bypass to the right coronary artery. Heart Surg Forum 2000;3:322–4.
22. Dogan S, Aybeck T, Westphal K, et al. Computer-enhanced totally endoscopic sequential arterial coronary artery bypass. Ann Thorac Surg 2001;72:610–1.
23. Kappert U, Cichon R, Schneider J, et al. Closed chest bilateral mammary artery grafting in double vessel coronary artery disease. Ann Thorac Surg 2000;70:1699–701.
24. Cichon R, Kappert V, Schneider J, et al. Robotically enhanced Dresden technique with bilateral internal

mammary artery grafting. Thorac Cardiovasc Surg 2000;48:193–7.

25. Falk V, Diegeler A, Walther T, et al. Endoscopic coronary artery bypass grafting on the beating heart using a computer enhanced telemanipulation system. Heart Surg Forum 1999;2:199–205.

26. Falk V, Grünenfelder J, Fann JI, et al. Total endoscopic computer-enhanced beating heart coronary artery bypass grafting. Ann Thorac Surg 2000;70:2029–33.

27. Kappert U, Cichon R, Schneider J, et al. Closed chest coronary artery bypass surgery on the beating heart with the use of a robotic system. J Thorac Cardiovasc Surg 2000; 120:809–11.

28. Kappert U, Cichon R, Schneider J, et al. Technique of closed chest coronary artery surgery on the beating heart. Eur J Cardiothorac Surg 2001;20:765–9.

29. Boehm DH, Reichenspurner H, Detter C, et al. Clinical use of a computer-enhanced surgical robotic system for endoscopic coronary artery bypass grafting on the beating heart. Thorac Cardiovasc Surg 2000;48:198–202.

30. Boyd WD, Rayman R, Desai ND, et al. Closed-chest coronary artery bypass grafting on the beating heart with the use of a computer-enhanced surgical robotic system. J Thorac Cardiovasc Surg 2000;120:807–9.

31. Falk V, Fann JI, Grünenfelder J, Burdon TA. Endoscopic Doppler for detecting vessels in closed chest bypass grafting. Heart Surg Forum 2000;3:331–3.

32. Falk V, Mintz D, Grünenfelder J, et al. Influence of 3D vision on surgical telemanipulator performance. Surg Endosc 2001;15:1282–6.

33. Chiu AM, Dey DD, Drangova M, et al. 3-D image guidance for minimally invasive robotic coronary artery surgery. Heart Surg Forum 2000;3:224–31.

34. Dogan S, Herzog C, Wimmer-Greinecker G, et al. Multidetector CT scan as a preoperative tool for totally endoscopic coronary artery bypass. Heart Surg Forum 2001; 4 Suppl I:80.

CHAPTER 14

ADVANCES IN CORONARY ARTERY SURGERY

ROBERT W. EMERY, MD, KIT V. AROM, MD, PhD, ARLEN R. HOLTER, MD, TIMOTHY J. KROSHUS, MD, PhD

Since the introduction of coronary artery bypass (CAB) surgery as a definitive therapy for atherosclerotic disease of this vessel, this procedure has become the most studied operation in the history of medicine and perhaps the most common surgical procedure performed on a global basis. Until late 1995, CAB surgery essentially represented one operation for all patients. Now termed "conventional," coronary revascularization surgery is completed with the patient placed on cardiopulmonary bypass (CPB) and the heart stopped by using surgeon-specific cardioplegic solution. This changed with the introduction of minimally invasive direct coronary bypass surgery (MIDCAB), which initiated a revolution in myocardial revascularization.[1–3] Although minimally invasive coronary surgery (MICS) can be difficult to define, the variations cited in Table 14-1 are considered MICS.[4] While conventional CAB surgery composes the majority of procedures performed, since 1995, variations of MICS have been devised to address the needs of the individual patient, resulting in an important paradigm change from one operation for all patients. Now, surgeons adjust the operation to the needs and comorbid risk factors of the individual patient. The original MIDCAB has come to occupy a small niche in all coronary revascularization procedures, at approximately 3%. MIDCAB approaches vary from left anterior thoracotomy to lateral thoracotomy, abdominal approaches, and right thoracotomy, depending on the vessel(s) to be bypassed, the commonality being that cardiopulmonary bypass is not used and pedicle conduits are necessary. Target revascularization or MIDCAB combined with stenting (hybrid procedure) has not gained support. Lessons learned from MIDCAB rapidly led surgeons to develop off-pump multivessel coronary surgery via sternotomy, a natural extension of MIDCAB, useful especially in patients at risk for cardiopulmonary bypass: the aged, those with significant comorbid risk factors, and those with markedly depressed ventricular function appear to particularly benefit.[5] In spite of forceful contradictory arguments, several trials have shown this surgery to be as safe as surgery done using conventional methods.[6–8] It is commonly accepted that avoiding CPB lessens the use of blood and blood products and decreases ventilator time; cost savings are a secondary benefit.[4,9,10] Graft patency has been excellent.[11] The Society of Thoracic Surgeons noted that off-pump coronary artery bypass (OPCAB) is an extension of accepted surgical techniques as opposed to a new procedure.[12] Currently, it is estimated that 25% of all CAB surgery is completed without CPB. The technologic advances listed in Table 14-2 place OPCAB in the realm of trained cardiac surgeons as opposed to the realm of a few surgeons with special technical ability.

Parallel to the development of OPCAB, HeartPort Inc. (now part of Johnson & Johnson Inc.) developed the instrumentation to allow peripheral cannulation and multivessel coronary bypass to be performed via a small left anterior thoracotomy with the heart stopped.[13] Although successful, the procedure proved to be difficult, time-consuming, and expensive, without specific advantage aside from a smaller incision. These procedures are undertaken rarely.

Lastly, computer-enabled (robotic) totally endoscopic CAB surgery (TECAB) was introduced, with two companies vying for dominance.[14,15] This concept is indeed a

TABLE 14-1. Components of Minimally Invasive Cardiac Surgery

Minimally invasive direct coronary bypass (MIDCAB)
Off-pump coronary bypass (OPCAB)
Port-access coronary bypass (PACAB)
Totally endoscopic (robotic) coronary bypass (TECAB)

TABLE 14-2. Technologic Advances Permitting OPCAB to Be Routinely Performed

Stabilizing systems (1996)
Intracoronary shunts (1997)
Mister blowing devices (1999)
Mechanical connectors (2001)

new operation, and special skills and training are necessary. Because of the experimental nature of this process and the extreme expense, such surgeries are only carried out at a few quaternary centers. This approach to coronary surgery is detailed in a separate chapter of the text.

New developments continue at a rapid rate and will further modify the surgical approach and concepts of myocardial revascularization. Several that have or soon will have clinical experience are listed in Table 14-3 and are discussed in the remainder of this chapter.

Facilitated Anastomoses

A giant step forward in the process of myocardial revascularization has been the recent introduction of devices to mechanically construct proximal and distal vascular anastomoses. These devices provide quality control and uniformity that are currently lacking in spite of the intensive training of cardiovascular surgeons. The advantages of these devices are several and include increased consistency and speed of construction, the elimination of the need for aortic clamping, and the ability to perform the proximal anastomoses first, without adding a pressure load to the ventricle by partial occlusion, with the benefit of immediate reperfusion of the grafted area upon completion of the distal suturing.

Currently, the St. Jude Medical Inc. (Little Canada, Minnesota) Symmetry device for proximal anastomoses is the only one clinically available in the United States (Figure 14-1). More than 10,000 implants have been accomplished since Symmetry's release in May 2001. There have been minimal problems, and most of the problems are associated with a learning curve for loading the vein onto the device and the positioning of the vein on the aorta.[16] Positioning of the vein on the aorta is particularly important because the connector requires that the grafts come off the aorta at 90° as opposed to the bevel to which surgeons are more accustomed. For example, the left-sided grafts have to be placed more laterally to lie against the pulmonary artery, and the right graft has to come off anteriorly, just distal to the right coronary following the path of the native artery (Figure 14-2). Lateral placement of the right graft can lead to kinking at the level of the anastomosis. The CorLink proximal anastomotic device (Figure 14-3) is under development by Ethicon, Inc., (Cornelia, GA), and is currently undergoing early experimental and clinical trials.

TABLE 14-3. Transition from Present to Future

Facilitated anastomosis

On-pump beating-heart surgery

Transmyocardial laser revascularization

Ventriculocoronary bypass (VACAB)

Postoperative adjuvant medical therapy

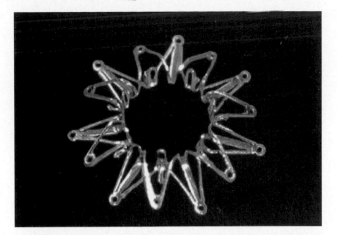

FIGURE 14-1. The deployed St. Jude Medical Inc. Symmetry device. With the vein loaded on stent barbs, the arms grasp the inside and outside of the aorta. This serves to secure the vein to the aorta and to trap endothelium of the aorta between the device's arms.

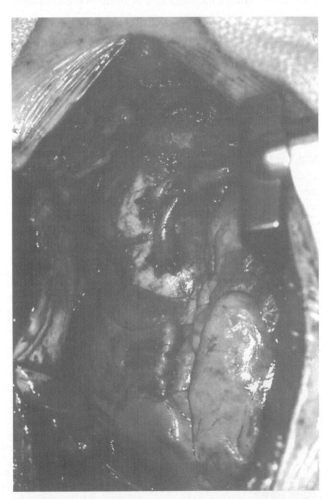

FIGURE 14-2. Operative photo of two left-sided grafts secured to the aorta with the St. Jude Medical Inc. Symmetry device. The proximal graft lies nicely at 90°, but the more distal graft is somewhat less than 90° and ideally could have been placed more laterally in the aorta, toward and resting against the pulmonary artery.

St. Jude Medical Inc. has also introduced a variant of the proximal mechanical device for use in distal anastomotic surgery. This device (Figure 14-4) creates an end-to-side distal anastomosis with ligation of the distal conduit in much the same fashion as Wolf used for early MIDCAB graft construction and evaluation.[17] This is the first device with early clinical experience, and the results are promising.[18] A unique device using magnetic connection is undergoing initial clinical testing, and an experimental study was presented at the International Society for Minimally Invasive Cardiac Surgery (Figure 14-5). Early human results are pending (verbal communication, David Adams). This device may offer great future potential, broadening MICS application.

Other innovative devices are in early engineering phases, and little information is available because of patent concerns. Other means of anastomotic completion without sutures, such as biologic glues and hybrid sutureless anastomosis, are also under investigation.[19,20]

Certainly these devices will change the way surgery is conducted. Smaller incisions can be used, as the ascending

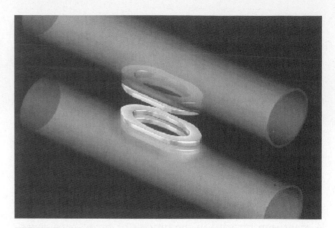

FIGURE 14-5. The Ventrica Inc. connector functions on the principle of magnetic attraction between the pieces placed in the artery and bypass conduit. Clinical results are not measurable.

aorta does not have to be accessed to provide room for an occluding clamp and hand suturing. These devices are likely to cause an increase in the application of OPCAB procedures and, when coupled with the improved stabilization systems, coronary shunts, and mister-blower devices, enable the OPCAB procedure to become a more universal application. By eliminating partial occlusion of the aorta, automated anastomotic connectors may also minimize the incidence of aortic dissection and particulate embolization that can occur with aortic cannulation and clamping, thus minimizing neurologic injury.[21,22]

Importantly, the limiting factor in the broader application of TECAB is the construction of a "perfect" anastomosis. While not addressing cost, mechanically coupled anastomosis places the surgical robot in the role of facilitating completion of the operation, rather than completing the operation itself. Consequently, such robotic devices can be developed more easily to expose rather than construct, allowing broader application and potentially leading truly to same-day heart surgery.

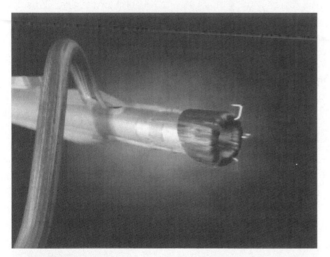

FIGURE 14-3. Corlink proximal connectors are being tested in early clinical trials. No results are currently published.

On-Pump Beating-Heart Surgery

While somewhat of an oxymoron in certain patients, procedures that the surgeon may want to do without perfusion, such as OPCAB surgery, may not be able to be completed in this fashion. Akins and colleagues have long performed bypass surgery on the warm fibrillating heart.[23] There have been concerns regarding subendocardial perfusion in this circumstance. Data, however, indicate a remarkably low rate of myocardial injury during short periods of regional myocardial ischemia in OPCAB procedures, which indicates that one does not need to stop the heart while on CPB.[4] By cannulating the aorta distal to the left carotid artery, cerebral emboli emanating from the cannulation site per se can be minimized.[22] Proximal aortic grafts can be completed off-pump using automatic mechanical connectors, and the patient can then be placed

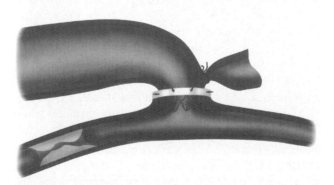

FIGURE 14-4. Schematic of the St. Jude Medical Inc. distal connector. This device also entraps the intima of the conduit and coronary artery.

on CPB. A left ventricular vent is placed via the right superior pulmonary vein. With the heart maximally decompressed and using beating-heart technology (see Table 14-2), the distal anastomoses can be rapidly and easily constructed with immediate reperfusion. There is no need for myocardial recovery time as the patient is kept warm and the heart beating, and bypass can be readily discontinued when the procedure is completed, minimizing CPB time. Table 14-4 shows the advantages of such an approach.

Since the FDA's approval of the St. Jude Medical Inc. Symmetry device, we have performed 21 such procedures, all in patients with significant comorbid risk factors, including extreme age, cardiomegaly, active congestive heart failure, obesity, and pulmonary hypertension. The procedures could not be completed off-pump. One patient died suddenly on postoperative day 3, and one patient had prolonged hospitalization due to multiorgan system dysfunction. There were no CVAs or other significant postoperative complications. We found this to be a useful alternative approach to completing revascularization, thus individualizing the operation to the patient. This methodology may also be of value in patients who do not tolerate cardiac manipulation, due to intense ischemia or left main disease; in patients with cardiomegaly, as well as patients with high filling pressures in whom the approach to areas other than anterior are difficult; and in obese or deep-chested patients who present difficult off-pump anatomy.

Transmyocardial Laser Revascularization

Laser therapy for ischemic cardiovascular disease has had a long and checkered history. Introduced more than 25 years ago, the mechanism of action is still unclear and the clinical results have been questioned. Yet, if one believes that prospective randomized trials are the gold standard of surgical therapeutic results, several separate trials have shown significant improvement in angina class after laser therapy.[24–26] Most recently, Horvath and associates published a 5-year result indicating the ongoing benefits of transmyocardial laser revascularization (TMLR) as sole therapy.[27] Unfortunately, such studies cannot be blinded, and this has been a major criticism. The eligible population for the use of TMLR as sole therapy is currently limited.

TABLE 14-4. Advantages of On-Pump Beating-Heart Surgery

Short cardiopulmonary bypass time

No aortic clamping

No cardioplegic delivery

No central cooling

Ease of visualization of target vessels

Minimized neurologic injury

In a prospective randomized trial in patients having incomplete CAB versus CAB + TMLR, Allen and associates demonstrated a significant decrease in operative mortality, early (1.5% vs 7.6%, $p = .02$) and at 1 year in patients having combined CAB and TMLR (as survival was 95% versus 89%, $p = .05$).[28]

This study was criticized for the expected high operative mortality, yet the patients enrolled were at higher risk because surgical revascularization was incomplete, consistent with the observation of others.[29] Additionally, two methods of expressed risk assessment were modeled. Aside from improved operative mortality, benefit was also gained in terms of diminished incidence of recurrent angina and prolonged time interval to recurrence in patients having combined procedures. This may be an important purview for the future.[28] Although use of TMLR is limited at this point in time, as surgeons we will be asked in the future to deal with patients who have recurrent coronary artery disease post multistenting. In our group's experience in 1998, 18% of our CAB procedures had prior intervention. However, 2 years later, 60% of all primary bypass operations had prior intervention (Cardiac Surgical Associates STS Based Registry). This is likely to increase further as the number of stents per patient and the number of arteries stented increase. Drug-eluting stents are likely to further enhance these applications. As disease progresses, such patients may have some bypassable vessels, but many will have no lumen for revascularization, having burned out or scarred arteries for which no direct revascularization can be achieved. It is this cohort of patients that may benefit from isolated or combined TMLR procedures, and continued search for innovative therapy for such patients must be ongoing. Certainly, other innovative therapies, such as myocardial or endothelial cell implant/transplant or gene therapy, may arise, but such applications are likely many years away. The use of TMLR is discussed at length in a separate chapter.

Ventriculocoronary Perfusion

The traditional physiologic thinking that perfusion of the heart may only effectively occur in diastole was recently challenged by the development of two devices (HeartStent Inc., Minneapolis, MN, and Percaria Inc.) designed to provide systolic coronary perfusion directly from the ventricle.[30–32] Older literature has provided provenance that systolic perfusion of the heart adequately supports myocardial function.[33] Patients having severe aortic insufficiency had valve replacement in the supracoronary position. No short- or long-term mortality was reported related to coronary insufficiency; in fact, enlargement of the coronary arteries was found. Three recent reports indicate that 46 to 74% of net coronary flow can be provided via ventricular coronary connection. Greater-than-normal flow occurs during systole, with net retrograde flow during diastole. One device creates a starling valve limitation to retrograde flow, which appears to increase net forward flow.[31] In the other study, only unidirectional flow (Figure 14-6) was tested. Baseline net flow was 74% of native coronary flow, and there was adequate perfusion to stress up to 40 kg/mm of dobutamine infusion.[30] There are no long-term data beyond 12 weeks. Advances in the design of devices to allow clinical application are ongoing.[32] Such devices may be valuable adjuncts to complete revascularization or, possibly, to promote coronary size growth. Applications for European ethics approval and limited US trials are pending.

Adjunctive Medical Therapy

Most advances in the surgery of coronary disease are technical in nature, but recently, focus has been on increasing the longevity of the operation. Complete arterial grafting has been one answer,[34] but because more than 80% of all bypass surgeries completed in the United States involve one or more saphenous vein grafts, attention has been directed at impacting the longevity of these conduits. It has long been known that aspirin improves the early patency of vein grafts.[35] Recent data indicate that aggressive cholesterol lowering using a statin agent further protects vein grafts over the longer term, as well as stabilizing plaque.[36] Progression of native arteriosclerosis in the face of competitive flow from bypass grafts is diminished as a result of aggressive cholesterol lowering in the postbypass period.[37] More powerful antiplatelet drugs are also being used in postoperative bypass patients, with improvement in graft patency.[38] The use of β-blocking agents decreases the incidence of major adverse cardiac events postoperatively, thereby improving long-term survival.[39]

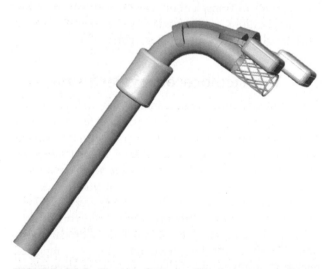

FIGURE 14-6. The HeartStent Inc. Ventriculo-coronary Bypass (VCAB) Device. This unidirectional device has an arm that traverses the ventricular wall to provide inflow directly from the ventricular chamber, and the other mesh-tipped end is inserted directly into the coronary artery. A stabilizing arm minimizes motion and endothelial trauma. A bi-directional device is being developed.

In our practice, patients are placed on a platelet inhibitor 6 to 8 h after surgery, when hemostasis has been assured. They are also given β-blocker and a statin cholesterol agent, pending cardiology preference and patient tolerance. The use of clopidogrel (Plavix), a more powerful platelet inhibitor, may become more prominent as further data accumulate.[38] This drug is given to all OPCAB patients in our practice for 60 days, starting on postoperative day 1.

Another innovative therapy to preserve saphenous vein graft (SVG) life expectancy is the use of E2F decoy, a vein endothelial coating. Recent data indicate experimental enhancement of graft longevity, and such therapy would be an added benefit to bypass surgery.[40] The ability to secure long-term disease-free patency of SVG represents an important goal.

Comment

The previous sections of this chapter were chosen to discuss both current and future innovative issues. The discussions are brief and certainly not inclusive. In the face of efforts to improve patient care, the profession is beset with the strife and controversy threatening the field of cardiovascular surgery.[41] Reimbursement continues to decrease, compounded by the loss of Medicare practice and training components, in addition to reduced conversion factors for relative value units. Practice volumes are decreasing nationwide due to innovative medical therapy, application of interventional procedures, and healthier lifestyles. Surgical volume decrease is expected to continue with the application of drug-eluting stents that are soon to be released. Our older, sicker patients[29,42] are being denied the cooperative care of our cardiology colleagues in the postoperative period by the US Department of Health and Human Services except by specific consultation, indicating that events have to occur to obtain consultative care in these higher-risk patients rather than be prevented by cooperative care. As a result, for the first time in 2001 all available fellowship positions in cardiovascular surgery did not fill. To continue the advance against cardiovascular disease requires more than dedication and research. As a profession, cardiac surgeons need to support the efforts of the Society of Thoracic Surgeons (STS) and the American Association for Thoracic Surgery (AATS) in government relations and maintain our communication and collegiality. As individuals, we need to become educated to the political process through the societal-initiated programs such as the Kennedy Government School Program. As individuals and statewide organizations (ie, regional STS chapters), we need to become involved in the political process, contributing time and dollars to candidates espousing views consistent with improved patient care. We need to visit, lobby, and become acquainted with our public officials and be a resource for future decisions. John McDonough noted that politics is the art of who gets what, when, and for whom; thus the impact can be great.[41] With the average age of our patients rising, we are, in effect, being converted as a profession to a one-payor system, the federal government, and we must have a voice in the process. As cardiovascular surgeons, we are trained to make evidence-based life-and-death decisions and are ideally suited for a role in policy determination and for having a voice in our own destiny.[43] We are, therefore, becoming social scientists as well as surgical scientists, a further advance in the therapy for coronary artery disease.

References

1. Robinson MC, Gross Dr, Zeman W, Stedje-Larsen E. Minimally invasive coronary artery bypass grafting: a new method using an anterior mediastinotomy. J Card Surg 1995;10(5):529–36.

2. Subramanian VA, Sani G, Benetti FJ, Calafiore AM. Minimally invasive coronary bypass surgery: a multi-center report of preliminary clinical experience. Circulation 1995;92 Suppl 2:645.

3. Calafiore AM, Di Giammarco G, Teodori G, et al. Left anterior descending coronary artery grafting via left anterior small thoracotomy without cardiopulmonary bypass. Ann Thorac Surg 1996;61:1658–63.

4. Emery RW, Flavin TF, Arom KV, et al. Minimally invasive coronary artery bypass surgery: state of the art. New Surg 2001;1:33–9.

5. Arom KV, Flavin TF, Emery RW, et al. Safety and efficacy of off-pump coronary artery bypass grafting. Ann Thorac Surg 2000;69:704–10.

6. Van Dijk D, Nierich AP, Jansen EW, et al. Early outcome after off-pump versus on-pump coronary bypass surgery: results from a randomized study. Circulation 2001;104:1761–6.

7. Bull DA, Neumayer LA, Stringham JC, et al. Coronary artery bypass grafting with cardiopulmonary bypass versus off-pump cardiopulmonary bypass grafting: does eliminating the pump reduce morbidity and cost? Ann Thorac Surg 2001;71:170–5.

8. Yacoub M. Off-pump coronary bypass surgery: in search of an identity. Circulation 2001;104:1743–5.

9. Arom KV, Emery RW, Flavin TF, Petersen RJ. Cost-effectiveness of minimally invasive coronary artery bypass surgery. Ann Thoracic Surg 1999;68:1562–6.

10. Lancey RA, Soller BR, Vander Salm TJ. Off-pump versus on-pump coronary artery bypass surgery: a case-matched comparison of clinical outcomes and costs. Heart Surg Forum 2000;3(4):277–81.

11. Mack MJ. Invited commentary. Midterm angiographic assessment of coronary artery bypass grafting without cardiopulmonary bypass [review]. Ann Thorac Surg 2000;70:850.

12. Policy statement: minimally invasive coronary artery bypass surgery. The Society of Thoracic Surgeons/American Association for Thoracic Surgery Committee on New Technology. Ann Thorac Surg 1998;66:1848–9.

13. Ribakov GH, Galloway AC, Grossi EA, et al. Port-access coronary artery bypass. In: Oz ME, Goldstein DJ, editors. Minimally invasive cardiac surgery. Totowa, NJ: Humana Press; 1999. p. 117–28.

14. Boyd WD, Rayman R, Desai ND, et al. Closed-chest coronary artery bypass grafting on the beating heart with the use of a computer-enhanced surgical robotic system. J Thorac Cardiovasc Surg 2000;120:807–9.

15. Kappert U, Cichon R, Schneider J, et al. Closed-chest coronary artery surgery on the beating heart with the use of a robotic system. J Thorac Cardiovasc Surg 2000;120:809–11.

16. Mack MJ, Emery RW, Ley LR, et al. Initial experience with one hundred thirty-nine consecutive proximal anastomoses performed with a mechanical connector. Ann Thorac Surg. [In press]

17. Wolf RK. The intraoperative assessment of coronary bypass grafts. In: Cohen RE, Mack MJ, Fonger JD, et al, editors. Minimally invasive cardiac surgery. St. Louis, MO: Quality Medical; 1999. p. 205–11.

18. Eckstein FS, Meyer B, Bonilla L, et al. First clinical results with a new mechanical connector for coronary artery anastomoses in CABG. Circulation 2001 Suppl II;104:II-362–3.

19. Gundry SR, Black K, Izutani H. Sutureless coronary artery bypass with biologic glued anastomoses: preliminary in vivo and in vitro results. J Thorac Cardiovasc Surg 2000;120:473–7.

20. Buijsrogge MP, Scheltes JS, Heikens M, et al. Sutureless coronary anastomoses using an anastomotic device and tissue adhesive in off-pump porcine coronary bypass surgery. Circulation 2001 Suppl II;104:II–362.

21. Chavanon O, Carrier M, Cartier R, et al. Increased incidence of acute ascending aortic dissection with off-pump aortocoronary bypass surgery? Ann Thorac Surg 2001;71:117–21.

22. Fearn SJ, Pole R, Wesnes K, et al. Cerebral injury during cardiopulmonary bypass: emboli impair memory. J Thorac Cardiovasc Surg 2001;121:1150–60.

23. Akins CW. Ischemic heart disease: coronary bypass: hypothermic ventricular fibrillation. In: Kaiser LR, Kron IL, Spray TL, editors. Mastery of cardiothoracic surgery. Philadelphia, PA: Lippincott-Raven Publishers; 1997. p. 395.

24. Frazier OH, March RJ, Horvath KA. Transmyocardial revascularization with a carbon dioxide laser in patients with end-stage coronary artery disease. N Engl J Med 1999;341:1021–28.

25. Allen KB, Dowling RD, Fudge TL, et al. Comparison of transmyocardial revascularization with medical therapy in patients with refractory angina. N Engl J Med 1999;341:1029–36.

26. Schofield PM, Charples LD, Caine N, et al. Transmyocardial laser revascularisation in patients with refractory angina: a randomized controlled trial. Lancet 1999;383:519–24.

27. Horvath, KA, Aranki SF, Cohn LH, et al. Sustained angina relief 5 years after transmyocardial laser revascularization with a CO_2 laser. Circulation 2001;104(12 Suppl 1):181–4..

28. Allen KB, Dowling RD, DelRossi AJ, et al. Transmyocardial laser revascularization combined with coronary artery bypass grafting: a multicenter, blinded, prospective,

randomized, controlled trial. J Thorac Cardiovasc Surg 2000;119:540–9.

29. Abramov D, Tamariz MG, Fremes SE, et al. Trends in coronary artery bypass surgery results: a recent 9-year study. Ann Thorac Surg 2000;70:84–90.

30. Suehiro K, Shimizu J, Yi GH, et al. Direct coronary artery perfusion from the left ventricle. J Thorac Cardiovasc Surg 2001;121:307–15.

31. Tweden KS, Eales F, Cameron JD, et al. Ventriculocoronary artery bypass (VCAB), a novel approach to myocardial revascularization. Heart Surg Forum 2000;3(1):47–55.

32. Emery RW, Eales F, Van Meter CH Jr, et al. Ventriculocoronary artery bypass results using a mesh-tipped device in a porcine model. Ann Thorac Surg 2001;72:1004S–8S.

33. Liddicoat JE, Bekassy SM, De Bakey ME. Double prosthetic aortic valve: case report. J Thorac Cardiovasc Surg 1975;69:763–6.

34. Tector AJ, Kress DC, Downey FX, Schmahl TM. Complete revascularization with internal thoracic artery grafts. Semin Thorac Cardiovasc Surg 1996;8:29–41.

35. Chesebro JH, Fuster V, Elveback LR, et al. Effect of dipyridamole and aspirin on late vein-graft patency after coronary bypass operations. N Engl J Med 1984;310:209–14.

36. Campeau L, Hunninghake DB, Knatterud GL, et al. Aggressive cholesterol lowering delays saphenous vein graft atherosclerosis in women, the elderly, and patients with associated risk factors. Circulation 1999;99:3241–7.

37. White CW, Gobel FL, Campeau L, et al. Effect of an aggressive lipid-lowering strategy on progression of atherosclerosis in the left main coronary artery from patients in the Post Coronary Artery Bypass Graft trial. Circulation 2001;104:2660–5.

38. Bhatt DL, Chew DP, Hirsch AT, et al. Superiority of clopidogrel versus aspirin in patients with prior cardiac surgery. Circulation 2001;103:363–8.

39. Chen J, Radford MJ, Wang Y, et al. Are beta-blockers effective in elderly patients who undergo coronary revascularization after acute myocardial infarction? Arch Intern Med 2000;160:947–52.

40. Mann MJ, Whittemore AD, Donaldson MC, et al. Ex vivo gene therapy of human vascular bypass grafts with E2F decoy: The PREVENT single-centre, randomised, controlled trial. Lancet 1999;354:1493–8.

41. Matloff JM. The practice of medicine in the year 2010: revisited in 2001. Ann Thorac Surg 2001;72:1105–12.

42. Avery GJ, Ley SJ, Hill JD, et al. Cardiac surgery in the octogenarian: evaluation of risk, cost and outcome. Ann Thorac Surg 2001;71:591–6.

43. Frist WH. Public policy and the participating physician. Ann Thorac Surg 2001;71:1410–4.

Chapter 15

Transmyocardial Laser Revascularization

Keith A. Horvath, MD

It has been more than a decade since the first patients were treated with transmyocardial laser revascularization as sole therapy for their end-stage coronary disease. Since then, more than 8,000 patients have been treated worldwide. Different wavelengths of laser light—CO_2 and Ho:YAG (holmium:yttrium-aluminum-garnet)—and different approaches—thoracotomy, thoracoscopy, and percutaneous—have been employed. The clinical experience, now that both short- and long-term results are available, indicates differences between the types of laser light and the delivery of that light to the tissue.

While the use of a laser to revascularize the heart is relatively new, the underlying concept is not. Before the advent of coronary artery bypass grafting (CABG) or percutaneous transluminal coronary angioplasty (PTCA), attempts were made to revascularize the heart by direct perfusion. These were first described by Beck in 1935, who, through a number of means, achieved at least superficial angiogenesis, primarily as a response to epicardial and pericardial inflammation.[1] Later, Vineberg demonstrated that direct perfusion was possible by implanting the internal mammary artery into the myocardium.[2] Results of this procedure led to neovascularization and collateral formation in some cases. In an effort to recreate the anatomy of the reptilian heart, Sen and colleagues and others performed direct perfusion by transmyocardial acupuncture.[3-5] Although these results yielded some success, they were not long-lasting, they were difficult to reproduce, and, more importantly, they were eventually overshadowed by the ability to perform CABG. Although most patients can be treated with conventional methods such as CABG or PTCA with stenting, there is a significant and growing number of patients who have exhausted the ability to undergo these procedures repeatedly, primarily because of the diffuse nature of their coronary artery disease. As a result of this severe disease, they have chronic disabling angina that is refractory to medical therapy. Transmyocardial laser revascularization (TMLR) was developed to treat these patients. Mirhoseini and associates and Okada and

colleagues used a laser to perform this type of revascularization in conjunction with coronary artery bypass grafting in the early 1980s.[6-8] After improvements in the laser that allowed TMLR to be performed as sole therapy on a beating heart, results from individual institutions and from multicenter trials were reported in 1995 through 1997.[9-13] Although the outcomes of these trials were encouraging, they lacked an appropriate control group. Four prospective randomized controlled trials comparing medical management versus TMLR in patients with severe angina have been published. These trials enrolled 837 patients and, by virtue of the one-to-one randomization, 418 of them were treated with the laser and the others continued on maximal medical therapy. All patients were followed for 12 months. One important similarity of these trials was that TMLR provided significant symptomatic improvement when compared with maximal medical therapy (for example, see Figure 15-1). The same improvement was not seen in recent trials using a laser percutaneously (percutaneous myocardial revascularization [PMR]). Although there are other similarities between these studies, there are also significant differences.

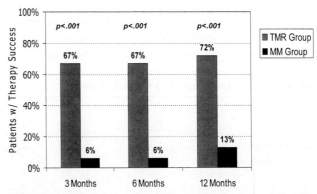

FIGURE 15-1. Success rate of CO_2 TMLR therapy as defined by decrease of two or more angina classes. MM Group = patients randomized to maximal medical therapy; TMR Group = patients randomized to CO_2 TMLR.

Methods

Patients

A review of the demographics of the enrollees from the randomized trials provides a picture of the type of patient who has TMLR. Table 15-1 lists the baseline characteristics of patients who underwent TMLR. Because the patients were equally randomized to the medical management group, there were no demographic differences between the groups for any of these trials. The average patient age was 61 years, and the majority were male. Most of the patients had severe angina and were in Canadian Cardiovascular Society (CCS) angina class IV. The ejection fractions for all of the patients were relatively well preserved at 50%. The majority of the patients had experienced a previous myocardial infarction and had undergone some type of previous attempt at revascularization, CABG, and/or PTCA.

The entry criteria were (1) the patients had to have refractory angina that was not amenable to standard methods of revascularization and (2) they had to have reversible ischemia based on myocardial perfusion scanning with ejection fractions > 25%.

Operative Technique

All patients underwent a small anterior lateral thoracotomy under general anesthesia. Figures 15-2 and 15-3 depict the operative techniques. Two different types of lasers were used: CO_2 and Ho:YAG. The CO_2 laser was used to create a 1 mm channel with a single 25 to 30 J pulse.[14,15] Transesophageal echocardiography was employed on all of these CO_2-treated patients to confirm transmural penetration of the laser. The Ho:YAG laser achieved a similar 1 mm channel by manually advancing a fiber through the myocardium while the laser was fired.[16,17] Typical pulse energies were 2 J for this laser, with 20 to 30 pulses required to traverse the myocardium. Confirmation of Ho:YAG transmural penetration was primarily by tactile and auditory feedback.

End Points

The principal subjective end point was a change in angina symptoms. This was assessed by the investigator and/or a blinded independent observer. In addition to assigning an

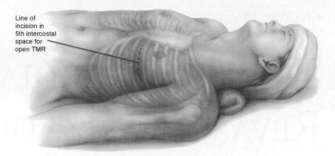

FIGURE 15-2. Transmyocardial laser revascularization performed as an open surgical procedure.

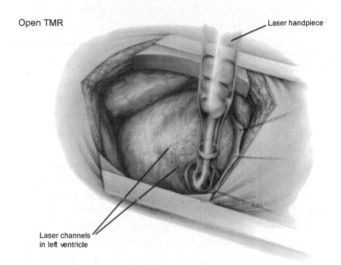

FIGURE 15-3. CO_2 laser handpiece placed against the epicardial surface. Channels are created, starting near the base of the heart and then progressing serially in a line approximately 1 cm apart toward the apex. Transesophageal echocardiography is employed to confirm transmural penetration of the laser energy.

angina class, standardized questionnaires such as the Seattle Angina Questionnaire, the Short Form 36 Questionnaire (SF-36), and the Duke activity status index were employed. These tests were used to detect changes in quality of life. Objective measurements consisted of repeated exercise tolerance testing as well as repeat myocardial perfusion scans. Patients were reassessed at 3, 6, and 12 months after randomization.

Results

Mortality

All the studies reported low perioperative mortality rates, ranging from 1 to 5%. One lesson learned was that patients who underwent TMLR less than 2 weeks after an episode of unstable angina requiring intravenous medications had a significantly higher perioperative mortality rate (22% for the unstable patients vs 1% for the stable patients). Predictably, the studies with more patients in

TABLE 15-1. Demographics of TMLR Patients

Average age (years)	61
Women	17%
Insulin-dependent diabetes mellitus	35%
Canadian Cardiovascular Society angina class III	35%
Canadian Cardiovascular Society angina class IV	65%
Ejection fraction % (mean ± SD)	49 ± 10
Previous myocardial infarction	72%
Previous CABG	91%
Previous PTCA	48%

CABG = coronary artery bypass grafting; PTCA = percutaneous transluminal coronary angioplasty; SD = standard deviation; TMLR = transmyocardial laser revascularization.

class IV or unstable angina patients had higher mortality rates.[14,16] Meta-analysis of the 1-year survival demonstrated no statistically significant difference between the patients treated with the laser (89%) and those patients who continued their medical therapy (87%).

Medications

The protocols were established such that the TMLR patients would continue on their maximum medical therapy and be weaned as tolerated. The frequencies of antianginal and cardiovascular drugs were similar between the two groups at baseline. At 12 months, the CO_2-treated patients had a decrease in nitrate use from 86% to 69%, as compared to the use of the medical management patients, which increased slightly, from 79% to 82%, in one study. The other CO_2 investigators reported a 60% decrease in nitrate use among the TMLR patients, whereas the medical management patients had a 22% increase in their use of nitrates. Ho:YAG investigators reported "little change in overall pattern of medications during the study" for both groups.

Angina Class

A blinded independent observer in all studies performed angina class assessment. This was done as either the only angina assessment or in comparison with the investigator's assessment. Significant symptomatic improvement was seen in all studies for patients treated with a laser. Using a definition of success of a decrease of two or more angina classes, all of the studies demonstrated a significant success rate for treatment with the laser, with success rates ranging from 25 to 76%. A smaller portion of patients in the medical management group also experienced symptomatic improvement, and the success rate for these patients ranged from 4 to 32%. The seemingly broad range of success is due to the differences between the baseline characteristics of the studies. The study that started with most of the patients in angina class III unsurprisingly showed the lowest success rate.[15] In contrast, the largest success rate for TMLR was seen in the trial in which all of the patients were in class IV at enrollment. Of note, the medical management group in this study also showed the largest success rate, at 32%.[16]

Quality of Life and Myocardial Function

The Seattle Angina Questionnaire, the SF-36, and the Duke activity status index all demonstrated significant improvement in the quality of life by all of these indices in the TMLR group versus the medical management group for each study. Global assessment of myocardial function by ejection fraction, using echocardiography or radionuclide multigated acquisition scans, showed no significant change in the overall ejection fraction of any of the patients, regardless of group assignment or study.

Hospital Admissions

Another indicator of the efficacy of the two treatments was demonstrated in the hospital admissions for unstable angina or cardiac-related events for all the patients. Meta-analysis of the data provided indicates that the 1-year hospitalization rate for patients in the laser-treated group was statistically significantly less than that for those treated medically. The odds ratio for 1-year hospitalization in the laser-treated group was 0.28 that of the 1-year hospitalization for the medically treated group, with an associated 95% confidence interval of 0.192 to 0.408.

Exercise Tolerance

Additional functional assessment by exercise tolerance testing was also performed. Treadmill testing employed the modified Bruce protocol, in which exercise intensity was increased every 3 min. Differences between TMLR-treated and medically managed patients were observed. One study reported a 70 s improvement over the baseline for the TMLR group and only a 5 s improvement for the medical management group at 12 months. Another study reported an average of a 65 s increase in the TMLR group at 12 months when compared with their baseline, with an average 46 s decrease in the medical management group over the same interval.

Myocardial Perfusion

As mentioned, myocardial perfusion scans were obtained preoperatively to verify the extent and severity of reversible ischemia. Postoperative scans were also obtained. The perfusion results from all of these studies are represented in Figure 15-4 and are expressed as changes in infarcted or ischemic myocardium at 1 year. It is at this point that the results differed dramatically depending on which wavelength of laser light was used (Figure 15-4A to D). Patients treated with the CO_2 laser showed a significant decrease in the number of ischemic segments at 1-year of follow-up without a significant increase in the infarcted segments. The medical management patients over that same period of time had significant increase in their ischemic and infarcted myocardium (see Figure 15-4A to D). In contrast, patients treated with the Ho:YAG laser showed no significant change in their ischemic segments. Not only did they not show an improvement in perfusion, but patients treated with the Ho:YAG laser showed no difference in their perfusion when compared with patients randomized to maximum medical therapy (see Figures 15-4C and D).

Morbidity

A comparative assessment for morbidity is difficult because the baseline demographics were not identical between the studies. Additionally, unlike mortality, the exact definition of the various complications varies from one study protocol to the next. However, review of the

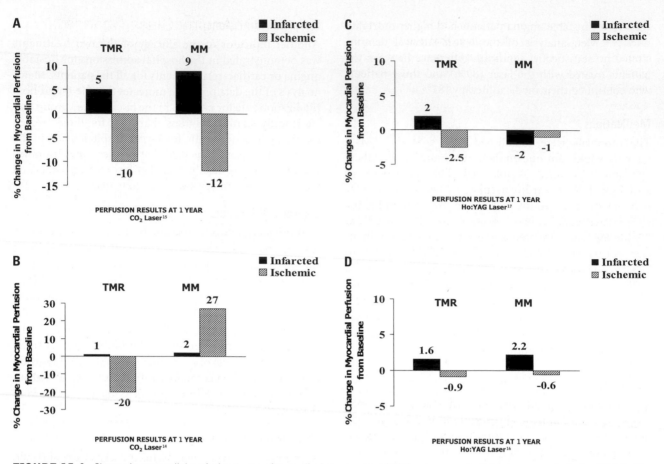

FIGURE 15-4. Change in myocardial perfusion 1 year after medical management (MM) or transmyocardial laser revascularization (TMLR). The percentage change is calculated as baseline perfusion results minus follow-up results, divided by the baseline results. Bars above the abscissa indicate an improvement in perfusion.

A, Significant improvement in perfusion of ischemic myocardium treated with CO_2 TMLR ($p < .05$) without a significant change in infarcted areas. Similar "improvement" in ischemic myocardium for MM patients is due to a concomitant change in infarcted myocardium.

B, Significant improvement in perfusion of ischemic myocardium treated with CO_2 TMLR, coupled with a significant worsening in perfusion of ischemic myocardium for MM patients ($p < .05$). No significant change in infarcted areas for either group.

C and *D*, Perfusion was not changed after Ho:YAG TMLR.

available rates of postoperative congestive heart failure, myocardial infarction, and arrhythmias demonstrated a higher rate of all of these complications for patients treated with the Ho:YAG laser.

Discussion

Almost 12 years have passed since the first patients were treated with a laser as sole therapy for their end-stage coronary artery disease. Since then, more than 8,000 patients have undergone the procedure around the world. In addition to patients who have undergone the procedure as sole therapy, an increasing number of patients are being treated with TMLR in combination with coronary artery bypass grafting.[18] A similar procedure, creating partial-thickness channels, has also been performed as PMR via peripheral arterial access.[19–26]

In evaluating the results, particularly in making comparisons, it is critical to determine whether the patients were treated with a CO_2 or Ho:YAG laser. On the surface, for all of the patients in all of the studies, there was a similar symptomatic response. This success rate in the relief of angina as a result of TMLR was accompanied by improvements in the quality of life for these patients. Interestingly, however, the perfusion results did not mirror these clinical outcomes. One would not expect an anatomic study (perfusion scan) to correlate perfectly with symptoms. For example, the size of a patient's reversible defect is not always reflected by the severity of the patient's symptoms. Be that as it may, a significant perfusion benefit was noted in CO_2-treated patients. A similar perfusion benefit was not seen in patients who underwent Ho:YAG TMLR. The argument is made that the present methods of perfusion imaging may not be sensitive enough; however, they appear sensitive enough to detect improvement in patients treated with the CO_2 laser. This may also indicate that the mechanism of action for Ho:YAG TMLR is not an increase in myocardial perfusion.

The lack of improvement in myocardial perfusion after Ho:YAG TMLR may be one reason that a recent report documented a loss of the long-term symptom relief in patients treated with a Ho:YAG laser.[27] Significant short-term angina relief was demonstrated at 1 year, as the average angina class fell from 3.5 ± 0.5 at baseline to 1.8 ± 0.8 at 1 year ($p < .01$). However, the average angina class at 3 years after Ho:YAG TMLR had significantly increased to 2.2 ± 0.7 ($p = .003$ at 1 year). Additionally, at 3 years, only 30% of the patients had a two-class angina improvement as compared to their baseline and 70% had a one-class improvement (Figure 15-5). Long-term results with a CO_2 laser were markedly different. As reported, these results demonstrated a decrease in angina class from 3.7 ± 0.4 at baseline to 1.5 ± 1.0 at 1 year ($p = .0001$). This was unchanged from the 1.5 ± 1.0 average angina classes at 1 year of follow-up ($p =$ not significant at 5 years).[28] Additionally, 68% of the patients at 5 years had two or more angina class improvement and 23% had a one-class improvement (Figure 15-6). This loss of clinical effectiveness seen with a Ho:YAG laser was also noted in a direct clinical comparison.[29,30] In a review of 460 patients treated by a single investigator who used the one device on some patients and the other device on others, the angina improvements seen with CO_2 were greater than with Ho:YAG.[30] At 12 months the majority of CO_2 patients were in class I or angina free, whereas the majority of the Ho:YAG patients were in class II.

This distinction in wavelengths of light between Ho:YAG and CO_2 may have increasing importance because PMR (which also employs a Ho:YAG laser) has failed to demonstrate a perfusion benefit and perhaps even a significant clinical benefit. PMR employs a Ho:YAG laser and a catheter-based delivery system in which the laser fiber is placed against the endocardium and fired, creating a nontransmural 3 to 4 mm depression in the

Ho:YAG Angina Class Change from Baseline to 3 Years

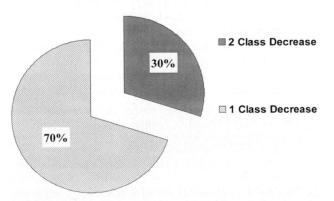

FIGURE 15-5. Distribution of Ho:YAG TMLR–treated patients by decrease in Canadian Cardiovascular Society angina class; baseline versus 3 years.

CO_2 Angina Class Change: from Baseline to 5 Years

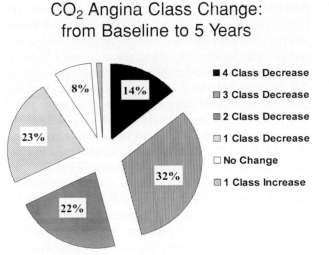

FIGURE 15-6. Distribution of CO_2 TMLR–treated patients by decrease in Canadian Cardiovascular Society angina class; baseline versus 5 years.

subendocardial layer.[19–26] In a randomized controlled trial comparing PMR and maximal medical therapy, the results at 12 months indicated a significant increase in exercise tolerance and a decrease in symptoms for PMR-treated patients.[24] However, the symptomatic improvement with PMR was not as great as had been seen with TMLR, with only 34% of the patients in angina class II or lower. As a result, the Food and Drug Administration (FDA) recently rejected PMR as a treatment for angina.

One advantage that PMR trials have over the surgical TMLR trials is the ability to perform a double-blind randomized placebo-controlled trial. The catheter may be placed against the subendocardium and the laser not fired. Recent reports of the 6-month data of such a trial have indicated that the placebo group had the same results as the PMR-treated group.[22] There was no difference in the exercise tolerance at 6 months between the groups, despite a significant increase in exercise tolerance for each group versus their baseline. Forty-two percent of the placebo group achieved a greater-than-two angina class reduction in symptoms at 6 months. As a result of the improvement in the PMR placebo group, it has been suggested that the placebo effect may be an important mechanism of surgical TMLR as well. Unfortunately, it is impossible to run a double-blind surgical trial. Patient expectations for the surgical procedure certainly may generate a placebo effect. However, the long-term benefits seen with the CO_2 laser argue against the placebo effect, and more salient and objective data have also been obtained. In addition to the symptomatic improvement, CO_2 TMLR has been demonstrated via numerous studies to improve myocardial perfusion, by nuclear single-photon emission computed tomography (SPECT) scans as well as position emission tomography (PET) scans.[9,12,14,15,31,32] A significant decrease in the number of reversible or ischemic myocardial defects without an increase in the number of fixed or infarcted areas has been demonstrated with CO_2 when compared to TMLR patients, both against their baseline and versus patients randomized to medical management.[14, 15] Further evaluation using other objective measures such as dobutamine stress echocardiography cineangiography (CINE) and contrast-enhanced magnetic resonance imaging (MRI) demonstrated improvement in myocardial function and decrease in myocardial ischemia without an increase in myocardial infarction in patients treated with CO_2 TMLR.[33,34] This evidence is not subject to the placebo effect and has been analyzed by readers blinded to the treatments that the patients received. A better understanding of the mechanisms whereby TMLR achieves its effect is needed and is the impetus for ongoing studies. Additionally, the enhancement of these results by combining laser revascularization with conventional revascularization (ie, CABG) as well as with other types of unconventional revascularization (eg, gene therapy) will undoubtedly be the focus of investigations of the future.

References

1. Beck CS. The development of a new blood supply to the heart by operation. Ann Surg 1935;102:801–13.
2. Vineberg A. Clinical and experimental studies in the treatment of coronary artery insufficiency by internal mammary artery implant. J Int Coll Surg 1954;22:503–18.
3. Sen PK, Daulatram J, Kinare SG, et al. Further studies in multiple transmyocardial acupuncture as a method of myocardial revascularization. Surgery 1968;64:861–70.
4. Goldman A, Greenstone SM, Preuss FS, et al. Experimental methods for producing a collateral circulation to the heart directly from the left ventricle. J Thorac Surg 1956;31:364–74.
5. Massimo C, Boffi L. Myocardial revascularization by a new method of carrying blood directly from the left ventricular cavity into the coronary circulation. J Thorac Surg 1957;34:257–64.
6. Mirhoseini M, Cayton M. Revascularization of the heart by laser. J Microsurg 1981;2:253–60.
7. Mirhoseini M, Shelgikar S, Cayton MM. New concepts in revascularization of the myocardium. Ann Thorac Surg 1988;45:415–20.
8. Okada M, Ikuta H, Shimizu K, et al. Alternative method of myocardial revascularization by laser: experimental and clinical study. Kobe J Med Sci 1986;32:151–61.
9. Frazier OH, Cooley DA, Kadipasaoglu KA, et al. Myocardial revascularization with laser: preliminary findings. Circulation 1995;92 Suppl II:II-58–65.
10. Horvath KA, Mannting F, Cummings N, et al. Transmyocardial laser revascularization: operative techniques and clinical results at two years. J Thorac Cardiovasc Surg 1996;111:1047–53.
11. Dowling RD, Petracek MR, Selinger SL, et al. Transmyocardial revascularization in patients with refractory, unstable angina. Circulation 1998;98 Suppl II:II-73–6.
12. Horvath KA, Cohn LH, Cooley DA, et al. Transmyocardial laser revascularization: results of a multicenter trial with transmyocardial laser revascularization used as sole therapy for end-stage coronary artery disease. J Thorac Cardiovasc Surg 1997;113:645–54.
13. Vincent JG, Bardos P, Kruse J, et al. End-stage coronary artery disease treated with the transmyocardial CO_2 laser revascularization: a chance for the "inoperable" patient. Eur J Cardiothorac Surg 1997;121:888–94.
14. Frazier OH, March RJ, Horvath KA. Transmyocardial revascularization with a carbon dioxide laser in patients with end-stage coronary artery disease. N Engl J Med 1999; 341:1021–8.
15. Schofield PM, Sharples LD, Caine N, et al. Transmyocardial laser revascularization in patients with refractory angina: a randomized controlled trial. Lancet 1999;353:519–24.
16. Allen KB, Dowling RD, Fudge TL, et al. Comparison of transmyocardial revascularization with medical therapy in patients with refractory angina. N Engl J Med 1999; 341:1029–36.
17. Burkhoff D, Schmidt S, Schulman SP, et al. Transmyocardial laser revascularization compared with continued medical therapy for treatment of refractory angina pectoris: a prospective randomized trial. Lancet 1999;354:885–90.
18. Trehan N, Mishra Y, Mehta Y, et al. Transmyocardial laser as an adjunct to minimally invasive coronary artery bypass grafting for complete myocardial revascularization. Ann Thorac Surg 1998;66:1113–8.
19. Kim CB, Kesten R, Javier M, et al. Percutaneous method of laser transmyocardial revascularization. Catheter Cardiovasc Diagn 1997;40:223–8.
20. Lauer B, Junghans U, Stahl F, et al. Catheter-based percutaneous myocardial laser revascularization in patients with end-stage coronary artery disease. J Am Coll Cardiol 1999a;34:1663–70.
21. Lauer B, Junghans U, Stahl F, et al. Catheter-based percutaneous myocardial laser revascularization in patients with end-stage coronary artery disease. J Am Coll Cardiol 1999b;33:381A.
22. Leon MB, Baim DS, Moses JW, et al. A randomized blinded clinical trial comparing percutaneous laser myocardial revascularization (using Biosense LV mapping) vs. placebo in patients with refractory coronary ischemia. Circulation 2000;102:II-565.
23. Oesterle SN, Reifart NJ, Meier B, et al. Initial results of laser-based percutaneous myocardial revascularization for angina pectoris. Am J Cardiol 1998;82:659–62.
24. Oesterle SN, Sanborn TA, Ali N, et al. Percutaneous transmyocardial laser revascularization for severe angina: the PACIFIC randomized trial. Lancet 2000;356:1705–10.
25. Shawl FA, Domanski MJ, Kaul U, et al. Procedural results and early clinical outcome of percutaneous transluminal myocardial revascularization. Am J Cardiol 1999;83: 498–501.
26. Stone GW, Rubinstein P, Schmidt D, et al. A prospective, randomized, multicenter trial of percutaneous transmyocardial laser revascularization in patients with non-recanalizable chronic total occlusions. Circulation 2000; 102:II-689.
27. De Carlo M, Milano AD, Pratali S, et al. Symptomatic improvement after transmyocardial laser revascularization: how long does it last? Ann Thorac Surg 2000;70:1130–3.

28. Horvath KA, Aranki SA, Cohn LH, et al. Sustained angina relief five years after transmyocardial revascularization with a CO_2 laser. Circulation 2001;104(12 Suppl I): I81–4.

29. Lansing AM. Transmyocardial revascularization: mechanism of action with CO_2 and Ho:YAG lasers. J Thorac Cardiovasc Surg 1998;115:1392.

30. Lansing AM. Transmyocardial revascularization: late results and mechanisms of action. J Ky Med Assoc 2000;98: 406–12.

31. Cooley DA, Frazier OH, Kadipasaoglu KA, et al. Transmyocardial laser revascularization: clinical experience with 12-month follow-up. J Thorac Cardiovasc Surg 1996;111:791–9.

32. Kadipasaoglu KA, Frazier OH. Transmyocardial laser revascularization: effective laser parameters on tissue oblation and cardiac perfusion. Semin Thorac Cardiovasc Surg 1999;11:4–11.

33. Donovan CL, Landolfo KP, Lowe JE, et al. Improvement in inducible ischemia during dobutamine stress echocardiography after transmyocardial laser revascularization in patients with refractory angina pectoris. J Am Coll Cardiol 1997;30:607–12.

34. Horvath KA, Kim RJ, Judd RM, et al. Contrast enhanced MRI assessment of microinfarction after transmyocardial laser revascularization. Circulation 2000;102:II-765.

CHAPTER 16

ANGIOGENESIS AND GENE THERAPY FOR THE TREATMENT OF CORONARY ARTERY DISEASE

ANDREW I. YEE, BS, TODD K. ROSENGART, MD, FACS

Percutaneous transluminal coronary angioplasty (PTCA) and coronary artery bypass grafting (CABG), the primary interventional therapies for the treatment of coronary atherosclerosis, remain of limited effectiveness because of the development over time of native vessel restenoses and graft occlusions. Partly as a consequence of these limitations, cardiovascular disease is still the leading cause of death in the United States. Moreover, an estimated 100,000 to 200,000 individuals with severe or widespread vascular pathology are not candidates for these interventions because of the severity or diffuse nature of their disease.[1] Based upon these considerations, angiogenic therapy, a strategy whereby ischemic tissues are induced to propagate an endogenous bypass neovasculature, may represent a promising alternative to conventional revascularization techniques.

Gene therapy describes a new technology that involves the insertion of functioning genetic material into selected cells of the body to treat inherited and acquired diseases.[2–4] Gene therapy is versatile and can be used to treat monogenic diseases (where one gene has been altered as in rare enzymatic diseases); acquired gene alteration diseases (eg, AIDS and cancer); and diseases that are spurred by the interaction of multiple genes in combination with environmental factors (eg, diabetes and coronary artery disease). This technique can be used, for instance, to replace or augment specific genes, to induce cell suicide or eliminate toxic genes, or to reinforce the immune system. Gene therapy may prove to be a particularly effective tool in the treatment of cardiovascular disease in that it can provide for the insertion of genes and sustained expression of the corresponding protein product in relatively inaccessible tissues, such as the heart.[5,6] Significantly, the duration of gene expression can be tailored to meet specific therapeutic requirements based on the type of delivery vehicle, or vector, used for gene transfer.

Therapeutic Angiogenesis

While vasculogenesis refers to growth of angioblast-mediated embryologic blood vessels or the in situ development of adult vasculature, angiogenesis is specifically defined as the sprouting of capillaries and small nonmuscular vessels from preexisting vessels.[7–10] Although elucidation of the mechanisms that induce and propagate angiogenesis is still incomplete, angiogenesis is believed to act through a cascade of events, beginning with the secretion of proteases that decompose the basement membrane and extracellular matrix of the endothelium lining the parent blood vessel (Figure 16-1). Subsequent endothelial cell proliferation, migration, and reattachment result in a conical complex that extends from the tip. This tip "seeks out" and merges with other blood vessels, thus generating a new source of blood flow.

Central to the angiogenic process is the capillary endothelial cell, which seems unique in its ability to express critical molecules essential for the construction of new microvascular networks. To establish such revascularization, the endothelial cells apparently collaborate with a number of other cells, such as monocytes, mast cells, lymphocytes, and pericytes. These cells are thought to contribute to angiogenesis by expressing growth factor proteins and cytokines that, in turn, induce the proliferation and migration of endothelial cells and other critical elements of the vascular wall. These critical mediators include intra- and extracellular integrins and adhesion molecules involved in cell–cell interaction, proteases that modify the composition and activities of the extracellular matrix which permits endothelial cell migration and the release of growth factors, and intracellular signaling moieties such as mitogen-activated protein kinase, which are integral for cell replication.

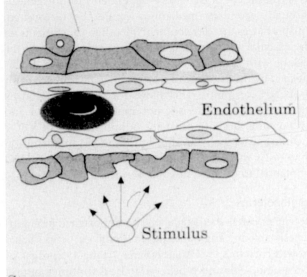

Smooth muscle cells

Basement membrane

Endothelium

Stimulus

Steps:
1. Degradation of matrix
2. Endothelial cell migration and invasion
3. Cell proliferation
4. Realignment and basement membrane formation

FIGURE 16-1. Schematic of cellular mechanisms involved in angiogenesis.

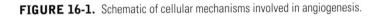

In addition to providing recovery from ischemia, angiogenesis occurs as a component of numerous biologic events, such as wound healing, reproductive growth, and the growth of neoplasms. In the setting of chronic myocardial ischemia, angiogenesis is thought to represent one of the primary mechanisms responsible for increased collateral blood flow.[5–11] The angiogenic process is, however, characteristically insufficient in completely restoring blood flow to ischemic tissue and ameliorating anginal symptoms. It has been hypothesized that inadequate local production of cytokines and other angiogenic factors or reduced sensitivity of atherosclerotic endothelium to growth factors is responsible for this inability of naturally occurring processes to adequately provide tissue reperfusion.[10,11] Thus, an alternative strategy, such as the delivery of additional quantities of exogenous angiogenic agents (therapeutic angiogenesis), may be useful in facilitating vascularization of the ischemic myocardium, as well as other tissues. It is interesting to note that although the process of angiogenesis is complex and intensely regulated, the upregulation of growth factor concentration alone appears to be sufficient to activate the angiogenic cascade. While more potent strategies may yet be determined, the initial success of therapeutic angiogenesis is predicated entirely on the potency of these growth factors, or angiogens, to stimulate angiogenic mechanisms.

Angiogenic Factors

Fibroblast Growth Factors

Among the number of growth factors that stimulate angiogenesis, the two prototypic members of the fibroblast growth factor (FGF) family, acidic and basic fibroblast growth factor (aFGF and bFGF; FGF-1 and -2), were among the first to be discovered.[12–14] FGF-1 and FGF-2 are heparin-binding proteins consisting structurally of 140 and 146 amino acids, respectively.[12–14] These two structurally and physiologically related family members have a 53% absolute sequence homology. Because of the widespread expression of FGF receptors, FGF-1 and FGF-2 are mitogenic for many types of cells, such as endothelial cells, smooth-muscle cells, fibroblasts, myocytes, and some tumor cells. With regard to angiogenesis, FGF-1 and FGF-2 are known to regulate many vital intra- and extracellular events. For instance, these growth factors are responsible for the upregulation of proteases like collagenase and plasminogen, which are critical in modulating the extracellular matrix; the activation of kinases important in replicative intracellular signaling pathways; and the regulation of platelet–endothelial cell adhesion molecules and other molecules involved in capillary tubule formation.

FGF-1 and FGF-2 administration augment the revascularization process in vivo in a number of models.

Nonischemic models in which this has been demonstrated include chick chorioallantoic membrane, rabbit cornea, vascular adventitia, and rat renal capsule; in addition, it has been demonstrated in peripheral, myocardial, and cerebral ischemic models.[14,15] Despite the demonstration of potent angiogenic properties by the FGFs, there exist concerns that administration of these growth factors may result in unwanted toxicities, including nephrotoxicity and hypotension.[14–16] Furthermore, because of the relatively indiscriminate mitogenic potential of these angiogens, unwanted growth of smooth-muscle cells (intimal hyperplasia) or fibroblasts (fibrosis) is an additional theoretical concern.

Vascular Endothelial Growth Factor

The vascular endothelial growth factor (VEGF) family of polypeptides has also been extensively studied.[17–20] VEGF (VEGF-A), also known as vascular permeability factor and vasculotropin, is a heparin-binding disulfide-linked dimeric glycoprotein weighing 34 to 46 kilodaltons that naturally exists in humans as isoforms of 121, 165, 189, and 206 amino acids. Each of these isoforms is a potent stimulator of angiogenesis and is able to upregulate the expression of proteases and other factors critical for the formation of vasculature. The VEGF isoforms bind heparin or cell surface heparin sulfate proteoglycan proportionately to their size, to such a degree that larger isoforms stay bound to targets in the extracellular matrix, while the smallest VEGF 121 isoform has no heparin-binding capacity. Aside from VEGF-A, various other structurally related angiogenic polypeptides have also been identified. These molecules, including VEGF-B, -C, -D, and -E, have overlapping biologic properties, including stimulation of lymphangiogenesis.

VEGF is believed to function early in the stages of vessel formation, during development of the vascular plexus. Upregulation of VEGF appears to be induced by a number of stimuli, including hypoxia. In this regard, expression of VEGF and its receptors is enhanced in ischemic tissues.[21] VEGF is also profoundly involved in native processes such as embryonic development, growth and differentiation, wound healing, reproduction, the pathogenesis of neoplasia, rheumatoid arthritis, and proliferative retinopathy.

Two unique features differentiate VEGF from other heparin-binding, angiogenic growth factors such as the FGF family. First, the growth factor interacts with cells through high-affinity tyrosine kinase receptors, flk-1/KDR and flt-1, which are confined almost exclusively to endothelial cells. As a consequence of this localization of its receptors to the crucial cellular constituent in angiogenesis, VEGF is thought to maintain selective mitogenic effects for the vasculature. Thus, there may be a low risk for undesirable induction of mitogenic activity in tissues or cells other than the vascular endothelium. However,

the theoretical possibility of fibrosis, smooth-muscle cell hyperplasia, or vasculature-dependent tumorigenesis through secondary mediations cannot be discounted. Furthermore, the development of other constituents of the vascular wall, such as smooth-muscle cells, may be lacking with isolated VEGF therapy. VEGF is also distinguished by the presence of a typical signal sequence prior to its NH_2 terminus. This allows for VEGF secretion by intact cells, a characteristic not applicable to FGF-1 and -2. Potential limitations of the administration of VEGF include a short half-life after intravenous administration (like FGF), the induction of hypotension (like FGF), and a potential to increase vascular permeability.

Angiopoietins

Recent research sheds light on the importance in angiogenesis of the angiopoietins, a family of endothelial growth cofactors.[22–24] Angiopoietin-1 (ang-1) consists of 498 amino acids and is believed to be a multimer, bound together by coiled–coil structures and disulfide crosslinks. Ang-1 is a 70-kD secreted glycoprotein that binds the endothelial cell-specific tyrosine kinase receptor tie-2. The role of ang-1 in vascular development is thought to be late in vessel generation, helping to mature and stabilize the vasculature. Ang-1 also appears able to counter the permeability effects of VEGF. Thus, the dual expression of VEGF and ang-1 may have additive angiogenic effect in producing leakage-resistant vasculature. However, ang-1 and the related tie-2 ligand angiopoietin-2 (ang-2) alone appear unable to induce neovascularization.

Ang-2, composed of 496 amino acids, acts as an antagonist for ang-1 by competing with ang-1 in binding to the tie-2 receptor on endothelial cells. With tie-2 inhibited, the vasculature is thought to become destabilized and more receptive to angiogenic factors, such as VEGF. Ang-2 activity appears to be greatest at the leading edge of vessel development, and its function in angiogenesis seems to be that of initiating neovascularization, possibly by destabilizing the vascular wall and allowing cell replication and migration.

Other Angiogenic Factors

Among many additional agents, other angiogens include angiogenin, hepatocyte growth factor, interleukin-8, platelet-derived growth factor, proliferin, transforming growth factors α and β, and tumor necrosis factor-α.[8–12] Studies indicate that nitric oxide and heparin also serve as angiogenic cofactors. Additionally, sheer stress, hypoxia, and ischemia are known to be associated inducers of the angiogenic process. Conversely, numerous inhibitors of angiogenesis, such as angiostatin, are also known to exist. Thus, the completion of the angiogenesis process is highlighted by the multiplicity of angiogenic growth factors and cofactors, and the interplay of numerous other cofactors and processes (Figure 16-2).

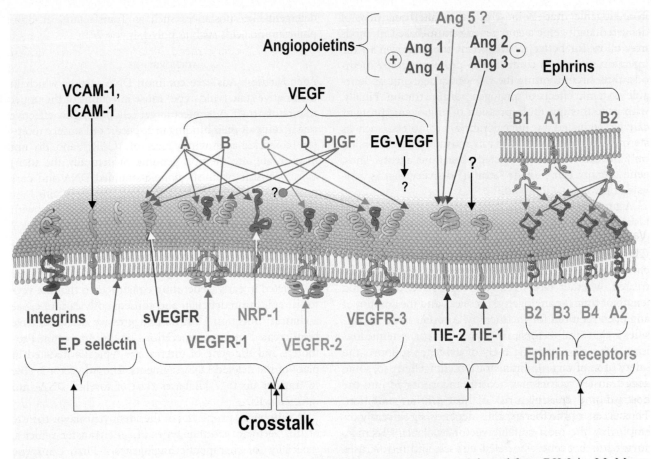

Adapted from RK Jain, LL Munn
Nature Medicine 6:131-132, 2000

FIGURE 16-2. Schematic of biochemical mechanisms involved in angiogenesis. ANG = angiopoietin; EG-VEGF = endocrine gland derived vascular endothelial growth factor; ICAM = intracellular adhesion molecule; NRP-1 = neuropilin; PIGF = placenta growth factor; sVEGFR = soluble vascular endothelial growth factor receptor; VCAM = vascular cell adhesion molecule; VEGF = vascular endothelial growth factor; VEGFR = vascular endothelial growth factor receptor.

Angiogenic Therapies and Delivery Strategies

Protein Therapy

Protein-based angiogenic therapy involves the administration of one of the number of growth factors known to include angiogenesis.[6,7,25,26] The potential advantage of this approach is its simplicity; unlike gene therapy, no gene needs to be inserted into the nucleus. Although it is not a proven prerequisite to stimulating angiogenesis, sustained growth factor expression may, however, be needed for optimal angiogenic effect, and this may be problematic with systemic protein delivery. To address this concern, a slow release of recombinant protein can be achieved by incorporating growth factor in bioabsorbable polymers or similar materials.[25] One disadvantage of protein therapy as compared to gene therapy, however, is that protein therapy may require the injection of relatively large amounts of angiogenic substance, which may leak and induce angiogenesis in tissues besides those targeted.

Gene Therapy

Gene therapy strategies involve the insertion of genetic material into selected cells of the body by means of transfer vectors, such as recombinantly modified viruses, which are made incapable of replication by deletion of critical viral genes responsible for the replicative process.[2,6,7] Gene delivery is customarily accomplished via a single administration of a modified vector containing the complementary deoxyribonucleic acid (cDNA) coding sequence of the growth factor to be transferred, in addition to controlling sequences such as a promoter to regulate gene expression, and stop signals to end translation and stabilize the messenger ribonucleic acid (mRNA).

There are a number of reasons to consider gene therapy–based strategies over protein therapy–based strategies. First, the amount of expressed angiogen produced in gene therapy–based methods may be much closer to physiologic concentrations than that delivered by protein therapy techniques. This difference in angiogen expression may not, of course, correspond to a significant difference in angiogenic yield. Because of the smaller quantities of delivered angiogenic agent, gene therapy–based methods may allow for better restriction of the angiogen to the injection sites when compared to protein therapy methods, thus circumventing the risk of leakage and undesirable systemic effects of angiogen administration. Finally, with gene therapy, the expression of angiogenic proteins can be regulated by incorporating promoters, such as steroids, into the vector that can activate gene expression only in the presence of selected exogenous agents. Thus, gene therapy can provide "stealth" delivery that is activated only upon command.[27]

A primary challenge in gene therapy treatment is the task of determining an optimal vector for transferring the gene. For example, the immunogenicity of the chosen vector must be evaluated. Factors to consider when choosing the vector include the organ system to be treated, whether target cells are replicative, the desired length of time for angiogen expression, and the amount of angiogen required for the therapy. Another issue to consider is that viral vectors may trigger local or systemic toxicity, although a growing body of evidence supports the safety of viral vector administration clinically. Also, some gene transfer vectors may become incorporated into the host genome, creating a risk of host genome mutation. The success of the therapy thus depends significantly on employing the most suitable vector available. Plasmids, adenoviruses, adeno-associated viruses, and retroviruses are among the vectors that have most commonly been utilized in cardiac gene therapy.

PLASMIDS

Plasmids are simple circular structures of DNA into which an expression cassette is covalently linked.[2,11] The cassette contains a promoter that activates transcription of the desired portion of the cDNA in the plasmid transgene. One advantage of plasmid vectors is that the size of the transgene is unrestricted, because the cDNA is able to enter cells without having been encapsulated in a separate vehicle for this purpose. Plasmid-mediated gene transfer occurs by simple *trans*-membrane transport. Upon entering the target organ, the plasmid cDNA is assimilated by endosomes, transported to lysosomes, and degraded. This processing accounts for the relative inefficiency of plasmids as transfection agents. Only 0.1 to 1% of the plasmid reaches the nucleus. To compensate for the low yield, large quantities of the vector must be administered. On the other hand, plasmids have the advantage of providing sustained levels of expression, which is likely because of their lack of immunogenicity, and appear to provide a degree of transfer expression sufficient to have a therapeutic effect. Furthermore, plasmid uptake can be enhanced through a number of methods, including simple contact, pressurized plasmid delivery, pellet-associated cell membrane penetration, strategies such as "gene guns," and incorporation into lipophilic or hydrophobic compounds such as liposomes, detergent-like substances such as Transfectam, or lipophilic amino acids such as poly-L-lysine.[28,29]

ADENOVIRUSES

Adenoviruses (Ads) are common DNA viruses which in their native state (wild-type) cause infections of the upper respiratory tract. Ads infect target cells at a highly effective rate because of their binding to a specific cell surface receptor (coxsackie-adenovirus receptor [CAR]) and do not incorporate into the host genome. Structurally, the adenovirus consists of linear, double-stranded DNA and core proteins surrounded by encapsulating capsid proteins.[30,31]

The 49 Ad serotypes are divided into 6 subgroups, with subgroup C being the most extensively studied. Types 2 and 5 in subgroup C are the backbone of the adenovirus vectors currently used for gene transfer. The E1a and E1b regulatory genes of Ad constructs used for gene transfer are deleted in early-generation constructs so that the vector is replication deficient and consequently cannot cause a clinical "infection," but more aggressive deletions have been created in later generations of the Ad vector. Promoters and the gene of interest are typically inserted in place of the deleted DNA segments. The Ad vector is able to transfer up to 7 kilobases (kb) of foreign DNA into infected cells.

A number of properties of the adenovirus favor the use of this vector over other types of gene transfer vehicles, especially for therapeutic angiogenesis. First, transgene expression is restricted to an interval of about 1 week, possibly because of host immune reactions to the virus. This important property may make the adenovirus vector well-suited for angiogenic gene therapy, because it would have the theoretical advantage of sufficiently stimulating blood vessel proliferation, while avoiding undesirably prolonged expressive angiogenic stimulation. Second, adenoviruses are likely nononcogenic because of their lack of chromosomal incorporation. Finally, recombinant adenovirus can be efficiently manufactured in mass quantities, as well as highly concentrated, without altering the cell infection capabilities of the Ad vector.

ADENO-ASSOCIATED VIRUSES

The adeno-associated virus (AAV) consists of single-stranded DNA and is a member of the family Parvoviridae and the wild-type genus *Dependovirus*.[32] Of the vectors used for gene therapy, AAV is the smallest in size. Wild-type virus integrates at chromosome 19, while replication-deficient vectors appear to exhibit random integration. The AAV vector can transduce dividing and nondividing cells. Moreover, AAV vectors seem not to cause host cellular immune responses or inflammatory reactions. Due to chromosomal interaction, the vector remains active for essentially the lifetime of the cell, and so it is able to mediate long-term in vivo gene expression. The main obstacle to widespread applicability of these vectors is their limited gene insertion capacity, at approximately 4.5 kb.

Unlike trials with plasmids and adenoviruses, AAV clinical trials only recently began and are focused on treating chronic diseases such as hemophilia, ophthalmic diseases such as diabetic retinopathy and macular degeneration, and central nervous system defects such as Parkinson's disease. For cardiovascular disease, AAV may be well suited for conditions requiring prolonged transgene expression, such as inotropic gene therapy in the setting of congestive heart failure.

RETROVIRUSES

Retroviruses are RNA viruses that carry a reverse transcriptase that converts viral RNA to pro-viral DNA.[33] Of the vectors employed for gene therapy clinical studies, retroviruses are the most widely used. Their popularity as a delivery method stems from their efficiency as infection agents, the simplicity of their design, and their versatility. They can facilitate gene transfer to an array of cell types and, like the AAV vector, stably integrate their genomes into host cell chromosomes, which confers long-term gene expression. As with AAV, there is an additional risk of mutagenesis associated with chromosomal integration. Retroviruses are rendered replication incompetent by excising relevant DNA segments, and the resulting vectors are able to accommodate about 8 kb of exogenous DNA. Because retroviruses require that host cells be actively replicating in order for chromosomal incorporation to occur, these vectors are not likely contributors for therapies requiring infection of nonreplicative myocytes. In response to these problems, lentiviral vectors that infect nondividing cells have recently been manufactured.

EX VIVO GENE THERAPY

Ex vivo gene therapy typically involves procurement of a cell or tissue sample from a living organism, transfecting these cells with a transgene in cell culture, and administering the cells back to the organism.[34] Although the ex vivo strategy provides an effective means of gene delivery, its applicability to treating coronary artery disease may be limited by its inherent cumbersomeness, costliness, and potential for exposing the organism and the heart to infection. One possible manner of using ex vivo strategies to treat coronary artery disease, however, may be in cardiac transplantation or vein graft therapies. In these cases, the targeted tissue is exposed to the vector before graft implantation. This process would allow for transfection of the heart or graft while avoiding the risks involved in systemic gene administration.

IN VIVO GENE THERAPY

In vivo therapy involves administration of vector into the host organism. A number of alternative in vivo delivery strategies are available. Simply classified, strategies for myocardial therapies include systemic (intravenous or intracoronary) and intramyocardial (endocardial or epicardial) approaches. Intracoronary and epicardial deliver-

ies are provided by conventional catheter and surgical (sternotomy or thoracotomy) techniques. A new series of endoventricular catheters allow endocardial delivery, generally by fluoroscopic or other means, such as electromechanical mapping.[35]

In general, local myocardial concentrations and systemic levels of expressed transgenes are inversely correlated, with intramyocardial delivery resulting in the greatest localization of transgene expression. This difference between myocardial expression levels following intracoronary versus intramyocardial delivery may be as great as one to two-log fold.[36] It has yet to be proven, however, whether these differences in myocardial angiogen concentrations translate into differences in therapeutic efficacy.

PRECLINICAL TRIALS

Investigations in a number of animal models have suggested the potential efficacy of gene therapy as a treatment of a number of cardiovascular diseases, including ischemic disorders and cardiomyopathies. This discussion focuses on the former application.

Ischemia in animal models is typically created in the canine or porcine model by placing an ameroid constrictor on the left circumflex or other coronary artery.[4–7] The ameroid, a steel ring encased by hydrophilic plastic with a lumen diameter matching that of the artery of interest, occludes the vessel gradually over approximately 20 days. In smaller animals, peripheral vessels, such as the femoral artery, are excised or ligated to create hind-limb ischemia. After induction of ischemia, a growth factor or other angiogen is injected into selected areas of the organism, such as the heart or skeletal muscle.

In general, evidence of angiogenesis and enhanced perfusion in these models have been equivalently demonstrated after delivery of a wide variety of angiogens via both protein and gene delivery techniques, and via both local and systemic administration. Enhancement of perfusion in these studies has been demonstrated by such studies as histology, angiography, microsphere perfusion, laser Doppler studies, hemodynamic studies, and other functional assays. In general, toxicity is seen in doses that approximate 100 times the therapeutic threshold.[37] As noted earlier, the most apparent toxicities include hypotension, hemangioma formation, edema formation (VEGF), and nephrotoxicity (FGF). Accelerated atherosclerosis has also been induced in specific models. Promising results from these animal studies have resulted in the initiation of a number of clinical studies.

CLINICAL TRIALS

To date, approximately 10 trials involving angiogenic therapy for the treatment of coronary artery disease have been reported (Table 16-1). Nearly the entire spectrum of putative therapeutic regimens has been investigated. More specifically, these trials included both protein- and gene-based strategies, intracoronary and intramyocardial (epicardial and endocardial) delivery, and use of VEGF and several of the FGF growth factors.[38–45] Additional trials underway include the use of other transgenes such as the transcription factor HIF (hypoxia inducible factor).

Most of the early trials reported thus far were non-randomized, unblinded phase I trials, and some were performed as an "adjunct to CABG," complicating definitive interpretation of safety and efficacy data from these studies. Several of these trials, however, were performed as randomized, blinded, placebo-controlled trials. Furthermore, even the nonrandomized trials yielded evidence suggesting efficacy when compared to placebo controls.

Based on this initial body of evidence, several trends appear to be emerging. First, appropriate dosing regimens of angiogenic agents, whether protein or gene based, do not appear to present evidence of significant toxicity, except for the cases of high-dose intravascular delivery of growth factor.[43] More specifically, although FGF-2–mediated nephrotoxicity and hematologic changes have been noted with intravascular delivery, as has hypotension with intravascular administration of both VEGF and FGF-2, neither hemangioma formation nor tumor progression has been observed in several hundred reported patients who received angiogenic therapy, with the exception of one clinical case of hemangioma formation.[46]

Evidence of efficacy is emerging from a number of clinical end points, including symptomatic improvement (at least two angina classes) and objective assessments of increased perfusion, as determined by such tests as improvement in exercise tolerance times (Figure 16-3), perfusion scanning, and echo. Importantly, there appears, in our opinion, to be a growing dichotomy between intra-coronary and intramyocardial delivery, with superior efficacy and fewer adverse side-effect results noted with the latter approach. As noted earlier, this finding seems consistent with the observation that significantly greater

TABLE 16-1. Summary of Clinical Cardiac Angiogenesis Trials

Angiogen	Trial	Agent	Delivery Route
FGF-1	Schumaker	Protein	Myocardial
FGF-2	Unger	Protein	Coronary
FGF-2	Simmons	Protein	Myocardial/CABG
FGF-2	Simmons	Protein	Coronary / IV
AdFGF-4	AGENT	Adeno	Coronary
rVEGF$_{165}$	VIVA	Protein	Coronary
pVEGF$_{165}$	Isner	Plasmid	Myocardial
pVEGF-2	Isner	Plasmid	Myocardial
AdVEGF$_{121}$	Rosengart	Adeno	Myocardial/CABG
AdVEGF$_{121}$	Rosengart	Adeno	Myocardial

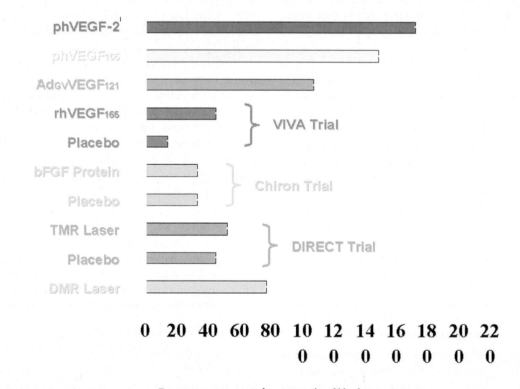

FIGURE 16-3. Composite of improvement in exercise treadmill times in angiogenesis and transmyocardial revascularization trials. (Personal communication, J. Isner.)

myocardial concentrations of angiogenic factors are obtained with direct local versus systemic delivery of angiogens.

Conclusion

Based on initial clinical data, it does appear likely that improvements in myocardial perfusion will be inducible via angiogenic therapies. It is not clear, however, whether clinical results in a diseased vasculature will prove it to be as robust as that seen in normal animal models, at least using current strategies. Furthermore, improvements in perfusion do not yet appear to be as great as those produced by interventions on the large epicardial vessels (as via CABG or PTCA). It is as yet also unclear whether angiogenic strategies mediated by the delivery of exogenous angiogens are superior to those generated by other putative angiogenic therapies, such as transmyocardial revascularization or enhanced external counterpulsation, although this may prove to be the case. Theoretically, these other "angiogenic" treatments may ultimately prove to represent indirect (and thus less efficient) means of increasing myocardial growth factor concentrations as a means of inducing angiogenesis.

The most effective method of administration for the angiogenic gene therapy has, of course, also not yet been determined, and optimal vectors, growth factors, and dosages have yet to be found. Furthermore, it is possible that the exogenous molecular strategies described in this chapter will need to be supplemented by delivery of exogenous or endogenously recruited cellular substrates, such as endothelial progenitor cells or stem cells. Furthermore, administering a combination of growth factors may also be the most efficacious manner to induce the desired amount of angiogenesis. It will be up to current and future clinical trials to more clearly define the bioactivity of growth factors, determine optimal delivery routes and methods, set safety parameters, and establish practical and proper applications for angiogenic gene therapy.

References

1. Mukherjee D, Bhatt DL, Roe MT, et al. Direct myocardial revascularization and angiogenesis—how many patients might be eligible. Am J Cardiol 1999;84:598–600.
2. Crystal RG. Transfer of genes to humans: early lessons and obstacles to success. Science 1995;270:404–10.
3. Rosengart TK, Hilledebrand K. Gene therapy for coronary artery disease. In: Karp R, Griffith B, Lakes H, editors. Advances in cardiac surgery. Vol.13. St. Louis: Mosby; 2001. p. 107–11.
4. Ehsan A, Mann MJ, Dzau VJ. Gene therapy for cardiovascular disease and vascular grafts. In: Templeton NS, Lasic DD, editors. Gene therapy: therapeutic mechanisms and strategies. New York: Marcel Dekker; 2000. p. 421–38.
5. Safi J Jr, Gloe TR, Riccioni T, et al. Gene therapy with angiogenic factors: a new potential approach to the treatment of ischemic disease. J Mol Cell Cardiol 1997; 29:2311–25.
6. Hamaway AH, Lee LY, Crystal RG, Rosengart TK. Cardiac angiogenesis and gene therapy: a strategy for myocardial revascularization. Curr Opin Cardiol 1999;14:515–22.
7. Rosengart TK, Patel SR, Crystal RG. Therapeutic angiogenesis: protein and gene therapy delivery strategies. J Cardiovasc Risk 1999;6:29–40.
8. Isner JM. Angiogenesis for revascularization of ischaemic tissues. Eur Heart J 1997;18:1–2.
9. Selke FW, Simon M. Angiogenesis in cardiovascular disease: current status and therapeutic potential. Drugs 1999; 58(3):391–6.
10. Schaper W, Ito WD. Molecular mechanisms of coronary collateral vessel growth. Circ Res 1996;79:911–9.
11. Losordo DW, Vale PR, Isner JM. Gene therapy for myocardial angiogenesis. Am Heart J 1999;138:S132–41.
12. Folkman J, Klagsbrun M. Angiogenic factors. Science 1987; 235:442–7.
13. Carmeliet P. Fibroblast growth factor-1 stimulates branching and survival of myocardial arteries: a goal for therapeutic angiogenesis? Circ Res 2000;87:176–8.
14. Lazarous DF, Shuo M, Scheinowitz M, et al. Comparative effects of basic fibroblast growth factor and vascular endothelial growth factor on coronary collateral development and the arterial response to injury. Circulation 1996;94:1074–82.
15. Lopez JJ, Edelman ER, Stamler A, et al. Basic fibroblast growth factor in a porcine model of chronic myocardial ischemia: a comparison of angiographic and coronary flow parameters. J Pharmacol Exp Ther 1997;282:385–90.
16. Unger EF, Banai S, Shou M, et al. Basic fibroblast growth factor enhances myocardial collateral flow in a canine model. Am J Physiol 1994;266:H1588–95.
17. Ferrara N, Alitalo K. Clinical applications of angiogenic growth factors and their inhibitors. Nat Med 1999;5: 1359–64.
18. Keck PJ, Hauser SD, Krivi G, et al. Vascular permeability factor, an endothelial cell mitogen related to PDGF. Science 1989;246:1309–12.
19. Dvorak HF, Brown LF, Detmar M, Dvorak AM. Vascular permeability factor / vascular endothelial growth factor, microvascular hyperpermeability, and angiogenesis. Am J Pathol 1995;146:1029–39.
20. Leung DW, Cachianes G, Kuang WU, et al. Vascular endothelial growth factor is a secreted angiogenic mitogen. Science 1989;246:1306–9.
21. Shweiki D, Itin A, Soffer D, Keshet E. Vascular endothelial growth factor induced by hypoxia may mediate hypoxia-initiated angiogenesis. Nature 1992;359:843–5.
22. Thurston G, Suri C, Smith K, et al. Leakage-resistant blood vessels in mice transgenically overexpressing angiopoietin-1. Science 1999;286:2511–4.
23. Peters KG. Vascular endothelial growth factor and the angiopoietins: working together to build a better blood vessel. Circ Res 1998;83:342–3.
24. Davis S, Yancopoulos GD. The angiopoietins: yin and yang in angiogenesis. Curr Top Microbiol Immunol 1999; 237:173–85.
25. Bailey SR. Local drug delivery: current applications. Prog Cardiovasc Dis 1997;40(2):183–204.

26. Sinnaeve P, Varenne O, Collen D, Janssens S. Gene therapy in the cardiovascular system: an update. Cardiovasc Res 1999;44:498–506.

27. Lee LY, Zhou X, Polce DR, et al. Exogenous control of cardiac gene therapy: evidence of regulated myocardial transgene expression after adenovirus transfer of expression cassettes containing corticosteroid response element promoters. J Thorac Cardiovasc Surg 1999;118: 26–35.

28. Stewart MJ, Plautz GE, Del Buono L, et al. Gene transfer in vivo with DNA-liposome complexes, safety and acute toxicity in mice. Hum Gene Ther 1992;3:267–75.

29. Pinnaduwage P, Schmitt L, Huang L. Use of a quaternary ammonium detergent in liposome mediated DNA transfection of mouse L cells. Biochem Biophys Acta 1989;985:33–7.

30. Guzman RJ, Lemarchand P, Crystal RG, et al. Efficient gene transfer into myocardium by direct injection of adenovirus vectors. Circ Res 1993;73:1202–7.

31. Hackett NR, Crystal RG. Adenovirus vectors for gene therapy. In: Templeton NS, Lasic DD, editors. Gene therapy: therapeutic mechanisms and strategies. New York: Marcel Dekker; 2000. p. 17–40.

32. Carter BJ. Adeno-associated virus and adeno-associated virus vectors for gene delivery. In: Templeton NS, Lasic DD, editors. Gene therapy: therapeutic mechanisms and strategies. New York: Marcel Dekker; 2000. p. 41–55.

33. Cannon PM, Anderson WF. Retroviral vectors for gene therapy. In: Templeton NS, Lasic DD, editors. Gene therapy: therapeutic mechanisms and strategies. New York: Marcel Dekker; 2000. p. 1–16.

34. Ozawa CR, Springer ML, Blau HM. Ex vivo gene therapy using myoblasts and regulatable retroviral vectors. In: Templeton NS, Lasic DD, editors. Gene therapy: therapeutic mechanisms and strategies. New York: Marcel Dekker; 2000. p. 61–76.

35. Vale PR, Losordo OW, Milliken CF, et al. Randomized, single-blind, placebo-controlled pilot study of catheter-based myocardial gene transfer for therapeutic angiogenesis using left ventricular mapping in patients with chronic myocardial ischemia. Circulation 2001;103: 2138–43.

36. Lee LY, Patel SR, Hackett NR, et al. Focal angiogen therapy using intramyocardial delivery of an adenovirus vector coding for vascular endothelial growth factor 121. Ann Thorac Surg 2000;69:14–24.

37. Patel SR, Lee LY, Mack CA, et al. Safety of direct myocardial administration of an adenovirus vector encoding vascular endothelial growth factor 121. Hum Gene Ther 1999; 10(8):1331–48.

38. Hendel RC, Henry TD, Rocha-Singh K, et al. Effect of intracoronary recombinant human vascular endothelial growth factor on myocardial perfusion: evidence for a dose-dependent effect. Circulation 2000;101:118–21.

39. Rosengart TK, Lee LY, Patel SR, et al. Six-month assessment of a phase 1 trial of angiogenic gene therapy for the treatment of coronary artery disease using direct intramyocardial administration of an adenovirus vector expressing the $VEGF_{121}$ cDNA. Ann Surg 1999;239:466–72.

40. Rosengart TK, Lee LY, Patel SR, et al. Angiogenesis gene therapy: phase I assessment of direct intramyocardial administration of an adenovirus vector expressing $VEGF_{121}$ cDNA to individuals with clinically significant severe coronary artery disease. Circulation 1999;100: 468–74.

41. Symes JF, Losordo DW, Vale PR, et al. Gene therapy with vascular endothelial growth factor for inoperable coronary artery disease. Ann Thorac Surg 1999;68:830–7.

42. Vale P, Losordo D, Dunnington C, et al. Direct myocardial injection of $phVEGF_{165}$ results of complete patient cohort in phase 1/2 clinical trial. Circulation 1999;100:1–4.

43. Schumacher B, Pecher P, von Specht BU, Stegmann T. Induction of neoangiogenesis in ischemic myocardium by human growth factors: first clinical results of a new treatment of coronary heart disease. Circulation 1998; 97:645–50.

44. Grines CL, Watkins MW, Helmer G, et al. Angiogenic gene therapy (AGENT) trial in patients with stable angina pectoris. Circulation 2002;105:1290–7.

45. Laham RJ, Sellke FW, Edelman ER, et al. Local perivascular delivery of basic fibroblast growth factor in patients undergoing coronary bypass: results of a phase 1 randomized, double-blind, placebo-controlled trial. Circulation 1999;100:1865–7.

46. Isner JM, Pieczek A, Schainfeld R, et al. Clinical evidence of angiogenesis after arterial gene transfer of $phVEGF_{165}$ in patient with ischemic limb. Lancet 1996;348:370–4.

Chapter 17

Minimally Invasive Cardiac Valve Surgery

Ram Sharony, MD, Eugene A. Grossi, MD, Greg H. Ribakove, MD,
Patricia Ursomanno, MA, F. Gregory Baumann, PhD,
Stephen B. Colvin, MD, Aubrey C. Galloway, MD

Lillehei and colleagues reported the first case of mitral valve repair in 1957, using femoral artery cannulation for cardiopulmonary bypass (CPB) and approaching the mitral valve through a right thoracotomy.[1] For the next 35 years, median sternotomy was the standard approach for valve repair or replacement. Single coronary artery bypass through a limited anterior thoracotomy incision was initially reported in 1980 by Benetti, but did not become increasingly used until the 1990s.[2] In the mid-1990s, however, cardiac surgeons began to explore several new methods of less-invasive surgery in an attempt to reduce the overall surgical trauma. With the development of less-invasive techniques for coronary bypass and the evolution of newer methods and visualization devices for laparoscopic surgery, a number of cardiac surgeons became interested in expanding the scope of less-invasive cardiac surgery to include multivessel revascularization and valve repair or replacement.

Beginning in 1994, experimental work performed in the laboratories at Stanford University and New York University (NYU) led to the introduction of a minimally invasive technique, termed port access, that utilized peripheral perfusion and a balloon catheter for aortic occlusion.[3-6] The first clinical cases using the port-access approach were performed in Europe in 1995 and in the United States in 1996.[7-9] At approximately the same time, Cosgrove, Gundry, Cohn, and others introduced several alternative minimally invasive approaches for valvular surgery, using either a minithoracotomy or a partial sternotomy incision with central cannulation.[10-14] Although the results with all these minimally invasive approaches have been quite good in selected centers, and less-invasive approaches for valvular surgery have been increasingly used throughout the world, many surgeons remain skeptical of minimally invasive cardiac surgery approaches and require more data before widely adopting them. Wherever these approaches are adopted, they must meet safety and efficacy standards equivalent to those of conventional surgery. Similarly, perioperative complications and late results must be evaluated in a scientific, comparative, nonbiased fashion.

This chapter highlights some of the existing data on the results of minimally invasive valve surgery and identifies gaps in the data as a basis for future needed studies. It will also pique the interest of practicing surgeons in these evolving technologies so that they may be evaluated and adopted appropriately.

Preoperative Evaluation of Minimally Invasive Surgical Candidates

The standard preoperative work-up used for conventional valve surgery also should be performed for minimally invasive valve surgery. A comprehensive medical history and physical examination are essential, particularly a vascular examination. Because the presence of severe peripheral vascular disease or abdominal aneurysm is considered a relative contraindication to femoral cannulation, peripheral vascular Doppler studies and transthoracic or transesophageal echocardiography (TEE) should be performed when peripheral vascular disease is suspected. The echocardiogram is the most valuable diagnostic tool because it demonstrates valvular pathology and ventricular function, and also evaluates the degree of atheromatous disease in the thoracic aorta and aortic arch. In patients considered for minimally invasive cardiac surgery at NYU over the last 5 years, severe peripheral or central aortic atherosclerotic disease was diagnosed in 9.2%, excluding these patients from approaches requiring peripheral cannulation.[15] In general, preoperative magnetic resonance imaging (MRI) or computed tomography (CT) scans have not proven necessary.[16] Cardiac catheterization is indicated prior to surgery to detect associated coronary artery disease in patients with angina or prior myocardial infarction, in those with a strong family history, and in most patients over 55 years of age.

Perfusion With Port-Access Technique

The percutaneous myocardial protection system was proposed independently by Peters and by Stevens, developed by industry (HeartPort Inc., Redwood City, California) and tested at Stanford University and New York University.[3–6,17,18] The port-access technology is an endovascular cardiopulmonary bypass system consisting of the following components (Figure 17-1): a Y-shaped femoral arterial return cannula, a femoral venous cannula for drainage of the right atrium, an endopulmonary vent catheter, and an endoaortic (Endoclamp) occlusion device. The Endoclamp is a 120 cm long, flexible, balloon-tip, triple-lumen catheter. The first lumen is used for Endoclamp balloon inflation, the second lumen enables monitoring of the aortic root pressure proximal to the balloon, and the third lumen facilitates contrast medium injections to secure the position of the catheter, cardioplegia delivery, and ascending aorta venting.

Prior to cannula insertion, arterial pressure should be monitored in both right and left radial arteries. This is essential to guard against the endoaortic occlusion balloon migrating and occluding the innominate artery, making repositioning of the endoaortic balloon necessary. When retrograde cardioplegia is used, an 8.5-French coronary sinus catheter is placed by the anesthesiologist through an introducer sheath in the right internal jugular vein and advanced into the coronary sinus under TEE or fluoroscopic guidance.[19] Alternatively, the coronary sinus catheter may be introduced through the chest port by a standard transatrial technique. Before placement of the coronary sinus catheter, the patient is systemically given heparin 100 U/kg to prevent clot formation on the catheter. Groin dissection is carried out simultaneously. After completion of full-dose systemic heparinization (300 U/kg), the femoral artery is cannulated through a transverse arteriotomy with a 23-French or 21-French dual-limb arterial cannula. The aorta can be occluded either internally by the Endoclamp or externally by direct aortic cross-clamping. When an Endoclamp is applied, the 10.5-French triple-lumen balloon endoaortic clamp is inserted through the side arm of the arterial return cannula and advanced over a guidewire by using the Seldinger technique. The Endoclamp is positioned in the ascending aorta under TEE guidance (Figure 17-2) and eventually placed 1 to 2 cm above the sinotubular ridge.

Venous drainage is achieved by advancing a 28-French or 21-French long venous cannula from the femoral vein into the right atrium under TEE guidance. The distal tip of the venous cannula is positioned in the superior vena cava, and venous drainage is augmented by vacuum assistance. Cardiopulmonary bypass is initiated, and the patient is cooled to 25° to 30°C. The Endoclamp is inflated, or, alternatively, the external cross-clamp is applied, and the heart is arrested by the delivery of cold-blood

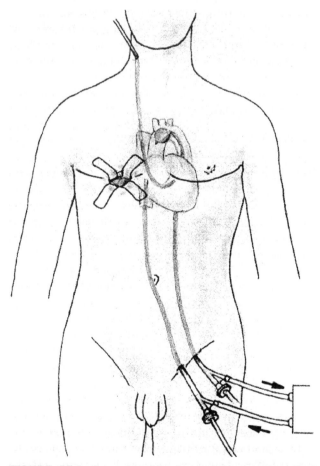

FIGURE 17-1. Set-up for minimally invasive port access mitral surgery. The port access technology is an endovascular cardiopulmonary bypass system consisting of a Y-shaped femoral arterial return cannula, a femoral venous cannula for drainage of the right atrium, an endopulmonary vent catheter, and an endoaortic (Endoclamp) occlusion device. (Illustration courtesy of Cardiovations Inc., Somerville, New Jersey.)

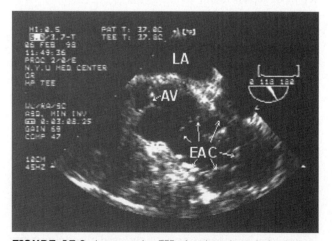

FIGURE 17-2. Intraoperative TEE of endoaortic occlusion balloon placement for minimally invasive mitral valve surgery. Longitudinal view of the ascending aorta shows the balloon of the endoaortic occlusion catheter (EAC) inflated 2 to 3 cm above the aortic valve (AV). The left atrium (LA) is also seen. Reproduced with permission from Korts et al.[24]

cardioplegia, either into the aortic root through the proximal port of the Endoclamp or through the coronary sinus catheter. Cold-blood cardioplegia is re-injected approximately every 30 min throughout the cross-clamp period.

The intracardiac procedures are conducted according to the standard techniques and accomplished using specially designed, long-shafted instruments.[20,21] After completion of the valve procedure, the Endoclamp is deflated or the external cross-clamp is released, and air is aspirated through the proximal catheter in the ascending aorta as monitored by TEE. Rewarming is completed, and the patient is weaned from bypass. The femoral cannulas are removed, and the femoral vessels are repaired. The pericostal incision is closed with absorbable suture, and the thoracotomy incision is closed in layers.

Alternatively, venous drainage is achieved using a right-angled cannula placed in the superior vena cava, in addition to the cannula that is placed from the femoral vein up to the inferior vena cava.[22] The vena cava can then be snared and the right atrium entered for atrial septal defect repair or for tricuspid valve procedures. In some centers, the aorta is cross-clamped directly through the incision. At NYU, direct aortic cross-clamping is used for aortic valve procedures and is performed through a right second or third intercostal space incision.

Visualization with Port-Access Technique

The port-access approach has been performed by using direct vision of the operative field for virtually all cases at NYU, although assisted vision through a thoracoscope is feasible. When applied, a 5 mm, two-dimensional (0°/30°) endoscope is inserted through the fourth or fifth intercostal space in order to achieve an axial view of the mitral valve. During the last several years, an evolution in thoracoscopic control has occurred, and manual direction of the tool by the surgeon has been replaced by a voice-activated system. High-definition imaging has been used through the endoscope to increase visual acuity. While these techniques give beautiful visualization, they have not proven necessary for proper visualization of the valve for port-access valve repair or replacement, and the surgeon has been able to complete the procedures under direct vision in all cases in our experience.

Echocardiography for Minimally Invasive Valve Surgery and Port-Access Technique

Every case of minimally invasive valve surgery should undergo routine intraoperative transesophageal echocardiography. In addition to evaluating valvular pathology and left ventricular function, the intraoperative TEE should evaluate (1) intraluminal aortic atherosclerotic pathology, (2) coronary sinus cardioplegia catheter placement, (3) femoral venous cannula positioning, (4) endoaortic catheter positioning (when used), (5) residual intracardiac air, and (6) the surgical result and postoperative cardiac function.[23,24]

Initially, the TEE probe (5.0 MHz omniplane or biplane) is placed, and a full TEE study is performed. To assess overall left ventricular function, a deep transgastric view is obtained at the midpapillary level. The probe is then withdrawn into the esophagus to view the other intracardiac structures in multiple planes, primarily for final evaluation of the valvular pathology and confirmation of the surgical plan. The presence and the degree of aortic insufficiency are assessed, as significant regurgitation precludes the use of closed antegrade cardioplegia through the proximal port of the Endoclamp. Previous studies have shown a relatively high incidence of intraoperative stroke in patients with protruding aortic arch atheromatous disease.[25,26] Therefore, special attention is given to identifying pathologic conditions of both the descending thoracic aorta and the aortic arch before the operation, as a positive finding might require alteration of the surgical approach. Finally, TEE is used exclusively for positioning of the catheters through the femoral vessels and for placement of the coronary sinus catheter. When difficulty is encountered passing the femoral catheters or coronary sinus catheter, fluoroscopy may be used as a back-up technique, although it is seldom necessary once the team has gained experience.

Prior to termination of cardiopulmonary bypass, a full TEE examination is performed to confirm de-airing and to assess left ventricular and right ventricular function and the results of the surgical procedure. After mitral valve procedures, we focus on valve competence and leaflet coaptation. In addition, it is important to calculate the mitral valve area and measure the gradient across the repaired valve, to exclude paravalvular leaks or prosthetic dysfunction following valve replacement, and to assess for possible systolic anterior motion of the anterior mitral leaflet after valve repair.

Minimally Invasive Aortic Valve Surgery

Operative Approaches

Several methods of operative access have been reported for minimally invasive valve surgery (MIVS) of the aortic valve. An upper sternal division using an "inverted T" ministernotomy was initially reported by Gundry.[11] Both Cosgrove and Byrne initially used parasternal incisions, extending the incision from the inferior border of the right second costal cartilage to the superior edge of the fifth costal cartilage, 3 cm lateral to the sternum.[12,22] The third and fourth cartilages were resected, and the right internal mammary artery (RIMA) was sacrificed. Later, Cosgrove converted from the parasternal to the ministernotomy approach and reported excellent results.[10] Like Arom, Cosgrove concluded that resection of the third and fourth costal cartilages occasionally resulted in instability in a portion of the anterior chest wall.[27] Other disadvantages of the parasternal approach included the sacrifice, in most cases, of the right internal thoracic artery. Subsequently, both Byrne and Gillinov reported that a partial upper sternotomy approach gave better exposure while allowing central cannulation and preservation of the internal mammary artery.[28,29]

Various related approaches also were proposed. Svensson described the "J"-shape partial sternal incision, extending from the first interspace or sternal notch into the right fourth intercostal space.[30] The "C" ministernotomy leaves intact the upper and lower ends of the sternum, while the "I" shape ministernotomy, from the second to the fifth intercostal spaces, preserves both mammary arteries.[31,32] The "T" shape partial lower sternotomy, reported by Doty, also provides adequate exposure for various types of valve operations.[33]

The currently used approach at NYU for aortic valve surgery takes advantage of direct-line vision to the aortic root, while avoiding both partial sternotomy and excision of cartilage. A small right anterior second or third intercostal incision is made to expose the aortic root. The ascending aorta is cannulated directly in most cases, and a small venous cannula is placed directly into the right atrium or, alternately, via the femoral vein. Cardiopulmonary bypass with vacuum-assisted drainage is initiated, and a vent is inserted through the right superior pulmonary vein. Carbon dioxide is routinely infused into the mediastinum through a small catheter. A direct external cross-clamp is applied to the aorta through the skin incision, and cardioplegia is given antegrade directly into the aortic root, via direct coronary cannulation, or retrograde through a percutaneous or transatrial coronary sinus catheter. Standard aortic valve replacement (AVR) techniques are employed.

Minimally Invasive Aortic Valve Results

Glower has described the early experience with the port-access minimally invasive technique, which included 252 patients undergoing aortic valve procedures.[34] Operative mortality was 4.4%. Causes of death were generally patient related and not a consequence of the minimally invasive approach. Gillinov from the Cleveland Clinic reported an operative mortality of 0.8% among 365 patients undergoing aortic valve procedures using the partial sternotomy approach.[29] Svensson reported an overall mortality of 4% in 54 patients, with no mortality among the 18 patients having reoperation.[35] Byrne, from the Boston group, reported 290 consecutive patients undergoing aortic root, valve, and ascending aortic surgery, with an operative mortality of 3.1% for aortic valve replacement.[36] Studies that compared minimally invasive with conventional median sternotomy demonstrated comparable early mortality (1.6 to 5.3%).[15,37,38]

Postoperative Course

Postoperative blood loss has been reported to be significantly lower after minimally invasive valve surgery than following the conventional sternotomy technique.[10,37–39] This may be a result of the smaller incision, the avoidance of continuous bleeding from the sternum, and from minimizing contact of blood with the open pericardial surface, with resultant less coagulopathy.[10] In addition, the less-invasive technique patients had earlier extubation and a lower incidence of postoperative supraventricular arrhythmias.[32,37,38,40,41] Postoperative pain has been reported to be milder after minimally invasive approaches in most reports, although this is difficult to measure comparatively.[32,42,43] Earlier hospital discharge after the minimally invasive approaches was also reported in several studies.[32,37] Szwerc, however, was unable to demonstrate any advantage in the above immediate postoperative parameters among patients undergoing MIVS.[14]

Byrne and his colleagues from Boston reported follow-up (mean, 12 ± 8 months) results for 250 patients who had undergone aortic MIVS.[28] Late complications included 0.8% nonfatal myocardial infarctions and 0.8% reoperations because of valve-related complications. There were five (2%) late deaths from congestive heart failure, pneumonia, hemorrhage, aneurysm, and cancer.

Table 17-1 summarizes the NYU experience with minimally invasive aortic surgery in 1,036 patients between July 1996 and December 2001. This experience includes 322 isolated aortic valve replacements and 160 aortic and mitral valve combined procedures. The operative mortality for isolated aortic valve replacement was 5.2%, with the vast majority of patients being older than 70 years of age. The advantages of avoiding a sternotomy incision were thought to be especially meaningful in this geriatric group of patients, particularly in terms of fewer pulmonary complications and infections.

Minimally Invasive Mitral Valve Surgery

Operative Approaches

Several types of less-invasive incisions for mitral valve surgery, using either partial sternotomy or a minithoracotomy, have been reported over the last several years. The

TABLE 17-1. NYU's Experience from July 1996 to December 2001 (Includes 1036 Patients Who Had Minimally Invasive Valve Surgery).

Procedure	Number of Patients	Mortality (%)
Mitral repair	378	1.0
Mitral replacement	133	6.0
Aortic replacement	322	5.2
Multivalve/combined	203	8.8

AVR = aortic valve replacement; MVP = mitral valve prolapse; MVR = mitral valve repair.

parasternal incision was initially used by the group from the Cleveland Clinic.[22] Subsequently they shifted to a partial upper sternotomy approach.[29] The subxiphoid approach was advocated by others to preserve the integrity of the chest wall by using a transverse skin incision over the superior rim of the xiphoid process, parallel to the skin crease.[44] Following skin undermining, an inverted J-type ministernotomy is carried out when using this approach.

At NYU, as in other centers, the port-access approach is used via a right anterolateral minithoracotomy incision.[45,46] For this approach, the patient is positioned supine and intubated with a single-lumen endotracheal tube. A 5 cm skin incision is made in the right infra-mammary groove, and the fourth intercostal space is entered. A soft-tissue retractor is inserted and the inter-space is gently spread. Alternatively, a right third inter-costal space incision, with the skin incision above the breast, is used. The third interspace approach is particu-larly useful in patients with peripheral vascular disease or obesity or whenever the surgeon prefers central can-nulation.

Port-Access Mitral Valve Surgery Results

The first report of the Port Access International Registry examined data on 1,063 patients from 121 centers, and demonstrated that port-access mitral valve operations could be performed safely, with morbidity and mortality rates similar to those associated with open-chest opera-tions.[8] Glower subsequently reported registry data on 491 patients undergoing port-access mitral valve repair and 568 patients with port-access mitral valve replacement.[34] Operative mortality was 1.6% for mitral valve repair and 5.5% for mitral valve replacement.

The group from Aalst, Belgium, reported its experience with 121 patients undergoing mitral valve surgery through a right anterolateral thoracotomy using the Port-Access system.[13] In their report, the mean preoperative New York Heart Association (NYHA) class was 2.5 ± 0.4, while during follow-up (mean, 31 months; range, 17 to 51 months), all patients significantly improved their NYHA class. Left ventricular end-diastolic and left ventricular end-systolic diameters decreased from 61 ± 7.3 mm to 53 ± 6.9 mm ($p < .01$) and from 37 ± 6.8 mm to 34 ± 6.9 mm ($p < .05$), respectively. Among the patients who had mitral valve repair, 88% had no or trivial mitral regurgitation (MR), and 12% had moderate MR (2+). There were two late valve replacements for endocarditis and no late deaths.

Felger and Chitwood studied 127 consecutive patients who underwent either manually directed ($n = 55$) or voice-activated robotically directed ($n = 72$), video-assisted, minimally invasive mitral valve operations and retrospectively compared this group with a consecutive group of 100 sternotomy mitral valve patients.[45] Although in the robotically directed group longer arrest times

(128.0 ± 4.5 min as compared to 90.0 ± 4.6 min, $p < .001$) and perfusion times (173.0 ± 5.7 min as compared to 144.0 ± 4.6 min, $p < .001$) were noted, these patients showed a significant decrease in blood loss, ventilator time, and length of hospitalization. Moreover, there was a low incidence of complications, including re-exploration for bleeding (2.4%) and stroke (0.8%). The 30-day mor-tality was 2.3%.

At NYU, 714 patients underwent mitral valve repair or replacement with the port-access minimally invasive approach between July 1996 and December 2001 (see Table 17-1). Operative mortality was 1.0% for isolated mitral repair and 3.8% for isolated mitral valve replacement. The average ventilation time was 11 h, the average intensive care unit (ICU) time was 19 h, and the median hospital stay was 6 d. Complications for all patients included permanent neurologic deficit (2.9%) and aortic dissection (0.3%), but no mediastinal infections (Table 17-2).

To evaluate early and intermediate-term results of MIVS, 100 consecutive patients undergoing minimally invasive mitral valve repair at NYU were compared with 100 patients who had mitral valve repair with a conven-tional sternotomy.[47] Both groups were similar in age and ejection fraction. There was 1% hospital mortality with the sternotomy approach and no deaths with the mini-mally invasive approach. No aortic dissections or neuro-logic injury occurred in either group. Freedom from any hospital morbidity was 88% for the sternotomy approach group and 91% for the minimally invasive approach group ($p > .05$). Echocardiographic follow-up (mean, 33 months) revealed that residual mitral insufficiency was similar in both groups, with a 1-year echocardiographic score of 0.79 and 0.77, respectively (0 to 3 scale). Likewise, the cumulative freedom from all valve-related complica-tions and reoperation was not significantly different (Fig-ure 17-3), and the late NYHA functional classification was equivalent between the two groups (Table 17-3).

TABLE 17-2. Minimally Invasive Mitral Valve Operations at NYU: Postoperative Morbidity for All Patients ($n = 714$)

Bypass time (min) (mean ± SD)	127 ± 43
Cross-clamp time (min) (mean ± SD)	92 ± 31
Median ventilation time (h)	11
Median ICU time (h)	19
Median total hospital stay (d)	6
Reoperation for bleeding or effusion	35 (4.9%)
Aortic dissection	2 (0.3%)
Permanent neurologic deficit	21 (2.9%)
Postoperative sepsis	21 (2.9%)
Mediastinal infection	0 (0.0%)
Leg wound infection	3 (0.4%)
Chest wall infection	6 (0.8%)
Renal failure	16 (2.2%)
Reoperation for valve failure	5 (0.7%)
Respiratory failure	51 (7.1%)
Any major complication excluding death	47 (6.6%)

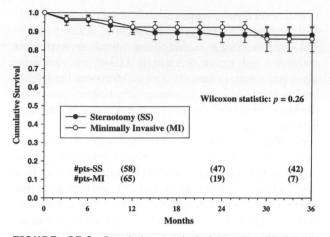

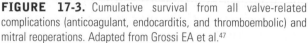

FIGURE 17-3. Cumulative survival from all valve-related complications (anticoagulant, endocarditis, and thromboembolic) and mitral reoperations. Adapted from Grossi EA et al.[47]

TABLE 17-3. Comparison of Minimally Invasive and Conventional Valve Repair: NYU Medical Center Experience

	Full Sternotomy Group (n = 100)	Minimally Invasive Group (n = 100)
Age (yr)	55	57
Hospital mortality	1%	0%
Residual MR	0.79	0.77
NYHA (1 yr)	1.6	1.3
Freedom from reoperation	93%	95%

Adapted from Grossi EA et al.[47]

MR = mitral regurgitation; NYHA = New York Hospital Association.

Subsequent late follow-up studies on the 376 patients undergoing minimally invasive valve repair in the NYU series demonstrated a 5-year cardiac survival of 97%, a 5-year freedom from reoperation of 96%, and a 5-year freedom from all valve-related complications of 94%. These results are equivalent to those previously reported after conventional valve repair.[20]

Data from various centers demonstrate that for teams that master the procedure, minimally invasive mitral valve surgery is comparable to conventional surgery in terms of survival, repair durability, and freedom from valve-related complications, yet the minimally invasive approach is associated with less need for blood, fewer short-term complications, and a shorter recovery time.

Complications of Minimally Invasive Valve Surgery

Stroke, Femoral Artery Injury, and Aortic Dissection

Inability to manipulate the entire heart and to manually remove air from the left ventricle during minimally invasive valve surgery was a source of concern about the potential for cerebrovascular accidents. Consequently, intraoperative computer-aided transcranial Doppler measurements were performed to measure cerebral microemboli in patients undergoing MIVS and conventional mitral valve operation. This study revealed no significant difference in the total number of detected cerebral microembolic signals between the groups.[48] To minimize neurologic complications, it is standard to apply TEE to carefully monitor the left ventricle for residual air prior to release of the aortic clamp or deflating the Endoclamp. Several groups flood the thoracic cavity with CO_2 in order to eliminate the danger of possible gas bubbles.[13,48] This approach, coupled with a transvalvular vent and a vent in the ascending aorta, appears to minimize the risk of air embolus. By using this strategy, Schroeyers reported a reduction of stroke rate from 1.4% in his first 70 cases to 0% in his last 105 cases.[13] Others reported stroke rates of 0 to 3.8 %.[13,28,34,45] Currently, there is no evidence of a higher perioperative stroke rate associated with the minimally invasive approach.

Groin cannulation for cardiopulmonary bypass carries the potential for direct femoral or iliac artery injury, aortic dissection, atheroembolism, and limb ischemia.[49] In addition, the endoaortic cross-clamp balloon might cause an aortic intimal tear leading to dissection. Mohr and colleagues published an initial experience with the port-access approach for mitral valve surgery that was characterized by significant morbidity, including a 4% incidence of acute retrograde aortic dissection.[50] Furthermore, endoaortic balloon migration can lead to cross-clamping dysfunction or innominate artery occlusion.

To minimize the risk of arterial injury, we recommend avoiding peripheral arterial cannulation when the femoral artery size is less than 21 French, when peripheral vascular occlusive disease is present, when the guidewire will not easily pass, in the presence of abdominal aortic aneurysms, and when significant thoracic aortic atheromatous disease is identified on the intraoperative TEE. An aortic diameter greater than 3.5 to 4.0 cm is also considered a relative contraindication to use of an Endoclamp catheter.[51] When any of the above findings are present, a central or axillary cannulation should be used or the operation should be converted to a sternotomy approach.[52]

Factors that minimize the risk of aortic dissection include advanced catheters with flexible guidewires, strict adherence to the Seldinger technique for catheter placement, conversion to an open-chest technique when the guidewire cannot pass, and conduction of vascular screening when peripheral vascular disease is suspected. In addition, long-standing experience with intraoperative TEE, greater familiarity with the Port-Access system, and adherence to the above "safety rules" have almost eliminated the incidence of aortic dissection, reducing it from 1.3% in the first half of our MIVS program to 0.18% in the most recent 532 patients.[53]

Groin wound infection, lymphocele, arteriovenous fistula, limb ischemia, and deep-vein thrombosis can be minimized by applying a limited groin skin incision for cannulation, by using Seldinger technique, by avoiding clamping of the femoral vessels, and by using the innominate vein as an alternative to femoral vein cannulation in selected cases.[13,54]

Benefits of Minimally Invasive Surgery to the Valve Patient

Several studies from NYU have evaluated potential differences in complication rates, pain, and recovery time after minimally invasive and after conventional cardiac surgery. Grossi reported results in a case-control study of 109 patients undergoing isolated aortic or mitral valve surgery using the port-access minimally invasive technique who were compared with 88 patients having conventional valve surgery.[15] Age, NYHA functional class, valve type, surgeon, previous cardiac surgery, and the presence of congestive heart failure were matched in the two groups. Hospital mortality was not significantly different, but, as Table 17-4 illustrates, the minimally invasive patients had a shorter hospital stay (7 vs 9 d, $p = .001$), a decreased number of combined septic, wound, and pulmonary complications (0.9% for minimally invasive vs 5.7% for sternotomy, $p = .05$), and significantly fewer blood transfusions ($p = .02$). Similar benefits were separately demonstrated in the geriatric population, in which the differences between surgical approaches appear to be even more profound.[55]

Similarly, postoperative pain, stress response, rapidity of recovery, and quality of life were compared in a study evaluating port-access minimally invasive coronary artery bypass graft surgery (CABG) versus conventional CABG.[43] Repeated measures analysis of variance showed lower pain scale ratings over the first four postoperative weeks in the minimally invasive group ($p < .001$); less muscle soreness, shortness of breath, fatigue, and loss of appetite at 1, 2, 4, and 8 weeks ($p < .05$); better pulmonary function at 1 and 3 days ($p < .03$); and lower norepinephrine levels at days 1, 2, and 3 ($p = .005$). The Duke Activity Scale questionnaire to evaluate functional recovery showed that the minimally invasive patients were better able to walk one to two blocks at 1 week, climb stairs at 1 and 2 weeks, perform light or moderate housework at 1 and 2 weeks, and engage in moderate recreational activities and perform heavy housework at 4 and 8 weeks ($p < .05$) than were conventional CABG patients. This study and other reports demonstrate that minimally invasive cardiac surgery through a minithoracotomy results in significantly less pain, better postoperative lung function, attenuation of stress response, improved early postoperative functional status, and a shorter recovery time than a conventional sternotomy approach.[56–58]

In contrast, other studies contend that smaller incisions are not necessarily less painful or associated with a shorter length of stay when compared with a median sternotomy approach.[59–61] A case of severe incision pain and long thoracic nerve injury has been reported in a patient after port-access minimally invasive mitral valve surgery that led to a prolonged hospitalization and rehabilitation period.[62] Whether damage to the long thoracic nerve occurred during insertion of the two catheters into the internal jugular vein or because of the large size (9 French and 11 French) of both catheters (coupled with their close proximity in the neck) is unknown.

Overall, the vast majority of larger clinical study series demonstrates that minimally invasive valve surgery using the port-access approach has a low morbidity and mortality and achieves functional and echocardiographic outcomes equivalent to those obtained with conventional surgery. Measurable patient benefits from case-matched control trials include less pain, fewer blood transfusions, fewer septic wound and pulmonary complications, a shorter recovery time, improved functional recovery, and a better cosmetic result.

In summary, minimally invasive surgical treatment of valvular heart disease has expanded exponentially over the last several years. Various minimally invasive approaches can be used routinely for both aortic valve replacement and mitral valve repair or replacement, as well as for many patients with multivalve pathology. Clinical studies demonstrate that minimally invasive valve surgery has numerous measurable patient benefits while achieving equal efficacy in terms of the valvular procedure. Minimally invasive valve surgery is highly successful in many centers that specialize in the treatment of valvular disease, and this technique should be increasingly used.

TABLE 17-4. Number of Blood Cell Transfusions, Including Autologous, and Incidence of Sepsis or Wound Complications among Port Access Minimally Invasive Valve Surgery and Standard Full Sternotomy Patients at NYU Medical Center 1996–1998

	Port Access Technique (n = 109)	Full Sternotomy (n = 88)	Statistical Value
Blood cell transfusion	3 ± 0.3	4.8 ± 0.7	$p = .02$
Incidence of sepsis or wound complications	0.9%	5.7%	$p = .06$

Adapted from Grossi EA et al.[15]

References

1. Lillehei CW, Gott VL, DeWall RA, Varco RL. Surgical correction of pure mitral insufficiency by annuloplasty under direct vision. Lancet 1957;77:446–9.
2. Benetti FJ. Direct coronary surgery with saphenous vein bypass without either cardiopulmonary bypass or cardiac arrest.
3. Pompili MF, Stevens JH, Burdon TA, et al. Port-access mitral valve replacement in dogs. J Thorac Cardiovasc Surg 1996;112:1268–74.
4. Schwartz DS, Ribakove GH, Grossi EA, et al. Single and multivessel port-access coronary artery bypass grafting

with cardioplegic arrest: technique and reproducibility. J Thorac Cardiovasc Surg 1997;114:46–52.

5. Schwartz DS, Ribakove GH, Grossi EA, et al. Minimally invasive mitral valve replacement: port-access technique, feasibility, and myocardial functional preservation. J Thorac Cardiovasc Surg 1997;113:1022–30; discussion 1030–1.

6. Schwartz DS, Ribakove GH, Grossi EA, et al. Minimally invasive cardiopulmonary bypass with cardioplegic arrest: a closed chest technique with equivalent myocardial protection. J Thorac Cardiovasc Surg 1996;111:556–66.

7. Falk V, Walther T, Diegeler A, et al. Echocardiographic monitoring of minimally invasive mitral valve surgery using an endoaortic clamp. J Heart Valve Dis 1996;5:630–7.

8. Galloway AC, Grossi EA, Applebaum RM, Colvin SB. Minimally invasive port-access valvular surgery: initial clinical experience. Circulation 1997;(suppl 1):508.

9. Colvin SB, Galloway AC, Ribakove G, et al. Port-access mitral valve surgery: summary of results. J Card Surg 1998;13:286–9.

10. Cosgrove DM 3rd, Sabik JF, Navia JL. Minimally invasive valve operations. Ann Thorac Surg 1998;65:1535–8; discussion 1538–9.

11. Gundry SR, Shattuck OH, Razzouk AJ, et al. Facile minimally invasive cardiac surgery via ministernotomy. Ann Thorac Surg 1998;65:1100–4.

12. Byrne JG, Mitchell ME, Adams DH, et al. Minimally invasive direct access mitral valve surgery. Semin Thorac Cardiovasc Surg 1999;11:212–22.

13. Schroeyers P, Wellens F, De Geest R, et al. Minimally invasive video-assisted mitral valve repair: short and midterm results. J Heart Valve Dis 2001;10:579–83.

14. Szwerc MF, Benckart DH, Wiechmann RJ, et al. Partial versus full sternotomy for aortic valve replacement. Ann Thorac Surg 1999;68:2209–13; discussion 2213–4.

15. Grossi EA, Galloway AC, Ribakove GH, et al. Impact of minimally invasive valvular heart surgery: a case-control study. Ann Thorac Surg 2001;71:807–10.

16. Ammar R, Porat E, Eisenberg DS, Uretzky G. Utility of spiral CT in minimally invasive approach for aortic valve replacement. Eur J Cardiothorac Surg 1998;14 Suppl 1: S130–3.

17. Peters WS. Minimally invasive cardiac surgery by cardioscopy. Australian J Cardiac Thorac Surg 1993;2:152–4.

18. Stevens JH, Burdon TA, Peters WS, et al. Port-access coronary artery bypass grafting: a proposed surgical method. J Thorac Cardiovasc Surg 1996;111:567–73.

19. Applebaum RM, Colvin SB, Galloway AC, et al. The role of transesophageal echocardiography during port-access minimally invasive cardiac surgery: a new challenge for the echocardiographer. Echocardiography 1999;16: 595–602.

20. Spencer FC, Galloway AC, Grossi EA, et al. Recent developments and evolving techniques of mitral valve reconstruction. Ann Thorac Surg 1998;65:307–13.

21. Galloway AC, Colvin SB, Baumann FG, et al. Long-term results of mitral valve reconstruction with Carpentier techniques in 148 patients with mitral insufficiency. Circulation 1988;78:I97–105.

22. Navia JL, Cosgrove DM 3rd. Minimally invasive mitral valve operations. Ann Thorac Surg 1996;62:1542–4.

23. Applebaum RM, Cutler WM, Bhardwaj N, et al. Utility of transesophageal echocardiography during port-access minimally invasive cardiac surgery. Am J Cardiol 1998; 82:183–8.

24. Kort S, Applebaum RM, Grossi EA, et al. Minimally invasive aortic valve replacement: echocardiographic and clinical results. Am Heart J 2001;142:476–81.

25. Katz ES, Tunick PA, Rusinek H, et al. Protruding aortic atheromas predict stroke in elderly patients undergoing cardiopulmonary bypass: experience with intraoperative transesophageal echocardiography. J Am Coll Cardiol 1992;20:70–7.

26. Stern A, Tunick PA, Culliford AT, et al. Protruding aortic arch atheromas: risk of stroke during heart surgery with and without aortic arch endarterectomy. Am Heart J 1999;138:746–52.

27. Arom KV, Emery RW. Minimally invasive mitral operations. Ann Thorac Surg 1997;63:1219–20.

28. Byrne JG, Hsin MK, Adams DH, et al. Minimally invasive direct access heart valve surgery. J Card Surg 2000;15:21–34.

29. Gillinov AM, Banbury MK, Cosgrove DM. Hemisternotomy approach for aortic and mitral valve surgery. J Card Surg 2000;15:15–20.

30. Svensson LG. Minimal-access "J" or "j" sternotomy for valvular, aortic, and coronary operations or reoperations. Ann Thorac Surg 1997;64:1501–3.

31. Aris A. Reversed "C" ministernotomy for aortic valve replacement. Ann Thorac Surg 1999;67:1806–7.

32. Chang YS, Lin PJ, Chang CH, et al. "I" ministernotomy for aortic valve replacement. Ann Thorac Surg 1999;68:40–5.

33. Doty DB, Flores JH, Doty JR. Cardiac valve operations using a partial sternotomy (lower half) technique. J Card Surg 2000;15:35–42.

34. Glower DD, Siegel LC, Frischmeyer KJ, et al. Predictors of outcome in a multicenter port-access valve registry. Ann Thorac Surg 2000;70:1054–9.

35. Svensson LG, Nadolny EM, Kimmel WA. Minimal access aortic surgery including re-operations. Eur J Cardiothorac Surg 2001;19:30–3.

36. Byrne JG, Karavas AN, Cohn LH, Adams DH. Minimal access aortic root, valve, and complex ascending aortic surgery. Curr Cardiol Rep 2000;2:549–57.

37. Liu J, Sidiropoulos A, Konertz W. Minimally invasive aortic valve replacement (AVR) compared to standard AVR. Eur J Cardiothorac Surg 1999;16 Suppl 2:S80–3.

38. Machler HE, Bergmann P, Anelli-Monti M, et al. Minimally invasive versus conventional aortic valve operations: a prospective study in 120 patients. Ann Thorac Surg 1999;67:1001–5.

39. Sun L, Zheng J, Chang Q, et al. Aortic root replacement by ministernotomy: technique and potential benefit. Ann Thorac Surg 2000;70:1958–61.

40. Marianeschi SM, Seddio F, McElhinney DB, et al. Fast-track congenital heart operations: a less invasive technique and early extubation. Ann Thorac Surg 2000;69:872–6.

41. Byrne JG, Karavas AN, Adams DH, et al. Partial upper re-sternotomy for aortic valve replacement or re-replacement after previous cardiac surgery. Eur J Cardiothorac Surg 2000;18:282–6.

42. Lee JW, Lee SK, Choo SJ, et al. Routine minimally invasive aortic valve procedures. Cardiovasc Surg 2000;8:484–90.

43. Grossi EA, Zakow PK, Ribakove G, et al. Comparison of post-operative pain, stress response, and quality of life in port access vs. standard sternotomy coronary bypass patients. Eur J Cardiothorac Surg 1999;16 Suppl 2:S39–42.

44. Karagoz HY, Bayazit K, Battaloglu B, et al. Minimally invasive mitral valve surgery: the subxiphoid approach. Ann Thorac Surg 1999;67:1328–32; discussion 1333.

45. Felger JE, Chitwood WR Jr, Nifong LW, Holbert D. Evolution of mitral valve surgery: toward a totally endoscopic approach. Ann Thorac Surg 2001;72:1203–8; discussion 1208–9.

46. Mohr FW, Onnasch JF, Falk V, et al. The evolution of minimally invasive valve surgery—2 year experience. Eur J Cardiothorac Surg 1999;15:233–8; discussion 238–9.

47. Grossi EA, LaPietra A, Ribakove GH, et al. Minimally invasive versus sternotomy approaches for mitral reconstruction: comparison of intermediate-term results. J Thorac Cardiovasc Surg 2001;121:708–13.

48. Schneider F, Onnasch JF, Falk V, et al. Cerebral microemboli during minimally invasive and conventional mitral valve operations. Ann Thorac Surg 2000;70:1094–7.

49. Hendrickson SC, Glower DD. A method for perfusion of the leg during cardiopulmonary bypass via femoral cannulation. Ann Thorac Surg 1998;65:1807–8.

50. Mohr FW, Falk V, Diegeler A, et al. Minimally invasive port-access mitral valve surgery. J Thorac Cardiovasc Surg 1998;115:567–74; discussion 574–6.

51. Glower DD, Clements FM, Debruijn NP, et al. Comparison of direct aortic and femoral cannulation for port-access cardiac operations. Ann Thorac Surg 1999;68:1529–31.

52. Bichell DP, Balaguer JM, Aranki SF, et al. Axilloaxillary cardiopulmonary bypass: a practical alternative to femoro-femoral bypass. Ann Thorac Surg 1997;64:702–5.

53. Galloway AC, Shemin RJ, Glower DD, et al. First report of the Port Access International Registry. Ann Thorac Surg 1999;67:51–6; discussion 57–8.

54. Zlotnick AY, Gilfeather MS, Adams DH, et al. Innominate vein cannulation for venous drainage in minimally invasive aortic valve replacement. Ann Thorac Surg 1999;67:864–5.

55. Grossi EA, Galloway AC, Ribakove GH, et al. Minimally invasive port access surgery reduces operative morbidity for valve replacement in the elderly. Heart Surg Forum 1999;2:212–5.

56. Blanc P, Aouifi A, Chiari P, et al. Minimally invasive cardiac surgery: surgical techniques and anesthetic problems [in French]. Ann Fr Anesth Reanim 1999;18:748–71.

57. Mishra YK, Malhotra R, Mehta Y, et al. Minimally invasive mitral valve surgery through right anterolateral mini-thoracotomy. Ann Thorac Surg 1999;68:1520–4.

58. Walther T, Falk V, Metz S, et al. Pain and quality of life after minimally invasive versus conventional cardiac surgery. Ann Thorac Surg 1999;67:1643–7.

59. Heres EK, Marquez J, Malkowski MJ, et al. Minimally invasive direct coronary artery bypass: anesthetic, monitoring, and pain control considerations. J Cardiothorac Vasc Anesth 1998;12:385–9.

60. Chaney MA, Durazo-Arvizu RA, Fluder EM, et al. Port-access minimally invasive cardiac surgery increases surgical complexity, increases operating room time, and facilitates early postoperative hospital discharge. Anesthesiology 2000;92:1637–45.

61. Liem TH, Williams JP, Hensens AG, Singh SK. Minimally invasive direct coronary artery bypass procedure using a high thoracic epidural plus general anesthetic technique. J Cardiothorac Vasc Anesth 1998;12:668–72.

62. Chaney MA, Morales M, Bakhos M. Severe incisional pain and long thoracic nerve injury after port-access minimally invasive mitral valve surgery. Anesth Analg 2000; 91:288–90.

CHAPTER 18

PULMONARY AUTOGRAFT

RONALD C. ELKINS, MD

The pulmonary autograft replacement of the aortic valve, the Ross operation, introduced in 1967 by Donald Ross, is a major contribution to the treatment of many children and young adults with aortic valve disease.[1] Initially championed by Ross, the operation has received increasing interest and study during the past 15 years and is now being performed in most developed countries. However, in many countries, its use is limited by the availability of allograft valves or another suitable alternative for reconstruction of the right ventricular outflow tract. The operation continues to be used by a limited number of surgeons (270 surgeons have submitted cases to the International Ross Registry[2]), and its total use represents only a small proportion of the total number of aortic valve replacements. However, in young children and in adults who wish to avoid using anticoagulates, it appears to be the operation of choice for many informed patients, parents, and physicians. The technical aspects of the operation have been refined during the past 15 years, and its use in the very young (neonates), as well as in patients in their sixth and seventh decades, has been reported, with results similar to those reported in younger adults.[3,4] The long-term outcome of the Ross operation by using present techniques is still unknown as the late results reported by Ross are composed primarily of patients operated on using the scalloped subcoronary technique and only included 20 patients with root replacement.[5] Recently, several series of more than 100 patients followed for more than 10 years were reported; these series are early indications of longer-term results in patients operated on by using the most commonly used technique, the root replacement.[3,6–8]

Our knowledge about aortic valve disease, particularly the prevalence of bicuspid aortic valve disease and its associated abnormalities of the ascending aorta, has expanded during the past decade. The widespread availability of echocardiography has led to earlier detection of aortic valve disease and associated aortic pathology, as well as to a more exacting postoperative evaluation of our early and late results of treatment. Better technical evaluation has enabled us to consider additional patient-related factors that affect late results and has led to several modifications of operative technique and postoperative treatment. As additional information is acquired from extended longitudinal evaluation of large series of patients, our patient indications, surgical techniques, and management will continue to evolve.

In 1999, David and colleagues identified autograft root dilation as a common cause of autograft valve dysfunction and the need for autograft valve reoperation.[9] In their series, this occurred more commonly in patients with congenital aortic valve disease (bicuspid or unicuspid aortic valve), which they attributed to an increased incidence of degenerative pathologic changes in the pulmonary artery of their patients. The authors suggest that in patients with congenital aortic valve disease, the Ross operation should be done as an intraaortic implant technique, and if a root replacement is used, the aortic annulus and sinotubular junction should be "fixed" with an external band of Dacron fabric. This concern about the anticipated results in patients with congenital aortic valve disease has led to many recent publications, some confirming the findings of David and colleagues, and some failing to demonstrate a difference in the incidence of degenerative changes in the pulmonary artery or the long-term outcome of root replacements in patients with congenital aortic valve disease as compared to patients with tricuspid aortic valve disease.[8,10–14] Continued careful surveillance of patients with annual echocardiographic evaluation over an extended time period will help to define the incidence of autograft root dilation and the late function of the pulmonary valve in the systemic circulation.

Interest in the pulmonary autograft as an aortic valve replacement remains high, as indicated by the number of recent reports of relatively large series of patients.[3,6,8,13] The International Ross Registry, established in 1989 to evaluate the performance of the Ross operation, shows a decline in the number of reported cases since 1997 and a more marked decline since the report of David in 1999.[2] Whether this is a true decrease in the number of Ross operations being performed or a decrease in interest of surgeons in reporting their cases is unclear. During this same time period, the number of pulmonary allografts obtained for use in Ross operations from one of the larger commercial tissue banks remains unchanged, averaging 600 to 650 per annum since 1996 (CryoLife, Inc., Kennesaw, GA, personal communication concerning number of allografts used for autografts, 2002). This exceeds the total number of Ross operations reported to the International Ross Registry in each year. This represents the pulmonary homograft use of one tissue valve bank, of which there are five in the United States. The number of allografts that have been provided for Ross operations by the remaining four is unknown. Worldwide, approximately 83,000 aortic valves were implanted in 2001: 50% were bioprosthetic valves, 43% were mechanical valves, and 7% were allograft valves, including Ross operations.[15]

Patient Selection

The Ross operation is a technically demanding operation, and the surgeon's experience with this operation and similar procedures does affect the decision-making process. Patient factors that affect this process include the patient's age, lifestyle, and coexisting cardiac and noncardiac disease. Pathologic abnormality of the aortic valve, ascending aorta, and the pulmonary valve affect the process, especially if the surgeon has limited experience. Table 18-1 outlines the patient factors, patient disease, and cardiac pathology that affect the decision process. Surgeons will modify this list based on their experience and the individual patient. The only absolute contraindications to the Ross operation are Marfan's syndrome (or other known genetic defects in fibrillin, elastin, or collagen), abnormal pulmonary valve, and probably significant immune complex disease as a coexisting disease, especially if it is the etiology of the aortic valve disease.

Operative Technique

The original operative technique described by Ross was the scalloped subcoronary implant, a technique developed for implantation of a homograft aortic valve. We, the cardiac surgery team at the Oklahoma University Health Sciences Center, initiated our experience with this technique but have evolved to the inclusion cylinder technique or the root replacement technique. The most common operative technique used by surgeons reporting their experience to the International Ross Registry is the root replacement. It

is the most versatile technique and appears to be associated with a decreased incidence of early and late failure.[16,17] In our experience, the Ross operation is associated with an increased incidence of autograft insufficiency and of late failure when it is used in patients with primary aortic valve insufficiency or dilatation of the aortic annulus and/or ascending aorta if this abnormal dilatation is not addressed at the original operation. Techniques for annular reduction have been developed, as have techniques for enlargement of the aortic annulus or an extended root replacement for patients who require an aortoventriculoplasty for subvalvar aortic obstruction.

Root Replacement

In patients with an aortic annulus diameter that is within the 70% confidence limits of the aortic annulus size predicted for the patient's body surface area,[18,19] the operation is done by using the following technique.

CANNULATION

Bicaval cannulation is used in all patients, with insertion of the superior vena cava cannula relatively high in the vena cava. This allows for excellent exposure of the aortic valve, avoids problems with an "air lock" when the outflow tract of the right ventricle is being reconstructed, and allows opening of the right atrium for direct cannulation of the coronary sinus if necessary. Ascending aortic cannulation is accomplished near the origin of the innominate artery unless the ascending aorta is dilated. If the ascending aorta is aneurysmal or significantly dilated, aortic cannulation is accomplished in the transverse aortic arch. A left ventricular vent is inserted through the right superior pulmonary vein.

MYOCARDIAL PROTECTION

Moderate systemic hypothermia is utilized (28 to 30°C) with cold antegrade blood cardioplegia for induction and intermittent retrograde blood cardioplegia for maintenance. Right ventricular protection is enhanced with ice saline slush. Myocardial temperature is maintained below 15°C.

TABLE 18-1. Candidate Factors for Ross Operation

Patient Factors	Good	Poor
Age	Young	> 60 yr
Lifestyle	Active	Sedentary
Ease of anticoagulation	Difficult	Relatively easy
Aortic valve pathology	Aortic stenosis	Aortic insufficiency
Aortic annulus	Small or normal size for body surface area	> Normal for body surface area
Ascending aorta	Normal	Aneurysmal
Pulmonary valve pathology	Normal or minor fenestration	Bicuspid or quadricuspid, multiple major fenestrations
Systemic disease	Minor effect on life expectancy	Marfan's syndrome, immune complex disease, connective tissue disorder
Coronary disease	Limited	Reduced life expectancy (< 20 yr)
Mitral valve disease	None or easily repaired	Requires replacement
Bacterial endocarditis	Involves only aortic valve	Extensive aortic valve and aortic annulus involvement

AUTOGRAFT HARVEST

With the heart arrested, the pulmonary artery is opened at the origin of the right pulmonary artery with a transverse arteriotomy (Figure 18-1). Careful visual inspection of the pulmonary valve should identify three leaflets with minimal fenestration (Figure 18-2). The presence of a bicuspid or quadricuspid pulmonary valve or the presence of large (greater than 5 mm) fenestrations or multiple (five or more) fenestrations preclude a Ross operation. In our experience, the incidence of an abnormal pulmonary valve is 2%. The main pulmonary artery and its normal contained valve is harvested by completing the transverse arteriotomy and beginning the dissection of the pulmonary artery in a posterior plane, staying adjacent to the pulmonary artery. The left main coronary artery, the anterior descending coronary artery, and the first septal perforator must be identified and protected. It may be helpful to open the aorta and place a flexible probe in the left main coronary artery in the reoperative patient or when the surgeon is beginning his experience. This dissection continues close to the pulmonary artery until septal musculature is encountered (Figure 18-3). The attachment of the pulmonary artery and the aorta at their common conal tissue may be difficult to dissect, and the surgeon should avoid injury to the autograft by dissecting into the aortic wall if necessary. When septal musculature is encountered, the surgeon, looking through the pulmonary valve into the right ventricle, identifies a point 3 to 4 mm below the pulmonary artery annulus and, using a right-angled clamp, elevates the free wall of the right ventricle and performs a ventriculotomy (Figure 18-4). With the pulmonary valve visualized, the right ventricle is divided 3 to 4 mm below the annulus. Where the right ventricle becomes adherent to the ventricular septum, the dissection is kept superficial, and only right ventricular musculature is divided to avoid injury to the first septal perforator of the anterior descending coronary artery (Figure 18-5). After completion of the dissection and harvesting of the autograft, it is prepared for implantation. When the autograft is used as a root replacement, all adventitia is left on the autograft and the proximal musculature attached to the pulmonary valve annulus is trimmed in a plane 3 to 4 mm below the nadir of the three coronary sinuses.

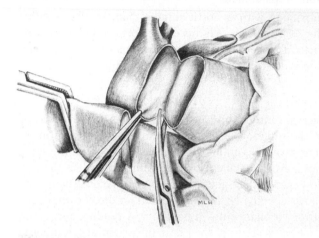

FIGURE 18-1. The distal pulmonary artery is incised at the origin of the right pulmonary artery. A transverse arteriotomy, adequate to allow careful inspection of the pulmonary artery, is made. Reproduced with permission from Elkins RC. Aortic valve: Ross procedure. In: Kaiser LR, Kron IL, Spray TL, editors. Mastery of cardiothoracic surgery. Philadelphia: Lippincott-Raven; 1997. p. 376–84.

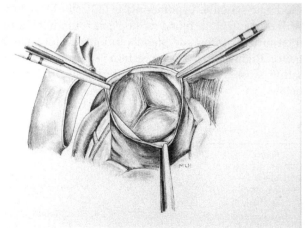

FIGURE 18-2. The normal trileaflet pulmonary valve with three equal sinuses and no significant fenestrations or other abnormalities of the leaflets. Reproduced with permission from Elkins RC. Aortic valve: Ross procedure. In: Kaiser LR, Kron IL, Spray TL, editors. Mastery of cardiothoracic surgery. Philadelphia: Lippincott-Raven; 1997. p. 376–84.

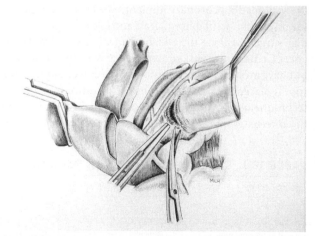

FIGURE 18-3. Dissection of the pulmonary autograft is initiated on the posterior aspect of the proximal pulmonary artery. Dissection is continued in this plane, adjacent to the pulmonary artery until septal myocardium is encountered. The left main coronary artery and left anterior descending coronary artery are protected. Reproduced with permission from Elkins RC. Aortic valve: Ross procedure. In: Kaiser LR, Kron IL, Spray TL, editors. Mastery of cardiothoracic surgery. Philadelphia: Lippincott-Raven; 1997. p. 376–84.

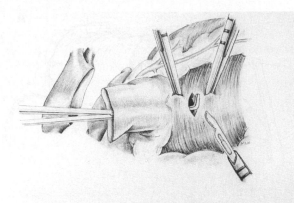

FIGURE 18-4. Identification of the anterior right ventriculotomy is facilitated by placing a right-angled clamp through the pulmonary valve and indenting the myocardium 3 to 4 mm below the pulmonary valve annulus. Reproduced with permission from Elkins RC. Aortic valve: Ross procedure. In: Kaiser LR, Kron IL, Spray TL, editors. Mastery of cardiothoracic surgery. Philadelphia: Lippincott-Raven; 1997. p. 376–84.

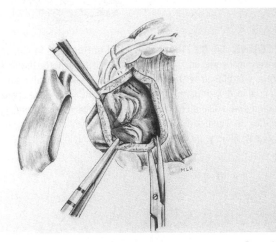

FIGURE 18-5. Completion of the posterior enucleation of the pulmonary autograft from the outflow tract of the right ventricle, the usual location of the first large septal perforating coronary artery. It arises adjacent to the first diagonal coronary artery of the left anterior descending and traverses the septal musculature toward the conal papillary muscle of the tricuspid valve. Reproduced with permission from Elkins RC. Aortic valve: Ross procedure. In: Kaiser LR, Kron IL, Spray TL, editors. Mastery of cardiothoracic surgery. Philadelphia: Lippincott-Raven; 1997. p. 376–84.

AUTOGRAFT IMPLANTATION

The aortotomy should be transverse and located about 2 cm above the origin of the right coronary artery. After careful excision of the aortic valve and any subvalvar obstruction, the aortic annulus is débrided, removing all calcification. The aortic annulus is sized with an aortic valve sizer or a calibrated dilator (Hegar uterine dilator). The left and right coronary arteries are then mobilized with large cuffs of aortic wall. Minimal dissection of the coronary arteries is usually required. The remaining proximal aorta is then excised to the level of the aortic

annulus in the nadir of the coronary sinuses and removal of the commissural attachment in the interleaflet triangle. The pulmonary autograft is positioned so the posterior sinus of the pulmonary valve becomes the left coronary sinus. Interrupted sutures of 4–0 polypropylene are placed between the nadir of the pulmonary sinuses and the nadir of the aortic sinuses unless the aortic annulus is markedly dysplastic. These sutures are used to trifurcate the aortic annulus, beginning with the first suture placed below the left coronary ostium, the second suture adjacent to the right coronary ostium, and the remaining suture trifurcating the aortic annulus (Figure 18-6). The three sinuses of the pulmonary valve are symmetric, and the proximal suture line should attempt to maintain this anatomic symmetry. In adult patients, the proximal suture line is interrupted and tied over a thin strip of pericardium. In children, in whom growth is anticipated, the suture line is running polyglyconate (Maxon, Davis+Geck, Manati, PR).

After completing the proximal suture line, the left coronary ostium is implanted to a 5-mm opening made in the midpoint of the neo-left coronary sinus (Figure 18-7). This suture line is running 5–0 polypropylene. (If the patient is a young child, a 4-mm opening is made, and the suture line is 6–0 polyglyconate.) Next, the autograft is trimmed for the distal suture line, leaving 4 to 5 mm of pulmonary artery distal to the sinotubular junction of the pulmonary artery. The distal suture line is then completed with a running 4–0 polypropylene suture. If the ascending aorta is dilated, a vertical aortoplasty is completed prior to completing the distal anastomosis (Figure 18-8A). The aorta should be reduced in size so that it approximates the

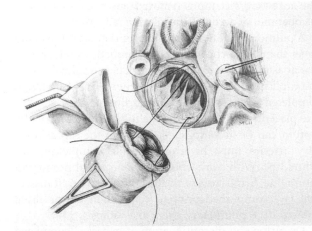

FIGURE 18-6. The pulmonary autograft is in an anatomic position with the posterior sinus of the autograft becoming the neo-left coronary sinus. (For clarity, the stay suture in this sinus is not shown.) The remaining sutures for orientation are placed to position the neo-right coronary sinus and to trifurcate the aortic annulus. Reproduced with permission from Elkins RC. Aortic valve: Ross procedure. In: Kaiser LR, Kron IL, Spray TL, editors. Mastery of cardiothoracic surgery. Philadelphia: Lippincott-Raven; 1997. p. 376–84.

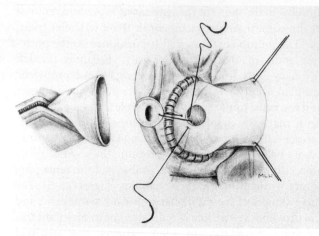

FIGURE 18-7. The left coronary artery is implanted with a continuous suture of polypropylene. Reproduced with permission from Elkins RC. Aortic valve: Ross procedure. In: Kaiser LR, Kron IL, Spray TL, editors. Mastery of cardiothoracic surgery. Philadelphia: Lippincott-Raven; 1997. p. 376–84.

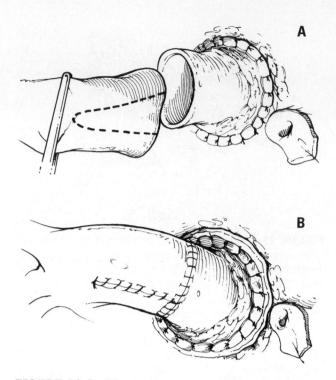

FIGURE 18-8. Elliptical vertical aortoplasty to correct non-aneurysmal aortic enlargement. After excision of aortic tissue (A), aortotomy is closed with a double row of polypropylene suture (B). Reproduced with permission from Elkins RC. The Ross operation in patients with dilation of the aortic annulus and of the ascending aorta. In: Cox JL, Sundt TM III, editors. Operative techniques in cardiac and thoracic surgery: a comparative atlas. Philadelphia: Saunders; 1997. p. 331–41.

size of the sinotubular junction of the pulmonary autograft (Figure 18-8*B*). If the ascending aorta is aneurysmal, the aorta is resected to the level of the innominate artery and replaced with a collagen-filled Dacron graft of appropriate size. In general, the Dacron graft should be the size of the aortic annulus or 2 to 3 mm smaller (Figure 18-9). After completing the distal anastomosis to the aorta, the autograft is distended with cardioplegia and the site for implanting the right coronary artery is selected, being careful to avoid kinking of this coronary artery. A 5-mm opening is made in the autograft, and after trimming the aortic cuff of the right coronary artery, it is sewn to this opening with a running suture of 5–0 polypropylene (Figure 18-10). The aortic cross-clamp is removed, and the remainder of the operation is accomplished during rewarming.

A pulmonary homograft of appropriate size, 4 to 6 mm larger than the aortic annulus, is trimmed, and the proximal anastomosis of the right ventricular outflow tract is accomplished with 4–0 polypropylene. This suture line is completed while cardiac activity is limited so that accurate placement of the suture line to the right ventricular septum can be accomplished. Injury to the septal coronary arteries must be avoided while completing this suture line. With completion of the proximal homograft suture line, hemostasis of the bed of the autograft dissection is accomplished prior to completion of the distal homograft to pulmonary artery anastomosis.

De-airing and discontinuation of bypass is completed after warming and establishment of adequate cardiac function.

Inclusion Cylinder

The operative technique for the inclusion cylinder is similar to that used for the root replacement. Cannulation, perfusion, myocardial protection, and harvesting the autograft

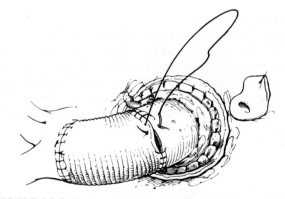

FIGURE 18-9. Replacement of an ascending aortic aneurysm with a knitted Dacron graft, similar in size to the size of the aortic annulus following annulus reduction. The graft is anastomosed to the pulmonary autograft 4 to 5 mm distal to the sinotubular junction of the autograft. This anastomosis is completed prior to implantation of the right coronary artery so that the autograft can be distended and the proper site for implantation of the right coronary can be selected. Reproduced with permission from Elkins RC. The Ross operation in patients with dilation of the aortic annulus and of the ascending aorta. In: Cox JL, Sundt TM III, editors. Operative techniques in cardiac and thoracic surgery: a comparative atlas. Philadelphia: Saunders; 1997. p. 331–41.

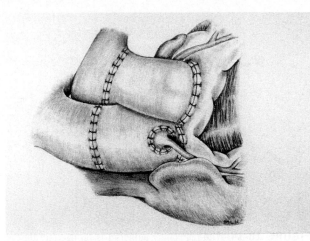

FIGURE 18-10. Completion of the pulmonary autograft root implantation, with selection of site of implantation of the right coronary artery with the autograft distended. The pulmonary homograft reconstruction of the outflow tract of the right ventricle is with two continuous suture lines. Reproduced with permission from Elkins RC. Aortic valve: Ross procedure. In: Kaiser LR, Kron IL, Spray TL, editors. Mastery of cardiothoracic surgery. Philadelphia: Lippincott-Raven; 1997. p. 376–84.

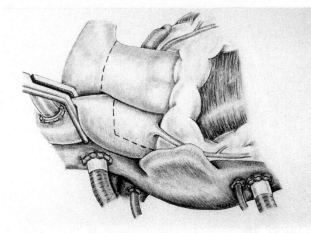

FIGURE 18-11. Cannulation: distal aorta, bicaval cannulation with superior vena caval cannula placed through a purse-string in the vena cava, left ventricular vent through the right superior pulmonary vein, and retrograde cardioplegia cannula through the right atrium. All illustrations are oriented from the perspective of a surgeon standing on the right side of the patient. Reproduced with permission from Elkins RC. Aortic valve: Ross procedure. In: Kaiser LR, Kron IL, Spray TL, editors. Mastery of cardiothoracic surgery. Philadelphia: Lippincott-Raven; 1997. p. 376–84.

are identical. The inclusion cylinder technique is used in patients with an aortic annulus between 22 and 25 mm in diameter, when this is an appropriate aortic annulus size for the patient's body surface area. When performing an inclusion cylinder, the transverse aortotomy is extended into the middle of the noncoronary sinus to the level of the aortic annulus. This provides excellent exposure of the aortic annulus (Figure 18-11). After harvesting the pulmonary autograft, all adventitia is trimmed from the autograft prior to its insertion, and the proximal myocardial rim below the pulmonary valve annulus is trimmed so that it is no more than 3 mm in length and thickness.

The proximal suture line is interrupted and is similar to the suture line of the root replacement technique (Figure 18-12). As the pulmonary valve has three sinuses that are equal in size and as the nadirs of these sinuses are 120° apart, the patient with a dysplastic or a bicuspid aortic valve and coronary arteries that are 180° apart presents a technically difficult problem for insertion using the inclusion cylinder technique. These patients should have a root replacement if the surgeon does not have extensive experience with this technique. After placement of the proximal sutures, the valve is seated and the sutures are tied, with the valve inverted into the left ventricular outflow tract (Figure 18-13).

The autograft is reverted and trimmed for the distal anastomosis, leaving 3 to 4 mm of pulmonary artery distal to the sinotubular junction. The site for attachment of the commissural fixation suture is selected by placing traction to elevate the commissure of the pulmonary autograft and the appropriate site on the host aorta so that equal tension is on both. A horizontal mattress suture

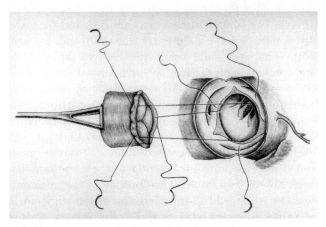

FIGURE 18-12. Placement of three polypropylene sutures to orient the pulmonary autograft. The posterior sinus of the pulmonary autograft becomes the neo-left coronary sinus. Reproduced with permission from Elkins RC. Aortic valve: Ross procedure. In: Kaiser LR, Kron IL, Spray TL, editors. Mastery of cardiothoracic surgery. Philadelphia: Lippincott-Raven; 1997. p. 376–84.

is placed through the pulmonary artery 2 mm above the commissure of the pulmonary artery and full thickness of the aorta at the previously identified point. This usually places the sinotubular junction of the pulmonary artery 5 mm or more above the sinotubular junction of the host aorta. The attachment of the commissures to the aorta affects the long-term autograft valve function, and therefore the placement of these sutures is very important. They should be very similar in height and should be 120° apart when they have been properly placed. These sutures are not tied until the coronary arteries have been

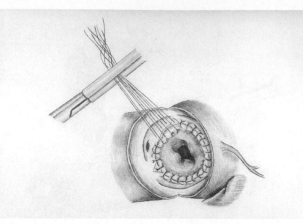

FIGURE 18-13. The autograft is inverted into the left ventricle, and the proximal sutures are tied and divided. Reproduced with permission from Elkins RC. Aortic valve: Ross procedure. In: Kaiser LR, Kron IL, Spray TL, editors. Mastery of cardiothoracic surgery. Philadelphia: Lippincott-Raven; 1997. p. 376–84.

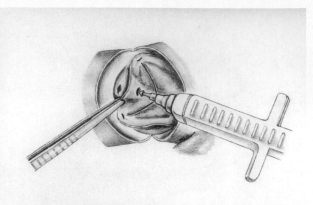

FIGURE 18-14. The pulmonary autograft is re-inverted; that is, horizontal mattress sutures are placed to secure the height and position of autograft (but not tied until the right and left coronary arteries are implanted). An aortic punch (4 or 5 mm) is used to create an opening in the autograft to allow attachment of the coronary artery ostia. Reproduced with permission from Elkins RC. Aortic valve: Ross procedure. In: Kaiser LR, Kron IL, Spray TL, editors. Mastery of cardiothoracic surgery. Philadelphia: Lippincott-Raven; 1997. p. 376–84.

implanted to the pulmonary autograft. The left coronary artery is sutured to a 5-mm opening in the midportion of the posterior sinus of the pulmonary autograft with a running suture of 5–0 polypropylene, followed by a similar technique for the right coronary anastomosis (Figure 18-14). The commissural sutures are tied, and the distal anastomosis of the pulmonary autograft and the host aorta is initiated at the commissure between the right and left coronary sinuses. This suture is placed through the pulmonary artery and the aorta, and tied outside the lumen of the aorta. The suture is then brought into the lumen of the aorta and a running technique is used. When the suture line approaches the aortotomy that has been extended into the noncoronary sinus, the suture line is not completed until this portion of the aortotomy has been closed. The closure of this portion of the aortotomy includes a limited full-thickness bite of the autograft in this sinus to insure fixation of the noncoronary sinus of the autograft to the aortic sinus. The distal suture line is then completed, and the remaining portion of the aortotomy is completed in the usual fashion (Figure 18-15).

Annulus Reduction and Fixation

In patients who have reached their adult size and who have an aortic annulus that is greater than their predicted size based on their body surface area by 2 mm or more, an aortic annulus reduction and fixation is accomplished as a modification of the Ross operation. After excision of the aortic valve and débridement of the aortic annulus if required, two purse-string sutures of heavy polypropylene (2–0 or 3–0) are placed in the left ventricular outflow tract. These sutures are 1 mm apart and are in the aortic annulus at the nadir of the coronary sinuses and below the aortic annulus in the interleaflet triangle (Figure 18-16). Between the commissure between the right and noncoronary sinus and the adjacent commissure between

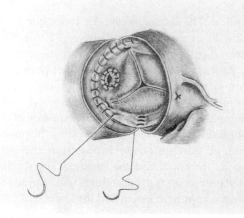

FIGURE 18-15. After completion of the coronary artery anastomosis, commissural stay sutures are tied and divided, and the distal suture line is initiated at the commissure between the left and right coronary artery. This is continued to the aortotomy extension into the noncoronary sinus. This portion of the aortotomy is closed with a running suture line, with the suture including a full thickness "bite" of the noncoronary sinus of the pulmonary autograft. Reproduced with permission from Elkins RC. Aortic valve: Ross procedure. In: Kaiser LR, Kron IL, Spray TL, editors. Mastery of cardiothoracic surgery. Philadelphia: Lippincott-Raven; 1997. p. 376–84.

the noncoronary and left coronary sinus, the reduction sutures are in the membranous septum, close to the aortic annulus, so as to avoid injury to the conduction system. These two sutures are passed external to the aorta in the midportion of the noncoronary sinus and through a Teflon felt pledget. A calibrated dilator (uterine dilator), sized to equal the expected mean size of the normal aortic annulus for this patient's body surface area, is passed

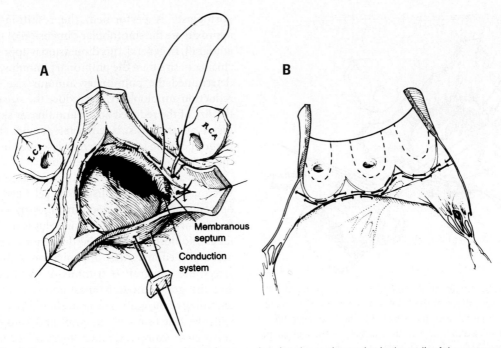

FIGURE 18-16. *A,* Two purse-string sutures of 2–0 polypropylene are placed at the aortic annulus in the nadir of the coronary sinuses, in the lateral fibrous trigone in the interleaflet triangle between the left and noncoronary sinus, in the muscle of the ventricular septum at the commissure between the left and right coronary sinuses, and in the membranous septum between the right and noncoronary sinus. The sutures are brought through the aortic annulus external to the aorta in the midpoint of the noncoronary sinus and passed through a felt pledget.
B, An opened view of the aortic annulus, showing the exact placement of the sutures. Notice the placement of the sutures in the membranous septum to avoid the conduction system. Reproduced with permission from Elkins RC. The Ross operation in patients with dilation of the aortic annulus and of the ascending aorta. In: Cox JL, Sundt TM III, editors. Operative techniques in cardiac and thoracic surgery: a comparative atlas. Philadelphia: Saunders; 1997. p. 331–41.

through the annulus into the left ventricle, and the sutures are tied snugly, reducing the aortic annulus to the size of the dilator (Figure 18-17). The Ross operation is accom-

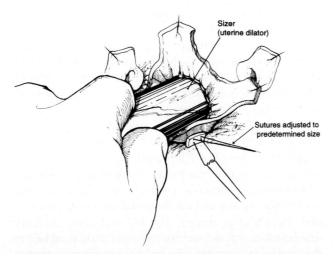

FIGURE 18-17. The two sutures are tied over the felt pledget with a graduated dilator in the aortic annulus of appropriate size for the patient. Reproduced with permission from Elkins RC. The Ross operation in patients with dilation of the aortic annulus and of the ascending aorta. In: Cox JL, Sundt TM III, editors. Operative techniques in cardiac and thoracic surgery: a comparative atlas. Philadelphia: Saunders; 1997. p. 331–41.

plished as a root replacement, and the proximal line of interrupted sutures is carefully placed so that it includes the sutures used to reduce the aortic annulus (Figure 18-18). The pulmonary autograft is "seated" into the reduced annulus, and the sutures of the proximal suture line are tied over an external cuff of woven Dacron material 2 to 3 mm thick (Figure 18-19). These sutures are carefully tied to ensure apposition of the aortic annulus and the autograft, keeping the Dacron cuff external to the anastomosis. The ends of the external Dacron cuff are secured with an additional suture to complete the "fixation" of the aortic annulus.

Many patients with aortic annulus dilatation also have significant dilatation of the ascending aorta, and in some there will be aneurysmal changes in the aorta. In these patients, the aortic cannula is placed in the transverse arch and the aortic cross-clamp is placed at the origin of the innominate artery. A decision whether to replace the ascending aorta or to reduce the aortic diameter with a vertical aortoplasty is based on the degree of dilatation and the pathologic appearance of the aortic wall. In either situation, the Ross operation proceeds with implanting the left coronary artery and then trimming the pulmonary autograft 3 to 4 mm distal to the sinotubular junction for attachment to the reduced aorta or to an interposition graft used to replace the ascending aorta. If a vertical

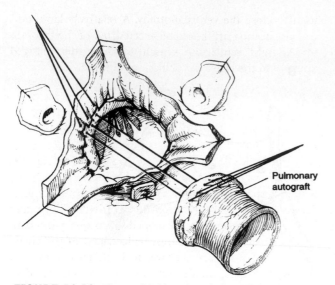

FIGURE 18-18. The proximal interrupted suture line includes the annulus reduction sutures at the level of the aortic valve annulus. Reproduced with permission from Elkins RC. The Ross operation in patients with dilation of the aortic annulus and of the ascending aorta. In: Cox JL, Sundt TM III, editors. Operative techniques in cardiac and thoracic surgery: a comparative atlas. Philadelphia: Saunders; 1997. p. 331–41.

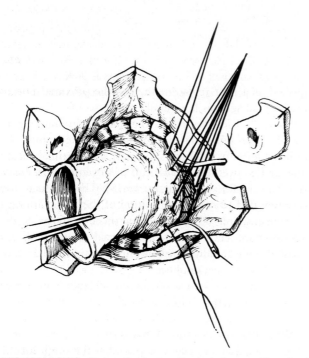

FIGURE 18-19. The proximal suture line is tied over a thin strip of woven Dacron graft, being careful to keep the Dacron material external to the autograft and not between the apposition line of the aortic annulus and the autograft. The two ends of the Dacron graft are tied together with the last two sutures to complete the "fixation" of the aortic annulus. Reproduced with permission from Elkins RC. The Ross operation in patients with dilation of the aortic annulus and of the ascending aorta. In: Cox JL, Sundt TM III, editors. Operative techniques in cardiac and thoracic surgery: a comparative atlas. Philadelphia: Saunders; 1997. p. 331–41.

aortoplasty is performed, the resulting aorta should approximate the sinotubular dimension of the pulmonary autograft. In general, this dimension is approximately 10% smaller in size than the pulmonary annulus,[20] and we have determined the pulmonary annulus size by our aortic reduction annuloplasty. We reduce the size of the aorta to the size of the reduced aortic annulus, or slightly less. The distal anastomosis is completed, and the remainder of the operation is completed as described in the section on the technique for root replacement.

If the aorta is aneurysmal, it is replaced with a knitted Dacron graft that is collagen or gel filled so that postoperative hemostasis is not difficult. A graft equal in size to the size of the reduced aortic annulus is used, and the distal anastomosis between the distal aorta and the graft is accomplished first. After implantation of the left coronary artery, the autograft is trimmed as previously described and the graft–autograft anastomosis is completed after trimming of the graft. The graft should be trimmed so that with the distension of the graft and autograft when the aortic cross-clamp is removed there will be no "kinking" of the autograft produced by a redundant graft. The site for implantation of the right coronary artery is always selected after completion of the ascending aortic reconstruction and distention of the autograft with cardioplegia so that the right coronary can be implanted without distortion.

Extended Root Replacement (Ross-Konno Operation)

Patients with left ventricular obstruction that involves the aortic valve, the aortic annulus, and the left ventricular outflow tract may require an aortoventriculoplasty to relieve their obstruction. Most patients in our experience with subvalvar obstruction and aortic valve disease require resection of the subvalvar obstruction and a left ventricular myomectomy with or without a limited annuloplasty for correction of their obstruction. In these patients, the Ross operation is usually accomplished as a root replacement. In patients with severe obstruction, or when complete relief of the obstruction is uncertain, an aortoventriculoplasty is performed.

The operation proceeds as a standard root replacement with cannulation, perfusion, and myocardial protection as previously described. The aortotomy includes an extension into the noncoronary sinus to allow good visualization of the left ventricular outflow tract. The aortic valve is carefully excised and all abnormal subvalvar endocardial thickening is excised. The left and right coronary arteries are mobilized and the proximal aorta is excised to the level of the annulus. The pulmonary artery is opened at the origin of the right pulmonary artery, and the pulmonary valve is inspected. If the pulmonary valve is normal, the pulmonary autograft is harvested in the usual fashion, except that the right ventriculotomy is initiated approximately 1 to 1.5 cm below the pulmonary annulus so that the anterior free wall of the right ventricle can be used to "patch" the ventriculotomy of the aortoventriculoplasty. After enucleation of the autograft with this segment of the anterior wall of the right ventricle, the ventriculotomy can be initiated in the right coronary sinus, adjacent to the commissure between the right and noncoronary sinus. The ventriculotomy is extended until complete relief of the outflow tract has been achieved. If additional subvalvar resection of obstructing septal muscle is necessary, it can be accomplished at this time. The autograft is then positioned so that the posterior sinus of the pulmonary valve will become the neo-left coronary sinus and the attached segment of the anterior wall of the right ventricle will be used to close the ventriculotomy. The proximal suture line of 5–0 Maxon is placed to attach the nadir of the left coronary sinus to the nadir of the posterior sinus of the autograft. A second suture is placed through the nadir of the noncoronary sinus and through the nadir of the right sinus of the autograft. A third suture is at the apex of the ventriculotomy and through the free wall of the right ventricle below the commissure between the right and left sinuses of the autograft. These three sutures orient the autograft properly. The suture at the left coronary sinus is tied, and a continuous suture line attaches the aortic annulus to the autograft posteriorly; this suture is tied to the suture in the noncoronary sinus of the aorta. The suture line is continued in the left and right coronary sinuses to the ventriculotomy suturing the aortic annulus to the autograft. The suture line between the ventriculotomy and the right ventricular wall is buttressed with a strip of pericardium (Figure 18-20), which completes the proximal suture line. The remainder of the autograft implantation is similar to the usual root replacement. Insertion of the pulmonary homograft requires the proximal suture line of the homograft to be sewn to the autograft where the right ventricular muscle has been used to close the ventriculotomy. A relatively large pulmonary homograft should be selected; use of the cryopreserved right ventricular muscle to close this enlarged opening in the right ventricle is not difficult.

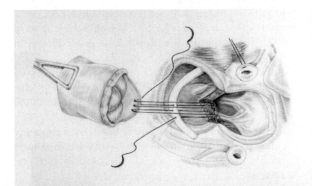

FIGURE 18-20. The pulmonary autograft is positioned in an anatomic position, with the anterior free wall of the right ventricle being used to close the ventriculotomy, and the pulmonary root is attached to the aortic annulus in the normal fashion. Reproduced with permission from Elkins RC. Valve repair and valve replacement in children, including the Ross procedure. In: Kaiser LR, Kron IL, Spray TL, editors. Mastery of cardiothoracic surgery. Philadelphia: Lippincott-Raven; 1997. p. 938–47.

Current Results

Ross reported his personal series of 339 patients in 1991, with 80% patient survival at 20 years and a freedom from reoperation of 85%. Freedom from valve-related complications was 70%.[21] These historical controls provide the reference standard for all subsequent reports and studies. Almost all patients in this exceptional series had their Ross operation performed as a scalloped subcoronary implant. The first pulmonary autograft replacement of the aortic valve as a root replacement was in 1974. This is now the most common technique used, and most subsequent data will be based on the experience with this technique.[22]

Survival

The operative risk for the Ross operation has steadily declined and is now similar to the risk for an aortic valve replacement. The 30-day mortality at the University of Oklahoma is 4.4% (23 of 518 patients), and during the past 8 years it has been reduced to 12 of 380. This includes neonates who are on an extracorporeal membrane oxygenator and patients with multiple concomitant procedures. The 30-day mortality, as reported to the International Ross Registry, is 3.6% (139 of 3,904 patients). Actuarial survival of the 518 patients is 90% ± 2% at 13 years, and actuarial freedom from autograft valve replacement is 90% ± 3% at 13 years.

Early Autograft Valve Failure

Autograft valve failure or dysfunction requiring replacement of the autograft valve at the time of operative insertion or reoperation within 6 months of the original Ross operation is rare. At our institution, this has only occurred once; the second patient in our operative series required autograft valve replacement. This event has not been reported in any significant numbers in the literature, and in the International Ross Registry, the incidence since 1990 is 0.7% (27 of 3,904 autograft valves explanted within 6 months of implantation).

Late Autograft Valve Degeneration

Autograft valve degeneration (severe autograft insufficiency not caused by infection, autograft reoperation not related to infection or obstruction, or valve-related death) has been used to assess operative and patient-related factors affecting late outcome of the Ross operation. At our institution, between August 1986 and June 2002, 518 patients had a Ross operation. Follow-up is available within the most recent 2 years on 91% of these patients, and 81% have had an echocardiogram in that time period. Actuarial freedom from autograft valve degeneration is

81% ± 4% at 10 years in the 495 operative survivors. In the 431 patients with a root replacement, the actuarial freedom from autograft degeneration is 85% ± 4% at 13 years, and in the 86 intraaortic implant patients, it is 80% ± 5% ($p = .03$). Eighteen patients have required operative replacement of their autograft valve, and an additional 17 patients underwent autograft repair for progressive autograft insufficiency, most commonly because of dilation of the aortic valve annulus or of the sinotubular junction. Autograft replacement occurred in 6 patients for autograft insufficiency associated with autograft root dilation, in 3 patients for an abnormal autograft valve (bicuspid in 2 and quadricuspid in the third), endocarditis in 3 patients, technical in 3 patients, lupus erythematosus in 1 patient, and prolapsed autograft leaflets in the remaining 2 patients (both intraaortic implants). Patients with a primary lesion of aortic insufficiency and patients who had a Ross operation as an intraaortic implant (scalloped subcoronary implant or an inclusion cylinder) were at higher risk of autograft degeneration. Age at operation, valve pathology (bicuspid or tricuspid), and annulus enlargement or dilation of the ascending aorta (if surgically repaired at the time of the Ross operation) did not affect the occurrence of autograft degeneration. In 165 patients with an ascending aortic aneurysm or dilation of the ascending aorta managed by resection of the ascending aorta when aneurysmal or a vertical aortoplasty in patients with dilation, the actuarial freedom from autograft degeneration is similar to that of the entire group at 5 years. Some patients who were not treated by surgical management for their mildly dilated aorta have developed increasing enlargement of the aorta. They are being carefully followed and may need reoperation for replacement of their ascending aorta. It is now known that 50 to 60% of patients with bicuspid aortic valve and with a normally functioning bicuspid aortic valve develop dilation of the ascending aorta and that 5% develop dissection of the aorta.[23] This strongly supports aggressive management of significant ascending aortic pathology at the time of a Ross operation.

Annular reduction plus fixation in 99 patients with aortic insufficiency as the primary lesion has appeared to decrease the early incidence of autograft degeneration when compared to the 70 patients with primary aortic insufficiency who were treated early in the series without annular reduction or fixation. However, two patients in the annular fixation group have required autograft valve reoperation, with successful repair in one and replacement in the other.

HOMOGRAFT VALVE FUNCTION

Pulmonary homograft valve reconstruction of the right ventricular outflow tract was used in 515 patients in our series. An aortic homograft was used in the remaining three patients because of availability of suitable homografts. In the 495 operative survivors, the actuarial free-
dom from reoperation on the homograft is 92% ± 2% at 13 years. This underestimates the incidence of homograft dysfunction, as 15 patients have severe pulmonary insufficiency and 38 have a peak instantaneous gradient across the pulmonary homograft of 40 mm Hg or more by follow-up echocardiography. These patients are being followed closely and will undergo reoperation if they develop significant right ventricular enlargement or dysfunction. In our patient series, interventional procedures by our cardiologists have had limited impact on the homograft obstruction. It is a general consensus that the homograft dysfunction is related to the immunologic response to the allograft valve, and it is hoped that additional knowledge will lead to homograft modifications that will improve long-term function.

LIFESTYLE

These patients have not required anticoagulation, and there have been no thromboembolic events. The patients have had minimal restrictions on their lifestyle, and the majority are on no cardiac medications. Actuarial freedom from replacement of the autograft valve in the 495 operative survivors is 90% ± 3% at 13 years, and their survival is 95% ± 2%. For the 190 children in this series, the actuarial freedom from replacement of the autograft valve is 94% ± 3% at 13 years and survival is 97% ± 2%.

The excellent long-term function of the Ross operation in our patients and similar results which are being reported by other investigators strongly suggest that in children and young adults, the Ross operation may be the preferred procedure for replacement of the aortic valve.

References

1. Ross DN. Replacement of aortic and mitral valves with a pulmonary autograft. Lancet 1967;2:956–8.
2. The International Registry for the Ross Procedure. http://www.rossregistry.com (accessed Aug 8, 2002).
3. Oswalt JD, Dewan SJ, Mueller MC, Nelson S. Highlights of a ten-year experience with the Ross procedure. Ann Thorac Surg 2001;71:S332–5.
4. Schmidtke C, Bechtel JF, Noetzold A, Sievers HH. Up to seven years of experience with the Ross procedure in patients >60 years of age. J Am Coll Cardiol 2000; 36(4):1173–7.
5. Chambers JC, Somerville J, Stone S, Ross DN. Pulmonary autograft procedure for aortic valve disease: long-term results of the pioneer series. Circulation 1997;96: 2206–14.
6. Elkins RC, Lane MM, McCue C, Ward KE. Pulmonary autograft root replacement: mid-term results. J Heart Valve Dis 1999;8:499–506.
7. Stelzer P, Weinrauch S, Tranbaugh RF. Ten years of experience with the modified Ross procedure. J Thorac Cardiovasc Surg 1998;115:1091–100.
8. Al Halees Z, Pieters F, Qadoura F, et al. The Ross procedure is the procedure of choice for congenital aortic valve disease. J Thorac Cardiovasc Surg 2002;123(3):437–41.

9. David TE, de Sa MPL, Ivanov J, et al. Dilation of the pulmonary autograft after the Ross procedure. J Thorac Cardiovasc Surg 2000;119:210–8.

10. Laudito A, Brook MM, Suleman S, et al. The Ross procedure in children and young adults: a word of caution. J Thorac Cardiovasc Surg 2001;122(1):147–53.

11. Luciani GB, Barozzi L, Tomezzoli A, et al. Bicuspid aortic valve disease and pulmonary autograft root dilatation after the Ross procedure: a clinicopathologic study. J Thorac Cardiovasc Surg 2001;122(1):74–9.

12. Schmidtke C, Bechtel M, Hueppe M, Sievers HH. Time course of aortic valve function and root dimensions after subcoronary Ross procedure for bicuspid versus tricuspid aortic valve disease. Circulation 2001;104(12 Suppl 1):I21–4.

13. Bohm JO, Botha CA, Hemmer W, et al. The Ross operation in 225 patients: a five-year experience in aortic root replacement. J Heart Valve Dis 2001;10(6):742–9.

14. Carr-White GS, Afoke A, Birks EJ, et al. Aortic root characteristics of human pulmonary autografts. Circulation 2000;102(19 Suppl 3):III15–21.

15. U.S. opportunities in heart valve disease management. Health Research International. Cleveland (OH): Health Research International; May 2002.

16. Elkins RC, Lane MM, McCue C. Pulmonary autograft reoperation: incidence and management. Ann Thorac Surg 1996;62:450–5.

17. Kouchoukos NT, Davila-Roman VG, Spray TL, et al. Replacement of the aortic root with a pulmonary autograft in children and young adults with aortic valve disease. N Engl J Med 1994;330:1–6.

18. Kirklin JW, Barratt-Boyes BG. Cardiac surgery. 2nd ed. New York: Churchill Livingstone; 1993.

19. Capps SB, Elkins RC, Fronk DM. Body surface area as a predictor of aortic and pulmonary valve diameter. J Thorac Cardiovasc Surg 2000;119:975–82.

20. David TE, Omran A, Webb G, et al. Geometric mismatch of the aortic and pulmonary roots causes aortic insufficiency after the Ross procedure. J Thorac Cardiovasc Surg 1996;112:1231–9.

21. Ross D, Jackson M, Davies J. Pulmonary autograft aortic valve replacement: long-term results. J Card Surg 1991; 6:529–33.

22. Gerosa G, McKay R, Ross DN. Replacement of the aortic valve or root with a pulmonary autograft in children. Ann Thorac Surg 1991;51:424–9.

23. Ward C. Clinical significance of the bicuspid aortic valve. Heart 2000;83:81–5.

CHAPTER 19

Surgical Management of Chronic Thromboembolic Pulmonary Hypertension

Michael S. Mulligan, MD

Each year in the United States, 500,000 to 600,000 symptomatic pulmonary emboli are diagnosed. These emboli account for or contribute to approximately 150,000 deaths annually.[1]

In the vast majority of patients, the clots resolve completely, and minimal irregularities or obstructions are left within the pulmonary arteries. However, in 0.1 to 0.5% of these patients, the resolution of the thromboembolism is incomplete and, ultimately, these patients progress to the development of chronic thromboembolic pulmonary hypertension (CTEPH).[2] From these statistics it can be inferred that between 500 and 2,500 new cases of CTEPH are generated each year in the United States. Only 150 to 175 operations are performed each year for CTEPH in North America, which implies that this disease is both underdiagnosed and grossly undertreated. It is difficult to identify patients at risk for developing CTEPH, because 90% of the patients have no discernible abnormality in coagulation. Approximately 10% of these patients have a lupus anticoagulant, and fewer than 1% of patients will have anti-thrombin[3] (AT[3]) deficiencies, protein C or S deficiencies, or other coagulopathies.[3]

Clinical Presentation

A history of prior symptomatic pulmonary embolus is not readily documented in many of these patients. Without that history, the diagnosis can be particularly difficult to make and is often quite delayed. Not uncommonly, however, a patient will provide a history of having had a large pulmonary embolus. Typically, the therapy for that event will have been entirely appropriate. Other patients may report that the diagnosis was not made until some months after the acute event or perhaps that therapy was suboptimal. After stabilization following the inciting embolic event, there is typically partial clinical improvement associated with partial clot lysis. At this stage, patients may, in fact, feel relatively well. This "honeymoon period" is characterized by minimal symptoms and may last months to years. Subsequently, however, patients begin to develop dyspnea on exertion.[4] Because there are a multitude of diagnoses associated with dyspnea on exertion and because CTEPH is less common, the diagnosis is not usually made at this stage. Patients then progress to hypoxemia and will ultimately manifest signs and symptoms of right-heart failure.[5] It was believed that the reason for this progression was recurrent pulmonary emboli. Although this certainly may be true, a number of these patients will progress with vena caval filters in place on appropriate anticoagulation. Repeated ventilation/perfusion scans will demonstrate persistent abnormalities but no new defects. In such patients, and in many of these patients in general, there appears to be a secondary fibroproliferative response within the pulmonary arteries and a plexogenic arteriopathy that develops, producing progressively more distal obstructions. Such arteriopathy can be found in regions of the pulmonary vascular bed that are distal to points of obstruction and also in segments that are not related to any obstructing lesion or thrombus. It is possible that the unobstructed segments are subjected to excessive flow, which, in turn, causes vascular injury. This could conceivably potentiate the development of such an obstructive arteriopathy. If this were entirely responsible, however, one would not see the arteriopathy in arterial segments that are distal to a point of anatomic obstruction.

The earliest symptom of CTEPH is exertional dyspnea that can at times be debilitating. In some patients, the minimal exertion associated with having a conversation in the clinic can produce significant hypoxemia. Younger patients may be relatively asymptomatic at rest but may become profoundly short of breath with minimal exercise.[5] Patients with coronary disease may present with angina. Alternatively, excessive right-heart strain can also produce angina, even in the absence of significant coronary obstructions.

Most patients will relate a history of light-headedness or of possible syncope if questioned carefully. This is more common following a cough or other maneuvers that elicit a forced expiration of air and produce a transient increase in pulmonary vascular resistance. Exercise produces a relative increase in pulmonary vascular resistance because it relates to systemic vascular resistance. In such a scenario, because the pulmonary vascular resistance is fixed, as oxygen demands increase with exercise and there is peripheral systemic vascular relaxation, patients are unable to mount an increase in cardiac output to compensate for dilation, and their blood pressure drops. Ultimately, this will result in lightheadedness and/or syncope.

The *physical examination* may be quite normal early in the course of the disease. However, the majority of patients will manifest some degree of lower extremity swelling. Because many patients' original problem was a deep venous thrombosis, some component of this may be secondary to a chronic postphlebitic syndrome.[6] However, with increasing right-sided pressures, tricuspid insufficiency worsens and venous hypertension will exacerbate the swelling. Ascites is present in approximately 40% of patients. The fluid wave may be subtle in some patients, but in others, it is quite pronounced. The subcutaneous vasculature is more prominent on the torso (although not nearly to the degree that one sees with a superior vena cava syndrome), and jugular venous distension is often obvious.[7] There is a fixed split of S2 with a loud pulmonic component. At times, a right ventricular heave is evident; less commonly, a right ventricular S3 can be detected. A murmur of tricuspid insufficiency is typically obvious; however, murmurs of pulmonary insufficiency are uncommon. While many of the findings described would also apply to pulmonary hypertension of other etiologies, one can also begin to distinguish CTEPH from small-resistance vessel disease on physical examination. Specifically, there are continuous machine-like murmurs heard over the lung fields.[8] These may not be appreciated until the patient is asked to hold the breath. The murmurs are caused by turbulent flow through recanalized partially obstructed vessels. In patients with primary pulmonary hypertension (PPH), such murmurs are not heard.

Diagnostic Evaluation

The diagnostic evaluation often begins long before the patient presents to a surgeon. Without attention, the evaluation can quickly become redundant or misdirected. Therefore, it is important to organize existing information and order further studies with three specific goals in mind:
1. To determine whether the patient has pulmonary hypertension and assess its severity.
2. To determine the etiology of that pulmonary hypertension.
3. To determine whether the patient's disease is surgically accessible.

Blood tests tend to be nonspecific. Findings are consistent with manifestations of chronic hypoxemia and a low cardiac output state. Some degree of secondary polycythemia is common. Nonspecific liver function test (LFT) abnormalities, presumably caused by hepatic congestion, are seen, and increased blood urea nitrogen (BUN) and urate levels are commonly associated with a low cardiac output. The partial thromboplastin time may also be slightly prolonged although the reasons for this are not entirely clear.[8]

Not surprisingly, the electrocardiography demonstrates right ventricular hypertrophy and right ventricular strain. Large P waves associated with significant right atrial enlargement may be evident. Often, however, the cardiogram is relatively normal.

On chest x-ray films, one lung field may appear to have areas of increased or decreased vascular markings associated with regional hyperperfusion or hypoperfusion. Furthermore, there may be obvious enlargement of the central pulmonary arteries, occasionally with some degree of asymmetry. Because of marked right-heart enlargement, the cardiac silhouette may also appear to obliterate the retrosternal space on the lateral view (Figure 19-1).

Pulmonary function testing is critical. More important than documenting any specific numbers or threshold values, one must be able to recognize the pattern of abnormalities. Specifically, the symptoms and gas exchange abnormalities are far greater than any spirometric

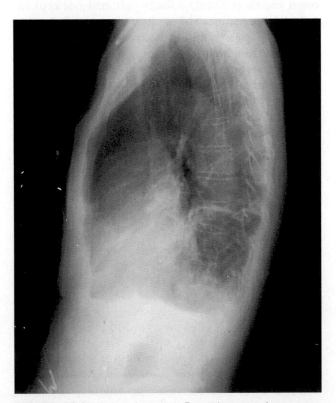

FIGURE 19-1. Lateral chest x-ray. Encroachment on the retrosternal space by right ventricular enlargement is notable.

defects.[9] There is often a significant reduction in diffusion capacity, and the patient's experience of dyspnea may be pronounced. However, there are typically less-restrictive or -obstructive defects. Chronic small pulmonary infarctions may result in some mild patchy peripheral pulmonary fibrosis that could produce a restrictive defect. With pulmonary arterial obstruction, there is a compensatory and often excessive development of bronchial collateral flow. As such, the bronchial mucosa may become quite congested, producing the mild, sometimes intermittent obstructive defect. Not surprisingly, with significant perfusion defects there is an increase in dead space and the minute ventilation may be significantly increased. If one sees primarily restrictive or obstructive defects, another explanation for the dyspnea may be present. Alternatively, patients with CTEPH may have other parenchymal lung disease that increases the risk of surgery or contraindicates it altogether.

The oxygen partial pressure (PO_2) on blood gas analysis is often low. If this is not the case at rest, there may be a precipitous decrease with exercise. This is partly caused by the patients' inability to increase their cardiac output adequately with exercise because of fixed obstructions to pulmonary blood flow. As they consume oxygen with exercise, their mixed venous oxygen content drops. Because reoxygenation is limited by inadequate cardiac output traversing functioning lung, progressive hypoxemia ensues. Furthermore, up to 25% of these patients have a patent foramen ovale.[10] With exercise, systemic vascular resistance drops and there is a rapid rise in pulmonary arterial and right-heart pressures. The resultant right-to-left shunting at the atrial level will further exacerbate any hypoxemia.

Echocardiography provides an estimate of pulmonary pressures and also screens for any coexistent cardiac pathology. Right atrial and ventricular enlargements are typically obvious (Figure 19-2), and both the atrial and ventricular septa may be displaced from right to left. The hypertensive right ventricle does not conform to the normally rounded left ventricle. Rather, as the ventricular septum is shifted from right to left, the left ventricle may assume a classic "D" shape (Figure 19-3). A patent foramen ovale is present in 25% of these patients; however, its detection may require an agitated saline contrast study. The tricuspid regurgitation is typically moderate to severe.[11] Once echocardiography has indicated the presence of pulmonary hypertension, the first goal of the diagnostic evaluation is essentially achieved. Next, one must try to discern the etiology of the pulmonary hypertension.

Ventilation/perfusion (V/Q) scanning typically demonstrates segmental or larger mismatched defects (Figure 19-4). With primary pulmonary hypertension, the defects may be patchy or subsegmental or the scan may be entirely normal. V/Q scanning better distinguishes between small-

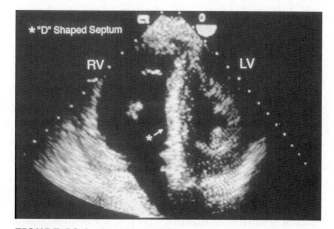

FIGURE 19-3. Significant right ventricular hypertension causes leftward shift of the intraventricular septum, producing the classic D-shaped left ventricle. LV = left ventricle; RV = right ventricle.

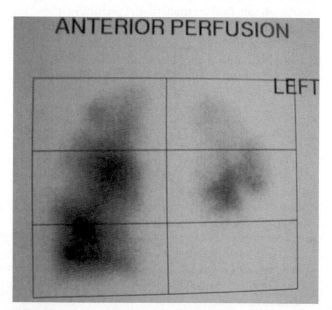

FIGURE 19-4. A significant defect in the left lower lobe is shown on perfusion scan.

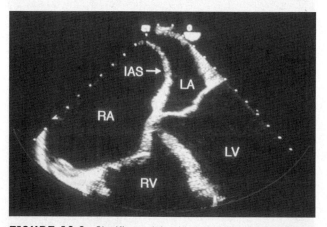

FIGURE 19-2. Significant right-sided chamber enlargement is obvious, and deflection of the interatrial septum (IAS) is shown. LA = left atrium; LV = left ventricle; RA = right atrium; RV = right ventricle.

resistance vessel disease and chronic thromboembolic pulmonary hypertension.[12] Unfortunately, V/Q scanning tends to underestimate the degree of central obstruction. Recanalized vessels may offer hemodynamic resistance to flow but still allow isotopes to reach the periphery. As a result, scans may look deceptively normal. Furthermore, V/Q scanning does not adequately demonstrate the magnitude, exact location, or proximal extent of the thickening of the diseased arterial wall.[8] Consequently, it is inappropriate to use V/Q scanning alone to select patients for operation. V/Q scanning is useful, however, as a screening tool to determine which patients should be referred for more invasive testing.

Once pulmonary hypertension has been documented by echocardiography and an etiology has been suggested by V/Q scanning, patients proceed to right-heart catheterization and pulmonary angiography. Although significant concerns linger about the safety of pulmonary angiography in these patients, those concerns largely relate to problems encountered in the past when ionic contrast was used and digital subtraction angiography was not available. It is best to wait at least several months after the initial inciting pulmonary embolus before proceeding with catheterization. This will allow for any potential resolution of thrombus that is likely to dissolve. One will therefore demonstrate the pathology that is likely to be encountered at surgery. The thrombus that remains may not have had time to become organized and fibrotic. This is critical as otherwise it may be too friable to be completely removed. Also, the risk of recurrent embolization with temporary cessation of anticoagulation is greatest during the first several months after an embolic event. Thus, it is prudent to defer invasive procedures until patients are out of that risk interval if there is high risk for recurrent thromboembolism.

Assessment of pulmonary pressures and pulmonary vascular resistance may require provocative exercise testing in order to demonstrate critical elevations.[8] This is particularly true in younger patients who are only symptomatic with exertion. Although there may be mild elevations in pulmonary pressures with exertion in many patients, patients with CTEPH typically demonstrate a steep rise in pressures with minimal exertion. This may be the only way to demonstrate that patients with relatively normal pressures at rest have a valid physiologic explanation for their symptoms.

Venous access is preferably obtained via the neck in order to avoid disturbing possible residual iliofemoral thrombus. Patients require careful monitoring in the radiology suite, and it is preferable to use one power injection with limited volume per side. Selective injections should be used only when absolutely necessary to provide detail important to operative decision making. The nature of their pathophysiology implies that these patients typically have significantly increased intravascular volume, and excessive use of contrasts can lead to cardiopulmonary

decompensation. To optimize the efficiency of the studies and to limit the number of injections, it is preferable for the surgeon to be present in the angiography suite in order to assist in the selection of quality views. Typical findings of CTEPH include pouch defects (produced by spherical filling defects), webs or bands, intimal irregularities, and/or abrupt narrowing of pulmonary branch vessels. Normal branching patterns should produce a gradual tapering of arterial caliber. In CTEPH, the caliber may narrow abruptly with loss of peripheral arborization or delayed filling of segmental and subsegmental vessels (Figures 19-5 and 19-6).[13]

Defining the proximal extent of disease is essential for determining surgical accessibility. As such, adjunctive studies are often used to confirm the site where thickening of the vessel wall or luminal irregularities begins. Intravascular ultrasonography has been used with limited experience but does appear to have reasonably good correlation with surgical findings. The limitation with this technology is that the probes are quite small and only provide information about the wall they are in contact with. With dilated central arteries, the views generated are very limited and far from circumferential. Pulmonary angioscopy[14] has been used at a single institution, but the techniques used are difficult to reproduce and the images

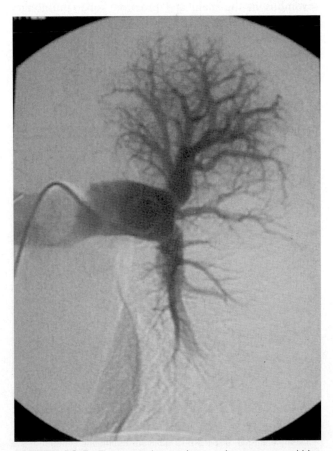

FIGURE 19-5. These arteriogram images demonstrate webbing and loss of proper arborization in the left lower lobe branches.

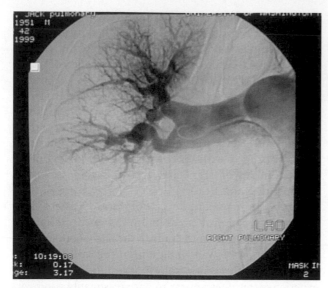

FIGURE 19-6. This pulmonary arteriogram also demonstrates areas of webbing, rapid tapering, post-stenotic dilatation, and a complete absence of perfusion to the right lower lobe.

generated can be troublesome to interpret. I currently employ spiral computed tomography (CT) scanning[15] with a pulmonary arterial–specific protocol in order to examine for thickening of the arterial walls and residual thrombus in the main and proximal lobar pulmonary arteries (Figure 19-7).

Any patient who presents with angina, men over the age of 40 years, and women over the age of 50 years typically undergo left-heart catheterization in order to rule out coexisting coronary artery disease. If significant coro-

nary disease is identified, revascularization is planned concurrently with pulmonary endarterectomy.

Surgical Selection

After the diagnostic examination is complete, proper selection of patients for surgical intervention can occur. Candidates for operation must have pulmonary vascular obstructive disease with significant hemodynamic and cardiopulmonary impairment. A pulmonary vascular resistance of at least 300 dyn/sec/cm^{-5} at rest or after exercise should be seen. The thrombi should also be surgically accessible. The recent development of a classification scheme of the anatomic distribution has been helpful in identifying appropriate patients. Type I disease is associated with obvious central thrombus. Type II disease demonstrates no major vessel thrombus but rather intimal thickening and webs at the main lobar and segmental level. Type III disease describes disease that is restricted to the segmental and subsegmental levels. Finally, type IV disease affects only very peripheral resistance vessels and is nonoperative. Types I and II disease are quite amenable to endarterectomy, but type III disease should be approached only by the surgeon experienced in pulmonary endarterectomy. Ideally, the proximal dissection plane should start in the main pulmonary artery (PA), but one would hope to see disease at least as proximal as the original lobar vessels. If disease starts in the lobar vessels or more distally, the plane has to be started with freehand knife dissection at that level. This is particularly hazardous because perforation at this level is exceedingly difficult to repair and may be associated with fatal hemorrhage.[10] As one would suspect, pulmonary resections for perforations beyond the lobar level are not tolerated well in this population.

Patients selected for endarterectomy should also have limited comorbidities. Significant parenchymal lung disease is a risk factor for prolonged postoperative mechanical ventilation, limited improvement in dyspnea, and mortality. Peripheral vascular disease is also a strong relative contraindication. Chronic renal insufficiency makes postoperative fluid management and establishment of a brisk and timely diuresis troublesome. Those with compromised renal function tend not to fare as well. When considering patients older than 80 years of age, one should be very selective.

Finally, patients must understand and accept the risks of surgery. In addition to complications that are relatively common to open heart surgery, there are added risks associated with circulatory arrest and operating on patients in advanced stages of right-heart failure. A generous amount of time should be spent with patients and their families, counseling them on the specifics of the operation, the anticipated postoperative course, and the potential complications. In general, patients are very enthusiastic about surgical intervention after the natural history of their

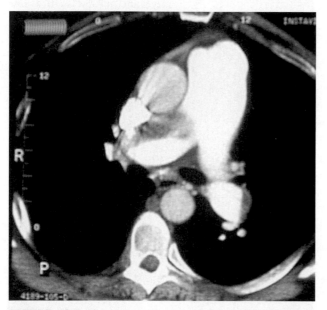

FIGURE 19-7. The central pulmonary arteries on this CT scan are markedly enlarged, and there is subacute thrombotic material in the proximal right main pulmonary artery (PA) as well as the left PA at the level of the lobar bifurcation.

disease has been explained. Once mean pulmonary arterial pressures exceed 30 mm Hg, the 5-year survival is only 30%. Once that pressure exceeds 50 mm Hg, the 5-year survival is only 10%.[16] The majority of the patients that I have cared for have had mean PA pressures averaging nearly 50 mm Hg, which infers a 90% risk of death over the next 5 years. Given the current perioperative survival rate of >90% at the University of Washington, the risks and extensive nature of this surgical operation are justified and seen as quite acceptable by my patients.

All patients must have a preoperative inferior vena cava (IVC) filter placed if anatomically possible; that is, if the IVC is not completely obstructed. The filter is extremely important in the prevention of recurrent thromboembolism.

Surgical Technique

The pulmonary arterial and bronchial arterial systems provide a unique dual blood supply to the lung tissue. When the pulmonary arterial system becomes obstructed, the nutrient bronchial flow maintains tissue viability. Accordingly, when the obstructions to pulmonary arterial flow are relieved, the lung can again participate in normal gas exchange. Unfortunately, however, bronchial collateral flow can also significantly obscure operative visualization (even on full cardiopulmonary bypass). Consequently, certain technical maneuvers must be undertaken to compensate for this.

This operation is not an embolectomy or the so-called Trendelenburg procedure, done for acute pulmonary emboli. The simple removal of residual central thrombus will not result in an effective reduction in pulmonary vascular resistance. Rather, the operation requires an actual endarterectomy with the dissection plane that is in the middle of the media.[17] A dissection plane that is too superficial will not achieve the appropriate hemodynamic result, and one that is too deep runs the risk of perforation.[10] A plane that is too deep yields a pink, raw appearance to the remaining vascular wall. This is the adventitia, and the dissection should be redirected to a more superficial plane.

The operation must be considered a bilateral procedure, even if angiography suggests a predominance of disease on one side. The obstruction must be relieved on both sides. This will allow for a optimal redistribution of pulmonary blood flow, improved oxygenation, and, ultimately, maximal perioperative and long-term survival. Therefore, the operation is conducted through a median sternotomy and not through a thoracotomy.[18]

To optimize visualization and counter the impaired visualization imposed by excessive bronchial collateral flow, the operation is performed using cardiopulmonary bypass and deep hypothermic circulatory arrest.

To expose the right pulmonary artery, extensive mobilization of the superior vena cava (SVC) is required. Using the cautery will limit bleeding at the end of the case, but great care must be taken to avoid injury to the phrenic nerve. Cardiopulmonary bypass is commenced with ascending aortic cannulation and venous drainage via the right atrium or bicaval access, depending on whether a patent foramen ovale has been detected on an agitated saline contrast echocardiogram. The left ventricle is vented via the right superior pulmonary vein. After the patient is cooled to 18°C, an aortic cross-clamp is applied and cardioplegia is administered. The SVC is retracted anteriorly and laterally, and the aorta is retracted medially to expose the main right PA. An incision is made in the right PA from underneath the aorta out toward the lower lobe division. This dissection is contained within the pericardium. In general, any central thrombus can be removed prior to circulatory arrest. After raising the endarterectomy plane in the main PA, it is carried out to the segmental and then on to the subsegmental vessels. Intermittent circulatory arrest is used, with arrest periods lasting no more than 20 min. Between arrest periods, cardiopulmonary bypass is recommenced for 10 min or until the mixed venous saturation returns to 90%. After completion of the right side, the vessel is closed with running 5–0 polypropylene suture, and the retraction on the aorta and SVC is released. Additional cardioplegia may be administered at this time. The heart is retracted anteriorly and to the right, and the left pulmonary artery is opened from the main PA into the left PA and extends to the pericardial reflection. An endarterectomy is then performed on that side, the patient is reperfused, and the left PA closed. The specimen is reconstructed on the back table and typically demonstrates some degree of acute or subacute thrombus, with the more mature fibrotic disease originating at the segmental level and beyond (Figures 19-8 and 19-9). If echocardiography demonstrated a patent foramen ovale, or if significant suspicion exists, the atrial

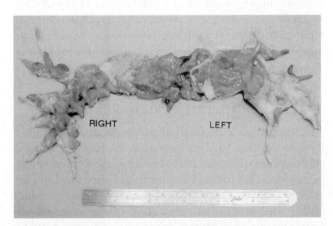

FIGURE 19-8. This specimen is from a 74-year-old woman with a chronic history of thromboembolic pulmonary hypertension. The peripheral material represents fibrocalcific plaques liberated from the segmental and subsegmental levels, while the more central material represents subacute on chronic thromboembolic material.

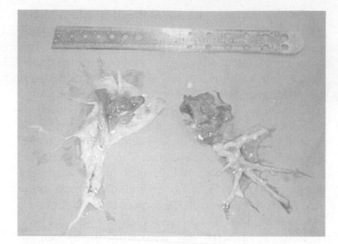

FIGURE 19-9. This specimen from a 50-year-old male athlete demonstrates the classic fibroproliferative obstructions which taper out nicely to the segmental and subsegmental levels. A more limited amount of subacute on chronic thromboembolic material is present centrally.

septum is inspected after rewarming has begun. Likewise, any revascularization or adjunctive procedures may be undertaken at this point if they were not completed during cooling. It is critical to use gradual cooling and warming so as to accomplish more uniform tissue temperatures and optimize metabolic protection. Maintaining an 8° to 10°C gradient while rewarming may also help limit reperfusion injury that would otherwise be exacerbated by a hyperthermic perfusate. Phenytoin was used with good effect for postoperative seizures that were observed early in the University of California, San Diego experience. Barbiturates are used to ensure the electroencephalographic silence after the patient is cooled to 18°C systemically.

Specific tricuspid valve repair is generally not required. There is marked resolution of the tricuspid regurgitation that occurs to a great degree in the operating room and continues postoperatively. This relates to right ventricular remodeling that occurs acutely after surgery. Valvular regurgitation is typically absent by 4 to 5 days postoperatively.[10]

Postoperative Management

In the past, patients received prostaglandin infusions.[10] These were associated with systemic hypotension and are not used currently. Similarly, concerns about mediastinal hemorrhage led to the abandonment of left atrial lines for pressor delivery. Every attempt should be made to minimize pulmonary vascular resistance. A target carbon dioxide partial pressure (Pco_2) on blood gas analysis of 30 to 35 mm Hg is desirable but permissive hypercapnia is acceptable when oxygenation is problematic. The fraction of inspired oxygen (F_IO_2) is minimized so long as oxygen saturations of 92% are maintained. Inhaled nitric oxide

may be helpful for potentiating the reductions in pulmonary vascular resistance that will develop over time, as well as for mitigating reperfusion injury. Inverse ratio and pressure control ventilation have at times been helpful, and minimizing plateau inspiratory pressures should be strongly considered. Subcutaneous heparin and the use of sequential compression devices are begun immediately postoperatively, and warfarin (Coumadin) or fractionated-heparin therapy is initiated 48 h after surgery and maintained for life. As mentioned, these patients generally have increased intravascular and interstitial volumes. With the abrupt reduction in pulmonary vascular resistance produced by surgery, they will typically require assisted diuresis beginning 24 h following surgery. This diuresis can be brisk and sustained.

Postoperative Complications

At the University of Washington, the 30-day mortality rate is 8%. Considerably higher mortality rates have been reported in the literature, and anecdotal institutional reports have revealed prohibitive perioperative mortality. Certainly, as institutional experience and, in particular, a single surgeon's experience is gained, mortality rates decline. The University of Washington's results are now on par with those of the most experienced centers.[19]

In a recent report from the University of California, San Diego, the most common cause of 30-day mortality was unrelieved pulmonary hypertension.[10] Less commonly, mediastinal hemorrhage, intraoperative cardiac arrest, and severe reperfusion pulmonary edema were cited. Cerebral vascular accidents accounted for several deaths, and cannulation site dissections resulted in two deaths.[10]

Complications that are not specific to pulmonary endarterectomy but which are associated with cardiac surgery in general include arrhythmias, atelectasis, wound infections, and phrenic nerve injury (particularly the right) because of the required SVC mobilization. Delirium or mental status changes occur in 10% of patients, but virtually all of these problems are transient. Pericardial infusions may develop late in the postoperative course. To prevent tamponade, the posterior pericardium can be fenestrated, or a closed suction drain can be left in place.

Reperfusion pulmonary edema develops in 10 to 25% of patients. It is often mild but may be hemorrhagic and fatal.[20] No preoperative factors reliably predict its development. It typically manifests within 8 to 12 h of operation but may not develop for up to 72 h. It only develops in previously obstructed segments and therefore may have a patchy appearance on x-ray film as compared to reperfusion injury, which may develop after lung transplantation. Therapy is generally supportive although a brief pulse of steroids may be helpful. Pulmonary arterial steal can also develop in 10 to 15% of patients and is associated with significant hypoxemia.[21] The diseased segments that underwent endarterectomy will have a lower resistance than will relatively nondiseased segments that were not manipulated. Unfortunately, because the manipulated (lower-resistance) segments are the only ones vulnerable to reperfusion injury, the preponderance of pulmonary blood flow may be directed to the most edematous. Much of the resultant hypoxemia will resolve over the first several days postoperatively, but 7 to 10 days of mechanical ventilation may be required. Ultimately, the pulmonary circulation patterns will normalize completely over 6 to 8 weeks, and patients should no longer require any supplemental oxygen.

Results

Significant improvements in cardiopulmonary hemodynamics are seen immediately after operation. Additionally, the pulmonary vascular resistance may continue to fall over the first few days or weeks after surgery. In the initial series at the University of Washington, the mean pulmonary arterial pressures fell from 48 mm Hg preoperatively to 22 mm Hg postoperatively (Figure 19-10).[22] Pulmonary vascular resistance fell dramatically (Figure 19-11), and the cardiac output nearly tripled (Figure 19-12). Tricuspid regurgitation resolved in virtually all patients (Figure 19-13), and New York Heart Association (NYHA) class improved from a mean of 3.7 to 1.3 postoperatively (Figure 19-14).

In addition to profound improvement in hemodynamics, lower extremity edema resolved or significantly improved in up to 90% of patients. Some lower extremity edema likely persisted because some of those patients had chronic postphlebitic syndrome from previous deep venous thromboses. Ascites likewise resolves in virtually all patients that achieve the desired hemodynamic result. Although up to 75% of patients may require supplemental oxygen at the time of discharge, nearly all patients are off of oxygen at follow-up 6 to 8 weeks later.

Pulmonary Vascular Resistance

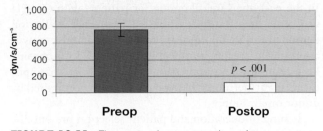

FIGURE 19-11. The mean pulmonary vascular resistance preoperatively was 760, which dropped to 120 postoperatively.

Cardiac Output

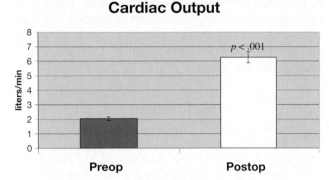

FIGURE 19-12. The cardiac output preoperatively averaged 2.0 L and rose to 6.2 L postoperatively.

Tricuspid Regurgitation

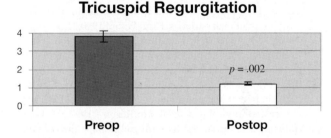

FIGURE 19-13. Tricuspid regurgitation was moderate to severe in all patients preoperatively, and trace to non-existent in the vast majority postoperatively.

Pulmonary Arterial Pressure

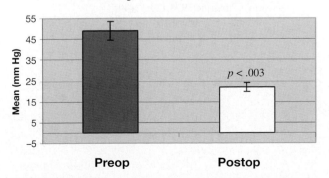

FIGURE 19-10. The preoperative mean pulmonary arterial pressure in the initial University of Washington experience was 48 mm Hg, which dropped to 22 mm Hg postoperatively.

NYHA Class

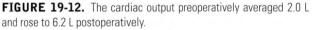

FIGURE 19-14. The New York Heart Association (NYHA) class was 3 to 4 in nearly all patients preoperatively and approached class I in most patients postoperatively. These results appear durable and are supported with at least 6 months of follow-up data for all patients.

Conclusion

In the past, the surgical option for patients with CTEPH was often lung transplantation.[23] If thorough evaluation demonstrates that pulmonary thromboendarterectomy is appropriate, treatment can obviate the need for chronic long-term immunosuppression and its associated complications. Furthermore, these operations are not limited by donor organ supply.

Timing of operation and patient selection present difficult issues. Acceptable morbidity and mortality have been achieved in a limited number of centers, however, largely due to the experience and skill of multidisciplinary teams that work together during patient evaluation, surgery, and postoperative care. Five-year survival in patients without operation is severely limited. With an acceptable 30-day mortality, pulmonary endarterectomy can convey a marked survival benefit to appropriately selected patients.

References

1. Dalen JE, Alpert JS. Natural history of pulmonary embolism. Prog Cardiovasc Dis 1975;17:257–70.
2. Benotti JR, Ockene IS, Alpert JS, Dalen JE. The clinical profile of unresolved pulmonary embolism. Chest 1983;84:669–78.
3. Auger WR, Permpikul P, Moser KM. Lupus anticoagulant, heparin use, and thrombocytopenia in patients with chronic thromboembolic pulmonary hypertension: a preliminary report. Am J Med 1995;99:392–6.
4. Presti B, Berthrong M, Sherwin RM. Chronic thrombosis of major pulmonary arteries. Hum Pathol 1990;21:601–6.
5. Moser KM, Auger WR, Fedullo PF. Chronic major-vessel thromboembolic pulmonary hypertension. Circulation 1990;81:1735–43.
6. Moser KM, Auger WR, Fedullo PF, Jamieson SW. Chronic thromboembolic pulmonary hypertension: clinical picture and surgical treatment. Eur Respir J 1992;5:334–42.
7. Mulligan MS. Initial results with pulmonary thromboendarectomy for chronic thromboembolic pulmonary hypertension. Proceedings of the Seattle Surgical Society; Jan 2000.
8. Fedullo PF, Auger WR, Channick RN, et al. Chronic thromboembolic pulmonary hypertension. Clin Chest Med 1995;16:353–74.
9. Morris TA, Auger WR, Ysrael MZ, et al. Parenchymal scarring is associated with restrictive spirometric defects in patients with chronic thromboembolic pulmonary hypertension. Chest 1996;110:399–403.
10. Jamieson SW, Auger WR, Fedullo PF, et al. Experience and results of 150 pulmonary thromboendarterectomy operations over a 29-month period. J Thorac Cardiovasc Surg 1993;106:116–27.
11. Chow LC, Dittrich HC, Hoit BD, et al. Doppler assessment of changes in right-sided cardiac hemodynamics after pulmonary thromboendarterectomy. Am J Cardiol 1988;61:1092–7.
12. Moser KM, Page GT, Ashburn WL, Fedullo PF. Perfusion lung scans provide a guide to which patients with apparent primary pulmonary hypertension merit angiography. West J Med 1988;148:167–70.
13. Auger WR, Fedullo PF, Moser KM, et al. Chronic major-vessel thromboembolic pulmonary artery obstruction: appearance at angiography. Radiology 1992;182:393–8.
14. Shure D, Gregoratos G, Moser KM. Fiberoptic angioscopy: role in the diagnosis of chronic pulmonary arterial obstruction. Ann Intern Med 1985;103:844–50.
15. Bergin CJ, Sirlin CB, Hauschildt JP, et al. Chronic thromboembolism: diagnosis with helical CT and MR imaging with angiographic and surgical correlation. Radiology 1997;204:695–702.
16. Riedel M, Stanek V, Widimsky J, Prerovsky I. Long term follow-up of patients with pulmonary embolism: late prognosis and evolution of hemodynamic and respiratory data. Chest 1982;81:151–8.
17. Daily PO, Johnson GG, Simmons CJ, Moser KM. Surgical management of chronic pulmonary embolism. J Thorac Cardiovasc Surg 1980;79:523–31.
18. Jamieson SW. Pulmonary thromboendarterectomy [editorial]. Heart 1998;79:118–20.
19. Jamieson SW, Kapelanski DP. Pulmonary endarterectomy. Curr Prob Surg 2000;37:165–252.
20. Levinson RM, Shure D, Moser KM. Reperfusion pulmonary edema after pulmonary artery thromboendarterectomy. Am Rev Respir Dis 1986;134:1241–5.
21. Olman MA, Auger WR, Fedullo PF, Moser KM. Pulmonary vascular steal in chronic thromboembolic pulmonary hypertension. Chest 1990;98:1430–4.
22. Mulligan MS. Early results with pulmonary thromboendarterectomy for chronic thromboembolic pulmonary hypertension. Proc Wash Am Coll Surg 2000. p. 15.
23. Dartevelle P, Fadel E, Chapelier A, et al. Pulmonary thromboendarterectomy with video-angioscopy and circulatory arrest: an alternative to cardiopulmonary transplantation and post-embolism pulmonary artery hypertension. Chirurgie 1998;123:32–40.

CHAPTER 20

UPDATE ON NEW TISSUE VALVES

W. R. ERIC JAMIESON, MD

Biologic (tissue) and mechanical prostheses have been used for valve replacement surgery for 30 years.[1,2] Although there have been extensive advancements over the years, residual problems still exist with both mechanical and biologic prostheses. These advancements were introduced to reduce or eliminate deterioration, thromboembolism, and anticoagulant-related hemorrhage, as well as to optimize hemodynamic performance.

The continuing problems with mechanical prostheses are thrombus formation from blood stasis and the resultant thromboembolic phenomena, despite anticoagulant therapy, which has an inherent risk of hemorrhage. Biologic prostheses, both porcine and pericardial, are at risk of structural failure over time, with leaflet degeneration and dystrophic calcification occurring either individually or in combination.[3–18]

The current generations of both biologic and mechanical prostheses were developed to address these complications. The present biologic valvular prostheses were developed with tissue preservation techniques to reduce structural failure, together with or without stent designs, contributing to preservation of the anatomic characteristics and biomechanical properties of the leaflets.

This chapter provides an update on modern cardiac biologic/tissue valvular substitutes that are new or relatively new to the United States market.[12,19] These biologic prostheses have been on the worldwide market for time intervals ranging from less than 1 year to 20 years.[19] The chapter also discusses investigational prostheses under regulatory control, as well as emerging technologies. The characteristics of these biologic prostheses are detailed to provide an informative understanding for cardiac surgeons and cardiologists. Special attention is given to the performance or anticipated performance of these prostheses.[20] The valve-related complications and the risk factors of these complications are discussed to support a rational approach for selection of biologic prostheses with consideration of comorbidity and factors affecting hemodynamic performance.[20] The emerging innovative investigational technologies will likely significantly improve the clinical performance of biologic prostheses in the future. The same can be said of the advancing technologies with mechanical rigid prostheses.[12] The future may see emerging tissue-engineered prostheses or mechanical flexible polymer prostheses.

The biologic valvular prostheses are formulated from porcine aortic valves or bovine (and, recently, equine) pericardium. Table 20-1 lists the biologic tissue prostheses considered of either current or new generation marketed in the United States. Table 20-2 lists the biologic prostheses marketed outside of the United States. Some of these prostheses are investigational or soon to be investigational under regulatory protocols.

The natural aortic porcine valve used to formulate both stented and stentless bioprostheses possesses unique architectural and material characteristics consistent with functional requirements. Porcine bioprostheses have had tissue preservation at high pressure, at low pressure, or pressure free, with glutaraldehyde to preserve bioprosthetic function and provide durability. This tissue preservation, together with stent designs, contributes to the anatomic characteristics and biomechanical properties of the leaflets. The first-generation porcine bioprostheses—Hancock standard and Carpentier-Edwards standard—had the porcine tissue fixed with glutaraldehyde at high pressure, 60 to 80 mm Hg.[12] The current-generation porcine prostheses are either low (< 2 mm Hg) pressure, low pressure followed by high pressure, or zero pressure glutaraldehyde-fixed prostheses.[19] The bovine pericardial prostheses have used pressure-free fixation with glutaraldehyde; the current generation has used advanced engineering to formulate the tissue-stent relationship.[19] The advanced-generation bovine bioprostheses are being formulated with alternative stent formulations or without a stent.[19]

TABLE 20-1. Bioprostheses: Current (United States and Worldwide)

Stented porcine (aortic and mitral)
  Hancock II porcine bioprosthesis
  Medtronic Mosaic porcine bioprosthesis
  Carpentier-Edwards SAV Supra-Annular porcine bioprosthesis (aortic only)

Stentless porcine (aortic)
  St. Jude Medical–Toronto SPV stentless porcine bioprosthesis
  Medtronic Freestyle stentless porcine bioprosthesis
  Edwards Prima Plus stentless porcine bioprosthesis

Stented pericardial (aortic and mitral)
  Carpentier-Edwards PERIMOUNT pericardial bioprosthesis

TABLE 20-2. Bioprostheses: Current or Investigational/Developmental (Worldwide)

Stented porcine (aortic and mitral)
St. Jude Medical Epic porcine bioprosthesis (St. Jude Medical–Biocor porcine bioprosthesis)
Carbomedics Synergy ST porcine bioprosthesis (Labcor porcine bioprosthesis)
AorTech Aspire porcine bioprosthesis
Carpentier–Edwards SAV Supra-Annular porcine bioprosthesis (mitral)

Stentless porcine (aortic)
Cryolife–O'Brien stentless porcine bioprosthesis
St. Jude Medical–Toronto SPV Duo Stentless Root porcine bioprosthesis
AorTech Aspire stentless porcine bioprosthesis
Shelhigh Skeletonized Super-Stentless aortic porcine bioprosthesis
Carbomedics Oxford stentless aortic bioprosthesis
St. Jude Medical–Biocor stentless porcine bioprosthesis
Labcor stentless porcine bioprosthesis
AorTech Elan stentless porcine bioprosthesis

Stented pericardial (aortic and mitral)
Carpentier-Edwards PERIMOUNT Magna pericardial bioprosthesis (only aortic)
Mitroflow Synergy PC pericardial bioprosthesis (only aortic)
St. Jude Medical–Biocor pericardial bioprosthesis
Sorin Pericarbon MØRE pericardial bioprosthesis
Labcor pericardial bioprosthesis

Stentless pericardial (aortic and mitral)
Sorin Pericarbon Freedom stentless pericardial bioprosthesis (aortic)
3F pericardial equine stentless bioprosthesis (aortic and mitral)
St. Jude Medical Quattro stentless bioprosthesis (mitral)
Edwards Alex flexible pericardial bioprosthesis (aortic)

Stentless porcine and pericardial (pulmonary)
Cryolife–Ross stentless porcine pulmonary bioprosthesis
Medtronic–Venpro Contegra pulmonary valved conduit
Shelhigh porcine pulmonary valve conduit
CryoSyner graft valve

Stentless porcine (mitral)
Medtronic physiologic mitral valve (PMV)

Allografts
CryoValve Aortic valve with/without conduit
CryoValve Pulmonary valve with conduit
CryoValve Mitral valve

Autografts
Pulmonary autograft for aortic root and pulmonary allograft for pulmonary root
Autologous pericardial aortic valve

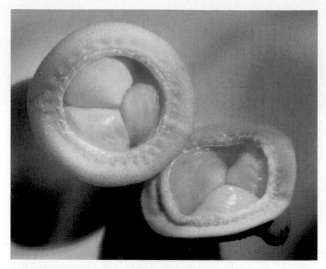

FIGURE 20-1. The Hancock II porcine bioprosthesis.

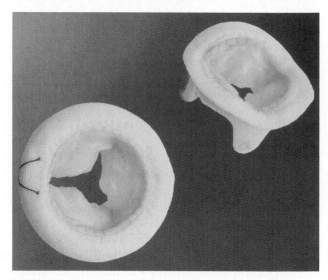

FIGURE 20-2. The Medtronic Mosaic porcine bioprosthesis.

Bioprostheses: Current (United States and Worldwide)

Stented Porcine (Aortic and Mitral)

The Hancock II porcine bioprosthesis (Medtronic, Inc., Minneapolis, MN) is a supra-annular prosthesis (Figure 20-1). The prosthesis has a Delrin stent, scalloped aortic sewing ring, and a reduced stent profile, and is fixed with glutaraldehyde at low pressure, subsequently, for a prolonged period at high pressure. The prosthesis is treated with sodium dodecyl sulfate to retard calcification.

The Medtronic Mosaic porcine bioprosthesis (Medtronic, Inc., Minneapolis, MN) is a third-generation prosthesis (Figure 20-2). The prosthesis has a supra-annular configuration with a Delrin stent, scalloped aortic sewing ring, and reduced stent profile. The tissue is pressure-free fixed with glutaraldehyde, and the aortic wall is predilated to reduce deformation of the commissures. The prosthesis is treated with alpha oleic acid to retard calcification.

The Carpentier-Edwards SAV Supra-Annular porcine bioprosthesis (aortic only) (Edwards Lifesciences, Irvine, CA) has a supra-annular configuration, mounted on a flexible Elgiloy wire frame for stress reduction (Figure 20-3). The prosthesis has a reduced stent profile, and the tissue is preserved with glutaraldehyde at low pressure (fixed at less than 4 mm Hg). The tissue is treated with the calcium mitigation agents polysorbate 80 and ethanol (XenoLogiX).

Stentless Porcine (Aortic)

The St. Jude Medical–Toronto SPV stentless porcine bioprosthesis (St. Jude Medical, Inc., St. Paul, MN) is a subcoronary stentless porcine bioprosthesis with an external surface, including muscle shelf covered with fine Dacron

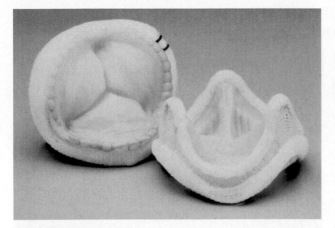

FIGURE 20-3. The Carpentier-Edwards SAV Supra-Annular porcine bioprosthesis (aortic).

mesh (Figure 20-4). The proximal sewing ridge is covered with fine Dacron. The porcine tissue is preserved with low-pressure glutaraldehyde fixation.

The Medtronic Freestyle stentless porcine bioprosthesis (Medtronic, Inc., Minneapolis, MN) is fashioned as a porcine aortic root for implantation using the subcoronary (allograft freehand-like), mini-root cylinder, or aortic root technique (Figure 20-5). Tissue is pressure-free-fixed with glutaraldehyde, and the aortic wall is pre-dilated to reduce deformation of the commissures. Tissue is treated with alpha amino oleic acid to retard calcification. Dacron mesh covers the muscle shelf and forms a fine proximal sewing cuff.

The Edwards Prima Plus is a stentless porcine bioprosthesis (Edwards Lifesciences, Inc., Irvine, CA) designed as a versatile cylinder without prefashioned coronary openings (Figure 20-6). The prosthesis has a Dacron

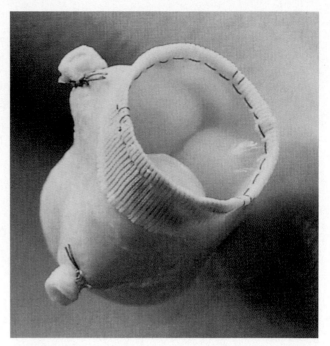

FIGURE 20-5. The Medtronic Freestyle stentless porcine bioprosthesis.

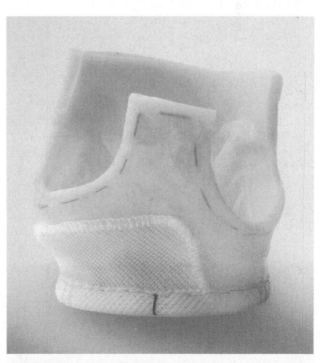

FIGURE 20-6. The Edwards Prima Plus is a stentless porcine bioprosthesis.

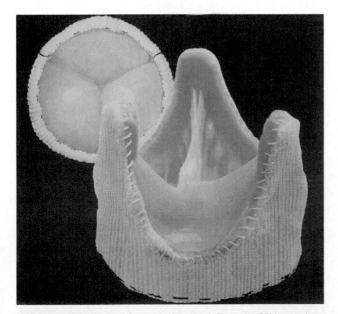

FIGURE 20-4. The St. Jude Medical–Toronto SPV stentless porcine bioprosthesis.

mesh that covers the muscle shelf and forms a thin proximal cuff. The porcine tissue is glutaraldehyde-fixed at low pressure with sinus-area dilatation. The prosthesis can be implanted using freehand subcoronary, mini-root cylinder, or aortic root replacement technique.

Stented Pericardial (Aortic and Mitral)

The Carpentier-Edwards PERIMOUNT pericardial bio-prosthesis (Edwards Lifesciences, Irvine, CA) is constructed with an Elgiloy stent at the orifice and commissures for flexibility and pericardium fixed without pressure in glutaraldehyde. Leaflets are produced by computer-aided design for optimal leaflet-to-stent matching (Figure 20-7 *A* and *B*). Leaflets achieve satisfactory coaptation without stent post sutures. The tissue is treated with the calcium mitigation agents polysorbate 80 and ethanol (XenoLogiX).

Bioprostheses: Current or Investigational/Developmental (Worldwide)

Stented Porcine (Aortic and Mitral)

The St. Jude Medical Epic porcine bioprosthesis (St. Jude Medical, Inc., St. Paul, MN) is a minimal-pressure glutaraldehyde-fixed porcine bioprosthesis (Figure 20-8). The prosthesis is formulated as a triple-composite design devoid of muscle bar and is a low-profile design in both

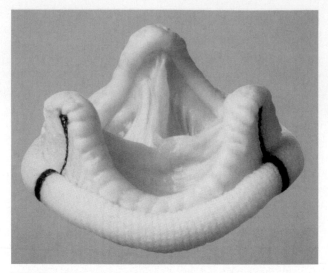

FIGURE 20-8. The St. Jude Medical Epic porcine bioprosthesis.

aortic and mitral positions. The stent posts and rails are covered with a rim of glutaraldehyde-preserved bovine pericardium. The prosthesis has a polyacetal stent and polyester sewing ring. In the Linx technology, ethanol is used to prevent calcification.

The St. Jude Medical–Biocor porcine bioprosthesis (St. Jude Medical, Inc., Belo Horizonte, MG, Brazil) is a zero-pressure glutaraldehyde-fixed porcine bioprosthesis (Figure 20-9). The prosthesis is formulated as a triple-composite design, with the leaflets devoid of a muscle bar. The stent posts and rails are covered with a rim of bovine glutaraldehyde-preserved pericardium. The design of the prosthesis includes a polyacetal stent and polyester sewing ring.

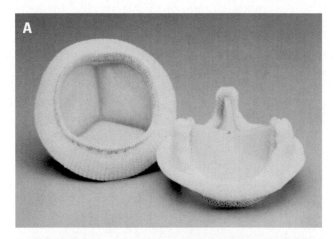

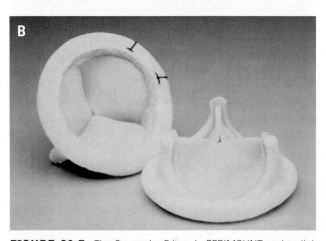

FIGURE 20-7. The Carpentier-Edwards PERIMOUNT pericardial bioprosthesis. *A,* aortic. *B,* mitral.

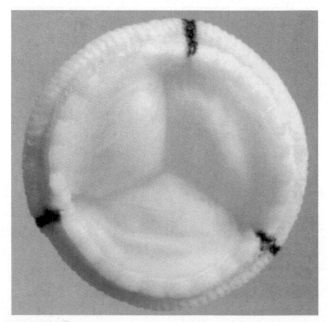

FIGURE 20-9. The St. Jude Medical–Biocor porcine bioprosthesis.

The Carbomedics Synergy ST porcine bioprosthesis (Carbomedics, Inc., Austin, TX) is a stented triple-composite supra-annular prosthesis of low-profile design (Figure 20-10). The triple-composite prosthesis has three noncoronary leaflets glutaraldehyde-preserved at zero-pressure fixation. The three noncoronary leaflets with no muscle shelf provide a large effective blood-flow area. The stent posts and stent rails are covered with glutaraldehyde-preserved pericardium. The porcine and pericardial tissue is treated with an advanced calcium mitigation therapy.

The Labcor stented porcine bioprosthesis (Labcor, Inc., Belo Horizonte, MG, Brazil) is a stented triple-composite prosthesis of low-profile design (Figure 20-11). The triple-composite prosthesis has three noncoronary leaflets glutaraldehyde-preserved at zero-pressure fixation. The three noncoronary leaflets with no muscle shelf provide a large effective blood-flow area.

The AorTech Aspire porcine bioprosthesis (AorTech, Bellshill, Scotland) is a low-pressure (< 2 mm Hg) glutaraldehyde-fixed stented porcine bioprosthesis (Figure 20-12). The bioprosthesis is formulated by a process of

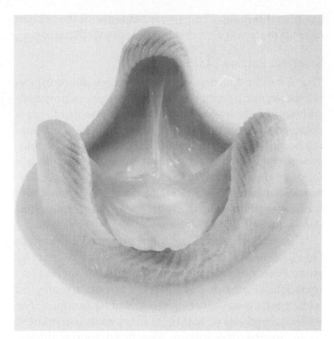

FIGURE 20-12. The AorTech Aspire porcine bioprosthesis.

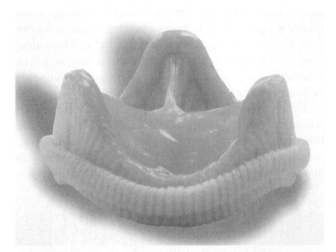

FIGURE 20-10. The Carbomedics Synergy ST porcine bioprosthesis.

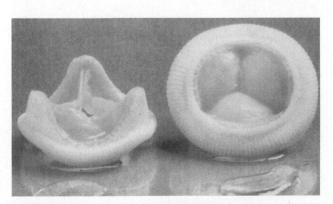

FIGURE 20-11. The Labcor stented porcine bioprosthesis.

"fresh mounting" to allow correct alignment of the commissures. Dilatation of the valve during preparation allows correct functional sizing. Dilation in conjunction with low-pressure fixation increases the angle of inclination of the leaflet and produces a reduction in open leaflet bending deformation. The valve tissue is selected to ensure minimal size of the muscle shelf.

The Carpentier-Edwards SAV Supra-Annular mitral porcine bioprosthesis (Edwards Lifesciences, Irvine, CA) has a supra-annular configuration, mounted on a flexible Elgiloy wire frame for stress reduction (Figure 20-13). The prosthesis has a reduced stent profile, and the tissue is preserved with glutaraldehyde at low pressure fixed at

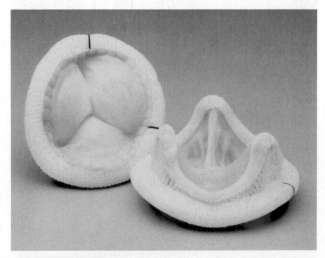

FIGURE 20-13. The Carpentier-Edwards SAV Supra-Annular porcine bioprosthesis (mitral).

less than 4 mm Hg. The tissue is treated with the calcium mitigation agents polysorbate 80 and ethanol (XenoLogiX).

Stentless Porcine (Aortic)

The CryoLife–O'Brien stentless porcine bioprosthesis (CryoLife, Inc., Kennesaw, GA) is a stentless prosthesis with composite leaflets (Figure 20-14). The prosthesis is designed only for distal suture-line implantation, above the annulus, in contrast to other stentless porcine bioprostheses that require two suture lines. The prosthesis is fixed in glutaraldehyde. The CryoLife–O'Brien stentless porcine bioprosthesis also is fashioned as an aortic root for implantation using the subcoronary, mini-root cylinder, or aortic root technique.

The AorTech Aspire stentless porcine bioprosthesis (AorTech, Bellshill, Scotland) is low-pressure (< 2 mm Hg) glutaraldehyde fixed, with aortic and pulmonary root formulations (Figure 20-15). The aortic roots are supplied with the anterior leaflet of the mitral valve intact. The inflow of both aortic and pulmonary roots is reinforced using porcine pericardium. The distal root is dilated, which facilitates the physiologic connection between the porcine implant and the patient aorta. The pulmonary root is also provided in a bifurcated fashion. The aortic root, pulmonary root, and pulmonary root bifurcated are provided in both adult and pediatric root configurations. The aortic prosthetic root can be implanted using subcoronary, cylinder, or root techniques.

The Shelhigh Skeletonized Super-Stentless (Shelhigh, Inc., Milburn, NJ) aortic porcine bioprosthesis is a com-

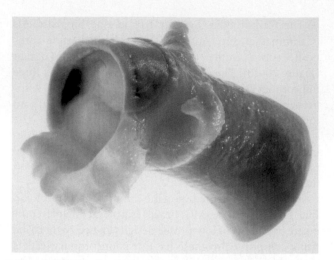

FIGURE 20-15. The AorTech Aspire stentless porcine bioprosthesis.

posite porcine bioprosthesis (Figure 20-16). The valve is mounted on a superflexible ring (skeleton), preserved with glutaraldehyde, detoxified, and heparin-treated with the No-React anticalcification treatment. The No-React treatment is a tissue detoxification and stabilization process that makes cross-linking permanent and prevents the toxic glutaraldehyde molecules from leaching out of the tissue. The Shelhigh Super-Stentless valve has stentless hemodynamics, and the implantation is as easy as that of a stented valve. The valve has a "volumeless" annulus that facilitates upsizing by one size.

The St. Jude Medical–Toronto SPV Duo Stentless Root porcine bioprosthesis (St. Jude Medical, Inc., Minneapolis, MN) is a new-generation porcine aortic root for implantation as a subcoronary free-hand valve insertion or as an aortic root replacement (Figure 20-17). The proximal sewing

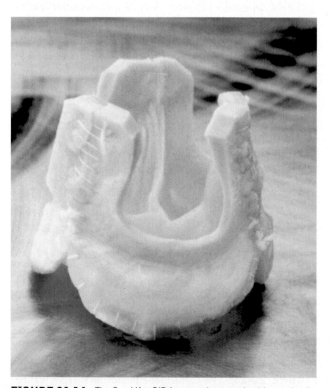

FIGURE 20-14. The CryoLife–O'Brien stentless porcine bioprosthesis.

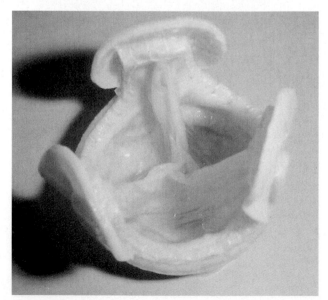

FIGURE 20-16. The Shelhigh Skeletonized Super-Stentless.

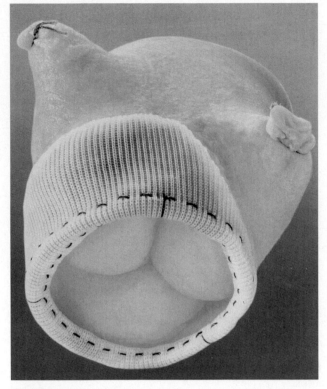

FIGURE 20-17. The St. Jude Medical–Toronto SPV Duo Stentless Root porcine bioprosthesis.

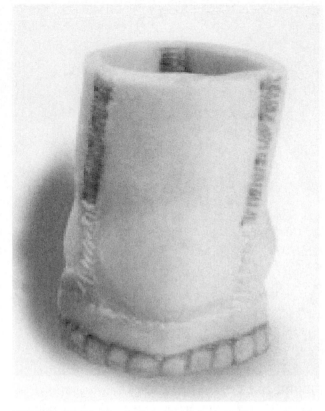

FIGURE 20-18. The Carbomedics Oxford stentless porcine bioprosthesis.

ridge is covered with fine Dacron, and the muscle shelf is also covered with fine Dacron mesh. The porcine tissue is preserved with low-pressure glutaraldehyde fixation. The tissue is treated with the BiLinx anticalcification technology, which reduces calcification on the aortic wall tissue as well as the aortic leaflet. The Toronto SPV Root is used in procedures where aortic root disease accompanies valve disease.

The Carbomedics Oxford stentless porcine bioprosthesis (Carbomedics, Inc., Austin, TX) is a triple-composite bioprosthesis formulated from three noncoronary porcine aortic cusps and adjacent aortic sinuses and aortic wall (Figure 20-18). Fabrication of the porcine root is formulated with the suturing of the three components to facilitate use as a subcoronary or aortic root implantation. The bioprosthesis may be introduced with glutaraldehyde preservation and advanced calcium mitigation therapy. The bioprosthesis may be re-introduced in the future with preservation of the porcine tissue conducted by collagen cross-linking by the dye-mediated photo-oxidation technique. Proximal suturing is to be formulated in a horizontal plane at the annular level and trimming of the root tissue for distal suturing in the subcoronary and commissural placement. The total root replacement is to be implanted with the same proximal suturing technique and coronary ostial aortic buttons for the coronary artery implantation.

The St. Jude Medical–Biocor stentless porcine bioprosthesis (St. Jude Medical, Belo Horizonte, MG, Brazil) is a stentless prosthesis with individual porcine cusps to mount a composite bioprosthesis, avoiding leaflets with muscular bands (Figure 20-19). The leaflets are treated under no pressure and tanned with different glutaraldehyde solutions for 3 months. The leaflets are sutured to a conduit of glutaraldehyde-treated bovine pericardium. The conduit is then shaped in a scalloped manner to mimic the natural aortic valve.

The Labcor stentless porcine bioprosthesis (Labcor, Inc., Belo Horizonte, MG, Brazil) is a stentless prosthesis of triple-composite design with three noncoronary leaflets (Figure 20-20). The leaflets are preserved in glutaraldehyde at no pressure. The triple-composite design provides a large effective blood-flow area.

The AorTech Elan stentless aortic porcine bioprosthesis (AorTech, Bellshill, Scotland) is a new-generation prosthesis in early stages of clinical evaluation (Figure 20-21).

Stented Pericardial (Aortic and Mitral)

The Mitroflow Synergy PC pericardial bioprosthesis (Carbomedics Mitroflow, Richmond, BC, Canada) is formulated with a acetyl homopolymer stent for flexibility and pericardium pressure-free fixed with glutaraldehyde (Figure 20-22). Pericardium is used as a single component without critical stent post sutures. The Dacron cloth of the prosthesis (current version) has the smooth, rather than ribbed, polyathylene terephthalate (PET) in contact with the pericardium.

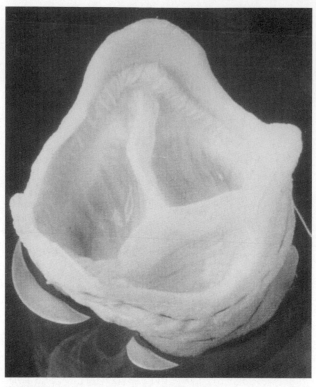

FIGURE 20-19. The St. Jude Medical–Biocor stentless porcine bioprosthesis.

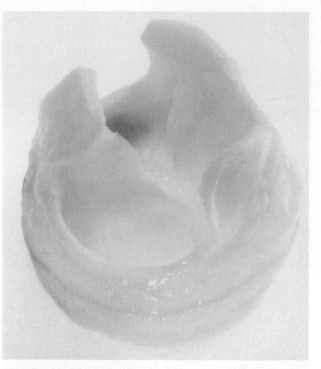

FIGURE 20-21. The AorTech Elan stentless aortic porcine bioprosthesis.

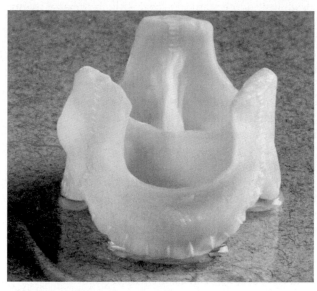

FIGURE 20-20. The Labcor stentless porcine bioprosthesis.

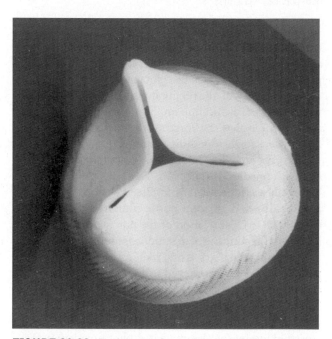

FIGURE 20-22. The Mitroflow Synergy PC pericardial bioprosthesis.

The Sorin Pericarbon MØRE pericardial bioprosthesis (Sorin Biomedica, Saluggia, Italy) is made with two sheets of pressure-free-fixed pericardium over a semiflexible polymeric stent covered with polyester fabric (Figure 20-23). One sheet forms the three cusps, with reduced stress on the commissures and a cylindrical shape in the open position. The other sheet coats the inner surface of the stent. The prosthesis is low profile and has a radio-

paque metal wire marker and a carbofilm-coated poly-ester fabric sewing ring (to control pannus overgrowth). The sewing ring in the aortic position is designed for supra-annular positioning. The tissue is submitted to postglutaraldehyde detoxification aimed at neutralizing residues of unbound aldehyde groups. The valve is stored in a solution free from aldehyde.

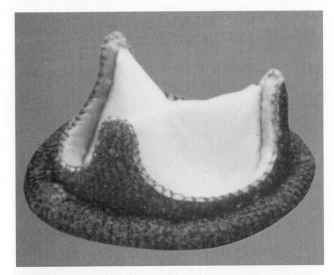

FIGURE 20-23. The Sorin Pericarbon MØRE pericardial bioprosthesis.

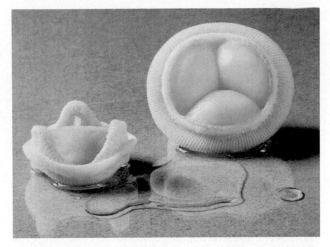

FIGURE 20-25. The Labcor stented pericardial bioprosthesis.

The St. Jude Medical–Biocor pericardial bioprosthesis (St. Jude Medical, Inc., Belo Horizonte, MG, Brazil) is a zero-pressure glutaraldehyde-fixed pericardial bioprosthesis with the stent posts and rails covered with pericardium (Figure 20-24). The design incorporates a polyacetal stent and polyester ring.

The Labcor stented pericardial bioprosthesis (Labcor, Inc., Belo Horizonte, MG, Brazil) is a triple-composite prosthesis with precisely determined individual cusp shape, with the tissue selected for mounting of uniformity and thickness (Figure 20-25). The prosthesis is formulated with a copolymer scalloped flexible stent to reduce stress on the tissue. The fabrication technique produces uniformity and consistency in valve function. The attachment of the pericardium at the stent post facilitates stress reduction and reinforces apposition of the leaflets. The prosthesis is also constructed to avoid contact of the pericardial membrane with the polyester and to reduce abrasion by means of pericardial padding of the inner surface of the valve at the post.

The Carpentier-Edwards PERIMOUNT Magna pericardial bioprosthesis (Edwards Lifesciences, Irvine, CA) (Figure 20-26) is constructed as a supra-annular prosthesis with an Elgiloy stent at the orifice and commissures for flexibility and pericardium fixed without pressure in glutaraldehyde. Leaflets are produced by computer-aided design for optimal leaflet-to-stent matching (see Figure 20-7). Leaflets achieve satisfactory coaptation without stent post sutures. The tissue is treated with the calcium mitigation agents polysorbate 80 and ethanol (Xeno-LogiX). The prosthesis has the sewing cuff below the

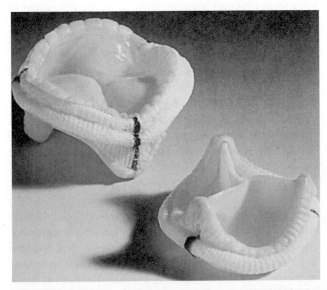

FIGURE 20-24. The St. Jude Medical–Biocor pericardial bioprosthesis.

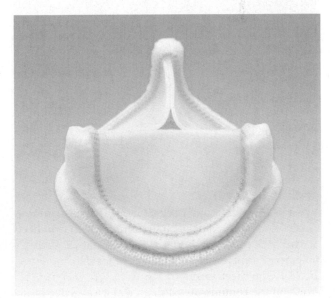

FIGURE 20-26. The Carpentier-Edwards PERIMOUNT Magna pericardial bioprosthesis (aortic).

prosthesis proper to facilitate supra-annular positioning to optimize hemodynamics in small annuli. The smaller sewing ring diameter, compared to the Carpentier-Edwards aortic PERIMOUNT, allows the valve to be implanted with total supra-annular positioning.

Stentless Pericardial (Aortic and Mitral)

The Sorin Pericarbon Freedom stentless pericardial bioprosthesis (Sorin Biomedica, Saluggia, Italy) is a stentless pericardial valve made of two separate sheets of low-pressure glutaraldehyde-treated bovine pericardium (Figure 20-27). The first sheet is shaped to form the three leaflets by means of a process of atraumatic tissue fixation without the use of molds and is then sutured to the second sheet using a carbofilm-coated suture. The suture line is designed especially to minimize the mechanical stress at the level of the commissures. The tissue is submitted to postglutaraldehyde detoxification aimed at neutralizing residues of unbound aldehyde groups. The valve is stored in a solution free from aldehyde.

The St. Jude Medical Quattro mitral bioprosthesis (St. Jude Medical, Inc., St. Paul, MN) is a stentless bovine pericardial mitral prosthesis (Figure 20-28). The pericardium is preserved with glutaraldehyde and treated with polyol technology to reduce calcification. The prosthesis is composed of a "D-shaped" sewing cuff with one large anterior leaflet and one posterior leaflet containing three scallops.

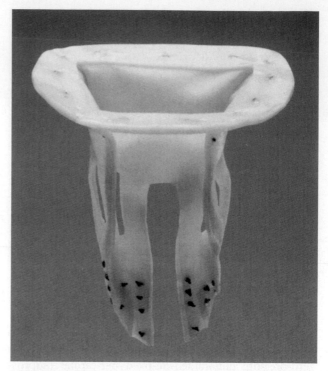

FIGURE 20-28. The St. Jude Medical Quattro mitral bioprosthesis.

Chordal support for both leaflets on the anterolateral (left) side of the prosthesis is brought together, forming one anterolateral papillary flap. Similarly, the chordae on the posteromedial (right) side are brought together to form another papillary flap. The valve components are held together by aligning stitches to form a four-leaflet stentless mitral prosthesis. The implantation technique incorporates the anchoring of each papillary flap to the corresponding papillary muscle with two horizontal or longitudinal pledgeted mattress sutures. The aligning sutures in the prosthesis sewing ring and papillary flaps guide the placement of sutures during implantation. The Quattro prosthesis is available in mitral sizes 26, 28, and 30 mm.

The 3F pericardial equine stentless bioprosthesis (aortic) (3F Therapeutics Inc., Lake Forest, CA) is composed of three equal sections of equine pericardium that have been processed by fixation with a buffered formulation of glutaraldehyde and that are assembled together to form a tubular structure (Figure 20-29A). The glutaraldehyde formulation is of a concentration low enough to preserve much of the flexibility of the raw material, and fully cross-link the collagenous structure to preserve its strength, minimize its immunogenic and thrombogenic potentials, and provide lengthened durability when implanted in the heart of the patient. In contrast with bovine pericardium, equine pericardium comes from a source that has not been implicated in transmissible spongiform encephalopathies. The inflow aspect of the bioprosthesis is fitted with a woven polyester cuff to facilitate suturing of the device to the orifice created by removal of the diseased

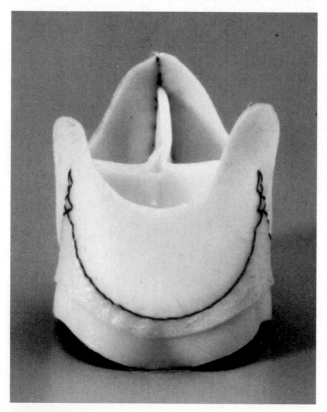

FIGURE 20-27. The Sorin Pericarbon Freedom stentless pericardial bioprosthesis (aortic).

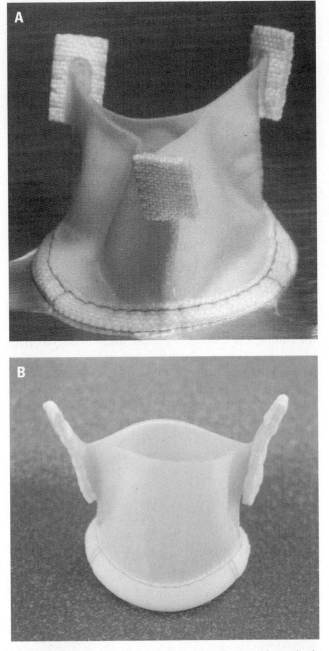

FIGURE 20-29. The 3F pericardial equine stentless bioprosthesis (aortic [A] and mitral [B]).

heart valve and allow fibrous ingrowth to help in the prevention of perivalvular leakage. The junctions of the three pericardial sections that form the leaflets become the three commissures of the bioprosthetic valve. These commissural attachment sites are integral tabs of pericardium backed by woven polyester material. The polyester material serves to reinforce the tissue and firmly affix the commissural attachment sites near the sinotubular junction of the native aorta during surgical implantation of the bioprosthesis. The 3F Therapeutics mitral bioprosthesis is composed of two leaflets of equine pericardium with

integral tabs of pericardium for papillary muscle attachment (Figure 20-29 B).

The Edwards Alex flexible pericardial aortic bioprosthesis (Edwards Lifesciences, Irvine, CA) is an investigational prosthesis. The design integrates the proven pericardial technology of the Carpentier-Edwards PERIMOUNT pericardial tissue valve into a flexible frame that conforms to the anatomy of the native aortic valve. The flexible frame allows contraction and expansion of the valve prosthesis at the aortic root and the commissures in concert with native aortic wall motion. The structural stent is highly flexible in a generally cylindrical configuration, with cusps and commissures permitted to move radially. The stent commissures are constructed so that the cusps are pivotally or flexibly coupled together at the commissures to permit relative movement. The stent is cloth covered and may be a single element or may be made in three separate elements for a three-cusp valve, each element having a cusp portion for each pair of adjacent stent elements combining to form the stent commissures. The cloth covering may incorporate an outward-projecting flap or connecting band that follows the cusps and commissures. The valve is connected to the natural tissue along the undulating connecting band. The connecting band is cloth-covered silicon to provide support to the stent and outer side of the valve at the commissures. The implantation will be supra-annular into the aortic wall above the native annulus, providing optimal coronary artery space in the coronary sinuses. The prosthesis incorporates a multi-legged holder used to implant the prosthesis and maintain its implant shape.

Stentless Porcine and Pericardial (Pulmonary)

The Cryolife–Ross stentless porcine pulmonary bioprosthesis (CryoLife International, Inc., Kennesaw, GA) is available in pediatric sizes (11 to 13 mm) and adult sizes (19 to 29 mm) (Figure 20-30). The porcine tissue is glutaraldehyde-fixed at low pressure (< 2 mm Hg). The stentless design with the symmetric muscle bar yields optional hemodynamics. The prosthesis has a potential increase in

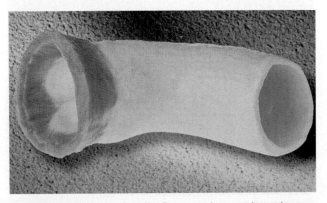

FIGURE 20-30. The Cryolife–Ross stentless porcine pulmonary bioprosthesis.

durability because of lower calcium content in pulmonary leaflets and wall, compared to aortic counterparts.

The Medtronic-Venpro Contegra pulmonary valved conduit (Venpro, Minneapolis, MN) is a bioprosthesis consisting of a heterologous bovine jugular vein having a trileaflet venous valve and possessing a natural sinus slightly larger in diameter than its lumen (Figure 20-31). The conduit is preserved in buffered glutaraldehyde in low concentration to preserve the flexibility of the leaflet material. The conduit is available in both unsupported and supported models. In the supported model, two external cloth-covered polypropylene rings provide additional support on either side of the valve. The available sizes are 12 to 22 mm.

The Shelhigh porcine pulmonic valve conduit (Shelhigh, Inc., Milburn, NJ) is a glutaraldehyde-fixed porcine pulmonic valve and pulmonary artery extension to formulate the conduit (Figure 20-32). The conduit is treated with the No-React tissue-detoxification process to reduce or delay the onset of calcification. The porcine pulmonic valve conduit has segments of bovine pericardial tissue to allow trimming to fit. The valve conduit is available in sizes 9 to 27 mm and, in the United States, up to 18 mm.

The CryoSyner graft valve (CryoLife International, Inc., Kennesaw, GA) is an acellular composite porcine-valve bioprosthesis (Figure 20-33). The valve contains three sized and symmetry-matched decellularized porcine non-coronary cusp units, each with aortic leaflet, anterior mitral leaflet, and aortic conduit. This construct contains no myocardium. Its inflow is created from pendant anterior mitral leaflets, and outflow is formed from the three segments of the aortic wall. The bioprosthesis is designed for right ventricular outflow tract reconstruction but also may be used for left ventricular outflow tract aortic root reconstruction. The acellular nonglutaraldehyde-prepared tissue facilitates repopulation with host fibroblastoid cells.

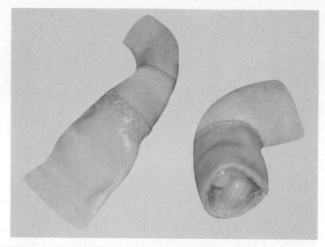

FIGURE 20-32. The Shelhigh porcine pulmonic valve conduit.

Stentless Porcine (Mitral)

The Medtronic physiologic mitral valve (Medtronic, Minneapolis, MN) is a prosthesis-in-development based on the platform of a stentless porcine mitral xenograft (Figure 20-34). The prosthesis is based on the concept that restoration of the native mitral valvular mechanics, caused by nonrepairable valvular disease, requires a complete functioning unit that includes both left ventricular and annular mechanics to ensure optimum valvular function.

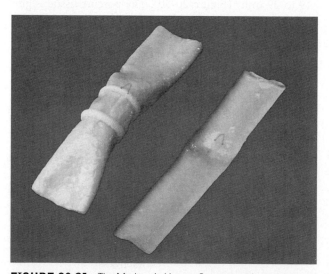

FIGURE 20-31. The Medtronic-Venpro Contegra pulmonary valved conduit.

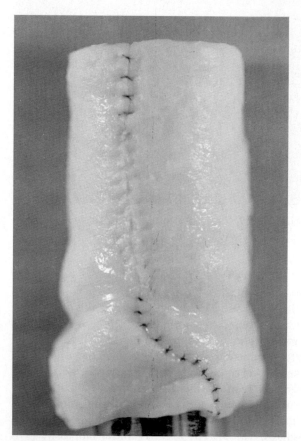

FIGURE 20-33. The CryoSyner graft valve.

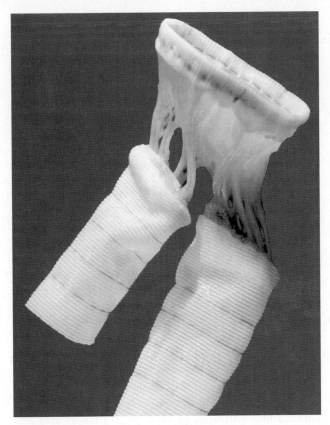

FIGURE 20-34. The Medtronic physiologic mitral valve.

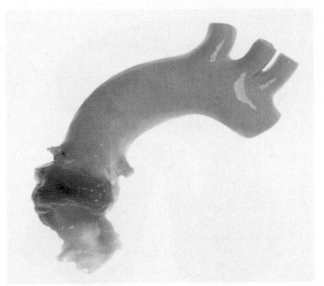

FIGURE 20-35. The CryoValve Aortic valve with or without conduits.

The valve is modified to facilitate implantation through the addition of sewing tubes attached along the three-dimensional axial direction of the strut chordae. Annular reinforcement is provided by either cloth or porcine pericardium. Markers are provided on the sewing tube in 5 mm increments to enable trimming. Annular markers delineate the commissures, as well as the short axis, of the valve annulus. Valve size is based on the linear intratrigonal distance. The valvular tissue is preserved with glutaraldehyde or another nonglutaraldehyde collagen cross-linking agent, such as carbodiimide. Zero-pressure fixation is used in situ within a portion of the porcine left ventricle to ensure maintenance of proper valvular geometry and leaflet biomechanics. Alpha amino oleic acid antimineralization treatment is provided to mitigate bioprosthetic calcification when the valve is processed using glutaraldehyde.

Allografts

The CryoValve Aortic valve with or without conduit (CryoLife International, Inc., Kennesaw, GA) is a cryopreserved human cadaveric aortic allograft for aortic root replacement or freehand aortic valve replacement (Figure 20-35). The aortic valve is transected from the left ventricle containing the muscle band with or without the anterior mitral leaflet. The aortic allograft (homograft) also is available from institutional or regional tissue banks. The allograft aortic valve is acceptable for pediatric and adult valve replacement, small aortic root, women of childbearing age, and infective endocarditis. The CryoValve Pulmonary valve with conduit is a cryopreserved human cadaveric pulmonary allograft for pulmonary root replacement (Figure 20-36).

The CryoValve Mitral valve (CryoLife International, Inc., Kennesaw, GA) is a cryopreserved mitral valve (Figure 20-37). The mitral valve is transected from the left ventricle containing the muscle band and anterolateral and posteromedial papillary muscles, with the chordae tendineae attached. The mitral valve prosthesis is used for both mitral and tricuspid valve replacements. The allograft valve is accepted for adult and pediatric valve replacement, women of childbearing age, infective endocarditis, and contraindication for anticoagulation therapy.

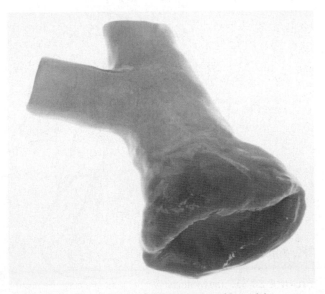

FIGURE 20-36. CryoValve Pulmonary valve with conduit.

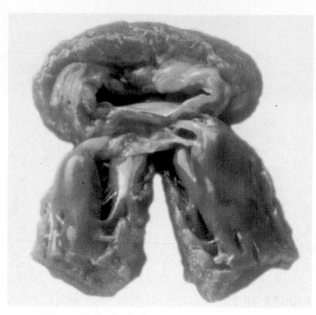

FIGURE 20-37. CryoValve Mitral valve.

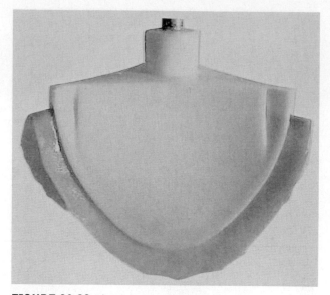

FIGURE 20-39. Autologous pericardial aortic valve.

Autografts

The pulmonary autograft is for the aortic root (and pulmonary allograft for the pulmonary root). The pulmonary autograft is used to replace and/or reconstruct the aortic root. Pulmonary allograft is usually used to replace the pulmonary root; stentless porcine root is another alternative (Figure 20-38).

An autologous pericardial aortic valve (CardioMed, Santa Barbara, CA) can be achieved by special instrumentation to formulate the stentless semilunar valve reconstruction with the autologous tissue (Figure 20-39). The autologous tissue is treated initially with a brief immer-sion in 0.625% buffered glutaraldehyde solution. The chemical treatment stiffens the tissue, makes it easier to handle, and prevents thickening and shrinkage. The instruments include a sizer to assess leaflet height and commissural symmetry in addition to annular diameter, an intraoperative tissue tester to assess the mechanical properties of the tissue before it is used, a tool to cut a precisely sized novel geometric pattern, and formers to hold the tissue in anatomic orientation during valve reconstruction. The concept of autologous pericardial aortic valve has been used on an institutional, not commercial, basis without advanced instrumentation.

Valve Replacement Surgery

Clinical Practice

The vast majority of patients having valve replacement surgery are older than 50 years of age.[21] The North American experience between 1991 and 1995, inclusive, from the Society of Thoracic Surgeons database revealed that 42% of patients were between the ages of 50 and 70 years and that 45% were older than 70 years of age.[22] During that time in the United States, mechanical prostheses were predominant in aortic valve replacement, as well as mitral valve replacement, when reconstructive procedures are not possible.[22] Since the latter part of the 1990s, there has been a significant resurgence of biologic prostheses for aortic valve replacement but not for mitral valve replacement.

Since the first edition of this textbook in 1999, the United States now has available second- and third-generation stented porcine bioprostheses, namely, the Hancock II, Carpentier-Edwards SAV, and Medtronic Mosaic bioprostheses.[12] The Hancock II and Carpentier-Edwards SAV have been available worldwide since the early 1980s. The Hancock standard, Carpentier-Edwards standard,

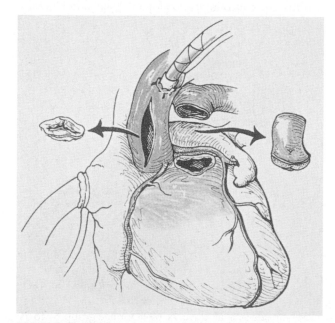

FIGURE 20-38. The pulmonary autograft for aortic root.

and Hancock modified-orifice first-generation porcine bioprostheses have fallen into disuse. The United States has the predominant worldwide stentless porcine bioprostheses, namely, the St. Jude Medical–Toronto SPV, Medtronic Freestyle, and Edwards Prima Plus stentless porcine bioprostheses.

During this same time frame, there has been a proliferation of stented and stentless bioprostheses in the worldwide market. This occurred because of a renewed confidence in biologic prostheses as advanced technologies are addressing durability, hemodynamic performance, and the potential of hemodynamic performance on survival. The optimization of hemodynamic performance is being addressed for the small aortic root by stentless aortic bioprostheses, and for medium-sized aortic roots by supra-annular porcine and pericardial bioprostheses.[23–33] The stented pericardial bioprostheses that will optimize hemodynamic performance in the small aortic root are the long-standing Mitroflow Synergy PC and the new Carpentier-Edwards PERIMOUNT Magna pericardial bioprostheses. A general commentary on bioprostheses would be incomplete without giving consideration to the South American triple-composite porcine bioprosthesis formulations, namely, the St. Jude Medical Epic (formerly Biocor porcine bioprosthesis) and the Carbomedics Synergy (formerly Labcor porcine bioprosthesis). The triple-composite prosthesis shows advanced durability in the mitral position for reduced commissural stress; at least one of the contributors to calcification may be an influential factor.[17]

Glutaraldehyde remains the collagen-linking nonimmunogenic agent for preservation of heterographic tissue for valvular bioprostheses.[34] Glutaraldehyde and mechanical stress have been implicated as causative factors of calcification.[35,36] It is felt that the toxicity from the leaching of the unbound glutaraldehyde or its polymers from the treated tissue, or the aldehyde storage solutions, give the tissue a propensity to develop calcification. There have been many measures over the past decade to control this glutaraldehyde toxicity.[35,36] Surfactants, particularly sodium dodecyl sulfate and polysorbate 80, were incorporated in the early part of the decade in the preservative process. The control of residual aldehydes with amino oleic acid has been extensively evaluated and is currently used in the Medtronic stented Mosaic porcine and stentless Freestyle porcine prostheses. Amino oleic acid is more effective in mitigation of calcification in the aortic cusps than aortic wall.[37] Ethanol and aluminium chloride are an additional method of preventing calcification of glutaraldehyde-preserved porcine tissue. The hypothesis of calcification inhibition is the interaction of membrane-lipid removal and ethanol-induced collagen structural changes. Ethanol has been incorporated with polysorbate 80 in the XenoLogiX technology of Edwards products. The St. Jude Medical–Toronto SPV Duo root porcine bioprosthesis utilizes ethanol in cusp preservation and aluminium and ethanol in aortic wall preservation.

Alternatives to glutaraldehyde cross-linking of collagen are available but have not been brought forward for clinical use.[35,36] The agents being evaluated either are incorporated into the tissue (eg, glutaraldehyde or epoxide) or act as promoters of the cross-linking process (eg, acyl azide, carbodiimide or dye-mediated photo-oxidation). The agent carbodiimide, leaves no cross-linking chemical as part of the bridge between polypeptide chains, but the process reduces calcification only in the valve cusps and not in the aortic wall, which could pose a problem with porcine root replacements. Dye-mediated photo-oxidation acts as a promoting agent of collagen cross-linking of porcine or pericardial tissue. The tissue is treated with an aqueous solution (including the photo-oxidation dye) and is light irradiated.[38]

Future bioprostheses will continue to be treated with glutaraldehyde and various agents to control active aldehyde residues, or possibly with the collagen cross-linking promoters, which help amino acid residues on adjacent chains to cross-link.

Results

Structural valve deterioration is the predominant valve-related complication with porcine and pericardial bioprostheses.[1,2] In 1988, Jamieson and colleagues[14] documented that the failure rate is greater for mitral prostheses than aortic prostheses and that the failure rate is less with each advancing decade of life. Jamieson and colleagues[13] further documented age as the predominant determinant for selection of porcine bioprostheses in 1991. The second-generation prostheses, namely, the Carpentier-Edwards Supra-Annular and the Hancock II, continue to be under evaluation to determine whether there are differences in durability as a result of tissue preservation.[5,8,9]

The freedom from structural valve deterioration (SVD) is best assessed within decades because various series have different mean ages.[13,14] The freedom from SVD should be reported by both actuarial and actual methodologies.[10,11,39] The actuarial method essentially means patients have immortality but is important to record for patients who reach designated time intervals, such as 15 and 20 years following implantation.[10,11,39] The actuarial method overestimates the incidence of SVD because of the assumption that a patient's life expectancy is essentially unlimited, but many patients die before the prosthesis fails.[10,11,39] The actual or cumulative incidence analysis may provide a better estimate of durability of tissue valves, especially in patients with limited survival.[10,11]

The actuarial freedom from SVD for aortic valve replacement with the Carpentier-Edwards SAV porcine bioprosthesis was, at 15 years, 69% for age group 61 to 70 years and 92% for > 70 years, while the actual freedom was 84% for age group 61 to 70 years and 97% for > 70 years.[9] The Hancock II porcine bioprosthesis probably has similar durability, but experience to 15 years is limited.[5,8] Jamieson and international colleagues[15] showed that in the mitral replacement, the Carpentier-Edwards PERIMOUNT pericardial bioprosthesis has superior durability to the Carpentier-Edwards SAV porcine bioprosthesis, considered to be a result of the low profile of the prosthesis and excessive commissural stress. The overall experience of the aortic and mitral Carpentier-Edwards PERIMOUNT pericardial bioprosthesis demonstrates excellent durability at 12 years, while 15-year performance is needed for further comparison of these second-generation bioprostheses.[3,16,18] Myken and co-investigators[17] reported on the triple-composite St. Jude Medical–Biocor porcine bioprosthesis, demonstrating advanced durability with the mitral prosthesis similar to the aortic prosthesis at 12 to 13 years. Comparison of noncomposite and triple-composite porcine bioprostheses needs extended evaluation. The durability of stentless porcine bioprostheses and the third-generation Medtronic Mosaic porcine bioprosthesis remains to be determined.[31]

The important objectives of aortic valve replacement are to minimize postoperative gradients and to optimize the normalization of left ventricular mass and function.[29] The most frequent cause of high postoperative gradients is being the effective prosthetic valve area is less than that of the normal human valve.[40,41] This is commonly known as patient–prosthesis mismatch, even in the presence of normally functioning valve prostheses.[40,41] Pibarot and colleagues[41] recommend that the effective orifice area index of < 0.85 to 0.90 cm^2/m^2 represents patient–prosthesis mismatch. Patient–prosthesis mismatch indicates that the reserve is being used for rest conditions and that left ventricular mass regression may not be a reality. The effect of mismatch on the incidence of sudden deaths and long-term survival is receiving consideration.[42]

The most important consideration is the hemodynamic performance of stentless bioprostheses and stented supraannular bioprostheses.[43] Yun and colleagues,[33] in comparing Medtronic Freestyle stentless bioprosthesis experience from Los Angeles to the Medtronic Mosaic stented experience from Vancouver, showed that the former had larger effective orifice areas (EOAs) and lower gradients. These authors found that 19% of stentless prostheses and 64% of stented prostheses had varying degrees of patient–prosthesis mismatch. Del Rizzo and coauthors,[29] reporting in 1999, with the combined multicenter trials experience of the Toronto SPV stentless bioprosthesis and the Medtronic Freestyle stentless bioprosthesis, found that at 3 years post aortic valve replacement, the mean gradient was 6.3 ± 5.0 mm Hg and the effective orifice area index (EOAI) was 1.2 ± 0.4 cm^2/m^2. The left ventricular mass commences to regress immediately after aortic valve replacement, with the maximal regression being completed by 6 months. Jamieson and coauthors found no difference between the

Carpentier–Edwards SAV porcine, Carpentier-Edwards PERIMOUNT pericardial, and Medtronic Mosaic porcine bioprostheses with regard to mean gradients by prosthesis size and to indexed effective orifice area by prosthesis size.[27] There was a tendency for an element of patient–prosthesis mismatch in sizes 19 to 23 mm, with mean gradients between 12 and 17 mm Hg. Thomson and the Canadian investigators[31] of the Medtronic Mosaic identified mean gradients of 10 to 13 mm Hg throughout the various prosthesis sizes. The tendency for patient–prosthesis mismatch in sizes 21 to 23 mm did not alter adequate achievement of appropriate indexed left ventricular mass regression for all valve sizes. Del Rizzo and colleagues reported that the major effect on LV mass regression was baseline left ventricular mass index (LVMI) and patient–prosthesis mismatch.[29] For patients with EOAI > 0.8 cm^2/m^2 to > 1.0 cm^2/m^2, the LVMI at 3 years was 75 to 80% of baseline and for patients with EOAI < 0.8 cm^2/m^2 was 96% of baseline.

The extended 5-year survival of the Hancock II stented and Medtronic Freestyle stentless bioprostheses from the respective multicenter regulatory trials revealed superiority for the stentless bioprosthesis for age groups < 60 years and 60 to 69 years, but similar survival for the age group 70 to 79 years.[42]

Autografts are now more commonly used while homografts are less commonly used.[44,45] The resting and exercise EOAs and gradients are essentially similar for autografts and homografts to native aortic valves.[41] The autograft has better durability than the cryopreserved allograft. The trend favoring the autograft over the allograft occurs at 8 years of evaluation.[46] The allograft is now primarily used in adults for management of native and prosthetic valve endocarditis. The concerns with the autograft procedure are late pulmonary allograft stenosis and late dilatation of the autograft involving root, sinuses of Valsalva, and sinotubular junction.

The Canadian investigators from Laval University have proposed a three-step algorithm that can be easily performed in the operating room to prevent patient–prosthesis mismatch.[40,47] The steps are as follows:

1. Calculate the patient's body surface area from weight and height.
2. From a published table, determine the minimal valve EOA required to ensure an EOAI > 0.85, > 0.80, or > 0.75 cm^2/m^2; the choice of EOAI is deemed to be the minimum requirement for a given patient.
3. Select the type and size of prosthesis that has reference values for EOA greater or equal to the minimal EOA value obtained in step 2. (The reference values provided by manufacturers and/or published by investigators may be in vivo or in vitro values.)

Prosthesis Indications

The prosthesis type options for aortic valve replacement by adult age groups are detailed in Table 20-3.[48,49]

TABLE 20-3.

Age Range (years)	Prosthesis Type
20 to 40	Pulmonary autograft (no contraindication [ie, annuloaortic ectasia]) Mechanical prosthesis Allograft (if contraindication to autograft or anticoagulation)
41 to 64	Mechanical prosthesis Stentless heterograft prosthesis Stented heterograft prosthesis Pulmonary autograft (to age 55 years if good candidate) Allograft Mechanical prosthesis
65 ≥	Stented heterograft—porcine or pericardial (specifically if large annulus) Stentless heterograft—subcoronary implantation Allograft or stentless porcine root (specifically if small annulus or calcified root) Mechanical prosthesis

The prosthesis type options for mitral valve replacement are more simplified in cases where reconstruction is not feasible or possible. Mechanical prostheses are used for age groups < 70 years and bioprostheses are used for ages > 70 years or younger if comorbid risk factors are considered to reduce survival.[48]

Innovative Technologies

The innovative technologies of the past have contributed to optimizing hemodynamic performance and to potentially reducing structural valve deterioration.

Tissue engineering strategies are commencing to evolve.[50–55] The premise is to create a living valve that will not be rejected by the patient's own immune system. Novel tissue-engineering approaches are being investigated as ways to improve replacement heart valve durability. These tissue-engineered techniques are focused on fabricating the intricate architecture of the valve leaflets. Scaffolds have been developed from synthetic and naturally occurring polymers and then cellularized from host endothelial cells in tissue culture.[51,52] Besides synthetic scaffolds, both heterograft and allograft valvular tissue can be decellularized and repopulated in vitro with the predetermined host cells.[51,52] Preoperatively, endothelial cells would be harvested from the patient. These cells would then be cultured and incorporated into the scaffold. A living valve with recipient-specific endothelial cells would then be implanted at the time of surgery.[56] On a theoretical basis, these approaches are the most attractive. They are, however, also the most complicated.

More recently, O'Brien and colleagues[56] developed stentless allograft bioprosthetic valves that were fabricated from acellular tissues, cryopreserved, and implanted as pulmonary root replacements in juvenile sheep. After 150 days the grafts showed intact leaflets with in-growth of host fibroblastoid cells in all explanted porcine valves and no evidence of calcification. Elkins and collaborators[50] have implanted porcine decellularized conduits in both the pulmonary and aortic outflow tracts in humans.

The decellularization process with heterografts replaces the use of glutaraldehyde for collagen cross-linking to limit xenograft antigenicity. The predominant issues with this modality of tissue engineering is the maintenance of balancing scaffold disappearance, interstitial cell reseeding, and supporting a desirable host cellular response not susceptible to antigenic recognition and immunologic rejection.[51,52]

The current status of achieving tissue-engineered heart valves with autologous cells is to have scaffolds of either biodegradable polymers or biologic extracellular matrices.[53–55] The polymeric scaffolds are biodegradable and are used for cell anchorage, cell proliferation, and cell differentiation. The thermoplastic biopolyesters that have been studied to mold a trileaflet valve scaffold are polyglycolic acid, polyhydroxy-alkanoate, and poly-4-hydroxybutrate.[54,55] The disadvantages of these synthetic polymers are stiffness, thickness, and nonpliability. The in vitro seeding to form a three-dimensional matrix is with fibroblasts, smooth-muscle cells, and endothelial cells. The xenogenic or allogenic biologic extracellular matrices may be the most promising with decellularization and cryopreservation followed by recellularization with autologous myofibroblasts and endothelial cells either in vitro or in vivo.[50,56] These modalities provide the opportunity for a physiologic environment that is nonimmunogenic without the propensity for calcification.

Given our current knowledge and understanding, it is not likely that commercially prepared tissue-engineered valves will be available for several years.

References

1. Jamieson WRE. Valvular surgery—mechanical and bioprosthetic aortic valve replacement. In: Edmunds LH Jr, editor. Cardiac surgery in the adult. New York: McGraw-Hill; 1996. p. 859–909.
2. Cohn LH, Reul RM. Mechanical and bioprosthetic mitral valve replacement. In: Edmunds LH, editor. Cardiac surgery in the adult. New York: McGraw Hill; 1997. p. 1025–1050.
3. Aupart MR, Sirinelli AL, Diemont FF, et al. The last generation of pericardial valves in the aortic position: ten-year follow-up in 589 patients. Ann Thorac Surg 1996;61: 615–20.
4. Burdon TA, Miller DC, Oyer PE, et al. Durability of porcine valves at fifteen years in a representative North American patient population. J Thorac Cardiovasc Surg 1992; 103(2):238–51.
5. David TE, Ivanov J, Armstrong S, et al. Late results of heart valve replacement with the Hancock II bioprosthesis. J Thorac Cardiovasc Surg 2001;121:268–77.

6. Fann JI, Miller DC, Moore KA, et al. Twenty-year clinical experience with porcine bioprostheses. Ann Thorac Surg 1996;62:1301–12.

7. Hammermeister K, Sethi GK, Henderson WG, et al. Outcomes 15 years after valve replacement with a mechanical versus a bioprosthetic valve: final report of the Veterans Affairs randomized trial. J Am Coll Cardiol 2000;36:1152–8.

8. Jamieson WRE, David TE, Feindel CM, et al. Performance of the Carpentier–Edwards SAV and Hancock II porcine bioprostheses in aortic valve replacement. J Heart Valve Dis 2002;11:424–30.

9. Jamieson WRE, Janusz MT, Burr LH, et al. Carpentier–Edwards supra-annular porcine bioprosthesis: second-generation prosthesis in aortic valve replacement. Ann Thorac Surg 2001;71 Suppl 5:S224–7.

10. Jamieson WRE, Miyagishima RT, Burr LH, et al. Carpentier–Edwards porcine bioprostheses: clinical performance assessed by actual analysis. J Heart Valve Dis 2000; 9:530–5.

11. Jamieson WRE, Burr LH, Miyagishima RT, et al. Actuarial versus actual freedom from structural valve deterioration with the Carpentier–Edwards porcine bioprostheses. Can J Cardiol 1999;15:973–8.

12. Jamieson WRE. Update on mechanical and tissue valves. In: Franco KL, Verrier ED, editors. Advanced therapy in cardiac surgery. Hamilton (ON): BC Decker; 1999. p. 201–12.

13. Jamieson WRE, Tyers GF, Janusz MT, et al. Age as a determinant for selection of porcine bioprostheses for cardiac valve replacement: experience with Carpentier–Edwards standard bioprosthesis. Can J Cardiol 1991;7:181–8.

14. Jamieson WRE, Rosado LJ, Munro AI, et al. Carpentier–Edwards standard porcine bioprosthesis: primary tissue failure (structural valve deterioration) by age groups. Ann Thorac Surg 1988;46(2):155–62.

15. Jamieson WRE, Marchand MA, Pelletier CL, et al. Structural valve deterioration in mitral replacement surgery: comparison of Carpentier–Edwards supra-annular porcine and PERIMOUNT pericardial bioprostheses. J Thorac Cardiovasc Surg 1999;118:297–304.

16. Marchand M, Aupart M, Norton R, et al. Twelve-year experience with Carpentier–Edwards PERIMOUNT pericardial valve in the mitral position: a multicenter study. J Heart Valve Dis 1998;7:292–8.

17. Myken P, Bech-Hanssen O, Phipps B, Caidahl K. Fifteen years follow-up with the St. Jude Medical–Biocor porcine bioprosthesis. J Heart Valve Dis 2000;9:415–22.

18. Pelletier LC, Carrier M, Leclerc Y, Dyrda I. The Carpentier–Edwards pericardial bioprosthesis: clinical experience with 600 patients. Ann Thorac Surg 1995;60 Suppl 2:S297–302.

19. Jamieson WRE. Current and advanced prostheses for cardiac valvular replacement and reconstructive surgery. Surg Tech Int 2002;1–29.

20. Edmunds LH Jr, Clark RE, Cohn LH, et al. Guidelines for reporting morbidity and mortality after cardiac valvular operations, Ad Hoc Liaison Committee for Standardizing Definitions of Prosthetic Heart Valve Morbidity. Ann Thorac Surgery 1996;62:932–35; J Thorac Cardiovasc Surg 1996;112:708–11.

21. Edwards FH, Peterson ED, Coombs LP, et al. Prediction of operative mortality after valve replacement surgery. J Am Coll Cardiol 2001;37:885–92.

22. Jamieson WRE, Edwards FH, Schwartz M, et al. Risk stratification for cardiac valve replacement. National Cardiac Surgery Database. Database Committee of the Society of Thoracic Surgeons. Ann Thorac Surg 1999;67:943–51.

23. Bach DS, Goldman B, Verrier E, et al. Eight-year hemodynamic follow-up after aortic valve replacement with the Toronto SPV stentless aortic valve. Semin Thorac Cardiovasc Surg 2001;13(4 Suppl 1):173–9.

24. David TE. The Toronto SPV bioprosthesis. Clinical and hemodynamic results at 6 years. Ann Thorac Surg 1999; 68 Suppl 3:S9–13.

25. David TE, Puschmann R, Ivanov J, et al. Aortic valve replacement with stentless and stented porcine valves: a case-match study. J Thorac Cardiovasc Surg 1998;116:236–41.

26. Doty DB, Cafferty A, Cartier P, et al. Aortic valve replacement with Medtronic Freestyle bioprosthesis: 5-year results. Semin Thorac Cardiovasc Surg 1999;11(4 Suppl 1):35–41.

27. Jamieson WRE, Janusz MT, MacNab J, Henderson C. Hemodynamic comparison of second- and third-generation stented bioprostheses in aortic valve replacement. Ann Thorac Surg 2001;71 Suppl 5:S282–4.

28. Jin XY, Pillai R, Westaby S. Medium-term determinants of left ventricular mass index after stentless aortic valve replacement. Ann Thorac Surg 1999;67:411–6.

29. Del Rizzo DF, Abdoh A, Cartier P, et al. Factors affecting left ventricular mass regression after aortic valve replacement with stentless valves. Semin Thorac Cardiovasc Surg 1999;11(4 Suppl 1):114–20.

30. Rao V, Christakis G, Sever J, et al. A novel comparison of stentless versus stented valves in the small aortic root. J Thorac Cardiovasc Surg 1999;117:431–8.

31. Thomson DJ, Jamieson WRE, Dumesnil JG, et al. Medtronic mosaic porcine bioprosthesis—mid-term investigational trial results. Ann Thorac Surg 2001;71:S269–72.

32. Walther T, Falk V, Langebartels G, et al. Prospectively randomized evaluation of stentless versus conventional biological aortic valve: impact on early regression of left ventricular hypertrophy. Circulation 1999;100 Suppl 1: II6–10.

33. Yun KL, Jamieson WRE, Khonsari S, et al. Prostheses–patient mismatch: hemodynamic comparison of stented and stentless aortic valves. Semin Thorac Cardiovasc Surg 1999;11(4–1):98–102.

34. Cunanan CM, Cabiling CM, Dinh TT, et al. Tissue characterization and calcification potential of commercial bioprosthetic heart valves. Ann Thorac Surg. 2001;71 Suppl 5:S417–21.

35. Myers D. New tissue-processing techniques. In: Piwnica A, Westaby S, editors. Stentless bioprostheses. Oxford: Isis Medical Media; 1997. p. 448–59.

36. Myers DJ, Gross J, Nakaya G. Stentless heart valves: biocompatibility issues associated with new antimineralization and fixation agents. In: Piwnica A, Westaby S, editors. Stentless bioprostheses. Oxford: Isis Medical Media; 1995. p. 100–17.

37. Girardot MN, Torrianni M, Girardot JM. Effect of AOA on glutaraldehyde-fixed bioprosthetic heart valve cusps and walls; binding and calcification studies. Int J Artif Organs 1994;17:76–82.

38. Moore MA, Bohachevsky IK, Cheung DT, et al. Stabilization of pericardial tissue by dye-mediated photo-oxidation. Biomed Mater Res 1994;28:611–8.

39. Grunkemeier GL, Jamieson WRE, Miller DC, Starr A. Actuarial versus actual risk of porcine structural valve deterioration. J Thorac Cardiovasc Surg 1994;108:709–18.

40. Pibarot P, Dumesnil JG. Hemodynamic and clinical impact of prosthesis–patient mismatch in the aortic valve position and its prevention. J Am Coll Cardiol 2000;36: 1131–41.

41. Pibarot P, Dumesnil JG, Jobin J, et al. Hemodynamic and physical performance during maximal exercise in patients with aortic bioprosthetic valve position and its prevention. J Am Coll Cardiol 1999;(34):1609–17.

42. Del Rizzo DF, Abdoh A, Cartier P, et al. The effect of prosthetic valve type on survival after aortic valve surgery. Semin Thorac Cardiovasc Surg 1999;11(4 Suppl 1):1–8.

43. Pibarot P, Dumesnil JG, Leblanc MH, et al. A comparison between stentless and stented valves with regard to the changes in left ventricular mass and function after aortic valve replacement. Can J Cardiol 1999;15 Suppl D:223d.

44. Chambers JC, Somerville J, Stone S, Ross DN. Pulmonary autograft procedure for aortic valve disease: long-term results of the pioneer series. Circulation 1997;96:2206–14.

45. Doty JR, Salazar JD, Liddicoat JR, et al. Aortic valve replacement with cryopreserved aortic allograft: ten-year experience. J Thorac Cardiovasc Surg 1998;115:371–80.

46. Yacoub M, Rasmi NRH, Sundt TM, et al. Fourteen-year experience with homovital homografts for aortic valve replacement. J Thorac Cardiovasc Surg 1995;110:186–94.

47. Pibarot P, Dumesnil JG, Cartier PC, et al. Patient–prosthesis mismatch can be predicted at the time of operation. Ann Thorac Surg 2001;71 Suppl 5:S265–8.

48. Jamieson WRE, Cartier PC, Canadian Primary Panel. Canadian consensus on surgical management of valvular heart disease. Can J Cardiol. [In Press]

49. Birkmeyer NJ, Birkmeyer JD, Tosteson AN, et al. Prosthetic valve type for patients undergoing aortic valve replacement: a decision analysis. Ann Thorac Surg 2000;70: 1946–52.

50. Elkins RC, Goldstein S, Hewitt CW, et al. Recellularization of heart valve grafts by a process of adaptive remodeling. Semin Thorac Cardiovasc Surg 2001;13(4 Suppl 1): 87–92.

51. Hoerstrup SP, Sodian R, Daebritz S, et al. Functional living trileaflet heart valves grown in vitro. Circulation 2000; 102(19 Suppl 3):III44–9.

52. Hoerstrup SP, Zund G, Lachat M, et al. Tissue engineering: a new approach in cardiovascular surgery—seeding of human fibroblasts on resorbable mesh. Swiss Surg 1998; Suppl 2:23–5.

53. Kim WG, Park JK, Park YN, et al. Tissue-engineered heart valve leaflets: an effective method for seeding autologous cells on scaffolds. Int J Artif Organs 2000;23:624–8.

54. Shinoka T. Tissue-engineered heart valves: autologous cell seeding on biodegradable polymer scaffold. Artif Organs 2002;26:402–6.

55. Sodian R, Sperling JS, Martin DP, et al. Fabrication of a trileaflet heart valve scaffold from a polyhydroxyalkanoate biopolyester for use in tissue engineering. Tissue Eng 2000;6:183–8.

56. O'Brien MF, Goldstein S, Walsh S, et al. The SynerGraft valve: a new acellular (nonglutaraldehyde-fixed) tissue heart valve for autologous recellularization—first experimental studies before clinical implantation. Semin Thorac Cardiovasc Surg 1999;11(4 Suppl 1):194–200.

CHAPTER 21

UPDATE ON STENTLESS VALVES

BERNARD S. GOLDMAN, MD, FRCSC, HARI MALLIDI, MD

The goals of aortic valve replacement (AVR) are the relief of symptoms from abnormal hemodynamics, prolonged survival, and improvement of left ventricular performance.[1] Aortic valvular disease produces left ventricular hypertrophy (LVH), secondary to pressure or volume overload.[2] Persistent LVH is known to be associated with poor survival.[3] Although significant improvement of LVH occurs after AVR, it is generally believed that incomplete regression affects ventricular function and late outcomes.[4] An ideal prosthesis for AVR should provide a large effective orifice area (EOA) with minimal transvalvular gradient, thereby allowing for the continued resolution of LVH.[5]

Tissue bioprostheses are commonly used in the elderly (> 65 years), in those with potential bleeding problems, and in younger patients (< 65 years) who do not wish anticoagulants. Conventional stented aortic bioprostheses, however, have relatively high transvalvular gradients, particularly in smaller sizes.[5] Thus, stented valves are inherently obstructive with detrimental leaflet stresses during the cardiac cycle. This ultimately produces tissue degeneration, calcification, leaflet tears, or cusp rupture.[6,7] Stent-mounted homografts are less durable than free hand-sewn homografts.[8]

Stentless xenografts for AVR were first reported in 1965 but did not gain favor because of the technical demands of implantation and the ready availability of improved commercial stented porcine valves.[9] David designed a subcoronary stentless porcine valve in 1985 and reported the initial clinical series in 1990.[10] Subsequently, different stentless valves have been introduced as an alternative to conventional stented bioprostheses. Clinical results have stimulated considerable interest and some controversy.

The design of stentless aortic valves was intended to reduce residual obstruction by maximizing the available flow area, that is, provide larger effective orifice areas and lower gradients than stented bioprostheses; excellent hemodynamics were soon reported.[2,11–16] The inherent flexibility of a stentless valve takes advantage of the dynamic nature of the aortic annulus, which may vary considerably during the cardiac cycle. Incorporation of the stentless valve within the native aortic root permits normal leaflet motion during systole and dampens mechanical stress during diastole.[5,7] This has suggested the potential for both enhanced durability with fewer valvular complications during follow-up.[6] Numerous clinical series are now approaching 10 years from first implant, providing considerable information on stentless valve function over time.[17–23]

Currently Available Stentless Aortic Valves

Several stentless aortic prostheses are available. They are described in the following paragraphs.

The Toronto Stentless Porcine Valve (TSPV, St. Jude Medical Inc., St. Paul, Minnesota) is a fully scalloped aortic valve fixed in glutaraldehyde at low pressure with the aortic sinuses and subannular tissue trimmed to 1.5 to 2.0 mm from the base of the cusps with the porcine aortic wall covered by a fine layer of Dacron. The valve is designed for subcoronary implantation.[24] No anticalcification agent is used. A root version treated with a new anticalcification agent is currently undergoing clinical trials (Figure 21-1).

The Freestyle Stentless Bioprosthesis (Medtronic Corp., Minneapolis, Minnesota) is a stentless porcine aortic root cross-linked in dilute glutaraldehyde solution at zero pressure, providing stress-free fixation for the valve leaflets. Treatment with amino-oleic acid reduces the potential for calcification. This valve provides the versatility to implant fully scalloped in a subcoronary position or as a modified subcoronary implant with retention of the donor noncoronary sinus, as a root inclusion within a dilated aorta, or as a full root replacement by using a modified Bentall technique.[25] The septal muscle bar only is covered with Dacron (Figure 21-2).

The Cryolife–O'Brien Stentless Valve (Cryolife Inc., Marietta, Georgia) is a composite design constructed of noncoronary leaflets obtained from three porcine valves without foreign material support and fully scalloped. The leaflets are carefully excised from valves already fixed in glutaraldehyde at low or near-zero pressure. Individual noncoronary leaflets are matched for size and symmetry to ensure synchronous opening and to promote maximal leaflet coaptation. The matched set of leaflets are sutured together along the free edges of the porcine aortic walls at the commissures. The valve is secured in a supra-annular position with a single suture line (Figure 21-3).[26]

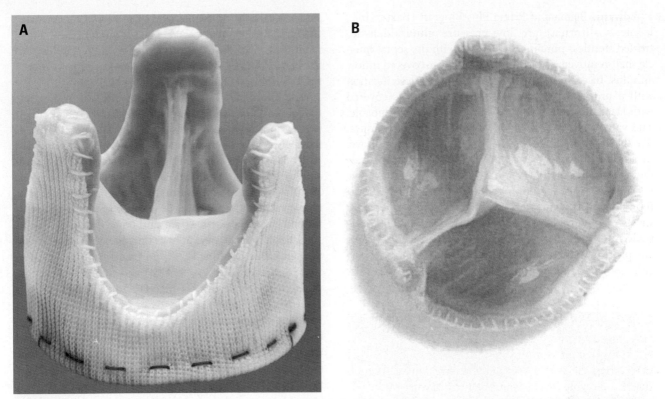

FIGURE 21-1. The Toronto Stentless Porcine Valve (TSPV, St. Jude Medical Inc., St. Paul, Minnesota). Lateral view (A) of the scalloped bioprosthesis and superior view (B), showing the large leaflet coaptation surfaces.

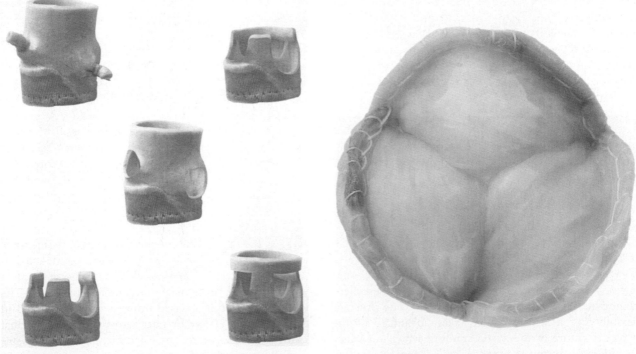

FIGURE 21-2. The Freestyle Bioprosthesis (Medtronic Inc., Minneapolis, Minnesota). Potential configurations: the xenograft root design is versatile, allowing implantation by the modified subcoronary technique, full scalloping of all three porcine sinuses, the miniroot method, or full aortic root replacement.

FIGURE 21-3. The Cryolife–O'Brien Stentless Valve (Cryolife Inc., Marietta, Georgia). A composite design of noncoronary leaflets obtained from three porcine valves, designed for supra-annular insertion with a single suture line.

Edwards Prima and Prima Plus Biograft (Baxter, Inc., Irvine, California) are low-pressure glutaraldehyde-treated stentless porcine aortic roots with the septal muscle shelf removed and a reinforced Dacron-covered inflow annulus. In each, the valve is treated for anticalcification with a proprietary agent. The septal muscle is covered with Dacron. The aortic wall is thick but soft and pliable. The valve may be implanted with different techniques, like the Freestyle Stentless Bioprosthesis discussed above. In addition, marker stitches facilitate subcoronary scalloping by the surgeon (Figure 21-4).[27]

The Sorin Pericarbon Stentless Aortic Valve (Sorin Biomedica, Saluggia, Italy) is made from two separate sheets of glutaraldehyde-treated pericardium. This thin-walled pericardial stentless valve is constructed without any prosthetic material and is much softer and more pliable than porcine stentless aortic valves. The pericardial stentless valve is implanted using a modified subcoronary technique. Care must be taken with commissural alignment because of the extreme flexibility and redundancy of the pericardium.[28] A new anticalcification process is currently employed (Figure 21-5).

The Biocor PSB Stentless Valve (Biocor Industriae, Pesquisa, Ltda, Belo Horizonte-MG, Belo Horzonte, Brazil) is a composite valve of selected individual porcine cusps fixed with glutaraldehyde at zero pressure and sutured to a strip of bovine pericardium shaped in the form of a conduit and scalloped above and below the insertion of the leaflets. The No-React anticalcification treatment is employed. The Biocor valve has been primarily used for implantations performed in Brazil, South Africa, and Italy.

Other stentless valves used mainly in South America are the Unique Suture Line (USL) porcine bioprosthesis (Bio-Sud SA, Buenos Aires, Argentina) and the Labcor porcine valve (Belo Horizonte-MG, Belo Horzonte, Brazil).

Two new valves were recently introduced. The Aortech Elan Stentless Aortic Valve (United Kingdom) is a glutaraldehyde-preserved porcine valve with a pericardial reinforced inflow tract, a scalloped outflow to reduce bulk, and no Dacron covering. The SAVR (Stentless Aortic Valve Replacement) bioprosthesis (BioSurg, United States) is a tubular structure of unique bioprosthetic material used during cardiac repair procedures. This valve is not yet in clinical trials.

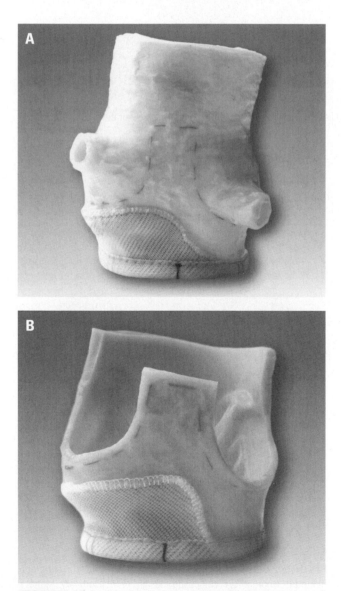

FIGURE 21-4. The Edwards Prima Biograft showing the full xenograft root (A) and marker stitches to facilitate scalloping (B).

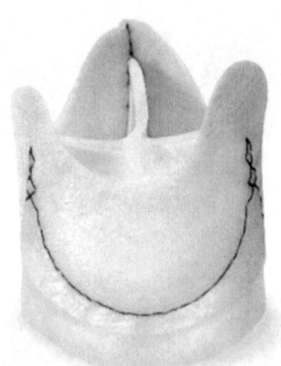

FIGURE 21-5. The Sorin Pericarbon Stentless Valve (Sorin Biomedica, Saluggia, Italy), constructed of two separate sheets of glutaraldehyde-treated pericardium and designed for a modified subcoronary implant technique.

Hemodynamics

The hemodynamic characteristics and clinical outcomes after stentless aortic valve implantation have been extensively documented over the past decade.[6,29-31] Stentless porcine xenografts function like aortic homografts with virtually identical flow characteristics.[11] Stentless aortic valves demonstrate low transvalvular pressure gradients and a progressive increase in calculated orifice areas over time. Left ventricular mass index (LVMI) and wall thickness approach normal between 6 and 12 months post operation. Mass regression continues beyond 2 years. Left ventricular (LV) remodeling, with changes in the outflow tract, is considered responsible for the increase in calculated valve area. Lower residual gradients remove the stimulus for persistence of LVH.[2,32] The resultant improved LV performance may be associated with a survival benefit.[33] David and colleagues, in a case-match study, showed improved cardiac survival in patients implanted with stentless valves compared to those with a stented bioprosthesis.[34]

The issue of valve sizes has influenced our understanding of the hemodynamic observations. David had noted, in his first clinical series, leaflet distraction and subsequent aortic insufficiency due to sinotubular ridge (STJ) dilatation, common in aortic valve disease. He suggested that subcoronary implants be sized to the STJ diameter, provided this was no more than 10% greater than the measured annulus, that is, one valve size larger than the annulus.[10] The concept of implanting larger stentless valves, as compared to implanting stented valves, is noted throughout early series and was considered one of the benefits of stentless valve implantation. However, more manufacturers' valve sizes and sizers recently have come under scrutiny because of a challenging study by Christakis and associates that revealed inaccurate and misleading information.[35] Among 403 patients operated upon for predominant aortic stenosis (AS), those 98 patients receiving a stentless valve (TSPV) had a larger mean internal diameter (ID 22.3 ± 1.9 mm) than did the 204 patients receiving a stented bioprosthesis (ID 20.9 ± 1.9 mm). But when the manufacturers' labeled sizes were considered, the results were even more exaggerated in favor of TSPV (26.3 ± 1.9 mm) when compared to the stented tissue valves (23.1 ± 2.1 mm). Thus, comparisons of hemodynamic differences between valve types based on implanted sizes may be erroneous and require careful interpretation. Walther also showed that exact sizing of the annulus after complete decalcification is crucial for further comparisons of different cohorts.[36]

Not withstanding this caveat, numerous studies demonstrate the excellent hemodynamics of stentless aortic valves. Del Rizzo reported serial echocardiography on 254 patients with TSPV during a 3-year follow-up: the mean gradient decreased by 35.8% from postoperation to 3 months and by 6.1% at each subsequent interval; effective orifice area increased 17.2% initially, and 4.4% thereafter. The mean gradient at 2 years was 3.3 mm Hg and the EOA 2.2 cm²; LVMI decreased by 15.2% from postoperation to 3 to 6 months.[2] David reported on 542 patients showing mean gradients at 3 to 6 months of 6.3 mm Hg decreasing to 3.0 mm Hg by 6 years. Valve area increased from 1.9 to 2.2 cm² and LVMI decreased from 153 to 118 g/m².[37]

Similar results have been obtained with the Medtronic Freestyle valve, with significant decreases in gradient noted early after AVR and with a further reduction by 3 to 6 months.[38] However, there was a difference in transvalvular gradients noted between the three different implantation techniques, subcoronary, root inclusion, or full root replacement. The mean gradients were 11.2, 9.5, and 6.2 mm Hg, respectively, at 4 weeks and 7.2, 6.2, and 4.8 mm Hg at 3 to 6 months, remaining relatively stable thereafter.[39] Medtronic summarized the trial data for 1,100 implants, showing a mean transvalvular gradient for all techniques of 5.9 mm Hg, with an EOA of 2.1 cm² at 7 years. The mean gradient for subcoronary implants was 9.4 mm Hg, 5.3 mm Hg for root inclusion, and 6.0 mm Hg for full root replacement.[40] The implant technique used was based on the aortic morphology. Konertz recently presented 4- to 5-year follow-up data on 116 patients with the Edwards Prima stentless valve, showing mean gradients ranging from 27.9 mm Hg for the 19 mm valve to 4.2 mm Hg for the 29 mm bioprosthesis. The majority of patients had 23, 25, and 27 mm valves, showing mean gradients of 9.9, 8.8, and 6.5 mm Hg, respectively.[41]

Five-year hemodynamic evaluation of the Cryolife–O'Brien stentless aortic valve (CLOB) also demonstrates a significant decrease in gradient and increased EOA from early postoperation to 6 months follow-up.[42] Similar results have been observed with the Biocor valve at a mean of 5.8 years.[43] Jin and Westaby compared the results of patients with the Sorin Biomedica Pericarbon Stentless Aortic valve to patients with the Freestyle porcine valve; at discharge, the EOA and mean transvalvular gradients did not differ between the two groups. However, the stentless porcine valve had a higher flow velocity at both the outflow tract and valve levels, a higher peak pressure gradient, and a higher mean systolic flow rate than did the stentless pericardial valves. Nonetheless, at 1 year, EOA, gradients, and outflow tract diameters were indistinguishable between the two valve types; systolic flow velocity and flow rate were no longer different. The more favorable results observed early with the pericardial valve were attributed to the thin-walled, soft and pliable material.[44]

Greve compared hemodynamic results between Freestyle, TSPV, and CLOB valves and found little difference, with the full-root Freestyle having the lowest pressure gradients and the subcoronary Freestyle having the highest, perhaps due to oversizing. The differences at 1 year were not significant, although the CLOB valve did have the lowest, and the subcoronary Freestyle the highest, gradients.[45] In summary, all current stentless bioprostheses demonstrate excellent early hemodynamics, which are sustained through medium-term follow-up.

Comparative Studies

The hemodynamic superiority of stentless aortic valves has been described in numerous papers that have compared them to stented bioprostheses. There are recognized difficulties with the interpretation of results because most studies are observational, some are retrospective, some are from trial databases, others are case-matched, and only a few are prospectively randomized with attention to the true annulus and valve dimensions. Cohen evaluated a consecutive series of TSPV versus stented-tissue-valve patients (Hancock II and Carpentier-Edwards (CE) Perimount). Although there was no difference in LVMI regression or decrease in gradients between groups, the increase in EOA was greater with the TSPV, and with fractional shortening and velocity of circumferential shortening also greater in the TSPV group at 3 to 6 months after AVR, suggesting early improved LV performance.[46] Gelsomino reported a retrospective study of stentless valves (CLOB) compared to both stented bioprostheses (CE porcine and pericardial) and mechanical valves after AVR in patients with severe AS and poor LV function (ejection fraction [EF] < 35%). He noted similar changes in all groups. Although EF increased in all patients postoperatively, at any given point in follow-up, the EF was higher for stentless valves, as was fractional shortening and the velocity of circumferential shortening. Meridional wall stress and circumferential wall stress also returned to normal for the stentless implants. The indexed EOA (EOAI) was higher for stentless valve patients, and ventricular volumes and LVMI were all significantly lower (as were the mean gradients) than those for the stented valve patients.[47]

Fries compared rest and exercise hemodynamics of a 23 mm stentless valve (Freestyle) to a 23-mm stented (CE supra-annular porcine) valve and also in healthy volunteers. Peak exercise-induced gradients were significantly less in the stentless (18 mm Hg) than in the stented (40 mm Hg) patients and similar to the normal patients' values.[48] However, Lee noted no difference in LVMI or exercise performance, despite significantly lower pressure gradients at rest and exercise, in stentless versus stented patients.[49] Maselli described better hemodynamic performance indices for homograft and stentless valves (both TSPV and Freestyle) when compared to a stented bioprosthesis (Medtronic Intact). The amount of absolute LVMI reduction was significantly greater in the homograft group than that of Intact and TSPV patients but without significant difference between the homograft and Freestyle valves.[50] Morsy studied exercise gradients in young patients (mean, 29.9 years of age) with TSPV as compared to patients with mechanical valves: peak pressure gradients rose 51.1% for TSPV but 101.7% for mechanical valves, without differences in EF or EOAI.[51]

Silberman made similar findings.[52] These studies suggest a hemodynamic advantage of stentless valves for young and active patients.

Hemodynamic improvement may be more significant in patients with aortic stenosis and small aortic roots. Milano and colleagues retrospectively compared the performance of stentless versus stented bioprostheses in patients with a measured 21 mm annulus (receiving either a 21 mm Perimount or a 23 mm TSPV) and a measured 23 mm annulus (receiving either a 23 mm Medtronic Mosaic or a 25 mm Edwards Prima).[53] Significant reductions of mean and peak gradients were more evident for TSPV versus Perimount and for Prima versus Mosaic. The EOA increased significantly for the TSPV group, and regression of LVMI was greatest for the Prima cohort. The authors concluded that for the increasing number of elderly patients presenting with small aortic roots, stentless valves have a more pronounced hemodynamic improvement. However, they conceded that the new generation of stented bioprostheses do, in fact, parallel the hemodynamic performance of the stentless group and thus appear to be valid alternatives, given the lower activity expectations of the elderly.

Walther evaluated LVH and mass regression in a prospective randomized study of stentless (Freestyle, TSPV) versus stented bioprostheses (Perimount). Although aortic annulus diameter indices were comparable, the authors noted that larger stentless valves were implanted due to the oversizing technique. Regression of LVH occurred in all patients but was significantly enhanced by 6 months after stentless valve implantation.[36] However, in a prospective randomized trial in which the annuli were sized for the optimal insertion of either TSPV or CE Perimount *before* randomization, Cohen and associates showed no differences in mean decrease of left ventricular outflow tract (LVOT) diameter or in actual mean valve size (based on internal valvular dimensions rather than manufacturer's labeled size). Although EOA increased and pressure gradients decreased in both groups over time, as did LV mass regression, there were no significant differences between the stentless and stented groups at rest, up to 1 year of follow-up. This was also true for any improvement noted in functional status.[54] Although the controversy remains unsolved and requires longer follow-up, there is a definite trend in most reported series regarding the hemodynamic superiority of stentless versus stented bioprostheses or mechanical valves, particularly in patients with small annuli or during exercise.

Clinical Events

Clinical outcomes after valve replacement are related not only to the type of implanted prosthesis but also to the cardiac status and other comorbidities present in the patient at the time of surgery or developing thereafter. While stentless valves have excellent hemodynamic function in early and mid-term follow-up, long-term structural durability and functional integrity are as yet unknown. Indeed, stentless valves may demonstrate improved longevity due to preservation of the aortic root and sinuses, which allows for normal leaflet motion, normal systolic flow, and dissipation of diastolic stresses. Despite longer operating times and a high percentage of patients in clinical trials who required concomitant coronary artery bypass (approximately 40%), actuarial survival at 6 to 8 years has been excellent (65 to 80%) and freedom from valve related death approximately 97.0%. Freedom from structural valve deterioration has been approximately 98%.[40,55] Reoperation rates within the 6- to 8-year window are gratifyingly low. Tables 21-1 through 21-4 show the adverse event rates during follow-up and actuarial freedoms from late valve-related complications for both TSPV (Tables 21-1 and 21-2) and Freestyle (Tables 21-3 and 21-4) valves.

Luciani compared outcomes in a nonrandomized retrospective study of stentless valves (TSPV, CLOB, Biocor) versus stented bioprostheses (Hancock II). Although the stentless patients were older and operating times longer, the stented patients usually had more complex associated surgery. The operative mortality for stentless versus stented patients was lower (2.7% vs 6.2%) with higher late survival at 7 years (81% vs 70%) due to fewer late cardiac deaths (4.1% vs 8.4%). Freedom from cardiac events at 7 years was 92% versus 85% for stentless versus stented valves, and freedom from valve-related deaths was 95% versus 79%.[56] It has been suggested, therefore, that stentless valves confer a survival advantage when compared with conventional stented biologic and mechanical valves. David showed significant improvement in actuarial survival in a case-controlled study in which the TSPV stentless valve patients were compared to the Hancock II stented bioprosthesis patients (91% vs 69% at 8 years), implying that valve design and thus cardiac performance had a significant effect on long-term patient survival after AVR.[34]

TABLE 21-1. Linearized Event Rates for Late Valve-Related Complications for the Toronto Stentless Porcine Valve

| | Early (< 30 days) | | Late (> 30 days) | |
Adverse Event	N	% of Patients	N	%/Patient-Years
Bleeding event	1	0.2	2	0.1
Endocarditis	0	0.0	6	0.3
Paravalvular leak	8	1.8	17	0.9
Embolism	6	1.3	18	1.0
RIND/CVA/peripheral embolism	5	1.1	7	0.4
Thrombosis	0	0.0	0	0.0
Structural deterioration	0	0.0	7	0.4
Reoperation (explant)	0	0.0	10	0.5
Death (all cause)	4	0.9	49	2.5
Death (valve-related)	2	0.4	9	0.5

From St. Jude Medical Clinical Report #3, August 2000.

TABLE 21-2. Actuarial Freedoms from Late Valve-Related Complications for TSPV

Adverse Event	At 7 Years (%)
Bleeding event	99.2
RIND/CVA/peripheral embolism	96.7
Endocarditis	98.5
Paravalvular leak	92.8
Structural deterioration	96.1
Structural deterioration implant age > 60 yr	98.0
Reoperation	95.2
Death	81.8
Valve-related death	96.9

TABLE 21-3. Linearized Rates for Late Valve-Related Complications for the Medtronic Freestyle Stentless Porcine Valve

Event	N	%/Patient-Years
Thromboembolism		
Permanent	28	1.1
Transient	33	1.2
Thrombosis	2	0.1
Major antithromboembolic-related hemorrhage	25	0.9
Primary paravalvular leak	13	0.5
Endocarditis	11	0.4
Primary hemolysis	0	0.0
Structural deterioration	2	0.1
Nonstructural dysfunction	1	0.04
Reoperation	12	0.5
Explant	9	0.3
Expiration	12	0.5

From Medtronic Inc., Seven-Year Clinical Compendium, October 2001.

TABLE 21-4. Actuarial Freedoms from Late Valve-Related Complications for the Medtronic Freestyle Stentless Bioprosthesis

| | Freedom from % | |
Event	At 7 Years (%)	Standard Error (%)
Thromboembolism		
Permanent	89.6	(4.8)
Transient	92.1	(4.0)
Thrombosis	99.7	(0.9)
Major antithromboembolic-related hemorrhage	93.2	(1.3)
Primary paravalvular leak	96.0	(3.0)
Endocarditis	97.4	(2.5)
Primary hemolysis	100.0	(0.0)
Structural deterioration	99.5	(1.1)
Nonstructural dysfunction	98.8	(0.8)
Reoperation	97.2	(2.5)
Explant	97.8	(2.2)
Expiration	97.4	(2.4)

Del Rizzo examined the databases for the Medtronic Freestyle (453 patients) and the Hancock II bioprosthesis (224 patients). Five-year actuarial survival was 86% for Freestyle and 77% for Hancock II. The survival advantage was greater in patients younger than 60 years of age, with a fivefold increase in the probability of death for those with a stented valve. With advancing age the benefits of the stentless valve were less notable.[57] Del Rizzo later examined the manufacturers' and institutional databases for a stentless cohort (Freestyle, TSPV) as compared to stented valves (Hancock II, CE supra-annular). The stented patients were older (70.6 vs 69.3 years of age), required more coronary artery bypass graft (CABG) surgery (45.8% vs 40.6%), and were generally sicker (New York Heart Association [NYHA] class III/IV, 82.2% vs 66.4%) with a higher proportion of patients with aortic stenosis. It is not surprising, therefore, that early mortality was better for the stentless cohort (3.5% vs 4.8%) as was the 5-year survival (isolated AVR, 84% vs 80%; AVR + CABG, 82% vs 77%). The stated benefits of the stentless valves (lower incidence of patient prosthesis mismatch, better hemodynamics, more complete resolution of LVH, and better coronary perfusion from laminar flow) were suggested as conferring a survival advantage for the stentless- over stented-valve patients. It is also likely that selection bias played a significant role in these results.[58] Nonetheless, overall morbidity in follow-up to almost 10 years appears reduced for stentless valves when compared to those stented bioprostheses reported.

Aortic Insufficiency

The development of aortic insufficiency has frustrated the long-term function of some aortic homografts and pulmonary autografts. Aortic insufficiency (AI) may appear early after implantation of a subcoronary stentless valve due to inadequate sizing, malalignment of the commissural posts, cusp injury, or inappropriate patient or prosthesis selection (dilated aortic root or ascending aorta). Techniques such as the modified subcoronary implant with retention of the donor noncoronary sinus wall, root inclusion, or full root replacement are less likely to show significant AI. Nonetheless, 95.2% of patients, early (< 3 months) after TSPV subcoronary implants, showed 0 or trivial to mild (1+) aortic insufficiency, and by 8 years this had only decreased to 86.4%.[22]

The late development of aortic insufficiency is thus of concern and may be due to primary tissue valve failure (cusp tear or perforation), endocarditis, or structural changes in the aortic root complex. Dilatation of the sinotubular junction pulls the commissures of the stentless aortic valve apart, preventing the cusps from coapting, thus causing central AI. Because they are relatively inelastic, glutaraldehyde-fixed aortic cusps cannot compensate for the dilatation; consequently, mechanical stress increases, with resulting premature valve failure. David reported 11% of 174 patients followed up to 8 years post implant who developed more than 1+ AI due to dilatation of the sinotubular junction (STJ).[59] Freedom from structural valve deterioration was 99% for patients without AI and 82% for those with AI at 8 years. Jin and Westaby

described the identical problem with the Medtronic Freestyle valve and noted progressively more severe AI as the STJ diameter increased postoperatively.[60] Shargall noted a small cohort of 6 younger patients (mean, 39.8 years of age) in the TSPV Food and Drug Administration (FDA) trial (447 patients) with congenital bicuspid aortic valves that required reoperation for severe AI after stentless valve implant due to late dilatation (mean, 6 years) of the STJ, aortic sinus, or ascending aorta.[55] Therefore, it is necessary to identify patients with the potential for aortic dilatation and to secure the STJ diameter by a prosthetic band equal in diameter to that of the implanted valve.[59] While full root replacement has been recommended to prevent postoperative AI, this technique is best reserved for patients with concomitant valvular and aortic root disease. Root occlusion or preservation of the donor noncoronary aortic wall may be appropriate for patients with sinus dilatation undergoing stentless aortic valve insertion.

The Small Aortic Root

Increasing numbers of elderly patients present with calcific aortic stenosis, many being females with a small aortic root. AVR in the small aortic root often poses technical and physiologic challenges (see chapter 25, "Management of the Small Aortic Root"). Difficult implantation may require annular enlargement. Implantation of a small prosthesis, or even an oversized prosthesis, may not effectively relieve the aortic obstruction. Residual obstruction may result in inadequate LV mass reduction. Issues regarding patient–prosthesis mismatch remain controversial (defined as EOAI < 0.85 cm^2/m^2). The reduced activity levels of elderly patients may not require a maximal or even optimal valve orifice. Recent studies have not shown significant differences in outcome for patients with residual obstruction and apparent mismatch. Hanayama showed no difference in outcome for patients with or without mismatch (defined in this study as indexed EOA < 0.59 cm^2/m^2) or abnormally high postoperative gradients (ninetieth-percentile mean gradient was > 22 mm Hg and peak gradient was 38 mm Hg).[62] Furthermore, he showed no difference in survival or NYHA functional class at 7 years for patients with or without incomplete mass regression (LVMI > 128 mg/m^2).[63] Gelsomino studied 68 patients with small-sized CLOB bioprostheses to determine the occurrence of patient–prosthesis mismatch and to evaluate its clinical and hemodynamic implications. Multivariant analysis revealed female sex and advanced age to be determinants of mismatch defined here as EOA < 0.85 cm^2/m^2. These patients had high mean gradients at discharge and at 6 months, but at 1 year there was no difference in mean gradient in patients with or without mismatch, and EOAI did not correlate with mean gradient. Survival and clinical status were not affected by apparent mismatch.[64] Full root replacement with a stentless bioprosthesis has been recommended for patients with AS and small aortic root, but this may be excessive in terms of surgical risk relative to patient needs. Sinteck described excellent hemodynamics, even in smaller sizes, by using Freestyle valves implanted free-hand in elderly patients with a small aortic root, thus avoiding the need for some aortic root enlargement procedures.[65]

Summary

The impetus for use of stentless aortic bioprostheses arises from the awareness that mechanical valves have important complications of hemorrhage and thrombosis, and that conventional stented bioprostheses have limitations of long-term durability and residual obstruction, which may impede complete LV mass regression. Detailed echocardiographic studies show that stentless porcine valves have gradients, mechanical energy loss at the valve, peak systolic pressure, and LV wall stress directly equivalent to an aortic homograft.[11] Implant times are indeed longer and do require an increased level of surgical skill. However, current methods of myocardial protection allow for more complex procedures with little effect on early or late outcome. The learning curve for the implant technique of stentless valves is usually short; nonetheless, many surgeons may still opt for the simplicity of a stented valve insertion. The selective use of stentless valves has a bias in favor of lower-risk patients, reflected in lower hospital and late mortality, with better overall survival and a lower incidence of valve-related and cardiac events. Westaby documented that the routine use of a stentless valve decreases surgical risk due to accumulated experience. He suggested that those early trial results that did show higher overall operative risks were likely due to the learning-curve impact.[66]

Subcoronary stentless bioprostheses are usually contraindicated in patients with shallow aortic sinuses, annular diameter > 30 mm, calcified aortic root, marked dilatation of the STJ, anomalous origin of coronary arteries, or mirror-image coronary arteries (180° apart) as in some cases of bicuspid aortic valves. Nonetheless, Markowitz demonstrated the feasibility of working within such abnormal or calcified aortic roots, and Westaby described the versatility of a full root stentless bioprosthesis in many such patients by tailoring the valve to the patients' anatomy.[66,67] Thus, currently available stentless valves, depending on implant technique, may be used in patients with valvular disease and any form of concomitant aortic pathology. Appropriate sizing of the stentless valves and fixation of the STJ to the diameter of the implanted stentless bioprosthesis is essential. Because aortic root insufficiency may result from aortic dilatation, definition of the aortic root, sinotubular, and ascending aortic diameters will dictate the method of stentless valve implantation. Elderly patients with a small aortic root may benefit from stentless valves, even in smaller sizes. Comparative studies in general favor the hemodynamic superiority of stentless valves over stented bioprostheses, but issues of sizing and patient selection may have biased these observations. Nonetheless, the external diameter of the sewing cuff of a stented bioprosthesis may cause difficult insertion and/or require root enlargement; in addition, exercise gradients rise sharply with stented valves, although this may be less important in elderly patients. The implications of residual obstruction in small sizes with apparent patient–prosthesis mismatch seem to have been overly exaggerated, and current studies suggest no or little effect on clinical outcomes.

Incorporation of stentless valves within the normal aortic root provides normal leaflet opening and normal systolic flow with dissipation of diastolic pressures by the aortic sinuses whereas the leaflets of stented tissue valves are subject to flexion and diastolic pressures, with ultimate calcification and tearing. Thus, stentless valves may demonstrate greater durability. Indeed, freedom from structural deterioration and reoperation at 8 to 10 years has been excellent; the hemodynamic improvements are maintained.[40,55] In the most recent report of TSPV (at 8 years), the mean gradient for all valve sizes was 4.3 mm Hg and the mean EOA was 2.4 cm. Mean LVMI at hospital discharge was 151.4 g/m^2, and at 8 years it was 125 g/m^2.[55] The dramatic improvements in LV dynamics reported for all stentless valves translate to improved LV performance. This may have a beneficial effect on patient survival by decreasing late mortality from the progressive fibrosis, failure, or arrhythmias associated with incomplete mass regression, and may thereby provide greatest benefit to patients with LV dysfunction. In addition, improved postoperative LV function may decrease mortality if reoperation is required at some later date.

Stentless aortic bioprostheses, therefore, have an important role in the treatment of aortic valvular disease. The authors believe that the benefits of the stentless concept are best realized with implantation of a fully scalloped subcoronary valve. Care must be taken to avoid impingement on coronary arteries, with proper alignment of commissural posts and detailed attention to annulus and sinotubular dimensions. Preservation of the noncoronary sinus aortic wall facilitates implantation and is indicated for abnormalities of the patient noncoronary sinus; similarly, root inclusion is also recommended for those patients with dilatation of the aortic root including all sinuses. However, donor aortic root is subject to calcification, which may negate one of the postulated benefits of stentless valves, that is, dissipation of diastolic pressures into normal sinuses. The full root technique is obviously indicated for patients with concomitant disease of the aortic valve, aortic root, and proximal ascending aorta, but calcification is an inherent risk, and ultimate replacement may be a formidable task.

Stentless bioprostheses are recommended when tissue valves are chosen for patients older than 65 to 70 years of age, and especially for those with small aortic root. There is increasing suggestion that stentless valves may be ideal for active middle-aged (35–65 years) patients due to excellent exercise hemodynamics and improved LV functional indices despite the possibility of reoperation. Stentless valves have been used as an alternative to a homograft in some cases of endocarditis. Stentless bioprostheses should be considered for AVR accompanied by marked LVH or LV dysfunction. Longer follow-up is required to document better event-free survival and improved valve durability when compared to stented tissue valves; carefully controlled prospective randomized trials will be important in this regard. The ready availability and versatility of stentless valves suggests an increasingly important role in the surgeon's armamentarium.

References

1. Ruygrok PN, Barrat-Boyes BG, Agnew TM, et al. Aortic valve replacement in the elderly. J Heart Valve Dis 1993;2(5):550–7.

2. Del Rizzo DF, Goldman BS, Christakis GT, David TE. Hemodynamic benefits of the Toronto stentless valve. J Thorac Cardiovasc Surg 1996;112(6):1431–45; discussion 1445–6.

3. Levy D, Garrison RJ, Savage DD, et al. Prognostic implications of echo cardiographically determined left ventricular mass in the Framingham Heart Study. N Engl J Med 1990;322:1561–6.

4. Jin XY, Zhang ZM, Gibson DG, et al. Effects of valve substitute on changes in left ventricular function and hypertrophy after aortic valve replacement. Ann Thorac Surg 1996;62(3):683–90.

5. Cohen G, Christakis GT, Buth KJ, et al. Early experience with stentless versus stented valves. Circulation 1997:96 Suppl 9:II-76–82.

6. Westaby S, Huysmans HA, David TE. Stentless aortic bioprostheses: compelling data from the Second International Symposium. Ann Thorac Surg 1998;65(1):235–40.

7. Vesely I, Mako WJ. Comparison of the compressive buckling of porcine aortic valve cusps and bovine pericardium. J Heart Valve Dis 1998;7(1):34–9.

8. Angell WW, Pupello DF, Bessone LN, et al. Effect of stent mounting on tissue valves of aortic valve replacement. J Card Surg 1991;6 Suppl 4:595–9.

9. Binet JP, Duran CG, Carpentier A, et al. Heterologous aortic valve transplantation. Lancet 1965;ii:1275.

10. David TE, Pollick C, Bos J. Aortic valve replacement with stentless porcine aortic bioprosthesis. J Thorac Cardiovasc Surg 1990;99(1):113–8.

11. Jin XY, Gibson DG, Yacoub MH, Pepper JR. Perioperative assessment of aortic homograft, Toronto stentless valve, and stented valve in the aortic position. Ann Thorac Surg 1995;60 Suppl 2:S395–401.

12. Sidiropoulos A, Hotz H, Tschesnow J, Konertz W. Stentless porcine bioprostheses for all types of aortic root pathology. Eur J Cardiothorac Surg 1997;11(5):917–21.

13. Westaby S, Amaresna N, Ormerod O, et al. Aortic valve replacement with the Freestyle stentless xenograft. Ann Thorac Surg 1995;60:S422–7.

14. Pillai R, Spriggings D, Amarasena N, et al. Stentless aortic bioprosthesis? The way forward: early experience with the Edwards valve. Ann Thorac Surg 1993;56:88–91.

15. Hvass U, Chatel D, Ouroudji M, et al. The O'Brien-Angell stentless valve: early results of 100 implants. Eur J Cardiothorac Surg 1994;42:36–9.

16. Kon ND, Westaby S, Amarasena N, et al. Comparison of implantation techniques using Freestyle stentless porcine aortic valve. Ann Thorac Surg 1995;59:857–62.

17. Goldman BS, Christakis GT, David TE, et al. Will Stentless valves be durable? The Toronto Valve (TSPV) at 5 to 6 years. Semin Thorac Cardiovasc Surg 1999;11:4 Suppl 1:42–9.

18. David TE, Feindel CM, Scully HE, et al. Aortic valve replacement with stentless porcine aortic valves: a ten-year experience. J Heart Valve Dis 1998;7:250–4.

19. Goldman BS, David TE, Wood JR, et al. Clinical outcomes after aortic valve replacement with the Toronto stentless porcine valve. Ann Thorac Surg 2001;71:S302–5.

20. Shargall Y, Peterson M, Goldman B, et al. Ten years experience with the Toronto SPV bioprosthesis explant and mortality analysis (abstracts 35 and 36). Stentless Bioprosthesis, Fourth International Symposium; 2001 May 3–5; San Diego, California.

21. Jin XY, Ratnatunga C, Pillai R, et al. Up to 8 year's performance of Edwards Prima stentless porcine aortic valve (abstract 48). Stentless Bioprosthesis, Fourth International Symposium; 2001 May 3–5; San Diego, California.

22. Bach DS, Goldman B, Verrier E, et al. Eight-year hemodynamic follow-up after aortic valve replacement with the Toronto SPV stentless aortic valve (abstract 51). Stentless Bioprosthesis, Fourth International Symposium; 2001 May 3–5; San Diego, California.

23. Dagenais F, Cartier P, Lemieux M, et al. A single-center experience with the freestyle Medtronic bioprosthesis: mid-term results at the Laval Hospital (abstract 47). Stentless Bioprosthesis, Fourth International Symposium; 2001 May 3–5; San Diego, California.

24. Cutrara CA, Goldman BS, Christakis GT. Preferred method for insertion of the Toronto stentless porcine valve. J Card Surg 1998;13:408–11.

25. Doty DB, Cafferty A, Kon ND, et al. Medtronic Freestyle aortic root bioprosthesis: implant techniques. J Card Surg 1998;13:369–75.

26. O'Brien MF. Implantation technique of the Cryolife-O'Brien xenograft aortic valve: the simple, rapid and correct way to implant and the errors to avoid. Semin Thorac Cardiovasc Surg 1999;11:121–5.

27. Konertz, WF, Sidiropoulos A, Liu J. Aortic valve replacement with the Edwards Prima Plus stentless bioprosthesis. Op Tech Thorac Cardiovasc Surg 2001;6:75–81.

28. Westaby S. Implant technique for the Sorin stentless pericardial valve. Op Tech Thorac Cardiovasc Surg 2001;6:101–15.

29. Bach DS, David T, Yacoub M, et al. Hemodynamics and left ventricular mass regression following implantation of the Toronto SPV valve. Am J Cardiol 1998;82:1214–9.

30. Doty DB, Cafferty A, Cartier P, et al. Aortic valve replacement with Medtronic Freestyle bioprosthesis: five-year results. Semin Thorac Cardiovasc Surg 1999;11 Suppl 1:35–41.

31. Pibarot P, Dumesnil JG, Jobin J, et al. Hemodynamic and physical performance during maximal exercise in patients with an aortic bioprosthetic valve: comparison of stentless versus stented bioprostheses. J Am Coll Cardiol 1999;34:1609–17.

32. Walther T, Falk W, Autschbach R, et al. Hemodynamic assessment of the stentless Toronto SPV bioprosthesis by echocardiography. J Heart Valve Dis 1994;3:657–65.

33. Westaby S, Horton M, Jin XY, et al. Survival advantage of stentless aortic bioprostheses. Ann Thorac Surg 2000;70:785–91.

34. David TE, Puschmann R, Ivanov J, et al. Aortic valve replacement with stentless and stented porcine valves: a case match study. J Thorac Cardiovasc Surg 1998;116:236–41.

35. Christakis GT, Buth KJ, Goldman BS, et al. Inaccurate and misleading valve sizing: a proposed standard for valve size nomenclature. Ann Thorac Surg 1998;66:1198–203.

36. Walther T, Falk V, Langebartels G, et al. Prospectively randomized evaluation of stentless versus conventional biological aortic valves: impact on early regression of left ventricular hypertrophy. Circulation 1999;100 Suppl II:II-6–10.

37. David TE, Feindel CM, Bos J, et al. The Toronto SPV bioprosthesis: clinical and hemodynamic results at 6 years. Ann Thorac Surg 1999;68:S9–13.

38. Cartier P, Dumesnil JG, Metras J, et al. Clinical and hemodynamic performance of the Freestyle aortic root bioprosthesis. Ann Thorac Surg 1999;67(2):345–9; discussion 349–51.

39. Kappetein AP, Braun J, Baur LHB, et al. Outcome and follow-up of aortic valve replacement with the freestyle stentless bioprosthesis. Ann Thorac Surg 2001;71:601–8.

40. Medtronic Inc. Freestyle aortic root bioprosthesis: 7-year clinical compendium (linearized rates and freedoms). Minneapolis, MN.

41. Konertz W, Sidiropoulos A, Vanezweu H, et al. Safety and effectiveness of aortic valve replacement with Edwards Prima Stentless Bioprosthesis Model 2500 (abstract 49). Stentless Bioprosthesis, Fourth International Symposium; 2001 May 3–5; San Diego, California.

42. Gelsomino S, Frassani R, DaCol P, et al. The Cryolife-O'Brien stentless porcine aortic bioprosthesis: 5-year follow-up. Ann Thorac Surg 2001;71:86–91.

43. Luciani GB, Santini F, Auriemma S, et al. Long-term results after aortic valve replacement with the Biocor PSB stentless xenograft in the elderly. Ann Thorac Surg 2001;71:S306–10.

44. Jin XY, Westaby S. Pericardial and porcine stentless aortic valves: are they hemodynamically different. Ann Thorac Surg 2001;71:S311–4.

45. Greve HH, Farah I, Everlien M. Comparison of three different types of stentless valves: full root or subcoronary. Ann Thorac Surg 2001;71:S293–6.

46. Cohen G, Christakis GT, Buth KJ, et al. Early experience with stentless versus stented valves. Circulation 1997;96 Suppl II:II-76–82.

47. Gelsomino S, Frassani R, Da Col P, et al. Early recovery of left ventricular function after stentless vs stented aortic valve replacement for pure aortic stenosis and severe cardiac dysfunction (abstract 41). Stentless Bioprosthesis, Fourth International Symposium; 2001 May 3–5; San Diego, California.

48. Fries R, Wendler O, Schieffer H, et al. Comparative rest and exercise hemodynamics of 23-mm stentless versus 23-mm stented aortic bioprostheses. Ann Thorac Surg 2000;69:817–22.

49. Lee J, Kim K, Song M. Comparative hemodynamics of stentless versus mechanical aortic valves through dobutamine stress echocardiogram and exercise testing (abstract 43). Stentless Bioprosthesis, Fourth International Symposium; 2001 May 3–5; San Diego, California.

50. Maselli D, Pizio R, Bruno LP, et al. Left ventricular mass reduction after aortic valve replacement: homografts, stentless and stented valves. Ann Thorac Surg 1999;67:966–71.

51. Morsy S, Zahran M, Usama M, et al. Hemodynamic performance of stentless porcine bioprosthesis and mechanical bileaflet prosthesis using dobutamine stress echocardiography (abstract 42). Stentless Bioprosthesis, Fourth International Symposium; 2001 May 3–5; San Diego, California.

52. Silberman S, Shaheen J, Merin O, et al. Exercise hemodynamics of aortic prostheses: comparison between stentless bioprostheses and mechanical valves. Ann Thorac Surg 2001;72:1217–21.

53. Milano AD, Blanzola C, Mecozzi G, et al. Hemodynamic performance of stented and stentless bioprostheses. Ann Thorac Surg 2001;72:33–8.

54. Cohen G, Christakis GT, Joyner CD, et al. Are stentless valves hemodynamically superior to stented valves? A prospective randomized trial. Thirty-seventh Scientific Sessions of the Society of Thoracic Surgeons; 2001 January 29–February 1; New Orleans, Louisiana,.

55. Shargall Y, Goldman B, Christakis GT, et al. Analysis of explants and causes of mortality during long-term follow-up of the Toronto stentless porcine valve (TSPV). Semin Thorac Cardiovasc Surg 2001;13:106–12.

56. Luciani GB, Auriemma S, Casali G, et al. A comparison of late outcome after stentless versus stented xenograft aortic valve replacement (abstract 44). Stentless Bioprosthesis, Fourth International Symposium; 2001 May 3-5; San Diego, California.

57. Del Rizzo DF, Abdoh A, Cartier P, et al. The effect of prosthetic valve type on survival after aortic valve surgery. Semin Thorac Cardiovasc Surg 1999;11 Suppl 1:1–8.

58. Del Rizzo DF, Freed D, Abdoh A, et al. Mid-term survival of stented versus stentless valves. Does concomitant CABG impact survival (abstract 46)? Stentless Bioprosthesis, Fourth International Symposium; 2001 May 3–5; San Diego, California.

59. David TE, Ivanov J, Eriksson MJ, et al. Dilation of the sinotubular junction causes aortic insufficiency after aortic valve replacement with the Toronto SPV bioprosthesis. J Thorac Cardiovasc Surg 2001;122:929–35.

60. Westaby S, Jin XY, Katsumata T, et al. Valve replacement with a stentless bioprosthesis: versatility of the porcine aortic root. J Thorac Cardiovasc Surg 1998;116:477–84.

61. Hvass U, Palatianos GM, Frassani R, et al. Multicenter study of stentless valve replacement in the small aortic root. J Thorac Cardiovasc Surg 1999;117:267–72

62. Hanayama N, Christakis GT, Mallidi HR, et al. Patient prosthesis mismatch is rare following aortic valve replacement: valve size may be irrelevant. Thirty-seventh Annual Scientific Sessions of the Society of Thoracic Surgeons; 2001 January 29–February 1; New Orleans, Louisiana.

63. Hanayama N, Mallidi HR, Rao V, et al. Incomplete regression of hypertrophy following AVR is not influenced by valve size nor patient prosthesis mismatch. 81st Scientific Sessions of the American Association for Thoracic Surgery; May 6–9, 2001.

64. Gelsomino S, Morocutti G, Da Col P, et al. Patient prosthesis mismatch after small size stentless aortic valve replacement (abstract 25). Stentless Bioprosthesis, Fourth International Symposium; 2001 May 3–5; San Diego, California.

65. Sintek CF, Fletcher AD, Khonsari S. Stentless porcine aortic root: valve of choice for the elderly patient with small aortic root? J Thorac Cardiovasc Surg 1995;109:871–6.

66. Westaby S, Johnsson A, Payne N, et al. Does the use of a stentless bioprosthesis increase surgical risk (abstract 45)? Stentless Bioprosthesis, Fourth International Symposium; 2001 May 3–5; San Diego, California.

67. Markowitz A. Utility of the full root bioprosthesis for complex aortic valve-ascending aortic disease (abstract 8). Stentless Bioprosthesis, Fourth International Symposium; 2001 May 3–5; San Diego, California.

CHAPTER 22

MITRAL VALVE REPAIR

CRAIG R. HAMPTON, MD, EDWARD D. VERRIER, MD

Mitral valve repair is the preferred treatment for mitral regurgitation and can be successfully performed in the majority of patients who require surgery, particularly for regurgitant mitral valves. When compared to prosthetic mitral valve replacement, repair is associated with lower operative mortality and decreased risk of long-term thromboembolic complications.[1,2] Moreover, mitral repair is associated with better flow dynamics across the mitral valve, better preservation of left ventricular function, and improved survival.[1,3-5] Accordingly, in patients who require surgical attention for mitral valve disease, surgical reconstruction of the valve is the standard treatment, with prosthetic replacement reserved for those in whom repair is not feasible.

Historical Perspective

The following historical perspective is condensed primarily from two sources and highlights the surgical developments contributing to the current operative strategy for repair of the mitral valve.[6,7]

Although Lauriston Shaw, in 1890, was the first to suggest that a diseased mitral valve could be surgically repaired, it was not until 1923 that the first account of a repair was reported. Elliot Cutler of Boston performed the first commissurotomy on a stenotic mitral valve on a bedridden teenage girl, who lived for 4.5 years with some clinical improvement. Following Cutler's initial attempt to repair a stenotic mitral valve, there were a limited number of attempts by him and others around the world for stenotic mitral valves—all with uniformly dismal results. These poor results, coupled with widespread skepticism among physicians about the feasibility of this surgical endeavor, led to a relatively stagnant period over the ensuing 25 years. In 1948, Charles Bailey, Dwight Harken, and Russell Brock performed the first successful digital commissurotomies in different parts of the world. Over the ensuing years, thousands of procedures were performed for stenotic mitral valves; effective surgical therapy for mitral regurgitation (MR), however, proved more challenging.

In 1945, Gordon Murray and his Toronto colleagues applied the techniques developed in the animal laboratory to a patient with MR, by using a transventricular subvalvular venous-tendon sling. This remarkable endeavor,

antecedent to Gibbon's introduction of extracorporeal circulation by 8 years, was soon applied to 10 very sick patients, 8 of whom lived with "fairly satisfactory" results. Although the ensuing years spawned varied interest in the surgical repair of mitral insufficiency, effective repair would not come until years later when open intracardiac surgery could be performed with the use of cardiopulmonary bypass. In 1957, Lillehei reported the use of posterior annuloplasty for mitral regurgitation, performed under direct vision using the pump-oxygenator.[8] The landmark report described the technique applied to four very ill patients without any operative or late mortality and with sustained clinical improvement up to 14 months postoperatively. That same year, Merendino reported similar treatment of two similar patients with mitral regurgitation through open cardiotomy.[9] Although these techniques were subsequently widely accepted and applied, there were increasing recurrences, proportional to the length of follow-up. Accordingly, in 1960, McGoon of the Mayo Clinic described a localized plication for a flail segment caused by ruptured chordae without the use of prosthetic materials, which he had applied to two patients.[10] In 1963, Kay and Egerton reported a series of 10 patients with MR, all successfully treated with tailored mitral valve repair.[11] The varied techniques included posterior leaflet suture annuloplasty, creation of neochordae with silk suture by tethering of the leaflets to either chordae or the papillary muscles, and annular plication. This classic paper emphasized a tailored surgical approach based on the intraoperative inspection of the mitral apparatus. Reed and colleagues described the asymmetric mitral annuloplasty in 1965, which also was associated with persistent and recurrent regurgitation.[12] It is important to note that, in addition to the usual challenges associated with novel surgical therapies, these early pioneers had limited diagnostic techniques for preoperative assessment, relying entirely on auscultation of the heart, electrocardiography, and chest roentgenography. Recognizing this, their remarkable accomplishments are considered even more extraordinary.

Although mechanical prostheses were first used in 1960 for valvular replacement, this technique had limited utility in the second and third world, where resources were scarce and anticoagulation management continues to be a challenge.[6] Thus, part of the impetus to find alternative therapies to mechanical valve replacement was the inability to perform this operation in many parts of the world where rheumatic heart disease was prevalent and affected a very young population. Accordingly, Carpentier and Duran made significant contributions to mitral valve repair in the 1970s by advocating a more systematic approach to mitral valve assessment and repair, including thorough evaluation of the mitral annulus, the tensor apparatus, and the leaflets.[13,14] Moreover, these pioneers refined the surgical techniques for mitral repair and clearly demonstrated their effectiveness. During this time, quadrangular resection of the posterior leaflet with a ring annuloplasty became an important aspect of repair. Furthermore, the techniques for repairing a diseased anterior leaflet were also established, including chordal shortening, chordal transfer, and leaflet apposition. Annuloplasty rings were routinely used with good results.[13] While Carpentier favored a rigid annuloplasty ring, Duran, recognizing the dynamic changes of the annulus during the cardiac cycle, advocated use of a flexible, more physiologic ring.[14] This concept evolved to implantation of a posterior C-shaped ring only (sparing the trigone), rather than a complete ring.

Mitral Valve Anatomy and Physiology

The mitral valve normally functions to prevent regurgitant flow into the left atrium during ventricular systole, while allowing unfettered flow into the left ventricle during diastole. Recently, based on observations made after the chordae tendineae were severed, it was suggested that the mitral valve also functions to maintain left ventricle morphology, geometry, and function. To these ends, normal function of the mitral valve results from finely orchestrated movements of its five components, including the mitral annulus, the leaflets, the mitral commissures, the chordae tendineae, and the papillary muscles. Collectively, these structures are referred to as the *mitral apparatus*.

Mitral Annulus

The mitral annulus is part of the fibrous skeleton of the heart that provides the rigid framework for the attachment of the valvular tissue and the muscular tissue of the atria and ventricles.[15] The fibrous skeleton of the heart is like a series of contiguous rings in the position of the four valves that converge centrally at the central fibrous core. The anteromedial third of the annulus is in continuity with the trigones of the heart and the left coronary aortic cusps. This portion of the annulus is relatively nondistensible, except in the rare patient with a severe connective-tissue disease such as Marfan's syndrome.[16] These observations support the assertion that reinforcement of the anterior annulus is not routinely needed when annuloplasty is performed, and partial posterior rings suffice.

The remaining two-thirds of the mitral annulus extends laterally from the left fibrous trigone around to the right fibrous trigone posteromedially. This portion of the ring is often incomplete and less well defined, owing to the propensity for mitral regurgitation to result from posterior abnormalities. This is the physiologic basis for using posterior partial annuloplasty rings, particularly for myxomatous mitral prolapse. The anterior and posterior portions of the annulus are in continuity at the right fibrous trigone, which is delimited by the anteromedial mitral leaflet on the left, the posterior aortic (noncoronary) cusp in front, the septal tricuspid leaflet on the right, and the membranous ventricular septum inferiorly.[16] The left fibrous trigone is less well developed and is bounded by the aortic root and the anteromedial mitral leaflet.

Mitral Leaflets

The mitral valve should be considered a continuous veil of fibroelastic tissue attached circumferentially to the mitral annulus.[17] The free edge of the veil contains two indentations, termed *commissures*, which conveniently divide the valve into anteromedial (or anterior or aortic) and posterolateral (or posterior or mural) leaflets. The commissural interruption is anatomically fairly constant and occurs in the anterolateral and posteromedial positions. The commissures are usually easily identified with simple inspection; however, in patients with rheumatic disease, they can be quite obscured because of thickening, calcification, and fusion of the leaflets and chordae. When this occurs, the commissures can be most readily identified by the unique commissural chords which arise from the adjacent papillary muscles as single stems which then radially branch into multiple fan-like cords prior to insertion into the leaflet edge.[18] Furthermore, when regurgitation results from elongated chordae, the commissural chordae are rarely affected and can serve as a guide for determining adequate chordae length prior to repair.

The anteromedial leaflet is triangularly shaped, with its base attached to the annulus while its apex extends hinge-like into the lumen of the left ventricle.[15] It measures 1.8 to 3.5 cm in height, nearly twice that of the posterolateral leaflet, which contributes to its increased mobility relative to the posterior leaflet.[15] Because of its shape, there is little redundancy of the anterior leaflet, thereby limiting resection of this leaflet to ≤ 20%. The leaflet has a ridge on its atrial surface that parallels the free edge, but is offset by 0.8 to 1 cm, thus defining the demarcation of the rough and clear zones (Figure 22-1).[18] During valve closure, the rough zone comes into apposition with its counterpart on the posterior leaflet. The anteromedial leaflet also forms an important boundary of the left ventricular outflow tract (LVOT), as it is contiguous with the left and posterior coronary cusps of the aortic valve. This anatomic position explains the LVOT obstruction that is consequent to systolic anterior motion (SAM) of the anterior mitral leaflet, a complication of mitral valve repair.

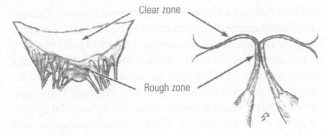

FIGURE 22-1. Mitral valve leaflet morphology.

The posterolateral leaflet is more quadrangular in shape and is much longer than it is wide, thereby limiting its mobility. Its base varies from 0.9 to 2.6 cm, while its height is 0.6 to 1.2 cm, only half that of the anterior leaflet.[18] In accord, the posterior leaflet encircles approximately two-thirds of the mitral orifice. The free edge of the posterior leaflet has a variable number of indentations that give it a scalloped appearance, most commonly tri-scalloped, and is often used to further subdivide the posterior leaflet.[18] Like the anterior leaflet, the posterior leaflet has a rough and a clear zone, demarcating the normal area of valve apposition during ventricular systole. The combined surface areas of both mitral leaflets is more than twice the area of the mitral orifice, permitting a large area of leaflet apposition during ventricular systole to effectively prevent mitral regurgitation.[15]

Tensor Apparatus

The tensor apparatus of the mitral valve comprises the papillary muscles, the adjacent left ventricular wall, and the chordae tendineae. There are usually two main papillary muscles in the left ventricular lumen, which lie in the anterolateral and posteromedial positions, subtending the leaflet commissures in these positions. The papillary muscles originate from the ventricular wall, one-third of the distance from the annulus to the apex. They may be bifid, trifid, or, less frequently, a row of muscles but are substantial structures and may make up to 25% of the left ventricular (LV) muscle mass.[15,16] The papillary muscles provide dynamic tethering of the valve leaflets via the chordae to withstand the stress of ventricular systole and prevent regurgitation. To this end, the papillary muscles receive neural input from the left bundle branch, which is patterned so that the papillary muscles are stimulated prior to the ventricle to allow mitral apposition prior to ventricular systole.[15]

The blood supply to the papillary muscles is of clinical interest and has been well described.[15] The anterolateral papillary muscle receives its blood from the left coronary artery (LCA), particularly the obtuse marginal (OM) branches of the circumflex artery and the diagonal branches of the left anterior descending (LAD) artery. The blood supply of the posteromedial papillary muscle is more variable but usually originates from the posterior descending artery. Nonetheless, the blood supply to the posteromedial papillary muscle is more tenuous, accounting for the higher frequency of infarction and rupture at this location.

The chordae tendineae are fibrous strings that originate from the tip of the papillary muscles, or, less commonly, directly from the ventricular wall. Beyond the origin of the chordae, there are significant interconnections between them, which increases structural integrity through effective force distribution between chordae. The chordae then insert onto the mitral leaflets. The chordal attachments into the posterior leaflet are in three layers: marginal (first order), which are attached to the leaflet edge; intermediate (second order); and mural (third order).[16] The attachments to the anterior leaflet are identical, excepting for an absence of third-order chordae. The presence of third-order chordae on the posterior leaflet also contributes to its decreased mobility relative to the anterior leaflet, which lacks this additional tethering. The chordae that tether the posterior leaflet are aligned parallel to each other, while the anterior leaflet chordae insert obliquely on either side of the leaflet.[19] Furthermore, the posterior leaflet chords are shorter (0.6 to 1.5 cm) and thicker (0.11 to 0.93 mm) than chords inserting into the anterior leaflet (length: 1.32 to 2.39 cm; thickness: 1.41 to 1.76 mm), further enhancing the increased mobility of the anterior leaflet.[19]

Important Anatomic Relationships

The mitral valve is positioned in close association with a number of important structures, including the atrioventricular (AV) nodal conduction fiber region, the AV nodal artery, the left and noncoronary cusps of the aortic valve, the septal cusp of the tricuspid valve, the coronary sinus that lies posterior to the posteromedial leaflet, and the circumflex artery (Figure 22-2).

The left and noncoronary cusps of the aortic valve are vulnerable to injury when placing sutures anteriorly, for example, during an annuloplasty with a complete ring. The conduction fibers are most vulnerable in the area of

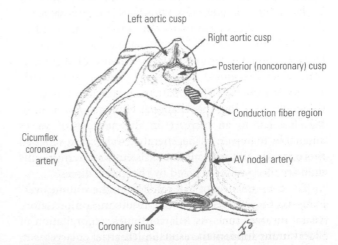

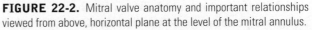

FIGURE 22-2. Mitral valve anatomy and important relationships viewed from above, horizontal plane at the level of the mitral annulus.

the right fibrous trigone and can be injured in a similar manner, leading to postoperative conduction disturbances. The circumflex artery is vulnerable to injury in its lateral and posterior course around the annulus. Of note, the vulnerability of the circumflex artery is increased in left and codominant systems because it lies closer to the annulus, averaging 4.1 mm in left dominance, 5.5 mm in codominance, and 8.4 mm in right dominance.[20]

Mitral Valve Physiology

In the course of the cardiac cycle, the mitral valve allows unfettered flow through the mitral orifice during diastole and completely seals the mitral orifice during ventricular systole. Despite fairly extensive inquiry, the exact cause and mode of mitral valve closure are not entirely clear. Contraction of the papillary muscles precedes ventricular systole to ensure adequate tethering of the mitral valve during ventricular systole.[21] As the intraventricular pressure rises, the rough zones of the leaflets firmly coapt, orienting in a near vertical direction, while the remainder of the leaflets bulge like a parachute into the left atrium.[21] Coincidentally, the area of the mitral orifice is reduced by 23 to 40%, primarily resulting from dynamic reduction of the posterior annulus during late atrial systole and ventricular systole.[16] To these ends, the mitral annulus is shaped like a saddle in the anteroposterior direction, the height of which is increased during ventricular systole, thereby contributing to the reduction in mitral orifice size and facilitating coaptation of the leaflets.[16] The coordination of these dynamic movements between the components of the mitral apparatus affects normal valve function as described and provides the basis for restoring physiologic valve function through surgical repair.

Mitral Regurgitation

In the United States, the etiology of mitral regurgitation requiring surgical intervention has changed dramatically in the last few decades. Over this time, the prevalence of degenerative disease has increased from 40% in the 1970s to 60% in the 1980s.[22,23] This change has been paralleled by a coincidental decline in the prevalence of rheumatic MR, which accounted for 46% of patients in the early 1970s but only for 15% of patients by the late 1980s.[23–25] Generally speaking, this changing etiologic spectrum of MR has led to an increase in the number of valves amenable to repair, as degenerative valves are repaired more readily and with more consistent long-term results than are those valves affected by rheumatic disease.

The consequences of MR result from the volume overloads of the left ventricle that result in compensatory dilatation over time. As MR continues, regurgitation of blood in the left atrium results in left atrial enlargement, which itself can worsen MR, illustrating the self-perpetuating course of severe MR and congestive heart failure (CHF). Although these compensatory structural changes may maintain cardiac output for some time, they eventuate in increased myocardial oxygen demand and increased transmural wall tension with subsequent myocardial decompensation, CHF, and an increased risk of sudden death.[26] Furthermore, long-standing MR may cause pulmonary hypertension and result in left atrial enlargement causing atrial fibrillation. Other complications of MR include endocarditis and ischemic cerebral events, likely from thromboembolism. Despite the obviously self-perpetuating course of MR, it is likely that many patients with mild MR remain asymptomatic and never require surgical attention, especially with improved medical therapy, including unloading agents (eg, angiotensin-converting enzyme [ACE] inhibitors), diuretics, and agents that enhance cardiovascular remodeling (eg, ACE inhibitors).[26]

Timing of Surgical Repair

Surgical repair of the regurgitant mitral valve is indicated when symptoms are present. The nature and severity of symptoms and signs of MR are quite varied and depend on the severity, the rate of progression, the associated cardiovascular conditions, and the level of pulmonary artery pressures. Patients can experience symptoms of left-heart failure, including orthopnea, dyspnea on exertion, and edema, or they can present with signs of heart failure or atrial fibrillation. Acute pulmonary edema, systemic embolization, and hemoptysis are infrequent. The strategy of operative intervention for symptomatic MR is based on the poor clinical outcome without surgery, with survival rates as low as 33% over 8 years and an average annual mortality of about 5%.[27] Most of these deaths result from heart failure although sudden cardiac death is not infrequent.

The natural history of asymptomatic patients with MR is varied and depends on myriad factors, including the etiology, rate of progression, presence of coronary artery disease, and the state of the myocardium. In asymptomatic patients with mitral valve prolapse, the natural history may be insidious with a low incidence of complications,[28] while other studies demonstrate that up to 28% of patients will require operation within 5 years.[29] In contrast, more than 90% of patients with mitral valve prolapse caused by flail leaflet either die or require surgery over 10 years.[30] Moreover, these patients are at risk of sudden cardiac death, irrespective of antecedent symptoms.[31] As a result, early surgical repair is indicated for MR caused by flail leaflet and likely decreases the incidence of sudden death.[31]

The indications for and timing of surgical repair in asymptomatic patients with MR are controversial. Indeed, there are no data available from randomized controlled trials guiding the optimal timing of surgical repair. Conceptually, the goal is to identify patients who have progressive MR and to prevent the irreversible structural changes outlined previously. To this end, echocardiography is a sensitive tool to discern early structural and functional changes resulting from MR. Echocardiographic determination of an ejection fraction (EF) of 0.60 or less and/or an end-systolic dimension of 45 mm or more may indicate early systolic dysfunction and identify those patients without symptoms who should be considered for mitral repair.[32] Correction of MR when these criteria are met will likely prevent further decreases in LV function and may improve survival.[33] Furthermore, in the absence of these criteria, the presence of atrial fibrillation or pulmonary hypertension in asymptomatic patients are also indications for mitral valve repair.

Preoperative Evaluation

Transthoracic echocardiography (TTE), and transesophageal echocardiography (TEE), are invaluable in the evaluation of MR preoperatively. Recognizing that general anesthesia and cardiopulmonary bypass reduce the afterload of the ventricles, thereby attenuating MR, it is important to fully evaluate MR preoperatively for optimal assessment. Echocardiography can accurately identify the mechanism of MR through evaluation of the structural components of the mitral apparatus.[34] Furthermore, the suitability of the valve for repair can be assessed to plan operative strategy. More importantly, echocardiography can assess the other cardiac valves and evaluate coincidental aortic or tricuspid pathology. We routinely obtain preoperative TEE in patients being considered for mitral valve surgery and in patients who are receiving a coronary artery bypass graft (CABG), when there is a question about the concurrent need for mitral repair. Despite the increasing accuracy of this imaging modality, confirmation with intraoperative inspection is mandated.

We perform cardiac catheterization in patients with known coronary artery disease (CAD), symptoms suggestive of CAD by history, or patients older than 40 years of age. There are few data available to guide the use of preoperative angiography prior to mitral valve repair, and its use should be individualized.

Operative Approach

The mitral valve is routinely approached via a median sternotomy although technologic advances have led to minimally invasive approaches through smaller limited incisions (eg, right or left anterior thoracotomy or partial sternotomy). Minimally invasive approaches may be enhanced by robotically assisted technologies.

Open repair of the mitral valve is approached with standard techniques of myocardial protection and cardiopulmonary bypass. Ample exposure of the mitral valve is absolutely imperative for satisfactory repair. To this end, there are four standard open incisions that may be used, two of which are commonly used. We prefer the biatrial transseptal approach through the right atrium, atrial septum, and left atrium as described by Smith (Figure 22-3).[35] This provides optimal exposure to the mitral valve, and we have not seen any significant incidence of sinus dysrhythmias postoperatively. The standard left atriotomy incision posterior and parallel to the intraatrial groove is used by many surgeons and provides adequate exposure of the mitral valve in most patients except those with small atria. The other two incisions are used less often and include the left atrial dome incision and the transatrial H-type incision.

Port-Access (Heartport, Inc., Menlo Park, CA) technology has been used by some surgeons with success.[36] This technique uses an endoluminal balloon for occlusion of the aorta, as well as for cardioplegia. The catheter/balloon is introduced through the groin, which allows smaller incisions to be used to expose the mitral valve (eg, anterior thoracotomy). A careful evaluation for peripheral vascular disease is mandated in these patients because there is a risk of thromboembolic complications with peripheral cannulation and catheter manipulation. Since this technology was first described, various minimally invasive incisions have been used, including anterior minithoracotomy, partial sternotomy, and, less frequently, paramedian sternotomy. The impetus for these minimally invasive techniques is the reduction of perioperative morbidity from incisional discomfort, perhaps leading to earlier patient mobilization, decreased postoperative pain, improved cosmesis, and less scarring in the anterior mediastinum, making reoperation less formidable. Early results of mitral repair using this technology suggest an operative mortality of 1.1% with excellent technical results, and patients may have a shorter recovery time.[36] More recently, intermediate-term results have been reported up to 4 years postoperatively, with results comparable to those in case-matched control patients.[37,38] However, no comparative data with the standard approaches are available, and long-term outcome data are needed.

Video and robotic-assisted mitral valve repair is also being evaluated by some surgeons and has been reviewed in detail.[39] Early results indicate that this is an effective technique for mitral valve repair. Again, however, there are no comparative data and long-term outcome data are not available.

Inspection of the Valve

A thorough inspection of the components of the mitral apparatus is performed once the valve is exposed, bearing in mind the Carpentier types of valve abnormalities (Figure 22-4). The presence of a jet lesion, usually seen by preoperative TEE, indicates prolapse of the opposite leaflet. The annulus is inspected for dilatation. A nerve hook is used to retract the leaflet and chordae to assess their pliability and document the presence of leaflet prolapse or restricted leaflet motion. This also allows inspection of the chordae tendineae to search for ruptured or elongated chords. A "reference point" for the proper plane of the leaflet may be established by identifying the commissures

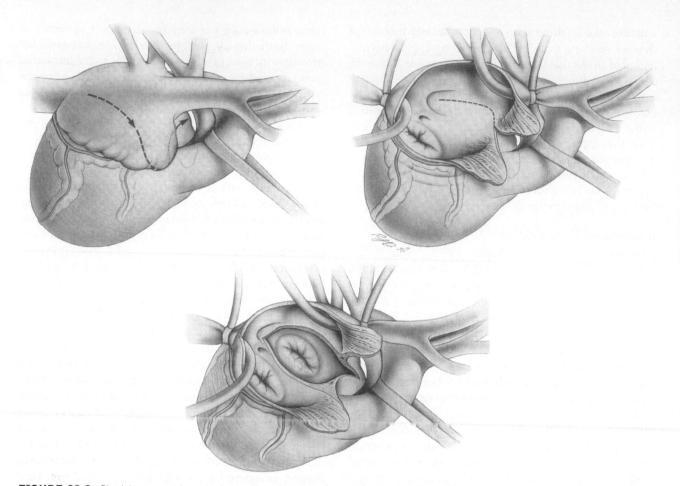

FIGURE 22-3. Biatrial transseptal approach seen from the surgeon's perspective, with the patient's head to the left. Reproduced with permission from Smith CR.[35]

and by checking the adjacent and contralateral leaflet edge. Injection of cold saline with a bulb syringe into the left ventricle to identify regurgitant sites can also be used. With the routine use of sophisticated and accurate preoperative imaging modalities, intraoperative inspection of the valve usually only confirms the preoperative impression and the appropriateness of the operative strategy for repair. However, on rare occasion, the plan for repair may change toward valve replacement when heavily calcified leaflets or commissures, or severely fibrotic/retracted chordae and subvalvular structures, are identified. Nevertheless, given the declining frequency of rheumatic MR, the frequency of this scenario is declining, and greater than 90% of regurgitant mitral valves in the United States are amenable to repair.

Functional Approach to Surgical Repair

Carpentier has divided mitral regurgitation into two functional anomalies: the motion of each leaflet may be either increased (ie, leaflet prolapse) or decreased (ie, restricted leaflet motion) (see Figure 22-4).[25] With this classification scheme, one must only determine if leaflet motion is normal (type I), increased (type II), or

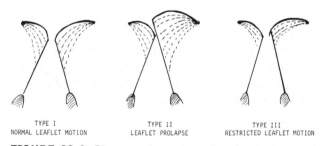

| TYPE I | TYPE II | TYPE III |
| NORMAL LEAFLET MOTION | LEAFLET PROLAPSE | RESTRICTED LEAFLET MOTION |

FIGURE 22-4. Diagrammatic representation of pathophysiologic leaflet classification. Reproduced with permission from Carpentier A.[25]

restricted (type III), which also helps in recognizing the structural lesions that produce these leaflet anomalies (Table 22-1). Mitral regurgitation associated with normal leaflet motion (type I) may be attributed to annular dilatation or leaflet perforation.[25] The most common type, increased leaflet motion (type II), may result from leaflet prolapse, chordal rupture, chordal elongation, papillary muscle rupture, or papillary muscle elongation. Restricted leaflet motion (type III) may result from chordal thickening and fusion, commissural fusion, or leaflet thickening.

TABLE 22-1. Classification of Structural Valve Abnormalities

Type	Abnormality
I	Normal leaflet motion
	Annular dilation
	Leaflet perforation
II	Leaflet prolapse
	Chordal rupture
	Chordal elongation
	Papillary muscle rupture
	Papillary muscle elongation
III	Restricted leaflet motion
	Commissure fusion
	Leaflet thickening
	Chordal fusion and thickening

Adapted from Carpentier A.[25]

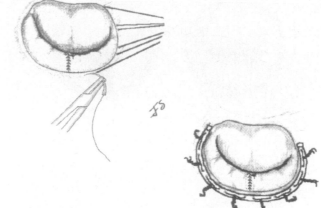

FIGURE 22-5. Technique for placement of a flexible partial annuloplasty ring.

Annuloplasty

Recognizing that the annulus is a dynamic structure that changes dramatically with the cardiac cycle, thereby facilitating a reduction in mitral orifice size to allow leaflet apposition, flexible annuloplasty rings have been developed.[14] Extending these observations, it is clear that the reduction in orifice size primarily results from the underdeveloped flexible posterior annulus, while the anterior part of the mitral annulus is fairly rigid.[16] Accordingly, flexible, partial annuloplasty rings were developed to optimally mimic the normal dynamics of the mitral valve, thereby preserving the physiologic saddle conformation during ventricle systole. Additional advantages to the posterior annuloplasty are the reduced risk of rare conduction abnormalities postoperatively by virtue of avoidance of the anterior annulus. This may also reduce the incidence of injury to the aortic cusps (left and noncoronary).

In animal studies and prospective randomized clinical trials, flexible rings have proven superior to rigid rings with respect to ventricular performance and preservation of annular dynamics.[40,41] In accordance with these data and the aforementioned physiologic principles, we believe that partial flexible posterior annuloplasty rings are adequate for most repairs (Figure 22-5). Using appropriate sizers, a flexible ring that simulates intertrigonal and height dimensions of the anterior leaflet is selected for implantation.

Posterior Leaflet Prolapse

Posterior leaflet abnormalities with annular dilatation most commonly underlie significant mitral regurgitation that requires surgical repair. Indeed, isolated posterior leaflet prolapse is the sole abnormality in up to 60% of patients in surgical series.[42] We believe the surgical approach to the posterior leaflet should be standardized and include quadrangular resection, with modified sliding leaflet plasty as needed (see below). Furthermore, we routinely include a flexible partial posterior annuloplasty ring as an important aspect of repair.

Quadrangular resection, which may include up to 30% of the posterior leaflet, is the mainstay for surgical repair of posterior leaflet prolapse. The abnormally prolapsing leaflet section is identified via valve inspection, and normal-appearing chordae are confirmed to be subtending the adjacent leaflet area. A rectangular incision is then made to resect this portion of the leaflet, radially oriented perpendicular to the annulus, extending to, but not including, the annulus. The redundant leaflet and flail chord are thus resected. The annulus is re-approximated with a pledgeted 3–0 braided polyester (Ti-Cron, Davis and Geck) mattress suture followed by leaflet re-approximation with simple interrupted 4–0 or 5–0 polypropylene sutures. Care should be taken to approximate the leaflet edges without wrinkling or kinking.

If the posterior leaflet is very large and redundant, or if the prolapse is determined to be greater than or equal to 1.5 cm beyond the horizontal plane of the commissures and normal leaflet coaptation, then a sliding leaflet plasty should be performed in addition to quadrangular resection (Figure 22-6). In this case, performing a quadrangular resection with sliding leaflet plasty will reduce the incidence of SAM of the anterior leaflet from approximately 10% to 0 to 2%.[43] After the quadrangular resection is performed, the posterior leaflet is sharply detached from the annulus toward the commissures until nonprolapsing leaflet is encountered. Annuloplasty sutures are placed, and the leaflet is anchored to the annulus with a running 4–0 or 5–0 polypropylene suture, including enough leaflet to adequately tether the repair and to ensure normal leaflet height. The leaflet edges at the site of quadrangular resection are then re-approximated as described. Placing the annuloplasty ring (see "Annuloplasty") completes the repair.

Anterior Leaflet Prolapse

In contrast to the posterior leaflet, very little leaflet tissue (ie, ≤ 15%) may be resected from the anterior leaflet

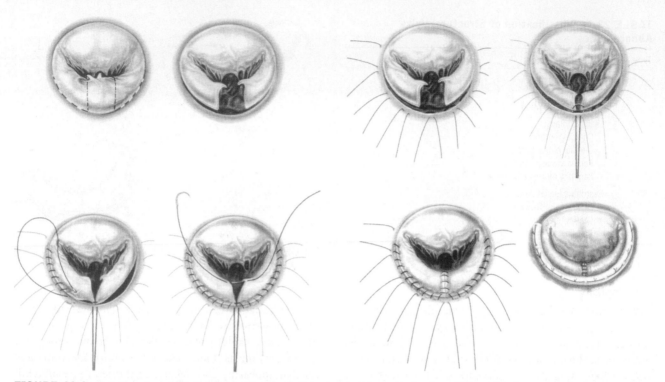

FIGURE 22-6. Technique for modified sliding leaflet plasty. Reproduced with permission from Gillinov AM, Cosgrove DM. Modified sliding leaflet technique for repair of the mitral valve. Ann Thorac Surg 1999;68:2356–7.

without excessively reducing leaflet area. Furthermore, because of the completeness and rigidity of the anterior part of the annulus, annular reduction with annuloplasty cannot adequately account for reduced leaflet area that leads to MR. Thus, repair of mitral regurgitation resulting from anterior abnormalities requires a more tailored surgical approach depending on the exact causative structural abnormality that has led to regurgitation.

CHORDAL ELONGATION OR RUPTURE

Anterior leaflet prolapse resulting from chordal elongation or rupture may be repaired with a variety of techniques, including chordal transposition, chordal shortening, attaching ruptured chordae onto adjacent secondary chordae, or the formation of neochords with PTFE (polytetrafluoroethylene) suture. Although most of these techniques have been used with success, we agree with others that chordal replacement is more reproducible and provides a more durable, superior repair relative to chordal shortening or transposition.[44–46]

We use 5–0 or 6–0 PTFE sutures for repair (Figure 22-7). The double-arm sutures are first passed through the fibrous papillary muscle two or three times. The sutures are then passed through the leaflet edge where the native chord was/is attached, about 5 mm from one another. After the appropriate length of PTFE is determined, through comparison of the adjacent and opposite leaflets, the sutures are passed back through the anterior leaflet, where they are tied on the ventricular side. This is repeated as needed to ensure adequate tethering of the anterior leaflet and sufficient distribution of tension. David and colleagues report a mean of 6.6 new chordae per patient (range, 2–16).[45] This technique provides excellent results, with actuarial freedom from reoperation at 10 years of 96% and freedom from severe mitral regurgitation of 93%.[45]

PAPILLARY MUSCLE RUPTURE

Rupture of the papillary muscles is an uncommon cause of mitral regurgitation. When present, the posteromedial papillary muscles are usually involved as a result of their more tenuous and inconsistent blood supply. If thought feasible after intraoperative inspection, the papillary muscle may be reattached to the ventricular free wall with pledgeted horizontal mattress 4–0 polypropylene suture. However, in the presence of an acute or extensive myocardial infarction, with edematous tissues and decompensated CHF, mitral valve (MV) replacement may be more prudent and is more often performed in this situation.[47,48]

Restricted Leaflet Motion

Restricted leaflet motion (Carpentier type III) is significantly less frequent than leaflet prolapse because of the decreasing frequency of rheumatic heart disease. Nonetheless, many of these lesions are amenable to surgical repair, and the required techniques should be part of the surgeon's armamentarium. There are four conditions that may restrict leaflet motion and are amenable to repair including commissural fusion, leaflet thickening, chordal thickening, and chordal fusion.[25]

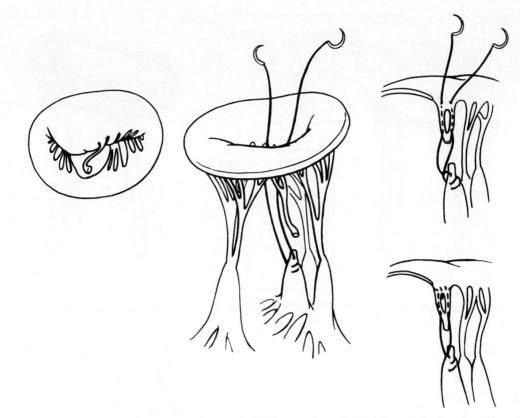

FIGURE 22-7. Technique of chordal replacement with expanded PTFE suture. Reproduced with permission from David T, et al.[45]

Chordal thickening and fusion is the major cause of restricted leaflet motion, often involving secondary chordae. These thickened chordae can be resected with their thick leaflet attachment to remobilize the posterior leaflet (Figure 22-8). When first-order, or marginal, chordae are restricting leaflet motion, they should be fenestrated by removing a pyramidal wedge of thickened fibrous tissue, thereby remobilizing the leaflet.[25] Resection of first-order chordae should be avoided because it results in leaflet prolapse. When commissural fusion underlies restricted leaflet motion, identification of the commissure can be difficult. Carpentier recommends placing traction with a nerve hook around the major chordae of the anterior leaflet to create a groove that delineates the line of commissurotomy (Figure 22-9).[25] This fused area is then carefully incised beginning 6 mm from the annulus and directed toward the central orifice, thus remobilizing the leaflets.

Bileaflet Prolapse and Barlow's Syndrome

Bileaflet prolapse and Barlow's syndrome are complex lesions that infrequently are the cause of MR. These conditions must be distinguished from the more frequent scenario of bileaflet prolapse without anterior chordal pathology. In this much more common situation, the anterior leaflet prolapses as a result of a lack of coaptation with the posterior leaflet, which is structurally abnormal. In these patients who have normal anterior leaflet chor-

dae, standard repair of the posterior leaflet with annuloplasty invariably corrects the anterior prolapse.[49]

In contrast, Barlow's syndrome, which is caused by myxomatous degeneration, is characterized by billowy prolapse of both leaflets, which prevents effective coaptation and results in MR. For these patients, we place a ring annuloplasty and perform a quadrangular resection, as necessary. A double-orifice repair (ie, the Alfieri repair) has been reported with excellent results, including freedom from reoperation of 90% at 5 years.[50] This technique is performed by approximating the margins of the leaflets at the site of regurgitation with a running 5–0 polypropylene suture (Figure 22-10). This creates a double-orifice valve with centrally coapted leaflets. As Alfieri describes, the two openings can be measured with Hagar dilators, and a total valve area of ≥ 2.5 cm is acceptable for typically sized patients.[50] For thin leaflet tissue, the suture line is reinforced with pledgets. This is nearly routinely supplemented with a partial flexible annuloplasty ring as previously described.

Postrepair Assessment

The adequacy of mitral valve repair can be assessed by distending the left ventricle with cold saline while still on cardiopulmonary bypass or with antegrade cardioplegia. Although this testing is not physiologic, valves that are competent with filling and distension of the left ventricle usually remain so after weaning from cardiopulmonary

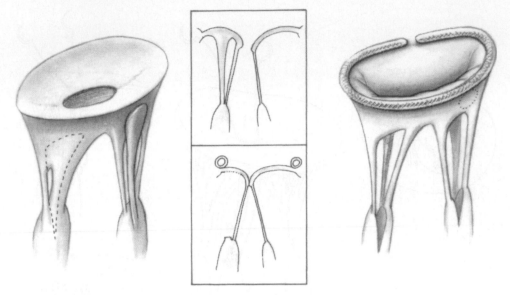

FIGURE 22-8. Leaflet mobilization by resection of secondary chordae. Reproduced with permission from Carpentier A.[25]

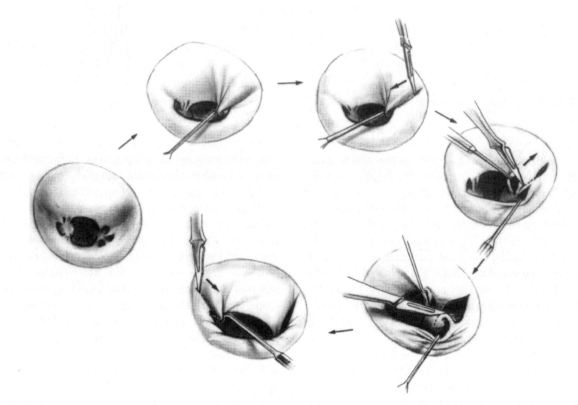

FIGURE 22-9. Leaflet mobilization by commissurotomy. Reproduced with permission from Carpentier A.[25]

bypass although dynamic testing with appropriate loading conditions is critical.

Intraoperative TEE with Doppler color flow measurement is the most valuable postrepair assessment tool and is only reliable after the patient is weaned from cardiopulmonary bypass. It is important to understand that intraoperative TEE evaluates the mitral valve when the ventricular afterload is dramatically reduced as a result of general anes-

thesia. Because ventricular afterload is one of the main variables affecting MR, the severity of MR is underestimated in these circumstances. For accuracy, volume loading and phenylephrine may be given to effect vasoconstriction, thereby increasing afterload to permit an accurate intraoperative assessment of mitral valve function and the competence of the repair. Additionally, TEE can accurately assess the anatomic features of the repair, assess the mitral

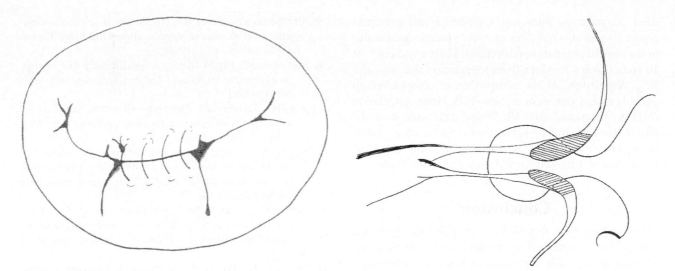

FIGURE 22-10. The double-orifice technique (ie, the Alfieri repair). The free edges of the leaflets may also be approximated with a "U-stitch" or with simple interrupted sutures. Reproduced with permission from Maisano F, Schreuder JJ, Oppizzi M, et al. The double-orifice technique as a standardized approach to treat mitral regurgitation due to severe myxomatous disease: surgical technique. Eur J Cardiothorac Surg 2000; 17(3):201–5.

valve area, measure transvalvular gradients, and determine ventricular function. In this regard, it is important to view the repair in multiple TEE views to exclude the presence of significant eccentric jets of regurgitation. Persistent moderate-to-severe regurgitation seen while the patient is anesthetized warrants exploration and revision of the repair because it will certainly worsen when the patient is awakened and the systemic vascular resistance increases.

SAM of the anterior mitral leaflet complicates mitral repair in 5 to 10% of patients and can cause dynamic LVOT obstruction. Although SAM is often diagnosed postoperatively, measurement of the pressure gradient across the LVOT with TEE may confirm its presence. It is treated with intravascular volume loading and avoidance of inotropic support that induces a hyperdynamic circulation. If this does not correct the condition, then surgical correction may be indicated.

Adjunctive Procedures

Cox-Maze Procedure for Atrial Fibrillation

Up to 40% of patients undergoing mitral repair for MR have chronic antecedent atrial fibrillation, and the majority remain in atrial fibrillation after valve repair.[51] In these patients, the risk of stroke without anticoagulation is 5 to 8% per year and is reduced significantly with chronic anticoagulation therapy.[52–54] However, chronic warfarin therapy has substantial associated costs and associated morbidity, particularly the risk of spontaneous hemorrhage.[53,55] Accordingly, there is interest in ablating atrial fibrillation with the Cox-Maze procedure, which effectively controls atrial fibrillation in 80% of patients, in those patients with atrial fibrillation who are undergoing mitral valve repair.

It was recently demonstrated that in patients undergoing mitral valve repair, the Cox-Maze procedure, especially with radiofrequency (RF) or cryoablation, does not seem to increase perioperative mortality.[51,56] Furthermore, in patients with atrial fibrillation undergoing mitral repair, there is a higher freedom from atrial fibrillation, freedom from stroke or anticoagulant-associated bleeding, and reduced continued need for chronic antiarrhythmic medications in those undergoing the Cox-Maze procedure at the time of mitral repair.[51,56] The efficacy at maintaining sinus rhythm approximates 80% after 2-year follow-up, even in those with chronic (ie, > 3 months) atrial fibrillation prior to the Cox-Maze procedure. For these reasons, we routinely perform the Cox-Maze procedure as an adjunct to mitral repair in patients with antecedent atrial fibrillation. In addition, recent modifications in ablative procedures seem to have dramatically reduced the incidence of heart block requiring pacemaker and have improved atrial transport and natriuretic function.

Complications

The complications most often seen following mitral valve repair are residual mitral regurgitation, mitral stenosis, and LVOT obstruction from SAM of the anterior mitral leaflet. With use of partial posterior annuloplasty rings, conduction disturbances infrequently complicate mitral valve repair.

Results

Mitral valve repair is associated with excellent short- and long-term outcomes. Perioperative mortality and need for reoperation are low, not exceeding 2% in most series.[57]

After 20 years of follow-up, Carpentier and associates report 20-year survival rates of 48%, which is comparable to the normal population with the same age structure.[57] At 10 and 20 years, freedom from reoperation was 94% and 92%, respectively. At the completion of observation, all patients except one were in New York Heart Association (NYHA) functional class I/II. These data underscore the effectiveness of mitral valve repair for treating mitral regurgitation and set a benchmark for long-term outcomes that all surgeons should endeavor to duplicate.

Conclusion

Mitral valve repair should be considered the preferred therapy for patients with symptomatic MR. Its superiority over mitral valve replacement has been established with improved long-term ventricular function and survival.[1] Of those patients requiring surgery for MR, application of the principles and techniques outlined above will lead to successful mitral reconstruction in greater than 90% of patients, with excellent outcomes. Given the outstanding results of mitral valve repair with low operative morbidity and mortality, coupled with more routine cardiac screening with echocardiography, the indications for mitral repair may continue to expand in favor of earlier repair.

References

1. Enriquez-Sarano M, Schaff HV, Orszulak TA, et al. Valve repair improves the outcome of surgery for mitral regurgitation. A multivariate analysis. Circulation 1995; 91(4):1022–8.

2. Perier P, Deloche A, Chauvaud S, et al. Comparative evaluation of mitral valve repair and replacement with Starr, Bjork, and porcine valve prostheses. Circulation 1984; 70(3 Pt 2):I187–92.

3. Goldman ME, Mora F, Guarino T, et al. Mitral valvuloplasty is superior to valve replacement for preservation of left ventricular function: an intraoperative two-dimensional echocardiographic study. J Am Coll Cardiol 1987; 10(3):568–75.

4. David TE, Burns RJ, Bacchus CM, et al. Mitral valve replacement for mitral regurgitation with and without preservation of chordae tendineae. J Thorac Cardiovasc Surg 1984;88(5 Pt 1):718–25.

5. Mohty D, Orszulak TA, Schaff HV, et al. Very long-term survival and durability of mitral valve repair for mitral valve prolapse. Circulation 2001;104(12 Suppl 1):I1–7.

6. Shumacker HBJ. The evolution of cardiac surgery. Bloomington, IN: Indiana University Press, 1992.

7. Spencer FC, Galloway AC, Colvin SB. Acquired disease of the mitral valve. In: Sabiston DC, Spencer FC, editors. Surgery of the chest. Philadelphia: Saunders; 1995. p. 1673–701.

8. Lillehei CW, et al. Surgical correction of pure mitral insufficiency by annuloplasty under direct vision. Lancet 1957; 77:446–9.

9. Merendino KA, Bruce RA. One hundred seventeen surgically treated cases of valvular rheumatic heart disease. JAMA 1957;164(7):749–55.

10. McGoon DC. Repair of mitral insufficiency due to ruptured chordae tendineae. J Thorac Cardiovasc Surg 1960; 39(3):357–62.

11. Kay JH, Egerton WS. The repair of mitral insufficiency associated with ruptured chordae tendineae. Ann Surg 1963;157(3):351–60.

12. Reed GE, Tice DA, Clauss RH. Asymmetric exaggerated mitral annuloplasty: repair of mitral insufficiency with hemodynamic predictability. J Thorac Cardiovasc Surg 1965;49(5):752–61.

13. Carpentier A, Deloche A, Dauptain J, et al. A new reconstructive operation for correction of mitral and tricuspid insufficiency. J Thorac Cardiovasc Surg 1971; 61(1):1–13.

14. Duran CMG, Pomar JL, Cucchiara G. A flexible ring for atrioventricular heart valve reconstruction. Cardiovas Surg 1978;19:417–20.

15. Silverman ME, Hurst JW. The mitral complex. Interaction of the anatomy, physiology, and pathology of the mitral annulus, mitral valve leaflets, chordae tendineae, and papillary muscles. Am Heart J 1968;76(3):399–418.

16. Lawrie GM. Mitral valve repair vs replacement. Current recommendations and long-term results. Cardiol Clin 1998;16(3):437–48.

17. Harken D, Ellis L, Dexter L. The responsibility of the physician in the selection of patients with mitral stenosis for surgical treatment. Circulation 1952;5:349.

18. Ranganathan N, Lam JH, Wigle ED, Silver MD. Morphology of the human mitral valve. II. The valve leaflets. Circulation 1970;41(3):459–67.

19. Lam JH, Ranganathan N, Wigle ED, Silver MD. Morphology of the human mitral valve. I. Chordae tendineae: a new classification. Circulation 1970;41(3):449–58.

20. Virmani R, Chun PK, Parker J, McAllister HA Jr. Suture obliteration of the circumflex coronary artery in three patients undergoing mitral valve operation. Role of left dominant or codominant coronary artery. J Thorac Cardiovasc Surg 1982;84(5):773–8.

21. Perloff JK, Roberts WC. The mitral apparatus. Functional anatomy of mitral regurgitation. Circulation 1972; 46(2):227–39.

22. Thomson HL, Enriquez-Sarano M. Echocardiographic assessment of mitral regurgitation. Cardiol Rev 2001; 9(4):210–6.

23. Grossi EA, Galloway AC, Miller JS, et al. Valve repair versus replacement for mitral insufficiency: when is a mechanical valve still indicated? J Thorac Cardiovasc Surg 1998; 115(2):389–94; discussion 394–6.

24. Luxereau P, Dorent R, De Gevigney G, et al. Aetiology of surgically treated mitral regurgitation. Eur Heart J 1991; 12 Suppl B:2–4.

25. Carpentier A. Cardiac valve surgery—the "French correction." J Thorac Cardiovasc Surg 1983;86(3):323–37.

26. Otto CM. Clinical practice. Evaluation and management of chronic mitral regurgitation. N Engl J Med 2001; 345(10):740–6.

27. Delahaye JP, Gare JP, Viguier E, et al. Natural history of severe mitral regurgitation. Eur Heart J 1991;12 Suppl B:5–9.

28. Freed LA, Levy D, Levine RA, et al. Prevalence and clinical outcome of mitral-valve prolapse. N Engl J Med 1999; 341(1):1–7.

29. Rosen SE, Borer JS, Hochreiter C, et al. Natural history of the asymptomatic/minimally symptomatic patient with severe mitral regurgitation secondary to mitral valve prolapse and normal right and left ventricular performance. Am J Cardiol 1994;74(4):374–80.

30. Ling LH, Enriquez-Sarano M, Seward JB, et al. Clinical outcome of mitral regurgitation due to flail leaflet. N Engl J Med 1996;335(19):1417–23.

31. Grigioni F, Enriquez-Sarano M, Ling LH, et al. Sudden death in mitral regurgitation due to flail leaflet. J Am Coll Cardiol 1999;34(7):2078–85.

32. ACC/AHA guidelines for the management of patients with valvular heart disease. A report of the American College of Cardiology/American Heart Association. Task Force on Practice Guidelines (Committee on Management of Patients with Valvular Heart Disease). J Am Coll Cardiol 1998;32(5):1486–588.

33. Enriquez-Sarano M, Tajik AJ, Schaff HV, et al. Echocardiographic prediction of left ventricular function after correction of mitral regurgitation: results and clinical implications. J Am Coll Cardiol 1994;24(6):1536–43.

34. Muratori M, Berti M, Doria E, et al. Transesophageal echocardiography as predictor of mitral valve repair. J Heart Valve Dis 2001;10(1):65–71.

35. Smith CR. Septal-superior exposure of the mitral valve. The transplant approach. J Thorac Cardiovasc Surg 1992; 103(4):623–8.

36. Spencer FC, Galloway AC, Grossi EA, et al. Recent developments and evolving techniques of mitral valve reconstruction. Ann Thorac Surg 1998;65(2):307–13.

37. Grossi EA, La Pietra A, Ribakove GH, et al. Minimally invasive versus sternotomy approaches for mitral reconstruction: comparison of intermediate-term results. J Thorac Cardiovasc Surg 2001;121(4):708–13.

38. Schroeyers P, Wellens F, De Geest R, et al. Minimally invasive video-assisted mitral valve surgery: our lessons after a 4-year experience. Ann Thorac Surg 2001;72(3): S1050–4.

39. Chitwood WR Jr. Video-assisted and robotic mitral valve surgery: toward an endoscopic surgery. Semin Thorac Cardiovasc Surg 1999;11(3):194–205.

40. David TE, Komeda M, Pollick C, Burns RJ. Mitral valve annuloplasty: the effect of the type on left ventricular function. Ann Thorac Surg 1989;47(4):524–7; discussion 527–8.

41. Spence PA, Peniston CM, David TE, et al. Toward a better understanding of the etiology of left ventricular dysfunction after mitral valve replacement: an experimental study with possible clinical implications. Ann Thorac Surg 1986;41(4):363–71.

42. Gillinov AM, Cosgrove DM, Blackstone EH, et al. Durability of mitral valve repair for degenerative disease. J Thorac Cardiovasc Surg 1998;116(5):734–43.

43. Gillinov AM, Cosgrove DM 3rd. Modified sliding leaflet technique for repair of the mitral valve. Ann Thorac Surg 1999;68(6):2356–7.

44. Phillips MR, Daly RC, Schaff HV, et al. Repair of anterior leaflet mitral valve prolapse: chordal replacement versus chordal shortening. Ann Thorac Surg 2000;69(1):25–9.

45. David TE, Omran A, Armstrong S, et al. Long-term results of mitral valve repair for myxomatous disease with and without chordal replacement with expanded polytetrafluoroethylene sutures. J Thorac Cardiovasc Surg 1998; 115:1279–86.

46. Kobayashi J, Sasako Y, Bando K, et al. Ten-year experience of chordal replacement with expanded polytetrafluoroethylene in mitral valve repair. Circulation 2000;102 (19 Suppl 3):III30–4.

47. Tavakoli R, Weber A, Vogt P, et al. Surgical management of acute mitral valve regurgitation due to post-infarction papillary muscle rupture. J Heart Valve Dis 2002;11(1): 20–5; discussion 26.

48. Chen Q, Darlymple-Hay MJ, Alexiou C, et al. Mitral valve surgery for acute papillary muscle rupture following myocardial infarction. J Heart Valve Dis 2002;11(1): 27–31.

49. Cho L, Gillinov AM, Cosgrove DM 3rd, et al. Echocardiographic assessment of the mechanisms of correction of bileaflet prolapse causing mitral regurgitation with only posterior leaflet repair surgery. Am J Cardiol 2000;86(12): 1349–51.

50. Alfieri O, Maisano F, De Bonis M, et al. The double-orifice technique in mitral valve repair: a simple solution for complex problems. J Thorac Cardiovasc Surg 2001; 122(4):674–81.

51. Handa N, Schaff HV, Morris JJ, et al. Outcome of valve repair and the Cox-Maze procedure for mitral regurgitation and associated atrial fibrillation. J Thorac Cardiovasc Surg 1999;118(4):628–35.

52. Preliminary report of the Stroke Prevention in Atrial Fibrillation Study. N Engl J Med 1990;322(12):863–8.

53. Ezekowitz MD, Bridgers SL, James KE, et al. Warfarin in the prevention of stroke associated with nonrheumatic atrial fibrillation. Veterans Affairs Stroke Prevention in Nonrheumatic Atrial Fibrillation Investigators. N Engl J Med 1992;327(20):1406–12.

54. The effect of low-dose warfarin on the risk of stroke in patients with nonrheumatic atrial fibrillation. The Boston Area Anticoagulation Trial for Atrial Fibrillation Investigators. N Engl J Med 1990;323(22):1505–11.

55. Gage BF, Cardinalli AB, Albers GW, Owens DK. Cost-effectiveness of warfarin and aspirin for prophylaxis of stroke in patients with nonvalvular atrial fibrillation. JAMA 1995;274(23):1839–45.

56. Raanani E, Alloage A, David TE, et al. The efficacy of the Cox/maze procedure combined with mitral valve surgery: a matched control study. Eur J Cardiothorac Surg 2001;19(4):438–42.

57. Braunberger E, Deloche A, Berrabi A, et al. Very long-term results (more than 20 years) of valve repair with Carpentier's techniques in nonrheumatic mitral valve insufficiency. Circulation 2001;104(12 Suppl 1):I8–11.

ROBOT-ASSISTED MITRAL VALVE SURGERY

W. RANDOLPH CHITWOOD JR, MD

Evolution toward Robotic Mitral Valve Surgery

To perform an ideal cardiac valve operation (Table 23-1), surgeons must operate in restricted spaces through tiny incisions, which requires assisted vision and advanced instrumentation. Although this goal has not been achieved widely yet, minimally invasive heart valve surgery (MIHVS) is evolving toward video-assisted and video-directed operations. New robotic methods now offer near endoscopic possibilities for mitral valve surgeons. Both video-assisted and direct-vision, limited access valve surgeries are within the reach of most cardiac surgeons. To be sure, robotic technology will evolve even more and should enable surgeons to reach intracorporeal pathology with much greater facility while damaging less natural tissue.

TABLE 23-1. Ideal Cardiac Valve Operation

Tiny incisions—endoscopic ports

Central antegrade perfusion

Tactile feedback

Eye–brain-"like" visualization

Facile, secure valve attachment

Intracardiac access

Dexterous topographic access
  Valve and subvalvular

No instrument conflicts

Minimal
  Cardiopulmonary perfusion
  Blood product usage
  Ventilation and intensive care unit care
  Hospitalization

Same or better quality
  Valve repairs in 60 to 80%
  Few reoperations (1 to 2%)
  Low mortality (1 to 2%)

Computerized surgical pathway memory

Instrument navigation systems

Minimally invasive cardiac surgery has not enjoyed a standard nomenclature. The terms *minimally invasive* and *limited access cardiac surgery* have connoted either the size of the incision, the avoidance of a sternotomy, use of a partial sternotomy, or abstention from cardiopulmonary bypass. However, the development of MIHVS may be considered analogous to a Mt. Everest ascent, embarking from a conventional or "base camp" operation and advancing progressively toward less invasiveness through experience and acclimatization. Table 23-2 shows a nomenclature that parallels this "mountaineering" analogy. In this scheme, entry levels of technical complexity are mastered premonitorily to advancing past small-incision direct-vision approaches (Level 1), toward more complex video-assisted procedures (Level 2 or 3), and, finally, to robotic valve operations (Level 4). With the constant evolution of new technology and surgical expertise, many established surgeons already have attained serial "comfort zones" along this MIHVS trek.

Level 1: Direct Vision Minimally Invasive Mitral Valve Surgery

Early MIHVS was based solely on modifications of previous incisions, and nearly all operations were done under direct vision. In 1996, the first truly minimally invasive

TABLE 23-2. Minimally Invasive Cardiac Surgery Classification

Level 1
  Direct vision
  Mini-incisions (10 to 12 cm)

Level 2
  Video assisted
  Micro incisions (4 to 6 cm)

Level 3
  Video directed and robot assisted
  Micro incisions or port incisions (1 cm)

Level 4
  Robotic telemanipulation
  Port incisions (1 cm)

aortic valve operations were reported.[1–3] At that time, surgeons found that minimal access incisions also provided adequate exposure of the mitral valve.[3–6] Using either ministernal or parasternal incisions, Cohn, Cosgrove, Gundry, Arom, and others showed encouraging results with low surgical mortality (1 to 3%) and morbidity for valve surgery.[1–8] In Cosgrove's first 50 minimally invasive aortic operations, perfusion and cardioplegia times approximated conventional operations, and his operative mortality was only 2%. More than 50% of the patients were discharged by postoperative day 5.[2] In early 1997, Cohn presented 41 minimally invasive aortic operations and first defined the economic benefits of these operations.[1]

In early 1996, the Stanford group performed the first minimally invasive mitral valve replacements, using direct vision, intraaortic balloon occlusion (Port-Access system), and cardioplegia.[9,10] Subsequently, surgeons at the University of Leipzig reported 24 mitral valve repairs done through a minithoracotomy using the Port-Access system.[11] This group later reported a high incidence of retrograde aortic dissections and neurologic complications, which seemed to be related to new catheter technology and limited surgeon experience.[11] By early 1997, Colvin and Galloway had performed 27 direct-vision Port-Access mitral repairs or replacements with a single death. They experienced no aortic dissections, and 63% of patients had mitral valve repairs with no reoperations for leakage.[12] By December 1998, Cosgrove had done 250 minimally invasive mitral valve operations using either a ministernotomy or parasternal incision with no mortality.[2] The successes of these early MIHVS procedures became the springboard to current direct-vision techniques described herein.

Level 2: Video-Assisted Minimally Invasive Mitral Valve Surgery

Avant-garde endoscopic surgical techniques of the 1980s became routine general, urologic, orthopedic, and gynecologic operations in the 1990s. This was related primarily to successes with extirpative endoscopic operations. In contrast, fine anastomotic and complex reparative procedures are the centerpieces of cardiac surgery. Because of difficulty in acquiring the fine video dexterity needed for these operations, cardiac surgeons are the last to explore the benefits of operative video assistance.

As mentioned, most Port-Access, sternal modification, and parasternal mitral valve operations have been done by using direct vision. In early 1996, Carpentier performed the first video-assisted mitral valve repair through a minithoracotomy by using hypothermic ventricular fibrillation.[13] Shortly thereafter, our team completed the first video-assisted mitral valve surgery through a minithoracotomy, using a new percutaneous transthoracic aortic clamp and retrograde cardioplegia.[14,15] This clamping and visualization technique was simple and cost-effective, and has remained the mainstay of isolated mitral valve operations at our center.

In 1997, Mohr reported 51 minimally invasive mitral operations, done by using Port-Access cardioplegia techniques, a 4-cm incision, and, for the first time, three-dimensional videoscopy.[16] In this series, three-dimensional (3-D) assistance aided mitral replacements; however, these surgeons found that less-complex reconstructions were significantly more difficult than when performed with sternotomy-based operations. At about the same time, Loulmet and Carpentier deployed an intracardiac "minicamera" for lighting and subvalvular visualization; however, they concluded that two-dimensional visualization was inadequate for detailed repairs.[17] Concurrently, our group reported 31 successful mitral operations done by using two-dimensional video assistance.[18] Complex repairs were possible and these included quadrangular resections, sliding valvuloplasties, chordal transfers, and synthetic chordal replacements. Our initial results were encouraging.

Level 3: Video-Directed and Robot-Assisted Minimally Invasive Mitral Valve Surgery

In 1997, Mohr first used the Aesop 3000 voice-activated camera robot in minimally invasive videoscopic mitral valve surgery.[16] Six months later, our team began using the Aesop 3000 to perform both video-assisted and video-directed minimally invasive mitral valve repairs (Figure 23-1).[19] We continue to use this device during most isolated mitral valve surgeries. This instrument provides surgeon camera site voice activation, precluding translation errors inherent with verbal transmission to an assistant. Camera motion is much smoother, more predictable, and requires less lens cleaning than during manual direction. Currently, if necessary, we can do more than 90% of a mitral repair under video direction with the Aesop 3000. Mohr termed this method "solo mitral surgery" and reported eight patients undergoing successful mitral repairs by using this robotic technique.[16] Since these early procedures, more than 1,500 videoscopic and robot-assisted mitral valve repairs have been done worldwide with excellent results. Table 23-3 shows the current indications for the video-assisted and robotic approach for mitral valve surgery.

Level 4: Telemanipulation and Robotic Minimally Invasive Mitral Valve Surgery

In June 1998, Carpentier and Mohr did the first true robotic mitral valve operations by using the da Vinci Surgical System.[20,21] In May 2000, the East Carolina University group performed the first da Vinci mitral repair in the United States (Figure 23-2).[22] This system provides both tele- and micromanipulation of tissues in small spaces. The surgeon operates from a console through end-affecter, micro wrist instruments, which are mounted on robotic arms that are inserted through the chest wall. These devices emulate human X-Y-Z axis wrist activity throughout a full seven degrees of manipulative excursion. These

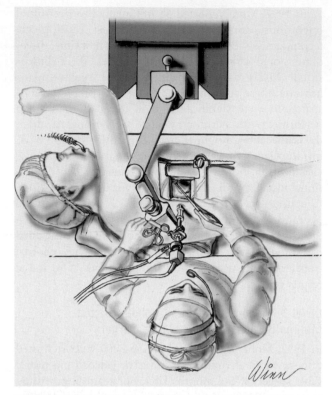

FIGURE 23-1. Robot-assisted (Aesop 3000) videoscopic mitral valve surgery. During minimally invasive video-assisted mitral surgery, the camera is voice activated and positioned by the surgeon using the Aesop 3000 robot. Operative maneuvers are made through the 5-cm incision, using long instruments and secondary vision. This illustrates how the surgeon manipulates the camera for accurate two-dimensional magnified vision on the video monitor.

TABLE 23-3. Current Patient Selection: Videoscopic or Video-Assisted Mitral Valve Surgery

Unsuitable candidates
  Highly calcified mitral annulus
  Severe pulmonary hypertension, especially with a small right coronary
  Significant untreated coronary disease
  Severe peripheral atherosclerosis
  Prior right chest surgery
Suitable candidates
  Patients with primary mitral valve disease
  Reoperative mitral valve patients
  Bileaflet and/or anterior leaflet disease
  Combined tricuspid and mitral operations
  Mild annular calcification
  Obese or large patients
  Elderly patients

motions occur through two joints that each affect pitch, yaw, and rotation. Additionally, arm insertion and rotation, as well as variable grip strength, give additive freedom to the operating "wrist." Mohr and Chitwood have the greatest experience in this area and independently have determined that this device is effective for perform-

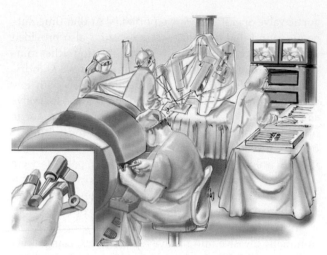

FIGURE 23-2. da Vinci robotic telemanipulation system. The operative console is in the foreground, and the instrument cart is at the operating table. The operating surgeon and the patient-side assistant are shown.

ing complex mitral valve repairs.[21,23] Grossi and associates used the Zeus system to perform a partial mitral valve repair but had limited ergonomic freedom.[24] Lange and associates, in Munich, were the first to perform a totally endoscopic mitral valve repair using only 1-cm ports and the da Vinci system.[25]

Robotic Technology for Minimally Invasive Mitral Valve Surgery

The Aesop 3000 robotic camera manipulator (Computer Motion, Inc., Santa Barbara, CA) is the pillar of robotic control during our minimally invasive video-assisted mitral surgery. Figures 23-3 and 23-4 show how this device is arranged during these operations. Even though video assistance with robotic vision control has proved valuable, surgeons still must operate with long instruments in a two-dimensional operative field (Figures 23-5 and 23-6).

The da Vinci Surgical System (Intuitive Surgical, Inc., Mountain View, CA) comprises three components: a surgeon console, an instrument cart, and a visioning platform (Figure 23-7; see also Figure 23-2). The operative console is removed physically from the patient and enables the surgeon to sit comfortably, resting the arms ergonomically with his or her head positioned in a 3-D vision array (Figure 23-8). The surgeon's finger and wrist movements are registered, through sensors, in computer memory banks, and these actions are transferred efficiently to an instrument cart, which operates the synchronous end effector instruments (Figure 23-9). Through 1-cm ports, instruments are positioned near cardiac operative sites in the thorax, and the camera is passed via a 4-cm working port used for suture and prosthesis passage (Figures 23-10 and 23-11). Every analog finger movement, along with

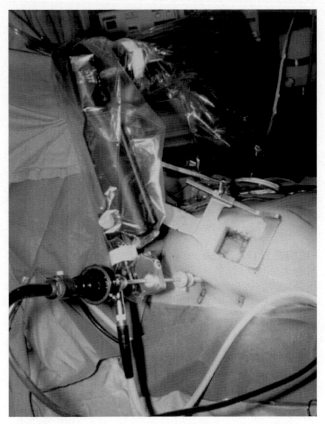

FIGURE 23-3. Operative preparation for robot-assisted videoscopic mitral valve surgery. Here the Aesop 3000 is attached to a 5-mm 0° two-dimensional telescope. For mitral valve surgery, the pericardial edges are retracted using transthoracic sutures.

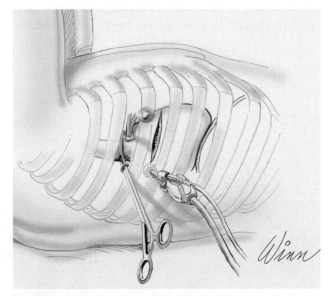

FIGURE 23-4. Right minithoracotomy for video access. The right minithoracotomy allows aortic access for the transthoracic clamp shown here, as well as for the video camera. With this arrangement, minimal rib spreading is needed to perform mitral surgery. The camera is attached to the Aesop 3000. The transthoracic cross clamp provides a safe easy method for cardiac arrest.

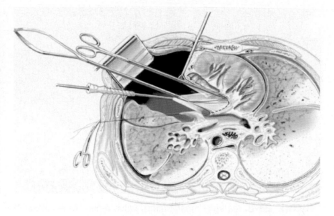

FIGURE 23-5. Cross section of the thorax during video-assisted mitral surgery. Pericardial edges are retracted using transthoracic retention sutures, and the interatrial septum is retracted using a transthoracic retractor.

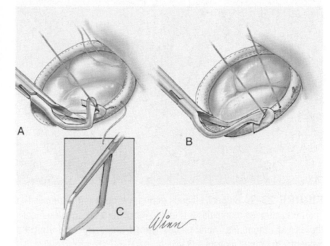

FIGURE 23-6. Mitral valve knot pusher (A), suture cutter (B), and handle for both devices (C). Specially designed instruments are used to perform these operations with speed and facility.

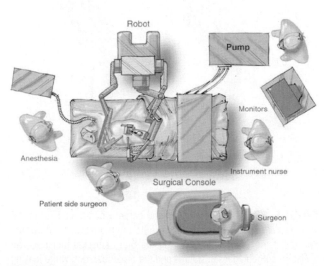

FIGURE 23-7. An aerial view of the da Vinci operating room arrangement for a robotic mitral valve operation.

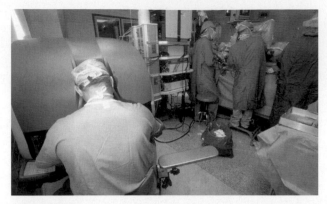

FIGURE 23-8. da Vinci robotic mitral valve repair. The instrument cart is placed on the left side of the tilted patient, with the robot's arms entering the right thorax. The surgeon's operative console is positioned about 10 feet from the operating table and instrument cart.

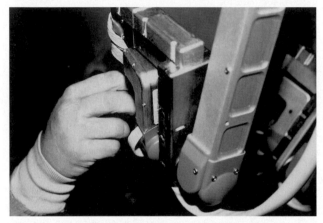

FIGURE 23-9. Surgeon's hands during a robotic mitral repair. The operating surgeon manipulates effecter instrument tips in the patient's thorax via ergonomic "hand-pieces" that transfer filtered digitized data into smoothed movements.

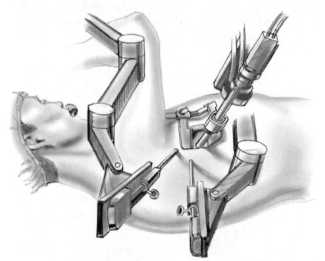

FIGURE 23-10. Robotic arms and camera positioned for mitral valve repair surgery. Each arm passes into the thorax via 1-cm trocars, and the camera is shown entering the 5-cm surgical incision. The assistant surgeon passes sutures and the prosthetic ring while looking at a two-dimensional slave monitor. The surgeon has true three-dimensional vision.

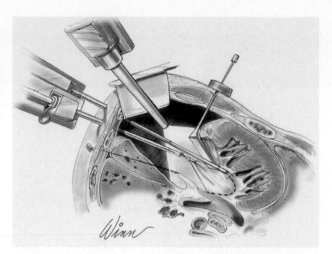

FIGURE 23-11. Thoracic cross section during a da Vinci mitral valve operation. This view shows how both instrument arms and the visual field converge at the operative plane to effect an unobstructed topographic view with full access to valvular and subvalvular structures.

inherent human tremor at 8 to 10 Hz/s, is converted to binary digital data, which are smoothed and filtered to increase microinstrument precision. Wristlike instrument articulation emulates precisely the surgeon's actions at the tissue level, and dexterity becomes enhanced through combined tremor suppression and motion scaling (Figure 23-12). This allows both increased precision and dexterity, with the surgeon becoming truly ambidextrous. A clutching mechanism enables readjustment of hand positions to maintain an optimal ergonomic attitude with respect to the visual field. This clutch acts very much like a computer mouse, which can be reoriented by lifting and repositioning it to reestablish unrestrained freedom of computer

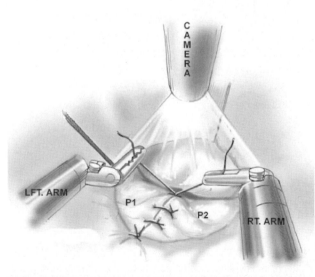

FIGURE 23-12. Camera and articulated instrument tips. The instrument tips have a full 7° of freedom and emulate the range of motion attendant in the human wrist. This allows a wide range of intraatrial and intraventricular mobility during mitral valve surgery.

activation. The 3-D digital visioning system enables natural depth perception with high-power magnification (×10). Both 0° and 30° endoscopes can be manipulated electronically to look either "up" or "down" within the heart. Access to and visualization of the internal thoracic artery, coronary arteries, and mitral apparatus have been shown to be excellent. The operator becomes ensconced in the 3-D operative topography and can perform extremely precise surgical manipulations, devoid of traditional distractions. Figure 23-13 (*A* through *E*) shows the surgeon's operative field during a da Vinci mitral valve repair surgery.

Current Status of Minimally Invasive Heart Valve Surgery

Level 1: Direct-Vision Mitral Surgery

Cosgrove and Gundry have been consistent proponents of using the ministernotomy for mitral surgery. They have considered the ministernotomy technique more reproducible for surgeons with variable experiences and abilities. Both complex replacements and repairs have been done through this incision, and to date, few operative failures have resulted from this exposure. Between 1996 and early 2002, Cosgrove and his Cleveland Clinic group performed 1,427 minimally invasive mitral operations by using direct vision, the upper hemisternotomy, and modified perfusion methods. As noted earlier, the extended atriotomy, used by Cosgrove, apparently has not resulted in significant atrial arrhythmias. Of these patients, 81% had degenerative and 9% had rheumatic disease. Of all mitral valves, 90% were insufficient and nearly all were repaired, with 98% having a band annuloplasty and 85% undergoing leaflet resections. Perfusion and aortic occlusion times averaged 80 and 60 min, respectively. These times are shorter than those of many experienced surgeons who use a full sternal approach. As seen earlier in their aortic operations, perfusion times have fallen more significantly than arrest times since 1996. This mitral valve series presents an impressive mortality (0.3%) and complication rate (bleeding [3.1%], strokes [1.8 %], respiratory insufficiency [0.8%]). Conversions to a full sternotomy have fallen at the Cleveland Clinic from 5% in 1997 to 0.5% in 2002 (1.5% overall), and most of these were related to poor exposure, not bleeding. Only 7% of patients were transfused, and the mean hospitalization was 6.5 days with 20% being discharged in less than 4 days.

After initially using a right parasternal incision with bicaval cannulation and left atrial entry via the interatrial septum, Cohn and associates now prefer modified hemisternal approaches for mitral valve surgery. Of the 411 mitral patients operated on between 1996 and early 2002, 201 had hemisternotomies and 201 had parasternal incisions, with 8 having a minithoracotomy. Myxomatous (81%), rheumatic (10%), and endocarditis (4%) were the most common etiologies. In 88% of these patients, repairs were done; in the remaining 12%, replacements were done using mechanical valves (84%). Their operative mortality was an impressive 0.2% with no deaths in the repair group. Bleeding occurred in 2%, and 38% were transfused with an average of one packed cell unit per patient. Strokes occurred in 2.2% of patients, and myocardial infarctions occurred in 1.0%. Patients were hospitalized for a mean of 6 days, and 8.3% required additional rehabilitation prior to discharge.

Grossi and associates at New York University compared 100 minimally invasive mitral operations, done through a 6- to 8-cm minithoracotomy by using direct vision and Port-Access methods, to a cohort of 100 conventional mitral operations.[26] They reported a perioperative mortality of 1.0%. In these patients, 80% had a posterior leaflet procedure and 30% had an anterior leaflet reconstruction. This ratio did not differ from their full sternotomy patients, nor did the status of repairs 1 year following surgery. Their results suggest minimally invasive mitral operations can be done safely by using Port-Access methods, with results similar to those obtained from conventional operations and with no added mortality or morbidity. At the same time, they had fewer transfusions, shorter lengths of stay, and less-septic complications, despite longer cardiopulmonary bypass times. In a multi-institutional analysis of 491 Port-Access mitral repairs from 104 centers, Glower reported that 86% of all valves were repaired with aortic occlusion times of 90 min and perfusion times of 137 min.[27,28] The overall mortality for repairs was 1.6% and was 5.5% for replacements. Age was the only independent predictor of strokes (2.7%) in these patients. Neurologic complications associated with early use of this technique have diminished with the advent of better devices and more experience. The overall length of stay for this large group of mitral patients was 7 days.

Levels 2 and 3: Video- and Aesop-Assisted and Aesop Mitral Surgery

In early 2001, the East Carolina University (ECU) group reported their 128 successful video- and robot-assisted mitral valve operations.[19] At first, patients with anterior leaflet pathology and annular calcification were avoided. However, we now consider these patients within the realm of video-assisted surgery. Table 23-3 details our current criteria for patient selection. In our series, repairs included quadrangular resections, annuloplasties, and complex chordal operations. The majority of patients had myxomatous disease, and 61% of the total group underwent a repair. Figure 23-14 shows a videoscopic bileaflet repair using two (P1 and P2) sliding plasties as well as a P2 segment transfer to A2 for type 2 anterior leaflet prolapse. When the early series is combined with the subsequent 100 video-assisted mitral operations, repairs have been done in

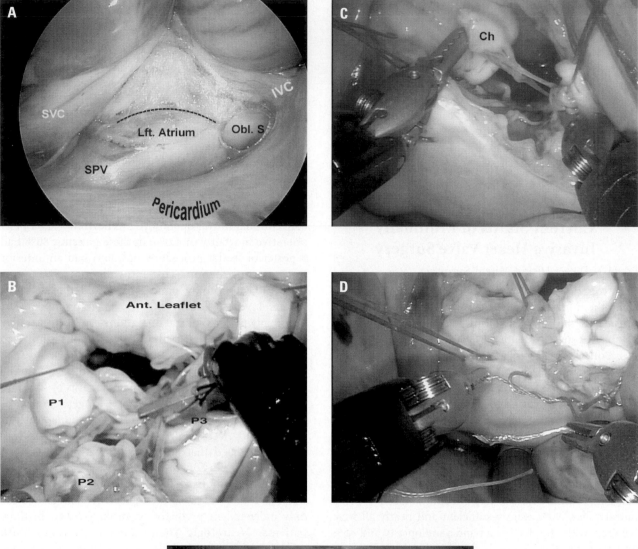

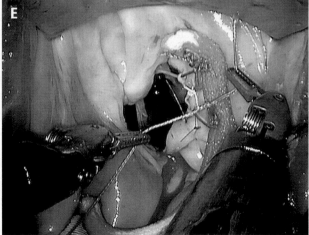

FIGURE 23-13. *A,* Videoscopic view of the operative approach during da Vinci robotic mitral surgery. IVC = inferior vena cava; Lft. Atrium = site of left atriotomy (dashed lines); Obl. S = oblique sinus behind the IVC; SPV = stentless porcine valve; SVC = superior vena cava. This view is provided by camera placement in the 4th interspace. *B,* da Vinci mitral valve repair. The P2 segment of the posterior leaflet is being resected by robotic micro-scissors. The annulus is reduced and both P1 and P3 are approximated. *C,* da Vinci chordal transfer from resected P2 to P1. Ch = chordal cluster with small valve segment. *D,* Robotic annular closure after a P2 resection. The gap is closed with a figure-of-eight braided (2–0) suture material. The surgeon is preparing to perform a sliding plasty of P3. *E,* da Vinci instrument tips are tying sutures to secure an annuloplasty band along the posterior annulus.

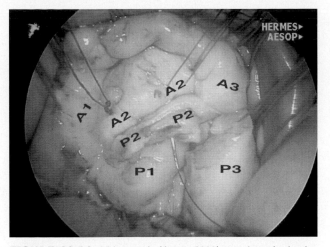

FIGURE 23-14. Videoscopic (Aesop 3000) complex mitral valve repair. Here both the anterior and posterior leaflets are redundant with severe type 2 prolapse. The posterior part of P2 is resected, leaving the anterior quarter of the leaflet with chords attached along the coapting edge. This segment of P2 is then transferred along the coapting edge of A2. Securing mattress sutures are being placed. Finally, a height-reducing sliding plasty is done for both P1 and P3 before central approximation. Lastly, a band annuloplasty is done. We find this method to be very effective for treating severe anterior prolapse minimally invasively.

81% of patients at ECU. The operative and 30-day mortalities for our entire series are 0.4% and 1.7%, respectively. After implementing the Aesop 3000 robot to voice-direct the endoscopic camera, cross-clamp and perfusion times fell secondary to improved visualization and reduced lens cleaning. However, in the latter half of the early series, cross-clamp (90 min) and perfusion times (143 min) still remained longer than conventional operations. Currently, cardiac arrest and perfusion times are 70 and 100 min, respectively. Interestingly, we see no difference in bleeding and transfusion requirements between our conventional and MIHVS patients. However, the hospital lengths of stays have averaged 4.9 days for MIHVS patients, as compared to 8 days for conventional operations. Of these 228 patients, there were 2 conversions to a sternotomy, 2 strokes, and no aortic dissections. We had one vena caval injury during cannulation in nearly 300 growing cannulations for cardiopulmonary bypass. Included in this series are 30 patients who have had either prior coronary or mitral surgery. These patients underwent video-assisted reoperations with a 3.5% mortality and markedly less blood loss than conventional reoperations.

Mohr and associates reported on 154 video-assisted mitral valve operations performed by using Aesop 3000 robotic camera control.[16,21,29] In these patients, the aortic cross-clamp and perfusion times were similar to Mohr's conventional operations, and the operative mortality was 1.2%. He considered three-dimensional visualization to be the key to excellent results during videoscopic valve reconstructions. In a study comparing the Port-Access technique to transthoracic clamping, Wimmer-Greinecker obtained similar repair results but with faster operations, less technical difficulties, and lower cost by using the clamping method.[30] In early 2002, Vanermen reported success in 187 patients undergoing totally endoscopic repairs by using the Port-Access method and no rib spreading. He used a holder-mounted two-dimensional endoscopic camera and performed complex repairs with excellent results at follow-up 19 months later.[31,32] The hospital mortality was 0.5%, and there were two conversions to a sternotomy for bleeding. Freedom from reoperation was 95% at 4 years. More than 90% of patients had minimal postoperative pain. Although this and other series have not been randomized, there are strong suggestions that mitral valve surgery has entered a new era and that video techniques can facilitate these operations.

Level 4: da Vinci Robotic (Telemanipulation) Mitral Surgery

At my institution, as part of phase I and II Food and Drug Administration trials, mitral repairs were performed in 48 patients by using the robotic da Vinci Surgical System.[22,23] Quadrangular leaflet resections, leaflet sliding plasties, chordal transfers, polytetrafluoroethylene (PTFE) chord replacements, and annuloplasty band insertions have been done with facility (see Figure 23-13). Difficult commissural and trigone sutures dissolved into simple efforts by using da Vinci. Robotic repair and total operating times decreased from 1.9 and 5.1 h, respectively, for the first 21 patients to 1.5 and 4.4 h, respectively, for the last 21 patients. Excepting times required to place annuloplasty bands, all time intervals decreased significantly with experience. In the last cohort, cross-clamp and perfusion times were 1.8 and 2.7 h, respectively. This time course paralleled improvements experienced with our videoscopic series reported above. We have had no major complications, and the mean length of stay has been 3.8 days. Two valves were replaced either because of hemolysis (19 days) or a new grade 3 leak (2 months). Mohr successfully has completed 22 mitral repairs in Leipzig with da Vinci.[21] As mentioned above, Lange in Munich has performed a totally endoscopic mitral repair using only 1-cm port incisions.[24] A multicenter da Vinci trial, enlisting approximately 120 patients, is nearing completion, and to date demonstrates efficacy and safety in performing these operations by multiple surgeons at various centers. To date, aortic and tricuspid valves have not held widespread interest for robotic surgeons. Additionally, our team is developing methods that will facilitate valve and annuloplasty ring attachment without the use of traditional sutures. Specialized clips are being used experimentally to attach annuloplasty rings and repair leaflets. Also, monofilament suture ultrasonic welding may hold promise for use during robotic valve operations.

Conclusion

The above information suggests that robotic mitral valve surgery is well on the way to reality. Although operative philosophies, patient populations, and surgeon abilities differ between centers, the compendium of recent results remains very encouraging. The advent of true three-dimensional vision with tactile instrument feedback will be the major bridge to truly "tele-micro-access" operations. Also, to perform these operations optimally, "extracorporeal" surgeons and engineers will need to improve methods by which instruments are directed by computers. Recent successes with direct vision, videoscopic, and robotic minimally invasive surgery all have reaffirmed that this evolution can be extremely fast, albeit through various pathways. In fact, catheter-based technology is even moving toward treating aortic valve disease, and mitral annuloplasties have been done experimentally through the coronary sinus.

Patient requirements, technology developments, and surgeon capabilities all must align to drive these needed changes. In addition, we must work closer with our cardiology colleagues in these developments. This is an evolutionary process, and even the greatest skeptics must concede that progress has been made. However, curmudgeons and surgical scientists alike must continue to interject their concerns. Caution cannot be overemphasized. Traditional valve operations enjoy long-term success with ever-decreasing morbidity and mortality, and remain our measure for comparison. Surgeons and cardiologists must remember that less-invasive approaches to treating valve disease cannot capitulate to poorer operative quality or unsatisfactory valve and/or patient longevity.

References

1. Cohn LH, Adams DH, Couper GS, Bichell DP. Minimally invasive aortic valve replacement. Semin Thorac Cardiovasc Surg 1997;9:331–6.

2. Cosgrove DM, Sabik JF. Minimally invasive approach for aortic valve operations. Ann Thorac Surg 1996;62:596–7.

3. Arom KV, Emery RW. Minimally invasive mitral operations. Ann Thorac Surg 1996;62:1542–4.

4. Arom KV, Emery RW, Kshettry VR, Janey PA. Comparison between port access and less invasive valve surgery. Ann Thorac Surg 1999;68:1524–8.

5. Koenertz W, Waldenberger F, Schutzler M, et al. Minimal access valve surgery through superior partial sternotomy: a preliminary study. J Heart Valve Dis 1996;5:638–40.

6. Navia JL, Cosgrove DM. Minimally invasive mitral valve operations. Ann Thorac Surg 1996;62:1542–4.

7. Cohn LH, Adams DH, Couper GS, et al. Minimally invasive cardiac valve surgery improves patient satisfaction while reducing costs of cardiac valve replacement and repair. Ann Surg 1997:226:421–6.

8. Gundry SR, Shattuck OH, Razzouk AJ, et al. Facile minimally invasive cardiac surgery via mini-sternotomy. Ann Thorac Surg 1998;65:1100–4.

9. Fann JI, Pompili MF, Stevens JH, et al. Port-Access cardiac operations with cardioplegic arrest. Ann Thorac Surg 1997;63 Suppl 6:35–9.

10. Fann JI, Pompili MF, Burdon TA, et al. Minimally invasive mitral valve surgery. Semin Thorac Cardiovasc Surg 1997;9:320–30.

11. Mohr FW, Falk V, Diegeler A, et al. Minimally invasive Port-Access mitral valve surgery. J Thorac Cardiovasc Surg 1998:115:567–74.

12. Spencer FC, Galloway AC, Grossi EA, et al. Recent developments and evolving techniques of mitral valve reconstruction. Ann Thorac Surg 1998;65:307–13.

13. Carpentier A, Loulmet D, Carpentier A, et al. Chirugie à coeur ouvert par vidéo-chirurgie et mini-thoracotomie - primier cas (valvuloplastie mitrale) opéré avec succès [First open heart operation (mitral valvuloplasty) under videosurgery through a minithoracotomy] [Fr]. Comptes Rendus De L'Academie des Sciences: Sciences de la vie 1996;319:219–23.

14. Chitwood WR, Elbeery JR, Moran JM. Minimally invasive mitral valve repair: using a minithoracotomy and transthoracic aortic occlusion. Ann Thorac Surg 1997;63:1477–9.

15. Chitwood WR, Elbeery JR, Chapman WHH, et al. Video-assisted minimally invasive mitral valve surgery: the "micro-mitral" operation. J Thorac Cardiovasc Surg 1997;113:413–4.

16. Falk V, Walther T, Autschbach R, et al. Robot-assisted minimally invasive solo mitral valve operation. J Thorac Cardiovasc Surg 1998:115:470–1.

17. Loulmet DF, Carpentier A, Cho PW, et al. Less invasive methods for mitral valve surgery. J Thorac Cardiovasc Surg 1998;115:772–9.

18. Chitwood WR Jr, Wixon CL, Elbeery JR, et al. Video-assisted minimally invasive mitral valve surgery. J Thorac Cardiovasc Surg 1997;114:773–80.

19. Felger JE, Chitwood WR, Nifong LW, Holbert D. Evolution of mitral valve surgery: toward a totally endoscopic approach. Ann Thorac Surg 2001;72:1203–8.

20. Carpentier A, Loulmet D, Aupecle B, et al. Computer assisted open-heart surgery. First case operated on with success. CR Acad Sci II 1998;321:437–2.

21. Mohr FW, Falk V, Diegler A, et al. Computer-enhanced "robotic" cardiac surgery: experience in 148 patients. J Thorac Cardiovasc Surg 2001;121:842–53.

22. Chitwood WR, Nifong LW, Elbeery JE, et al. Robotic mitral valve repair: trapezoidal resection and prosthetic annuloplasty with the da Vinci Surgical System. J Thorac Cardiovasc Surg 2000;120:1171–2.

23. Nifong LW, Chitwood WR, Chu VF, et al. Complete robotic mitral valve repair: experience with the da Vinci system. Ann Thorac Surg 2002. [In press]

24. Grossi E, Lapietra A, Applebaum RM, et al. Case report of robotic instrument-enhanced mitral valve surgery. J Thorac Cardiovasc Surg 2000;120:1169–71.

25. Mehmanesh H, Henze R, Lange R. Totally endoscopic mitral valve repair. J Thorac Cardiovasc Surg 2002;123:96–7.

26. Grossi E, LaPietra A, Ribakove GH, et al. Minimally invasive sternotomy approaches for mitral reconstruction: comparison of intermediate term results. J Thorac Cardiovasc Surg 2001;121:708–13.

27. Glower DD, Siegel LC, Galloway AC, et al. Predictors of operative time in multicenter Port-Access valve registry: institutional differences in learning. Heart Surg Forum 2001;4:40–6.

28. Glower DD, Siegel LC, Frischmerer KL, et al. Predictors of outcome in a multicenter Port-Access valve registry. Ann Thorac Surg 2000;70:1054–9.

29. Autschbach R, Onnasch JF, Falk V, et al. The Leipzig experience with robotic valve surgery. J Card Surg 2000;15: 82–7.

30. Aybek T, Dogan S, Wimmer-Greineker G, et al. The micro-mitral operation comparing the Port-Access technique and the transthoracic clamp technique. J Card Surg 2000;15:76–81.

31. Schoeyers P, Wellens F, De Geest R, et al. Minimally invasive video-assisted mitral valve surgery: our lessons after a 4-year experience. Ann Thorac Surg 2001;72:S1050–4.

32. Casselman FP, van Slyche S, Dom H, et al. Totally endo-scopic mitral valve repair: feasible, reproducible, and durable. J Thorac Cardiovasc Surg 2002. [In press]

CHAPTER 24

SURGICAL MANAGEMENT OF HYPERTROPHIC OBSTRUCTIVE CARDIOMYOPATHY

CHAD E. HAMNER, MD, HARTZELL V. SCHAFF, MD

Since its initial description more than 40 years ago, hypertrophic cardiomyopathy (HCM) has interested clinicians as a diverse but incompletely defined disease process. Early attempts to delineate the clinical characteristics and management of HCM produced a varied nomenclature of descriptive terms including idiopathic hypertrophic subaortic stenosis, muscular subaortic stenosis, diffuse subaortic stenosis, congenital subaortic stenosis, asymmetric septal hypertrophy, and hypertrophic obstructive cardiomyopathy (HOCM).[1]

Left ventricular hypertrophy (LVH) with no underlying cardiac or systemic etiology, such as valvular disease or hypertension, is the key feature of the disorder, and in 1996, the World Health Organization adopted the term *hypertrophic cardiomyopathy* to describe this disease process. However, the discovery of multiple disease-causing genetic mutations in the last decade, and the absence of identifiable LVH in as many as 20% of gene carriers,[2] have stimulated new debate as to whether HCM is a single disease or a group of related disorders.[1]

Molecular Basis

Hypertrophic cardiomyopathy is a familial myocardial disease inherited in an autosomal dominant pattern with variable penetrance; sporadic proband cases have been identified. Approximately 100 mutations, mostly of the missense type, in 9 different genes encoding for sarcomere constituent proteins have been implicated in a process that leads to impaired actin-myosin cross-bridging and abnormal force generation.[3,4] Involved proteins include the β-myosin heavy chain; myosin-binding protein C; the essential and regulatory light chains; cardiac actin; α-tropomyosin; troponins C, I, and T; and titin. Although the prevalence of each mutation among affected individuals varies, more than 50% of all reported cases involve

mutations for those genes encoding β-myosin heavy chain, myosin-binding protein C, and troponin T.[4]

Factors such as cardiac morphology, prevalence, natural history, and risk of sudden death vary widely among mutations.[4] Despite a strong genetic basis for HCM, no more than half of all cases have a known mutation, and the clinical significance of all known genes is not yet determined. Therefore, the applicability of genetic testing to family members of affected individuals remains limited.[4]

Myocardial Morphology

Ventricular morphologies of patients with HCM vary as widely as the genetic defects underlying them (Figure 24-1). As stated previously, some degree of LVH is the

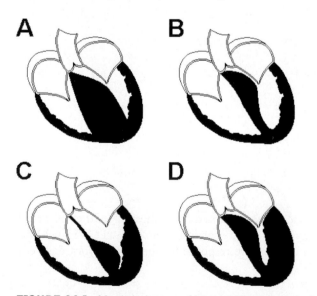

FIGURE 24-1. Morphologic types of hypertrophic cardiomyopathy. *A,* Asymmetric septal hypertrophy; *B,* subaortic septal hypertrophy; *C,* apical hypertrophy; and *D,* diffuse left ventricular hypertrophy.

predominant feature, but other structural abnormalities are recognized, especially in connective-tissue elements such as the mitral valve and intramural arterioles.[1,5]

Hypertrophy usually involves only the left ventricle but is often asymmetric, affecting the interventricular septum, diffusely or segmentally, and the left ventricular free wall.[1,5] Left ventricular wall thickness in affected individuals ranges widely from 13 to 60 mm (normal ≤ 12 mm), and an increased risk of sudden death has been correlated to greater degrees of hypertrophy (≥ 35 mm).[1] Abnormal cellular organization is a prominent feature seen in varying degrees within the septum or free ventricular wall of most individuals who die from HCM. This myocardial cellular disarray is characterized by chaotic patterns of cells or groups of cells oriented at oblique and perpendicular angles to one another with multiple intercellular connections.[1] Foci of disorganized cells may serve as an arrhythmogenic stimulus by impairing normal electrical conduction, thereby promoting the development of reentry circuits within the myocardium.[1]

Mitral valve malformations can occur independent of the underlying myocardial morphology, including various patterns of leaflet enlargement[1,5] or anomalous insertion of the papillary muscles, and may have some impact on obstruction of the left ventricular outflow tract (LVOT).[5] Finally, intramural arterioles may have unusual architecture because of increased quantities of intimal and medial collagen producing wall thickening and luminal narrowing; this finding has been referred to as the "small-vessel disease" of HCM.[1,5]

Many patients with HCM acquire ventricular hypertrophy in a progressive fashion, but the underlying stimulus for this progression has not been defined. Substantial LVH is rarely identified in infants and young children, and when the disease is manifest at this early age, prognosis is poor. Most frequently, left ventricular wall thickness increases disproportionately, occurring during adolescence, and further substantial increases in left ventricular wall thickness are uncommon once full somatic growth and maturation have occurred.[1] Paradoxically, regression of LVH occurs in as many as 15% of adults referred with a diagnosis of HCM and can represent an "end stage" in the natural history of the disease.[1] In these patients, left ventricular remodeling leads to thinning of the wall to normal or mildly increased thickness, dilation of the ventricular chamber, and varying degrees of systolic functional impairment.[1,6]

The most accepted hypothesis for the observed changes in the left ventricle in HCM is that LVH develops as a maladaptive response by abnormal myocardial cells to a perceived excessive afterload, resulting in short-term improvements in wall tension and oxygen demand.[3] "End stage" remodeling likely occurs by a combination of factors leading to myocardial ischemia, cell death, and fibrosis, including increased oxygen demand created by

marked muscular hypertrophy, small-vessel disease with reduced vasodilator capacity and myocardial capillary density, and increased coronary vascular resistance produced by increased diastolic wall tension.[1,3]

Pathophysiology

A triad of pathophysiologic features are responsible for the recognizable clinical manifestations of HCM: diastolic dysfunction, LVOT obstruction, and late systolic dysfunction. Most patients have some degree of diastolic dysfunction, likely related to the increased stiffness and reduced relaxation of the hypertrophied left ventricular wall. There is, however, no precise correlation between the degree of diastolic dysfunction and the degree or pattern of hypertrophy.[1,5]

Left ventricular outflow obstruction is present in approximately 25% of patients with HCM.[1,6] Initially, subaortic outflow gradients in HCM were attributed to contraction of a sphincter ring,[7] but echocardiography has clearly demonstrated that obstruction is produced by the combination of LVOT narrowing by ventricular septal hypertrophy and systolic anterior motion of the mitral valve leaflets against the interventricular septum, with leaflet coaptation occurring at the body and not the tip of the leaflets.[5] Abnormal mitral leaflet coaptation and septal contact is associated with varying degrees of mitral regurgitation, producing a sequence of ejection, obstruction, and valve leakage during systole.[5]

Systolic gradients can also occur in the midventricle at the level of the papillary muscles and is common in the setting of apical hypertrophy.[5] In its most severe form, midventricular obstruction with severe apical hypertrophy may lead to subendocardial infarction and pouch-like apical aneurysms. Rarely, a small aneurysm can be the site of thrombus formation or an arrhythmogenic focus. Unlike subaortic obstruction, midventricular obstruction does not cause mitral regurgitation.[7] Each of these pathophysiologic features appear to be interrelated and vary among patients with HCM.[1]

Systolic function of the left ventricle can be normal or hyperdynamic with supernormal fractions[5] and reduced stroke volume augmentation with exercise.[8] If ventricular remodeling produces the "end stage" manifestations of HCM, systolic function becomes impaired with reduced ejection fraction and increased end systolic volume.[7]

Clinical Spectrum

As may be expected from the genetic and morphologic diversity of HCM, the clinical features at presentation vary substantially among affected individuals. In a population-based study in Olmsted County, MN, the estimated age and sex-adjusted prevalence of HCM was 19.7 per 100,000 people, with an incidence of 2.5 per 100,000 person-years;

this incidence appears to be increasing over time, likely related to better awareness and diagnostic capabilities.[9] More recent echocardiographic studies determined that the prevalence may be higher, approaching 0.2% in the general population.[1,2,6] However, such estimates based on referral populations may not be valid in the general population.[4,6]

Within the same population in the Olmsted County study, a new diagnosis of HCM occurred at a median age of 59 years (range, 1 week to 92 years), and the vast majority (87%) did not come to the attention of physicians until after 40 years of age.[10] A slight majority of patients (58%) had symptoms; unfortunately, 14% of patients were not identified until after death, and 9% died suddenly and unexpectedly.[10] Most common symptoms included angina (43%), dyspnea (16%), syncope (11%), and clinical heart failure (16%). Arrhythmias, mostly supraventricular in nature, were documented in 5%.[10]

Diagnosis

Physical examination in asymptomatic patients with HCM who do not have LVOT obstruction may be normal. When marked LVH has developed, cardiac examination may reveal a displaced and forceful apical impulse; occasionally, the fourth heart sound may be palpable.[5] The presence and quality of a systolic murmur varies, from only a faint (1/6) systolic murmur at the apex in latent disease to a palpable apical thrill (3 to 4/6) with left sternal border and axillary radiation (from mitral regurgitation) in patients with subaortic obstruction at rest.[5] A systolic apical murmur is also evident in midventricular obstruction, but the intensity is usually less (2 to 3/6) than that seen in subaortic obstruction.[5]

Provocative testing typically does not increase the intensity of a systolic murmur in patients without obstructive HCM.[5] Individuals with latent subaortic obstruction usually respond with slight increases in intensity of the systolic murmur to provocative maneuvers, such as Valsalva's maneuver, upright posture, or amyl nitrate inhalation.[5]

Other auscultatory findings that may be demonstrated in subaortic obstruction include reversed splitting of the second heart sound, a double or triple systolic apex beat, mitral diastolic inflow murmur, or a mitral valve leaflet-septal contact sound.[5] With midventricular obstruction, a split-second heart sound and a long mitral diastolic murmur may be heard, while a mitral leaflet-contact sound is never heard.[5]

Pulse examination may also be normal in asymptomatic HCM patients without LVOT obstruction. However, those with obstruction gradients will typically demonstrate pulsus bisferiens. This is characterized by a brisk rise early in systole, a midsystolic decline as the gradient develops, and a secondary upstroke late in systole as the gradient is overcome.[11] Examination of the jugular venous pulsation may reveal a prominent a wave. This finding reflects reduced right ventricular compliance that can occur from impaired relaxation of the hypertrophied interventricular septum.[11]

At a minimum, an echocardiogram and an electrocardiogram should be obtained if HCM is suspected; however, other diagnostic studies, including magnetic resonance imaging, coronary catheterization and angiography, electrophysiologic evaluation, and genetic testing, may be useful for risk stratification or to clarify the diagnosis.

Transthoracic echocardiography and Doppler examination are crucial in the diagnosis of HCM, as well as the screening of family members of patients with known disease. These studies can delineate cardiac morphology, including the degree and distribution of LVH, presence of mitral valve abnormalities, and size estimation of the left atrium.[5] Systolic and diastolic function can be quantified, and the severity and location of LVOT obstruction can be determined.[5] Transesophageal Doppler echocardiography is rarely necessary for diagnosis but is used routinely for intraoperative monitoring and assessment of surgical outcome.[5]

The majority of patients with HCM manifest some abnormality on their electrocardiograms; however, up to 25% of individuals can have completely normal studies, usually in the setting of mild to moderate localized LVH.[5,12] Certain patients have even been found to have abnormal electrocardiograms without echocardiographic evidence of LVH.[5] For individuals with abnormalities, those most commonly reported occur in the ST segment and T wave and are typically of a nonspecific nature.[12,13] Changes consistent with LVH may be seen, with abnormally high R and S wave voltage (≥ 25 mm) manifested in the precordial leads.[12] Pronounced Q waves have been documented in up to 50% of patients, often in the inferior and precordial leads.[13] These Q waves may reflect septal hypertrophy and an imbalance between the relative contributions of the right and left ventricles to the electrical forces of depolarization;[5] however, they do not directly correlate to the degree of septal hypertrophy[13] and may even be mistaken for Q waves associated with myocardial infarction.[5] The apical variant of HCM often is accompanied by giant negative T waves in the precordial leads, referred to as the "giant T-negativity syndrome."[5] Other changes that can be demonstrated include left axis deviation, abnormal P waves consistent with left atrial enlargement, atrioventricular and interventricular conduction delay, and a prolonged Q–Tc interval.[14]

A variety of disturbances of cardiac rhythm have been documented on ambulatory Holter monitoring and may pose a threat of sudden death.[1,14–16] Ventricular arrhythmias can occur in more than 75% of HCM patients, with 25% demonstrating runs of ventricular tachycardia; however, sustained ventricular tachycardia is uncommon.[16] The presence of ventricular tachycardia is considered a marker for subsequent sudden death, but its predictive value in this respect remains limited.[15] Supraventricular arrhythmias are present in up to half of patients with HCM.[16] The most common of these, atrial fibrillation, may occur in up to 30% of patients and is more common in adults than in children.[15]

Chest radiographs may be normal or show enlargement of the cardiac silhouette, especially the area pertaining to the left ventricle.[13] Mitral valve regurgitation may produce enlargement of the left atrial shadow, and pulmonary vasculature markings may be increased[5] as a result of retrograde extension of increased left ventricular filling pressures. On rare occasion, a prominent bulge may be discernible between the left atrial and left ventricular shadows as a consequence of anteroseptal hypertrophy.[5]

Natural History

The natural history of HCM is benign in the majority of patients, and the annual mortality rate varies depending upon the population under study, for example, as high as 3 to 6% in referral centers.[1,10,11,15] However, more recent reports from population-based studies indicate that the annual mortality rate is likely closer to 1%,[1,6,10,15] similar to survival of the general population.[1,10]

Disease progression varies substantially and may be age related. Rapid progression of LVH has been documented in adolescents, but hypertrophy is usually stable in adults and rarely (if ever) progresses.[1,5] Interestingly, adult patients frequently develop worsening left ventricular outflow obstruction over time even though ventricular morphology changes minimally. As many as 15% of adult patients, however, will develop thinning of the ventricular wall and dilation of the left ventricular cavity, with systolic failure in the end stage of the disease.[6,15] The clinical progression does not necessarily correlate with these changes in the myocardial morphology, and substantial symptomatic progression can occur with age.[10,15,17] One report estimated that 23% of patients had some degree of deterioration in their clinical course, and that another 5% developed congestive heart failure, over a time course of many years.[17] Complications, including arrhythmias, stroke, syncope, myocardial infarction, systemic embolization, and cardiac arrest requiring internal defibrillator placement, have occurred in more than 75% of patients in certain studies.[10]

Sudden Death

The most serious complication of HCM is sudden death.[6,10,15,17] Indeed, sudden death may be the only presenting feature in an otherwise asymptomatic and healthy individual.[1,10,17] Sudden death rarely occurs in the first 10 years of life and is most commonly encountered in adolescents and young adults although the age range is wide (12 to 35 years).[1,5,6] Among young competitive athletes, HCM is the most common cause of sudden death, identi-fied as the etiology in 36% of cases, and occurs just after vigorous physical exertion.[1]

Debate still exists regarding the risk factors associated with sudden death, but the greatest risk is seen in patients with the following characteristics: young age, family history of sudden death (two or more sudden deaths in young family members), previous cardiac arrest, documented sustained ventricular tachycardia or prolonged episodes of nonsustained ventricular tachycardia (more than 5 episodes or a run of 10 or more beats) by Holter monitor, high-risk genetic mutation, recurrent syncope, and massive LVH ($\geq$ 35 mm thickness) in the presence of other risk factors.[6] When the risk of sudden death is determined to be substantial by the presence of one or more of these factors, prophylactic therapy with an implantable cardioverter defibrillator is warranted.[1,6]

Treatment Alternatives

Management of patients with HCM depends upon the severity of symptoms, the presence or absence of LVOT obstruction and pressure gradients, and the risk of sudden death. For the purpose of discussion, it is common to cluster patients with LVOT obstruction in a subcategory of HCM known as HOCM. The diverse nature of the clinical and underlying genetic and pathophysiologic mechanisms for the entire spectrum of HCM makes it difficult to devise precise guidelines for therapy, and treatment must be individualized.

Asymptomatic

Therapies for asymptomatic patients are aimed at preventing sudden death, but these measures can have application in symptomatic patients as well. Participation in competitive sports and intense physical activity are discouraged in HCM patients,[1] especially when high-risk clinical features are present.

High-risk patients are also considered for antiarrhythmic medication and/or an implantable cardioverter defibrillator;[1,6] administration of other medications (β-blockers or calcium channel blockers) to reduce risk is no longer advised.[1,6,18] Long-term amiodarone therapy may be beneficial in preventing sudden death, but empiric use of the drug is associated with a number of fatal events, mainly in patients displaying ventricular tachycardia;[19] some believe that amiodarone increases risk of postoperative complications in patients undergoing septal myectomy,[20] but this has not been our experience.

An increasing number of patients are receiving implantable cardioverter-defibrillators.[21] With current technology, complications of implantation and device failures are uncommon,[22] and indications for device implantation have become more liberal. Certainly, patients with HCM and a strong family history of sudden death should be considered for defibrillators.[21]

Mild to Moderate Symptoms

The presence of mild to moderate symptoms warrants medical therapy, and standard treatment includes either a β-blocker or calcium channel blocker (verapamil) although no general consensus exists as to which one should be used first.[1,6] Combination therapy is used often, but little evidence is available to demonstrate effectiveness.[6] Some patients who fail β-blocker therapy get significant relief changing therapies to verapamil.[1,5,23] Disopyramide is preferred by some institutions to verapamil, specifically in patients with LVOT obstruction;[23] however, initial clinical and hemodynamic benefits of this drug diminish over time.[5,23]

The benefit of β-blockers on dyspnea, angina, and reduced exercise tolerance appears to be related to negative inotropic effect and prolongation of left ventricular filling.[24] Medical therapy can reduce LVOT gradients in patients with HOCM, but this effect often diminishes with time. Further, improvement in symptoms is observed in only a third to two-thirds of patients, and, indeed, some studies have failed to show any appreciable improvement in exercise capacity with medical treatment.[23,25]

Most investigations of calcium channel blockers have focused on verapamil, but nifedipine and diltiazem have been used to treat HCM. Verapamil appears to produce its effects by increasing diastolic filling through a combination of improved myocardial relaxation, reduced asynchronous regional diastolic motion, and improved regional myocardial blood flow.[26,27] In HOCM patients, verapamil, like β-blockers, may reduce LVOT gradients during exercise, and one study suggests superiority of verapamil over propranolol for relief of symptoms, improved exercise tolerance, and improved hemodynamic indices in these patients.[25] However, in the presence of a substantial gradient or markedly elevated pulmonary pressures, verapamil has resulted in serious complications from its vasodilatory effects, including hypotension, pulmonary edema, and sudden death.[1,5,28]

Severe or Refractory Symptoms

When drug therapy fails to control symptoms, or when side effects further interfere with lifestyle, subsequent treatment depends upon the presence or absence of LVOT gradients. Those patients who develop end-stage systolic heart failure should be transitioned to the standard congestive heart failure regimens,[6] and a few will be candidates for cardiac transplantation.[29] Patients with the obstructive form of hypertrophic cardiomyopathy who progress to this stage have a wider variety of treatment options available to them, including, in addition to septal myectomy, permanent dual-chamber pacing and alcohol septal ablation.

Surgical Alternatives

Cleland described the first procedure for relief of left ventricular outflow obstruction in patients with HOCM 40 years ago.[30] Since that time, several different surgical approaches have been described (Table 24-1). Today, the most commonly employed technique is the transaortic septal myectomy (Morrow procedure), in which a portion of the basal interventricular septum is excised following exposure through an aortotomy. Transatrial (left atrium) or transventricular (left or right ventricle) approaches have been used and may be helpful in special circumstances; however, the transaortic approach is safe, effective, and highly reproducible.[31,32] Other procedures such as mitral valve replacement or insertion of left ventricular apicoaortic conduits are rarely necessary.

Surgical Technique

The surgical technique for transaortic left ventricular septal myectomy at the Mayo Clinic includes standard cardiopulmonary bypass at normothermia. Myocardial protection is achieved by antegrade cold-blood potassium cardioplegia, and the initial volume for most patients is 1,000 cc to insure adequate arrest and cooling of the hypertrophied ventricle. A repeat infusion of 400 cc of cardioplegia is given after 20 min if the period of aortic occlusion extends beyond this interval. Transesophageal echocardiography is employed in all patients, and special attention is given to the degree of systolic anterior motion of the anterior leaflet of the mitral valve, the degree of mitral valve regurgitation, the thickness of the subaortic septum, and the point of apposition of the anterior mitral valve leaflet with the septum.

Prior to instituting cardiopulmonary bypass, it is important to directly measure LVOT gradient, which is best accomplished with simultaneous insertion of needles into the aorta and left ventricle. Accurate documentation

TABLE 24-1. Surgical Techniques for Outflow Obstruction in HCM

Surgeon	Year	Procedure
Cleland	1956	Transaortic ventriculomyotomy
Morrow	1961	Transaortic ventriculomyectomy
Kirklin	1961	Transaortic transapical myectomy
Lillihei	1963	Transatrial myectomy, detachment MV
Dobell	1964	Transatrial myectomy, MV repair
Johnson	1964	Transatrial myectomy, MV replacement
Julian	1965	Transapical myectomy
Stinson	1968	Cardiac transplantation
Cooley	1970	MV replacement without myectomy
Rastan Konno	1975	Aortoventriculoplasty
Bernhard Cooley	1975	Apicoaortic conduit
Vouhe	1984	Trans-RV myectomy
Alvarez-Diaz	1984	Trans-RV myectomy, patch
Schulte	1987	Extended myectomy

MV = mitral valve; RV = right ventricle.

of the outflow gradient before myectomy is critically important so that there is a value to compare against when postmyectomy pressures are measured (Figure 24-2). If conditions of general anesthesia reduce the left ventricular outflow gradient to a value of less than 30 mm Hg, we stimulate the ventricle by incremental doses of isoproterenol (Figure 24-3), or by inducing premature ventricular contractions to obtain postextrasystolic potentiation of left ventricular pressure.

Following induced asystole with cold cardioplegia, the septum is exposed through a low transverse aortotomy that is extended into the noncoronary aortic sinus; the aortic valve cusps are gently retracted to expose the subaortic area. Visualization of the hypertrophied septum is facilitated by two maneuvers. The first and most important technique is to have the first assistant displace the left ventricle posteriorly, using a sponge in a forceps or similar instrument. This rotates the septum into view through the aortic valve. Second, it may be helpful to grasp and pull down on the septal endocardium with a hook to deliver the septum into the aortic outflow area as much as possible.

Resection begins with an upward incision in the septum (using a No. 10 blade) beginning a few millimeters to the right of the nadir of the right aortic sinus. As the blade reaches the necessary depth, it is turned leftward, and muscle is excised over to the anterior mitral valve leaflet. Rarely is removal of this initial segment of septum sufficient. The area of excision should be deepened and lengthened toward the apex to ensure that all obstructing muscle has been removed. Often, septal excision is extended to the level of the heads of the papillary muscles, and, in this region, removal of thick trabeculations may further relieve outflow obstruction.[32] Adequacy of septal excision is gauged visually and with palpation. The most common reason for residual gradients is inadequate length of septectomy, and visualization of the distal extent

of excision requires wide excision of the immediate subaortic area.

Upon completion of myectomy, the ventricle is irrigated with cold saline solution to remove any particulate debris, and the surgeon should inspect the aortic valve to be certain there has been no injury to the cusps. The aortotomy is then closed with two layers of 4–0 polypropylene suture, and the aortic clamp is slowly released as air is aspirated through an aortic tack vent. During reperfusion, it is important to defibrillate the heart as early as possible and to maintain perfusion pressure at or above 80 mm Hg. After separating the patient from cardiopulmonary bypass, pressure measurements are then repeated in the left ventricle and ascending aorta to ensure the adequacy of resection. Postbypass transesophageal echocardiography should include assessment of mitral function and aortic valve function; as many as one-third of patients will have some degree of new aortic regurgitation after myectomy.[33] Doppler echocardiography is helpful also in quantifying and localizing any residual left ventricular outflow gradient and excluding the presence of a ventricular septal defect.

Following adequate myectomy, most patients will have no residual gradient and little or no residual systolic anterior motion. We would resume bypass and remove additional muscle if the measured gradient is more than 15 to 20 mm Hg, especially if this increases after a premature ventricular contraction or after stimulation with isoproterenol.

Surgical Results

The major indications for operation in patients with HOCM are persistent symptoms and a left ventricular outflow gradient despite optimal medical therapy, intolerance to medical regimens, and persistence of high (≥ 50 mm Hg) gradients in patients with risk factors for

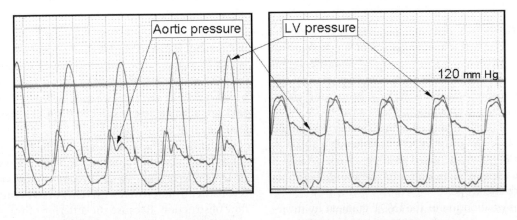

Premyectomy   **Postmyectomy**

FIGURE 24-2. Left ventricular outflow gradient measured intraoperatively both before (*left panel*) and after (*right panel*) septal myectomy. Both aortic and left ventricular (LV) pressures are simultaneously depicted. The reference line lies at 120 mm Hg of pressure. Successful myectomy abolishes the outflow gradient.

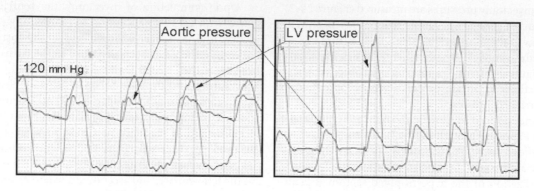

A

Premyectomy

Rest   Isuprel

B

Postmyectomy

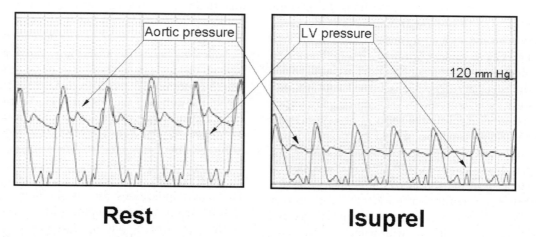

Rest   Isuprel

FIGURE 24-3. Effect of isoproterenol (Isuprel) upon left ventricular outflow gradient measured intraoperatively both *A,* pre- and *B,* post myectomy. Both aortic and left ventricular (LV) pressures are simultaneously depicted. The reference line lies at 120 mm Hg of pressure. Note the substantial gradient increase produced by isoproterenol prior to septal myectomy, which is abolished following a successful procedure.

sudden death such as documented ventricular arrhythmias, syncope, or strong family history of sudden cardiac death and HCM.[1,5,31,34] Some authors advocate septal myectomy for children with a gradient higher than 100 mm Hg because of the poor natural history of HCM when it is detected in childhood.[34]

Operative mortality rates of approximately 3% can be achieved and, in the most experienced hands, can be as low as 1 to 2%.[5,31,35,36] Increased postoperative mortality is associated in some studies with combined surgical procedures and advanced age.[31,35,36]

Reduction or abolition of the LVOT gradient by myectomy is achieved in more than 90% of patients,[31,35–37] and mitral valve regurgitation is eliminated or greatly improved in as many as 75% of patients.[31,37] Long-term improvement in symptoms and exercise capacity 5 years or more from surgery has been seen in more than 70% of patients,[31,35,36] with some centers reporting rates as high as 90%.[31] Surgery

has shown even more benefit than medication in improving exercise tolerance in HOCM patients.[25] However, the effect of surgery on overall survival in these patients remains unclear.[34,35] Procedure-related complications can occur, including ventricular septal defects, cardiac perforation, and complete heart block,[31,32] but in experienced centers, these are uncommon.[31]

As stated previously, mitral valve regurgitation caused by systolic anterior motion is common in patients referred for septal myectomy, and valve leakage is consistently improved with relief of left ventricular outflow obstruction. Because the anterior mitral valve leaflet participates in LVOT obstruction, some surgeons advocate valve replacement as primary surgical treatment for HOCM. We believe, as Roberts pointed out almost 30 years ago, that because of the liabilities of prosthetic valves, mitral replacement should be used rarely.[38] There may be some patients who have intrinsic mitral valve disease and HOCM who would benefit from replacement, but for simple problems such as associated ruptured chordae tendineae, we favor septal myectomy combined with mitral valve repair.[39]

Experience at the Mayo Clinic

Since 1959, more than 600 patients have had septal myectomy for HOCM at the Mayo Clinic. McCully and colleagues[36] recently reviewed the contemporary surgical experience, focusing on 65 patients, aged 20 to 70 years, who underwent operation between 1986 and 1992. Preoperatively, all but one were symptomatic, and 95% had New York Heart Association (NYHA) functional class III or IV disability. Preoperative mean peak resting LVOT gradient was 66 mm Hg (highest was 180 mm Hg) while provoked LVOT gradient was 89 mm Hg (highest was 196 mm Hg).

Septal myectomy alone was performed in 45 patients (69%) while the remaining patients underwent myectomy plus additional procedures, including mitral valve repair or replacement (7 patients), coronary artery bypass grafting (4 patients), aortic valve repair or replacement (4 patients), right ventricular myectomy (1 patient), resection of left atrial myxoma (1 patient), anomalous papillary muscle (1 patient) or tricuspid valve papilloma (1 patient), and implantation of cardioverter-defibrillator (1 patient). Emergency procedures were performed in three patients who had pulmonary edema caused by HOCM and flail mitral valve leaflets.

Initial septal resection was successful in 95%, while three patients required additional septal resection when intraoperative pressure measurements showed a residual LVOT gradient following initial resection. In this series, there were no perioperative deaths in patients undergoing isolated septal myectomy.

Clinically significant (> 50%) symptomatic improvement was reported by 90% of patients, and almost half (47%) felt their symptoms had completely resolved. Symptom-specific improvement (Figure 24-4), defined as a perceived change from moderate or severe preoperative symptoms to mild or no symptoms postoperatively, was noted in 67% of patients with dyspnea and 90% of patients with angina. Those experiencing near-syncope and syncope preoperatively had complete relief of these symptoms in 67% and 100% of cases, respectively. NYHA functional class improved within the first postoperative year in 88% of patients, with 89% of early survivors occupying class I or II.

On subsequent follow-up, 5-year survival was 92%, and the one death beyond the postoperative period was a result of pulmonary embolus 3 years after myectomy while receiving chronic hemodialysis unrelated to the patient's cardiac disease. Reoperation-free survival at 5 years was 80%; one patient underwent mitral valve replacement 6 years after myectomy, and another had aortic valve replacement 4 years after myectomy for severe valve regurgitation.

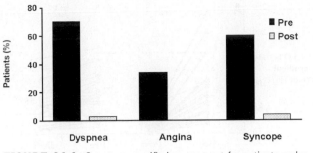

FIGURE 24-4. Symptom-specific improvement for patients undergoing septal myectomy for hypertrophic obstructive subaortic stenosis. Myectomy profoundly reduces the percentage of patients reporting moderate or severe dyspnea, angina, and syncope.

Nonsurgical Alternatives

Dual-Chamber Pacing

The mechanism by which dual-chamber (DDD) pacing reduces LVOT gradients is uncertain; pacing causes uncoordinated septal contraction and paradoxical septal motion,[40,41] which may decrease projection of the basal septum into the LVOT during systole. Other alterations in myocardial physiology that may play a role in this improvement include late activation of the basal septum, decreased left ventricular contractility, asynchronous ventricular contraction and relaxation, or long-term remodeling and thinning of the ventricular wall.[40,42]

Initial studies of dual-chamber pacing in HOCM showed a 50% reduction in gradients and improvement of symptoms in almost 90% of patients, plus a significant beneficial effect on exercise capacity.[40] However, more recent and carefully controlled investigations have found less favorable responses.[43] The average gradient reduction during pacing is only 25%, and this varies substantially among patients.[43] Symptomatic improvement is seen in 30 to 80% of patients,[43] but the degree of symptomatic benefit does not necessarily correlate to the amount of gradient reduction. Early improvement in symptoms may not persist, particularly in young patients with very active lifestyles.[43] Some studies of exercise capacity show little difference between patients with or without pacing, suggesting that short-term symptomatic improvement may be a placebo effect.[43] At this time, long-term benefits of pacing remain unknown.[5]

A recent study from the Mayo Clinic suggests that surgery is superior to pacing in both short-term objective and subjective parameters;[44] among patients treated with DDD pacing, 26% had almost complete relief of left ventricular outflow obstruction, and 47% had improvement in their symptoms. In contrast, 90% or more of surgical patients experienced these benefits (Figures 24-5 and 24-6). Exercise performance, both duration and maximal oxygen consumption, was significantly better in surgical patients compared to those having pacing (Figures 24-7 and 24-8). In current practice, implantation of a dual-

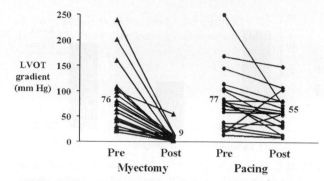

FIGURE 24-5. Change in Doppler-derived resting left ventricular outflow gradient (LVOT) following septal myectomy and dual-chamber ventricular pacing. Both groups experience a substantial reduction in LVOT, but gradient reduction is significantly greater in those undergoing myectomy ($p = .03$). Numbers given represent the group average at each time point. Reproduced with permission from Ommen SR et al[44] and Elsevier Science Inc.

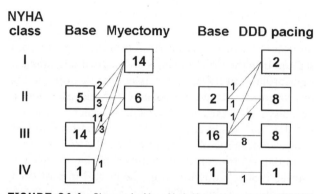

FIGURE 24-6. Change in New York Heart Association (NYHA) classification from baseline to follow-up for patients undergoing septal myectomy and dual-chamber (DDD) ventricular pacing. Both groups experience a significant improvement in their NYHA classification, but the improvement is significantly greater for those undergoing myectomy ($p = .0006$). Reproduced with permission from Ommen SR et al[44] and Elsevier Science Inc.

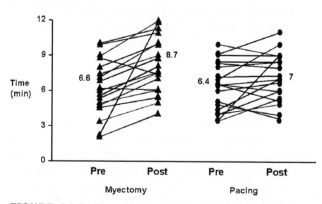

FIGURE 24-7. Change in treadmill exercise duration following septal myectomy and dual-chamber ventricular pacing. Myectomy patients experience a significant improvement in exercise duration ($p = .0003$) not observed in pacing patients ($p = NS$). The degree of improvement is significantly greater for myectomy patients ($p = .05$). Numbers given represent group averages at each time point.

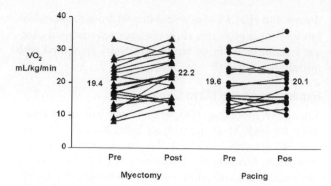

FIGURE 24-8. Change in peak oxygen consumption (VO$_2$) during exercise following septal myectomy and dual-chamber ventricular pacing. Myectomy patients experience a significant improvement in VO$_2$ ($p < .005$) not observed in pacing patients ($p = NS$). The degree of improvement is significantly greater for myectomy patients ($p = .04$). Numbers given represent group averages at each time point.

chamber pacemaker is used for patients who are poor surgical candidates or those who refuse myectomy.[44]

Septal Alcohol Ablation

Percutaneous transluminal septal myocardial ablation (PTSMA) was performed first by Sigwart; approximately 900 cases have been performed worldwide.[45,46] In experienced centers, PTSMA produces satisfactory reduction in the LVOT gradient in up to 90% of patients, and most patients report improvement in symptoms.[45–49] A recent report combining the experience of the Mayo Clinic and Baylor College of Medicine, Houston, TX, compared PTSMA to surgical myectomy. In this nonrandomized study, patients had similar hemodynamic and symptomatic improvements at 1 year, suggesting PTSMA may be a viable alternative to surgery.[50] It is important to note that the morbidity related to heart block and need for permanent pacing was higher in patients having alcohol septal ablation (22% vs 2%). Other series have shown heart block requiring permanent pacemaker placement as the most common complication following PTSMA, with trifascicular block seen in as many as 60% and bundle branch blocks (mostly right-sided) occurring in up to 50% of cases.[50] Other reported complications of PTSMA are myocardial ischemia[48] and ventricular free-wall infarction, ventricular septal defect, cerebral embolism, and dissection of the left anterior descending artery.[45]

Conclusion

The clinical features and morphologic subtypes of hypertrophic cardiomyopathy vary widely. For patients with associated left ventricular outflow obstruction, surgical myectomy is highly effective in relieving gradients and symptoms of angina, dyspnea, and syncope. The procedure can be performed in patients < 65 years of age with low operative risk (1%), and with current methods, complications of heart block and iatrogenic ventricular septal defect are rare. Operation should be considered for young patients who remain symptomatic despite medical therapy and for patients who are intolerant of medications. An important subgroup are those patients with severe LVOT obstruction and predominant septal hypertrophy; these patients have little diastolic dysfunction after successful myectomy, and operation may be the preferred first-line treatment.

It should be emphasized that relief of left ventricular outflow obstruction, no matter how complete, does not prevent sudden death in patients at high risk for this complication. For these patients, we advise myectomy and implantation of a transvenous cardioverter-defibrillator.

References

1. Maron BJ. Hypertrophic cardiomyopathy. Lancet 1997;350: 127–33.
2. McKenna WJ, Spirito P, Desnos M, et al. Experience from clinical genetics in hypertrophic cardiomyopathy: proposal for new diagnostic criteria in adult members of affected families. Heart 1997;77:130–2.
3. Mohiddin S, Fananapazir L. Advances in understanding hypertrophic cardiomyopathy. Hosp Prac 2001;36:23–5, 29–30, 33–6.
4. Fananapazir L. Advances in molecular genetics and management of hypertrophic cardiomyopathy. JAMA 1999; 281:1746–52.
5. Wigle ED, Rakowski H, Kimball BP, et al. Hypertrophic cardiomyopathy: clinical spectrum and treatment. Circulation 1995;92:1680–92.
6. Spirito P, Seidman CE, McKenna WJ, et al. The management of hypertrophic cardiomyopathy. N Engl J Med 1997;336:775–85.
7. Criley JM. Unobstructed thinking (and terminology) is called for in the understanding and management of hypertrophic cardiomyopathy. J Am Coll Cardiol 1997; 29:741–3.
8. Firoozi S, Sharma S, McKenna WJ. The role of exercise testing in the evaluation of hypertrophic cardiomyopathy. Curr Card Rep 2001;3:152–9.
9. Codd MB, Sugrue DD, Gersh BJ, et al. Epidemiology of idiopathic dilated and hypertrophic cardiomyopathy. A population-based study in Olmsted County, Minnesota, 1975–1984. Circulation 1989;80:564–72.
10. Cannan CR, Reeder GS, Bailey KR, et al. Natural history of hypertrophic cardiomyopathy. A population-based study, 1976 through 1990. Circulation 1995;92:2488–95.
11. Wynne J, Braunwald E. The cardiomyopathies and myocarditides. In: Braunwald E, Zipes D, Libby P, editors. Heart disease: a textbook of cardiovascular medicine. Philadelphia (PA): WB Saunders; 2001. p. 1751–806.
12. Maron BJ, Mathenge R, Casey SA, et al. Clinical profile of hypertrophic cardiomyopathy identified de novo in rural communities. J Am Coll Cardiol 1999;33:1590–5.
13. Maron BJ. Hypertrophic cardiomyopathy. Curr Probl Cardiol 1993;18:639–704.
14. Pelliccia F, Cianfrocca C, Cristofani R, et al. Electrocardiographic findings in patients with hypertrophic cardiomyopathy. Relation to presenting features and prognosis. J Electrocardiol 1990;23:213–22.
15. McKenna WJ, Behr ER. Hypertrophic cardiomyopathy: management, risk stratification, and prevention of sudden death. Heart 2002;87:169–76.
16. Stewart JT, McKenna WJ. Management of arrhythmias in hypertrophic cardiomyopathy. Cardiovasc Drugs Ther 1994;8:95–99.
17. Ishiwata S, Nishiyama S, Nakanishi S, et al. Natural history of 82 patients with hypertrophic cardiomyopathy: follow-up for over ten years [Japanese]. J Cardiol 1991; 21:61–73.
18. Louie EK, Edwards LC III. Hypertrophic cardiomyopathy. Prog Cardiovasc Dis 1994;36:275–308.
19. Fananapazir L, Leon MB, Bonow RO, et al. Sudden death during empiric amiodarone therapy in symptomatic hypertrophic cardiomyopathy. Am J Cardiol 1991;67: 169–74.
20. Kupferschmid JP, Rosengart TK, McIntosh CL, et al. Amiodarone-induced complications after cardiac operation for obstructive hypertrophic cardiomyopathy. Ann Thorac Surg 1989;48:359–64.
21. Fananapazir L, McAreavey D. Hypertrophic cardiomyopathy: evaluation and treatment of patients at high risk for sudden death. Pacing Clin Electrophysiol 1997;20: 478–501.
22. Nunain SO, Roelke M, Trouton T, et al. Limitations and late complications of third-generation automatic cardioverter-defibrillators. Circulation 1995;91:2204–13.
23. Gilligan DM, Chan WL, Joshi J, et al. A double-blind, placebo-controlled crossover trial of nadolol and verapamil in mild and moderately symptomatic hypertrophic cardiomyopathy. J Am Coll Cardiol 1993;21:1672–9.
24. Thompson DS, Naqvi N, Juul SM, et al. Effects of propranolol on myocardial oxygen consumption, substrate extraction, and hemodynamics in hypertrophic obstructive cardiomyopathy. Br Heart J 1980;44:488–98.
25. Losse B, Loogen F, Schulte HD. Hemodynamic long-term results after medical and surgical therapy of hypertrophic cardiomyopathies. Z Kardiol 1987;76 Suppl 3:119–30.
26. Anderson DM, Raff GL, Ports TA, et al. Hypertrophic obstructive cardiomyopathy. Effects of acute and chronic verapamil treatment on left ventricular systolic and diastolic function. Br Heart J 1984;51:523–9.
27. Bonow RO, Dilsizian V, Rosing DR, et al. Verapamil-induced improvement in left ventricular diastolic filling and increased exercise tolerance in patients with hypertrophic cardiomyopathy: short- and long-term effects. Circulation 1985;72:853–64.
28. Epstein SE, Rosing DR. Verapamil: its potential for causing serious complications in patients with hypertrophic cardiomyopathy. Circulation 1981;64:437–41.
29. Shirani J, Maron BJ, Cannon RO III, et al. Clinicopathologic features of hypertrophic cardiomyopathy managed by cardiac transplantation. Am J Cardiol 1993;72:434–40.
30. Cleland WP. The surgical management of obstructive cardiomyopathy. J Cardiovasc Surg (Torino) 1963;4:489–91.
31. Schulte HD, Bircks W, Losse B. Techniques and complications of transaortic subvalvular myectomy in patients

with hypertrophic obstructive cardiomyopathy (HOCM). Z Kardiol 1987;76 Suppl 3:145–51.

32. Mohr R, Schaff HV, Danielson GK, et al. The outcome of surgical treatment of hypertrophic obstructive cardiomyopathy: experience over 15 years. J Thorac Cardiovasc Surg 1989;97:666–74.

33. Sasson Z, Prieur T, Skrobik Y, et al. Aortic regurgitation: a common complication after surgery for hypertrophic obstructive cardiomyopathy. J Am Coll Cardiol 1989; 13:63–7.

34. Fiddler GI, Tajik AJ, Weidman W, et al. Idiopathic hypertrophic subaortic stenosis in the young. Am J Cardiol 1978;42:793–9.

35. Robbins RC, Stinson EB. Long-term results of left ventricular myotomy and myectomy for obstructive hypertrophic cardiomyopathy. J Thorac Cardiovasc Surg 1996; 111:586–94.

36. McCully RB, Nishimura RA, Tajik AJ, et al. Extent of clinical improvement after surgical treatment of hypertrophic obstructive cardiomyopathy. Circulation 1996; 94:467–71.

37. Brunner-La Schonbeck MH, Rocca HP, Vogt PR, et al. Long-term follow-up in hypertrophic obstructive cardiomyopathy after septal myectomy. Ann Thorac Surg 1998;65:1207–14.

38. Roberts WC. Operative treatment of hypertrophic obstructive cardiomyopathy. The case against mitral valve replacement. Am J Cardiol 1973;32:377–81.

39. Zhu WX, Oh JK, Kopecky SL, et al. Mitral regurgitation due to ruptured chordae tendineae in patients with hypertrophic obstructive cardiomyopathy. J Am Coll Cardiol 1992;20:242–7.

40. Fananapazir L, Epstein ND, Curiel RV, et al. Long-term results of dual-chamber (DDD) pacing in obstructive hypertrophic cardiomyopathy. Evidence for progressive symptomatic and hemodynamic improvement and reduction of left ventricular hypertrophy. Circulation 1994;90:2731–42.

41. Erwin JP III, Nishimura RA, Lloyd MA, et al. Dual-chamber pacing for patients with hypertrophic obstructive cardiomyopathy: a clinical perspective in 2000. Mayo Clin Proc 2000;75:173–80.

42. Nishimura RA, Hayes DL, Ilstrup DM, et al. Effect of dual-chamber pacing on systolic and diastolic function in patients with hypertrophic cardiomyopathy. Acute Doppler echocardiographic and catheterization hemodynamic study. J Am Coll Cardiol 1996;27:421–30.

43. Nishimura RA, Trusty JM, Hayes DL, et al. Dual-chamber pacing for hypertrophic cardiomyopathy: a randomized, double-blind, crossover trial. J Am Coll Cardiol 1997; 29:435–41.

44. Ommen SR, Nishimura RA, Squires RW, et al. Comparison of dual-chamber pacing versus septal myectomy for the treatment of patients with hypertrophic obstructive cardiomyopathy: a comparison of objective hemodynamic and exercise end points. J Am Coll Cardiol 1999;34: 191–6.

45. Seggewiss H. Current status of alcohol septal ablation for patients with hypertrophic cardiomyopathy. Curr Cardiol Rep 2001;3:160–6.

46. Sigwart U. Non-surgical myocardial reduction for hypertrophic obstructive cardiomyopathy. Lancet 1995;346: 211–4.

47. Seggewiss H, Gleichmann U, Faber L, et al. Percutaneous transluminal septal myocardial ablation (PTSMA) in hypertrophic obstructive cardiomyopathy: acute results and 3-month follow-up in 25 patients. J Am Coll Cardiol 1998;31:252–8.

48. Ruzyllo W, Chojnowska L, Demkow M, et al. Left ventricular outflow tract gradient decrease with non-surgical myocardial reduction improves exercise capacity in patients with hypertrophic obstructive cardiomyopathy. Eur Heart J 2000;21:770–7.

49. Gietzen FH, Leuner CJ, Raute-Kreinsen U, et al. Acute and long-term results after transcoronary ablation of septal hypertrophy (TASH). Catheter interventional treatment for hypertrophic obstructive cardiomyopathy. Eur Heart J 1999;20:1342–54.

50. Nagueh SF, Ommen SR, Lakkis NM, et al. Comparison of ethanol septal reduction therapy with surgical myectomy for the treatment of hypertrophic obstructive cardiomyopathy. J Am Coll Cardiol 2001;38:1701–6.

CHAPTER 25

MANAGEMENT OF THE SMALL AORTIC ROOT

DAVID C. MCGIFFIN, MD, JAMES K. KIRKLIN, MD

The dilemma of the "small aortic root" in patients undergoing aortic valve replacement has permeated the surgical literature for many years. The crux of the issue is the adequacy of the aortic annulus to accept a valve replacement device that would not be "unacceptably obstructive," implying a resultant reduction in duration of survival and/or exercise capacity. This chapter reviews the anatomy of the "aortic annulus" (an issue of relevance when considering enlargement of the aortic annulus), discusses issues involved in characterizing the small aortic root, and outlines one approach to the small aortic annulus, recognizing that many surgeons have equally justifiable approaches (together with surgical strategies).

Anatomy of the Aortic "Annulus"

There are three important points:

1. There is an anatomic ventriculoaortic junction that is distinct from the hemodynamic ventriculoaortic junction (Figure 25-1) that is defined by the attachment of the leaflets of the aortic valve.

2. The impression that the fibroskeleton of the heart is a well-defined structure of the attachment of all four cardiac valves is erroneous.[1] The fibroskeleton really consists of the fibrous continuity between the aortic and mitral valves, each end being thickened to form the left and right fibrous trigones (Figure 25-2), the right fibrous trigone being continuous with the membranous component of the ventricular septum to form the central fibrous body.

3. Although the term *aortic annulus* is embedded in the surgical lexicon, it is the attachment of the aortic valve leaflets to both the aortic wall and left ventricular muscle that precludes the possibility of a true annular ring structure.

Conditions Associated with a Small Aortic Annulus

The small aortic annulus is most likely to occur in elderly female patients with calcareous aortic stenosis of a trileaflet aortic valve and rheumatic aortic valve disease.

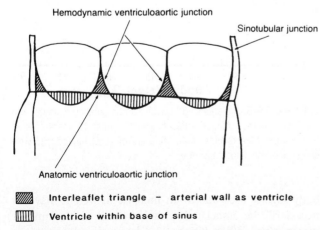

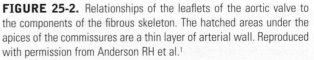

FIGURE 25-1. The anatomic and hemodynamic ventriculoaortic junctions are distinct and the hemodynamic ventriculoaortic function is defined by the attachments of the aortic valve leaflets. Reproduced with permission from Anderson RH et al.[1]

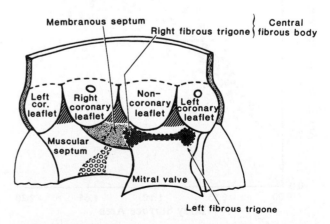

FIGURE 25-2. Relationships of the leaflets of the aortic valve to the components of the fibrous skeleton. The hatched areas under the apices of the commissures are a thin layer of arterial wall. Reproduced with permission from Anderson RH et al.[1]

In patients with congenitally bicuspid aortic valve disease the aortic annulus is frequently larger than normal. It is not uncommon for elderly patients with aortic stenosis to have associated subvalvar stenosis due to asymmetric septal hypertrophy.

Issues Inherent in Surgery Associated with a Small Aortic Root

The Relationship between Body Size and Aortic Valve Dimension

The practice of indexing valve area to body surface area is widely used in the angiographic and echocardiographic assessment of the degree of aortic stenosis to adjust for differences in body size, a technique that is also used for assessing prosthetic valve area. However, the use of body surface area as a means of allowing for difference in body size has been challenged, since the relationship between body surface area and aortic annulus diameter is non-linear (Figure 25-3).[2] Although the relationship between aortic annulus diameter and body height is linear (Figure 25-4), it is the nonlinearity of the relationship between aortic annulus diameter and body weight (Figure 25-5) that is responsible for the nonlinear relationship between aortic annulus diameter and body surface area.[2] The linear relationship between aortic valve annulus and height suggests that during development, growth of the aortic annulus dimension is primarily due to skeletal growth.[2] With body surface areas greater than 1.0 m², the major determinant of body surface area is weight as opposed to height (Figure 25-6); hence, it could be assumed that beyond a body surface area of 1.5 m², increases in

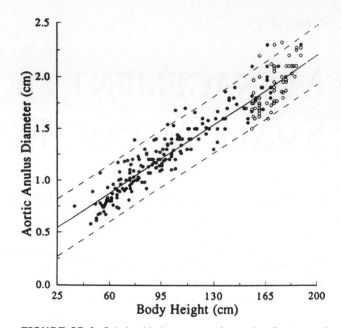

FIGURE 25-4. Relationship between aortic annulus diameter and body height. (• = normal subjects younger than 18 years of age; ○ = normal subjects older than 18 years of age.) Reproduced with permission from Nidorf SM et al.[2]

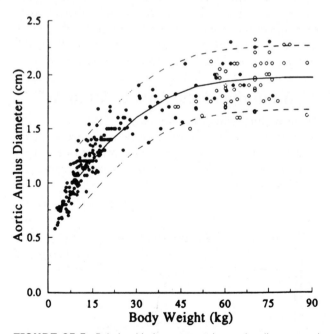

FIGURE 25-5. Relationship between aortic annulus diameter and body weight. (• = normal subjects younger than 18 years of age; ○ = normal subjects older than 18 years of age.) Reproduced with permission from Nidorf SM et al.[2]

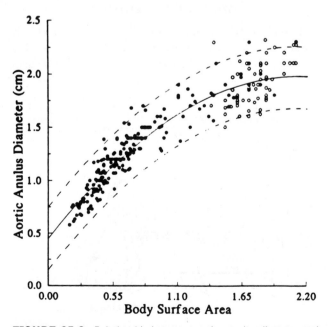

FIGURE 25-3. Relationship between aortic annulus diameter and body surface area. (• = normal subjects younger than 18 years of age; ○ = normal subjects older than 18 years of age.) Reproduced with permission from Nidorf SM et al.[2]

body surface area due to an increase in weight may not necessarily be associated with increased aortic annulus dimensions.[2] When Figure 25-3 is examined, it appears that beyond a body surface area of 1.5 m², the nonlinearity of the relationship may become important. An example of how this relationship might be important is, for

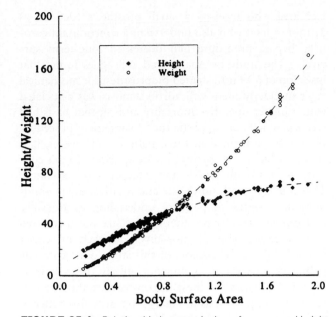

FIGURE 25-6. Relationship between body surface area and height and weight. As body surface area increases beyond 1.0, the major determinant of body surface area is weight rather than height. Reproduced with permission from Nidorf SM et al.[2]

example, in a short, obese patient (with a body surface area of 2.2 m[2]) who has a 21 mm mechanical valve implanted in the aortic position, and about whom there are postoperative concerns about a patient–prosthesis mismatch. If an effective orifice area was determined and then indexed to body surface area, it could be falsely assumed that the prosthesis was too small. This issue may also be of importance in predicting postoperative hemodynamic performance using indexed prosthetic valve area in an individual patient. It should be mentioned that the relationship between aortic valve dimensions measured at autopsy and body surface area is weak, which further suggests that relating valve area to body surface area ("valve area index") is erroneous, particularly in an attempt to predict the adequacy of a prosthetic device in an individual patient given the wide individual variation in adult aortic valve diameters.[3,4]

What Is a Small Aortic Root?

The fundamental problem in the small aortic root is that the size of the device used to replace the aortic valve is inadequate rather than the aortic annulus being too small; consequently, the definition of the small aortic root is rather artificial and should be related to the valve replacement device to be implanted (because the aortic annulus is the size that it needs to be).[5] A small aortic root is implied by the suggestion that a 19 mm valve should not be implanted in a patient with a body surface area of 1.7 m[2], effective orifice area of less than 1.2 cm[2]/m[2], or 1.4 cm[2]/m[2], or where an anticipated orifice area index of a prosthesis is below 0.80 cm[2]/m[2].[5–9] These are but a few

of the many definitions of a small aortic root, most of which embody the prosthetic valve size of controversy, that is, insertion of a 19 mm or 21 mm mechanical or stented bioprosthesis (Figure 25-7).

The crux of the issue is that all mechanical and stented bioprostheses have a smaller effective orifice area than that of a normal human aortic valve, and, as pointed out by Rahimtoola, the relationship between aortic valve area and the mean systolic gradient is exponential.[10] By using as examples several types of noncontemporary mechanical and bioprosthetic valves, it can be demonstrated that these valves are on the transition point of the curve, indicating that small decreases in valve area may result in large increases in gradient (Figure 25-8). More recently, the same exponential relationship between indexed effective orifice area and mean gradient for contemporary aortic bioprostheses was determined by using a pulse duplicator, this relationship being accentuated by increases in stroke volume (Figure 25-9).[11]

Determining Whether an Aortic Root (and the Aortic Prosthesis) Is Too Small

There are a number of ways in which the putative impact of valve replacement in the setting of small aortic root could be determined.

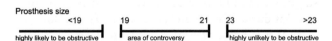

FIGURE 25-7. The definition of the small aortic root is not absolute and involves a size region of controversy, that is, insertion of a mechanical or stented bioprosthesis of size 19 or 21 mm.

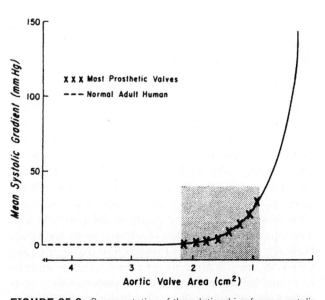

FIGURE 25-8. Representation of the relationship of mean systolic gradient to the aortic valve area, assuming the cardiac output and velocity of flow are constant. Reproduced with permission from Rahimtoola SH.[10]

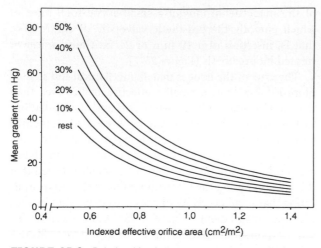

FIGURE 25-9. Relationships between mean transprosthetic pressure gradients and indexed effective orifice areas for aortic bioprostheses studied in vitro in a physiologic pulse duplicator system, assuming a normal cardiac index of 3.0 L/min/m^2 at rest (systolic ejection period 285 ms) and 10 to 50% increases in stroke volume, as may occur during maximal upright exercise. Reproduced with permission from Dumesnil JG et al.[11]

A number of studies attempted to investigate whether insertion of a "small prosthesis" (most studies focused on a 19 mm or 21 mm mechanical valve or stented bioprosthesis) influences short- and long-term *survival*. However, survival is a very insensitive determinant of prosthetic valve performance. Early and late survival after aortic valve replacement is principally determined by the structure and function of the left ventricle and the presence of comorbidity (including coronary artery disease).[12] Given this important caveat, it is not surprising that most studies have not found a relationship between early and late survival and aortic valve prosthesis size.[13–15] The study by Medalion and colleagues, with survival as the end point and using multivariable methods to allow for valve device selection factors (mechanical, stented xenograft, and allograft valves were used) and prevalent risk factors for death, was unable to detect an adverse impact on survival of moderate patient–prosthesis mismatch, and in a few patients, even at a Z-value (number of standard deviations the diameter of the device departed from the mean normal native valve size for a given body surface area) of −4.[16] Despite this finding and the sophistication of the methods, this study should not be regarded as an endorsement of a disregard for the postoperative prosthetic gradient, given the insensitivity of survival as an end point. However, there are studies that did find that aortic valve prosthesis size is a determinant of survival. The study by Kratz and colleagues suggested that patients with a body surface area of greater than 1.9 m^2 who received St. Jude valves sized 19 mm or 21 mm had a greater probability of late sudden death.[17] The study of He and colleagues found that (by multivariable methods) patients with a body sur-

face area who received a small prosthesis (defined as 21 mm or less) who also underwent a concomitant coronary bypass procedure had decreased long-term survival.[18] The study by Adams and colleagues found that insertion of a 19 mm stented bioprosthesis or mechanical valve in elderly men with aortic stenosis was associated with a higher operative mortality and on that basis had recommended that an aortic root enlargement procedure should be performed in these patients.[19] However, it is very possible that these findings are spurious. In this context, the study by Morris and colleagues is germane.[20] They found by both univariate and multivariate methods that, in a series of patients undergoing aortic valve replacement, smaller prosthetic valve size was associated with increased risk of mortality. However, on closer examination, as the authors of this study quite correctly point out, survival was better not only in those patients receiving a 23 mm prosthesis as compared to those receiving a 21 mm prosthesis or smaller, but was also better in patients receiving a prosthesis larger than 25 mm as compared to those patients receiving a 23 mm prosthesis, a situation in which unacceptable postoperative prosthetic valve gradients is highly unlikely to be an issue. Consequently, using survival as an end point for studying the impact of small prosthetic valves does carry the risk of producing spurious findings.

The degree of *regression of left ventricular hypertrophy* may be a more sensitive indication of the adequacy of an implanted aortic valve prosthesis. Preoperative left ventricular hypertrophy is a well-validated risk factor for decreased long-term survival after aortic valve replacement.[12,20] Regression of left ventricular mass has been demonstrated, with most of the regression occurring within the first few weeks or months after surgery.[21–25] It is unproven, although highly likely, that regression of left ventricular hypertrophy after aortic valve replacement is associated with improved long-term survival. It is interesting to note that this regression is incomplete, which could be the result of residual postoperative aortic valve prosthetic gradients, as well as of a hypertrophy process and an accompanying fibrosis that may be immutable.[24,25] Of particular interest is the degree of regression of left ventricular hypertrophy associated with different valve sizes; however, the information is unclear. Some authors found that regression associated with 19 mm and 21 mm stented and mechanical valves was similar to that of patients receiving larger-sized valves.[25,26] On the other hand, the data of Sim and colleagues suggested that the regression of left ventricular hypertrophy was less in patients receiving a 19 mm stented bioprosthesis or mechanical valve when compared with that in patients receiving larger valve sizes.[27] The regression of left ventricular hypertrophy as a means of assessing the adequacy of the implanted aortic valve prosthesis could be useful, but is confounded by other factors, including postoperative medical therapy to promote regression and the presence of concomitant fibrosis and extreme hypertrophy for which substantial regression is unlikely to occur.

Patient–prosthesis mismatch is a useful concept but, in practice, it is often difficult to confirm its presence in an individual patient. Rahimtoola defined patient–prosthesis mismatch as follows: "mismatch can be considered to be present when the effective prosthetic valve area, after insertion into the patient, is less than that of a normal human valve."[10] Applying that definition, patient–prosthesis mismatch should be present after virtually every aortic valve replacement, but when a surgeon is choosing a prosthesis, especially when the size of the prosthesis to be inserted may be inadequate, it is worthwhile conceptualizing the problem as, for example, in aortic stenosis, trading severe native valve disease for mild or moderate aortic stenosis. Rahimtoola indicated that severe aortic stenosis is present with an aortic valve area index of 0.75 cm^2/m^2.[10] The aortic valve area of a 19 mm and a 21 mm St. Jude medical prosthesis is 0.86 cm^2/m^2 and 1.08 cm^2/m^2, respectively.[28] Because of the curvilinear shape of the relationship between a prosthetic valve gradient and valve area, a relatively modest improvement in the aortic valve area produces a proportionately greater reduction in valve gradient. Symptomatic patient–prosthesis mismatch, implying an inadequate-sized prosthesis, is usually very difficult to confirm because postoperative heart failure caused by patient–prosthesis mismatch is difficult to distinguish from other mechanisms such as left ventricular systolic and diastolic dysfunction (although any combination may be present). Therefore, symptomatic patient–prosthesis mismatch is a very unreliable and insensitive indication of implantation of an inadequate-sized aortic prosthesis.

The measurement of *Doppler gradients* across prosthetic valves is a useful means both for determining prosthetic valve function and, potentially, for determining the adequacy of the prosthesis in the small aortic root. At the outset it should be recognized that although there is good relationship between catheter-derived gradients and Doppler-derived gradients across bioprosthetic and some mechanical valves, Doppler gradients across bileaflet valves may be overestimated. These potential inaccuracies occur from (1) early pressure recovery downstream (as a result of decreased flow velocity) and (2) nonuniform local velocities (with a higher velocity between the two leaflets as a result of the partitioning of the blood flow through the valve by the two leaflets).[29,30] Dobutamine-stress Doppler echocardiography has been used to determine flow velocity across the aortic valve prostheses under the circumstances of increased cardiac output to simulate an exercise gradient.[26,31] With dobutamine stress, mean gradients across 19 mm and 21 mm St. Jude medical and Medtronic-Hall prostheses have been reported as between 35 and 40 mm Hg.[29,32] Although these gradients are described as "normal" or "within a clinically acceptable range" (although dopamine stress

gradients appear to be higher than that of exercise gradients), the clinical significance of gradients of this magnitude (particularly in regard to the long-term structure and function of the left ventricle) is unknown. Gradients of this magnitude do reflect the compromise inherent in valve surgery, substituting native valve obstruction with devices that are, despite decades of progress, still obstructive, a feature that is particularly evident in the small aortic root.

Prosthetic Valve Sizing and the Small Aortic Root

It has been pointed out on a number of occasions that the labeling of prosthetic valves (both mechanical and bioprosthetic) and valve sizers does not bear a consistent relationship to the internal diameter of the valve orifice, which is the dimension that is probably the most hemodynamically significant in terms of postoperative gradients.[33,34] For example, the internal diameter of the St. Jude standard mechanical aortic valve, which is labeled as 21 mm, is 16.7 mm, and the internal diameter of the Modified Orifice Hancock II porcine aortic valve, which is labeled as 21 mm, is 18.0 mm.[33] This discrepancy between the labeled size and the true internal diameter is particularly germane to the insertion of mechanical bioprosthetic valves in the small aortic root, where prostheses with a small internal orifice diameter may be unwittingly inserted in the small aortic root, resulting in excessive postoperative prosthetic valve gradients. Furthermore, comparison of the hemodynamic performance between different prosthetic valves when implanted in the small aortic root become difficult to judge.

A Strategy for Dealing with the Small Aortic Root

The fact that surgery involving the small aortic root is still controversial implies incomplete information and the confounding of the issue by a number of imponderables (as previously outlined). However, because prosthetic valves are inherently obstructive and because there is at least some evidence that residual left ventricular outflow tract obstruction may have deleterious long-term consequences, placement of a valve replacement device with the lowest possible gradient seems prudent. Therefore, our strategy is to not use either a 19 mm mechanical or stented bioprosthesis or a 21 mm mechanical or stented bioprosthesis in patients with a body surface area of greater than 1.9 m^2. Because in the light of current information this strategy is discretionary, increasing the aortic root dimension to accommodate a larger prosthesis must be achieved with minimal or no increase in operative mortality. Consequently, this policy is not employed in patients for whom the surgeon determines that the risk of an annulus-enlarging procedure would increase the operative risk more than a minimal degree, and this particularly applies to frail, elderly patients in whom the putative long-term advantages of a lower postoperative prosthetic valve gradient would not be seen.

Surgical Strategies for the Small Aortic Annulus

The fundamental goal of this surgical strategy is avoidance of implantation of a 19 mm or 20 mm mechanical or stented bioprosthesis. The surgical options are as follows: (1) *Mechanical dilatation of the small aortic root.* Although mechanical dilatation of the aortic root with Hegar metal dilators has been described in only one patient, its simplicity does make it appealing and worthy of future investigation.[35] (2) *Implantation of stentless tissue valves.* Allograft aortic valves inserted by either the subcoronary technique or inclusion technique are well known to have a postoperative transvalvar gradient that is lower than that of the mechanical or stented bioprosthetic valve. Similarly, the stented xenograft valves have the same excellent hemodynamics (a superior effective orifice area to that of a stented bioprosthesis) and, because of the flexibility of the valve, may allow for some oversizing and accommodation of an even larger valve in the small aortic root.[36] Furthermore, there is also the suggestion that the postoperative orifice area of the implanted stentless xenograft may increase over the first postoperative year.[37] Stentless xenograft valves do offer the solution to the problem of limited availability of allograft aortic valves. Allograft valves and stentless xenograft valves do appear to offer a very satisfactory option for the small aortic root. (3) *Supra-annular positioning of a valve replacement device.* Because the noncoronary sinus at its nadir may be lower than the nadir of the left and right aortic sinuses, a prosthesis can be implanted in the supra-annular position within the noncoronary sinus. The prosthesis is sutured along the aortic annulus in the left and right coronary sinuses but attached by pledgeted mattress sutures (the pledgets being outside the aorta in the noncoronary sinus). This technique usually allows implantation of a prosthesis that is one valve size larger than the size of the aortic annulus. (4) *Nicks procedure.* The Nicks procedure allows for implantation of a prosthesis that is usually two sizes larger than the measured size of the aortic annulus and is the simplest of the annulus-enlarging procedures to be performed. The Nicks procedure involves extension of the aortotomy into the noncoronary sinus at its nadir, through the aortic annulus and the aortic-mitral septum to the attachment of the left atrium (Figure 25-10A).[38] An autologous pericardial patch is fashioned in a teardrop shape, and this patch must be at least 4 cm in its transverse diameter. The pericardial patch is sutured along the incision through the aortic-mitral septum and aortotomy with continuous 4–0 polypropylene (Figure 25-10B). The prosthesis is sutured to the aortic annulus, and in the region of the patch, the prosthesis is secured with pledgeted mattress sutures passed from the prosthesis outward through the patch and tied over felt pledgets (Figure 25-10C). The remainder of the aortotomy is then closed (Figure 25-10D). The operative risk may be increased (in one series, 3.5% without annulus enlargement to 7.1% with annulus enlargement, $p = .1$; but this may be explained by factors other than the procedure).[39]

Manouguian Procedure

The Manouguian procedure, like the Nicks procedure, is a posterior annular enlargement procedure, but it produces on average a 5.4 mm increase in annular size.[40,41] The aortotomy is carried through the aortic annulus at the commissure between the left and noncoronary cusps (as opposed to the nadir of the noncoronary cusp with the Nicks procedure) (Figure 25-11). The incision is carried through the aortic-mitral septum and on to the anterior leaflet of the mitral valve for up to 2 cm (and this opens the roof of the left atrium). A pericardial patch (or Dacron patch as in Manouguian's original description) is sutured along the mitral valve incision, aortic-mitral septum, and the aortotomy, and, as with the Nicks procedure, the prosthesis is secured to the patch with horizontal mattress sutures. The roof of the left atrium is then repaired

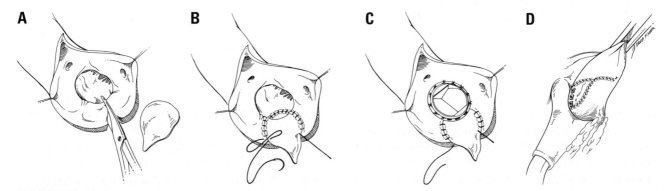

FIGURE 25-10. The Nicks procedure. *A,* Extension of the aortotomy through the noncoronary sinus and nadir of the annulus and aortic and mitral septums. A teardrop-shaped autologous pericardial patch is fashioned. *B,* The pericardial patch is sutured to the aortic-mitral septum and aortotomy with continuous 4–0 polypropylene. *C,* The prosthesis is sutured along the annulus and to the pericardial patch with mattress sutures through the prosthesis and pericardial patch with pledgets on the outside of the pericardial patch. *D,* The remainder of the aortotomy is closed.

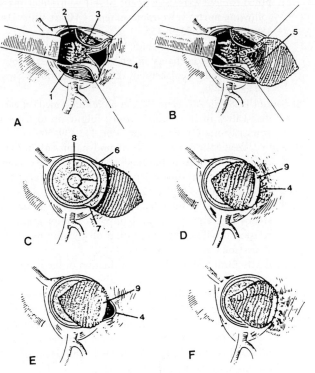

FIGURE 25-11. Manouguian procedure: (1) left coronary cusp; (2) anterior leaflet of the mitral valve; (3) noncoronary cusp; (4) left atrial wall; (5) patch; (6 and 7) enlargement of the aortic valve ring; (8) aortic valve prosthesis; (9) sewing ring of the prosthesis. *A*, The incision; *B*, initial suture of patch; *C*, implantation of prosthesis; *D*, suture of the left atrium and patch to the sewing ring with the same suture in small atriotomies; *E* and *F*, separate suture of larger left atriotomy following larger posterior enlargements. Reproduced with permission from Manouguian S et al.[40]

by suturing the cut edge to the patch or, as is often necessary, with a pericardial patch. The remainder of the aortotomy is then closed. Both the Nicks and the Manouguian procedures can be used to facilitate implantation of a larger-sized allograft aortic valve. The use of the Manouguian procedure should be rare as the other options, such as the Nicks procedure, on insertion of an allograft or stentless xenograft valve, are usually perfectly adequate solutions.

Radical Solutions to the Small Aortic Root

The Konno procedure (aortoventriculoplasty) is mentioned for completeness, but its use in the small aortic root associated with aortic valve disease is exceedingly rare.[42] Its role is really for complex left ventricular tract obstruction. It is an anterior enlargement procedure that involves a longitudinal aortotomy that is carried through the anterior wall of the aortic root and into the ventricular septum and free wall of the right ventricle. The procedure involves patch repair of the interventricular septum

and patch closure of the defect created in the right ventricle. Similarly, left ventricular apicoabdominal aortic conduits have been used but should be a procedure of the last resort, particularly in patients with no other identifiable option in the setting of multiple previous procedures on the aortic root.

Conclusion

There is abundant evidence that the structure and function of the left ventricle after aortic valve replacement is an important determinant of long-term survival and symptoms of heart failure, and, although unproven, the goal of facilitating the regression of left ventricular hypertrophy after aortic valve replacement seems important. The definition of the small aortic root (and the aortic prostheses) and its management seems less important than an overall strategy for aortic valve replacement that embodies the concept that the lowest possible transvalvar prosthetic gradient possible is the most desirable. However, except in unusual situations in which the prosthesis selected (without root enlargement) is likely to reduce late survival or impair desired activity level, the surgical methods used to minimize the transvalvar prosthetic gradient should not significantly increase the operative risk above that of standard aortic valve replacement. There are now available several surgical options that should facilitate this strategy and, it is hoped, make the small aortic root a less controversial issue.

References

1. Anderson RH, Devine WA, et al. The myth of the aortic annulus: the anatomy of the subaortic outflow tract. Ann Thorac Surg 1991;52:640–6.
2. Nidorf SM, Picard MH, Triulzi MO, et al. New perspectives in the assessment of cardiac chamber dimensions during development and adulthood. J Am Coll Cardiol 1992; 19:983–8.
3. Westaby S, Karp RB, Blackstone EH, Bishop SP. Adult human valve dimensions and their surgical significance. Am J Cardiol 1984;53:552–6.
4. Hutchins AM, Araya OA. Measurement of cardiac size, chamber volumes, and valve orifices at autopsy. Johns Hopkins Med J 1973;133:96–106.
5. Chambers J. Echocardiography and the small aortic root. J Heart Valve Dis 1996;5 Suppl III:S264–8.
6. Schaff HV, Borkon AM, Hughes C, et al. Clinical and hemodynamic evaluation of the 19-mm Bjork-Shiley aortic valve prosthesis. Ann Thorac Surg 1981;32:50–7.
7. Davidson WR, Pasquale MJ, Fanelli. A Doppler echocardiographic examination of the normal aortic valve and left ventricular outflow tract. Am J Cardiol 1991;67:547–9.
8. Singh B, Mohan JG. Doppler echocardiographic determination of aortic and pulmonary valve orifice areas in normal adult subjects. Int J Cardiol 1992;37:73–8.
9. Dumesnil JG, Honos GN, Lemieux M, Beauchemin J. Validation and applications of indexed aortic prosthetic

valve areas calculated by Doppler echocardiography. J Am Coll Cardiol 1990;16:637–43.

10. Rahimtoola SH. The problem of valve prosthesis-patient mismatch. Circulation 1978;58:20–4.

11. Dumesnil JG, Yoganathan AP. Valve prosthesis hemodynamics and the problem of high transprosthetic pressure gradients. Eur J Cardiothorac Surg 1992:6 Suppl 1:S34–8.

12. McGiffin DC, O'Brien MF, Galbraith AJ, et al. An analysis of risk factors for death and mode-specific death after aortic valve replacement with allograft, xenograft, and mechanical valves. J Thorac Cardiovasc Surg 1993;106: 895–911.

13. Fiore AC, Swartz M, Grunkemeier G, et al. Valve replacement in the small aortic annulus: prospective randomized trial of St. Jude with Medtronic Hall. Eur J Cardiothorac Surg 1997;11:485–92.

14. Sawant D, Singh AK, Feng WC, et al. Nineteen-millimeter aortic St. Jude medical heart valve prosthesis: up to sixteen years' follow-up. Ann Thorac Surg 1997;63:964–70.

15. Medalion B, Lytle BW, McCarthy PM, et al. Aortic valve replacement for octogenarians: are small valves bad? Ann Thorac Surg 1998;66:699–706.

16. Medalion B, Blackstone EH, Lytle BW, et al. Aortic valve replacement: is valve size important? J Thorac Cardiovasc Surg 2000;119(5):963–74

17. Kratz JM, Sade RM, Crawford FA Jr, et al. The risk of small St. Jude aortic valve prostheses. Ann Thorac Surg 1994; 57:1114–9.

18. He GW, Grunkemeier GL, Gately HL, et al. Up to thirty-year survival after aortic valve replacement in the small aortic root. Ann Thorac Surg 1995;59:1056–62.

19. Adams DH, Chen RH, Kadner A, et al. Impact of small prosthetic valve size on operative mortality in elderly patients after aortic valve replacement for aortic stenosis: does gender matter? J Thorac Cardiovasc Surg 1999; 118:815–22.

20. Morris JJ, Schaff HV, Mullany CJ, et al. Determinants of survival and recovery of left ventricular function after aortic valve replacement. Ann Thorac Surg 1993;56:22–30.

21. St. John Sutton M, Plappert T, Spiegel A, et al. Early postoperative changes in left ventricular chamber size, architecture, and function in aortic stenosis and aortic regurgitation and their relation to intraoperative changes in afterload: a prospective two-dimensional echocardiographic study. Circulation 1987;76:77–89.

22. Henry WL, Bonow RO, Borer JS, et al. Evaluation of aortic valve replacement in patients with valvular aortic stenosis. Circulation 1980;61:814–25.

23. Christakis GT, Joyner CD, Morgan CD, et al. Left ventricular mass regression early after aortic valve replacement. Ann Thorac Surg 1996;62:1084–9.

24. De Paulis R, Sommariva L, De Matteis GM, et al. Extent and pattern of regression of left ventricular hypertrophy in patients with small size Carbomedics aortic valves. J Thorac Cardiovasc Surg 1997;113:901–9.

25. Kahn SS, Siegel RJ, DeRobertis MA, et al. Regression of hypertrophy after Carpentier-Edwards pericardial aortic valve replacement. Ann Thorac Surg 2000;69:531–5.

26. Anderson WA, Ilkowski DA, Eldredge J, et al. The small aortic root and the Medtronic Hall valve: ultrafast computed tomography assessment of left ventricular mass following aortic valve replacement. J Heart Valve Dis 1996;5 Suppl III:S329–35.

27. Sim FKW, Orszulak TA, Schaff HV, Shub C. Influence of prosthesis size on change in left ventricular mass following aortic valve replacement. Eur J Cardiothorac Surg 1994;8:293–7.

28. Sawant D, Singh AK, Feng WC, et al. St. Jude medical cardiac valves in small aortic roots: follow-up to sixteen years. J Thorac Cardiovasc Surg 1997;113:499–509.

29. Kadir I, Izzat MB, Birdi I, et al. Hemodynamics of St. Jude medical prostheses in the small aortic root: in vivo studies using dobutamine Doppler echocardiography. J Heart Valve Dis 1997;6:123–9.

30. Baumgartner H, Schima H, Tulzer G, Kühn P. Effect of stenosis geometry on the Doppler-catheter gradient relation in vitro: a manifestation of pressure recovery. J Am Coll Cardiol 1993;21:1018–25.

31. Izzat MB, Birdi I, Wilde P, et al. Evaluation of the hemodynamic performance of small CarboMedics aortic prostheses using dobutamine-stress Doppler echocardiography. Ann Thorac Surg 1995;60:1048–1052.

32. Fiore AC, Swartz M, Grunkemeier G, et al. Valve replacement in the small aortic annulus: prospective randomized trial of St. Jude with Medtronic Hall. Euro J Cardiothorac Surg 1997;11:485–92.

33. Christakis GT, Buth KJ, Goldman BS, et al. Inaccurate and misleading valve sizing: a proposed standard for valve size nomenclature. Ann Thorac Surg 1998;66: 1198–203.

34. Bartels C, Leyh RG, Bechtel JFM, et al. Discrepancies between sizer and valve dimensions: implications for small aortic root. Ann Thorac Surg 1998;65:1631–3.

35. Bartels C, Sievers HH. Successful dilatation of the small aortic root for implantation of a larger valve prosthesis. J Heart Valve Dis 1999;8:507–8.

36. Walther T, Falk V, Diegeler A, et al. Stentless bioprostheses for the small aortic root. J Heart Valve Dis 1996;5 Suppl III:S302–7.

37. Sintek CF, Fletcher AD, Khonsari S. Small aortic root in the elderly: use of stentless bioprosthesis. J Heart Valve Dis 1996;5 Suppl III:S308–13.

38. Nicks R, Cartmill T, Bernstein L. Hypoplasia of the aortic root—the problem of aortic valve replacement. Thorax 1970;25:339–46.

39. Sommers KE, David TE. Aortic valve replacement with patch enlargement of the aortic annulus. Ann Thorac Surg 1997;63:1608–12.

40. Manouguian S, Seybold-Epting W. Patch enlargement of the aortic valve ring by extending the aortic incision into the anterior mitral leaflet—new operative technique. J Thorac Cardiovasc Surg 1979;78:402–12.

41. Demmy TL, Magovern GJ. Aortic root enlargement procedures: In: Emery RW, Arom KV, editors. The aortic valve. Philadelphia: Hanley & Belfus, 1991.

42. Konno S, Imai Y, Iida T, et al. A new method for prosthetic valve replacement in congenital aortic stenosis associated with hypoplasia of the aortic valve ring. J Thorac Cardiovasc Surg 1975;70:909–17.

CHAPTER 26

Apicoaortic Conduits for Left Ventricular Outflow Tract Obstruction

Denton A. Cooley, MD

Although left ventricular outflow tract (LVOT) obstruction can sometimes be treated nonsurgically by means of a balloon valvotomy, this condition often requires surgical repair or replacement of the aortic valve. When extensive repair is needed, the patient may undergo patch grafting or the Rastan-Konno procedure or one of its variants.[1–3] Alternatively, the surgeon may create a new outflow tract by extending a valved conduit from the left ventricular apex to the abdominal aorta. The Texas Heart Institute helped pioneer apicoaortic bypass grafting in the mid-1970s, but the procedure was so technically difficult that it was never widely adopted.[4,5] Nevertheless, this author and colleagues continued to believe that apicoaortic conduits were valuable in selected cases. Lately, we began to use a simplified transthoracic approach for implanting these conduits in patients with LVOT lesions not readily treatable by other techniques.[6] Such lesions involve fibrous tunnel formation, calcific aortic stenosis, hypoplasia of the aortic annulus, tubular hypoplasia of the ascending aorta, or significant recurrent aortic valve stenosis unrelieved by aortic root repair or a valvotomy. This chapter describes our transthoracic technique for implanting apicoaortic conduits to treat complex LVOT obstruction.

Materials and Methods

Apicoaortic Conduit

Our apicoaortic conduit consists of a woven Dacron tube that has a rigid, right-angled connector with an attached sewing ring on its proximal end (Medtronic Hancock Left Ventricular Connector, Medtronic Inc., Minneapolis, Minnesota). In our early cases, the tube contained a Björk-Shiley tilting-disc valve. Later, when our stock of Björk-Shiley conduits ran out, we began using conduits that contained a St. Jude valve (St. Jude Medical, St. Paul, Minnesota).

Operative Procedure

After being anesthetized, the patient is intubated so that the left lung can be collapsed when the pleural cavity is entered. The patient is placed in the right lateral decubitus position, as appropriate for a transthoracic incision. The left groin is exposed to allow later cannulation of the femoral vessels for cardiopulmonary bypass. An incision is made in the fifth intercostal space, and the left lung is deflated and retracted cephalad. After the pleura has been incised over the distal descending aorta, a partial occluding clamp is applied to the aorta. An aortotomy is performed, and a continuous 3–0 or 4–0 polypropylene suture is used to anastomose the distal end of the valve-containing conduit to the aorta (Figure 26-1A). The conduit is clamped, and the partial occluding clamp is removed from the aorta.

Full heparinization is induced, and the left femoral vessels are cannulated for cardiopulmonary bypass. The right atrium is entered with a long venous cannula. The pericardium is opened, exposing the left ventricular apex. Pledgeted 3–0 sutures are applied around the target anastomosis site and pacing wires are attached. Electrical fibrillation is performed to decrease ventricular ejection. An apical plug is then removed with a coring device, and the opening is enlarged, as necessary, with a No. 15 scalpel.[7] The semirigid inlet conduit is then inserted into the ventricular cavity, and the sewing ring is affixed to the apex with interrupted 3–0 sutures. The circumference of the conduit is circled with a continuous 3–0 suture (Figure 26-1B). Temporary occluding clamps are then placed on the grafts. The heart is defibrillated and allowed to pump so that any bleeding vessels can be detected. The two grafts are anastomosed (end to end) (Figure 26-1C). The resulting conduit is tailored so as to curve gently above the left hemidiaphragm. Residual air is evacuated from the conduit proximal and distal to the valve, as well as

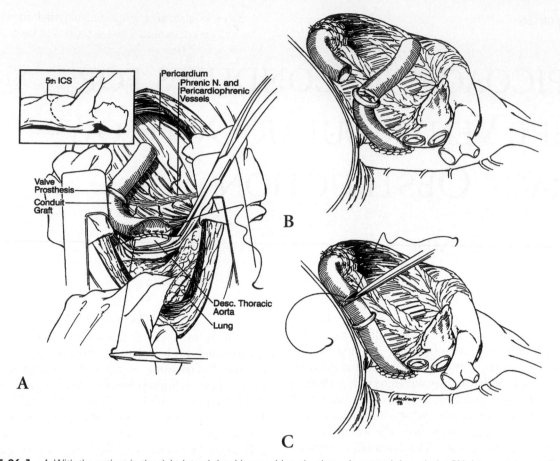

FIGURE 26-1. *A,* With the patient in the right lateral decubitus position, the thorax is entered through the fifth intercostal space (inset). The descending aorta is partially occluded, and the valved conduit is anastomosed with a continuous 3–0 or 4–0 polypropylene suture. *B,* During cardiopulmonary bypass, the rigid prosthesis is attached to the apex of the left ventricle with interrupted pledgeted mattress and continuous sutures. Induced ventricular fibrillation is used to facilitate the ventricular attachment. Temporary occluding clamps are used on the grafts during anastomoses. *C,* After tailoring, the prostheses are connected with a continuous suture. Air is evacuated, and cardiac function resumes. Ventricular countershock may be necessary to restore sinus rhythm. Reproduced with permission from Cooley D A et al.[6]

from the left ventricle and ascending aorta. The temporary occluding clamps are then released from the grafts, and the left lung is re-inflated. Protamine sulfate is given to reverse the effects of heparin, and the cannulas are withdrawn from the femoral artery and vein. Pressures are then measured in the left ventricle, in the conduit proximal and distal to the valve, and in the ascending aorta. We usually occlude the ascending aorta temporarily to evaluate the effect on the systemic circulation. Ordinarily, the blood pressure decreases by about 20%, after which the systemic pressure returns to normal. (As a result, if necessary, the conduit could handle the entire left ventricular output.) After the chest is closed, a chest tube is inserted and is connected to an underwater sealed drainage reservoir.

Antibiotic coverage is given during the early postoperative period. If the conduit contains a heterograft valve, long-term anticoagulation is rarely needed. In some patients, a regimen of aspirin and dipyridamole is initiated on the third day after surgery. If the conduit contains a Björk-Shiley convexoconcave valve, sodium warfarin is used for anticoagulation. If a mechanical valve is already in place, sodium warfarin therapy is simply continued.

Comments

The apicoaortic conduit relieves the signs and symptoms of LVOT obstruction in both children and adults. It corrects the left ventricular aortic gradient, preserves or improves left ventricular function, reverses hemolysis, and results in normal blood-flow distribution through both the coronary and systemic circulations. The amount of blood that flows through the conduit depends on the extent of the obstruction. The procedure is well tolerated and does not hinder normal growth or exercise in children and young adults.

This author's institution has considerable long-term experience in using apicoaortic conduits to relieve LVOT obstruction.[8–10] We began to perform this procedure in 1975 and a year later reported nine cases.[4,5] In 1980, we described 14 patients whose average flow gradient decreased from 100 mm Hg preoperatively to 22 mm Hg postoperatively; on average, 36% of the left ventricular outflow was ejected through the conduit.[11] Later that same year, we published an updated report concerning 27 patients whose flow gradient decreased by 85%.[7] By 1986, our series included 38 patients, whose 5-year survival rate was 78%.[12]

In all of these early cases, we used a sternotomy incision. The aortic anastomosis usually involved the supraceliac abdominal aorta or, occasionally, the ascending aorta. If necessary, saphenous vein bypass grafts were extended to the coronary arteries. Despite a lack of routine formal exercise testing, our patients had no exercise-related symptoms or physical restrictions. This experience showed that creating a double-outlet left ventricle was both feasible and effective, but the operation was technically difficult and was abandoned in favor of the Rastan-Konno procedure and its modifications.[1–3] Also, in some of our patients, the conduit's porcine valve degenerated and was replaced.

Recently, we adopted a simpler approach consisting of a left lateral thoracotomy, which gives direct access to the descending aorta, avoids a redo sternotomy, and could possibly be performed without cardiopulmonary bypass. The lateral incision is easier for the surgeon and seems better tolerated by the patient. We have used this approach in seven patients, five of whom survived and recovered completely. One of the nonsurvivors, who had severe congestive heart failure and multiple comorbidities, sustained a fatal cardiac arrest at the end of an otherwise uneventful apicoaortic procedure; the other nonsurvivor had a history of severe chronic pulmonary congestion, which led to respiratory insufficiency 2 weeks postoperatively.

Although an apicoaortic conduit is commercially available, we initially used prostheses that had been in our inventory for more than 5 years. We could fabricate the valved portion of the conduit with the valve of our choice. The choice of a biologic versus a mechanical valve depends on the needs of each individual patient. Whichever type of valve is selected, the commercial rigid apical connector should be used.

The above-described technique offers a practical surgical alternative for patients with severe LVOT. The technique is not only simple to perform but also avoids injuring major coronary arteries, the conduction system, and other valves. The left lateral thoracotomy is particularly suitable for repairing a porcelain aorta, as aortic cross-clamping might otherwise lead to dissection, hemorrhage, or embolization. This incision may also be appropriate for patients who have complications (infection, false aneurysm formation, etc.) from a previous operation.

With apicoaortic conduits, potential late problems include infection, thromboembolism, failure of the porcine valve, detachment of the conduit from the ventricular apex, and obstruction of the conduit at its insertion into the ventricle. Two of our early patients died suddenly because of a pseudoaneurysmal rupture that produced no symptoms; if the rupture had been detected earlier, these patients might have been saved. To prevent apex-conduit disruption, optimal follow-up may need to include echocardiography, computed tomography, or even contrast ventriculography.

Summary

When LVOT obstruction is refractory to conventional surgical techniques, implantation of an apicoaortic conduit can relieve the severe left ventricular aortic pressure gradient, preserve or improve left ventricular function and aortic hemodynamics, and allow normal blood-flow distribution to the body. This operation is well tolerated and, in children, is compatible with normal development and activity.

References

1. Konno S, Imai Y, Iida Y, et al. A new method for prosthetic valve replacement in congenital aortic stenosis associated with hypoplasia of the aortic valve ring. J Thorac Cardiovasc Surg 1975;70:909–17.
2. Rastan H, Koncz J. Aortoventriculoplasty. J Thorac Cardiovasc Surg 1976;71:920–7.
3. Reddy VM, Rajasinghe HA, Teitel DF, et al. Aortoventriculoplasty with the pulmonary autograft: the "Ross-Konno" procedure. J Thorac Cardiovasc Surg 1996;111:158–67.
4. Cooley DA, Norman JC, Mullins CE, Grace RR. Left ventricle to abdominal aorta conduit for relief of aortic stenosis. Cardiovasc Dis Bull Tex Heart Inst 1975;2:376–83.
5. Cooley DA, Norman JC, Reul GJ Jr, et al. Surgical treatment of left ventricular outflow obstruction with apicoaortic valved conduit. Surgery 1976;80:674–80.
6. Cooley DA, Lopez RM, Absi TS. Apicoaortic conduit for left ventricular outflow tract obstruction: revisited. Ann Thorac Surg 2000;69:1511–4.
7. Norman JC, Nihill MR, Cooley DA. Valved apicoaortic composite conduits for left ventricular outflow tract obstruction. Am J Cardiol 1980;45:1265–71.
8. Carrell A. On the experimental surgery of the thoracic aorta and the heart. Ann Surg 1910:52–83.
9. Bailey CP, Glover RP, O'Neill THE, Ramirez HPR. Experiences with the experimental surgical relief of aortic stenosis: a preliminary report. J Thorac Surg 1950;20:516–41.
10. Sarnoff SJ, Donovan TJ, Case RB. The surgical relief of aortic stenosis by means of apical aortic valvular anastomoses. Circulation 1955;11:564–74.
11. Nihill MR, Cooley DA, Norman JC, et al. Hemodynamic observations in patients with left ventricle to aorta conduit. Am J Cardiol 1980;45:573–82.
12. Sweeney MS, Walker WE, Cooley DA, Reul GJ. Apicoaortic conduits for complex left ventricular outflow obstruction: a 10-year experience. Ann Thorac Surg 1986;42:609–11.

CHAPTER 27

PROSTHETIC VALVE ENDOCARDITIS

BRUCE W. LYTLE, MD

The occurrence of prosthetic valve endocarditis (PVE) is a major complication of cardiac valve replacement. In the early years of the cardiac surgical era, treatment of PVE was rarely successful. Today, because of advances in diagnostic techniques, increased surgical experience, and effective antimicrobial agents, most patients will survive an episode of PVE. However, the long-term outcomes after treatment of PVE do not match those following elective valve replacement, and the treatment of PVE continues to challenge the judgment and skill of the physicians caring for these patients.

Incidence of PVE

The peak incidence of PVE in patients receiving a standard mechanical or xenograft heart valve prosthesis appears to occur between 3 and 6 weeks after operation, after which it declines to a low constant rate that appears to last indefinitely. The incidence of PVE within the first postoperative year in series from the 1970s and 1980s appeared to be 1.5 to 3%.[1,2] Recent (1992 to 1997) Cleveland Clinic Foundation data reviewed 7,043 patients undergoing valve replacement or repair and documented 74 (1%) cases of PVE within the first postoperative year.[3] In our studies, my colleagues and I have classified PVE identified within the first postoperative year as early endocarditis and those cases appearing more than 1 year after operation as late.[3,4] Patients receiving aortic valve allografts and undergoing valve repairs have a decreased incidence of early PVE whereas standard xenografts and mechanical valves appear to have the same incidence.[3,5] Factors that have been identified as increasing the risk of PVE include multivalve operations, aortic root replacement with a synthetic graft, and operation for active native valve endocarditis.[3,5,6]

For patients without native valve infections as an indication for valve replacement, early PVE appears to be a nosocomial infection based on intraoperative contamination or bacteremia in the postoperative phase. Studies of patients with prosthetic valves known to have had a bacteremia have documented an incidence of subsequent PVE of 10 to 24% and have identified the most common portals of entry as intravascular catheters and skin infections.[7,8] The distribution of microorganisms causing early PVE is representative of nosocomial infection. In The Cleveland Clinic Foundation series, bacteria included coagulase-negative staphylococci (52%), *Staphylococcus aureus* (10%, with half being methicillin-resistant organisms), enterococci (8%), *Streptococcus viridans* (5%), and gram-negative organisms (6%). Fungi accounted for 10% (*Candida albicans*, 8 of 10), and 2 cases were culture negative.

Once past the early phase, the incidence of late PVE appears to be about 0.5 to 1% per year.[5,6,9,10] Hammermiester and colleagues followed patients for 11 years postoperatively and noted an incidence of PVE ranging from 7% for patients with a mechanical aortic valve to 17% for those with mitral valve bioprostheses, although those differences were not statistically significant.[9] In following patients after aortic valve replacement (AVR), my colleagues and I noted an incidence of 0.91% per patient-year for patients with bioprostheses versus 0.42% per patient-year for those with mechanical valves.[10] The increased risk for patients with bioprostheses is a trend also cited by Agnihotri and colleagues.[5] The distribution of organisms causing late PVE is similar to that of those accounting for early PVE, but most series of patients with late PVE usually have a higher incidence of *Staphylococcus aureus* and *Enterococcus* infections. Nosocomial infection also causes late PVE, particularly for patients with prosthetic heart valves and associated medical conditions that require frequent hospitalization, such as the need for dialysis, patients post organ transplantation, or other conditions involving recurrent bacteremia and/or immunosuppression.

Pathology

The pathology created by PVE infections is related to the organism, the prosthesis, and the length of time the infection is present. Early PVE usually involves the interface of the prosthesis and the native valve annulus. Infection in that location often creates a periprosthetic leak, and further invasion causes progressive tissue destruction and abscess formation. Aortic PVE often extends into the fibrous trigone of the heart and may displace the anterior leaflet of the mitral valve inferiorly, creating abscess cavity. In the areas of the septum, extensive infection may erode into the right ventricle or into the right atrium in the region of the membranous septum, creating intracardiac fistulae. Mitral prosthetic valve endocarditis often extends posteriorly and may cause atrial ventricular separation or may extend anteriorly, involving the fibrous trigone. It is important to remember that PVE with extensive annular involvement may be present without causing either a periprosthetic leak or fistula formation. Concomitant with annular involvement, the valve leaflets often become involved with vegetations that may serve as a source for emboli and cause formation of distant abscesses.

Patients acquiring PVE late after operation may exhibit the same annular and leaflet pathology noted with early-onset endocarditis. However, patients with bioprostheses may also acquire late PVE that only involves the valve leaflets, at least initially. This type of PVE is important to recognize as it may be treatable with antibiotics alone, at least over the short term. Infection involving only the prosthetic leaflets is uncommon as early PVE. In our studies of surgical patients, my colleagues and I have classified the anatomic varieties of infections into those involving the prosthesis alone, those involving the prosthesis–native annular junction (annular infection), and those causing tissue destruction beyond the annulus (extensive infection).[4] A further subgrouping that is important is the distinction between active and healed endocarditis. In our surgical series, the definition of active PVE included the demonstration of organisms, either with preoperative blood cultures, cultures from the surgical specimen, or microscopic examination of the explanted valve. Cases where organisms cannot be demonstrated are classified as healed.[4,11]

Clinical Syndromes and Diagnosis of PVE

The diagnosis of PVE is based on evidence for systemic infection, usually with the documentation of bacteremia or fungemia, combined with anatomic evidence that localizes that infection to a prosthetic heart valve. Thus, the investigations that establish the diagnosis are blood cultures and cardiac imaging, usually echocardiography.[12,13] Accuracy in diagnosis is extremely important because therapies for PVE are expensive and involve some risk whereas failure to make the diagnosis potentially compromises outcomes.

The most common clinical presentations for patients with PVE are fever, embolization, new periprosthetic leak, a documented bloodstream infection, or some combination of these events. Most patients with PVE have fever, and the investigation of a fever in patients with a pros-

thetic heart valve is important. Any febrile illness in a patient with a prosthetic heart valve is an indication for drawing blood cultures, and the decision to place a patient with a prosthetic heart valve on antibiotic therapy for any reason other than prophylaxis is a major one and should not be taken lightly. Nonspecific oral antibiotic treatment of patients with a prosthetic heart valve with a fever risks progression of infection because of inadequate antibiotic therapy and may compromise the likelihood of identifying the organism.

The documentation of a bloodstream infection in a patient with a prosthetic heart valve is an indication for echocardiography and usually for transesophageal echocardiography (TEE). If echocardiography is negative, the bacteremia alone is an indication for prolonged intravenous antibiotic therapy as multiple studies have shown that patients with a bacteremia and without obvious PVE have a substantial risk (16% in a multicenter study by Fang and colleagues) of subsequently developing PVE.[8]

If echocardiography demonstrates new anatomic valvular abnormalities characteristic of PVE, including vegetations, periprosthetic leak, intracardiac fistulae, or abscess formation in association with a systemic infection, the diagnosis of PVE is as secure as it can be, short of examination of specimens removed at reoperation. However, a negative echocardiogram does not exclude the diagnosis of PVE, and even annular infection may not be initially visible on TEE prior to the development of periprosthetic leak. In these situations, magnetic resonance imaging (MRI) may identify abnormal tissue consistency in the annulus, aiding in the diagnosis. For patients with anatomic abnormalities of prosthetic valves, comparison of current studies with previous echocardiograms can be valuable.

In addition to fever, initial manifestations of PVE may be new periprosthetic leak and/or embolization. Both of these events are indications for blood cultures and transesophageal echocardiography. Although fever usually accompanies these events for patients with PVE, patients may be afebrile, particularly if the organism is not virulent. The possibility of PVE should be strongly considered for patients with bioprostheses who experience embolic phenomenon.

Although the diagnosis of PVE is often obvious, patients with a suggestive clinical syndrome but without positive blood cultures or clear anatomic abnormalities of a prosthetic valve present difficult problems. Such patients often have had multiple valves replaced, which causes shadowing during echocardiography; have received aortic root replacements with prosthetic valve-graft combinations, which makes a periprosthetic leak impossible; or have had homograft or autograft aortic valve replacements. Repeated echocardiographic or MRI studies may be needed to make the diagnosis, and persistent suspicion is important. It is also wise, if possible, to delay antibiotic therapy until an organism can be identified because having a specific organism to treat is very helpful in trying to cure a patient of PVE.

Once the patient has a documented bloodstream infection combined with an anatomic prosthetic valve abnormality, it is highly likely that reoperation will be needed. However, the timing of operation often remains an issue. Patients with bioprostheses who have a late infection that appears to be limited to the leaflets may sometimes receive a full course of antibiotic therapy that sterilizes the valve.[4] Those leaflet infections usually cause premature bioprosthetic failure and aortic insufficiency, but operation may not be needed over the short term. Operation for these patients is usually indicated by progressive aortic insufficiency and can be carried out electively.

Patients with annular or more extensive PVE will almost all need reoperation in the acute or subacute phase, and the issue tends to be the optimal length of preoperative antibiotic therapy. For patients with PVE, the goals of prolonged antibiotic therapy are (1) to decrease the virulence of the infecting organism, perhaps decreasing the risk of reinfection, and (2) to allow treatment of coexisting acute conditions that may increase the risk of reoperation. Included in these conditions may be acute renal failure, stroke, pneumonia, operations to treat complications of embolization, clotting abnormalities, and a myriad of other conditions caused by PVE or by the conditions that led to PVE. However, there are often many potential disadvantages of delaying operation, including ongoing risks of (1) progression of hemodynamic derangement, (2) ongoing systemic sepsis, (3) recurrent embolization, and (4) progressive cardiac tissue destruction. Patients with PVE are varied and complex, and it is difficult to be too dogmatic about the timing of operation. However, there are some good general rules to follow: (1) some antibiotic therapy is better than no antibiotic therapy; (2) there is no absolute contraindication to reoperation for patients with uncontrolled PVE; (3) for the continuation of antibiotic nonoperative therapy to make sense, the patient must demonstrate control of systemic infection and show no evidence of progression of infection, either locally or systemically. What does this last rule mean? For patients with PVE, the burden of proof lies with the advocate of nonoperative therapy. Once antibiotics are started, fever and tachycardia must resolve. Serial echocardiography must show no anatomic progression of valvular insufficiency, evidence of tissue invasion (abscess cavity, fistula, etc) or vegetations. Any recurrence of systemic symptoms such as fever or anatomic progression by echocardiography is an indication for operation.

Stroke in association with PVE is relatively common, occurring in 10 to 25% of patients, and the timing of surgery relative to the occurrence of a stroke is often an issue. Most strokes are embolic and occur early in the course of the PVE illness, and the risk of subsequent stroke appears to decrease with antibiotic therapy. However, residual vegetations > 1 cm in diameter represent a relative indication for operation. Embolic stroke can be associated with cerebral hemorrhage, raising concern that immediate operation for valve re-replacement might risk further hemorrhage resulting in a worsening of a neurologic deficit. In practice, worsening of stroke is usually not seen after operations for PVE, and if a strong indication for surgery exists, operation is usually the best choice. However, if indications for surgery are not compelling, logic would seem to dictate that in the face of cerebral hemorrhage that has already been demonstrated, delaying operation might decrease neurologic risk.

Other preoperative issues for patients with PVE include investigation of coronary anatomy and the possibility of metastatic infection. Many patients with PVE have coronary artery disease, and some have undergone previous bypass surgery. It is always an advantage to understand the coronary anatomy, and for patients with previous revascularization operations, it is important. Coronary angiography for patients with isolated mitral valve PVE is safe, and even with aortic valve PVE, graft angiography can usually be carried out safely. Because angiography involving the native coronary vessels in situations of aortic valve PVE does have some risk, judgment must be exercised in these situations.

Metastatic infection caused by PVE may also influence outcome. Abdominal symptoms should trigger preoperative computed tomography (CT) scanning to investigate the possibility of splenic or hepatic abscesses. These conditions do not preclude valve reoperation and are not clear indications for concomitant abdominal surgery, but it is helpful to know that abdominal abscesses exist. Failure of hepatic or splenic abscesses to improve postoperatively on antibiotic therapy may be an indication for splenectomy or drainage of hepatic abscess. Continued signs of systemic infection after valve replacement should raise the suspicion of continued seeding of infection from a metastatic abscess.

Surgery for Prosthetic Valve Endocarditis

The outcomes of combined medical-surgical therapy for PVE have improved because of multiple factors, including (1) increased experience of surgeons; (2) effective myocardial protection; (3) component transfusion therapy and biologic adhesives to control bleeding; (4) intraoperative TEE; (5) the use of aortic valve homografts, autologous pericardium, and glutaraldehyde-treated bovine pericardium for intracardiac reconstruction; (6) aggressive débridement of infected tissue and prosthetic material; and (7) effective and varied antibiotics. Operations for PVE are often time-consuming extensive procedures, and the increased surgical experience has not identified many effective shortcuts.

The surgeon should be prepared to operate on all cardiac chambers, valves, and coronary arteries regardless of the preoperative echo findings. Thus, most operations for PVE are best approached through a full median sternotomy. The risk of injury during the reoperative median sternotomy is increased by right-heart enlargement, multiple atherosclerotic vein grafts, a patent right internal thoracic artery graft, a previous aortic graft, or an aortic false aneurysm, and in these situations, we will obtain arterial and venous access before reopening the sternotomy. In difficult situations, a small right thoracotomy allows dissection of the cardiac structures from beneath the sternum prior to a repeat median sternotomy.

Cannulation for cardiopulmonary bypass involves arterial return via the aorta or a peripheral vessel (usually the axillary artery) and bicaval cannulation. Inferior vena cava cannulation via the femoral vein and direct cannulation of the superior vena cava (SVC) or the innominate vein are options for venous cannulation that keep the surgical field uncluttered. SVC cannulation close to the innominate vein allows division of the SVC to enhance exposure of the mitral valve and fibrous trigone of the heart. The use of vacuum-assisted venous drainage allows small cannulae (20 to 22 French) to be used, and if it is difficult to control and occlude the cavae because of multiple previous operations, vacuum-assisted drainage allows open venous drainage. A transatrial retrograde cardioplegia cannula is placed.

Myocardial protection is crucial during these long operations. Using antegrade and retrograde substrate-enhanced cardioplegia as described by Buckberg my colleagues and I give induction cardioplegia for at least 3 min and subsequently give 2-min maintenance doses at least every 15 to 20 min.[14] Retrograde cardioplegia delivery is very helpful for these patients who may have significant coronary stenoses and/or areas supplied by bypass grafts.

The steps in surgery for PVE are as follows: (1) remove the infection, the prosthetic valve, the neighboring infected tissue, and all prosthetic material; (2) close the holes in the heart created by removing the infection, and use biologic material such as autologous or bovine pericardium to do so; (3) replace the valves; (4) correct any negative change in coronary anatomy created by the operation.

Aortic Valve PVE

For patients with isolated aortic valve PVE, the intention is to replace the infected valve with a cryopreserved aortic valve homograft, almost always implanted as an aortic root replacement.[11,15,16] The infected aortic prosthesis is removed, and Teflon pledgets and suture material are débrided along with any neighboring infected cardiac tissue. Once the infected tissue is removed it is usually necessary to develop some mobility of the coronary ostia to allow implantation into the homograft. This can be difficult if the coronaries border severely infected tissue.

In patients with aortic valve PVE, the most common area of abscess formation is in the area of the fibrous trigone beneath the left and noncoronary cusps. An abscess cavity in this area will often displace the mitral valve inferiorly. If the mitral valve is competent on preoperative TEE, it is usually possible to débride the edges of this abscess cavity, and the mitral valve usually does not need replacement. When the abscess occurs in this area, it is usually not necessary to close the cavity separately when implanting a homograft, as the anterior leaflet of the homograft mitral valve can be used to bridge the gap between the level of the annulus and the superior edge of the anterior leaflet of the mitral valve. In septal areas of the annulus, it is often necessary to close abscess cavities, either to create an annulus to sew the new valve to or to close a fistula. These abscess cavities and/or fistulae are closed with autologous pericardium or bovine pericardium prior to implantation of the homograft.

Once the débridement of infection is completed and the holes are closed, a homograft is implanted. Because most commercially available homografts range in size from 19 to 21 mm, the cross-sectional area of the aortic root may be substantially larger than the annulus of the homograft, particularly once débridement of the host aortic root is completed. There are multiple ways of compensating for a size difference between the homograft and the aortic root where it is to be implanted, including (1) leaving the entire anterior leaflet of the mitral valve attached to the homograft, thus increasing its surface area; (2) avoiding the débridement of the septal muscle from the homograft; and (3) sewing a strip of autologous pericardium around the base of the homograft to add bulk and to prevent needle hole bleeding from the muscle. This last strategy (Figure 27-1) is often a good idea even if there is not a tremendous size difference as it adds strength and pliability to the homograft muscle. Strategies that can be used at primary operations for reducing the size of the recipient annulus, such as closing commissures and circumferential annuloplasty sutures, are usually ineffective in situations of PVE because of the rigidity and friability of the infected aortic root.

PVE and aortic insufficiency will sometimes create holes in the anterior leaflet of the mitral valve, so-called drop lesions. These perforations can usually be closed with pericardial patches and do not represent an indication for mitral valve replacement. Native mitral valve replacement is usually needed only for severe insufficiency caused by leaflet and chordal destruction from active infection.

After débridement of the aortic root is complete, the aortic root may seem somewhat distorted. Orientation of the homograft is usually best accomplished by matching the homograft mitral valve to the native mitral valve (Figure 27-2). The edges of the mitral valve define approximately a third of the annulus. Bisecting the remainder of the homograft and native annulus will divide both into thirds that help in the accurate spacing of suture placement.

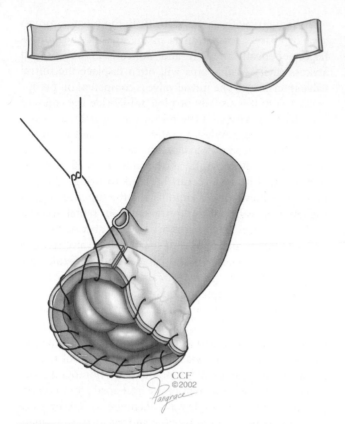

FIGURE 27-1. Sewing of a pericardial skirt around the base of the homograft with a 5–0 monofilament suture prior to implantation is helpful during homograft aortic root replacement. This strategy bulks up the homograft, establishing a better size match if the annulus is larger or distorted. In addition, when the anastomotic sutures pass through the homograft and pericardium, hemostasis is very secure.

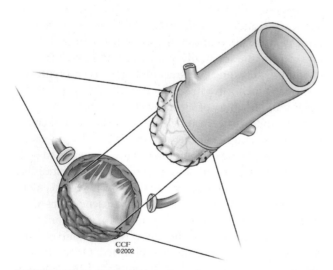

FIGURE 27-2. During homograft aortic root replacement for PVE, the aortic root is extensively débrided and coronary buttons are created. Matching the homograft mitral valve to the native mitral valve is a reliable way to orient the homograft in a distorted aortic root. The most common location for an annular abscess is in the area of the anterior leaflet of the mitral valve, as seen here. Reproduced with permission from Lytle BW.[17]

We use 4–0 monofilament sutures for the homograft implantation usually with a simple interrupted technique or interrupted figure of 8 sutures if there is a large discrepancy between the size of the native annulus and the size of the homograft. All the sutures are placed through the annulus and through the homograft, the homograft is lowered into place, and the aorta of the homograft is inverted while sutures are tied. The homograft aortic valve itself is not inverted during suture tying (Figure 27-3). Completion of the proximal suture line reconstructs abscess cavities in the region of the patient's mitral valve with the homograft mitral valve (Figure 27-4).

After the homograft is tied into place, buttons for the coronary anastomoses are removed from the right and left coronary sinuses, and the coronary patches are sewn into those sinuses with a continuous 5–0 monofilament suture (Figure 27-5).

After these anastomoses are completed, the homograft aorta is measured and sewn end-to-end to the host aorta with continuous 4–0 monofilament suture. If patent vein-to-coronary grafts are attached to the host aorta, they usually can be left in place with only a short segment of the host aorta being removed. Remnants of the aorta are not closed around the homograft. Early in our homograft experience my colleagues and I used some subcoronary and root inclusion techniques for the treatment of endocarditis; however, we have entirely switched to aortic root replacement because of the very low rate of early aortic valve insufficiency with this technique and because we are able to avoid the potential for enclosed infection between the aorta and the homograft.

Aortic valve homografts are our first choice in the surgical management of PVE because of their versatility in aortic root reconstruction and the low rate of reinfection and reoperations (see "Results of the Treatment of PVE").[11] However, it is possible to successfully treat PVE by using standard procedures, and prior to the availability of homografts, we achieved reasonable outcomes by reconstructing damaged areas of the aortic annulus by using pericardium and inserting standard prostheses.[4] If a surgeon has little experience with homografts on an elective basis, a difficult reconstruction in a patient with active endocarditis may be best accomplished with more familiar techniques.

When implanting a standard mechanical or bioprosthesis for a patient with PVE and annular destruction, it may be helpful to open the pulmonary artery, right ventricle, or right atrium, to allow placement of sutures through the annulus and tying down within those cardiac structures (Figure 27-6). There has not been demonstration of a clear advantage for either mechanical or standard bioprostheses in terms of avoiding reinfection or reoperation, but prior to the homograft era, my colleagues and I usually employed bioprostheses in situations of PVE because of a more forgiving sewing ring and the opportunity to avoid anticoagulation in the early postoperative period for these often critically ill patients.

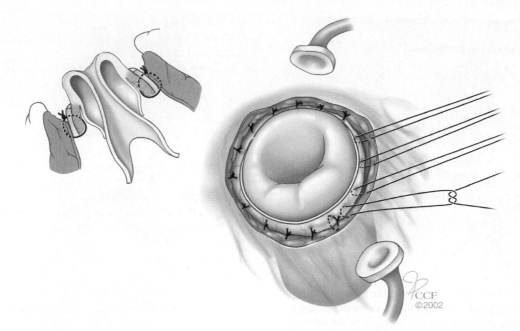

FIGURE 27-3. Once all the 4–0 monofilament sutures are placed in the annulus, the homograft aorta is inverted and the sutures are tied.

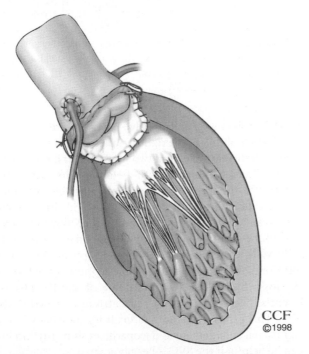

FIGURE 27-4. One strategy for management of an abscess cavity as seen in Figure 27-2 is to use the homograft mitral valve as an extension, sewing it to the superior rim of the native mitral valve. This allows the homograft to bridge the gap created by the abscess cavity. Reproduced with permission from Lytle BW.[17]

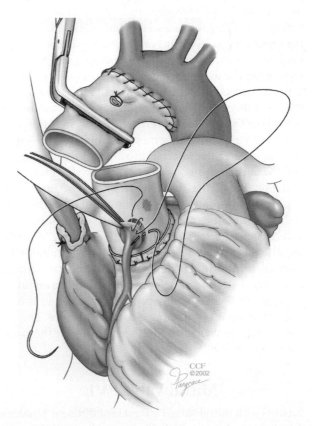

FIGURE 27-5. Infections involving aortic valve PVE combined with a previous ascending aortic graft are best treated with replacement of all prosthetic material, sometimes requiring two homograft segments. Here the arch anastomosis of an ascending aortic graft has been replaced with a homograft with the aid of circulatory arrest, and that homograft segment has been clamped, allowing rewarming while the aortic root reconstruction is being completed.

Infected Aortic Composite Grafts

PVE involving a composite graft to replace the aortic valve, root, and ascending aorta (Bentall operation) presents special problems. First, the diagnosis may be difficult to make because a periprosthetic leak between the Dacron

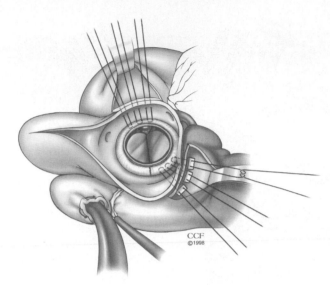

FIGURE 27-6. When placing a standard aortic valve prosthesis to treat PVE, it may help to open the right atrium and/or the pulmonary artery to allow suture placement through the prosthesis and the annulus. Reproduced with permission from Lytle BW.[17]

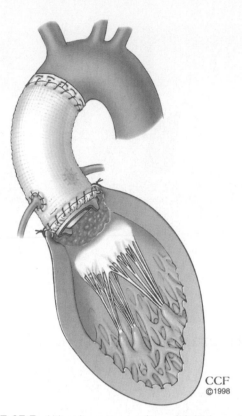

FIGURE 27-7. Although most composite graft infections primarily involve the valve–annulus interface, they usually extend along the length of the graft, requiring removal of the entire graft. Reproduced with permission from Lytle BW.[17]

graft and the valve cannot happen. Thus, the infection often becomes far advanced, and until a false aneurysm develops, the diagnosis may be obscure. Second, although the infection usually begins at the prosthesis-aortic annulus interface, it may extend all along the graft, requiring replacement of the entire ascending aortic graft, a distance that may be too long for a single homograft to suffice (Figure 27-7). To extend the homograft that is inserted into the aortic root to an anastomosis in the aortic arch, it is often effective to use a second homograft containing an imperfect valve. After the infected prosthetic graft is removed and the aortic valve is completely removed from the second homograft, the distal anastomosis of the second homograft to the aorta takes place at the level of the aortic arch with the aid of deep hypothermia, circulatory arrest, and retrograde cerebral perfusion (see Figure 27-5). After the distal anastomosis is completed with continuous 4–0 monofilament suture material, the systemic circulation is restarted, the homograft is clamped, and rewarming is accomplished while the proximal reconstruction is done with a homograft containing a competent valve. The two homografts are then sewn together to complete the procedure (Figure 27-8).

Mitral Valve PVE

Patients with mitral valve PVE present different problems than those with aortic PVE. First, mitral valve homografts do not provide the same reliable reconstruction and failure from reinfection and reoperation documented for aortic valve homografts. Second, exposure of the mitral valve is often more difficult than aortic valve exposure, particularly if multiple previous operations have been performed.

The problems of mitral valve exposure are related to achieving mobility of the right atrium and venae cavae; we approach these problems in two ways. The first is to divide the SVC and combine it with a standard left atriotomy anterior to the right superior pulmonary vein that then can be extended toward the aortic root. This incision has the advantage of avoiding the sinus node, allowing extension to the aortic root and providing good exposure, even if the right atrium is small. The second approach is a right atriotomy that extends through the septum at the level of the fossa ovalis, then out the dome of the left atrium, essentially leaving a cuff of right atrium attached to the SVC. This exposure is more difficult for patients without right atrial enlargement and jeopardizes sinus rhythm but can be helpful if the SVC is heavily scarred.

Once exposure of the mitral valve is accomplished, the infected valve and all prosthetic material are removed. Abscess formation extending posteriorly and some degree of atrial ventricular separation are common (Figure 27-9). Attempting to pull the ventricle back to join the atrium by the use of sutures alone often fails over the long term because the rigid fixed tissue resists being pulled together and the sutures pull through the tissue. It is usually a better strategy to débride the valve and bridge the defect with a pericardial patch (Figure 27-10) and then to sew the new valve prosthesis to this reconstructed annulus

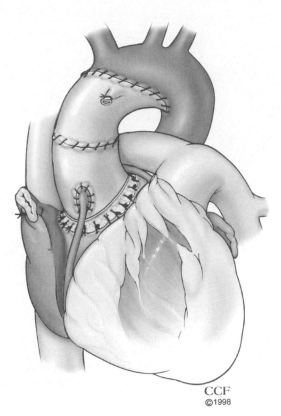

FIGURE 27-8. After the distal homograft is implanted into the aortic arch and the proximal reconstruction is complete, the two homografts are sewn together to complete the operation.

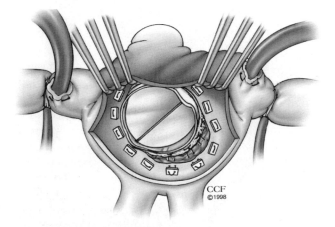

FIGURE 27-9. Mitral valve PVE may produce an abscess cavity separating the left atrium, left ventricle, and prosthesis. Reproduced with permission from Lytle BW.[17]

(Figure 27-11). In most situations, we prefer to use a bioprosthesis because of the larger softer sewing ring and to avoid anticoagulation.

Fibrous Trigone Infection

Extension of PVE into the fibrous trigone of the heart may lead to the need to replace both aortic and mitral valves, leaving little tissue between them. Rather than compro-

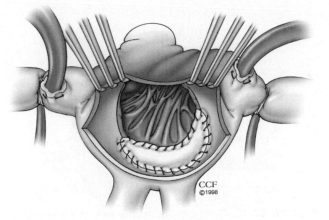

FIGURE 27-10. Following débridement of foreign material, the abscess cavity is closed with pericardium before implantation of a new prosthesis. Reproduced with permission from Lytle BW.[17]

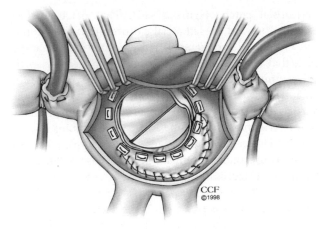

FIGURE 27-11. The mitral valve is replaced using the pericardium as part of the annulus. Thus, the abscess cavity is closed before the valve is implanted. Reproduced with permission from Lytle BW.[17]

mise on the débridement of infection in this area or sew two prostheses together, we think it is safer to replace the fibrous trigone with autologous or bovine pericardium with that material then being used to help secure the new prosthesis.[17] To obtain exposure of the fibrous trigone, the SVC is divided and a left atriotomy is extended from the left atrium anterior to the right superior pulmonary vein to the aortic root (Figure 27-12). This exposure allows the left atriotomy to be carried up through the aortic valve and allows débridement of both the aortic and mitral valves, as well as the fibrous trigone, and provides good exposure for reconstruction. After the infection is débrided and the defects of the remaining annulus repaired, the mitral valve prosthesis is implanted into the two-thirds to three-fourths of the mitral valve annulus that is still intact. A long triangular segment of autologous or bovine pericardium is then sewn to the cardiac tissue on each side of the mitral valve prosthesis, and horizontal mattress sutures are used to secure that prosthesis to the

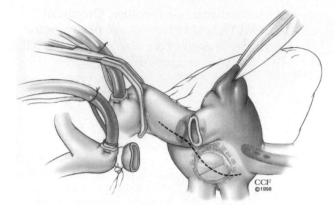

FIGURE 27-12. Division of the superior vena cava allows exposure of the aortic root, mitral valve, and fibrous trigone. (\Reproduced with permission from Lytle BW.[17]

pericardial patch (Figure 27-13). That patch is then extended toward the left atrial closure site with continuous Prolene suture material, as well as toward the aorta, such that it creates a third to a fourth of the new aortic valve annulus. Either a standard aortic valve prosthesis or an aortic valve homograft then can be used to replace the aortic valve, again using the pericardial replacement of the fibrous trigone as part of the aortic valve annulus (Figure 27-14). The patch is then extended to complete the left atrial closure and, if a standard prosthesis is used, the aortic closure (Figure 27-15).

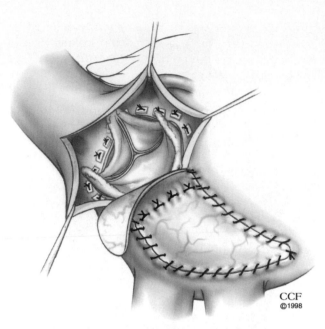

FIGURE 27-14. Once the mitral valve prosthesis is in place, the aortic valve prosthesis is secured throughout most of the annulus. The pericardial patch recreates the medial part of the aortic valve annulus, and the aortic valve is sewn to that patch. Reproduced with permission from Lytle BW.[17]

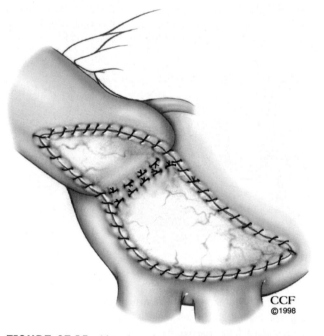

FIGURE 27-15. After the valve replacements are complete, the pericardial patch is extended to finish the closure of the aorta and the left atrium. Reproduced with permission from Lytle BW.[17]

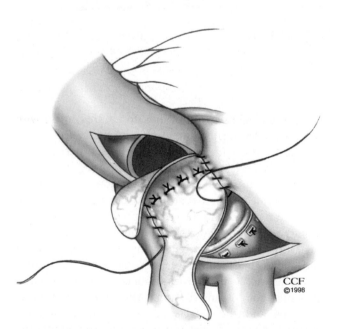

FIGURE 27-13. The new prosthetic mitral valve is sewn to the annulus posteriorly, medially, and laterally, but the superior portion of the mitral valve annulus is reconstructed by an elongated pericardial patch that replaces the fibrous trigone, and the valve is sewn to this patch with horizontal mattress sutures. Reproduced with permission from Lytle BW.[17]

Results of the Treatment of PVE

For patients with PVE, the treatment choices are antibiotic therapy alone or long-term antibiotic therapy combined with surgery (combined therapy). Most patients with PVE receive initial antibiotic therapy followed by valve replacement, and most decision making usually revolves around the timing of that reoperation.

How likely is it that antibiotic therapy alone will cure PVE? No randomized studies of medical versus combined medical-surgical treatment exist. In studies of medically treated patients prior to the availability of echocardiography, we have to accept some imprecision in those diagnoses, and some patients considered to have received successful medical treatment of PVE may not have actually had PVE. We do know that antibiotic treatment can sterilize bioprosthetic valves when infection of only the leaflet exists. And we know that antibiotic treatment occasionally appears to sterilize a valve, even in the presence of some degree of periprosthetic leak, but that favorable outcome is probably not common.

Most patients with PVE who are treated with only antibiotics do not have good outcomes. Ivert and colleagues documented a mortality rate of 70% with only antibiotic therapy, and Calderwood and colleagues found that of patients with complicated PVE (involving a new heart murmur, congestive heart failure, electrocardiogram conduction abnormalities, or evidence of an abscess), only 21% survived even the hospital stay.[18,19] These are older series, but even in a more recent era, Yu and colleagues noted a survival rate of 44% over a 1-year follow-up for medical therapy alone, as compared to 77% with combined medical-surgical therapy.[20] John and colleagues reported a series of patients with *S. aureus* PVE treated medically with only 7 of 19 patients surviving 90 days with antibiotic treatment alone.[21] Thus, despite improved antibiotics, outcomes are still poor without reoperation, particularly for patients with early endocarditis and with annular involvement.

In the past, the combined medical-surgical treatment has not been a panacea. Reported in-hospital mortality rates from experienced centers include 23% from Stanford (1982),[22] 23% from Massachusetts General Hospital (1986),[19] and 20% in our own pre-1984 series from The Cleveland Clinic Foundation.[4] However, surgical treatment has improved. We found that our in-hospital mortality rate dropped from 20% to 10% from the 1971 to 1984 time frame to the 1985 to 1992 time frame.

The use of homograft aortic root replacement is a step forward in the treatment of active aortic valve PVE. During the years 1988 to 2000, my colleagues and I reoperated on 103 patients with aortic PVE, using homograft aortic root replacement. These patients represented complicated PVE—cultures were positive in 90%, abscess formation had occurred in 78%, and 68% had congestive heart failure. In 27 patients the ascending aorta had been replaced previously in addition to the aortic valve. Four patients (3.9%) died in hospital, all presenting with early, active aortic valve PVE. Complete heart block occurred in 31 patients (30%). Four additional patients underwent reoperation for suspected recurrent PVE, three experiencing

prolonged survival after re-reoperation. Overall late survival was 90%, 73%, and 56% at 1, 5, and 10 postoperative years, respectively. Reports from Haydock and McGiffin and colleagues also note improved outcomes associated with the use of aortic valve allografts (Figure 27-16) although not all patients in these reports had PVE, some cases of native valve endocarditis being included.

Few studies have followed patients with PVE over the long term, but those that have clearly show that long-term survival is unfavorable when compared with patients undergoing valve surgery for noninfectious pathology. For example, David and colleagues noted a 67% 5-year survival rate for patients treated surgically for active PVE.[23] In our overall series of patients undergoing reoperation for active and healed PVE, the late survival and reoperation-free survival rates were 83% and 76% at 5 years, respectively. Most of that experience antedated our extensive use of homografts, and although those 5-year outcomes are favorable, not all patients in that series had active endocarditis, and those figures do not include in-hospital mortality. In our opinion, the results of the homograft aortic root strategy for the treatment of aortic PVE have produced a better early and late survival than has so far been noted for patients with such complicated PVE and represents our strategy for all patients with isolated aortic valve PVE.

The Ross operation (pulmonic valve autotransplantation) has also been reported as a surgical approach to aortic PVE, and in experienced hands it appears to have been a successful treatment.[24] Whether this concept has advantages over the use of homografts is not yet clear.

The success of homografts in the aortic position has led to attempts to use mitral valve homografts to treat mitral valve PVE. Few cases have been reported, and the outcomes of that strategy are at present not known.

Fungal endocarditis represents a special group of patients. For patients with aortic valve fungal endocarditis, aortic root homograft replacement, combined with

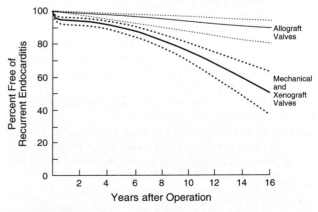

FIGURE 27-16. Parametric estimate of freedom from recurrent endocarditis for patients with mechanical and xenograft valves versus allograft aortic valves, with 70% confidence limits (*dotted lines*). Reproduced with permission from McGiffin DC et al.[15]

2 months of intravenous antifungal therapy and followed by indefinite oral antifungal therapy, has resulted in consistent cures.[25] In our series, the only patients with fungal aortic valve PVE for whom this strategy failed were those patients whose organism was not sensitive to antifungal therapy.

For all patients undergoing surgery for PVE, prolonged postoperative treatment with intravenous antibiotics is important. We treat patients with evidence of active endocarditis for at least 6 weeks after the date of operation with intravenous antibiotics, and all patients are followed up with postoperative transesophageal echo studies. There is some logic in treating patients with bacterial PVE with lifelong oral antibiotics, our current strategy for fungal PVE. However, for many bacteria there are no effective oral antibiotics that are available.

The improvements in the treatment of PVE have come during a period where a few resistant organisms have existed. Despite the importance of effective surgery, effective antibiotics are necessary for the consistently successful treatment of PVE, and the emergence of resistant organisms would represent a serious problem.

References

1. Blackstone EH, Kirklin JW. Death and other time-related events after valve replacement. Circulation 1985;72: 753–67.

2. Calderwood SB, Swinski LA, Waternaux CM, et al. Risk factors for the development of prosthetic valve endocarditis. Circulation 1985;72:31–7.

3. Gordon SM, Serkey JM, Longworth DL, et al. Early onset prosthetic valve endocarditis: The Cleveland Clinic experience 1992–1997. Ann Thorac Surg 2000;69: 1388–92.

4. Lytle BW, Priest BP, Taylor PC, et al. Surgical treatment of prosthetic valve endocarditis. J Thorac Cardiovasc Surg 1996;111:198–210.

5. Agnihotri AK, McGiffin DC, Galbraith AJ, O'Brien MF. The prevalence of infective endocarditis after aortic valve replacement. J Thorac Cardiovasc Surg 1995;110: 1708–24.

6. Grover FL, Cohen DJ, Oprian C, et al. Determinants of the occurrence of and survival from prosthetic valve endocarditis. Experience of the Veterans Affairs Cooperative Study on valvular heart disease. J Thorac Cardiovasc Surg 1994;108:207–14.

7. Keys TF. Early onset prosthetic valve endocarditis. Cleve Clin J Med 1993;60:455–9.

8. Fang G, Keys TF, Gentry LO, et al. Prosthetic valve endocarditis resulting from nosocomial bacteremia. A prospective, multicenter study. Ann Intern Med 1993; 119:560–7.

9. Hammermeister KE, Sethi GK, Henderson WG, et al. A comparison of outcomes in men 11 years after heart-valve replacement with a mechanical valve or bioprosthesis. N Engl J Med 1993;328:1289–96.

10. Lytle BW, Cosgrove DM, Taylor PC, et al. Primary isolated aortic valve replacement: early and late results. J Thorac Cardiovasc Surg 1989;97:675–94.

11. Sabik JF, Lytle BW, Blackstone EH, et al. Aortic root replacement with cryopreserved allograft for prosthetic valve endocarditis. Ann Thorac Surg. [In press]

12. Durack DT, Lukes AS, Bright DK. New criteria for diagnosis of infective endocarditis: utilization of specific echocardiographic findings. Am J Med 1994;96:200–9.

13. Stewart WJ, Shan F. The diagnosis of prosthetic valve endocarditis by echocardiography. Semin Thorac Cardiovasc Surg 1995;7:7–12.

14. Buckberg GD. Studies of controlled reperfusion after ischemia. I. When is cardiac muscle damaged irreversibly? J Thorac Cardiovasc Surg 1986;92:483–7.

15. McGiffin DC, Galbraith AJ, McLachlan GJ, et al. Aortic valve infection. Risk factors for death and recurrent endocarditis after aortic valve replacement. J Thorac Cardiovasc Surg 1992;104:511–20.

16. McGiffin DC, Kirklin JK. The impact of aortic valve homografts on the treatment of aortic prosthetic valve endocarditis. Semin Thorac Cardiovasc Surg 1995;7:25–31.

17. Lytle BW. Prosthetic valve endocarditis. In: Vlessis AA, Bolling SF, editors. Endocarditis: a multidisciplinary approach to modern treatment. Vol 14. Armonk (NY): Futura Publishing; 1999. p. 339–75.

18. Ivert TS, Dismukes WE, Cobbs CB, et al. Prosthetic valve endocarditis. Circulation 1984;69:223–32.

19. Calderwood SB, Swinski LA, Karchmer AW, et al. Prosthetic valve endocarditis: analysis of factors affecting outcome of therapy. J Thorac Cardiovasc Surg 1986;92:776–83.

20. Yu VL, Fang GD, Keys TF, et al. Prosthetic valve endocarditis: superiority of surgical valve replacement versus medical therapy only. Ann Thorac Surg 1994;58:1073–7.

21. John MD, Hibberd PL, Karchmer AW, et al. Staphylococcus aureus prosthetic valve endocarditis: optimal management and risk factors for death. Clin Infect Dis 1998;26: 1302–9.

22. Baumgartner WA, Miller DC, Reitz, BA, et al. Surgical treatment of prosthetic valve endocarditis. Ann Thorac Surg 1983;35:87–104.

23. David TE, Bos J, Christakis GT, et al. Heart valve operations in patients with active endocarditis. Ann Thorac Surg 1990;49:701–5.

24. Joyce F, Tingleff J, Pettersson G. The Ross operation: results of early experience including treatment for endocarditis. Eur J Cardiothorac Surg 1995;9(7):384–92.

25. Muehrcke DD, Lytle BW, Cosgrove DM. Surgical and long-term antifungal therapy for fungal prosthetic valve endocarditis. Ann Thorac Surg 1995;60:538–43.

CHAPTER 28

CARDIAC REOPERATIONS IN ADULTS WITH CONGENITAL HEART DISEASE

WILLIAM G. WILLIAMS, MD, FRCSC, DAVID A. ASHBURN JR, MD, GARY D. WEBB, MD, FRCPC

Patients with congenital heart disease require life-long medical care, and as adults they may need cardiac reoperation. At present, 50% of patients with congenital heart disease (CHD) are older than age 18 years; in the future, the majority of patients with CHD will be adults.[1] In Canada, there are nearly 100,000 adults with CHD, and the population will continue to grow. In the United States, there are more than 800,000 adults with CHD.[2]

Organization of Adult Congenital Cardiac Care

Medical care for the adult with congenital heart disease should be organized so that regional centers provide specialized tertiary level care and support for smaller specialist centers, referring cardiologists, and community physicians.[3] Tertiary adult congenital cardiac heart disease (ACHD) centers should serve a minimum population of 5 to 10 million.[4] The tertiary centers must provide a comprehensive team of experts who are capable of providing professional care and advice in specialties such as cardiology, electrophysiology, cardiac surgery, anesthesia, exercise physiology, obstetrics, and vocational counseling. All cardiology and cardiac surgery programs should be affiliated with an ACHD center, which, in turn, should be affiliated with a tertiary pediatric cardiac service.

Cardiac Reoperations

Adults with congenital heart disease may present without prior intervention, but that population is diminishing. In contrast, there is a growing population of adults with previous surgery who need reoperation. The trend in adult congenital surgery is illustrated by our experience (Figure 28-1). Since 1972, we have operated on 1,267 adults (1,336 operations) with CHD, including 442 who required reoperation. Over the entire experience, reoperations account for 36% of all ACHD operations and for 54% during the past 10 years. Mean age at reoperation is 33.4 years (range, 16.5 to 72.6 years).

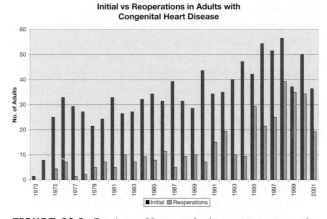

FIGURE 28-1. Trend over 28 years of primary versus reoperative cardiac surgery in adults with congenital heart disease. Reoperation accounts for 34% of all adult congenital operations and, in recent years, it accounts for 54%.

Among these 442 adults, there were 485 reoperations. The majority of reoperations (329) followed a previous intracardiac repair (Table 28-1), and these patients are the focus of this chapter. These types of previous repairs are listed in Table 28-2. The other reoperations were preceded by previous extracardiac palliation or repair. Among the adults with previous extracardiac repair, the majority (25 of 33 [76%]) had a previous coarctation repair, and the remainder had a variety of other lesions.

Sternal Reentry

Sternal reentry is fraught with the risk of cardiac injury. The loss of pericardial integrity from previous cardiac

TABLE 28-1. Previous Surgery in 442 Adults with CHD Requiring Reoperation.

Previous Surgery	% of Total
Palliation	25
Extracardiac repair	7
Intracardiac Repair	68

TABLE 28-2. Initial Diagnosis in Reoperated Adults with Prior Intracardiac Repair of CHD

Diagnosis at Previous Repair	N	% of Total
Tetralogy repair	139	42
Subaortic stenosis*	31	9
Fontan	30	9
ASD repair†	29	9
VSD repair	20	6
Coarctation repair	5	2
Other	75	23
Total	329	100

*16 with HOCM, 11 fibromuscular, and 4 other LVOT obstruction.

†20 with previous AVSD repair, 7 secundum atrial defects, and 2 sinus venosus defects.

ASD = atrial septal defect; AVSD = atrioventricular septal defect; HOCM = hypertrophic obstructive cardiomyopathy; LVOT = left ventricular outflow tract; VSD = ventricular septal defect.

surgery enables the cardiac structures to adhere to the sternum and chest wall. Patients with enlarged or hypertensive right-heart structures are at increased risk of injury. In addition, morphologic anomalies and/or altered physiology increase the risk of penetrating injuries of the aorta and right ventricle at reentry. For example, patients with complete transposition postatrial repair have adherence of the systemically pressurized right ventricle to the sternum. The ascending aorta in these patients, and in those patients with congenitally corrected transposition, is positioned anteriorly in contact with the sternum. There is similar risk of aortic injury in patients with tetralogy of Fallot or double-outlet right ventricle in whom there is marked dextrorotation of the aorta resulting in apposition of the aorta to the sternum. Another example of potential cardiac injury at sternal reentry is the patient with heart failure in whom the right ventricle may be both enlarged and hypertensive or who has developed right atrial enlargement and increased atrial pressure. Previous implants, such as extracardiac conduits and even pledget material, may increase the risk of cardiac injury at sternal reentry.

Although some patients may be identified to be at increased risk of cardiac injury, one should assume that every patient is at risk of death or serious morbidity at sternal reentry. The entire team of nurses, anesthetists, perfusionists, and surgeons must understand the mechanisms of injury and the protocols to be followed for a coordinated effective response.

Sternal Reentry Technique

Careful dissection under the sternum proceeds by direct vision from the linea alba. We resect the previous sternotomy scar and save the sternal wires by untwisting them so they can be used to provide traction and to gauge the depth of the cut by the sternal saw. The retrosternal dissection extends laterally on both sides of the midline in a moving V-shape. The point of the V is the center of the sternotomy and is never less than a 90° angle. As the plane behind the sternum is cleared, an oscillating saw is used to divide four of the five layers of the sternum; that is, the external periosteum, external cortex, marrow, and internal cortex. The internal periosteum is divided with straight Mayo scissors under direct vision. Division of the sternum proceeds stepwise in a cephalad direction in lengths of 2 to 4 cm. Each sternal cut provides access to further dissection laterally and cephalad, thereby moving the "V" cephalad. Bleeding from the chest wall can usually be controlled by cautery or suture ligation. Bleeding from the right coronary artery can usually be controlled by manual pressure and repaired once on cardiopulmonary bypass.

Judgment as to when dissection behind the sternum should be abandoned in favor of peripheral cannulation with support of the circulation by cardiopulmonary bypass is based upon experience tempered by an assessment of each individual patient's risk. The femoral artery and vein or alternate vessels should be available in the sterile field and exposed if there is serious concern about the safety of retrosternal dissection. In addition, the patient is fully heparinized at the initiation of the retrosternal dissection to avoid delay if emergent cannulation is required. On balance, peripheral cannulation is a lesser evil than persisting with a difficult dissection. Adding Y connectors to the arterial and venous pump lines permits transfer of perfusion cannulae after the heart is exposed, an important consideration in lengthy operations to lessen the complications of peripheral cannulation.

Complications of Sternal Reentry

It is important to have a protocol to manage the potential complications of dissecting the adherent cardiac structures from the chest wall. To do this, one must understand the mechanisms by which cardiac injury results in morbidity and mortality. Cardiac arrhythmia and bleeding are the major risks of sternal reentry.

Cardiac arrhythmia may develop from mechanical or electrical stimulation of the heart, especially with electrocautery. The surgeon and assistant should monitor cardiac rhythm by observing each heart beat within the chest and by listening to the pulse Doppler signal. The electrocardiogram (ECG) monitor is less helpful because the electrocautery will interfere with the electrical signal. Therefore, the surgeon should detect a rhythm change before the anesthetist. Ventricular tachycardia or fibrillation requires defibrillation. A defibrillator and its paddles, both external and internal types, should be immediately available. Defibrillator pads positioned on the chest wall prior to draping will simplify and expedite defibrillation. Supraventricular tachycardia may also require cardioversion.

Patients with pacemakers should be tested preoperatively to determine their underlying rhythm and intrinsic rate. After anesthetic induction, the pacemaker should be reprogrammed to fixed rate mode (VOO) at a rate of 80 to 100 bpm to prevent inappropriate cautery-induced pacemaker inhibition. Reprogramming to backup demand pacing will be required later during the operation, relying on temporary external atrial and ventricular leads to control postbypass rate and rhythm.

Bleeding from inadvertent injury to cardiac and vascular structures is the most serious complication of sternal reentry. Bleeding may be venous (from injury to the right ventricle, right atrium, innominate vein, or, rarely, the pulmonary artery) or arterial (from injury to the mammary arteries, right coronary artery, or aorta). The source of bleeding, whether venous or arterial, has critical implications. It is important to understand that bleeding per se is not usually fatal; rather, it is the complications that result from the bleeding or its management.

When massive bleeding occurs, cardiopulmonary bypass should be initiated immediately. Suction lines from the pump are used to return blood lost from the chest to the venous reservoir. Control of perfusion parameters is essential as discussed below.

If the bleeding is venous, the dissection may proceed with cardiopulmonary bypass support and modest hypothermia (35°C). Lacerations in the right heart can usually be repaired easily when the circulation is supported, and tension on the area of the laceration can be relieved by freeing up adjacent adhesions. It is essential that the central venous pressure be maintained positive, ideally +4 to +6 mm Hg. If a negative venous pressure is allowed to develop, air will be entrained into the heart and venous return line, thereby creating an airlock that will stop inflow to the pump. More importantly, any patient with an intracardiac shunt is at risk of systemic air embolism and irreversible brain damage.

If the bleeding is arterial, the site is compressed (for example, by clamping the partially open sternum with a towel clip) and cardiopulmonary bypass with cooling to profound hypothermia is initiated immediately. Further dissection should *not* proceed until the heart arrests, at which point the perfusion rate can be decreased to facilitate exposure. Opening the sternum while the heart is beating in the presence of an aortic laceration must be avoided because air will enter the aorta with each diastole and cause irreversible brain injury. In addition, it is most unlikely that the laceration can be controlled while the heart is ejecting. Carefully controlled perfusion cooling, not allowing perfusate temperature to fall below 15°C, and maintenance of optimal venous and arterial pressures should allow the heart to continue beating until the core temperature is less than 20° or 25°C. With the heart arrested by hypothermia and the core temperature low, bypass flow rates can be adjusted to allow control of the laceration. Circulatory arrest should be unnecessary and would complicate the control of air within the circulation.

Operative Risk for Reoperation

In our patients, there were 15 operative deaths (4.5%) following reoperation after previous intracardiac repair. During the same period the operative mortality for adults with congenital cardiac lesions and no previous surgery was 2.7%. The operative risk for reoperation decreased from 6.1% during the first half of this experience to 3.1% more recently. The trend in operative mortality is illustrated by the Cusum method (Figure 28-2). Long-term survival 10 years after reoperation in our patients with previous intracardiac repair is 79% (± 4 %).

Summary

Safe sternal reentry requires an experienced and integrated team, with all members understanding the mechanisms of injury and the protocol to provide a coordinated response to deal with every possible situation.

Management of Specific Lesions

Adults with CHD requiring reoperation may have almost any primary or secondary cardiac diagnosis. It would be impractical to describe the management of all possible lesions, and limited experience with the infrequent lesions precludes meaningful generalization. Therefore, we will describe two of the more prevalent lesions seen in the adult with CHD presenting for reoperation.

Tetralogy of Fallot

The adult with repaired tetralogy may present with either right- or left-sided lesions. The "unnatural history" late after repair depends upon residual lesions. All patients after tetralogy repair have either residual right ventricular outlet stenosis and/or pulmonary valve insufficiency. Either is usually well tolerated for many years, but there is accumulating evidence that the adult with repaired tetralogy is at increasing risk of developing symptoms after age 30 years.

Symptoms develop with decompensation of the right ventricle, usually from dilation and reduced ventricular contractility, and if there is stenosis, increasing hypertrophy. Branch pulmonary stenosis accelerates the rate of right ventricular decompensation. The right ventricle may become electrically unstable due to fibrosis or regional ischemia and become the site of origin of ventricular tachycardia or fibrillation. Gatzoulis and colleagues identified

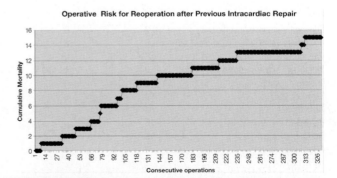

FIGURE 28-2. Cusum plot of operative mortality. The operative mortality declined from 6.1% during the first half of the experience to 3.1% since 1991.

the QRS width (> 0.180 s) and prolonged QT dispersion as risk factors for late sudden death.[5]

Progressive right ventricular failure may lead to dilation of the tricuspid annulus and distortion of the tricuspid papillary muscle support, resulting in tricuspid regurgitation. Severe tricuspid regurgitation aggravates right-heart failure, and the accompanying right atrial dilation predisposes to atrial flutter or fibrillation.

Residual ventricular or atrial septal defects will compromise the late results after tetralogy repair. An important ventricular septal defect (VSD) would almost certainly be resolved during childhood, but a small VSD may compound the effects of right ventricular outflow tract (RVOT) lesions.

Left-sided lesions seem to occur in older patients whose initial repairs were at an older age. The aortic root may dilate and progress to aortic valve insufficiency and an aortic root aneurysm.

CLINICAL EXPERIENCE

Adults with repaired tetralogy of Fallot are the most prevalent congenital cardiac group requiring reoperation. Tetralogy accounted for 139 of the 329 (42%) reoperations in patients with previous intracardiac repair. A total of 132 adults with tetralogy (mean age, 33.4 years) underwent reoperation, including 6 who had 7 further reoperations as adults (Table 28-3). The mean interval between these seven reoperations is 11.3 years (range, 2.1 to 17.7 years).

The indications for reoperation late after tetralogy of Fallot repair are outlined in the Canadian Consensus Conference on Adult Congenital Heart Disease (Table 28-4).[6] In our series, right ventricular outlet lesions are the dominant primary pathology and account for 76% of the reoperations. Most patients had more than one lesion. Although arrhythmia was the primary diagnosis leading to reoperation in only 3 patients, important atrial or ventricular arrhythmia was present before reoperation in 55 patients.

Tricuspid valve insufficiency was present in 31 patients. Left-sided lesions account for 5% of the reoperations.

Table 28-5 lists the primary operative procedures at reoperation. Most patients had more than one procedure at reoperation; the average was 2.9 procedures per patient. Pulmonary valve replacement was part of the reoperation in the majority, 121 of 139 reoperations (87%). Concomitant procedures included pulmonary arterioplasty in 59 reoperations, arrhythmia ablation in 43, tricuspid valve repair or replacement in 31, closure of a residual VSD in 12, and aortic root surgery in 7. The technique of pulmonary valve replacement was orthotopic placement of the largest porcine valve (usually 29 to 33 mm), accommodated by patch enlargement of the annulus and main pulmonary artery.

Operative survival following reoperation is 97.8%. Two of the three deaths occurred in patients requiring combined pulmonary valve replacement and aortic root replacement, and the third occurred 13 days post pulmonary valve replacement due to perforation of the esophagus by a vascular ring consisting of an aberrant subclavian artery used in a remote Blalock-Taussig shunt.

TABLE 28-4. Canadian Consensus Conference: Indications for Reoperation in Tetralogy of Fallot

Residual pulmonary stenosis: RV pressure > two-thirds systemic pressure

Free pulmonary insufficiency: with RV enlargement, worsening tricuspid insufficiency, sustained arrhythmia, or progressive symptoms

Residual VSD: shunt > 1.5:1

Aortic insufficiency: symptomatic and/or progressive LV enlargement or dysfunction

Aortic root dilatation: 5.5 cm or greater

RV outflow tract aneurysm: rapid enlargement, or evidence of infection or pseudoaneurysm

Major cardiac arrhythmias (atrial flutter or fibrillation, ventricular tachycardia), which may reflect hemodynamic deterioration

Combined mild-moderate residual VSD, pulmonary stenosis, and regurgitation leading to RV enlargement/dysfunction or symptoms

LV = left ventricular; RV = right ventricular; VSD = ventricular septal defect.

TABLE 28-3. Diagnosis at Reoperation in 132 Adults with Prior Intracardiac Repair of Tetralogy of Fallot

Diagnosis at Reoperation	N	% of Total
Pulmonary insufficiency	61	44
Pulmonary stenosis/insufficiency	9	6
Pulmonary valve/subvalvular stenosis	8	6
Prosthetic valve/conduit failure	27	19
Pulmonary artery stenosis	2	1
Tricuspid insufficiency	5	4
Residual VSD	9	6
Arrhythmia*	3	2
Re-repair	5	4
Aortic pathology	6	4
Mitral insufficiency	1	1
AV fistula	3	2
Total Reoperations	139	100

*Fifty-seven patients had associated preoperative arrhythmia.

AV = arterion nous; VSD = ventricular septal defect.

TABLE 28-5. Reoperative Procedures in Adults with Prior Intracardiac Repair of Tetralogy of Fallot

Primary Procedure	N
Pulmonary valve replacement	106
VSD repair	8
Revision of RVOT	6
AVR/ascending aorta	5
Tricuspid repair/replacement	5
Arrhythmia ablation	3
Takedown of previous shunt	3
Re-repair	2
Mitral valve repair	1
Total reoperations	139

AVR = aortic valve replacement; RVOT = right ventricular outflow tract; VSD = ventricular septal defect.

The number of previous operations may increase risk, although there were no deaths among the six patients who required a second, and in one patient, a third, reoperation as adults. The number of intraoperative concomitant procedures did not seem to affect operative risk, nor did the individual procedures, except perhaps aortic root surgery, where there were 2 deaths among 7 patients as compared to 1 death among the 132 without aortic root surgery. There was no operative mortality among the 30 patients having repair ($n = 26$) or replacement ($n = 4$) of the tricuspid valve. There were three late deaths, 4 months to 8 years after tricuspid surgery. Arrhythmia ablation was associated with 1 death among 43 patients (2.3%), which is not a different rate than that among those not having an ablation.

Late follow-up of these patients is important, and various aspects of their outcome have been published.[7–10] Pulmonary valve replacement inevitably requires subsequent further replacement, although we have estimated valve survival in this population to be 90% at 10 years after implant.[11] Among the 121 adults undergoing pulmonary valve replacement there were three re-replacements at 3, 12, and 18 years after implant. There is symptomatic improvement following pulmonary valve replacement, but it is more difficult to obtain objective evidence of functional improvement.[12] It may be as Therrien suggests: these patients have irreversible damage to the right ventricle and are too late to derive hemodynamic benefit from valve replacement. We have shown that the risk of reoperation late after tetralogy repair is reasonably low, and earlier intervention should be considered to obtain maximal functional ability for the adult with tetralogy.

Arrhythmia and Reoperation in the Adult after Previous Repair of Congenital Heart Disease

As patients with CHD age, either with or without previous intracardiac repair, they are at increasing risk of arrhythmia.[13] The mechanisms accounting for the increasing prevalence of arrhythmia with age include dilation of atrial or ventricular chambers, surgical incisions and scars, intramyocardial fibrosis, and ischemia.[5,14,15]

Operative Techniques for Arrhythmia Ablation

The operative technique for ventricular tachycardia (VT) requires electrophysiologic mapping after programmed electrical stimulation to induce VT. The patient must be prepared for cardiopulmonary bypass prior to inducing VT. If the site of VT is multiple or the VT cannot be induced, then ablation is not possible.

If induction is successful, epicardial and endocardial mapping identifies the site of origin.[16] After cardioplegic arrest of the heart, the site of origin and reentry circuit is frozen to –60°C for 2 min. Generally, three to six overlapping cryolesions are sufficient. Postcryolesion induction

of VT is attempted intraoperatively and repeated prior to hospital discharge.

For supraventricular tachycardia, ablation techniques vary with the type of arrhythmia. For atrial flutter, we place three to five overlapping cryolesions with a 15 mm probe between the inferior vena cava, tricuspid valve, and atrial septum, rightward of the coronary sinus orifice. For atrial fibrillation secondary to right-sided cardiac lesions, we use a right-sided maze operation as described by Danielson.[17] However, if the left side of the heart is involved, a complete bilateral maze is used.

Reentry tachycardias due to accessory atrioventricular antegrade or retrograde bypass tracts are divided by using the techniques described by Sealy.[18]

Clinical Experience

Among the 329 reoperations late after previous intracardiac repair of congenital lesions, 72 (22%) had important clinical arrhythmia prior to reoperation.

Supraventricular tachycardia (SVT) was present in 43 patients and ventricular tachycardia in 37, with 8 patients having both arrhythmias. Patients with SVT were older at reoperation than those with VT (39.5 vs 34.2 years). All VT patients had tetralogy of Fallot, whereas among those with SVT, 29 had tetralogy of Fallot and the others had a variety of pathology: six had univentricular heart; two had atrioventricular discordance; three had atrial septal defects; one had ventricular septal defect; and one had pulmonary atresia with intact septum. One patient had an anatomically normal heart and Wolff-Parkinson-White syndrome.

The operative risk among patients with arrhythmia was 1.4% as compared to 5.6% among those without arrhythmia. Ablation was performed in 55 patients with 1 death (1.8%), and there were no operative deaths among the 17 patients in whom arrhythmia was present but not ablated.

Table 28-6 lists the ablation techniques used. For atrial flutter ($n = 29$) cryoablation of the atrial isthmus between the inferior vena cava, tricuspid valve, and atrial septum was our treatment of choice. In treating atrial fibrillation ($n = 14$), a right atrial maze was used if the cardiac lesion was entirely right-sided and a full maze if the cardiac lesion affected both sides of the heart.[16]

The location of the VT circuit was the junction of the infundibular septum and parietal band along the upper margin of the VSD repair in 23 of the 29 patients in whom the location could be identified during intraoperative electrophysiologic mapping. In four patients, it was multifocal. In one patient, VT was localized in the anterior wall of the right ventricular outflow tract, and in another patient it was located at the base of the anterior papillary muscle. In eight patients, intraoperative mapping was unsuccessful because VT could not be induced. The site of VT was treated by cryotherapy in 28 patients and resection in one. There were no early deaths among the patients with ventricular tachycardia.

TABLE 28-6. Intraoperative Ablative Techniques for Tachyarrhythmias in Adults with Prior Congenital Heart Disease Repair

Technique	SVT	VT
Cryothermy*	24	24
RA maze	11	0
Full maze	2	0
None	4	13
Fontan conversion	2	0
Total	43	37

*Of eight patients with both SVT and VT, five had cryothermy of both arrhythmias and three had cryothermy of SVT alone.

RA = right atrial; SVT = supraventricular tachycardia; VT = ventricular tachycardia.

Discussion

Our initial experience in managing adults with tachyarrhythmia at reoperation after previous intracardiac repair indicates that intraoperative electrophysiologic mapping of the arrhythmia and ablation techniques can be done safely. Both early and late mortality may be better after ablation. Late follow-up of these patients is needed to determine the long-term efficacy of arrhythmia ablation and whether some ablation techniques yield better results than others. Among patients with VT, repair of the associated cardiac lesions will decrease the late prevalence of arrhythmia either with or without concomitant ablation.[19] However, successful repair of associated lesions is not sufficient to alleviate postoperative arrhythmia in patients with SVT, and ablation techniques are particularly important in this group of patients.

Summary of Reoperations in Adults with Congenital Heart Disease

As children with congenital heart disease mature into adults, they continue to need life-long expert medical and surgical care. The prevalence of congenital heart disease in the adult is increasing. The aging adult is at increasing risk of deterioration from residual lesions or of developing new lesions that may require reoperation. Reoperation after previous intracardiac repair of congenital cardiac lesions can be offered at low risk in most adult patients. Reoperation provides substantial improvement in their quality of life and longevity.

References

1. Webb GD, Williams RG. Thirty-second Bethesda Conference. Care of the adult with congenital heart disease: introduction. J Am Coll Cardiol 2001;37:1166–9.
2. Warnes CA, Liberthson R, Danielson GK, et al. Task Force 1: the changing profile of congenital heart disease in adult life. J Am Coll Cardiol 2001;37:1170–5.
3. Connelly MS, Webb GD, Somerville J, et al. Canadian consensus conference on adult congenital heart disease 1996. Can J Cardiol 1998;14:395–402.
4. Landzberg MJ, Murphy DJ, Davidson WR, et al. Task Force 4: organization of delivery systems for adults with congenital heart disease. J Am Coll Cardiol 2001;37:1187–93.
5. Gatzoulis MA, Till JA, Somerville J, Redington AN. Mechano-electrical interaction in tetralogy of Fallot: QRS prolongation relates to right ventricular size and predicts malignant ventricular arrhythmias and sudden death. Circulation 1995;92:231–7.
6. Therrien J, Gatzoulis M, Graham T, et al. Canadian Cardiovascular Society consensus conference 2001 update: recommendations for the management of adults with congenital heart disease—Part II. Can J Cardiol 2001;17:940–59.
7. Bove EL, Kavey RE, Byrum CJ, et al. Improved right ventricular function following late pulmonary valve replacement for residual pulmonary insufficiency or stenosis. J Thorac Cardiovasc Surg 1985;90:50–5.
8. Ilbawi MN, Idriss FS, DeLeon SY, et al. Long-term results of porcine valve insertion for pulmonary regurgitation following repair of tetralogy of Fallot. Ann Thorac Surg 1986;41:478–82.
9. Oechslin EN, Harrison DA, Harris L, et al. Reoperation in adults with repair of tetralogy of Fallot: indications and outcomes. J Thorac Cardiovasc Surg 1999;118:245–51.
10. Williams WG, Harris L, Downer E, et al. Reoperation late after repair of tetralogy of Fallot; indications, timing and outcome. In: Gatzoulis MA, Murphy DJ Jr, editors. The adult with congenital heart disease. New York: Futura Publishing; 2001. p 81–91.
11. Yemets IM, Williams WG, Webb GD, et al. Pulmonary valve replacement late after repair of tetralogy of Fallot. Ann Thorac Surg 1997;64:526–30.
12. Therrien J, Siu SS, McLaughlin PR, et al. Pulmonary valve replacement in adults late after repair of tetralogy of Fallot: are we operating too late? J Am Coll Cardiol 2000;36:1670–5.
13. Silka MJ, Hardy BG, Menashe VD, Morris CD. A population-based prospective evaluation of risk of sudden cardiac death after operation for common congenital heart defects. J Am Coll Cardiol 1998;32:245–51.
14. Bharati S, Lev M. Conduction system in cases of sudden death in congenital heart disease many years after surgical correction. Chest 1986;90:861–8.
15. Shen WK, Holmes DR, Porter CJ, et al. Sudden death after repair of double-outlet right ventricle. Circulation 1990;81:128–36.
16. Downar E, Harris L, Kimber S, et al. Ventricular tachycardia after surgical repair of tetralogy of Fallot: results of intraoperative mapping studies. J Am Coll Cardiol 1992;20:648–55.
17. Theodoro DA, Danielson GK, Porter CJ, Warnes CA. Right-sided maze procedure for right atrial arrhythmias in congenital heart disease. Ann Thorac Surg 1998;65:149–54.
18. Sealy WC, Anderson RW, Gallagher JJ. Surgical treatment of supraventricular tachyarrhythmias. J Thorac Cardiovasc Surg 1977;73:511–22.
19. Harrison DA, Harris L, Siu SC, et al. Sustained ventricular tachycardia in adult patients late after repair of tetralogy of Fallot. J Am Coll Cardiol 1997;30:1368–73.

CHAPTER 29

THE MINIMALLY INVASIVE MAZE PROCEDURE

JAMES L. COX, MD

The standard Maze procedure has proven to be extremely effective in curing atrial fibrillation.[1–3] However, as originally described, it required a median sternotomy and cardiopulmonary bypass. Both factors have limited the use of the Maze procedure either as a stand-alone operation or as an adjunctive measure in patients undergoing other types of cardiac surgery.

After establishing the safety and efficacy of the Maze procedure in the 1980s and then realizing that it would not be widely applied by others because of its complexity, I set out to develop a minimally invasive version of the procedure. As its usage has evolved in cardiac surgery, the term "minimally invasive" has no consensus single definition and is applied equally to cardiac surgery patients who have small skin incisions but who avoid cardiopulmonary bypass (eg, minimally invasive direct coronary artery bypass, [MIDCAB]) and to patients who have full median sternotomies without cardiopulmonary bypass (eg, off-pump coronary artery bypass [OPCAB]). Likewise, as the minimally invasive Maze procedure evolved, two versions were developed: one that required a median sternotomy but with minimal, and occasionally no, cardiopulmonary bypass support, and one that

required only a small (7-cm) incision but always with the aid of cardiopulmonary bypass.

Median Sternotomy with Limited or No Cardiopulmonary Bypass

Technical Considerations

To avoid the use of cardiopulmonary bypass, it was obvious that the atrial incisions used to create the Maze pattern would have to be replaced by some other type of lesion that would block electrical conduction in the desired locations. Because I had used cryosurgery to treat cardiac arrhythmias for many years,[4–6] I modified our available cryoprobes so that linear cryolesions could by created on the atria (Figure 29-1). I had learned years before that it is essentially impossible to attain a permanent transmural cryolesion in the atrium by placing cryoprobes on the epicardial surface because of the "heat sink" effect of the blood within the atrium, which prevents the endocardium from being permanently frozen. To circumvent this problem, I placed purse string sutures in the atrial wall, passed the linear cryoprobe through

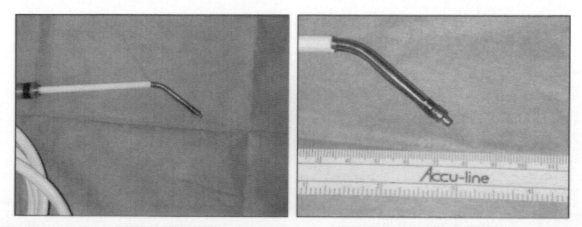

FIGURE 29-1. Linear cryoprobe (CooperSurgical, Inc., Shelton, CT) used to create atrial lesions instead of atrial incisions. This probe uses internally expanding nitrous oxide as a coolant and cools the myocardium to −60°C. Cell death is attained after 2 min at that temperature.

them to the inside of the atrium, and then lifted up on the cryoprobe, thereby making direct contact between the cryoprobe and the atrial endocardium with no warm blood interface.[7] This allowed the atrial wall to be frozen from the inside out to assure a permanent transmural lesion.

After the ablative technique had been established, it was simply a matter of replacing the surgical incisions with linear cryolesions to accomplish this off-pump type of "minimally invasive" Maze procedure. This was a relatively simple conversion for the right-sided lesions. However, the septal and left atrial lesions required additional modifications of the original procedure. For example, it was apparent that it would be much easier to encircle the right pulmonary vein orifices separately from the left pulmonary vein orifices, as opposed to encircling the four of them together. However, this necessitated that the separate pulmonary vein encircling lesions be "connected" to prevent macro-reentrant circuits from forming around the new lesions. I chose to place this additional lesion between the two inferior pulmonary veins. In addition, it was no longer desirable to excise the left atrial appendage; as a result, its base was encircled circumferentially and then tied off or stapled shut from outside the heart. Later, it became apparent that it was just as effective to place a single linear lesion from the tip of the left atrial appendage to its base as it was to encircle its entire base. This observation greatly simplified the left-sided lesions. These technical modifications in the procedure, so that it could be performed "off-pump," maintained the maze concept but resulted in slight changes in the anatomic pattern of the atrial lesions in comparison to the standard Maze 3 pattern of lesions (Figure 29-2).

Surgical Technique

RIGHT ATRIAL LESIONS

A median sternotomy is performed. A purse-string suture is placed in the posterior–lateral right atrium, and a linear cryoprobe is inserted through the purse-string into the inside of the right atrium (Figure 29-3). A cryolesion is placed superiorly to the superior vena cava (SVC). Using the same purse-string suture, a second cryolesion is placed down to the inferior vena cava (IVC) to complete the longitudinal lesion from the SVC to the IVC (Figure 29-4). The first purse-string suture is tied down and a second is placed near the atrioventricular (AV) groove. The cryoprobe is inserted through this second purse-string suture, and the "T" lesion is placed across the lower right atrium (Figure 29-5). Using the same purse-string suture, the "T" linear cryolesion is extended down to the level of the tricuspid valve annulus (Figure 29-6). The second pursestring suture is tied down, and a third purse-string suture is placed in the right atrial appendage. A lateral right atrial cryolesion is then placed, leaving at least 3 cm between its tip and the "T" cryolesion (Figure 29-7). Using the same purse-string suture in the right atrial appendage, a cryolesion is placed from the appendage down to the anteromedial tricuspid valve annulus (Figure 29-8). The interatrial groove is then dissected completely, and the right superior and right inferior pulmonary veins are dissected free anteriorly and posteriorly.

LEFT ATRIAL AND SEPTAL LESIONS

The interatrial groove is then dissected completely, and the right superior and right inferior pulmonary veins are dissected free anteriorly and posteriorly. One linear cryoprobe is placed posterior to the right pulmonary veins as they enter the left atrium (Figure 29-9). A second identical cryoprobe is placed on the anterior surface of the veins in the same plane. Cardiopulmonary bypass is usually instituted at this point. The cryoprobes are then "squeezed" together firmly, resulting in a circumferential transmural cryolesion around the orifices of the right pulmonary veins (Figure 29-10). Purse-string sutures are then placed in the posterior right atrium and in the posterior left atrium. (Figure 29-11). Two linear cryoprobes are placed through these purse-string sutures on either side of the atrial septum and "squeezed" together to create the atrial septal lesion (Figure 29-12).

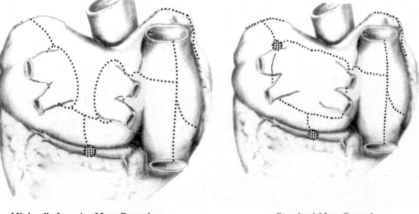

Minimally Invasive Maze Procedure   **Standard Maze Procedure**

FIGURE 29-2. Comparison of pattern of atrial lesions in the minimally invasive cryosurgical procedure and the standard Maze 3 procedure.

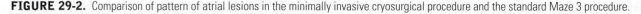

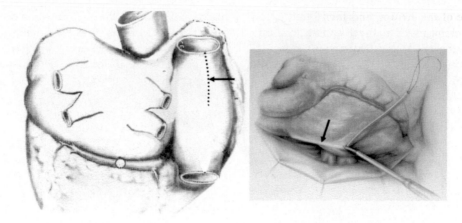

Posterior View   **Surgeon's View**

FIGURE 29-3. Lesion to the superior vena cava.

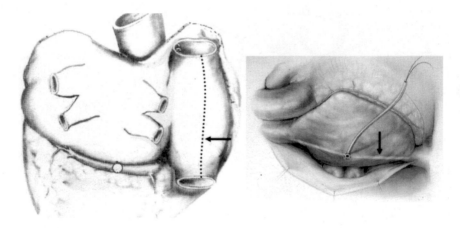

Posterior View   **Surgeon's View**

FIGURE 29-4. Lesion to the inferior vena cava.

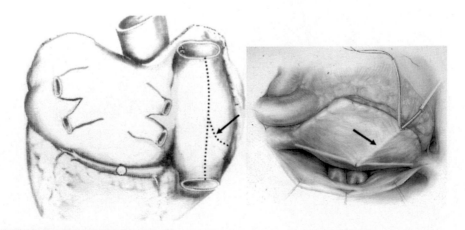

Posterior View   **Surgeon's View**

FIGURE 29-5. Right atrial free-wall portion of the "T" lesion.

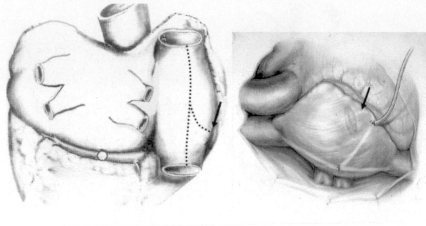

Posterior View **Surgeon's View**

FIGURE 29-6. Completion of the "T" lesion down to the tricuspid valve annulus.

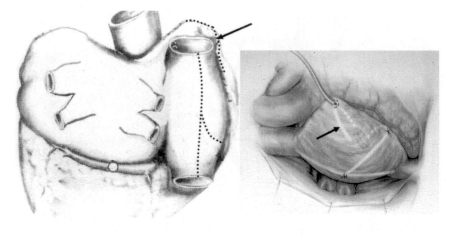

Posterior View **Surgeon's View**

FIGURE 29-7. Lateral right atrial free-wall lesion placed through a purse-string suture in the atrial appendage.

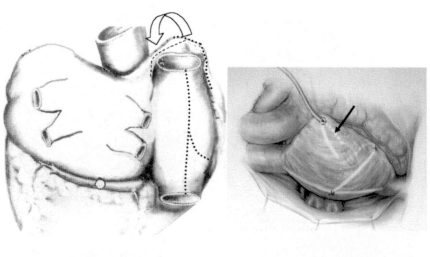

Posterior View **Surgeon's View**

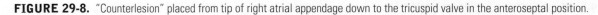

FIGURE 29-8. "Counterlesion" placed from tip of right atrial appendage down to the tricuspid valve in the anteroseptal position.

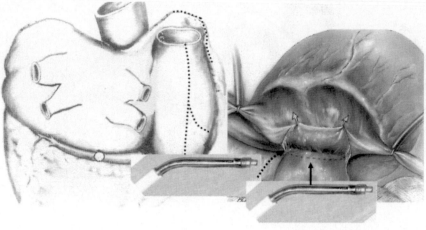

Posterior View

Surgeon's View

FIGURE 29-9. Placement of two linear cryoprobes on the left atrium simultaneously, one posterior and the other anterior to the orifices of the right pulmonary veins, in order to encircle them.

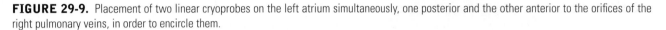

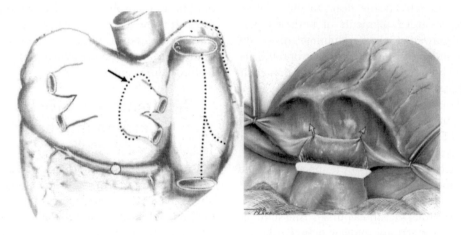

Posterior View

Surgeon's View

FIGURE 29-10. Circumferential cryolesion isolating the orifices of the right pulmonary veins.

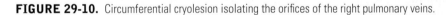

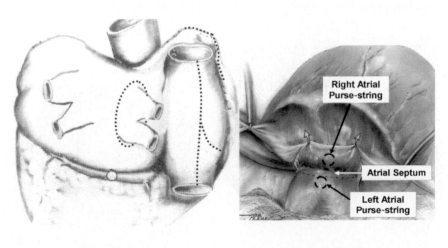

Posterior View

Surgeon's View

FIGURE 29-11. Purse-string sutures on either side of the atrial septum through which two linear cryoprobes are passed simultaneously to create the atrial septal cryolesion.

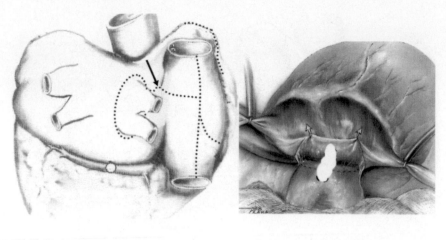

Posterior View

Surgeon's View

FIGURE 29-12. Epicardial extent of the atrial septal cryolesion.

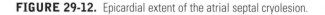

The surgeon then retracts the heart to the right to expose the intrapericardial segments of both left pulmonary veins (Figure 29-13). After minimal dissection around the left pulmonary veins, the two cryoprobes are "clamped" around both left pulmonary veins as they enter the left atrium posteriorly. This results in a circumferential transmural cryolesion around the orifices of the left pulmonary veins (Figure 29-14). A purse-string suture is then placed in the tip of the left atrial appendage, and a linear cryoprobe is inserted inside the atrial appendage. A cryolesion is placed from the tip of the appendage to the left superior pulmonary vein orifice (Figure 29-15).

The apex of the heart is retracted in a cephalad direction out of the pericardial sac, and a purse-string suture is placed in the posterior atrium, midway between the left and right inferior pulmonary veins. Cryolesions are then placed from this purse-string suture into the individual inferior pulmonary veins to "connect" their orifices (Figure 29-16). Using this same purse-string suture, a curved

but linear cryoprobe is placed down to (actually, "up to") the mitral valve annulus (Figure 29-17). Finally, an epicardial cryolesion is placed on the coronary sinus in the same plane as the lesion to the mitral annulus to complete the procedure (Figure 29-18).

Minimally Invasive Incision with Cardiopulmonary Bypass

Technical Considerations

The major problem with using a standard small right thoracotomy to perform the Maze procedure is that it is impossible to excise the left atrial appendage safely. Thus, the first modification of the original Maze procedure that was necessary in order to perform it through a small right thoracotomy was to isolate and close its orifice rather than excise it. This was accomplished with cryoprobes, as described above. Because it is not possible to perform the entire cryosurgical procedure from outside the heart via a

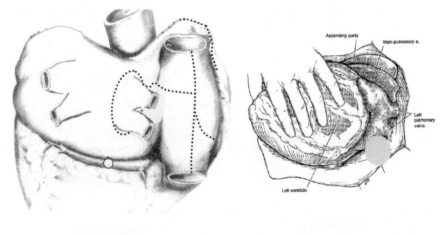

Posterior View

Surgeon's View

FIGURE 29-13. Exposure of the left pulmonary veins.

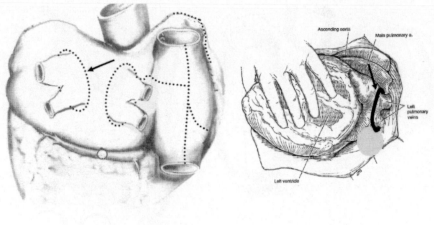

Posterior View

Surgeon's View

FIGURE 29-14. Circumferential cryolesion isolating the orifices of the left pulmonary veins.

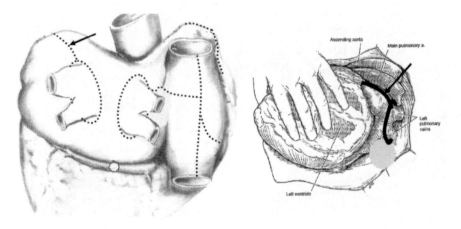

Posterior View

Surgeon's View

FIGURE 29-15. Cryolesion extending from the orifice of the left atrial appendage to its tip, thus preventing macro-reentry around the base of the appendage.

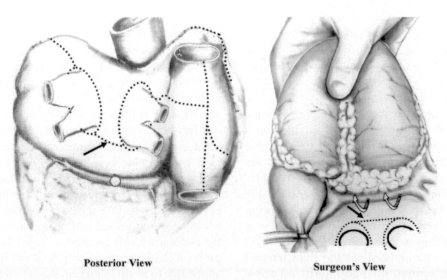

Posterior View

Surgeon's View

FIGURE 29-16. "Connection" of the two inferior pulmonary vein orifices with a linear cryolesion to prevent macro-reentry around their encircling lesions.

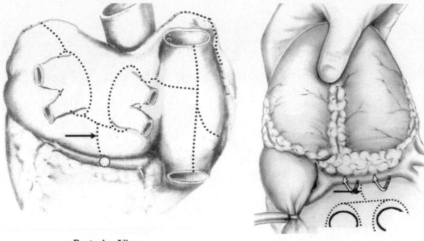

Posterior View

Surgeon's View

FIGURE 29-17. Placement of the critical lesion down to the level of the mitral valve annulus.

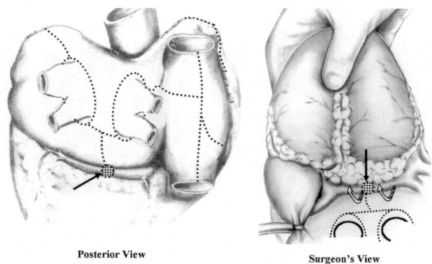

Posterior View

Surgeon's View

FIGURE 29-18. Cryoablation of the coronary sinus.

small right thoracotomy, the major difference between the above "minimally invasive" procedure and the one now described is in the method of placing the left atrial lesions.

Surgical Technique

The patient is positioned in the right anterior oblique position, with the right arm at the side. A 7-cm incision is placed in the fourth intercostal space. A wide malleable retractor is placed beneath the lower blade of a Tuffier retractor to keep the right hemidiaphragm retracted inferiorly. The pericardium is opened 3 cm anterior to the right phrenic nerve to expose the right atrium. Following systemic heparinization, the right femoral artery and vein are cannulated. Tourniquets are passed around the SVC and IVC. The SVC is cannulated via the right internal jugular vein. The IVC cannula tip is positioned just below the level of the diaphragm. The right atrial lesions are placed exactly as described above. In most instances, they

can be placed prior to initiating cardiopulmonary bypass.

Following completion of the right atrial lesions, cardiopulmonary bypass is instituted and the right pulmonary veins are encircled as described above (see Figures 29-9 and 29-10).

The aorta is then cross-clamped and the heart is cardioplegically arrested. A standard left atriotomy is performed, and the atrial septum is cryoablated between two rigid linear cryoprobes (Figure 29-19).

The superior and inferior ends of the standard left atriotomy are then "extended" with the linear cryoprobes rather than by cutting. The left superior pulmonary and left inferior pulmonary vein orifices are cryoablated from the endocardial side by using a large round 2.5-cm cryoprobe. A linear cryolesion is placed out into the left atrial appendage to its tip to prevent macro-reentry from occurring around the base of the appendage postoperatively. The inferior pulmonary veins are "connected" by placing a

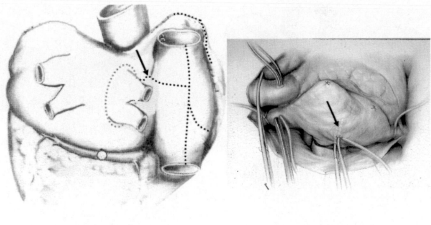

Posterior View **Surgeon's View**

FIGURE 29-19. The atrial septal cryolesion when performing the Maze procedure through a small right anterior thoracotomy using cardio-pulmonary bypass and cardioplegic arrest.

linear cryolesion between the two. For this lesion, the cryoprobe is placed on the epicardial surface of the posterior left atrium so that the transmurality of the lesion can be visualized as it occurs (Figure 29-20). The lesion from the pulmonary veins down to the posterior mitral valve annulus, which includes cryoablation of the coronary sinus, is created by placing the linear cryoprobe externally and then cryoablating separately in the same line but on the endocardial surface of the left atrium (Figure 29-21). The left atriotomy is then closed. This completes the procedure.

Results

The minimally invasive approach has resulted in a significant decrease in the time to extubation following surgery and was found to be an independent predictor for early extubation, after a review of all the patients.[8] In addition,

the length of stay in the intensive care unit and the length of stay in the hospital have decreased as a result of using this new approach. The only other differences in the results in comparison with the standard Maze 3 procedure are less need for permanent pacemakers postoperatively, a lower rate of perioperative atrial arrhythmias, and a higher incidence of right phrenic nerve paralysis. The safety and efficacy of these minimally invasive approaches compare most favorably with those of the proven standard Maze 3 procedure (Tables 29-1 and 29-2).

Summary

The major deterrent to the widespread application of the standard Maze procedure, despite its proven efficacy and relative safety, is that it is a major open heart procedure that is considered by many to be too invasive to treat most

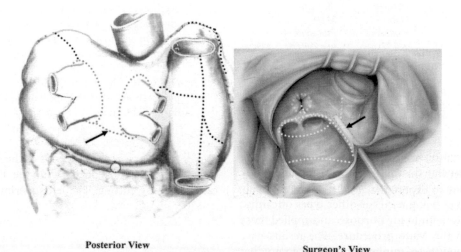

Posterior View **Surgeon's View**

FIGURE 29-20. Placement of the left atrial lesions inside the left atrium when performing the Maze procedure through a small right thoracotomy.

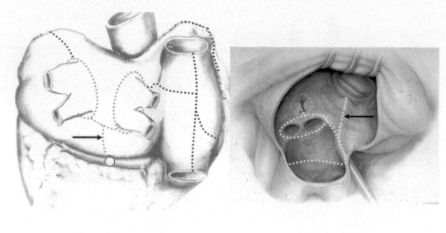

Posterior View   Surgeon's View

FIGURE 29-21. Placement of the lesion down to the mitral valve annulus and cryoablation of the coronary sinus when performing the Maze procedure through a small right thoracotomy.

TABLE 29-1. Early Complications of the Minimally Invasive and Standard Maze Procedures

	Minimally Invasive Maze Procedure (n = 72) (%)	Standard Maze Procedure (n = 290) (%)	p Value
Atrial arrhythmias	22	42	< .05
Bleeding	6	3	NS
Deep vein thrombosis	1.5	0	< .05
Fluid retention	1.4	4	NS
Paralyzed diaphragm (temporary)	11	0.4	< .05
Postoperative pacemaker	5.5	20	< .05
Stroke	1.4	0.7	NS
TIA	1.4	0.4	NS

NS = not significant; TIA = transient ischemic attack.

TABLE 29-2. Late Complications of the Minimally Invasive and Standard Maze Procedures

	Minimally Invasive Maze Procedure (n = 72) (%)	Standard Maze Procedure (n = 290) (%)	p Value
Arrhythmia recurrence	2	2.2	NS
Stroke	0	0	NS
TIA	0	0.9	NS

NS = not significant; TIA = transient ischemic attack.

References

1. Cox JL. The surgical treatment of atrial fibrillation: IV. Surgical technique. J Thorac Cardiovasc Surg 1991;101: 584–92.
2. Cox JL, Jaquiss RD, Schuessler RB, Boineau JP. Modification of the Maze procedure for atrial flutter and atrial fibrillation. II. Surgical technique of the Maze III procedure. J Thorac Cardiovasc Surg 1995;110:(2):485–95.
3. Cox JL, Schuessler RB, Lappas DG, Boineau JP. An 8.5 year clinical experience with surgery for atrial fibrillation. Ann Surg 1996;224(3):267–75.
4. Holman WL, Ikeshita M, Lease JG, et al. Elective prolongation of atrioventricular conduction by multiple discrete cryolesions: a new technique for the treatment of paroxysmal supraventricular tachycardia. J Thorac Cardiovasc Surg 1982;84:554–62.
5. Cox JL, Holman WL, Cain ME. Cryosurgical treatment of atrioventricular node reentry tachycardia. Circulation 1987;76:1329–36.
6. Holman WL, Ikeshita M, Douglas JM, et al. Ventricular cryosurgery: short-term effects on intramural electrophysiology. Ann Thorac Surg 1983;35:386–94.
7. Cox JL. The minimally invasive maze procedure. Operative techniques in thoracic and cardiovascular surgery. 2000; 5(1):79–92.
8. Ad N, Cox JL. The minimally invasive maze procedure for the treatment of atrial fibrillation. J Thorac Cardiovasc Surg. [Submitted]

patients with atrial fibrillation. In an effort to minimize the morbidity associated with the Maze procedure, I took advantage of some of the recently popularized minimally invasive techniques being used for other types of cardiac surgery, modified them to my purpose, and applied those modifications to the Maze procedure. The results have been gratifying, and these "minimally invasive" approaches now represent the techniques of choice when performing the Maze procedure.

CHAPTER 30

RADIOFREQUENCY AND MICROWAVE ABLATION FOR ATRIAL FIBRILLATION

DAVID C. KRESS, MD

Background

Atrial arrhythmias lend themselves to ablative procedures directed toward either the elimination of a trigger, interruption of reentrant pathways, or atrioventricular (AV) nodal modification for rate control. Procedures that were initially developed using surgical incisions or cryoablation to implement ablative lesions have now been modified to make use of radiofrequency (RF) energy, which can be applied by transvenous catheter electrodes. For example, AV nodal ablation, interruption of Wolff-Parkinson-White (WPW) syndrome accessory pathways, and atrial flutter ablation can all be accomplished using RF in the electrophysiology lab.[1–3]

The percutaneous ablation of atrial fibrillation (AF) has been more challenging for a variety of reasons. Approaches that seek to ablate identified trigger sites of AF in the pulmonary veins are appropriate for paroxysmal AF but not for the more common persistent or permanent AF. Accurately placed linear ablation lesions are difficult to achieve using current imaging techniques and generally require trans-septal puncture to access the left atrium. Finally, the left atrial appendage is a potential source of both triggers and thrombi and cannot be excluded at the present time using percutaneous methods.

An approach that applies ablative energy to surgically identified sites has the advantage of precise anatomic localization of the site of ablation, shorter application time, and the ability to remove or exclude the left atrial appendage. This chapter describes the use of radiofrequency and microwave energy for surgical ablation of atrial fibrillation. Following a discussion of the principles of hyperthermic cardiac ablation and a brief review of the results of ablation by other centers, techniques developed in Milwaukee by this author and colleagues to perform cardiac ablation using a left atrial lesion pattern derived from studies in animals with chronic atrial fibrillation are described.

Basic Science of Hyperthermic Cardiac Ablation

It is generally agreed that the cellular injury that follows from the application of radiofrequency current or microwave radiation is primarily due to tissue heating rather than to direct ionic effects of the actual energy source.

Temperature Effect on Cardiac Conduction

Nath and associates have demonstrated that the heating of isolated guinea pig papillary muscle in a tissue bath to temperatures greater than approximately 50° to 55°C for 60 s results in the irreversible loss of excitability (Figure 30-1).[4] The heating of such muscle segments to a slightly lower temperature results in reversible loss of excitability. In clinical practice, when heat is applied to the atrial wall at either

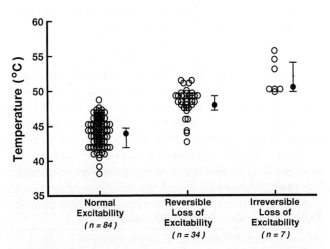

FIGURE 30-1. Chart showing the effect of temperature on cardiac excitability. Strips of isolated guinea pig papillary muscle were incubated in tissue baths of various temperatures for 60 s. Reproduced with permission from Nath S et al.[4]

the endocardial or epicardial surface, the entire wall thickness must reach the threshold temperature to reliably achieve the same electrical isolation as a surgical incision.

All surgical ablation probes have strengths and weaknesses; a list of desirable features in the "ideal" surgical ablation probe is given in Table 30-1. What follows is a description of the two currently available hyperthermic energy sources, their mechanism of action, and surgical considerations when applying them to cardiac ablation.

Radiofrequency Ablation

Radiofrequency ablation applies an alternating current to tissue, in the range of 350 to 1 MHz. Unlike direct current, which creates cellular injury via electrolytic dissociation of tissue fluids, alternating current causes tissue damage from heat via protein denaturation, blood coagulation, and fluid evaporation.[5,6] It is similar to electrocautery but generally less destructive because of the larger surface area of the surgical probe and the regulation of power delivery via probe thermistor measurement of tissue temperature.

MECHANISM OF TISSUE HEATING

Radiofrequency energy heats tissue in two main ways. First, *ohmic heating* occurs on the surface by a mechanism in which the myocardium in direct contact with the coil or probe acts as a resistor. This heating falls off by the fourth power of distance from the electrode in unipolar systems and typically penetrates only 1 mm.[7] Second, *conductive heating* occurs, in which this surface heat is transferred to increasingly deeper tissue; conductive heating accounts for the majority of the lesion depth.

RF can be applied either in *unipolar* fashion from a tissue electrode source to a grounding pad serving as the indifferent electrode, or between two *bipolar* tissue electrodes. Bipolar RF systems intended for surgical use apply two linear electrodes that gently squeeze together on either side of the cardiac tissue; this creates two opposing surfaces of ohmic heating and improves the efficiency with which the conductive heating occurs.

DETERMINANTS OF RF LESION SIZE

RF electrode temperature is a better predictor of RF lesion size than delivered energy or current.[8] Monitoring of electrode temperature is typically carried out with one or more thermistors. The maximal lesion size from conductive heating is determined primarily by the electrode surface area and electrode–tissue contact temperature, and is achieved at a rate that is a reverse exponential decay with half-time of 7 to 9 s.[7,9–11]

TABLE 30-1. Ideal Surgical Ablation Tool

Malleable, with variable lesion length and single-sided delivery surface

Produces rapid, narrow, visible, linear lesions of predictable depth without gaps

Achieves epicardial ablation through connective tissue and fat

Preserves tissue architecture

Lesion size is also influenced by time, irrigation of the electrode, impedance rise, and convective cooling. The duration of energy delivery has a diminishing effect on reaching maximal lesion size after 20 s.[11] Electrode irrigation results in deeper lesions.

Impedance rise during RF application is more common in power-controlled RF systems such as used in transvenous applications; it reduces transfer of RF energy to the tissue and is associated with endocardial disruption and formation of thermal blood coagulum. Impedance rises with increased power, increased electrode–tissue pressure, and repeat applications. Saline is protective against impedance rises when compared to blood.[12]

Convective cooling due to circulation within the tissue itself tends to be minimized by the coagulation of microvessels in the zone of injury; experimentally, myocardial RF lesion size is the same with and without intramyocardial perfusion.[7,13] Convective cooling from adjacent circulating blood pools can be significant when the ablated tissue is adjacent to an epicardial coronary artery (eg, an endocardial mitral valve connecting lesion that crosses the circumflex coronary artery during cold cardioplegia delivery), or when an epicardial lesion is delivered to a cardiac chamber with circulating blood. Convective cooling of the left atrial endocardium during epicardial ablation increases as blood temperature falls; it may occur to a greater degree in the beating heart than in the unloaded heart on bypass.

The Boston Scientific/EP Technologies Cobra system (San Jose, California) is currently the only radiofrequency system approved for use in the United States for general surgical tissue ablation (Figure 30-2). The electrosurgical unit (ESU) generates a 500 kHz sine wave. The surgical probe is a flexible single-use probe consisting of seven coagulating electrodes; six of the seven are 12.5 mm coiled electrodes spaced 2 mm apart, and the seventh is an 8 mm

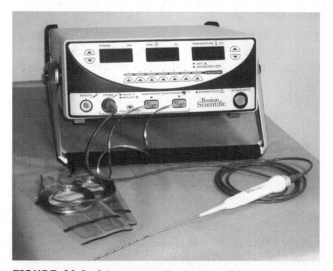

FIGURE 30-2. Cobra seven-coil unipolar radiofrequency ablation probe, grounding pads, and electrosurgical unit.

distal-tip electrode. Active coils are selected on the ESU prior to the delivery of each lesion. Two skin grounding pads are required to serve as indifferent electrodes.

Finite element simulation of RF ablation using these coil electrodes shows maximal current density at the coil ends, with 2 mm extension of the 50°C tissue heat isotherm from the coil ends.[14] Each electrode coil contains two temperature-sensing thermistors. One is located 180° apart at each coil end, where resistive heating is greatest. In vitro testing at 80°C shows all lesions from adjacent coils to be contiguous, although this is only true in 75% of lesions made at 70°C.[14]

Microwave Ablation

Microwave energy for tissue ablation is usually supplied at 915 MHz or 2.45 GHz. Although solid-state microwave (MW) generators are available, they are more commonly used in low-power electronic communication devices such as cellular phones. Tissue-ablation microwave generators typically generate the electromagnetic field using a magnetron, such as is used in microwave ovens.

The mechanism of thermal injury in microwave ablation is *dielectric heating*.[15] Body tissue contains various polar molecules, of which water is the most abundant and has an exceptionally high polarity. At microwave frequencies, electromagnetic radiation causes rotation of molecular dipoles; heat is created as these movements are opposed by intermolecular bonds and thus represents dissipation of part of the energy of the electromagnetic field in the form of molecular friction. Energy absorption is affected by the presence of electrolytes and other polar molecules such as amino acids in tissue water.[16] Conductive heating is a comparatively minor contributor to tissue heating.

The AFx system (Afx, Inc., Freemont, California) is currently the only microwave system approved for use in the United States for cardiac tissue ablation. The system consists of a magnetron-powered 2.45 GHz generator with power and timer settings, and a hand-held surgical probe that has an antenna at the end through which the electromagnetic radiation is emitted. The Flex-2 is a surgical probe with a 2 cm rigid antenna. The Flex-4 probe has both a bendable shaft and a 4 cm flexible antenna (Figure 30-3). The antennas have the desirable feature of being shielded on one side. This ensures that only one side of the antenna delivers the ablation energy, an advantage for epicardial ablation, as is discussed later.

Gaps and Nontransmural Lesions

A gap usually refers to a complete lack of thermal lesion in a particular location, whereas a nontransmural lesion is one in which there appears to be a lesion present on visual inspection, but the lesion is not of full thickness. Gaps are created when there is a failure to achieve continuity in the application of contiguous RF lesions. Ordinarily, RF delivery during simultaneous use of adjacent coils will create a single continuous lesion due to the overlap of the

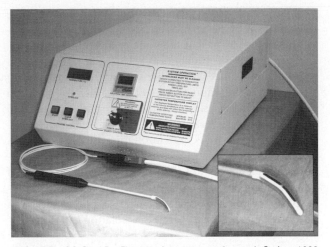

FIGURE 30-3. AFx Flex-4 microwave probe and Series 1000 generator. Grounding pads are not required. Inset: Black line on the white shielded side of the probe indicates the position of the 4 cm antenna.

lesion border zone of adjacent electrodes. A gap usually occurs in this setting because of poor tissue contact, either because of trabeculated endocardium, a curve made in the probe that makes tissue pressure inadequate, or local differences in the underlying floppiness of the open atrial wall. The interior of the left atrial appendage is the most trabeculated structure in the left atrium in addition to being quite thick in some patients.

When coils are applied sequentially to create a linear lesion, gaps can be created if there is not a slight overlap of the coils. This is most likely to occur during placement of ablation lesions in difficult-to-visualize areas.

Nontransmural lesions occur either when lesion delivery is suboptimal, when the atrial muscle is thicker than maximal lesion depth as predicted by dosimetry, or when conditions are present that inhibit full tissue penetration. The site of nontransmural injury is the atrial surface opposite the active electrode in unipolar systems, but in the mid-myocardium in bipolar systems.

Proper lesion delivery in unipolar systems depends on both the probe and atrial wall being held motionless with suitable pressure to ensure a slight indentation of the tissue by the probe. Movement of the coil will result in a wider but shallower lesion. In practice, the more coils that are simultaneously activated during lesion formation, the more difficult it is to achieve optimal conditions on each individual coil.

The presence of blood on the RF coils during endocardial ablation can create convective cooling but can also cool the coil thermistor and paradoxically lead to a deeper lesion due to a greater power output by the generator. Char often develops in the presence of blood. It can prevent proper coil contact and should be wiped clean from the coils or probe tip between each application.

In epicardial ablation, transmurality is influenced by the presence of blood in the underlying atrial chamber;

this convective cooling effect is more pronounced when the ablation is performed off-pump than during cardiopulmonary bypass at the same body temperature.

Assessment of transmurality is easiest to perform when lesions isolate a structure such as the left atrial (LA) appendage or pulmonary veins (PVs). Electrograms can be achieved using a simple hand-held probe connected to a strip recorder. Preablation and postablation electrograms are compared; the elimination of conducted LA activity into the PV muscle sleeve or LA appendage indicates complete isolation (Figure 30-4). Demonstration of failure to capture the left atrium from pacing of the isolated structure can also be used as an end point, although far field capture despite electrical isolation can occur.[17]

DRAG LESIONS

Drag lesions refer to the movement of an active single electrode-tip catheter or probe to create a linear lesion. Drag lesions were first described in percutaneous procedures in which atrial ablation is carried out under fluoroscopic, intracardiac echo, or mapping guidance. The main disadvantage of drag lesions in transcatheter procedures is the occurrence of gaps and nontransmural lesions, due in part to the lack of visual feedback during lesion delivery. The rate of probe tip movement and changes in point-to-point probe application pressure influence lesion depth reproducibility even in open heart applications. The Medtronic Cardioblate Surgical Ablation Pen (Medtronic, Inc., Minneapolis, Minnesota), which is now available in Europe, is an example of a surgical ablation tool that creates drag lesions. It has a saline-irrigated tip and can be used to trace a lesion pattern on the atrium.

Complications of Hyperthermic Left Atrial Ablation

Collateral damage refers to unintended ablation of structures that lie adjacent to the left atrium. It can occur during both hyperthermic and cryothermic ablation, although cryothermic damage is usually limited to late coronary intimal hyperplasia, acute coronary artery narrowing, or phrenic nerve paralysis.[18–21]

During endocardial ablation the esophagus and left phrenic nerves are most vulnerable to conductive heat transfer beyond the confines of the atrial wall. The circumflex coronary artery is also vulnerable if a connecting lesion from the left pulmonary veins (or LA appendage) to the mitral annulus is performed.

During epicardial ablation, any structure that ordinarily lies against the left atrium and comes into contact with a nonshielded ablation probe is potentially at risk, such as adjacent great vessels and the esophagus. The use of shielded probes for epicardial ablation, such as the AFx microwave antennas, will potentially prevent this form of collateral damage. Precise application of the ablation probe will avoid lesion delivery to unintended areas such as the AV groove during left PV isolation or the sinus node during right PV isolation. Placement of a dry sponge under the left atrial appendage during epicardial microwave ablation is discussed below.

Esophageal Injury

Injury to the esophagus has been described as a result of endocardial radiofrequency ablation during open heart surgery.[22] The etiology of the injury has been difficult to generalize as it has occurred using devices from different manufacturers, and in different surgical centers that use different lesion patterns. Such injuries can lead to fatal esophageal perforation.

The middle third of the esophagus is vulnerable to such injury for several reasons. The esophagus crosses behind the left atrium between the pulmonary veins (Figure 30-5), separated only by the oblique sinus and the pericardial reflection between the oblique and transverse sinuses. There is relatively little insulating mediastinal fat overlying the esophagus, particularly in cachectic patients. Unlike the nearby aorta, which is cooled by the blood it circulates, the esophagus has no ability to effectively dissipate heat. A transesophageal echo probe could

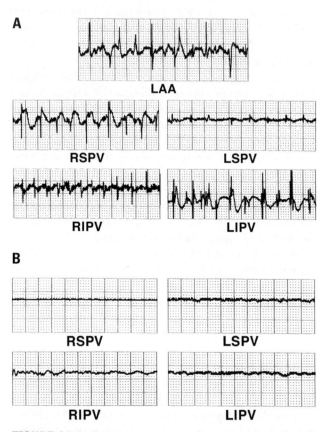

FIGURE 30-4. Pulmonary vein electrograms (*A*) preablation and (*B*) postablation. Tracings are made using a handheld surgical probe attached to a standard ICD programmer chart recorder. The LA appendage has been removed in *B*. LAA = left atrial appendage; LIPV = left inferior pulmonary vein; LSPV = left superior pulmonary vein; RIPV = right inferior pulmonary vein; RSPV = right superior pulmonary vein.

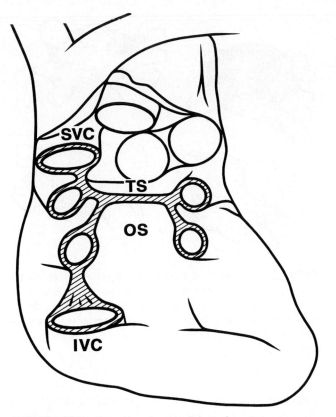

FIGURE 30-5. Illustration of pericardial attachments to vena cavae and pulmonary veins. Prior to epicardial ablation, the attachments that reflect onto the posterior left atrium must be taken down to achieve circumferential pulmonary vein isolation; IVC = inferior vena cava. OS = oblique sinus; SVC = superior vena cava; TS = transverse sinus.

serve to push the anterior esophageal wall toward the left atrium, and combined with the use of a probe in which pressure is exerted, the esophagus and left atrium could be "sandwiched" together. Consequently, lesions in this area require careful application.

Pulmonary Vein Stenosis

Pulmonary vein stenosis is a reported complication of percutaneous focal pulmonary vein ablation.[23] It is more likely to occur in PV branches than in the entire PV. It has not been described as a complication of surgical ablation employing either circumferential pulmonary vein isolation or the type of pulmonary vein connecting lesions described by Kottkamp.[24] In an interesting study of six single-lung transplant patients, two patients had pulmonary vein anastomosis pressure gradients of 8 to 12 mm without adverse effects on graft function.[25]

Coronary Artery Injury

The circumflex coronary artery may be at risk when a connecting lesion is performed from one of the left pulmonary veins to the mitral annulus, although there have been no reports of such injury, perhaps because of the common practice to administer cardioplegia during this

lesion. Coronary artery injury has been reported as a complication of transcatheter radiofrequency ablation.[26,27]

Lesion Patterns for Intraoperative Ablation

Maze 3

The Maze 3 lesion pattern usually is considered the model of a well-studied lesion pattern. It evolved from earlier concepts of left atrial isolation only, left atrial transection, and the Maze 1 and Maze 2.[28–30] It involves surgical incision lesions and cryoablation lesions of both the left and right atrium. Results of the Maze 3 vary by institution but range from 49% freedom from AF at mean 45-month follow-up in patients undergoing other cardiac procedures, to 98% freedom from AF at 8.5-year follow-up in all patients.[31,32] Recent changes to the Maze 3 involve more extensive use of cryoablation, elimination of right atrial appendectomy, and separate pulmonary vein isolation with a posterior left atrial connecting lesion.[33]

Patwardhan has successfully used a 7 mm bayonet-tipped bipolar electrocautery forceps at 45 to 55 watts (W) (and selective cryoablation) to create the Maze 3 lesion pattern in 18 patients.[34] The lesion time to achieve transmurality is shorter using bipolar RF, but the relative disadvantage of requiring one electrode on either side of the atrial tissue makes this more suitable to open exposure ablation via atriotomy. Sinus rhythm was restored in 80% of 15 survivors at mean 5-month follow-up.

Chen has also applied a modified Maze 1 using a power-controlled RF catheter at 30 to 50 W for 30 s and cryoablation in 12 patients.[23] Of the survivors, 80% were in sinus or ectopic atrial rhythm at 6-month follow-up.

Left Atrial Lesion Patterns

There are reasons to consider a procedure directed at the left atrium for the curative ablation of atrial fibrillation. A clinical series by Graffigna, based on earlier work by Williams, reported on 100 patients that underwent left atrial isolation.[28,35] Eighty-eight percent of the patients were successfully isolated and 81% had restoration of sinus rhythm, which persisted in 72% of patients at 14-month follow-up. Atrial fibrillation was confined to the left atrium in 56% of the patients. This study suggests that atrial fibrillation arises from the left atrium in the majority of patients.

Other more recent studies have documented pulmonary vein triggers in paroxysmal AF (Figure 30-6) and left atrial appendage triggers in mitral valve disease (Figure 30-7).[36,37] Autopsy studies have identified muscle sleeves that extend from the left atrium onto the pulmonary veins, extensive cross-connection of muscle bundles across the posterior left atrium (Figure 30-8), and HNK-1 antigen expression in the myocardium around the PVs in human embryonic tissue.[38–40]

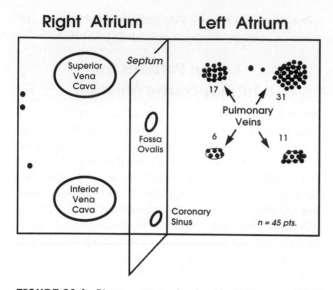

FIGURE 30-6. Diagram representing the sites of 69 paroxysmal AF foci in 45 patients undergoing mapping in electrophysiology lab. Note clustering of foci, indicated by black dots, in the pulmonary veins. Reproduced with permission from Haissaguerre M et al.[42]

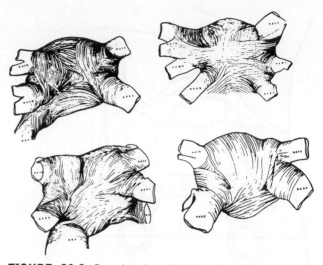

FIGURE 30-8. Posterior view of left atrium, representing the four predominant patterns of muscle fascicle organization in 16 postmortem studies. Note the extension of muscle sleeves onto the pulmonary veins and the complex crossing connections between pulmonary veins in some patients. Reproduced with permission from Nathan H et al.[38]

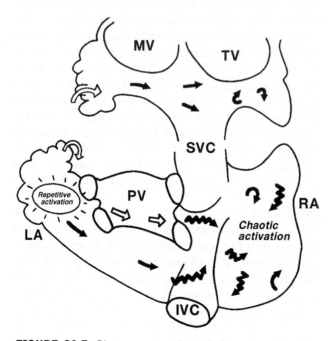

FIGURE 30-7. Diagram representing typical location of repetitive activation in LA appendage during mapping of patients with chronic AF undergoing mitral valve procedures. IVC = inferior vena cava; LA = left atrium; MV = mitral valve; PV = pulmonary veins; RA = right atrium; TV = tricuspid valve. Reproduced with permission from Harada A et al.[36]

LEFT ATRIAL MAZE 3

The earliest approach to a left atrial lesion pattern was simply performing the left atrial portion of the Maze 3 procedure.[37] Eleven patients underwent LA appendectomy and a cryoablation lesion pattern that isolated the pulmonary veins and connected to the LA appendage and

mitral annulus and pulmonary veins during mitral valve procedures. Of these patients, 91% were in sinus rhythm at 11-month mean follow-up.

PV ISOLATION

Melo has performed bilateral pulmonary vein isolation using the Cobra RF probe in 65 patients with atrial fibrillation, most with concomitant mitral valve procedures.[41] At 6-month follow-up, 52% of the patients were free of atrial fibrillation. seven of the 65 patients had epicardial PV isolation, and three of these seven cases were performed off-pump. The author used set temperatures of 70°C for endocardial lesions and 75°C for epicardial lesions.

CONNECTING LESIONS ONLY

A lesion pattern has been reported that connects the pulmonary veins sequentially to one another and then to the mitral annulus.[43] Circumferential isolation of the PVs is not performed; the left atrial appendage is not isolated. Kottkamp has reported 18 patients undergoing this procedure using the Osypka RF probe (Dr. Osypka, Grenzach-Wyhlen, Germany), which is a single-thermistor/single-electrode T-shaped rigid probe available in Europe.[24] At mean follow-up of 11 months, 55% of 11 survivors were free of atrial fibrillation or flutter. Knaut reports 46 patients undergoing this pattern using the Flex-2 microwave antenna during mitral valve surgery (with an additional right atrial isthmus lesion) and coronary artery bypass grafting (CABG).[44] At 6-month follow-up, 64% of mitral valve patients and 70% of CABG patients were in sinus rhythm.

PV ISOLATION WITH CONNECTING LESIONS

Benussi has reported a procedure during mitral valve procedures using the Cobra RF probe in which the pulmonary veins are isolated epicardially on bypass (75°C for 2 min) and then connecting lesions to the mitral valve and between the PVs are placed endocardially on bypass (65° to 70°C for 2 min).[45] The LA appendage is oversewn but not electrically isolated. At mean follow-up of 11.6 months, 77% of patents were in sinus rhythm.

PV AND LA APPENDAGE ISOLATION WITH CONNECTING LESIONS

A lesion pattern that (1) removes pulmonary vein and LA appendage triggers and (2) interrupts macroreentrant circuits with connecting lesions (Figure 30-9) has been validated in a chronic canine model of atrial fibrillation, and used both endocardially and epicardially in patients.[46,47] The following section describes this author and colleagues clinical experience with this lesion pattern using both radiofrequency and microwave ablation.

Surgical Technique of Current Procedures

Our clinical experience with radiofrequency ablation is greater than our experience with microwave ablation, which was introduced more recently in the United States. Following the establishment of our lesion pattern and

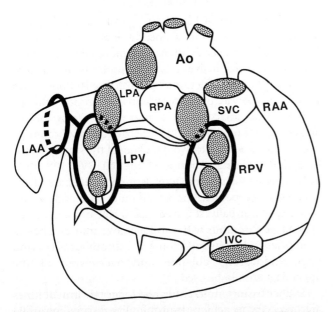

FIGURE 30-9. Left atrial lesion pattern developed in Milwaukee for surgical ablation of atrial fibrillation. The left atrial appendage and both pairs of pulmonary veins are electrically isolated. Two connecting lesions are also made. AO = aorta; IVC = inferior vena cava; LAA = left atrial appendage; LPA = left pulmonary artery; LPV = left pulmonary veins; RAA = right atrial appendage; RPA = right pulmonary artery; RPV = right pulmonary veins; SVC = superior vena cava. Reproduced with permission from Kress DC et al.[46]

dosimetric studies with the Cobra probe, we began performing endocardial ablation in patients undergoing mitral valve procedures who were already undergoing atriotomy. We subsequently performed the first epicardial radiofrequency ablation procedure in North America on December 7, 1999, during coronary artery bypass grafting and continued to offer this to patients with atrial fibrillation undergoing cardiopulmonary bypass without atriotomy. Our current series of patients undergoing off-pump epicardial microwave ablation began on June 13, 2001, with the first such procedure in North America. This has now become our procedure of choice to apply the lesion pattern in patients, whether off-pump or on-pump, with or without atriotomy.

Endocardial Ablation

RADIOFREQUENCY

Two standard grounding pads are applied to the back and attached to the ESU prior to skin prepping. Once the heart is arrested, RF ablation is carried out prior to valve repair or replacement to avoid possible contact with sutures or the prosthesis. In reoperations, an existing prosthesis is removed before ablation. The pericardium overlying the left phrenic nerve should be separated from the left atrial appendage in reoperations. It is important to pull back the transesophageal echo probe before lesions are delivered; this can be confirmed by palpating the esophagus through the posterior left atrial wall.

The ESU is set at 80°C and each lesion is delivered for 60 s. The lesion time begins when the probe reaches approximately 80°C, which is generally within 5 to 10 s. In theory, all seven electrodes can be simultaneously activated in the delivery of a long lesion but, in practice, good tissue contact becomes difficult to maintain when more than two or three electrodes are used. Lesion transmurality can be assessed by inspecting the epicardial surface of the LA after application of the right PV encircling lesion at the corners of the atriotomy (if the standard atriotomy is performed). In patients with unusually thin atrial walls, 70°C lesions are adequate for transmurality. Figure 30-10 shows the dosimetry data for the Cobra surgical probe.

Because electrode pressure against the tissue has an effect on lesion depth, the atrium should be slightly stretched by the application of the probe. If a lesion does not appear uniform after removal of the probe and a gap is suspected on visual inspection, a repeat application should be done with a single electrode to the area.

PULMONARY VEIN ISOLATION

The pulmonary veins are ablated in pairs, the left and right sides separately. Lesions are placed on the LA, 1 cm away from the PV orifice. A connecting lesion is placed between the two encircling lesions at the level of the lower PVs where the atrial wall is relatively thin.

An alternative method to isolate the PVs is to create a single encircling linear lesion that includes a line that

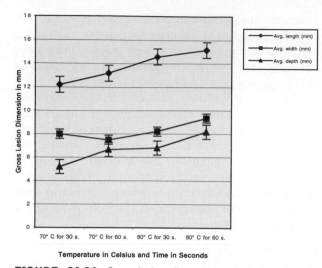

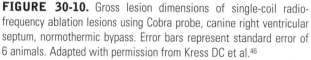

FIGURE 30-10. Gross lesion dimensions of single-coil radio-frequency ablation lesions using Cobra probe, canine right ventricular septum, normothermic bypass. Error bars represent standard error of 6 animals. Adapted with permission from Kress DC et al.[46]

extends from 1 cm above the right superior pulmonary vein to the left superior pulmonary vein across the dome of the atrium, and another one that extends from 1 cm below the right inferior pulmonary vein to the left inferior pulmonary vein. This method has the disadvantages of (1) ablating a relatively thick area of LA tissue in the dome and (2) isolating 30% of the entire LA, which may affect LA contractility.[38,48]

LA APPENDAGE ISOLATION

The base of the LA appendage is everted if possible and the base is ablated so that the line of isolation lies within the appendage base, not the LA. This allows the appendage to be oversewn more easily after it is restored to a non-everted state. If the appendage cannot be inverted, single-coil applications are usually required to ablate within it. In reoperations, it is important to free the LA appendage from the pericardium prior to ablation because of its proximity to the left phrenic nerve.

CONNECTING LESIONS

The two connecting lesions are (1) a lesion between the two PV encircling lesions, described above, and (2) a lesion between the left PV encircling lesion and the LA appendage-isolating lesion. This second isolating lesion may not be necessary, in practice, if the LA appendage is sufficiently near the left superior PV. In this event, the LA appendage-isolating lesion and left PV encircling lesion share a common border.

OVERSEW LA APPENDAGE

The LA appendage is oversewn with a double suture line of 3–0 Prolene. The opening of the appendage is usually oval and this is easiest to accomplish along its major axis.

The appendage is oversewn only after all ablation lines have been delivered to the LA appendage, the region of the left superior PV, and the connecting lesion has been made between the LA appendage and left PV.

MICROWAVE

The above endocardial ablation procedure can be accomplished with microwave energy using either the rigid antenna Flex-2 or flexible antenna Flex-4 probes (AFx, Inc., Freemont, California). Grounding pads are not necessary with microwave ablation. The Flex-2 is set at 45 W and applied for 25 s; the Flex-4 is set at 65 W and applied for 45 s. The Flex-4 is less malleable than the Cobra radiofrequency probe and delivers a 4 cm lesion; therefore, the Flex-2 is easier to use when the LA appendage cannot be everted or in a smaller atrium.

Efficient energy transmission from the antenna requires tissue contact. Mild heating of the antenna, probe, and cable will occur during even normal lesion delivery, and is not injurious; nevertheless, as a rule, the patient's skin is covered with drapes or towels. The generator should not be turned on if the antenna is not in contact with tissue, because doing so will cause the microwave energy to be reflected back to the generator, create significant cable heating, and eventually trigger an automatic generator shutoff. The probe can be tested, if necessary, by applying it to a wet gauze pad off-field.

Epicardial Ablation

RADIOFREQUENCY

The lesion pattern in Figure 30-9 can be applied epicardially by using the Cobra probe; cardiopulmonary bypass is necessary, however, in order to achieve adequate exposure to ensure that active coils of the probe are not in contact with adjacent structures. Pericardial reflections attach to the venae cavae, pulmonary veins, and roof of the left atrium; these must be divided to allow access for the ablation probe (see Figure 30-5). Separate bicaval cannulation is recommended to avoid kinking of the superior vena cava (SVC) during exposure of the left PVs. Left atrial appendectomy is preferable to ablation of the base of the LA appendage, because this area is quite thick and tedious to ablate epicardially. It is essential to rule out a left atrial appendage thrombus with intraoperative transesophageal echo prior to LA appendectomy. If a thrombus is present, open endocardial ablation and oversewing of the appendage should be used.

Higher tissue temperatures and longer treatment times are necessary to achieve transmurality during epicardial ablation. The ESU is manually ramped from an initial setting of 80°C for 30 s, then 85°C for 30 s, and finally 90°C for 2 min. The gradual increase in temperature avoids a sudden impedance rise, which would result in automatic ESU shutoff.

To achieve adequate tissue contact with the RF coils, fat must be cleaned off of the left atrial epicardium. This is usually necessary in the regions of the atrial septal groove and the dome of the left atrium, but in obese patients, fatty infiltration can be extensive. Fat is a relative insulator to RF current.

Pulmonary vein electrograms are recorded preablation and postablation to assess circumferential transmurality and lack of gaps (see Figure 30-4). Fatty tissue may need to be cleaned off of the pulmonary veins to get an adequate signal. Occasionally, there is no atrial activity present on the baseline recording because of the absence of a muscle sleeve on one or more of the veins.[38]

MICROWAVE

The Flex-4 microwave probe has two features that make it ideally suited for *off-pump epicardial ablation* using the lesion set in Figure 30-9. The first feature is the shielding that ensures that only one side of the microwave antenna applies the ablative energy. This allows the probe to slide under the left atrium and its inactive side to be in contact with adjacent structures without risk of collateral damage. Retraction of the heart can be less severe than with the unshielded RF probe because only identification of the ablation sites and safe initial placement of the probe need to be accomplished.

The second feature is related to the difference between electromagnetic radiation and alternating current. Microwave energy does not require electrodes and therefore the generator does not require safety power shutoffs, which are necessary with RF generators due to occasional nonfunctioning thermistors, sudden impedance rises, poor electrode contact, or high grounding pad current. Satisfactory microwave lesions require only proper orientation of the microwave antenna and tissue contact.

The AFx Flex-4 antenna is used at a power setting of 65 W for 90 s. In canine studies in our lab, epicardial lesions at this setting and duration, delivered off-pump to the right ventricular free wall, had an average length (mean ± SD) of 48 ± 3.1 mm, a width of 9.7 ± 2.0 mm, and a depth of 5.8 ± 1.1 mm.

The procedure is similar to on-pump epicardial RF ablation, with the exception that retraction of adjacent tissues away from the microwave antenna is not necessary during lesion delivery. Brief cardiac retraction to place the antenna under the LA is required for posterior lesions. One hand then holds the probe steady during lesion delivery while a finger of the other hand is used to ensure the antenna is flat against the left atrium. Safe lesion delivery under the left atrium requires determination that the active side of the proximal antenna is against the LA, by seeing the black line that is present on the inactive side of the probe (see Figure 30-3). As with RF lesion delivery, it is important to prevent movement of the antenna to minimize lesion width and maximize lesion depth.

The pericardial reflections of the venae cavae and of the superior pulmonary veins are opened similar to the epicardial RF procedure. Fatty tissue is removed from sites of ablation. PV electrograms are recorded pre- and postablation to determine electrical isolation. Heparin is given prior to ablation. Right PV ablation is first carried out. Following this, the right pleura is slit 1 cm away from the diaphragm to the level of the phrenic nerve. A vaginal pack is sutured to the oblique sinus pericardium to create two straps that can be used to pull the heart partially into the right chest.[49] This is usually adequate to expose the left pulmonary veins and LA appendage; in a patient with dilated left ventricle (LV), the more cephalad strap helps hold the base of the heart back.

During placement of the connecting lesion to the lateral LA appendage, MW energy can be transmitted through both walls of the appendage and onto the heart if the appendage is squeezed flat by the probe and allowed to lie on the left ventricle. This is easily avoided by placing a dry sponge between the appendage and the heart during this lesion and trying not to compress the lateral and medial walls of the appendage together. A small amount of thermal blood coagulum can occasionally occur inside the trabeculated tip of the appendage, despite the use of heparin. The appendage is therefore not manipulated prior to excision.

The stump of the LA appendage following appendectomy can be secured in several ways ranging from a purse string, a staple line, or oversewing it with pericardial reinforcement. This author and colleagues have found that using a TA-30 stapler at the base of the appendage is often associated with bleeding sites and have therefore adopted the use of a Beck vascular clamp to control the stump while it is oversewn with a double suture line of 4–0 Prolene with pericardial reinforcement. Lowering left atrial pressure either with reverse Trendelenburg or a vasodilator makes compression of the appendage less traumatic. In patients undergoing valvular surgery, it may be advisable to cannulate immediately prior to LA appendectomy; if a difficult appendectomy is anticipated, it can more simply be performed once on-pump.

The posterior connecting lesion between the left and right PV encircling lesions can be accomplished by placing the table in Trendelenburg and briefly lifting the heart to place the antenna. The right encircling lesion can be seen even though the inferior vena cava (IVC) makes visualization of the right PVs difficult. One or two lesions are delivered after the heart is let down.

In general, two types of situations may arise that make off-pump epicardial ablation difficult to accomplish. The first is seen in patients with chronically enlarged right atria, in which the IVC can be quite foreshortened, dilated, and thin-walled; in these patients, access to the oblique sinus to palpate the position of the antenna when ablating around the posterior right PVs may be quite difficult. The second situation is in patients with aortic and mitral insufficiency. Valvular insufficiency tends to worsen upon rotation of the heart to the right in exposing the left pulmonary veins, and may be difficult for the patient to tolerate even for brief periods. In these patients, beating-heart epicardial ablation is performed once on cardiopulmonary bypass prior to valve repair or replacement.

Perioperative Care

Right atrial temporary electrodes on the lateral wall are placed in all patients to allow for (1) atrial pacing at 10 beats per minute above the intrinsic sinus rate to prevent atrial fibrillation, (2) postoperative atrial electrograms for the diagnosis of atrial dysrhythmias, and (3) rapid overdrive pacing of postoperative atrial flutter. Postoperative fluid retention is not seen in these patients, even if the left atrial appendage is removed. Coumadin is empirically given for 6 weeks following both endocardial and epicardial ablation. In general, there is more significant endothelial injury from endocardial ablation, and therefore a greater relative indication for anticoagulation, than with epicardial ablation.

Reverse atrial remodeling refers to a reversal of electrical and structural atrial muscle abnormalities due to atrial fibrillation after sinus rhythm is restored. In animal studies, the ultrastructural and anatomic abnormalities lag behind electrical properties in returning to normal.[50] The time course of reverse atrial remodeling is unknown but is likely to vary between patients, depending on factors such as chronicity, atrial dilation, atrial wall hypertrophy, presence of endocardial fibrosis, and even active rheumatic carditis.

Perioperative atrial fibrillation or atrial flutter is not unusual in patients undergoing radiofrequency or microwave ablation of atrial fibrillation. Cox and co-workers report an approximately 40% incidence of perioperative atrial fibrillation in the first 3 months following the Maze procedure.[51] Atrial fibrillation "begets atrial fibrillation," meaning that the longer a patient remains in atrial fibrillation the less likely it will spontaneously terminate; elective cardioversion within 24 h for early postoperative atrial fibrillation is performed, with outpatient cardioversion as warranted.[52] Perioperative β-blocker is given to reduce the incidence of postoperative atrial fibrillation, as in any open heart patient. Amiodarone is routinely given for the treatment of early postoperative atrial dysrhythmias. We prefer to taper its dosage to 200 mg po qd and discontinue it after 3 months. Sotalol has also been used in lieu of amiodarone and β-blocker, but may be poorly tolerated in patients with low ejection fraction.

Current Results of Lesion Pattern

Endocardial RF ablation was carried out in 23 patients, with 1 operative death unrelated to the procedure.[53] There have been no strokes or ablation-related complications. In the 14 patients followed more than 3 months, all 14 (100%) are in sinus rhythm, with 1 patient requiring a dual-mode, dual-pacing, dual-sensing (DDD) pacemaker for AV dissociation. In the 8 surviving patients followed less than 3 months, the rhythms were sinus in 5 (63%) and

atrial fibrillation in 3. Combining all patients, at mean follow-up of 8 months, 100% of 18 patients with LA diameter less than 6 cm are in sinus rhythm.

Eight patients underwent epicardial RF ablation, seven during CABG and one during aortic valve replacement. Seven of eight patients were in sinus rhythm (88%) at a mean follow-up of 38 weeks; the other patient remained in atrial fibrillation. There were no strokes or ablation-related complications.

Eight patients underwent epicardial microwave ablation. All underwent concurrent mitral, tricuspid, or aortic valve procedures. Five patients tolerated off-pump ablation prior to cannulation for bypass, and three patients were ablated on pump. Of the five patients with over 3 months' follow-up, four (80%) were free of atrial fibrillation or flutter.

Future Goals

Sole Therapy

It is safe to say that the majority of patients with atrial fibrillation would prefer nonoperative treatment whenever possible, and that as a corollary, any operative procedure offered to patients has to minimize discomfort and morbidity while maximizing efficacy. Patient selection can help differentiate those patients most likely to benefit from operative ablation, sparing patients the prospect of a surgical failure.

Several authors have shown improved success of the Maze 3 operation with patients that either have AF of shorter duration or have limited left atrial enlargement.[54,55] A left atrial dimension of 7 cm is associated with successful early return to sinus rhythm in this author's own patients undergoing endocardial RF ablation; as indicated above, the patients with left atria less than 6 cm as a group remained in sinus rhythm at 6-month follow-up.[56] Increased age is also an independent predictor of failure of a modified Maze 3 procedure.[55]

Off-pump epicardial microwave ablation has been thus far accomplished in five of eight patients undergoing valvular surgery, many with cardiomegaly and cardiomyopathy. If long-term results show an 80 to 90% efficacy in unselected patients, not unlike that of the Maze 3 in many series, it is reasonable to offer sole therapy to selected patients, for example, patients with a LA diameter less than 6 cm, and patients who have chronic AF for less than 1 year.[57–59]

Minimally Invasive Approach

The demonstration that the lesion pattern in Figure 30-9 can be carried out epicardially off-pump leads to the natural question of whether it requires a median sternotomy to accomplish. Preliminary cadaver studies using the intuitive DaVinci robotic system demonstrate that left- and right-sided thoracoscopic approaches each have particular strengths and weaknesses. The interatrial groove and the pericardial reflections of the superior and inferior vena cava are readily accessed from a right-sided approach. The left atrial appendage and lateral left pulmonary veins are accessible from a left-sided approach. The transverse sinus allows access to the pericardial reflection at the cephalad end of the oblique sinus, and entrance into the oblique sinus is feasible from the left. A sequential left and right thoracoscopic approach using single-lung ventilation and robotic assist will require an ablation catheter that avoids collateral damage, such as a shielded microwave catheter, and a tissue stapler that can facilitate left atrial appendectomy without bleeding from the staple line. Bilateral robotic assist may be facilitated by a ceiling mounted system.

References

1. Natale A, Wathen M, Wolfe K, et al. Comparative atrioventricular node properties after radiofrequency ablation and operative therapy of atrioventricular node reentry. Pacing Clin Electrophysiol 1993;16:971–7.
2. Jackman WM, Wang XZ, Friday KJ, et al. Catheter ablation of accessory atrioventricular pathways (Wolff- Parkinson-White syndrome) by radiofrequency current. N Engl J Med 1991;324:1605–11.
3. Fischer B, Haissaguerre M, Garrigues S, et al. Radiofrequency catheter ablation of common atrial flutter in 80 patients. J Am Coll Cardiol 1995;25:1365–72.
4. Nath S, Lynch C 3rd, Whayne JG, Haines DE. Cellular electrophysiological effects of hyperthermia on isolated guinea pig papillary muscle. Implications for catheter ablation. Circulation 1993;88:1826–31.
5. Jones JL, Proskauer CC, Paull WK, et al. Ultrastructural injury to chick myocardial cells in vitro following "electric countershock." Circ Res 1980;46:387–94.
6. Erez A, Shitzer A. Controlled destruction and temperature distributions in biological tissues subjected to monoactive electrocoagulation. J Biomech Eng 1980;102:42–9.
7. Haines DE. The biophysics of radiofrequency catheter ablation in the heart: the importance of temperature monitoring. Pacing Clin Electrophysiol 1993;16:586–91.
8. Hindricks G, Haverkamp W, Gulker H, et al. Radiofrequency coagulation of ventricular myocardium: improved prediction of lesion size by monitoring catheter tip temperature. Eur Heart J 1989;10:972–84.
9. Haines DE, Watson DD, Verow AF. Electrode radius predicts lesion radius during radiofrequency energy heating. Validation of a proposed thermodynamic model. Circ Res 1990;67:124–9.
10. Blouin LT, Marcus FI. The effect of electrode design on the efficiency of delivery of radiofrequency energy to cardiac tissue in vitro. Pacing Clin Electrophysiol 1989;12:136–43.
11. Wittkampf FH, Hauer RN, Robles de Medina EO. Control of radiofrequency lesion size by power regulation. Circulation 1989;80:962–8.
12. Ring ME, Huang SK, Gorman G, Graham AR. Determinants of impedance rise during catheter ablation of bovine myocardium with radiofrequency energy. Pacing Clin Electrophysiol 1989;12:1502–13.
13. Haines DE, Watson DD. Tissue heating during radiofrequency catheter ablation: a thermodynamic model and observations in isolated perfused and superfused canine right ventricular free wall. Pacing Clin Electrophysiol 1989;12:962–76.
14. Panescu D, Fleischman SD, Whayne JG, et al. Radiofrequency multielectrode catheter ablation in the atrium. Phys Med Biol 1999;44:899–915.
15. Whayne JG, Nath S, Haines DE. Microwave catheter ablation of myocardium in vitro. Assessment of the characteristics of tissue heating and injury. Circulation 1994;89:2390–5.
16. Thury, J, Grant E. Microwave: industrial, scientific, and medical applications. Boston: Artech House; 1992. p. 1160.
17. Taylor GW, Walcott GP, Hall JA, et al. High-resolution mapping and histologic examination of long radiofrequency lesions in canine atria. J Cardiovasc Electrophysiol 1999;10:1467–77.
18. Holman WL, Ikeshita M, Ungerleider RM, et al. Cryosurgery for cardiac arrhythmias: acute and chronic effects on coronary arteries. Am J Cardiol 1983;51:149–55.
19. Iida S, Misaki T, Iwa T. The histological effects of cryocoagulation on the myocardium and coronary arteries. Jpn J Surg 1989;19:319–25.
20. Berreklouw E, Bracke F, Meijer A, et al. Cardiogenic shock due to coronary narrowings one day after a MAZE III procedure. Ann Thorac Surg 1999;68:1065–6.
21. Sueda T, Shikata H, Mitsui N, et al. Myocardial infarction after a maze procedure for idiopathic atrial fibrillation. J Thorac Cardiovasc Surg 1996;112:549–50.
22. Gillinov AM, Pettersson G, Rice TW. Esophageal injury during radiofrequency ablation for atrial fibrillation. J Thorac Cardiovasc Surg 2001;122:1239–40.
23. Yu WC, Hsu TL, Tai CT, et al. Acquired pulmonary vein stenosis after radiofrequency catheter ablation of paroxysmal atrial fibrillation. J Cardiovasc Electrophysiol 2001;12:887–92.
24. Kottkamp H, Hindricks G, Hammel D, et al. Intraoperative radiofrequency ablation of chronic atrial fibrillation: a left atrial curative approach by elimination of anatomic "anchor" reentrant circuits. J Cardiovasc Electrophysiol 1999;10:772–80.
25. Ross DJ, Vassolo M, Kass R, et al. Transesophageal echocardiographic assessment of pulmonary venous flow after single lung transplantation. J Heart Lung Transplant 1993;12:689–94.
26. Hope EJ, Haigney MC, Calkins H, Resar JR. Left main coronary thrombosis after radiofrequency ablation: successful treatment with percutaneous transluminal angioplasty. Am Heart J 1995;129:1217–9.
27. Chatelain P, Zimmermann M, Weber R, et al. Acute coronary occlusion secondary to radiofrequency catheter ablation of a left lateral accessory pathway. Eur Heart J 1995;16:859–61.
28. Williams JM, Ungerleider RM, Lofland GK, Cox JL. Left atrial isolation: new technique for the treatment of supraventricular arrhythmias. J Thorac Cardiovasc Surg 1980;80:373–80.
29. Cox JL, Schuessler RB, D'Agostino HJ Jr, et al. The surgical treatment of atrial fibrillation. III. Development of a

definitive surgical procedure. J Thorac Cardiovasc Surg 1991;101:569–83.

30. Cox JL, Boineau JP, Schuessler RB, et al. Modification of the maze procedure for atrial flutter and atrial fibrillation. I. Rationale and surgical results. J Thorac Cardiovasc Surg 1995;110:473–84.

31. Izumoto H, Kawazoe K, Eishi K, Kamata J. Medium-term results after the modified Cox/Maze procedure combined with other cardiac surgery. Eur J Cardiothorac Surg 2000;17:25–9.

32. Cox JL, Schuessler RB, Lappas DG, Boineau JP. An 8 1/2-year clinical experience with surgery for atrial fibrillation. Ann Surg 1996;224:267–73;discussion 273–5.

33. Cox JL. The minimally invasive Maze-III procedure. Operative Techniques in Thoracic and Cardiovascular Surgery. A comparative atlas. 2000;5:79–92.

34. Patwardhan AM, Dave HH, Tamhane AA, et al. Intraoperative radiofrequency microbipolar coagulation to replace incisions of Maze III procedure for correcting atrial fibrillation in patients with rheumatic valvular disease. Eur J Cardiothorac Surg 1997;12:627–33.

35. Graffigna A, Pagani F, Minzioni G, et al. Left atrial isolation associated with mitral valve operations. Ann Thorac Surg 1992;54:1093–7;discussion 1098.

36. Harada A, Sasaki K, Fukushima T, et al. Atrial activation during chronic atrial fibrillation in patients with isolated mitral valve disease. Ann Thorac Surg 1996;61: 104–11; discussion 111–2.

37. Sueda T, Nagata H, Shikata H, et al. Simple left atrial procedure for chronic atrial fibrillation associated with mitral valve disease. Ann Thorac Surg 1996;62:1796–800.

38. Nathan H, Eliakim M. The junction between the left atrium and the pulmonary veins. An anatomic study of human hearts. Circulation 1966;34:412–22.

39. Saito T, Waki K, Becker AE. Left atrial myocardial extension onto pulmonary veins in humans: anatomic observations relevant for atrial arrhythmias. J Cardiovasc Electrophysiol 2000;11:888–94.

40. Blom NA, Gittenberger-de Groot AC, DeRuiter MC, et al. Development of the cardiac conduction tissue in human embryos using HNK-1 antigen expression: possible relevance for understanding of abnormal atrial automaticity. Circulation 1999;99:800–6.

41. Melo J, Adragao P, Neves J, et al. Endocardial and epicardial radiofrequency ablation in the treatment of atrial fibrillation with a new intra-operative device. Eur J Cardiothorac Surg 2000;18:182–6.

42. Haissaguerre M, Jais P, Shah D, et al. Spontaneous initiation of atrial fibrillation by ectopic beats originating in the pulmonary veins. N Engl J Med 1998;339:659–66.

43. Hindricks G, Mohr FW, Autschbach R, Kottkamp H. Antiarrhythmic surgery for treatment of atrial fibrillation —new concepts. Thorac Cardiovasc Surg 1999;47 Suppl 3:365–9.

44. Knaut M. Microwave. Read at the Surgical Treatment of Atrial Fibrillation: New Techniques and Technologies; 2000 June 7; Atlanta, Georgia.

45. Benussi S, Pappone C, Nascimbene S, et al. A simple way to treat chronic atrial fibrillation during mitral valve surgery: the epicardial radiofrequency approach. Eur J Cardiothorac Surg 2000;17:524–9.

46. Kress DC, Krum D, Chekanov V, et al. Validation of a left atrial lesion pattern for intraoperative ablation of atrial fibrillation. Ann Thorac Surg 2002;73:1160–8.

47. Kress D, Krum D, Sra J. Clinical results of left atrial radiofrequency linear ablation during open heart surgery: endocardial and epicardial approach [abstract]. Circulation 2000;102:II-444.

48. Tsui SS, Grace AA, Ludman PF, et al. Maze 3 for atrial fibrillation: two cuts too few? Pacing Clin Electrophysiol 1994;17:2163–6.

49. Bergsland J, Karamanoukian HL, Soltoski PR, Salerno TA. "Single suture" for circumflex exposure in off-pump coronary artery bypass grafting. Ann Thorac Surg 1999; 68:1428–30.

50. Everett TH 4th, Li H, Mangrum JM, et al. Electrical, morphological, and ultrastructural remodeling and reverse remodeling in a canine model of chronic atrial fibrillation. Circulation 2000;102:1454–60.

51. Ad N, Pirovic EA, Kim YD, et al. Observations on the perioperative management of patients undergoing the Maze procedure. Semin Thorac Cardiovasc Surg 2000;12: 63–7.

52. Allessie MA. Atrial electrophysiologic remodeling: another vicious circle? J Cardiovasc Electrophysiol 1998;9: 1378–93.

53. Kress DC, Sra J, Krum D, et al. Radiofrequency ablation of artial fibrillation during mitral valve surgery. Semin Thorac Cardiovasc Surg 2002. [In press]

54. Kamata J, Kawazoe K, Izumoto H, et al. Predictors of sinus rhythm restoration after Cox Maze procedure concomitant with other cardiac operations. Ann Thorac Surg 1997;64:394–8.

55. Kawaguchi AT, Kosakai Y, Isobe F, et al. Surgical stratification of patients with atrial fibrillation secondary to organic cardiac lesions. Eur J Cardiothorac Surg 1996; 10:983–9; discussion 989–90.

56. Kress D, Sra J, Krum D, et al. Clinical experience with endocardial radiofrequency ablation of atrial fibrillation during mitral valve procedures [abstract]. Europace Suppl 2000;1:D266

57. Raanani E, Albage A, David TE, et al. The efficacy of the Cox/Maze procedure combined with mitral valve surgery: a matched control study. Eur J Cardiothorac Surg 2001;19:438–42.

58. Handa N, Schaff HV, Morris JJ, et al. Outcome of valve repair and the Cox Maze procedure for mitral regurgitation and associated atrial fibrillation. J Thorac Cardiovasc Surg 1999;118:628–35.

59. McCarthy PM, Gillinov AM, Castle L, et al. The Cox-Maze procedure: the Cleveland Clinic experience. Semin Thorac Cardiovasc Surg 2000;12:25–9.

CHAPTER 31

PRINCIPLES OF CEREBRAL PROTECTION DURING OPERATIONS ON THE THORACIC AORTA

JAMES J. KLEIN, MD, M. ARISAN ERGIN, MD, PhD

A period of interruption or temporary exclusion of the cerebral circulation has proved to be an indispensable technical addition in surgery of the thoracic aorta in general, and of the aortic arch in particular. This maneuver is necessary not only during open anastomosis and reconstruction of the arch vessels but also during dissection and mobilization of these structures in preparation for the anastomosis, in order to prevent particulate embolization to the brain during such manipulation. The neurologic outcome of these operations ultimately depends on the quality of the central nervous system protection during this critical period of interruption or exclusion of the cerebral circulation. The introduction of deep hypothermic circulatory arrest (DHCA) for this purpose has revolutionized the surgical treatment of thoracic aortic pathology in the last two decades.[1] However, cumulative clinical experience also shows that the protection afforded by DHCA alone is not quite perfect. Therefore, the search for an ideal strategy of cerebral protection continues. This search and the application of the currently available methods of protection are contingent upon a thorough understanding of the principles of cerebral protection. This chapter is a synopsis of our current state of knowledge of the pertinent physiology of brain protection, as well as the principles, rationale, and application of the current clinical methods of cerebral protection.

Physiology

Energy Generation

The adult brain constitutes 2% of the body mass but uses 15% of the total energy generated by body metabolism. The brain metabolic rate at rest is seven times that of the remainder of the body. The main source of neuronal energy, adenosine triphosphate (ATP), is generated through aerobic glycolysis. Complete breakdown of one molecule of glucose to H_2O and CO_2 in the aerobic cycle produces 38 molecules of ATP to power the neurons. Anaerobic glycolysis produces only two molecules of ATP for each molecule of glucose. Anaerobic glycolysis in the brain, unlike in other tissues such as muscle or liver, cannot sustain required energy demands. Persistence of anaerobic glycolysis and accumulation of lactate as its by-product in the brain tissue proves to be fatal to the neurons by rapidly lowering the intracellular pH.

Blood Flow and Autoregulation

Although glucose is its primary substrate for energy generation, the brain has no glucose or glycogen stores. To sustain active metabolism the brain, therefore, requires a constant supply of glucose, oxygen, and a regulated blood flow to maintain appropriate function; 60 mg of glucose and 3 to 4 mL of oxygen per 100 g of brain tissue is required to meet the demand every minute. This is supplied by a blood flow of about 50 mL/100 g of brain tissue per minute. Changes in metabolic demand are met by appropriate changes in blood flow. This coupling of blood flow to metabolic demand is controlled by autoregulation of the cerebral circulation.[2] Automatic adjustment of the cerebral vascular resistance maintains the ratio of cerebral blood flow to oxygen use at approximately 20 over a wide range (50 to 130 mm Hg) of perfusion pressures. Conditions such as advanced age, diabetes, and hypertension (common in patients with thoracic aortic pathology), in addition to other anesthesia and perfusion-related conditions associated with these operations, alter the autoregulation of cerebral blood flow. Perfusion pressures need to be adjusted according to predicted changes in autoregulation in order to avoid under- or overperfusion. As Table 31-1 illustrates, preexisting patient-related conditions or physiologic changes induced by anesthetic management alter the autoregulation of the cerebral blood flow. Perfusion pressures during cardiopulmonary bypass and cerebral perfusion have to be adjusted according to these

TABLE 31-1. Modifiers of Autoregulation of the Cerebral Blood Flow

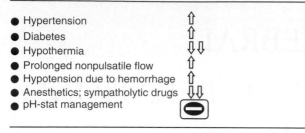

● Hypertension ⇑
● Diabetes ⇑
● Hypothermia ⇓⇓
● Prolonged nonpulsatile flow ⇑
● Hypotension due to hemorrhage ⇑
● Anesthetics; sympatholytic drugs ⇓⇓
● pH-stat management ⊖

predicted changes to avoid cerebral under- or overperfusion. Maintenance of cerebral autoregulation of blood flow during cardiopulmonary bypass in general, and during application of selective cerebral perfusion methods in particular, has an important protective role. During deep hypothermia, autoregulation is maintained at perfusion pressures as low as 30 mm Hg. Impaired autoregulation leads to purely pressure-driven brain blood flow, uncoupled from metabolic demand. Autoregulation is also lost with pH-stat management of the acid base balance during anesthesia. Nonpulsatile flow increases the cerebral vascular resistance over a period of time. Higher pressures may be required for effective perfusion toward the end of a long bypass period (and immediately thereafter) to avoid underperfusion in the presence of upward "re-regulated" autoregulation. Experimental use of pulsatile assistance has been shown to ameliorate these changes in the cerebral vascular resistance.[3]

Luxury Perfusion

The impairment of autoregulation creates extra blood flow exceeding the metabolic need: a state of "luxury perfusion." Under the artificial conditions of extracorporeal circulation and low pressure (low-flow hypothermic perfusion), the relatively large proportion of the pump flow reaching the brain exposes the brain to higher macro- or microembolic loads due to overperfusion.[4,5] Luxury perfusion per se under these circumstances may be injurious to the brain.[6] This mechanism of brain injury attains special importance in older patients, who are prone to enhanced luxury cerebral perfusion due to age-related changes in the autonomic vasomotor tone during hypothermia and nonpulsatile flow. Luxury perfusion may partly explain the higher incidence of strokes seen in older patients.[7]

Ischemic-Anoxic Brain Injury

There are two basic mechanisms that lead to ischemic cerebral injury during operations on the thoracic aorta that require temporary exclusion of the cerebral circulation. Global ischemia due to interrupted or inadequate flow leads to subtle brain injury that manifests itself as the clinical syndrome that we have called "temporary neuro-logic dysfunction." This condition, commonly believed to be self-limited and benign, has permanent functional sequelae detectable with detailed neuropsychological testing, especially of the memory function. It is a direct consequence of inadequate cerebral protection. In its extreme form, it results in anoxic brain injury. The second type of injury that has traditionally received the most attention (because of its devastating consequences) is represented by localized strokes caused by ischemic infarcts. These infarcts, detectable by conventional imaging techniques, are due to embolic events and were generally thought to be independent of the method of brain protection used. Recent studies regarding methods of cerebral perfusion have stimulated great discussion regarding the latter issue.

Pathogenesis

Neurotransmitter Toxicity

The importance of the failure of the neurotransmitter transport mechanism and the toxicity of excitatory neurotransmitters as common pathways in the pathogenesis of many neurologic disorders (including ischemic cerebral injury) has been well demonstrated.[8] Glutamate and aspartate are the primary messengers used by neurons for interneuronal communication. After release into the intercellular space, glutamate rapidly is converted to glutamine and then reenters the neuron ready to be used for the next message. Any cause that interrupts conversion of glutamate to glutamine will lead to accumulation of glutamate in the intercellular space, where in increasing concentrations it acts as a potent neurotoxic substance. It opens calcium channels, leading to an influx of calcium, which starts the catastrophic intracellular activation of several enzyme systems in a vicious "biochemical cascade," ultimately leading to neuronal autodigestion and cell death. Currently, there is a substantial amount of basic and pharmacologic research being conducted toward modification of the biochemical reactions that follow the failure of the neurotransmitter transport mechanism. Some information gained from these studies has already been incorporated into current preventive and therapeutic approaches.[8] There is also an intense search for appropriate pharmacologic agents to enhance the current cerebral protective methods. Certainly, more insight into these reactions is needed for effective clinical intervention.

Phases of Ischemic Cerebral Injury

The brain will tolerate an acute reduction in blood flow down to about 40 to 50% of normal during normothermia. Below that, functional and cellular biochemical changes that start with depletion of ATP stores, and progress to eventual impairment of glutamate transport, occur quite rapidly (Figures 31-1 and 31-2).[9] These changes ultimately lead to the unrelenting biochemical cascade that ends with the death of the neuron.[8]

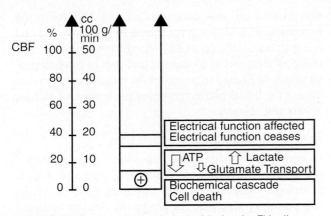

FIGURE 31-1. Thresholds of cerebral ischemia. This diagram illustrates the effect of reduced cerebral blood flow (CBF). Data are from awake primate experiments and show that at normothermia, a gradual reduction of the blood flow in the middle cerebral artery leads to cessation of function and reversible paralysis at around 50% reduction in the regional blood flow. At about 20 cc/100 g/min cerebral blood flow, cell death is a function of time, with rapid onset of the biochemical changes that lead to ultimate loss of the neuron. ATP = adenosine triphosphate. Reproduced and modified with permission from Jafar JJ et al.[9]

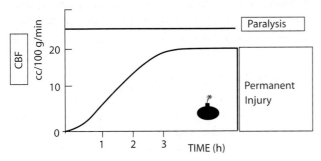

FIGURE 31-2. Thresholds of cerebral ischemia. This diagram illustrates the time course of the effect of reduced cerebral blood flow (CBF). Data from awake primate experiments and show that at normothermia, a gradual reduction of the blood flow in the middle cerebral artery leads to cessation of function and reversible paralysis at around 50% reduction. At about 20 cc/100 g/min cerebral blood flow, cell death and permanent injury is a function of time. With further reduction in flow, neurons are lost exponentially earlier, reaching down to about 5 to 8 minutes at zero flow. Reproduced and modified with permission from Jafar JJ et al.[9]

The pathogenesis of ischemic cerebral injury follows a set sequence of events in three distinct phases.

PHASE 1: DEPOLARIZATION

Depolarization is the first phase of this process. Lack of adequate oxygen to support aerobic metabolism rapidly leads to depletion of ATP and to accumulation of adenosine monophosphate (AMP), adenosine, and nitric oxide—all potent vasodilators—in the intercellular space. At the same time, glucose that is available is shunted into the anaerobic pathway. Vasodilatation makes more glucose

available for anaerobic glycolysis. The process is accelerated in the presence of hyperglycemia, and there is ample clinical evidence to suggest that hyperglycemia compounds ischemic cerebral injury. The inability of the brain to use lactate (the metabolic byproduct of anaerobic glycolysis), and the lack of adequate blood flow to carry it away, rapidly leads to its accumulation and the eventual decrease in the intracellular pH. This decrease in pH is a potent stimulator for the release of the neurotransmitters glutamate and aspartate. These substances accumulate in the interneuronal spaces because there is insufficient ATP available for their conversion to glutamine before they can reenter the neuron. All events in this phase are reversible, and current clinical protective methods are aimed at delaying or preventing the sequence of these events, which ultimately leads to the failure of the neurotransmitter transport mechanism at the end of the depolarization phase. As Table 31-2 illustrates, all events in this phase are reversible. They are either completely preventable or can be ameliorated and delayed by currently available protective modalities. Hypothermia and continued antegrade perfusion are the most effective measures to maintain aerobic glycolysis in the presence of reduced flow. Hypothermia and retrograde cerebral perfusion (RCP) are effective in delaying the depletion of ATP in zero antegrade flow state. Circulatory arrest helps reduce anaerobic glycolysis and accompanied acidosis by eliminating continued glucose supply to fuel the pathway. The trickle flow supplied by RCP supplies substrate to maintain anaerobic glycolysis, yet at the same time may help to remove acid metabolites. Depending on how effective the RCP flow is, the net effect of RCP may be marginally superior to DHCA alone.

PHASE 2: BIOCHEMICAL CASCADE

The collapse of the neurotransmitter transport mechanism starts the vicious cycle that constitutes the second phase, the biochemical cascade. Accumulation of neurotransmitters in the intercellular space opens up the calcium channels, leading to massive calcium influx and activation of several intracellular enzyme systems, with catastrophic consequences. This self-sustaining biochemical reaction ultimately results in neuronal autodigestion

TABLE 31-2. Phase 1 of Ischemic Injury: Depolarization Sequence and Preventive Measures

Phase 1: Depolarization	Prevention
1. ⇓ Aerobic glycolysis	Perfusion, hypothermia
2. **ATP** depletion	Hypothermia, RCP
3. ⇑ Anaerobic glycolysis Hyperglycemia Trickle flow	Arrest, RCP
4. ⇑ Lactate, acidosis	Hypothermia, RCP
5. ⇓ Neurotransmitter transport	Hypothermia

ATP = adenosine triphosphate
RCP = retrograde cerebral perfusion

and permanent loss of the cell. There are some promising experimental pharmacologic approaches (neurotransmitter-antagonists, neurotransmitter-receptor blockers, and calcium channel blockers) to the modification or prevention of the failure of the neurotransmitter mechanism and of the events of the biochemical cascade.[8,10] Currently, however, there is no practical pharmacologic remedy ready for clinical application for brain protection during aortic surgery. As Table 31-3 illustrates, these events cannot be reversed by currently available modalities. The search for effective inhibitors of neurotransmitter release and neurotransmitter receptor blockers continues. There are promising compounds in phase three clinical trials. There is experience with calcium channel blockers with mixed clinical results. Aminosteroids show promise in countering the toxic effects of free fatty acids, especially arachidonic acid. Suppression of apoptosis offers a new venue for prevention of delayed neuronal loss. It is hoped that ischemic injury can be substantially modified to preserve neuronal integrity by the discovery of the effective compounds aimed at the sequence of the biochemical cascade. The combination of these compounds may be an integral part of brain protection during surgery of the thoracic aorta in the near future.

PHASE 3: REPERFUSION INJURY

The last phase of ischemic brain injury occurs during reperfusion. Although the reperfusion injury, especially in the context of the present methods of cerebral protection, may be the most important phase in the pathogenesis of ischemic cerebral injury, our current understanding of its mechanism is rudimentary. Maintenance of adequate oxygen delivery during this vulnerable period is of paramount importance, especially following hypothermic circulatory arrest. In addition, leukocyte infiltration and cytokine-mediated inflammatory reactions are known to play an important role during this phase. In recent animal studies, leukocyte-depleting filtration seemed to mitigate reperfusion injury in the brain.[11] Currently, we employ leukocyte filtration in all of our hypothermic circulatory arrest cases. Local release of nitric oxide (NO) in response to ischemia is a protective mechanism designed to increase blood flow through vasodilatation. However,

overproduction and accumulation of NO following hypothermic arrest has been shown to be neurotoxic and is implicated in the genesis of reperfusion injury.[12,13] The principal elements of all current methods of cerebral protection are designed to interrupt the pathogenetic process during the initial phase, aiming at prevention of cellular anoxia and acidosis.

Apoptosis and Delayed Neuronal Loss

Increasing knowledge of the importance of programmed cell death in the pathogenesis of heart failure and chronic neurologic disorders recently led to exploration of the role that apoptosis plays in producing delayed neuronal loss and the associated delayed decline in cognitive function following acute ischemic cerebral injury. It has been shown that sublethal cellular injury sustained during acute ischemia can trigger apoptotic pathways that result in delayed loss of neurons.[14] Neurons that are not lost immediately by necrosis cover a wide spectrum of pathologic and physiologic states, from absolute viability and function to one of various stages of "suspended animation," apoptosis, and variable function or nonfunction.[15] The possibility that effective pharmacologic intervention may salvage some of these cells undergoing apoptosis and ameliorate the extent of delayed neuronal loss and late sequelae of hypothermic circulatory arrest is intriguing (see Table 31-3).

Selective Vulnerability and Location of Injury

Different regions of the brain have a substantial variation in energy requirements. Gray matter uses more energy than white matter, the cortex more than the basal ganglia, and active neurons more than quiescent ones. Some regions of the brain, therefore, are clearly more vulnerable to ischemic or anoxic injury. The earliest manifestation of such injury occurs in the regions of the brain with higher metabolic rates and activities that persist even under profound hypothermia. In experimental models, the earliest histopathologic signs of ischemic injury can be found anatomically in the hippocampus.[16] It is well known that this region of the brain is the locus for acquisition of new information and is particularly sensitive to anoxic or ischemic injury because of its high metabolic rate.[17] As a clinical corollary of this pathologic finding, the subtlest sign of brain injury following DHCA is represented by the deficits of memory function that can be detected by neuropsychological evaluation.[18] It is quite likely that the impairment of memory function in adults with prolonged DHCA is related to neuronal injury in the hippocampus. Recent evidence suggests strongly that the early postoperative syndrome of "temporary neurologic dysfunction" correlates significantly with the long-term deficits seen in memory and motor function following prolonged periods of DHCA.[19] Identification of a reliable biochemical marker for neurologic injury has remained elusive. Most such marker evidence regarding neurologic

TABLE 31-3. Phase 2 of Ischemic Injury: Biochemical Cascade and Modification of Injury

Phase 2: Biochemical Cascade	Modification
1. ⇧ Neurotransmitter release	Inhibitors, blockers
2. ⇧ Calcium influx	Ca^{2+} channel blocker
3. ⇧ Protease and lipase	Steroids
4. ⇧ Arachidonic acid	Aminosteroids
5. ⇧ Free radicals	Steroids, scavengers
6. Neuronal autodigestion	
7. Apoptosis	Caspase supressors

injury surrounds the study of astrocyte protein S-100β. Increased levels of S-100β have been measured after routine cardiopulmonary bypass and recovery of shed mediastinal blood with pump suckers. In some studies elevated levels have been shown to correlate with adverse cerebral events.[20] However, the utility of S-100β in assessing the efficacy of adjuncts for cerebral protection has not been proven.

Cerebral Protection

Currently, there is no practical way of completely turning off the functional component of the brain's activity to reduce the energy demands to the bare minimum required to maintain cellular viability during the critical periods of interruption or exclusion of the cerebral circulation. The objective of all current clinical methods of cerebral protection is prevention of cellular anoxia and acidosis in order to preserve the integrity of the central nervous system. These methods have evolved into three principal applications or their combinations. Hypothermic circulatory arrest, and the presence of no flow, rely on drastic reductions of oxygen demand with profound hypothermia, whereas methods that depend on continuous selective antegrade cerebral perfusion (SCP) or RCP aim at preserving oxygen supply while at the same time reducing oxygen demand with the aid of varying degrees of hypothermia.

Deep Hypothermic Circulatory Arrest

Hypothermia is the principal element of all current methods of brain protection in general and of DHCA in particular.

General Considerations

The protective effect of hypothermia primarily is based on the temperature-related reduction of intracellular enzymatic reactions. Proportionately, the need for oxygen delivery and, therefore, blood flow requirements, is reduced. Although the metabolic effects of drugs that are active depressants of neuronal function are comparable to hypothermia, experimentally hypothermia affords better protection against cerebral anoxia.[21] The cerebral protective effect of hypothermia is multifaceted in addition to temperature-related metabolic suppression. Hypothermia specifically preserves the tissue pH and ATP.[22] It also prevents release of excitatory neurotransmitters and delays the onset of the biochemical cascade that eventually leads to cell death due to ischemia (Figure 31-3).

Metabolic Suppression and "Safe Period of Arrest"

Michenfelder and colleagues have expressed the relationship between the temperature and the cerebral metabolic rate for oxygen ($CMRO_2$) as the temperature coefficient Q_{10} for $CMRO_2$. Q_{10} reflects an exponential function for

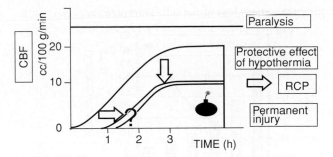

FIGURE 31-3. Protective effect of hypothermia. This diagram, in relation to Figure 31-2, summarizes the known effects of deep hypothermia on preservation of the brain during circulatory arrest or at low flow states. Hypothermia delays the onset of permanent cellular injury during arrest. Clinical and experimental evidence points that a safe period of arrest may extend up to 40 minutes at an esophageal temperature of 10° to 12°C. There is increasing risk of permanent ischemic injury if this limit is exceeded. Hypothermia also reduces the blood flow requirements during perfusion. A blood flow of 10 cc/100 g/min, or 20% of the resting cerebral blood flow at normothermia, is adequate to preserve cerebral integrity for prolonged periods of time in the presence of hypothermia. Whether the addition of RCP adds any further protection over that afforded by hypothermia remains largely unproven (?). CBF = cerebral blood flow. RCP = retrograde cerebral perfusion.

the rate of reduction in the metabolism over a 10°C temperature range within a clinically relevant temperature limit of 38° to 14°C. Q_{10} is reported to be between 2.0 and 3.0.[23] Recent studies in puppies show that the reduction of the cerebral metabolic rate for oxygen is substantially more modest than what had been reported earlier. There is 39% of the baseline metabolic activity still present at 18°C, a temperature generally thought to be safe for prolonged periods of clinical circulatory arrest. In the same study, quantitative electrocardiography (EEG) also showed significant slow-wave activity at 18°C, whereas EEG silence was present at 13°C and 8°C.[24] We have recalculated Q_{10} for the adult human brain, based on direct measurement of $CMRO_2$ during DHCA.[25] Based on this clinical study, the safe period of arrest is calculated to be about 30 min at 15°C and 40 min at 10°C. Beyond these time limits, anoxic cellular injury is inevitable at these temperatures (Figure 31-4).

As pointed out earlier, such injury is detected in its subtlest form in the function of the regions of the brain most vulnerable to anoxia. Clinical studies in infants undergoing correction of congenital heart defects using DHCA show subclinical seizure activity on EEG, with subtle abnormal neurologic examinations at 1 year following surgery.[26] These studies also confirm that prolonged durations of DHCA correlate with lower IQ scores in later childhood.

There is insufficient information of this nature regarding the adult population undergoing DHCA. In our initial review of 200 patients who underwent DHCA during

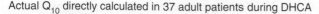

Actual Q$_{10}$ directly calculated in 37 adult patients during DHCA

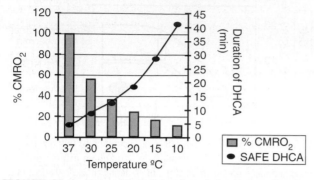

FIGURE 31-4. Limits of "safe" duration of circulatory arrest. Q$_{10}$ for the adult brain is calculated from direct measurement of CMRO$_2$ in 37 adult patients undergoing thoracic aortic operations with DHCA. The temperature-related reduction in the metabolic rate and the calculated "safe periods of arrest" are shown. CMRO$_2$ = cerebral metabolic rate for oxygen; DHCA = deep hypothermic circulatory arrest. Data from McCullough JN et al.[25]

operations on the thoracic aorta the incidence of "temporary neurologic dysfunction" was 19%. This significantly correlated with the duration of the arrest time and with patient age. The significant relationship between "temporary neurologic dysfunction" and the arrest time raised a flag of caution although the progress of most patients appeared to be quite benign following recovery from what was thought to be a self-limited syndrome of altered neurologic function. As a result of this finding, even at that early time in our experience, we recommended that every effort should be made to limit arrest times, especially in older patients.[7] To further investigate whether DHCA in the adult is associated with long-term neuropsychological deficits, a detailed study was conducted to compare patients undergoing "routine" cardiac surgery with cardiopulmonary bypass to those having surgery of the thoracic aorta with periods of DHCA. This study showed that circulatory arrest times longer than 25 min and advanced age were significant predictors of poor performance at 6 weeks for the memory and fine motor domains.[18] Recent evidence strongly suggests that the early postoperative syndrome of "temporary neurologic dysfunction" correlates significantly with long-term deficits in memory and motor function following prolonged periods of DHCA, and confirms the belief that this clinical syndrome is a manifestation of subtle brain injury due to inadequate cerebral protection.[19] Duration of DHCA, on the other hand, has no influence on mortality or occurrence of permanent neurologic injury caused by embolic strokes.[7]

There is now a consensus that affirms that temperatures colder than previously thought to be safe are necessary if prolonged periods of arrest are anticipated. Similarly, the duration of the arrest even at these cold temperatures should not exceed 40 (preferably 30) min at 12° to 15°C. Durations of circulatory arrest exceeding 60 min are universally regarded as risky, but success has been reported.

Current Clinical Application

Monitoring

Adequate and uniform cooling, and the demonstration of suppression of brain metabolic activity by monitoring of function and metabolism, is of paramount importance before the initiation of DHCA. In many circumstances, cerebral electrical function and activity by means of EEG and auditory- and sensory-evoked potentials are monitored.[27] Studies show that evoked potentials are a better guide than EEG alone and usually take longer to disappear, whereas EEG silence occurs quite variably at shorter durations of cooling and at relatively higher brain temperatures.[28] Because oxygen extraction is the most readily monitored parameter reflecting the metabolic state of the brain, we routinely measure jugular bulb venous oxygen saturations and continue cooling until these are well above 95%. At this level we are confident that brain metabolism is suppressed adequately to allow a period of 30 to 40 min of arrest safely.[25] Our current clinical practice closely follows the guidelines enumerated in the published reviews.[29,30] The following is a summary of the pertinent, and what we believe are the clinically important, features of hypothermic circulatory arrest.

COOLING

Surface cooling, which was routinely used early in our experience, currently is reserved for specific indications only (ie, in cases when the risk of aortic entry during sternotomy is high). In these situations, surface cooling adds a measure of increased safety by removing substantial amounts of heat from the whole body, prior to urgent institution of hypothermic circulatory arrest. This is especially valuable in the presence of aortic regurgitation, where rapid core cooling will invariably lead to ventricular fibrillation and left ventricular distension before adequate decompression of the heart or the application of the aortic cross-clamp is possible.

It is generally agreed that too short a period of cooling may result in neurologic damage due to uneven and inadequate lowering of the brain temperature, and that packing the head in ice during prolonged periods of circulatory arrest improves the outcome by maintaining cranial hypothermia.[31,32] Therefore, prior to the institution of prolonged periods of hypothermic circulatory arrest, we insist on cooling down to esophageal temperatures of 12° to 15°C. This is accompanied by EEG and evoked potential silence and/or jugular venous bulb oxygen saturations of higher than 95% as indicators of adequate suppression of cerebral function and metabolism. This active cooling period in an adult commonly takes at least 30 min or longer.

WARMING

This may well be the most crucial phase of perfusion. The critical postischemic period that was clearly seen in the experimental models at 2 h following hypothermic circulatory arrest, where impaired autoregulation and increased cerebrovascular resistance is pronounced, probably starts with reperfusion and warming in clinical practice. At this stage, $CMRO_2$ continues at reduced blood flows, and oxygen extraction is increased to meet the demand. Any further drop in oxygen delivery will be poorly tolerated. Therefore, it is important to proceed slowly with warming and never exceed a 10°C gradient between the perfusate temperature and the core temperature, as increased gradients may be associated with the formation of gas emboli. We stop warming at 36°C esophageal or 34°C bladder temperatures and do not allow perfusate temperature to exceed 37°C. Higher perfusion pressures are maintained by fine-tuning the hemodynamics throughout the initial 16 h of postarrest recovery. The patients usually leave the operating room relatively cold, which gives an additional margin of protection in this critical postischemic period. Much research regarding the effects of postischemic cerebral temperature strategies after circulatory arrest has been done. In an animal model, hyperthermia was associated with persistent deterioration of neurologic and behavioral outcome. Histologic assessment has confirmed the adverse effects of increased temperature and has been correlated with significant injury in the brain. Conversely, post-ischemic hypothermia has been shown to significantly improve outcome relative to hyperthermia, with a reproducible trend toward improved neurobehavioral and histologic outcomes.[33]

METABOLIC MANAGEMENT

The issue of how pH should be managed during cooling remains controversial. As blood is cooled, pH changes in an alkaline direction. Cerebral perfusion unequivocally is enhanced by pH-stat management (actively adding carbon dioxide), which abolishes cerebral autoregulation.[34] Cerebral vasodilatation due to increasing levels of CO_2 favors more thorough cooling, and it likely improves oxygen availability by counteracting the leftward shift of oxyhemoglobin induced by hypothermia. This is important in the early cooling phase, when the brain is warm but the blood is cold.[35] However, pH-stat management undoubtedly exposes the brain to an increased embolic load because of the "luxury perfusion" that accompanies cerebral vasodilatation. pH-stat management is also associated with intracellular acidosis and alterations in enzyme function during the arrest time. Alpha-stat management (allowing the pH to drift), on the other hand, preserves autoregulation even at lower temperatures and limits the flow to meet the metabolic demand diminished by hypothermia. This provides for improved intracellular enzyme function. It results in perfusion at a higher pH and eliminates "luxury perfusion" and the associated risk of an increased embolic load.[36] However, this reduction in cerebral blood flow may result in greater neurologic impairment, as suggested by the histologic injury seen in

animal studies.[37] As recently suggested, optimal management may involve initiating cooling with pH-stat management and then using alpha-stat principles to guide the perfusion prior to the arrest.[36,38]

There is substantial experimental and clinical evidence showing that hemodilution is important in limiting cerebral injury following hypothermic circulatory arrest by improving cerebral blood flow at low temperatures. Because the effects of affinity of hemoglobin to oxygen at these low temperatures determines that most O_2 delivery to the tissues is by oxygen in solution, the effective O_2-carrying capacity of the blood is changed little by the reduction of the red cell mass by hemodilution. On the other hand, the improvement in the blood flow by hemodilution, with prevention of hypothermia-related hemoconcentration and sludging, is, without a doubt, an essential element.[30]

The hypothermia-induced release of catecholamines and administration of steroids produce a significant tendency to hyperglycemia in the pre- or post-arrest periods.[39,40] High blood glucose levels in these periods are known to have an adverse effect on the intracellular pH and the neurologic outcome.[41] The overabundance of glucose drives the anaerobic glycolysis cycle and leads to faster accumulation of lactate and intracellular acidosis during the arrest interval. Therefore, hyperglycemia should aggressively be treated prior to and following hypothermic circulatory arrest. We use intravenous insulin drips liberally.

Among the many pharmacologic adjuncts thought to be effective in modifying ischemia and reperfusion-related cerebral responses that lead to injury, we continue to use steroids and mannitol. Steroids are used in all patients as membrane stabilizers and also to reduce cerebral edema.[40] In all patients with anticipated arrest times greater than 30 min, 1 g of methylprednisolone is given prior to arrest. It is continued in the first 48 h post arrest (125 mg q6h for 24 h; then 125 mg q12h for the next 24 h). Mannitol, besides reducing cerebral edema and intracranial pressure, has an important effect as a free radical scavenger and is given in standard doses both during the cooling and rewarming periods.[42]

We have all but abandoned the routine use of barbiturates as an adjunct to our approach, because of the associated myocardial depression and uncertain efficacy in this setting. There is experimental and some clinical indication that cerebral-specific calcium channel blockers and glutamate receptor antagonists are beneficial following ischemic cerebral insult.[8] Cerebral ischemia causes a rapid shift of calcium from the extracellular space into the cells. Some authors have favored the use of nicardipine, which directly reduces this influx.[43] Others have incorporated the use of lidocaine as an adjunct in reducing cerebral metabolism. Under normothermic circumstances, lidocaine reduces cerebral metabolism by blocking sodium channels, thus abolishing synaptic electrical activity. During hypothermia, it can further reduce brain metabolism by inhibiting ion leaks and, therefore, reducing the energy requirement for ionic homeostasis by the Na+- K+ and ATPase pumps. In an animal study, the average number of ischemic neurons in multiple sections of brain tissue was significantly less in the group receiving a continuous lidocaine infusion than in the control group.[44] We have not yet incorporated any of these new approaches in our management. When the efficacy and safety of these agents are proven, they will be considered in the protective protocol.

REPERFUSION

The possibility that some of the injury associated with DHCA may occur during reperfusion or thereafter has prompted studies suggesting that a brief period of cold perfusion following DHCA may be beneficial in prevention of cerebral vasoconstriction that results from immediate resumption of rewarming with reperfusion.[45] The use of pharmacologic agents for this same purpose (to regulate the cerebral vasomotor tone during reperfusion and to minimize injury related to reperfusion) is also an intense area of investigation. Perhaps this period of cerebral vasoconstriction is related to the impairment of nitric oxide production after DHCA. The loss of nitric oxide (a cerebral vasodilator) may be partly responsible for the reduction in cerebral perfusion during the recovery period. In an animal model, the stimulation of nitric oxide production with L-arginine significantly improved the recovery of cerebral blood flow after the arrest period.[46] On the other hand, excessive production of nitric oxide has been found to be neurotoxic.[13]

Some authors advocate the use of modified ultrafiltration in an attempt to improve oxygen use by the brain. Possible mechanisms in animal studies include decreased cerebral edema, removal of toxic substances, alteration of leukocyte-mediated injury, and hemoconcentration.[47]

Selective Cerebral Perfusion

Rationale

Before the introduction of hypothermic circulatory arrest, selective perfusion of the arch branches was used for cerebral protection, in many forms and permutations, with less-than-ideal results.[48,49]

There is little question that the concept of selective antegrade cerebral perfusion has a sound physiologic basis, especially in systems that take advantage of autoregulation of the cerebral blood flow and aim at predetermined target perfusion pressures rather than fixed flow rates. Although deep hypothermia is not an essential component, the addition of hypothermia makes the method safer by reducing the flow requirements and pressures. As the clinical experience indicates, it can be applied successfully at moderate degrees of hypothermia with equally good results.[50]

Probably the most important advantage of this method is that it provides the luxury of time to allow for an unhurried repair of the pathology. This luxury, however, comes at a price. To perfuse the brain evenly in the face of unknown cerebral vascular anatomy in a given patient, multiple cannulae are required for at least two, and preferably for all three, arch branches. These multiple cannulations clutter the field and may increase the risk of embolization from manipulations as well as cannula-related mishaps during the procedure. When the procedure is carried out during only moderate hypothermia, continued perfusion of the lower body is essential. Absence of lower body perfusion at these relatively higher temperatures leaves the spinal cord vulnerable to ischemic injury, especially during protracted cerebral perfusion periods. In this case, provisions for control of the descending aorta to maintain a bloodless field further complicate the exposure and prolong the operation.

Clinical Application and Results

There are some significant differences in the application of selective perfusion in larger clinical series. Potential for over- or underperfusion exists with any of these systems. The current trend is to perfuse at least the innominate and left carotid arteries with a dedicated pump in an autoregulated system with flows determined by target pressures measured at distal sites. Optimal cerebral perfusion and prevention of perfusion mismatch can be best achieved by continuous monitoring of jugular venous bulb O_2 saturations. This is an indispensable monitoring tool for selective cerebral perfusion methods. Alternative use of transcutaneous near-infrared spectroscopy (NIS) for hemoglobin saturation is gaining wider acceptance as a gauge of oxygen delivery to the brain. In one study, regional cerebrovascular saturation (rSO_2) was measured continuously throughout surgery. Patients receiving SCP had significant rSO_2 recovery while those receiving RCP showed a constant and sustained decrease.[51] NIS monitors that can measure the redox state of the mitochondrial cytochrome 3 aa are a more reliable indicator of cellular oxygen uptake than are the competing systems that can only measure the intravascular saturation. Other areas of research have integrated the use of somatosensory-evoked potentials (SSEPs) as an indicator of adequate cerebral blood flow.

Frist and associates used preoperative studies of the circle of Willis to determine patency and perfused the innominate artery only (superselective) through a Y connection off the main arterial line from a single pump.[50] This system relies on autoregulation of the cerebral blood flow, and pressure in the right radial artery is used to determine the pump flow rate. The descending aorta was occluded with a balloon catheter, and the perfusion of the lower body continued at 26°C.

Matsuda and colleagues reported 34 patients with perfusion of both the innominate and the left carotid arteries via separate pumps and with fixed predetermined flows at 16° to 20°C.[52] Balloon occlusion of the descending aorta from below was used. The system again depended on autoregulation of the cerebral blood flow; however, the presence of separate pumps necessitated pressure monitoring at both temporal arteries as well as the lower body. The operative mortality was 9%, with one serious neurologic complication. The impressive finding in this series, however, was the apparently well-tolerated periods of prolonged selective cerebral perfusion, the longest being 214 min, with complete neurologic recovery.

Bachet and colleagues further modified the method and introduced the intriguing term "cerebroplegia."[53] He used two pumps and two heat exchangers to perfuse the brain (through the innominate and the left carotid arteries) at 6° to 10°C with low flow and the rest of the body at 28°C. The period of selective cerebral perfusion was well within the limits that would be considered safe for hypothermic circulatory arrest. The report included 54 patients with an operative mortality of 13%, and 3 serious neurologic complications, one resulting in death. In general, the reported results of selective cerebral perfusion in other hands are similar to these three original series.

Perhaps one of the most improved surgical techniques in aortic arch reconstruction and cerebral protection can be attributed to Kazui. It involves a fairly new flexible perfusion cannula (which also contains a lumen for pressure monitoring), which can be used to separately cannulate the arch vessels and allow for selective cerebral perfusion. A multilimbed branched graft is then used to reconstruct the arch. Kazui used this method in 50 consecutive patients with atherosclerotic arch aneurysms and reported a 2% operative mortality, a 4% incidence of temporary neurologic dysfunction, and a 4% permanent stroke rate. These results are without equal in the literature.[54,55]

Because of the enhanced risk of embolization, we are not very enthusiastic about the routine use of SCP and reserve it only for cases requiring total arch replacement. Cannulation of the right axillary artery simplifies the routine application and maintenance of SCP in these cases but requires pressure monitoring distally. In the past, in an attempt to reduce the arrest times to less than 30 to 40 min, we had developed a simplified technique for SCP and used it in patients with anticipated complex repairs requiring longer arrest times. After cooling, during a period of arrest, we isolated the island of aortic tissue containing the origins of the head vessels. A beveled (often 18 mm) Dacron graft was sewn into this island, and flow was reestablished to all three arch branches with the perfusate temperature at 10°C. The flow rate was adjusted to achieve a perfusion pressure of about 50 mm Hg monitored at the right radial artery. At the end of the reconstruction of the remainder of the aorta, this beveled graft containing the orifices of the cerebral vessels was sewn to the rest of the aortic graft. This maneuver simply accomplished selective cerebral perfusion without the need to manipulate cerebral vessels individually. It also established prompt antegrade perfusion of the aorta at the end of the reconstruction.[29] Currently, for total arch replacement, we prefer a modification of the Kazui method with initial cannulation of the right axillary artery and separate sequential grafts to innominate, left carotid, and left subclavian arteries, with individual control of these vessels while maintaining antegrade cerebral perfusion through the right axillary and innominate artery and then via the other branches as they are individually anastomosed. This technique eliminates the need for individual cannulation of the brachiocephalic branches and limits the brain ischemia time to a bare minimum.

Retrograde Cerebral Perfusion

Rationale

The limitations of DHCA (particularly, time, pressure, and the complexity of selective cerebral perfusion methods) led to the exploration of alternative methods of cerebral protection. The concept of retrograde perfusion for cerebral protection has its roots in the description of its use in clearing massive air embolisms during cardiopulmonary bypass.[56] Lemole used brief periods of retrograde cerebral perfusion for cerebral-protective purposes during insertion of intraluminal grafts in the distal ascending aorta.[57] Ueda and colleagues described for the first time the planned use of retrograde cerebral perfusion as a simpler alternative to selective cerebral perfusion methods.[58,59] The main argument of the proponents of this method is that in application, it is as simple as hypothermic circulatory arrest and is safer over longer periods of arrest because the brain is being supplied by oxygenated blood, albeit in a retrograde manner.

Laboratory and Clinical Evidence

RCP gained widespread clinical acceptance prior to any serious experimental demonstration of its effectiveness and its mode of action. This, in part, may have occurred because RCP is difficult to study in the laboratory. There are substantial differences in anatomy and physiology of the cerebral venous circulation among species commonly used in laboratory investigations. The use of different species and different methods of delivery of RCP has yielded confusing and often conflicting experimental data. The available information does not produce a clear picture of whether RCP, in fact, is effective and, if so, how it works.[60,61] The two most striking and clinically relevant findings emerging from the laboratory investigation of RCP are (1) very little of the retrograde perfusate actually reaches the brain tissue and (2) RCP is highly effective in maintaining cranial hypothermia during the arrest period.

It is likely that effective maintenance of cranial hypothermia is not the only mechanism that explains the effect of RCP. Venovenous shunting, experimentally shown in primates and confirmed in humans by anatomic studies, explains why only a small fraction of the retrograde flow reaches the brain.[60,62] With RCP via the superior vena cava, less than 5% of the retrograde flow returns from the arch branches, and the portion actually returning from the brain may be substantially less than 5%. The effective fraction of the flow can be enhanced experimentally by using special techniques to eliminate the influence of the valves in the jugular venous system or the delivery of the flow directly into the sagittal sinus at high perfusion pressures. Clinical relevance of these experiments is dubious at best. Pressurizing the entire body venous system similarly enhances retrograde flow to the brain clinically. This, however, is associated with unacceptable fluid retention and the associated risk of cerebral edema. The amount of flow, even when enhanced, is far too little to meet the ongoing metabolic needs of the brain even in the presence of deep hypothermia.[31] However, some uptake of nutrients does seem to occur because the blood returning to the arch is desaturated, and the depletion of high-energy phosphates and the decline of the intracellular pH (as assessed by magnetic resonance [MR] spectroscopy) are less severe than with DHCA alone.[63] It is possible that the trickle flow supplied by RCP may allow the removal of some metabolites, delay the onset of acidosis in the ischemic brain, and help modestly prolong the safe period of protection afforded by DHCA alone. However, it is also clear that retrograde cerebral perfusion, especially when it is effective, gradually leads to the development of cerebral edema at a rate directly related to the perfusion pressure. Even at the minimum pressures required for effective RCP, development of cerebral edema clearly limits the safe duration of RCP to only slightly longer times than comparable safe periods with DHCA alone.[64,65]

There is experimental evidence indicating that the trickle RCP flow may help prevent debris and air from reaching the terminal vessels of the brain and may in fact clear them from the major arteries.[66] This might be the major beneficial effect of RCP, but the use of RCP has yet to make a significant clinical impact on the incidence of embolic strokes following these operations. There is evidence that it may in fact increase the incidence of temporary neurologic dysfunction.[67] Studies following serum S-100β as a marker for detection of brain injury revealed that RCP does not provide improved cerebral protection over DHCA alone.[20]

Clinical Application and Results

Despite the relative lack of substantial evidence proving the efficacy of RCP, a dearth of knowledge regarding its physiologic consequences, and continuing uncertainty regarding the best method for its implementation, some surgeons have adopted the method for routine clinical use in aortic surgery.[68,69] There is no uniformity in the literature regarding the mode of application, method of cannulation, or choice of perfusate temperature or pressure during application of RCP. Originally, Ueda used a shunt between the arterial and venous pump lines to perfuse a single cannula in the superior vena cava retrogradely at 15° to 18°C while the rest of the body was not perfused.[58]

Since then, others have employed this modality in different configurations—by using a separate heat exchanger and pump to perfuse the superior vena cava, or by simple elevation of the central venous pressure. Each of these systems incorporates deep hypothermia as an integral part of the method. Additional retrograde perfusion of the whole body has also been used in an attempt to preserve the spinal cord and distal organs during operations on the arch and the thoracic aorta.

Although the application of retrograde cerebral perfusion varies from center to center, there is sufficient experimental, clinical, and anatomic data to suggest that the most effective retrograde perfusion of the brain is achieved when the entire venous system is pressurized. This finding reflects the important role the valve-free azygos system plays as a connection between the central nervous system veins and the systemic venous plexus.[62] In our practice, RCP is initiated at a core temperature of 12° to 15°C by perfusion of either one or both venae cavae at a flow rate to maintain the superior vena cava pressure between 15 and 20 mm Hg and certainly not to exceed 20 mm Hg. Snaring both caval cannulae prevents cardiac distension. We do not favor using continuous RCP for prolonged periods because the occurrence of brain edema (especially at the higher end of the recommended perfusion pressures) is a distinct risk and may, in itself, be injurious to the brain.[70] We currently reserve the use of RCP primarily for prevention of neurologic injury in patients at high risk for embolic strokes (those with thrombus or atheroma present in the aorta). RCP is used for brief periods, particularly prior to resumption of antegrade flow and reperfusion, to wash out debris from the cerebral vessels. We do not rely on RCP for the purpose of global cerebral protection beyond the time limits allowed by DHCA alone, and certainly under no circumstances would we use it without accompanied deep hypothermia.

Cerebral Protection

Current Integrated Application

Table 31-4 summarizes the desired properties of the "ideal" brain protection and how the current methods measure up to these criteria. The method should allow enough time for an unhurried repair without compromising protection. It should keep the operation simple and the operative field free of clutter. It should, at best, totally avoid manipulation of the head vessels or at least minimize such manipulation in order to reduce the risk of embolization. It should be effective without the need for prolonged deep hypothermia and associated prolongation of cardiopulmonary bypass times. Currently, only selective perfusion provides flow and the luxury of time and

TABLE 31-4. Comparative Characteristics of the Methods of Cerebral Protection

Requirements	DHCA	SCP	RCP
• Simple and easy application	+ +	− −	+
• Flow to support metabolism	− −	+ +	−
• Provide luxury of time	− −	+ +	−
• Limit pump time	− −	+	− −
• Limit manipulation of arch branches	+ +	− −	+ +
• Reduce or eliminate "embolic load"	−	− −	+ +

DHCA = deep hypothermic circulatory arrest; RCP = retrograde cerebral perfusion; SCP = selective cerebral perfusion.

potentially can be used with moderate hypothermia; it will, therefore, limit the pump time, but it suffers from required manipulation of the arch branches and therefore has the potential to increase the risk of embolization. On the other hand, RCP is simpler to apply and may extend the safe limit modestly, but it certainly does not provide the luxury of time that SCP does. It might, however, minimize emboli. If time limits are observed, DHCA remains the simplest form of protection. We have tried to incorporate the advantages of each method into an integrated approach to cerebral protection. This approach is guided by the following principles:

1. Initiate DHCA only after adequate metabolic (Saturation of oxygen in the jugular vein [$SJvO_2$] > 95%) and/or functional (EEG-evoked potential silence) evidence of suppression exists, usually at 12° to 15°C core temperatures.
2. Maintain cranial hypothermia during arrest period.
3. Keep cerebral ischemia times to less than 40 min at 12°C.
4. Cannulate the right axillary artery, anastomose the brachiocephalic vessels first, and restart antegrade SCP to limit cerebral ischemia time. The rest of the body remains arrested until the reconstruction of the descending aorta is completed.
5. During SCP, regulate flow to maintain pressures at 40 to 50 mm Hg, measured at the right carotid artery (simple autoregulated flow).
6. Do not rely on RCP to prolong the "safe arrest period."
7. Use RCP in selected cases with a high risk of stroke (age > 60, "dirty aorta"), prior to resumption of antegrade flow.
8. When using RCP, occlude the inferior vena cava for maximum effect.
9. Avoid continuous RCP at high perfusion pressures (keep the central venous pressure < 20 mm Hg in order to minimize cerebral edema).
10. Avoid femoral perfusion, particularly in patients with diseased descending aortas if at all possible; if this is not avoidable, then do not manipulate the descending aorta during cooling.
11. Cannulate the right axillary artery instead. This prevents retrograde embolization from perfusion of a diseased descending aorta. It is also useful in prevent-

ing malperfusion in complex acute dissections of the aorta.
12. Always resume perfusion in an antegrade fashion during rewarming.
13. Maintain adequate oxygen delivery during reperfusion and in the immediate recovery period.
14. Avoid perioperative hyperglycemia.

Future Prospects

Worldwide, all the centers actively treating thoracic aortic pathology are reporting improving overall results. Besides efforts to prevent embolic strokes, there is more emphasis in optimizing long-term neuropsychological outcome. Without question, this is the result of increasing expertise in dealing with these cases, rather than the superiority of one particular protection method. Realization of the absolute limits of arrest times, with or without the addition of RCP, emphasizes the importance of reducing the duration of zero-flow periods. Further simplification of the SCP methods and their wider application should lead to better outcomes. The attempts at modification of the events during the second phase of ischemic injury and reperfusion are subjects of intense research and may hold the promise of improved neurologic outlook for these patients. Table 31-3 (see above) summarizes the developing pharmacologic approach. The strokes due to embolic infarcts remain a difficult and persistent problem. The promise of RCP remains unfulfilled. It remains to be seen whether the wider application of SCP coupled with separate anastomosis of the brachiocephalic branches as reported by Kazui will have a significant impact on the incidence of stroke.[55]

References

1. Griepp RB, Stinson EB, Hollingsworth JF, Buehler D. Prosthetic replacement of the aortic arch. J Thorac Cardiovasc Surg 1975;70:1051–63.
2. Lassen NA. Autoregulation of cerebral blood flow. Circ Res 1964;15:1201–4.
3. Watanabe T, Miura M, Orita H, et al. Brain tissue pH, oxygen tension, and carbon dioxide tension in profoundly hypothermic cardiopulmonary bypass. Pulsatile assistance for circulatory arrest, low-flow perfusion, and moderate-flow perfusion. J Thorac Cardiovasc Surg 1990;100:274–80.
4. Matsuda H, Sasako Y, Nakano S, et al. Determination of optimal perfusion flow rate for deep hypothermic cardiopulmonary bypass in the adult based on distributions of blood flow and oxygen consumption. J Thorac Cardiovasc Surg 1992;103:541–8.
5. Fox LS, Blackstone EH, Kirklin JW, et al. Relationship of brain blood flow and oxygen consumption to perfusion flow rate during profoundly hypothermic cardiopulmonary bypass. An experimental study. J Thorac Cardiovasc Surg 1984;87:658–64.
6. Smith PLC, Newman SP, Ell PJ, Griepp EB. Cerebral consequences of cardiopulmonary bypass. Lancet 1986;1:823.

7. Ergin MA, Galla JD, Lansman SL, et al. Hypothermic circulatory arrest in operations on the thoracic aorta. Determinants of operative mortality and neurologic outcome. J Thorac Cardiovasc Surg 1994;107:788–97; discussion 797–9.

8. Lipton SA, Rosenberg PA. Excitatory amino acids as a final common pathway for neurologic disorders. N Engl J Med 1994;330:613–22.

9. Jafar J, Crowell R. Focal ischemic thresholds. In: Wood J, editor. Cerebral blood flow: physiologic and clinical aspects. New York: McGraw Hill; 1987. p. 449–57.

10. Lipton P. Ischemic cell death in brain neurons. Physiol Rev 1999;79:1431–568.

11. Rimpilainen J, Pokela M, Kiviluoma K, et al. Leukocyte filtration improves brain protection after a prolonged period of hypothermic circulatory arrest: a study in a chronic porcine model. J Thorac Cardiovasc Surg 2000; 120:1131–41.

12. Tseng EE, Brock MV, Lange MS, et al. Neuronal nitric oxide synthase inhibition reduces neuronal apoptosis after hypothermic circulatory arrest. Ann Thorac Surg 1997; 64:1639–47.

13. Tseng EE, Brock MV, Lange MS, et al. Nitric oxide mediates neurologic injury after hypothermic circulatory arrest. Ann Thorac Surg 1999;67:65–71.

14. Narula J, Baliga R. What's in a name? Would that which we call death by any other name be less tragic? Ann Thorac Surg 2001;72:1454–6.

15. Hagl C, Tatton NA, Khaladj N, et al. Involvement of apoptosis in neurological injury after hypothermic circulatory arrest: a new target for therapeutic intervention? Ann Thorac Surg 2001;72:1457–64.

16. Ye J, Yang L, Del Bigio MR, et al. Neuronal damage after hypothermic circulatory arrest and retrograde cerebral perfusion in the pig. Ann Thorac Surg 1996;61:1316–22.

17. Ginsberg MD, Graham DI, Busto R. Regional glucose utilization and blood flow following graded forebrain ischemia in the rat: correlation with neuropathology. Ann Neurol 1985;18:470–81.

18. Reich DL, Uysal S, Sliwinski M, et al. Neuropsychologic outcome after deep hypothermic circulatory arrest in adults. J Thorac Cardiovasc Surg 1999;117:156–63.

19. Ergin MA, Uysal S, Reich DL, et al. Temporary neurological dysfunction after deep hypothermic circulatory arrest: a clinical marker of long-term functional deficit. Ann Thorac Surg 1999;67:1887–90; discussion 1891–4.

20. LeMaire SA, Bhama JK, Schmittling ZC, et al. S100beta correlates with neurologic complications after aortic operation using circulatory arrest. Ann Thorac Surg 2001;71: 1913–8; discussion 1918–9.

21. Michenfelder JD, Theye RA. The effects of anesthesia and hypothermia on canine cerebral ATP and lactate during anoxia produced by decapitation. Anesthesiology 1970; 33:430–9.

22. Swain JA, McDonald TJ Jr, Griffith PK, et al. Low-flow hypothermic cardiopulmonary bypass protects the brain. J Thorac Cardiovasc Surg 1991;102:76–83; discussion 83–4.

23. Michenfelder JD, Milde JH. The relationship among canine brain temperature, metabolism, and function during hypothermia. Anesthesiology 1991;75:130–6.

24. Mezrow CK, Midulla PS, Sadeghi AM, et al. Evaluation of cerebral metabolism and quantitative electroencephalography after hypothermic circulatory arrest and low-flow cardiopulmonary bypass at different temperatures. J Thorac Cardiovasc Surg 1994;107:1006–19.

25. McCullough JN, Zhang N, Reich DL, et al. Cerebral metabolic suppression during hypothermic circulatory arrest in humans. Ann Thorac Surg 1999;67:1895–9; discussion 1919–21.

26. Bellinger DC, Wernovsky G, Rappaport LA, et al. Cognitive development of children following early repair of transposition of the great arteries using deep hypothermic circulatory arrest. Pediatrics 1991;87:701–7.

27. Guerit JM, Verhelst R, Rubay J, et al. The use of somatosensory evoked potentials to determine the optimal degree of hypothermia during circulatory arrest. J Card Surg 1994;9:596–603.

28. Coselli JS, Crawford ES, Beall AC Jr, et al. Determination of brain temperatures for safe circulatory arrest during cardiovascular operation. Ann Thorac Surg 1988;45:638–42.

29. Ergin MA, Griepp EB, Lansman SL, et al. Hypothermic circulatory arrest and other methods of cerebral protection during operations on the thoracic aorta. J Card Surg 1994;9:525–37.

30. Griepp EB, Griepp RB. Cerebral consequences of hypothermic circulatory arrest in adults. J Card Surg 1992;7:134–55.

31. Midulla PS, Gandsas A, Sadeghi AM, et al. Comparison of retrograde cerebral perfusion to antegrade cerebral perfusion and hypothermic circulatory arrest in a chronic porcine model. J Card Surg 1994;9:560–74; discussion 575.

32. Bellinger DC, Jonas RA, Rappaport LA, et al. Developmental and neurologic status of children after heart surgery with hypothermic circulatory arrest or low-flow cardiopulmonary bypass. N Engl J Med 1995;332:549–55.

33. Shum-Tim D, Nagashima M, Shinoka T, et al. Postischemic hyperthermia exacerbates neurologic injury after deep hypothermic circulatory arrest. J Thorac Cardiovasc Surg 1998;116:780–92.

34. Aoki M, Nomura F, Stromski ME, et al. Effects of pH on brain energetics after hypothermic circulatory arrest. Ann Thorac Surg 1993;55:1093–103.

35. Jonas RA. pH strategy for deep hypothermic circulatory arrest in adults. Perfusion 2001;16:180.

36. Skaryak LA, Chai PJ, Kern FH, et al. Blood gas management and degree of cooling: effects on cerebral metabolism before and after circulatory arrest. J Thorac Cardiovasc Surg 1995;110:1649–57.

37. Jonas RA. Optimal pH strategy for hypothermic circulatory arrest. J Thorac Cardiovasc Surg 2001;121:204–5.

38. Hiramatsu T, Miura T, Forbess JM, et al. pH strategies and cerebral energetics before and after circulatory arrest. J Thorac Cardiovasc Surg 1995;109:948–57; discussion 957–8.

39. Firmin RK, Bouloux P, Allen P, et al. Sympathoadrenal function during cardiac operations in infants with the technique of surface cooling, limited cardiopulmonary bypass, and circulatory arrest. J Thorac Cardiovasc Surg 1985;90:729–35.

40. Griepp RB, Ergin MA, Lansman SL, et al. The physiology of hypothermic circulatory arrest. Semin Thorac Cardiovasc Surg 1991;3:188–93.

41. Anderson RV, Siegman MG, Balaban RS, et al. Hyperglycemia increases cerebral intracellular acidosis during circulatory arrest [published erratum appears in Ann Thorac Surg 1993;55(4):1054]. Ann Thorac Surg 1992;54:1126–30.

42. Traystman RJ, Kirsch JR, Koehler RC. Oxygen radical mechanisms of brain injury following ischemia and reperfusion. J Appl Physiol 1991;71.1185–95.

43. Hirotani T, Kameda T, Kumamoto T, et al. Protective effect of thiopental against cerebral ischemia during circulatory arrest. Thorac Cardiovasc Surg 1999;47:223–8.

44. Wang D, Wu X, Zhou Y, et al. Lidocaine improving the cerebral protection by retrograde cerebral perfusion. Chin Med J (Engl) 1998;111:885–90.

45. Jonassen AE, Quaegebeur JM, Young WL. Cerebral blood flow velocity in pediatric patients is reduced after cardiopulmonary bypass with profound hypothermia. J Thorac Cardiovasc Surg 1995;110:934–43.

46. Tsui SS, Kirshbom PM, Davies MJ, et al. Nitric oxide production affects cerebral perfusion and metabolism after deep hypothermic circulatory arrest. Ann Thorac Surg 1996;61:1699–707.

47. Skaryak LA, Kirshbom PM, DiBernardo LR, et al. Modified ultrafiltration improves cerebral metabolic recovery after circulatory arrest. J Thorac Cardiovasc Surg 1995; 109:744–51; discussion 751–2.

48. Cooley DA, Mahaffey DE, De Bakey ME. Total excision of the aortic arch for aneurysm. Surg Gynecol Obstet 1955; 101:667.

49. DeBakey ME, Henly WS, Cooley DA, et al. Aneurysms of the aortic arch. Factors influencing operative risk. Surg Clin North Am 1962;42:1543–54.

50. Frist WH, Baldwin JC, Starnes VA, et al. A reconsideration of cerebral perfusion in aortic arch replacement. Ann Thorac Surg 1986;42:273–81.

51. Higami T, Kozawa S, Asada T, et al. Retrograde cerebral perfusion versus selective cerebral perfusion as evaluated by cerebral oxygen saturation during aortic arch reconstruction. Ann Thorac Surg 1999;67:1091–6.

52. Matsuda H, Nakano S, Shirakura R, et al. Surgery for aortic arch aneurysm with selective cerebral perfusion and hypothermic cardiopulmonary bypass. Circulation 1989;80:I243–8.

53. Bachet J, Guilmet D, Goudot B, et al. Cold cerebroplegia. A new technique of cerebral protection during operations on the transverse aortic arch. J Thorac Cardiovasc Surg 1991;102:85–93; discussion 93–4.

54. Kazui T. Simple and safe cannulation technique for antegrade selective cerebral perfusion. Ann Thorac Cardiovasc Surg 2001;7:186–8.

55. Kazui T, Washiyama N, Muhammad BA, et al. Improved results of atherosclerotic arch aneurysm operations with a refined technique. J Thorac Cardiovasc Surg 2001;121:491–9.

56. Mills NL, Ochsner JL. Massive air embolism during cardiopulmonary bypass. Causes, prevention, and management. J Thorac Cardiovasc Surg 1980;80:708–17.

57. Lemole GM, Strong MD, Spagna PM, Karmilowicz NP. Improved results for dissecting aneurysms. Intraluminal sutureless prosthesis. J Thorac Cardiovasc Surg 1982; 83:249–255.

58. Ueda Y, Miki S, Kusuhara K, et al. Surgical treatment of aneurysm or dissection involving the ascending aorta and aortic arch, utilizing circulatory arrest and retrograde cerebral perfusion. J Cardiovasc Surg (Torino) 1990;31:553–8.

59. Ueda Y, Miki S, Kusuhara K, et al. Deep hypothermic systemic circulatory arrest and continuous retrograde cerebral perfusion for surgery of aortic arch aneurysm. Eur J Cardiothorac Surg 1992;6:36–41; discussion 42.

60. Boeckxstaens CJ, Flameng WJ. Retrograde cerebral perfusion does not perfuse the brain in nonhuman primates. Ann Thorac Surg 1995;60:319–27; discussion 327–8.

61. Imamaki M, Koyanagi H, Hashimoto A, et al. Retrograde cerebral perfusion with hypothermic blood provides efficient protection of the brain: a neuropathological study. J Card Surg 1995;10:325–33.

62. de Brux JL, Subayi JB, Pegis JD, Pillet J. Retrograde cerebral perfusion: anatomic study of the distribution of blood to the brain. Ann Thorac Surg 1995;60:1294–8.

63. Filgueiras CL, Winsborrow B, Ye J, et al. A 31p-magnetic resonance study of antegrade and retrograde cerebral perfusion during aortic arch surgery in pigs. J Thorac Cardiovasc Surg 1995;110:55–62.

64. Usui A, Oohara K, Liu TL, et al. Determination of optimum retrograde cerebral perfusion conditions. J Thorac Cardiovasc Surg 1994;107:300–8.

65. Yoshimura N, Okada M, Ota T, Nohara H. Pharmacologic intervention for ischemic brain edema after retrograde cerebral perfusion. J Thorac Cardiovasc Surg 1995;109: 1173–81.

66. Yerlioglu ME, Wolfe D, Mezrow CK, et al. The effect of retrograde cerebral perfusion after particulate embolization to the brain. J Thorac Cardiovasc Surg 1995;110: 1470–84; discussion 1484–5.

67. Okita Y, Takamoto S, Ando M, et al. Mortality and cerebral outcome in patients who underwent aortic arch operations using deep hypothermic circulatory arrest with retrograde cerebral perfusion: no relation of early death, stroke, and delirium to the duration of circulatory arrest. J Thorac Cardiovasc Surg 1998;115:129–38.

68. Coselli JS. Retrograde cerebral perfusion via a superior vena caval cannula for aortic arch aneurysm operations. Ann Thorac Surg 1994;57:1668–9.

69. Bavaria JE, Pochettino A. Retrograde cerebral perfusion (RCP) in aortic arch surgery: efficacy and possible mechanisms of brain protection. Semin Thorac Cardiovasc Surg 1997;9:222–32.

70. Griepp RB, Juvonen T, Griepp EB, et al. Is retrograde cerebral perfusion an effective means of neural support during deep hypothermic circulatory arrest? Ann Thorac Surg 1997;64:913–6.

CHAPTER 32

SURGERY FOR MARFAN SYNDROME

JOHN R. DOTY, MD, DUKE E. CAMERON, MD

Etiology

Marfan syndrome was first described by the French pediatrician Antoine Marfan in 1896.[1] The disease is the most common inherited connective-tissue disorder and affects approximately 1 in 10,000 adults.[2,3] It results from mutations in the gene for fibrillin-1 (*FBN1*), located on chromosome 15.[4] More than 125 different mutations have been identified for the *FBN1* gene, of which 75% are inherited and 25% are sporadic.[3,5,6] These mutations cause faulty synthesis of fibrillin, the core protein of microfibrils, and result in abnormal formation of the elastic components of the body. In the aorta, this is manifest as disorganized elastic fibers and premature cystic medial degeneration.[7] The disorder is also associated with ocular, musculoskeletal, central nervous system, and pulmonary abnormalities.

Aneurysm of the ascending aorta in the context of Marfan syndrome was first reported by Baer and Taussig in 1943, at the Johns Hopkins Hospital.[8] Comprehensive description of Marfan syndrome and its cardiovascular manifestations is generally credited to McKusick's paper in 1955.[9] Nearly 75% of patients with Marfan syndrome have aortic root dilation, which might or might not be associated with aortic valve regurgitation.[10] Aortic dilation increases wall tension according to the law of Laplace and may accelerate the premature degenerative process and lead to aortic dissection. Most patients with Marfan syndrome die from cardiovascular events, the majority from complications of aortic root dilation, including aortic dissection and aortic rupture.[10,11] Appropriately timed surgical intervention can prevent these complications and increase survival in patients with Marfan syndrome.[12,13]

Screening for Aortic Disease in Marfan Syndrome

Traditionally, aneurysmal disease of the aorta is evaluated and followed by either serial computed tomography or ultrasonography, with particular emphasis on size and location of the aneurysm, as well as rate of expansion.

More recently, magnetic resonance imaging (MRI) has assumed a growing role. In general, once the aorta reaches a diameter of 5 cm or expands at a rapid rate between imaging studies (> 1 cm per year), the aorta is considered to be at increased risk for dissection and rupture, and elective prophylactic surgery is undertaken. However, in patients with Marfan syndrome, acute dissection may occur in the absence of marked dilation of the aorta, particularly in patients with a family history of aortic catastrophe.[14,15,17] Genetic testing may be useful in patients with a family history of Marfan syndrome to help characterize the severity of an individual's disease and stratify risk, but it is not suitable as a screening tool in patients without the typical phenotype.[3,6,18]

Indications for Surgery

Patients with Marfan syndrome are at risk for life-threatening complications of dilation of the aortic root. Aortic root replacement should be performed when the diameter of the aortic root reaches 5.5 to 6.0 cm.[10,12,19] Patients with a family history of acute dissection or rupture should undergo surgery earlier, preferably when the aortic root reaches 5 cm in diameter, as there is evidence that aortic dissection can occur without marked dilation of the aortic root in these patients.[14,19] Other indications for surgery are aortic dissection (acute or chronic), severe aortic regurgitation, progressive dilation of the aorta on serial imaging, and aortic root diameter twice that of the normal aorta.[14,19–21]

It is now well documented that elective surgery for Marfan disease of the aorta is the preferred method of treatment. Emergent operation for aortic dissection or rupture in these patients carries an unacceptably high mortality and morbidity.

Operative Technique

Surgery for Marfan disease of the aorta is typically aortic root replacement with or without aortic valve replacement. Late complications of dissection in the distal aorta constitute the second most common cause for operation. Surgery is planned with recognition that the disease is not confined to the ascending aorta and that many patients will require additional surgery in the future.

Dilation of the aortic root can result in aortic regurgitation, which may require repair or replacement of the aortic valve. Key to successful surgery of the aortic root in Marfan syndrome is the understanding that the disease is most severe in the aortic sinuses, and therefore, removal of all aortic sinus tissue is vital to a favorable early outcome as well as for prevention of later complications such as dissection and pseudoaneurysm. Replacement of the aortic valve and separate supracoronary ascending aorta with a synthetic graft leaves behind vulnerable aortic sinus tissue and is inadequate treatment for patients with Marfan syndrome.

Several surgical approaches are now available for treatment of Marfan patients, allowing the surgeon to tailor the operation to the individual patient. These operations include composite replacement of the ascending aorta and aortic valve (Bentall operation), valve-sparing replacement of the ascending aorta, combined replacement of the ascending aorta and arch (elephant trunk procedure), and single-stage repair of the ascending aorta and arch (arch-first technique).

Composite Replacement of the Ascending Aorta and Aortic Valve (Bentall Operation)

Bentall and De Bono first described the technique for combined replacement of the ascending aorta and aortic valve in 1968.[22] After establishment of cardiopulmonary bypass and cardioplegic arrest, the ascending aorta is resected to a point of normal diameter (Figure 32-1). The aortic valve is excised, and the coronary arteries are mobilized with small collars of aortic tissue. The remainder of aortic sinus tissue is trimmed to the level of the aortic annulus. A composite graft consisting of a mechanical aortic valve within a woven synthetic tube graft is then sutured to the aortic annulus. The coronary arteries are anastomosed in anatomic position to small windows in the graft. Finally, the distal end of the graft is anastomosed to the transected ascending aorta in an end-to-end fashion.

The Bentall operation has become the gold standard for patients with concomitant disease of the aortic valve and aortic root and is particularly applicable to patients with Marfan disease. In 1999, Gott and associates reported a 1.5% operative mortality in patients undergoing elective aortic root replacement for Marfan disease of the ascending aorta.[23] Ten-year survival in this series of patients was 75%; the most common causes of late death were dissection or rupture of the residual aorta and congestive failure. Other reports have confirmed the safety and efficacy of this technique, which is suitable for nearly all patients with Marfan syndrome, especially those with aortic regurgitation.[24,25]

Valve-Sparing Replacement of the Ascending Aorta

Many patients with Marfan sinus aneurysms have competent aortic valves and do not require prosthetic valve replacement. In addition, there are patients, such as children and young adults, for whom anticoagulation mandated by a mechanical valve may be undesirable. These are the same patients for whom bioprostheses have limited durability. Reconstruction of the aortic root and remodeling of the aortic annulus in this setting can restore the native aortic valve to normal function and competence and can eliminate the need for anticoagulation and minimize the risk of endocarditis.

Correction of severe aortic annular dilatation is an important part of valve-sparing root surgery. Depending on the degree of dilation at the sinotubular junction and at the aortic annulus, a prosthetic graft can be tailored to adjust these dimensions back to a normal state. Doty described several methods of graft size selection and modification to remodel the aortic root in valve-sparing operations.[26] Figure 32-2 illustrates the method used when both the sinotubular junction and the aortic annulus are dilated.

Techniques for valve-sparing replacement of the aortic root were developed independently by Yacoub in London and David in Toronto.[27,28] As with the Bentall operation, the ascending aorta and sinus tissue are excised, leaving the mobilized coronary ostia with buttons of aortic tissue. The aortic valve is inspected for normal leaflet mobility and absence of degenerative changes, and the diameter of the aortic annulus is recorded, at which point normal coaptation could be expected to occur.

Several iterations of valve-sparing root replacement have been described. The David I, or implantation technique, slides a tubular Dacron graft around the valve apparatus, anchoring the low end of the graft below the nadir of the three sinuses by interrupted mattress sutures placed from within the left ventricular outflow tract outward (Figure 32-3). The top of each of the three commissures is then fixed to the graft at the appropriate height to promote leaflet coaptation. The annulus, along with a small rim of sinus tissue, is then sutured inside the graft with continuous 4–0 polypropylene suture. Holes are cut in the graft opposite the coronary "buttons," which in our practice are encircled with Teflon felt "lifesaver" pledgets and anastomosed to the graft, also with 4–0 polypropylene. The distal end of the Dacron graft is anastomosed end-to-end to the distal ascending aorta. Placement of a left ventricular vent is useful during the early stages of resuscitation of the heart, to prevent left ventricular dilatation and to assess residual aortic insufficiency.

The David II, or remodeling procedure, is similar to Yacoub's technique (Figure 32-4). In the David II, a synthetic graft that is the same diameter as the remodeled aortic annulus is selected, and three "tongues" of graft are created for reconstruction of the aortic sinuses. The length of each tongue is approximately two-thirds the

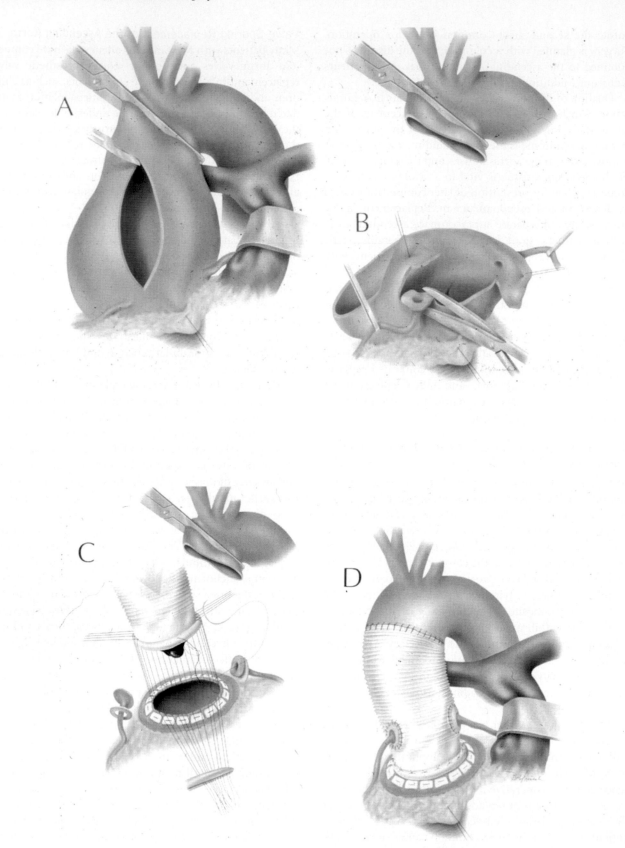

FIGURE 32-1. The Bentall procedure for aortic root replacement. *A,* On cardiopulmonary bypass, the aorta is cross-clamped and the aneurysm opened. *B,* The aneurysm is excised, and the coronary arteries are mobilized with a small collar of sinus tissue. *C,* The prosthesis is secured to the annulus with interrupted pledgeted horizontal mattress sutures and the coronary arteries encircled with Teflon felt "lifesaver" pledgets before anastomosis to side holes in the graft. *D,* The completed prosthesis.

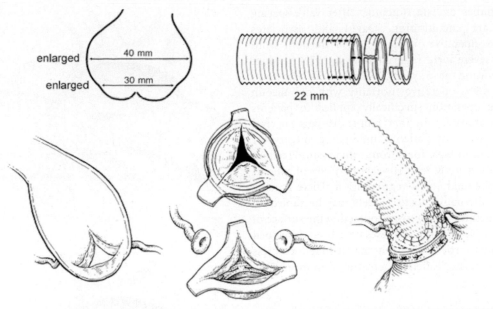

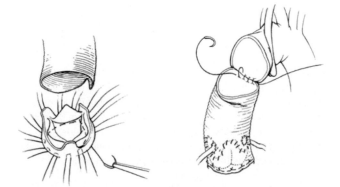

FIGURE 32-2. Method for restoring normal aortic root dimensions in aortic valve-sparing operations. A vascular graft 10% less than the desired diameter of the aortic annulus is chosen. Small strips of the graft are used to reduce the aortic annulus to five-sixths of the circumference of the left ventricular outflow tract. The remainder of the graft is then the appropriate size at the sinotubular junction. Reproduced with permission from Doty DB, Arcidi JM Jr.[26]

FIGURE 32-3. Valve-sparing aortic root replacement reimplantation technique (David I procedure). After excision of the sinus tissue and mobilization of the coronary arteries, horizontal mattress sutures are placed below the aortic annulus from inside outward and then through a Dacron graft. The aortic valve commissures are suspended at the appropriate height within the graft, and the annulus is secured to the graft wall with continuous suture before the coronary arteries are reimplanted and the distal graft anastomosis completed. Reproduced with permission from David TE, Feindel CM.[28]

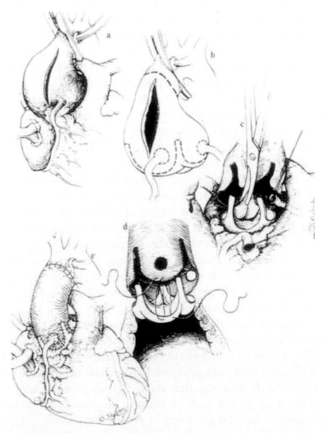

diameter of the graft. The graft is then sewn to the aortic annulus with continuous 4–0 polypropylene. We find external reinforcement with a thin strip of Teflon felt is helpful for hemostasis. The coronary ostia are reimplanted on the graft just as in the David I, and the distal end of the graft is anastomosed to the transected ascending aorta in an end-to-end fashion.

FIGURE 32-4. Valve-sparing aortic root replacement remodeling technique (David II or Yacoub procedure). The graft is trimmed to fit the excised sinuses, and the coronary arteries are reimplanted onto the graft. Reproduced with permission from Yacoub MH et al.[27]

Recent studies on late outcomes after valve-sparing operations are encouraging. David and associates reported low operative mortality, 90% freedom from moderate or severe aortic regurgitation, and 97% freedom from reoperation at 5 years.[29] Birks and associates described a 4.9% operative mortality with the Yacoub valve-sparing operation specifically applied to patients with Marfan disease.[30] In that report, 10-year survival ranged from 64% for patients undergoing surgery for acute dissection to 94% for chronic aneurysm. Freedom from reoperation was 83% at 10 years, and 79% of patients had no or only mild aortic regurgitation. There is some concern that the native aortic leaflets may be subject to stress and repetitive injury from contacting the surface of the prosthesis. New graft prostheses have been developed with preformed aortic sinuses that may help reduce stress on the native aortic leaflets by creating a more normal root architecture.[31]

Combined Replacement of the Ascending Aorta, Arch, and Descending Aorta (Elephant Trunk Procedure)

In some patients, dilation of the aorta extends into the aortic arch and descending aorta. Because patients with Marfan syndrome have a higher risk of rupture and dissection, resection of all aneurysmal aorta should be attempted. Borst first described the two-stage approach for extensive aneurysmal disease of the aorta, known as the elephant trunk procedure.[32] This technique traditionally requires a period of hypothermic circulatory arrest to complete the distal anastomosis and attachment of the arch vessels, although use of right axillary arterial cannulation and snaring of the neck vessels can substantially shorten arrest time. In the first stage, the ascending aorta and arch are resected just beyond the origin of the left subclavian artery, leaving the arch vessels on an island of aortic tissue. A prosthetic graft is sewn to the internal orifice of the descending aorta, leaving a short 4 to 6 cm cuff that is intussuscepted into the lumen of the descending aorta (Figure 32-5). The arch vessels are then reimplanted along the superior surface of the graft. Cardiopulmonary bypass is resumed after inserting the arterial cannula into the graft. A second graft is then used to replace the ascending aorta, and the two grafts are anastomosed end-to-end to complete the first stage of the repair.

The second stage is performed after adequate patient recovery. A thoracoabdominal incision is made, and the descending aorta is dissected to expose the remainder of the aneurysmal disease, as well as to expose the distal end of the graft from the first stage. Partial or full cardiopulmonary bypass with or without circulatory arrest is employed according to surgeon preference, and the distal end of the graft is clamped. The descending aortic aneurysm is then opened and the "elephant trunk" identified, which is the short cuff of graft that was intussuscepted into the descending aorta during the first stage.

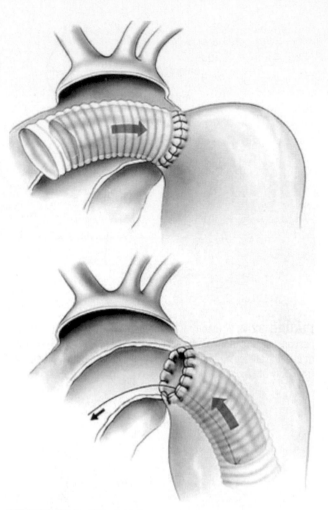

FIGURE 32-5. The elephant trunk technique. The original method as described by Borst is depicted in the top panel, in which the distal "trunk" portion is pushed into the descending aorta after completion of the anastomosis. Crawford's modification is depicted in the bottom panel, in which the proximal portion of the graft is inverted into the descending aorta and then retrieved after completion of the anastomosis. Reproduced with permission from Heinemann HK et al.[35]

A prosthetic graft is anastomosed to the "elephant trunk" proximally, intercostal islands are implanted into the body of the graft, and the distal end of the graft is anastomosed to the aorta beyond the aneurysm.

This is a formidable operation; mortality and morbidity are expectedly higher than isolated root replacement. However, Safi and associates reported low operative mortality rates of 5.1% and 6.2% for first and second stages of the operation, respectively.[33] Most deaths occurred from aortic rupture, either during the interval between stages or in patients who did not return for the second stage. Schepens and associates described a hospital mortality of 8% and permanent neurologic damage in 4%.[34] Heinemann and associates reported an operative mortality of 12.5%; only one-third of patients completed the second stage of the operation.[35]

Single-Stage Repair of the Ascending Aorta, Arch, and Descending Aorta (Arch-First Technique)

In a subset of patients with extensive marked dilation of the ascending aorta, arch, and descending aorta, the aneurysmal disease of the descending aorta prevents application of a staged repair such as the elephant trunk technique. In these patients, single-stage repair using hypothermic circulatory arrest can be employed to replace the entire aorta in one setting. This approach is best suited for patients in whom the aorta distal to the subclavian artery is greater than 4.5 to 5.0 cm in diameter and the aneurysm does not extend to the abdominal aorta. It is also useful in patients requiring reoperation for recurrent aneurysm or chronic dissection.

In Kouchoukos' arch-first technique, the arch vessels are reimplanted first to allow for early restoration of cerebral perfusion via a small side graft, illustrated in Figure 32-6.[36] The distal aortic anastomosis is completed during a period of hypothermic low flow, and the proximal aorta anastomosis is completed during rewarming. Although this is a technically challenging operation, Kouchoukos and colleagues reported a 6.2% operative mortality rate without a single stroke or spinal cord injury.[37] In that series, all patients were alive and well at a mean follow-up of 13 months.

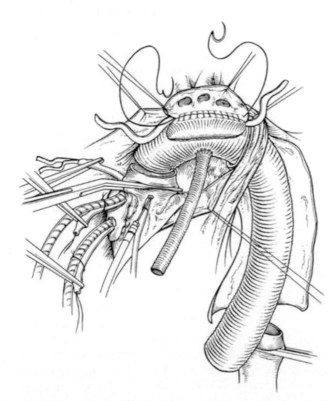

FIGURE 32-6. Single-stage replacement of the ascending aorta, arch, and descending aorta, using the arch-first technique. Hypothermic circulatory arrest is used to implant the arch vessels first. The distal aortic anastomosis is completed during a hypothermic low-flow state, and the proximal aortic anastomosis is completed during rewarming. Reproduced with permission from Rokkas CK, Kouchoukos NT.[36]

Conclusion

In summary, Marfan disease of the aorta is a pathologic entity with lethal implications because of the risk of rupture and dissection. Surgical intervention at the appropriate time can prevent these complications, save lives, and provide excellent quality of life. Complications from surgery are infrequent if performed in the elective setting, and most patients can anticipate good long-term results from any of the operations currently available for managing this disease.

References

1. Marfan AB. Un cas de déformation congénitale des quatre membres, plus prononcée aux extrémités, caractérisée par l'allongement des os avec un certain degré d'amincissement. Bull Soc Hop Paris 1896;13:220–6.
2. Pyeritz RE. The Marfan syndrome. In: Royce PM, Steinman B, editors. Connective tissue and its heritable disorders. New York: Wiley-Liss; 1993. p. 437.
3. Vincent GM. Role of DNA testing for diagnosis, management, and genetic screening in long QT syndrome, hypertrophic cardiomyopathy, and Marfan syndrome. Heart 2001;86:12–4.
4. Loeys B, Nuytinck L, Delvaux I, et al. Genotype and phenotype analysis of 171 patients referred for molecular study of the fibrillin-1 gene FBN1 because of suspected Marfan syndrome. Arch Intern Med 2001;161:2447–54.
5. Milewicz DM, Michael K, Fisher N, et al. Fibrillin-1 (FBN1) mutations in patients with thoracic aortic aneurysms. Circulation 1996;94:2708–11.
6. Pereira L, Levran O, Ramirez F, et al. A molecular approach to the stratification of cardiovascular risk in families with Marfan's syndrome. N Engl J Med 1994;33:148–53.
7. Robbins SL, Cotran RS, Kumar V. Blood vessels. In: Robbins SL, Cotran RS, Kumar V, editors. Pathologic basis of disease. 3rd ed. Philadelphia: WB Saunders; 1984. p. 503.
8. Baer RW, Taussig HB, Oppenheimer EH. Congenital aneurysmal dilation of aorta associated with arachnodactyly. Bull Johns Hopkins Hosp 1943;72:309–31.
9. McKusick VA. Cardiovascular aspects of Marfan's syndrome: heritable disorder of connective tissue. Circulation 1955;11:321–42.
10. Marsalese DL, Moodie DS, Vacante M, et al. Marfan's syndrome: natural history and long-term follow-up of cardiovascular involvement. J Am Coll Cardiol 1989;14:422–8.
11. Murdoch JL, Walker BA, Halpern BL, et al. Life expectancy and cause of death in the Marfan syndrome. N Engl J Med 1972;286:804–8.
12. Finkbohner R, Johnston D, Crawford ES, et al. Aortas/pulmonary arteries: Marfan syndrome: long-term survival and complications after aortic aneurysm repair. Circulation 1995;91:728–33.
13. Silverman DI, Burton KJ, Gray J, et al. Life expectancy in the Marfan syndrome. Am J Cardiol 1995;75:157–60.
14. Gott VL, Cameron DE, Pyeritz RE, et al. Composite graft repair of Marfan aneurysm of the ascending aorta: results in 150 patients. J Card Surg 1994;9:482–9.

15. Kornbluth M, Schnittger I, Eyngorina I, et al. Clinical outcome in the Marfan syndrome with ascending aortic dilatation followed annually by echocardiography. Am J Cardiol 1999;84:753–5.

16. Groenink M, Rozendaal L, Naeff MSJ, et al. Marfan syndrome in children and adolescents: predictive and prognostic value of individual aortic root growth for screening for aortic complications. Heart 1998;80:163–9.

17. Rozendaal L, Groenink M, Naeff MSJ, et al. Marfan syndrome in children and adolescents: an adjusted nomogram for screening aortic root dilatation. Heart 1998;79:69–72.

18. Keating MT, Sanguinetti MC. Molecular genetic insights into cardiovascular disease. Science 1996;272:681–5.

19. Gott VL, Cameron DE, Reitz BA, Pyeritz RE. Current diagnosis and prescription for the Marfan syndrome: aortic root and valve replacement. J Cardiac Surg 1994;9 Suppl:177–81.

20. Donaldson RM, Emanuel RW, Olsen EG, Ross DN. Management of cardiovascular complications in Marfan syndrome. Lancet 1980;2(8205):1178–81.

21. Svensson LG, Crawford ES, Coselli JS, et al. Impact of cardiovascular operation on survival in the Marfan patient. Circulation 1989;80 (3 Pt 1):I233–42.

22. Bentall HH, De Bono A. A technique for complete replacement of the ascending aorta. Thorax 1968;23:338–9.

23. Gott VL, Greene PS, Alejo DE, et al. Replacement of the aortic root in patients with Marfan's syndrome. N Engl J Med 1999;340:1307–13.

24. Mingke D, Dresler C, Pethig K, et al. Surgical treatment of Marfan patients with aneurysms and dissection of the proximal aorta. J Cardiovasc Surg 1998;39:65–74.

25. Bachet J, Goudot B, Dreyfus G, et al. Current practice in Marfan's syndrome and annuloaortic ectasia: aortic root replacement with a composite graft over a twenty-year period. J Card Surg 1997;12 Suppl 2:157–66.

26. Doty DB, Arcidi JM Jr. Methods for graft size selection in aortic valve-sparing operations. Ann Thorac Surg 2000;69:648–50.

27. Yacoub MH, Gehle P, Chandrasekaran V, et al. Late results of a valve-preserving operation in patients with aneurysms of the ascending aorta and root. J Thorac Cardiovasc Surg 1998;115:1080–90.

28. David TE, Feindel CM. An aortic valve-sparing operation for patients with aortic incompetence and aneurysm of the ascending aorta. J Thorac Cardiovasc Surg 1992;103:617–21.

29. David TE, Armstrong S, Ivanov J, et al. Results of aortic valve-sparing operations. J Thorac Cardiovasc Surg 2001;122:39–46.

30. Birks EJ, Webb C, Child A, et al. Early and long-term results of a valve-sparing operation for Marfan syndrome. Circulation 1999;100:II-29–35.

31. Zehr KJ, Thubrikar MJ, Gong GG, et al. Clinical introduction of a novel prosthesis for valve-preserving aortic root reconstruction for annuloaortic ectasia. J Thorac Cardiovasc Surg 2000;120:692–8.

32. Borst HG, Walterbusch G, Schaps D. Extensive aortic replacement using "elephant trunk" prosthesis. Thorac Cardiovasc Surg 1983;31:37–40.

33. Safi HJ, Miller CC 3rd, Estrera AL, et al. Staged repair of extensive aortic aneurysms: morbidity and mortality in the elephant trunk technique. Circulation 2001;104:2938–42.

34. Schepens MA, Dossche KM, Morshuis WJ, et al. The elephant trunk technique: operative results in 100 consecutive patients. Eur J Cardiothorac Surg 2002;21:276–81.

35. Heinemann HK, Buehner B, Jurmann MJ, Borst HG. Use of the "elephant trunk technique" in aortic surgery. Ann Thorac Surg 1995;60:2–6.

36. Rokkas CK, Kouchoukos NT. Single-stage extensive replacement of the thoracic aorta: the arch-first technique. J Thorac Cardiovasc Surg 1999;117:99–105.

37. Kouchoukos NT, Masetti P, Rokkas CK, Murphy SF. Single-stage reoperative repair of chronic type A aortic dissection by means of the arch-first technique. J Thorac Cardiovasc Surg 2001;122:578–82.

CHAPTER 33

VALVE-SPARING OPERATIONS FOR DILATED AORTIC ROOT

RICHARD P. COCHRAN, MD, KARYN S. KUNZELMAN, PhD

Overview

As surgical techniques have improved over the last two decades and the complications of prosthetic valves have been realized, valve-sparing operations have become increasingly popular. Initially, the efforts and success in valve sparing were seen in treatment of mitral and tricuspid valvular disease. However, during the last decade, there has been increased interest in valve-sparing procedures for the aortic valve, particularly in diseases like aortic annuloectasia that involve dilatation of the "aortic root" as opposed to those only involving the aortic valve. This is logical and appropriate, in that intrinsic aortic valve disease precludes the benefit of valve sparing. As such, the majority of technical advances in this area have dealt with valve sparing in diseases that affect the aortic root as a composite structure. This chapter discusses the currently used techniques for valve sparing in aortic root disease, their advantages and disadvantages, and what the authors believe is the best available operative technique.

When this topic of varying techniques was reviewed a few years ago, aortic valve–sparing operations were not new concepts, but they had not yet gained wide acceptance.[1] Since that time, there has been a significant increase in interest in this type of procedure. Rather than only three or four centers advocating this approach, now multiple centers in North America, Europe, and Asia are reporting their series of successful procedures.[2–10] There has also been a significant reevaluation of the various techniques, and some interesting controversy has arisen. Whereas previously there were four or five variations on the theme of aortic valve–sparing operations for ascending aortic aneurysmal disease, now there are two or three variations in clinical use. Currently, the primary discussion regarding differences of technique focuses on fixing the annulus below the aortic valve versus carrying out a supravalvular repair. Consequently, this chapter addresses only the currently advocated techniques.

Because the mechanical interaction of the aortic root components is essential to long-term durability, the biomechanical considerations of each repair technique are also discussed. Although there is increasing enthusiasm for the procedure, there is not any greater degree of agreement as to the best approach. In addition, there is significant variation and, often, difference of opinion as to the anatomic terms and definitions that apply to this region of reconstruction known as the aortic root. Furthermore, many of the biomechanical concepts are not familiar to practicing surgeons. As such, some clarifications are necessary in both areas. Prior to beginning a meaningful discussion of the actual technical aspects of the procedures used in this area of cardiac surgery, some background explanation and standardization of terminology is necessary.

Anatomy

The aortic root has fascinated anatomists, physicians, and surgeons for centuries. Leonardo da Vinci illustrated the aortic root quite accurately as early as 1513.[11] Although the term *aortic root* is familiar and well understood, it is not defined in *Stedman's* or *Dorland's* dictionaries, nor is it addressed in *Gray's* or *Grant's* anatomy texts.[12–15] Fortunately, this lack of formal definition has not prevented the tremendous strides made in the last two decades in surgical treatment of aortic root disease. The vagueness in terminology, however, does require that some definitions be established prior to discussion of surgical interventions. For this chapter, the aortic root (Figure 33-1) is defined as the region that begins at the left ventricular outflow tract, at what the authors consider the aortic "annulus." The annulus is one of the controversial aspects of the aortic root. In fact, some argue that no true annulus exists. However, because any aortic reconstruction must involve the origin of the aorta, and the origin has been traditionally called the annulus, the term will be used. For this discussion, the authors favor the subvalvular aortic annulus described by anatomists. This defines the annulus as a

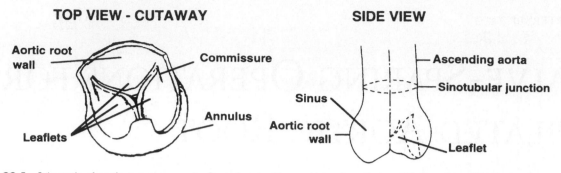

FIGURE 33-1. Schematic of aortic root components. Reproduced with permission from Cochran RP, Kunzelman KS. Aortic valve sparing in aortic root disease. In: Karp D, Laks H, Wechsler AS, editors. Advances in cardiac surgery. Vol. 8. St. Louis (MO): Mosby-Year Book; 1996. p. 81–107.)

circular orifice, not the crown-shaped annulus described by some surgeons.[14,16] Distal to the annulus, the aortic root includes the aortic valve leaflets, the aortic wall, the sinuses of Valsalva, and the coronary ostia. The aortic root terminates just distal to these structures at the sinotubular junction. The portion of the aorta just distal to the sinotubular junction is considered the ascending aorta. These definitions of the aortic root are chosen to aid in addressing the complex interactions that occur in this region, as well as to aid in tailoring surgical interventions that best recreate normal anatomy.

Although at first glance the aortic root appears relatively simple in a structural sense, it is in reality a complex geometric structure with balanced biomechanical interactions that are just beginning to be fully understood. It is the interaction of all of the aortic root components that maintains forward blood flow from the left ventricle and assures coronary perfusion. In addition, the resultant biomechanical forces are balanced in a manner that makes the aortic root efficient and durable. The complex biomechanical interactions of the aortic root are both its strength and its potential weakness. Disruption of any geometric component of the aortic root by disease processes such as aortic annuloectasia affects all the other components and can alter the biomechanics of the whole system. Prior to the understanding of this concept of interdependence in the aortic root, diseases were viewed as originating from the structural component that ultimately failed, not from the components that started the disruption of the interaction. Since geometric disruption of any root component may alter valve function, historically, all aortic root problems were simply presumed to be valve related. As such, for 30 years, the primary solution to all aortic root problems was to replace the valve. Recently, this simplistic approach has been questioned. Regarding all aortic root problems as valve related oversimplified the problem and delayed understanding of the complex interaction of the components, thus delaying development of appropriate surgical intervention. Understanding the biomechanics of the aortic root is necessary for surgeons to become more adept at addressing this once intellectually elusive anatomic region.

Biomechanics

The normal aortic root carries out its biomechanical functions very efficiently and with great durability. A complex biomechanical system of stress sharing allows the aortic root to tolerate large pressure changes and significant stress alterations during the cardiac cycle, as well as accommodate a fair amount of pathologic alteration. The critical mechanical components of the aortic root include a physiologically appropriate annulus, a valve with pliable leaflets, sinuses of Valsalva of appropriate depth, and a well-formed sinotubular junction. These components all work in concert to accomplish the roles of the aortic root. The composite functional outcomes of their interaction are numerous. The first is the maintenance of unidirectional forward flow with minimal resistance. The second is the creation of eddy formations within the flowing blood during ventricular ejection. This eddy formation aids in two more functions; one is valve closure, and the other is aiding or assuring coronary ostial perfusion (Figure 33-2). In addition to these physiologic benefits from the aortic root configuration, there is significant mechanical benefit from the anatomic configuration. The curvilinear attachment between the aortic valve leaflets and aortic root wall allows for stress sharing. This arrangement enables the high stresses carried by each leaflet during closure to be shared with the aortic root wall (Figure 33-3). Further mechanical benefit is realized in this interactive system. During appropriate valve closure, leaflet coaptation allows for compressive support for each leaflet from its adjacent leaflets, both at the point of closure and in the commissural regions. This stress sharing reduces tensile stresses in each individual leaflet. Understanding these interactions gives insight into the beauty of this complex biomechanical system. Unfortunately, this complexity of interaction has proven difficult to simulate. Even more unfortunate is that historically, surgeons and engineers adopted a more simplified view of the aortic root for surgical intervention. This simplification did allow surgical interventions to begin where previously none had existed, but the simplified approach also created some misunderstanding. This simplification may have actually slowed the evolution toward a more anatomically and physiologically appropriate surgical approach.

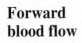
Forward blood flow

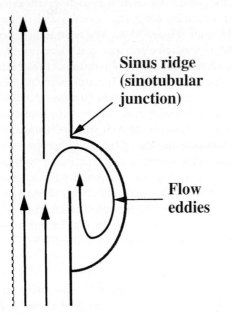

Sinus ridge (sinotubular junction)

Flow eddies

FIGURE 33-2. Schematic of aortic valve and root demonstrating the role of the sinus ridge in creation of eddy currents for enhanced valve closure and coronary perfusion. Reproduced with permission from Cochran RP, Kunzelman KS. Aortic valve sparing in aortic root disease. In: Karp D, Laks H, Wechsler AS, editors. Advances in cardiac surgery. Vol. 8. St. Louis (MO): Mosby-Year Book; 1996. p. 81–107.

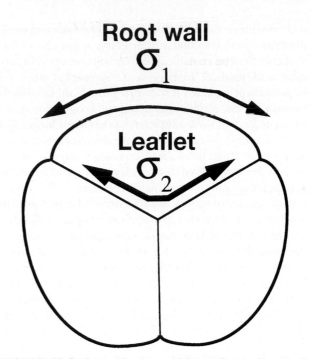

Root wall σ_1

Leaflet σ_2

FIGURE 33-3. Schematic of stress (σ) in leaflets and root wall. Because the leaflets are thinner, the leaflet stresses (σ_1) are higher than the root wall stresses (σ_2). However, the curvilinear attachment at the sinuses enables the high leaflet stress to be partially transferred to the root wall, thereby decreasing the stress on the leaflets. Reproduced with permission from Cochran RP, Kunzelman KS. Aortic valve sparing in aortic root disease. In: Karp D, Laks H, Wechsler AS, editors. Advances in cardiac surgery. Vol. 8. St. Louis (MO): Mosby-Year Book; 1996. p. 81–107.

Historical Perspective

Historically, cardiac surgery developed as an operative effort to treat disease processes that were considered fatal if the abnormality was not corrected. As such, early developments for correction of cardiac abnormalities were directed at expedient reproducible operative techniques. Unfortunately, not all life-threatening problems lent themselves to expedient surgical interventions. Two areas where expeditious solutions were not readily available involved aortic root problems, specifically, aneurysms and dissections. As a result, evolution of therapeutic intervention for aortic root problems often followed divergent routes.

One technique for treating dilatated aortic roots that was developed in an effort to provide an expedient solution for these problems was the Bentall procedure.[17] Although the Bentall procedure did offer expedience, it sacrificed geometric and anatomic accuracy. In addition, this technique included a prosthetic valve with the associated complications, most notably, lifelong risks of both thromboembolism and anticoagulation.[18–20] These complications have previously been described as "simply the exchange of one disease for another" when a diseased valve is replaced.[21] With this definition, in cases of dissection or aneurysm where an anatomically normal aortic valve may be involved, valvular replacement may be viewed as introduction of a new disease where formerly none existed.

Because of these concerns with prosthetic complications, resuspension of the aortic valve was described early in surgical treatment of ascending aortic dissections. These early efforts at valve sparing in proximal aortic dissections proved successful in both the short and long term. This opened the conceptual window for valve sparing in other aortic root processes, particularly aneurysm. However, before extensive valve sparing could be undertaken, advances in other aspects of surgical intervention were necessary.

Concurrent to the efforts of valve resuspension in dissections, the field of cardiac surgery was rapidly advancing. Advances were made in surgical technique, materials technology, and surgical and medical management. These advances made extensive aortic root reconstruction and complex aortic valve–sparing procedures a possibility. Advances in surgical technique included refinement of valve suspension techniques, such as those used in homograft and autograft placement. In addition to these technical advancements, a better understanding of the aortic root, its biomechanics, and its disease processes was gained. Materials technology improved and has resulted in the production of nonporous conduits. These conduits offer several advantages; they eliminate additional time for preclotting and reduce bleeding complications, both resulting in shortening of operative time. Probably the most notable improvements occurred in surgical and medical management. Significant areas of improvement included myocardial protection, cardiopulmonary bypass, cardiac anesthesia, and coagulation management. Each of these advancements has made longer and more complex procedures more tolerable. As a result of the advances in these three areas, reparative surgery for the aortic valve has evolved to a new level and should now be considered a viable alternative to replacement. This evolution of reparative surgery for the aortic valve is similar to the evolution of mitral valve repair techniques, only it has occurred a decade later. Aortic valve sparing is becoming the procedure of choice for many diseases of the root, treatment for which formerly included valve replacement as a component. As such, the remainder of this chapter deals with the valvular challenge of this new millennium, which is when and how the aortic valve should be spared.

Techniques of Aortic Valve–Sparing Operations for Diseases of the Aortic Root

The development of aortic valve-sparing techniques has clearly been an evolutionary process, particularly as improvements in surgical technique, materials technology, and surgical and medical management continue. Each technique described in this chapter has been part of this evolutionary process. The remainder of the chapter reviews rationale for and surgical approach of each technique and evaluates the strengths and weaknesses of each. The final section details how aortic valve sparing with pseudo-sinus creation is done and why the authors think that it is the best anatomic and physiologic solution for these patients.

Valve Resuspension for Aortic Dissections

RATIONALE

Aortic valve regurgitation caused by leaflet prolapse is a well-recognized complication of aortic dissection and constitutes a major cause of morbidity and mortality if uncorrected in these patients. Successful surgical treatment of commissural disruption and leaflet prolapse in patients with aortic dissection was reported as early as the 1960s.[22] Two trends emerged in the surgical treatment of these patients. The first technique, popular for speed and reproducibility, was replacement of the aortic root with a composite tube graft and aortic valve.[23–25] The second technique required more technical judgment in that it coupled preservation (resuspension) of the native aortic valve with repair of the dissection.[26–28] These early efforts at valve sparing were the first acknowledgment that composite replacement sacrificed a normal valve when treating aortic wall abnormalities.

TECHNIQUE

Although there was substantial variability in the techniques used, the general operative approach was the same. The dissected ascending aorta was resected and replaced with a tubular graft (Figure 33-4). The technical challenge of the procedure was valve resuspension. Valve resuspension in a dissected aorta required obliteration of the false lumen and appropriate repositioning (resuspension) of the disrupted valve commissures. An additional aspect that limited use of this technique was the recreation of the sinuses of Valsalva. When more than one commissure is disrupted, the sinuses of Valsalva are also disrupted, and appropriate valve sparing necessitated sinus reconstruction as well as commissural repositioning. The challenge of resuspension of one, two, or three of the aortic commissural posts in an appropriate orientation and the reconstruction of one or more sinuses of Valsalva were the limiting factors to wide acceptance of this very appealing procedure.

EVALUATION

These early techniques of valve resuspension had two very appealing aspects. First, all the techniques spared the

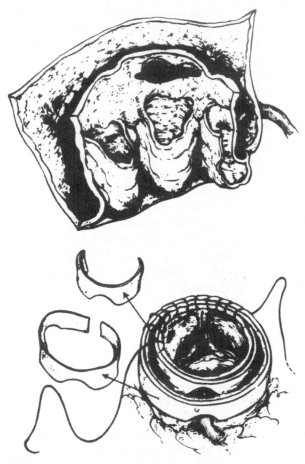

FIGURE 33-4. Key components of valve resuspension for aortic dissection, illustrating resuspension of commissural posts and buttressing with external and internal felt strips. Reproduced with permission from Miller DC. Surgical management of acute aortic dissection: new data. Semin Thorac Cardiovasc Surg 1991;3:225–37.

aortic valve and, as such, hopefully avoided valve-related complications. Second, and more compelling, as facility was gained with valve resuspension, these techniques actually shortened the operative intervention in a complex high-risk patient population.

Unfortunately, there are potential drawbacks with these techniques. Valve resuspension in the dissected aorta does not remove all of the abnormal tissue, particularly in the sinuses of Valsalva. This remaining tissue represents a continued risk for further dissection or aneurysm formation. One further limitation to widespread acceptance of this procedure was that in the era during which this technique was first described, the procedure was not applied to aneurysmal disease in the ascending aorta. Instead, the technique used for aneurysmal disease was either composite valve–conduit replacement or supracoronary graft replacement with or without valve replacement. The latter technique of supracoronary conduit replacement neglected the fact that any aortic wall tissue left in place was subject to recurrent aneurysmal disease, particularly evident in the sinuses of Valsalva.

Valve Resuspension in a Tubular Conduit

RATIONALE

As techniques for dissections evolved, it was recognized that similar aortic valve-sparing techniques also might be applicable for aneurysmal disease. In 1992, David reported an aortic valve-sparing technique for aortic insufficiency

in both aneurysm and dissection.[29] The rationale was that valve replacement was unnecessary if the valve leaflets were anatomically normal. More simply stated, if the pathology was confined to the aortic wall, only that tissue needed to be excised. He proposed that the valve could be resuspended within a Dacron conduit, similar to the techniques cited above. However, an additional and crucial feature was that the conduit size and configuration were used to restore a normal annular diameter. This aspect of annular fixation is one of the critical aspects of treating the diseased aortic root and attaining durable long-term results.

TECHNIQUE

In this technique, the ascending aorta is transected just beyond the aneurysmal dilatation, and all three sinuses of Valsalva are excised, leaving 5 to 7 mm of arterial wall attached to the aortic valve and a small button of arterial wall attached to the coronary ostia (Figure 33-5). Sutures are then placed from inside to outside of the left ventricular outflow tract, immediately below the valve, at the level of the annulus. A Dacron graft is sized and then trimmed to remove a scalloped segment, which corresponds to the commissural post between the right and left leaflets. The previously placed subvalvular, or "annular," sutures are passed through the end of the graft in such a way to correct the annular dilatation by fixing the size of the annulus to the size of the tube graft. The graft is then cut to 2 to 3 cm above the commissures, and the valve is resuspended

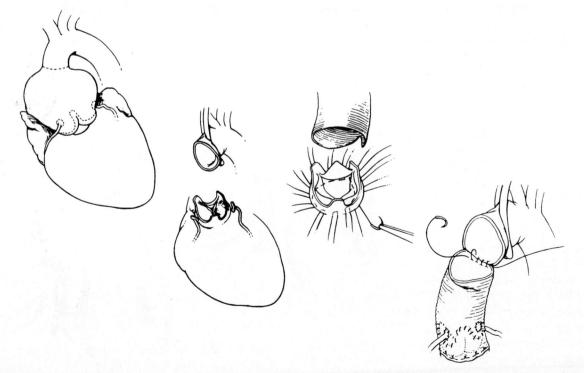

FIGURE 33-5. Valve resuspension in a tubular conduit. The dotted lines indicate lines of resection. The aortic valve and coronary buttons are left intact, and horizontal mattress sutures are placed subvalvularly. The valve is then resuspended within the graft, and the distal end is anastomosed. Adapted and reproduced with permission from David TE, Feindel CM.[29]

within the graft, similar to valve resuspension or freehand homograft techniques. Recently, David reported several modifications to this technique.[30] These modifications do not include subvalvular stitch placement, but they excise and reconstruct the sinuses selectively, so that "remodeling" of the sinuses may be addressed individually (Figure 33-6).

EVALUATION

This operation, as originally described, is theoretically very appealing albeit somewhat technically formidable. It offers the possibility of "cure" of the disease process by complete excision and/or stabilization of the diseased aortic wall. Furthermore, because the base of the graft is placed in a sub-valvular or "annular" position, the technique offers long-term fixation of the aortic annulus. This point is important because connective-tissue diseases that involve the aortic root theoretically involve the endoskeleton of the heart. Thus, a procedure such as this, which treats the aneurysmal disease from a subvalvular level up through the ascending aorta, cannot be criticized for leaving diseased tissue untreated. As such, one major appeal of this procedure as originally described is that recurrence of aneurysmal disease is unlikely. This appeal is lost in the modified procedures that do not include subvalvular stitch placement.

The greatest theoretical drawback of the original procedure is that the durability of the "normal" aortic valve in an abnormal environment remains to be seen. David acknowledges that a straight tubular graft, without sinuses of Valsalva, may have detrimental effects during leaflet opening and may also result in elevated stresses in the leaflets. In addition, because the native valve is to be spared, the relationship of the graft size and shape to the size of the leaflets may have significant effects on valve

closure, leaflet stress, and longevity of the repair. Thus, it is essential to have an understanding of the relationship of native aortic root size and shape to leaflet size and shape to effectively accomplish this procedure. Although this is a very appealing procedure, the technical demands, the required geometric understanding, and the necessary operative time have limited the use of this procedure. For these reasons, surgeons again sought more expeditious and simplified procedures.

The modification recently described by David that excludes subvalvular stitch placement in favor of "tailoring" the sinuses (David II) is more expedient but less theoretically appealing. This modification may benefit the operative time but abandons one of the original benefits of the procedure, fixation of the annulus. As the annulus is a subvalvular structure, it will not be subject to fixation by a supravalvular suture line. David has addressed this potential problem with the David II procedure by including an additional modification to the procedure, which is partial or complete annuloplasty. He has described both suture annuloplasty and a partial felt-reinforced annuloplasty. Both approaches add some fixation to the annulus.

Recently, David reported comparative data for the two types of repairs ("remodeling" [David II] vs "re-implantation" [David I]). At 6 years post operation, only 75% percent of patients with remodeling procedures were free from aortic insufficiency (AI), as compared to 90% in the reimplantation group.[31] Additionally, the annular and the sinus of Valsalva dimensions are significantly increased in the remodeling group versus the reimplantation group. Thus, David is once again recommending some form of reimplantation for the valve-sparing procedures.[32]

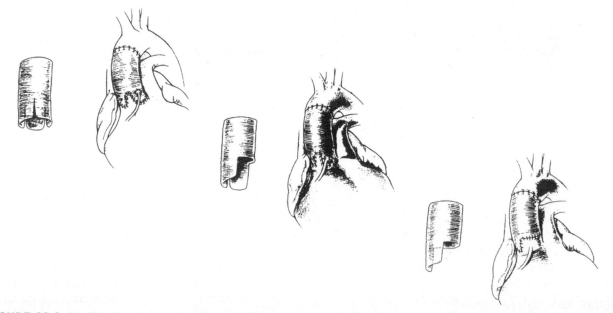

FIGURE 33-6. Modifications of valve resuspension in a tubular conduit. The conduit is cut to replace one, two, or three individual sinuses. Adapted and reproduced with permission from David RE et al.[30]

Conduit Tailoring in a Supravalvular Position

RATIONALE

Sarsam and Yacoub reported an alternative valve-sparing approach in 1993.[16,33] This technique offers an innovative anatomically based description of how to replace all of the aortic wall tissue above the valve. The aim of this procedure is to replace the diseased aortic wall tissue and, in the process, to reshape the anatomic "annulus" (as described in the paper) back to its normal geometry to restore valve competence and to preserve the valve leaflets. The primary focus of this technique is to tailor the conduit to match the asymmetric details of the human aortic sinuses of Valsalva. It should be noted, however, that the "annulus" cited in the title of this paper refers to the semilunar attachment of the leaflets (anatomic annulus), rather than the ringlike junction of the aortic wall and ventricle (surgical annulus). This is an example of the difference in terminology cited in the introduction in that by the terms preferred by the authors, "surgical" and "anatomic" annulus are reversed. In spite of this terminology difference, this is an insightful and remarkably descriptive paper that reviews some fundamentals of aortic root anatomy.

TECHNIQUE

The most appealing aspect of this procedure is that, similar to the procedure described by David, all possible aortic wall is excised, sparing only the remnants necessary to preserve the coronary ostia and the valve leaflets. The procedure differs from the original David procedure but is similar to David's own modifications (David II) in management of the conduit. The base of a prosthetic graft is incised longitudinally at three points corresponding to the anatomic location of the commissures, and the length of the incision is determined by the desired height of the commissural post (Figure 33-7). The graft is then cut in a "crown" shape, the commissural posts are fixed, the graft is attached to the aortic remnant above the valve leaflets, and, finally, the coronary buttons are anastomosed.

EVALUATION

There are several appealing aspects of this technique. First, the unique crown-shaped incisions may allow for anatomic variations of the sinus of Valsalva regions in individual patients. Second, the shape may theoretically allow "bulging" of the graft that may simulate the shape of the natural sinuses. As such, this technique may be particularly applicable to conditions such as "isolated" aneurysm of the sinuses of Valsalva. Third, the greatest appeal of this procedure is that there is only one suture line necessary at the valvular level, and accordingly, the operative time may be decreased, compared to other procedures.

However, there also are several drawbacks to this technique. The limitations to this procedure are similar to those in the modified David II procedures. As described, the Yacoub technique assumes that the aortic root pathol-

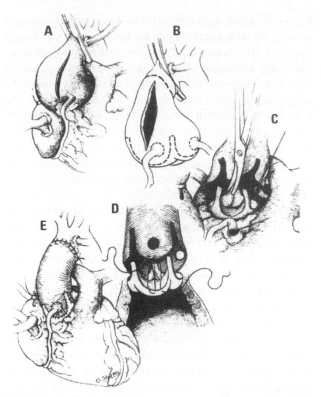

FIGURE 33-7. Conduit tailoring in a supravalvular position. The graft is prepared in a crown shape, tailored to individual sinuses of Valsalva anatomy, and is sutured to the aorta, with reimplantation of coronary arteries. Reproduced with permission from Yacoub MH, Sundt TM, Rasmi N, et al. Management of aortic valve incompetence in patients with Marfan syndrome. In: Hetzer R, Gehle P, Ennker J, editors. Cardiovascular aspects of Marfan syndrome. New York: Springer Verlag; 1995. p. 75.

ogy is restricted to the aortic tissue in the sinuses and does not address the endoskeleton of the heart. This is a premise that we do not support in aortic root disease. As a supravalvular procedure, if the disease is also present at the level of the subvalvular annulus, this technique will not suffice to remodel aortic tissue at that level, and subsequent dilatation is possible. Thus, this technique is not as globally applicable to aortic root disease as the one that encompasses and constrains or "fixes" in its treatment both the anatomic and surgical annulus. In a recent publication, our concerns were supported by the occurrence of late moderate AI in one-third of the patients undergoing this procedure.[34]

Conduit Tailoring with Pseudo-sinus Creation

RATIONALE

This procedure is based on maintaining the aortic root as a complex system that relies on a balanced interaction of all the components to attain efficient and durable function. The sinuses of Valsalva are crucial components for normal function of the aortic valve and root. As such, valve, sparing techniques must keep in mind the role of the sinuses of Valsalva and, if possible, try to re-create them. The sinuses, in concert with the sinotubular junction, create eddy currents behind the valve leaflets, which initiate valve closure and promote coronary blood flow. This eddy formation assists in leaflet coaptation assuring early and coordinated closure of all three aortic leaflets. In addition, the curvilinear configuration created by the unique attachment of the aortic leaflets to the sinuses of Valsalva allows for stress sharing between the valve leaflets and aortic wall. Any aortic reconstruction that ignores and disrupts this complex stress-sharing configuration will result in increased leaflet stress, increased fatigue, and decreased durability of the valve.

In designing a procedure that treats aortic wall disease and offers the best chance of long-term durability, four principles for re-creation of the complex aortic root interaction must be kept in mind. First, the aortic valve, once accessed and deemed salvageable, is spared and resuspended in as near a normal environment as possible. Second, all abnormal tissue that can be excised is excised. Third, any remaining abnormal annular or valvular tissue must be secured to prosthetic material to prevent future dilation. Fourth, and most important, the sinuses of Valsalva and the sinotubular junction must be reestablished. This last aspect is the most crucial because it assures that valve closure with its stress sharing is accomplished and that coronary perfusion is maintained as close to normal as possible. An additional aspect of reestablishment of the sinuses' configuration is the curvilinear orientation between leaflet and conduit wall that is also stress reducing. To accomplish these goals, the authors have coupled concepts from the previously described surgical techniques with a means of re-creating the sinuses of Valsalva.[35] The surgically created pseudo-sinus shape approximates the natural configuration. These pseudo-sinuses are designed to simulate and re-create the natural protective stress-sharing patterns that promote long-term durability of the native valve.

Creation of the pseudo-sinuses was based theoretically on increasing the proximal circumference of the conduit and then reducing its new increased length by fixation to the annulus, which, if appropriately sized, would be smaller. Fixation of the proximal end of the conduit and the commissural post results in "bulging" of the excess length of the conduit due to the increased circumference, resulting in creation of pseudo-sinuses. In addition to appropriate pseudo-sinus formation and orientation, the commissural post fixation assures re-creation of a sinotubular junction. Prior to clinical application of this technique, mathematical support for this concept was derived. The actual derivation has been reported previously.[35]

TECHNIQUE

For the modified technique, the conduit was trimmed, creating three symmetric scallops in the "annular" end of the Dacron conduit, each scallop with a maximal height of 5 to 7 mm, depending on conduit size. Other than the difference in trimming of the base of the conduit, the technique of insertion is similar to the technique initially described by David. A critical concept must be followed, which is subvalvular suture placement. To attain fixation of the endoskeleton of the heart, the horizontal mattress stitches are placed in the plane of the subvalvular annulus and do not follow the curve of the surgical or crown-shaped annulus in any of the commissural regions (Figure 33-8). Other than scalloping of the conduit, the techniques are very similar, with fixation of the annulus, placement of the subvalvular stitches along the proximal end of the scalloped conduit, resuspension of the valve within the conduit, and reimplantation of the coronary arteries (Figure 33-9).

EVALUATION

The creation of pseudo-sinuses was confirmed intraoperatively by visual inspection and postoperatively by echocardiography.[35] In the first patient in whom the author (RPC) undertook valve sparing for aortic aneurysmal disease with the technique originally described by David, there was no evidence of sinus formation on echocardiography. In contrast, in patients in whom the modified pseudo-sinus technique was performed, the constructed pseudo-sinuses were clearly apparent. In addition, the leaflets appeared to retract naturally without contact to the conduit walls.

We feel that this pseudo-sinus procedure is superior to the other valve-sparing procedures in that it adheres to the four goals established for best results in re-creation of the aortic root. It allows for sparing of any salvageable valves. It removes the maximal amount of diseased tissue. It "fixes" all remaining tissue so that further dilation cannot occur. Finally, and most significantly, it returns the spared aortic valve to a more natural environment that allows for the natural stress-sharing mechanisms of the aortic root to be re-created. However, this procedure shares one potential drawback with all the other techniques. Presently, all the aortic valve-sparing reconstructions use a synthetic conduit; unfortunately, all the available synthetic conduits have mechanical properties that are significantly different from the native aorta. Because all the available synthetic conduits are much less compliant, they will not expand as the native aorta would; this difference in compliance may, in and of itself, change the stress patterns in the valve. Because of the unknown impact of the difference in mechanical properties of synthetic conduits versus aorta, the long-term durability of all of these techniques is yet to be determined.

New Conduit Design

Two new conduit designs that facilitate the aortic valve-sparing operations were recently described. One conduit, designed by Thubrikar, has radially compliant sinuses attached to a longitudinally compliant conduit (Figure 33-10).[36] The graft is designed solely for the supravalvular techniques as described by Yacoub and by David in his

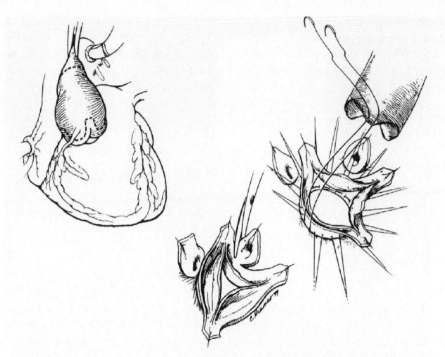

FIGURE 33-8. *Left*, Dashed lines represent incisions for valve-sparing aneurysm resection. *Center*, The spared aortic valve and preparation of coronary ostial buttons. *Right*, Subvalvular horizontal mattress sutures with initial stitch in scalloped conduit.

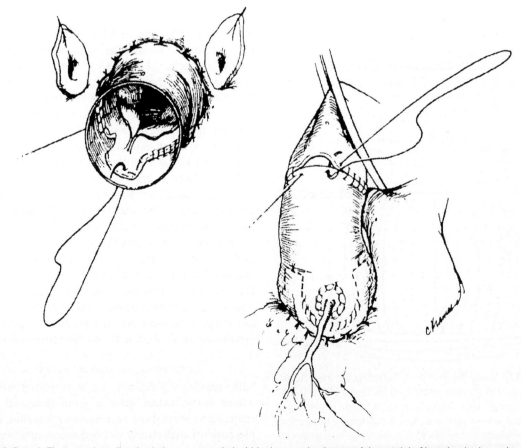

FIGURE 33-9. *Left*, The spared aortic valve being resuspended within the pseudo-sinuses of the conduit. Note that both running and horizontal mattress sutures can be used. *Right*, Completion of the distal anastomosis after pseudo-sinus creation and valve resuspension and coronary implantation.

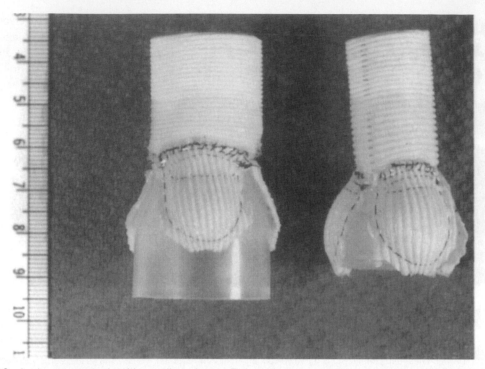

FIGURE 33-10. Aortic root prosthesis with compliant sinuses. The prosthesis is made by attaching three sinus-shaped flaps to a tubular Dacron graft. Reproduced with permission from Thubrikar MJ et al.[36]

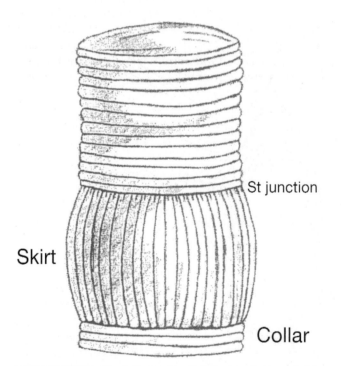

FIGURE 33-11. Newly designed graft. Skirted section has a height equal to the given graft diameter and is stated to have a 25% distensibility in the horizontal plane. The collar is cut out when performing a remodeling type of valve-sparing procedure, is trimmed to a minimum in the case of a reimplantation procedure, or is maintained for a prosthetic valve attachment in case of a Bentall procedure. Reproduced with permission from DePaulis R et al.[37]

(St = sinotubular.)

remodeling techniques.[16,30] The other conduit is designed by DePaulis, and it allows for subvalvular stitch placement into a fixed collar (Figure 33-11).[6,37] It then has a supra-annular bulging portion (similar to Thubrikar's, this is also radially compliant) that will allow for resuspension of the valve in a "sinuslike" environment. At the distal end of the bulging portion, there is attachment of a longitudinally compliant conduit. This distal junction reestablishes the sinotubular junction. Although standardization of height and sinus depth to appropriate annular size is not proven in either conduit, they both should allow expedient operative correction of the dilatation and also allow some form of sinus formation. We clearly favor the graft designed by DePaulis in that it allows the possibility of accomplishing all four goals of aortic root reconstruction that have been discussed earlier. The ability to affix the annulus to a stable Dacron collar, allowing long-term prevention of later dilatation, is a very appealing aspect of the DePaulis conduit. At present, there are no reports of long-term follow-up with either conduit, so their benefits are still theoretical.

CANDIDATES FOR AORTIC VALVE SPARING

Valve-sparing operations are best suited for patients whose aortic valves have a good potential of being returned to normal (or near normal) function. For example, patients with clearly isolated acute aortic wall disease, such as an acute dissection, are ideal. In addition, patients with aneurysmal disease, but with an aortic valve that is structurally intact and undamaged, are also appropriate for valve-sparing procedures. It is in this group of patients with dilated aortic roots, in particular, that the authors advocate early treatment rather than the "watchful waiting" that has been the historical approach to intervention for aortic aneurysms. The longer the aneurysm is present, the longer the period of abnormal stress, which may subsequently damage the leaflets, negating the opportunity for valve sparing.

In contrast to patients with dissection or aneurysm where the valves are relatively normal, patients with stenotic valvular lesions that require significant leaflet tissue mobilization or replacement remain poor candidates for valve-sparing operations. The literature to date supports this statement, in that the reported attempts at sparing the stenotic aortic valve have not shown good results, even in the short term. An additional concern about the present state of valve sparing for stenosis is that the nature of the reparative techniques has varied, and the indications have not been made clear in the published reports. At present, we cannot advocate sparing the valve in these patients.

In spite of this fairly rigorous patient restriction, the number of patients anatomically and physiologically suited for aortic valve–sparing operations is increasing. From 1965 to 1975, the prevalence of annular dilatation in patients operated on for pure aortic insufficiency was 17%.[38] In 1980, the reported incidence of annular dilatation increased to 37%; in 1990 it increased to 50%, making annular dilatation the single most common cause of AI in North America.[39,40] As such, there is and will be a greater demand for cardiac surgery that is appropriate for these patients.

In the patients with aortic root dilatation, two principle groups emerge, based on age. The first group consists of patients who are in the first six decades of life and who usually have Marfan syndrome or another connective-tissue abnormality. The second group consists of those patients in the last three decades of life who have age-related degenerative problems. Valve-sparing procedures are very appealing to both groups but for different reasons. The younger patients generally have a strong desire to maintain an active lifestyle and have a greater life expectancy; as such, they usually prefer to avoid the anticoagulation required with mechanical valves. These younger patients also want to avoid the obligatory reoperation necessitated in most biologic valve options. For these patients, a valve-sparing procedure offers an attractive alternative. In the older age group, valve-sparing procedures are popular for the avoidance of anticoagulation and its complications. Particularly as these patients enter the eighth and ninth decades of their lives, when there is an increase in complications due to anticoagulation, they prefer to avoid these complications if possible. Both of these patient groups are increasing in size as a result of earlier diagnosis of the connective-tissue diseases and of the increasing age of the population. Consequently, both groups of patients are increasingly referred for surgical consideration for aortic insufficiency and aortic root dilatation, and more of the patients that are referred are interested in aortic valve–sparing operations.

Unfortunately, not all of the patients who are referred for aortic valve–sparing operations are good candidates for this type of procedure. Ultimately, the appropriateness of an aortic valve–sparing operation is limited by the state of the aortic leaflet tissue; that is, there must be normal or near-normal tissue present. This is similar to the limitations now encountered with mitral valve repair. Hopefully, with an increased understanding of disease processes and aortic valve and root system biomechanics as well as customized materials design, the indications for aortic valve–sparing procedures will be extended to include many more patients. At present, for the patients who are currently selected for valve sparing, several potential techniques have been described. We feel strongly that the best long-term results will be attained by re-creating an environment as near to normal as possible for the "spared" aortic valve. For this reason, we feel that the procedure of choice remains aortic valve sparing coupled with creation of pseudo-sinuses. As it is designed, the procedure is simple and reproducible and has had gratifying results with both short and intermediate follow-up. That said, if DePaulis's new conduit proves to have a good size match versus the diameter, as well as height and depth of sinus, this may make the pseudo-sinus procedure even more reproducible. Only with careful investigation and clinical experience will anyone know whether the new conduit is beneficial; until then, we will continue to advocate the pseudo-sinus procedure.

CONCLUSION

The sparing of the aortic valve in selected cases of aortic insufficiency is an excellent alternative to procedures that require valve replacement—mechanical or biologic. The ideal procedure and the ideal materials for reconstruction of the aortic root continue to evolve. As the incidence of aortic root abnormalities increases, it is requisite that cardiac surgeons become facile in the management of this previously formidable region. If current trends continue, the next decade promises to significantly increase the need for this type of surgical option. Unfortunately, the long-term durability of the aortic valve that is spared by any technique in an artificial conduit is still undetermined. It seems intuitive that as valve-sparing procedures more closely approximate the natural anatomic arrangement, the resultant biomechanics and long-term durability will improve. As described, the introduction of a simple scalloped modification of the prosthetic graft end allows for creation of pseudo-sinuses adjacent to the valve leaflets. We believe that for patients with aortic root aneurysms and dissections, with normal or near-normal aortic valves, this modified aortic valve–sparing aortic root replacement is the procedure of choice.

References

1. Cochran RP, Kunzelman KS. Valve sparing operations for aortic annulo-ectasia. In: Franco KL, Verrier ED, editors. Advanced therapy in cardiac surgery. Hamilton (ON): BC Decker; 1999. p. 280–91.

2. Doty DB, Arcidi JM. Methods for graft size selection in aortic valve sparing operations. Ann Thorac Surg 2000; 69:648–50.

3. David TE, Armstrong S, Ivanov J, et al. Results of aortic valve-sparing operations. J Thorac Cardiovasc Surg 2001;1221:39–46.

4. Gowdamarajan A, Cohen DM, Rowland DG, et al. Valve sparing operation in a child with aneurysmal disease of the ascending aorta. Ann Thorac Surg 1999;67:1151–2.

5. Leyh RG, Schmidtke C, Bartels C, Sievers H. Valve-sparing aortic root replacement (remodeling/reimplantation) in acute type A dissection. Ann Thorac Surg 2000;70:21–4.

6. Bassano C, DeMatteis GM, Nardi P, et al. Mid-term follow-up of aortic root remodeling compared to Bentall operation. Eur J Cardiothorac Surg 2001;19:601–5.

7. Pretre R, Turina MI. Aortic valve-sparing operation in dilatation of the ascending aorta. J Card Surg 2000;15:434–6.

8. Guilmet D, Bonnet S, Bonnet N, Bachet J. Preservation of the native aortic valve in the treatment of aortic aneurysmal dilatation. Arch Mal Coeur Vaiss 1999;92:1181–7.

9. Ninomiya M, Takamoto S, Kotsuka Y, et al. Midterm results after aortic valve-sparing operation. Jpn J Thorac Cardiovasc Surg 2001;49:706–10.

10. Ito T, Otsubo S, Norita H, et al. Aortic valve sparing operation and selection of operative technique. Jpn J Thorac Cardiovasc Surg 1998;46:153–5.

11. Robicsek F. Leonardo da Vinci and the sinuses of Valsalva. Ann Thorac Surg 1991;52:328–35.

12. Stedman's medical dictionary. Baltimore (MD): Williams and Wilkins; 2000.

13. Agnew LRC. Dorland's illustrated medical dictionary. Philadelphia (PA): WB Saunders Company; 2000.

14. Gray's anatomy. Philadelphia (PA): Lea and Febiger; 1973.

15. Anderson J. Grant's atlas of anatomy. Baltimore (MD): Williams and Wilkins; 1983.

16. Sarsam MA, Yacoub M. Remodeling of the aortic valve anulus. J Thorac Cardiovasc Surg 1993;105:435–8.

17. Bentall H, De Bono A. A technique for complete replacement of the ascending aorta. Thorax 1968;23:338–9.

18. Angell WW, Oury JH, Shah P. A comparison of replacement and reconstruction in patients with mitral regurgitation. J Thorac Cardiovasc Surg 1987;93:665–74.

19. Perier P, Deloche A, Chauvaud S, et al. Comparative evaluation of mitral valve repair and replacement with Starr, Bjork, and porcine valve prostheses. Circulation 1984;70:I187–92.

20. Bernal J, Rabasa JM, Cagigas JC. Valve related complications with the Hancock I porcine bioprostheses: a twelve- to fourteen-year follow-up study. J Thorac Cardiovasc Surg 1991;101:871–80.

21. Antunes MJ. Techniques of valvular reoperation. Eur J Cardiothorac Surg 1992;6:54S–8S.

22. Groves LK, Effler DB, Hank WA, et al. Aortic insufficiency secondary to aneurysmal changes in the ascending aorta: surgical management. J Thorac Cardiovasc Surg 1964;48:362–79.

23. Kouchoukos NT, Karp RB, Blackstone EH, et al. Replacement of the ascending aorta and aortic valve with a composite graft. Ann Surg 1980;192:403–13.

24. Massimo CG, Presenti LF, Marronci P, et al. Extended and total aortic resection in the surgical treatment of acute type A aortic dissection. Ann Thorac Surg 1988;46:420–1.

25. DeBakey ME, McCollum CH, Crawford ES, et al. Dissection and dissecting aneurysms of the aorta: twenty-year follow-up of five hundred twenty-seven patients treated surgically. Surgery 1982;92:118–34.

26. Miller DC. Aortic dissection, aneurysm, and trauma and congenital disease of the aorta. Curr Opin Cardiol 1989; 4:693–704.

27. Miller D, Stinson E, Oyer P, et al. Operative treatment of aortic dissection. J Thorac Cardiovasc Surg 1979;78:365–82.

28. Najafi H, Dye WS, Javid H. Acute aortic regurgitation secondary to aortic dissection. Ann Thorac Surg 1972;14:474–82.

29. David TE, Feindel CM. An aortic valve-sparing operation for patients with aortic incompetence and aneurysm of the ascending aorta. J Thorac Cardiovasc Surg 1992; 103:617–22.

30. David TE, Feindel CM, Bos J. Repair of the aortic valve in patients with aortic insufficiency and aortic root aneurysm. J Thorac Cardiovasc Surg 1995;109:345–52.

31. David T. Aortic valve sparing: remodeling or reimplantation. Rocky Mountain Valve Symposium; 2001 Aug 15; Missoula, MT.

32. David T. Aortic valve-sparing operations for aortic root aneurysms. Semin Thorac Cardiovasc Surg 2001;13: 291–6.

33. Yacoub M, Halim M, Radley Smith R, et al. Surgical treatment of mitral regurgitation caused by floppy valves: repair versus replacement. Circulation 1981;64:II210–6.

34. Yacoub M, Gehle P, Chardasekaran V, et al. Late results of a valve-preserving operation in patients with aneurysms of the ascending aorta and root. J Thorac Cardiovasc Surg 1998;115:1080–90.

35. Cochran RP, Kunzelman KS, Eddy AC, et al. Modified conduit preparation creates a pseudosinus in an aortic valve-sparing procedure for aneurysm of the ascending aorta. J Thorac Cardiovasc Surg 1995;109:1049–57.

36. Thubrikar MJ, Robicsek F, Gong GG, Fowler BL. A new aortic root prosthesis with compliant sinuses for valve-sparing. Ann Thorac Surg 2001;71:S318–22.

37. DePaulis R, DeMatteis GM, Nardi P, et al. Opening and closing characteristics of the aortic valve after valve-sparing procedures using a new aortic root conduit. Ann Thorac Surg 2001;72:487–94.

38. Davies MH. Pathology of cardiac valves. Toronto: Butterworths; 1980. p. 37–61.

39. Olson LJ, Subramanian R, Edwards WD. Surgical pathology of pure aortic insufficiency: a study of 225 cases. Mayo Clin Proc 1984;59:835–41.

40. Dare AJ, Veinot JP, Edwards WD, et al. New observations on the etiology of aortic valve disease: a surgical pathologic study of 236 cases from 1990. Hum Pathol 1993;24: 1330–8.

CHAPTER 34

ANEURYSMS OF THE AORTIC ARCH

JAN D. GALLA, MD, PHD

Perhaps no other 12-cm segment of the thoracic aorta stimulates as much concern and trepidation as the aortic arch. Despite the complexity of the aortic root or, within the retroperitoneum, the compact organization of the suprarenal aorta, the possibility of a catastrophic complication following what appears to be a "textbook" repair of the top of the thoracic aorta remains both real and finite. As a result, the development of procedures to deal with aneurysms of the aortic arch have a long, rich, and continually evolving history. The reader is directed to any of the several excellent and entertaining reviews of these developments that have been published.[1–3] Consequently, this chapter does not reiterate the history of the treatment of arch aneurysms; instead, it provides a succinct, comprehensive review of methods of approaching this condition so that when faced with a patient with this condition, a safe repair does not seem too formidable a task. Additionally, newer approaches to the reconstruction of the aortic arch are presented, as well as the initial forays into the use of intravascular stenting for the treatment of arch aneurysms.

Etiology and Presentation

Aneurysms of the aortic arch, isolated to the arch (Figure 34-1), are unusual and more commonly encountered as a continuum of aneurysm disease in the ascending and/or the descending aortae. They may arise from a variety of causes, including atherosclerotic or degenerative diseases, trauma, dissection, connective tissue disorders, or infection. Aortic pathology arising from dissection is discussed in Chapters 33 and 37 of this text, as is aortic reconstruction peculiar to the Marfan's patient. For these reasons, discussions in this chapter primarily focus on those aneurysms of atherosclerotic or degenerative origin. However, many of the surgical principles and techniques presented within this chapter are directly applicable to a variety of pathologies, including those discussed in more detail elsewhere.

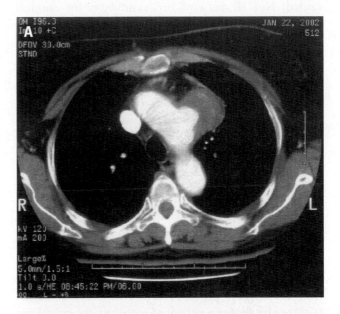

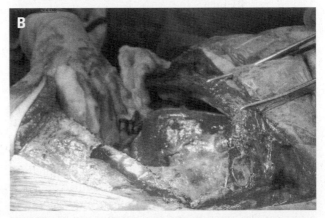

FIGURE 34-1. *A*, CT scan of a saccular aneurysm of aortic arch. Note the small intraluminal protrusion into the larger thrombus of the aneurysm sac. The surrounding arch neck is normal in size and free from disease, suggesting the possibility of primary repair of this arch. *B*, Intraoperative photograph of the aneurysm imaged in *A*. The patient's head is to the viewer's right; chest is away from the viewer. The vagus nerve is readily visualized coursing over the aneurysm.

Many patients with arch aneurysms are entirely asymptomatic and discover their conditions serendipitously, usually in the course of a routine examination or during evaluation of some other condition. Occasionally, arch aneurysms may manifest themselves by causing a change in voice quality, increasing pulmonary symptoms, dysphagia, or chest discomfort. The presence of these symptoms is less frequent, however, than the incidental discovery of an aneurysm by routine chest x-ray, which is usually confirmed by computed tomography (CT) scanning. Thoracic surgical consultation usually rapidly follows, as aneurysms remain of great concern to most practicing physicians. The thoracic surgeon, however, should reassure the patient, explaining the nature and prognosis of their condition, as well as the need for additional diagnostic tests if surgical intervention is warranted. Not all patients are candidates for surgical resection, however, as those with limited life expectancy, extreme comorbid conditions, or religious/personal beliefs contravening surgery might not be considered for repair. Patients may express fear of the procedure or of the possible complications of surgery; these fears are quite normal and can usually be assuaged with careful and considerate counseling. The variety of surgical options available affords the thoughtful surgeon a considerable armamentarium with which an appropriate patient may be safely treated.

Preoperative Assessment

As part of the routine preoperative assessment, a complete history and physical examination is conducted, paying particular attention to any preexisting neurologic, cardiac, or hematologic condition. While not a contraindication to surgery, previous cerebrovascular accidents (CVAs) may render a patient at more risk for neurologic complications following hypothermic circulatory arrest (HCA), and a history of transient ischemic attacks (TIAs) may portend more serious neurologic problems. Similarly, undiagnosed bleeding diatheses may manifest themselves only as intra- or postoperative hemorrhage, and are potentially preventable situations if dealt with in an appropriate manner. Cardiac conditions may similarly be occult; negative electrocardiograms (ECGs) or stress tests are not uncommonly found among the information provided during the initial assessment. Because cardiopulmonary bypass (CPB) is almost universally required for the treatment of arch aneurysms, a full cardiac catheterization is highly recommended prior to surgery, both to assess cardiac function and to determine the presence of hitherto unknown coronary artery disease (CAD) or valvular dysfunction. It makes little sense to electively place a patient on CPB to fix one problem, yet leave other problems behind; the repair of other cardiac conditions adds little time to the complete repair as coronary artery bypass grafting (CABG) or valve repair/replacements can

be performed while the patient is being cooled for HCA. The substitution of combinations of other cardiologic examinations (echocardiograms, myocardial perfusion studies, etc) for cardiac catheterization has occasionally led to unfortunate, and usually preventable, unfavorable results, and is no longer practiced in our institution.

Occasionally, a patient will be referred for whom no CT or magnetic resonance imaging (MRI) scan is available. It is highly desirable to obtain one of these two diagnostic examinations prior to surgery to fully assess the extent of the resection required. Although some idea of the amount of aortic resection required might be obtained from the cardiac catheterization, the anatomy of the thoracic aorta is better visualized with these other two tests. The CT/MRI is also useful for comparative purposes following the repair and for future reference when following the patient postoperatively. Despite the need for additional exposure to ionizing radiation and nephrotoxic dyes, CT scans seem yet to be the favored test; as quality and surgeon comfort with MRI scans increase, it is likely that this modality may replace the CT scan as the test of choice. Limited access to this examination, however, may hinder development of MRI as the more common test. Implicit in the recommendation for these examinations is their availability in the operating room; with the increasingly common practice of "filmless" radiology departments, the ability to view the scans in the operating room might be limited, making availability of "hard copies" of these exams a necessity.

Operating Room Management

Preparation of the patient about to undergo arch aneurysm repair is dictated partially by the approach to be used. Both median sternotomy and thoracotomy approaches offer good visualization of the aortic arch: the former is more useful if intracardiac or proximal aortic procedures are to be included in the procedure, the latter if descending aortic resection is anticipated. Coronary revascularization, including use of the internal mammary artery (IMA), can also be performed from the left chest, especially during the interval of cooling or HCA. A functional combination of these two approaches, the thoracosternotomy incision, allows extended repairs of both the heart and proximal descending aorta with good visualization. Whichever incision is used, appropriate positioning and padding of the patient helps limit postoperative complications of the extremities.

Arterial pressure monitoring is placed in accordance with proposed cannulation techniques in mind. For routine ascending aortic or arch cannulation, radial artery cannulation on either side may be used. If axillary/subclavian artery cannulation is planned, an ipsilateral radial arterial pressure tracing will be compromised during the period that the pump cannula is occluding the arterial flow peripherally, and alternative, preferably contralateral, pressure monitoring sites should be used. In select cases, especially if extended periods of regional hypoperfusion are planned, both right- and left-sided tracings or upper and lower body tracings are useful.

Pulmonary artery (PA) catheters are routinely placed via the left internal jugular vein, and at the same time as the PA catheter insertion, a jugular venous bulb (JVB) catheter is placed. Monitoring of JVB sample saturations affords a measure of cerebral activity, with higher saturations indicative of decreased metabolic activity. During the cooling interval preceding HCA, a JVB saturation of > 95% is sought. Topical head cooling, by packing the head in ice, also helps keep cerebral activity minimized.

Intraoperative transesophageal echocardiography (TEE) is also routinely employed. Assessment of myocardial wall motion, both pre- and post-CPB, allows judicious volume loading to maximize cardiac function. Valve repairs may be assessed with the TEE, and evaluation of the aorta can detect dissection and luminal flow abnormalities (as in malperfusion of the branch arteries).

Pharmacologic supplementation of the patient for HCA is limited to adding 2 g Solu-Medrol to the CPB circuit. Postoperative steroid taper, over 2 days, is only used if HCA time exceeds 30 min. Barbiturates, formerly routinely used, are no longer administered. Anesthetic management is in accordance with routine cardiac protocols.

Surgical Techniques

Basic Tenets

Exposure of the aorta is as per routine approach. Once the aorta is visualized and a limited mobilization is accomplished, cannulation for bypass is undertaken. From a sternal approach, the right atrium and aorta may be cannulated as in routine cardiac procedures. Increasingly, the use of the right axillary/subclavian artery has been suggested to limit the possibility of neurologic complications, to allow unimpeded access to the field, and to potentially limit the intervals of HCA. This arterial cannulation site may be used from either of the main approaches, although access to the left subclavian artery may be precluded by a large, relatively fixed distal arch aneurysm. Arch or descending aortic cannulation can also be used, replacing the arterial cannula into the graft if necessary. Femoral arterial cannulation, once almost exclusively used, is used with increasingly less frequency. Indeed, many aortic surgeons have come to favor subclavian and axillary artery cannulation, believing these routes to be associated with fewer embolic complications. Venous cannulation, when working via a left thoracotomy approach, is best obtained with placement of a right atrial cannula, inserted over a guidewire from the left common femoral vein. Correct intraatrial positioning may be guided with the TEE. An alternative site, although less frequently used, is the PA, positioning the cannula across the pulmonic valve and into the right ventricle. Left ventricular venting

is sometimes required, especially when working from the left chest and aortic cross-clamping is difficult or undesirable. Although venting via the left atrium is possible, adequate decompression of the ventricle, especially with a competent mitral valve, may not be possible; in these cases, direct venting of the ventricle via the apex of the heart is preferable.

Once CPB is established, cooling is initiated immediately. As the duration of HCA is often indeterminate prior to completion of the repair, liberal use of profound hypothermia (< 15°C) is used. Hypothermia is supplemented with topical cold applied to the heart throughout the procedure for myocardial preservation. Selective antegrade cerebral perfusion is intermittently used in accordance with the repair employed; retrograde cerebral perfusion is no longer routinely used. (For a full discussion of the effects of these two perfusion techniques, see Chapter 31, "Cerebral Protection during Operations on the Thoracic Aorta.")

Primary Repair

In a very few instances, a primary repair following resection of an arch aneurysm is possible (Figures 34-1 and 34-2). Aneurysms offering this possibility of repair are very localized and of (usually) moderate size or less. Full mobilization of both proximal and distal segments of the arch must be possible to allow a tension-free anastomosis; Teflon felt is routinely used to reinforce the outside of the native aorta.

Suture repair is with 3–0 polypropylene.

Occasionally, an arch defect may be repaired with only a patch, as in those instances when a pseudoaneurysm may be excised at its neck. A patch of coated Dacron (eg, Hemashield) yields a very strong, durable repair with little likelihood of leak. Other materials (Gortex, reinforced pericardium, homografts) have also been used with acceptable results.

"Classic" Arch Repairs

As originally described by Griepp and colleagues, arch replacement is performed as illustrated in Figure 34-3.[4] After establishing HCA, the diseased segments are resected, leaving the arch vessels on a cap of native aorta. An appropriately sized graft is selected and sutured end-to-end with the descending aortic stump. An orifice is created to correspond to the size of the arch cap, which is reattached as illustrated. Following reattachment of the arch cap, CPB may be reinstituted, either by retrograde perfusion via the femoral vessels by reinserting the arterial cannula into the arch component of the graft, or by antegrade flow through the subclavian/axillary artery cannula. The graft is flushed of air or entrained debris, both by vigorously shaking the arch cap and its vessels as well as aspirating liberally. When the vessels have been completely flushed, the proximal segment of the graft is clamped and full antegrade flow to the upper body is

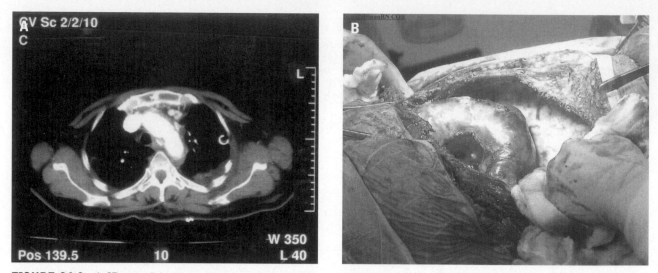

FIGURE 34-2. *A*, CT scan of the resected aneurysm shown in Figure 34-1*A*. The aortic arch is slightly shortened in length; the narrowing in midarch is the intussuscepted distal segment. *B*, Intraoperative photograph of the repaired arch aneurysm shown in Figure 34-1*B*. Note the smooth contour of the primarily reconstructed arch (patient's head is to the viewer's right).

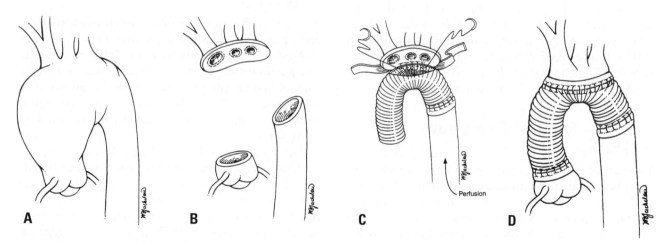

FIGURE 34-3. *A*, Diagram of aortic aneurysm. Note continuation of ascending aneurysm into the aortic arch. *B*, Complete resection of aneurysmal segments of aorta, leaving a cap of the aortic arch containing the arch vessels. *C*, "Classic" repair of aortic arch. The distal end of the aortic graft has been sewn end-to-end to the descending aortic stump, an oval opening corresponding to the site of reimplantation of the arch cap is created, and the cap is being sewn to the graft with a running polypropylene suture. Note the felt reinforcement of the suture lines. In this repair, perfusion is from the femoral artery, a technique largely abandoned for other cannulation sites. *D*, The completed "classic" repair, showing the three suture lines, which are all reinforced with felt.

reestablished, maintaining the perfusate temperature below 20°C. The proximal anastomosis is then completed in routine fashion, and the patient is rewarmed and separated from CPB as normal. Note that all aortic suture lines are reinforced with felt to insure a secure, watertight repair; the felt also lessens the tension on the diseased aortic tissue. This technique readily lends itself to extended repairs of the aorta, as in the "elephant trunk" extension into the descending aorta or any of the reconstructive techniques for the aortic root, and rapidly became the standard for aortic arch surgery.[4–10]

As experience mounted with the arch cap repair, evaluation of the technique suggested that difficulties in reconstruction were associated with increased tendency to severe neurologic complications. Ultimately, it was found that there existed a direct correlation between the interval of HCA and the incidence of CVA, and efforts to reduce the amount of circulatory arrest increased. In 1994, Ergin and colleagues described a technique whereby the arch cap was reconstructed first, allowing relatively rapid reperfusion of the head and upper body, thereby permitting a more leisurely approach to completion of the remainder of the repair.[11] This technique was further expanded by Kouchoukos and colleagues and came to be known as the "arch-first" technique, as illustrated in Figure 34-4.[12]

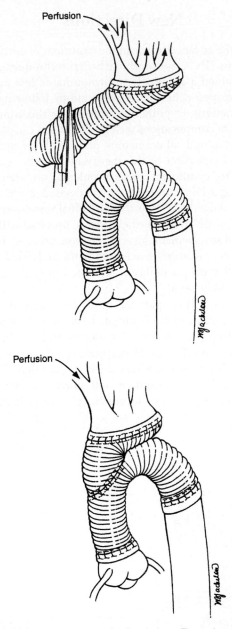

A

Perfusion

B

Perfusion

FIGURE 34-4. *A*, The "arch-first" technique. The arch cap has been reconstructed with a beveled graft, again reinforcing the suture line with felt. Arterial perfusion has been resumed via the axillary artery after flushing the reconstructed arch and clamping the distal end of the graft; alternatively, the graft may be recannulated directly through a separate incision proximal to the arch cap or via the open end of the graft, tying the free end of the graft around the arterial cannula. Once upper body/head reperfusion has been restarted, the ascending to descending graft is sutured. *B*, The completed "arch-first" repair. The arch graft has been sewn to the ascending to descending graft in an end-to-side fashion by using either a side-biting graft on the larger ascending aortic graft or a second short period of HCA.

The arch-first technique is performed following establishment of HCA. The arch cap is removed as previously described, and a segment of graft, usually 16 to 20 mm in diameter, is opened longitudinally for an appropriate

length and sutured to the undersurface of the arch cap. Perfusion of the upper body and head can then be reinstituted via the axillary artery, as illustrated in Figure 34-4*A*, by placing the arterial cannula into a stab incision of the graft or by inserting the cannula into the open end of the graft. The distal graft is occluded after the reconstructed arch has been appropriately deaired, permitting reestablishment of flow to the upper body after a minimal amount of HCA. Flows are maintained to achieve perfusion pressures of ~ 60 mm Hg and temperatures are kept cold (20°C). Following reconstruction of the other segments of resected aorta with a separate, larger tube graft, the arch graft can be connected in an end-to-side manner to the larger graft by using a second, short (~ 5 to 10 min) interval of HCA. Full-body perfusion is then reestablished (see Figure 34-4*B*), rewarming is completed, and the patient is separated from CPB in the routine fashion. As in the previous technique, it is preferable to reinforce the outside of the native aorta at the suture lines with strips of felt. With this technique, HCA intervals of 15 to 20 min are routinely encountered when reconstructing the aortic arch, and decreased incidence of neurologic complications have been reported.[9,10]

The arch-first technique can also be used from the left thoracotomy position to reconstruct the arch and descending aorta simultaneously. This technique is also useful for those patients who had previously sustained, and had repaired, type A dissections, leaving an ascending aortic graft as part of the previous repair. For the patients undergoing repair via a left thoracotomy, CPB cannulation may be accomplished in several ways: arterial cannulation can be via the arch or descending portions of the aorta, the left subclavian artery, the left femoral artery, or via the right axillary artery, if the patient is either positioned appropriately or the dissection and cannulation are performed prior to opening the left chest. Venous cannulation is most easily performed via the left common femoral vein (or the saphenous vein as it joins the common femoral), by using a long 32 to 34 French wire-reinforced atrial cannula; TEE can be useful in positioning the tip of the cannula at the vena caval/right atrial junction. Alternatively, the PA may be cannulated, with the tip of the cannula extending across the pulmonic valve into the right ventricle. This latter method requires some experience in dealing with the PA, because the PA tends to be somewhat more prone to tearing and disruption than the structures normally encountered in cannulation. The right atrium can also be cannulated from the left chest, albeit with great difficulty; this technique is best kept for historical reference only.

Once CPB has been established, it is quite commonly necessary to vent the left ventricle. It is probably best to vent via the apex, fixing the vent cannula to the apex with a (large) pledgetted suture and Rommel tourniquet. The left atrium can also be easily cannulated, but ventricular decompression is not so easily assured, particularly if the mitral valve is competent. Similarly, the pulmonary veins, both of which are readily accessible from the thoracotomy, may be cannulated for left ventricular decompression, but a similar caveat as for the left atrial drainage should be understood.

Cooling is as described before, but if retrograde pump flow into the arch is present, as in femoral or aortic cannulation, no manipulation of the aorta should be performed until HCA is started. The process of moving the aorta can dislodge material that becomes readily embolized, thereby increasing the likelihood of neurologic sequelae. After circulatory arrest is established, the aorta can be repositioned with more impunity, although the surgeon should still respect the ease with which intraaortic debris can become instilled into the arch vasculature.

The arch cap is transected, shaped, and reconstructed as described above. The arterial inflow cannula is repositioned as demonstrated in Figure 34-4B, CPB is again reinstituted, and the remainder of the repair is completed. The reinitiation of CPB should be with cold perfusate and maintained until the repair is completed. The extra time spent cold affords additional protection for the brain. Attempts to shorten the operative time by early warming frequently land the surgeon in an unforgiving position that can compromise the patient's outcome.

New Directions

Despite the advances made in the treatment of aortic arch aneurysms (HCA, no touch, arch-first techniques), there still remained a seemingly insurmountable few patients that developed neurologic complications following their reconstructions. Hypothesized reasons for this continued low level of complications include prolonged use of HCA, calcification and atheromatous disease of the arch cap itself, and extension of the aneurysm into the arch cap vessels. To counteract these problems, an alternative method of arch reconstruction was devised, avoiding the arch cap altogether.[13–15] As the individual vessels seem less commonly involved in the disease process, with less aneurysm involvement, less calcification, and less atheromatous accumulation than is seen in the arch itself, it was thought that the possibility of fewer neurologic complications would be seen.

The trifurcation graft technique is described below. After CPB and cooling is initiated, the graft is prepared. Using a length of 14-mm Hemashield graft as the base, side arms of 10-mm Hemashield graft are sutured end-to-side to openings created with an ophthalmic electrocautery, using a running 4–0 polypropylene stitch (Figure 34-5A and B). Sidearm lengths are left long to

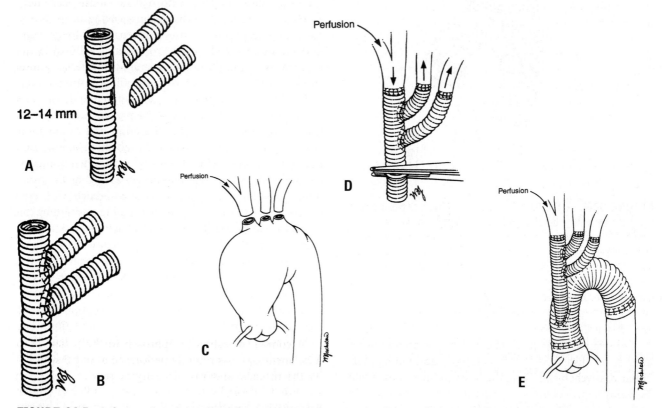

FIGURE 34-5. *A,* Construction of the trifurcation graft for arch reconstruction. Two tangentially positioned 10-mm sidearm grafts are sewn obliquely to a larger 12- to 14-mm main trunk graft. *B,* The completed trifurcated graft. *C,* The arch aneurysm with the arch vessels transected. Perfusion had been established via the right axillary artery. *D,* The arch vessels have been sequentially sutured to their respective grafts, flushed, and upper body/head reperfusion restarted after clamping the distal main graft. *E,* The completed repair. The trifurcation arch graft has been sewn to the ascending to descending graft; the operation is competed in routine fashion.

accommodate any anatomic abnormalities encountered, trimming them to length as needed.

When appropriate conditions are reached, HCA is induced and the arch vessels are transected from the top of the arch (Figure 34-5C). An end-to-end anastomosis of innominate artery to the 14-mm graft is performed with continuously running 4–0 polypropylene; the suture is tightened gingerly as the arch vessels can easily tear. The remaining two vessels are sutured sequentially to their respective sidearm grafts. Each graft takes between 5 and 10 min to accomplish; the order of vessel reconstruction may be reversed if exposure so dictates. When the last graft is completed, the head vessels may be reperfused, either via the axillary arterial cannula, as illustrated in Figure 34-5D, or by the methods described above in the arch-first technique. Flows are initially begun at low (~ 500 cc/min) rates to flush the vessels of air and embolic material, and liberal use of aspiration of the grafts and limbs is made. The distal end of the main (14-mm graft) trunk is occluded and reperfusion of the upper body is resumed, maintaining perfusion pressures of 50 to 60 mm Hg, allowing blood temperatures to drift upward, but not actively cooling at this time.

The arch is then reconstructed by using a separate graft to connect the descending aorta to the proximal segment of the ascending vessel. If an elephant trunk reconstruction of the descending aorta is planned, it may be performed at this time, giving the surgeon the option of adding a second arterial cannula into the reconstructed descending aorta and perfusing the remainder of the body while any proximal aortic pathology is addressed.[4,5] Care is taken to identify, mobilize, and avoid traumatizing the recurrent laryngeal nerve that encircles the aorta at this point. The anastomosis is performed with running 3–0 polypropylene suture, reinforcing the outside of the native aorta with a strip of Teflon felt. This gives an extremely hemostatic repair, favored in this site where later repair of a suture leak may be extraordinarily difficult. An ascending aneurysm or aortic root reconstruction may thus be performed while the entire body is on CPB, maintaining the heart with the surgeon's preferred myocardial preservation technique. Alternatively, after creating the distal anastomosis, a simple proximal anastomosis completes ascending to descending continuity. As before, the anastomosis is performed with running 3–0 polypropylene, reinforcing the outside of the native aorta with a strip of Teflon felt.

Completion of arch–aorta continuity is accomplished after gently distending the ascending to descending graft, either passively by allowing the heart to fill and manually expelling ventricular blood into the graft, or by instilling cardioplegic solution into the graft directly. This gives the surgeon a sense of spatial orientation of the larger graft so that the 14-mm graft may be stretched into position and transected at an appropriate length. An ovoid hole is created in the larger graft with an ophthalmic electro-cautery and an end-to-side, graft-to-graft anastomosis is performed with running 2–0 polypropylene. Upper-body perfusion need not be interrupted for this anastomosis; if the surgeon prefers, a short (5- to 10-min) second period of HCA may be used. With completion of this final anastomosis, active rewarming is initiated. Meticulous inspection of all suture lines is undertaken, placing individual sutures to secure any bleeding points. De-airing is performed in the surgeon's usual fashion, keeping the patient in steep Trendelenburg position until no visible air is recovered and TEE shows no further intracardiac or intraaortic air. Defibrillation is performed when appropriate temperatures are reached and the patient separated from CPB in the usual fashion. The completed repair is shown in Figure 34-5E.

New Approaches

Despite the numerous alternatives available for arch reconstruction, there still remains risk of neurologic compromise, resulting from HCA, embolization of air or particulate matter, or surgical misadventure. In addition to these risks, there still remain risks associated with CPB, median sternotomy, and open surgical procedures. The development of intravascular stenting technology in the coronary and peripheral circulations was stimulated, in part, to avoid exposing patients to the risks involved with open revascularization procedures, as well as to make the repairs of vascular diseases a more readily acceptable therapy. Stenting technology has been well developed in the treatment of abdominal aortic conditions and is now being attempted in a variety of thoracic aortic pathologies.[16,17] The application of stent therapies to aortic arch aneurysms has been limited by the necessity of maintaining perfusion to the arch vessels; alignment of holed stents has been too imprecise to reliably use in a clinical situation, and sidearm stent graft technology is not yet available for use. Thoracic stent graft treatments for the aortic arch have been described, but these efforts have been limited to the distal arch or combined with traditional arch reconstructions using CPB and HCA.[18–20] These limitations have not halted the development of alternative surgical approaches to the treatment of arch aneurysms, however, and the use of combined open and percutaneous therapies may represent an alternative approach to the patient thought too high risk for the use of conventional arch reconstruction.

A combined technique approach to the patient with arch aneurysm was recently performed at our institution by the thoracic and vascular surgery services, following the initial report by Kato and colleagues.[21] The patient presented with the arch aneurysm seen in CT scans depicted in Figure 34-6A and B. Initially, the patient underwent a translocation of the arch vessels to a graft arising from the ascending aorta. This procedure was performed via a median sternotomy, but CPB was not

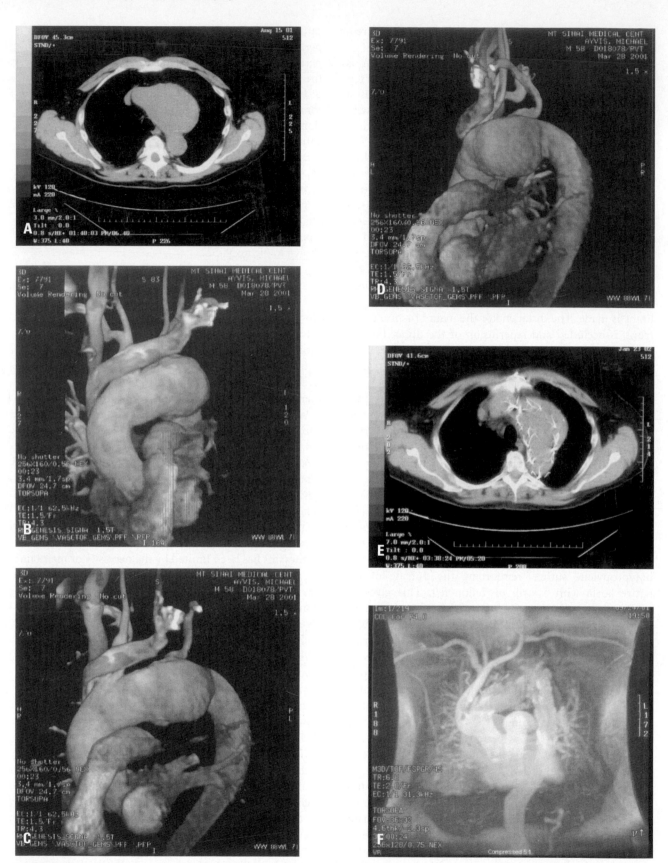

FIGURE 34-6. *A*, CT scan of aortic arch aneurysm, extending over the entire length of the arch. *B* to *D*, Three-dimensional CT scan of aneurysm imaged in *A*, in rotational projections. Note the detailed anatomic relationships between intrathoracic structures. *E*, CT scan of stented arch aneurysm, following translocation of the arch vessels. *F*, Three-dimensional scan of completed, off-pump arch aneurysm repair. The translocated arch vessels' graft is seen arising from the right lateral aspect of the ascending aorta, and the arch stents are seen across the aneurysm.

required. After the proximal anastomosis was created at the ascending aorta, each arch vessel was grafted sequentially. This allowed continuous perfusion of the head and upper body, obviating the need for circulatory arrest. The stumps of the transected arteries were oversewn, effectively denuding the top of the arch of all its vessels. After the arch vessels had been effectively translocated to the side of the ascending aorta, a coated stent graft was positioned across the arch aneurysm via a sidearm graft previously sutured to the ascending aortic graft. The stent was anchored, the guide withdrawn, and the sidearm suture ligated. The patient was closed in routine fashion and initially had an uneventful recovery. Reexploration on postoperative day 1 was required for bleeding from the graft to aorta suture site but he otherwise did well, being discharged on postoperative day 7 with normal neurologic function. The postreconstruction images are displayed in Figure 34-6C to E.

Although the patient still required an open procedure to address his arch aneurysm, the need for CPB and HCA was avoided. The ability to treat all arch aneurysms awaits the development of newer technology stents and techniques that enable stenting of the arch vessels as well. Although currently in development, these technologies are not yet available for clinical application. Additionally, the observation of late endoleaks in the abdominal and early thoracic experiences has given investigators pause before entering newer and potentially more dangerous applications. It is likely, however, that the development of the necessary devices and skills for percutaneous repair of arch aneurysms is but several years away and offers the promise of less invasive and risky treatments for these conditions.

New Diagnostics

Although the development of new surgical approaches to the treatment of aortic arch aneurysms is of great interest, stimulating aggressive new procedures and techniques by both thoracic and vascular surgeons, interventional radiologists, and interventional cardiologists, the need for earlier and more readily accessible diagnostic modalities has also been noted. By treating the arch aneurysm before complications related to its size (airway compromise, recurrent laryngeal nerve involvement, dysphagia and weight loss, etc) arise, the prognosis for recovery and quality of life is, theoretically, improved. Because many arch aneurysms are only discovered incidentally or when symptoms related to aneurysm size manifest themselves, the need for earlier diagnosis is self-evident.

Among the primary diagnostic techniques used for thoracic aortic disease is CT scanning.[22] The rapid development of CT scanning over the past two to three decades has allowed imaging such as that seen earlier in Figures 34-1A, 34-2A, and 34-6A and E to be available in virtually every hospital. As sophistication of the techniques increased and enhanced computing power became avail-

able, more-detailed images became available, similar to those seen in Figure 34-6B to D. The ability to isolate structures, rotate the images, and project them in various planes, gives the surgeon a greater appreciation of the interrelationships of the adjacent structures and allows the surgeon to structure the surgical approach accordingly. This potentially offers the ability to avoid complications arising from unknown anatomic relationships, improving the patient's chances for an uneventful procedure. The cost of the ability to make these advanced images is more powerful and rapid CT scanners and their associated computing stations, as well as the software capable of rendering these projections. The amount of computer time necessary for the projection of these images is also increased but is partially offset by the power of the newer computers. These advanced devices, however, require a greater capital investment by the hospital/radiology unit, which can only be made up by increasing either costs to the patient or the number of patients imaged. The increased awareness by primary caregivers of thoracic aneurysm disease has led, in major medical centers, to the more aggressive use of CT scanning for symptoms suggestive of aneurysm disease, resulting in holding down patient cost for these more current imaging techniques.

In parallel with the advances in CT scanning, MRI has developed alternative methods for imaging the thoracic aorta. This particular imaging technique is especially useful for those patients in whom significant allergies to the intravenous contrast material used in CT scanning exist, or for those patients in whom renal function is compromised. The ability of the MRI and MRA (angiography) scans to isolate, highlight, and variably project structural images has proven to be very useful in dissecting, radiographically, vascular structures and their intrathoracic relationships. This has proved especially useful in evaluation of intravascular structures, as in dissection disease, but also provides very detailed and striking images to evaluate the success of one's procedures (see Figure 34-6E). The use of color highlights to further augment projection of the desired structures adds an even greater clarity to the studied structures (Figure 34-7).

Use of MRI/MRA and/or high-speed CT scanning has all but obviated the need for angiography, by enabling the physician to assess the intrathoracic aorta without the need for intraarterial diagnostics. Still, the need to transport patients to radiologic suites, the exposure to ionizing radiation, patient discomfort with confined MRI chambers, and remuneration issues have stimulated efforts to develop yet other diagnostic tests. Familiarity of many internist, cardiologists, and emergency room doctors with echocardiography and sonography, as well as the accessibility of the equipment, offered the promise of easy, noninvasive arch aneurysm diagnosis. While the promise of echocardiography held much hope, its use for evaluation of the aortic arch has been less forthcoming, primarily because much of the aortic arch exists in an acoustic dead

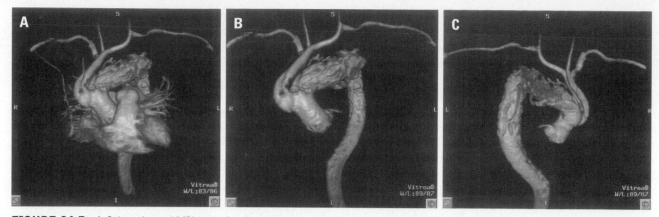

FIGURE 34-7. *A,* Color-enhanced MRI scan of arch stent repair shown in Figure 34-6. Note placement of arch stent immediately distad to the translocated arch vessels' graft and the relationships of intrathoracic structures. *B,* Subtraction, color-enhanced MRI scan shown in *A,* with heart, pulmonary artery (PA), and lungs removed. *C,* Aortic image of *B* rotated 180 degrees.

space created by the air column of the trachea. This air window interferes with the visualization of much of the aortic arch, limiting the usefulness of this technique for surgical analysis and planning. TEE is, however, a useful adjunct to fluoroscopy during distal arch and thoracic stent graft placement.[23]

Surgical Results

Patients undergoing repair of arch aneurysms may expect good outcomes with acceptable rates of postoperative complications. The reported results vary, as might be expected, with the institution reporting, the techniques employed, the experience of the surgeons involved, and the long-term follow-up. In a recent review of aortic arch surgery, Griepp and Ergin summarized their institution's experience over a 10-year period (1985 to 1995) in 427 patients.[2] Overall mortality was 11.3%, but a marked difference was discovered when comparing the early half of their experience to the later half (16% versus 7%). The incidence of neurologic dysfunction was similar between the two groups, however, with 10% of the former and 8% of the more recent patients sustaining stroke or other permanent neurologic dysfunction. Hagl and colleagues updated this institution's data by examining 717 patients undergoing ascending aorta–aortic arch reconstructions requiring HCA.[24] Mortality over the 15-year period reported by Hagl and colleagues was 10%, and permanent stroke was observed in 5.7% of the patients. An additional 3.3% of the patients sustained a transient stroke, defined as stroke characteristics that resolved prior to discharge from the hospital.

In other large series, investigators have reported similar results.[25–30] Svensson and colleagues observed a 10% mortality in 656 patients undergoing arch replacement, with a stroke rate of 7%.[25] Crawford and colleagues had earlier reported a mortality of 9% in a large series of 717 patients, but these included both aneurysm and dissec-

tion patients.[26] Similarly, Coselli and colleagues showed an early mortality of 6% and a late mortality of 9% in 227 patients, but only a 3% stroke rate.[27] Laas and colleagues reported a somewhat higher mortality of 14%, with a stroke rate (9%) comparable to these other groups.[28] In examining the results he obtained by using retrograde cerebral perfusion and HCA, Ueda found a hospital mortality of 12% and a late mortality of 16% in his cohort of 207 patients, and Kawahito and colleagues, who used antegrade selective cerebral perfusion in a series of 99 patients, reported 11% hospital mortality.[29]

Summary

The development of techniques and protocols for the surgical management of aortic arch aneurysms has both progressed tremendously over the past 25 years as well as highlighted many areas in which our management of these patients' conditions can yet be improved. The increasing awareness of primary care practitioners of the presence and natural history of arch aneurysm disease, coupled with their readiness to use the generation of new diagnostic modalities, makes early diagnosis of arch aneurysm a more common occurrence. The possibility of earlier, safer intervention can be offered to these patients, using a variety of surgical repairs, most of which are familiar to the active cardiac surgeon. Development of better neurologic protection strategies offers the promise of lessened risk for stroke or transient neurologic dysfunction, although much work remains to be done in this area. Still ahead is the promise of percutaneous therapies, via endovascular techniques, of complete arch aneurysm repair without the need for HCA, CPB, or possibly even sternotomy. Although, in select cases, complete off-pump reconstruction of arch aneurysms (using combined therapies) may be considered and safely performed, the extent of the aneurysm frequently dictates the amount of resection/repair required. Until stent technology improves tremendously, the lure of percutaneous treatment of these conditions will remain an elusive goal. As many patients will not have the luxury of waiting until these therapies of the future are available, the surgeon should become familiar with the available options and knowledgeable in their safe application.

References

1. Westaby S. Landmarks in cardiac surgery. Oxford: Isis Medical Media Ltd; 1997. p. 223–52.

2. Griepp RB, Ergin MA. Aneurysms of the aortic arch. In: Edmunds LH Jr, editor. Cardiac surgery in the adult. New York: McGraw-Hill; 1997. p 1197–226.

3. Lansman SL, Griepp RB. Resection of aortic arch aneurysms using hypothermic circulatory arrest. In: Kaiser LR, Kron IL, Spray TL, editors. Mastery of cardiothoracic surgery. Philadelphia: Lippincott-Raven; 1998. p. 472–78.

4. Griepp RB, Stinson EB, Hollingsworth JF, Buehler D. Prosthetic replacement of the aortic arch. J Thorac Cardiovasc Surg 1975;70:1051–63.

5. Borst HG, Walterbusch G, Schaps D. Extensive aortic replacement using "elephant trunk" prosthesis. Thorac Cardiovasc Surg 1983;31:37–40.

6. Bentall H, DeBono A. A technique for complete replacement of the ascending aorta. Thorax 1968;23:338–9.

7. Kouchoukos NT, Marshall WG, Wedigie-Strecher T. Eleven-year experience with composite graft replacement of the ascending aorta and aortic valve. J Thorac Cardiovasc Surg 1986;42:691–705.

8. Cabrol C, Pavie A, Gandjabakhch I, et al. Complete replacement of the ascending aorta with reimplantation of the coronary arteries. J Thorac Cardiovasc Surg 1981;81:309–15.

9. David TE. Aortic valve-sparing operations for aortic root aneurysm. Semin Thorac Cardiovasc Surg 2001;13:291–6.

10. Sommerville J, Ross D. Homograft replacement of aortic root with reimplantation of coronary arteries. Br Heart J 1982;47:473–82.

11. Ergin MA, Griepp EB, Lansman SL, et al. Hypothermic circulatory arrest and other methods of cerebral protection during operations of the thoracic aorta. J Card Surg 1994;9:525–37.

12. Kouchoukos NT, Masetti P, Rokkas CK, Murphy SF. Single-stage reoperative repair of chronic type A aortic dissection by means of the arch-first technique. J Thorac Cardiovasc Surg 2001;122:578–82.

13. Kazui T, Washiyama N, Muhammad BAH, et al. Total arch replacement using aortic arch branched grafts with the aid of antegrade selective cerebral perfusion. Ann Thorac Surg 2000;70:3–9.

14. Kuki S, Taniguchi K, Masai T, Endo S. A novel modification of elephant trunk technique using a single four-branched arch graft for extensive thoracic aortic aneurysm. Eur J Cardiothorac Surg 2000;18:246–8.

15. Spielvogel D, Griepp RB. Aortic arch aneurysm. In: Yang SC, Cameron D, editors. Current therapy in thoracic and cardiovascular surgery. Orlando, FL: Harcourt; [In press].

16. Dake MD, Miller DC, Semba CP, et al. Transluminal placement of endovascular stent-grafts for the treatment of descending thoracic aortic aneurysms. N Engl J Med 1994;331:1729–34.

17. Dake MD. Endovascular stent-graft management of thoracic aortic diseases. Eur J Radiol 2001;39:42–9.

18. Miyairi T, Kotsuka Y, Morota T, et al. Paraplegia after open surgery using endovascular stent graft for aortic arch aneurysm. J Thorac Cardiovasc Surg 2001;122:1240–3.

19. Burks JA Jr, Faries PL, Gravereaux EC, et al. Endovascular repair of thoracic aortic aneurysms: stent-graft fixation across the aortic arch vessels. Ann Vasc Surg 2002;16:24–8.

20. Suzuki T, Shimono T, Kato N, et al. Extended total arch replacement by means of the open stent-grafting method to treat intimal tears after transluminal stent-graft placement for a ruptured acute type B aortic dissection. J Thorac Cardiovasc Surg 2002;123:354–6.

21. Kato M, Kaneko M, Kuratani T, et al. New operative method for distal aortic arch aneurysm: combined cervical branch bypass and endovascular stent-graft implantation. J Thorac Cardiovasc Surg 1999;117:832–4.

22. Adachi H, Nagai J. Three-dimensional CT angiography. Boston: Little, Brown; 1995.

23. Moskowitz DM, Kahn RA, Konstadt SN, et al. Intraoperative transoesophageal echocardiography as an adjuvant to fluoroscopy during endovascular thoracic aortic repair. Eur J Vasc Endovasc Surg 1999;17:22–7.

24. Hagl C, Ergin MA, Galla JD, et al. Neurological outcome after ascending aorta–aortic arch operations: effect of brain protection technique in high-risk patients. J Thorac Cardiovasc Surg 2001;121:1107–21.

25. Svensson LG, Crawford ES, Hess KR, et al. Deep hypothermia with circulatory arrest: determinants of stroke and early mortality in 656 patients. J Thorac Cardiovasc Surg 1993;106:19–28.

26. Crawford ES, Svensson LG, Coselli JS, et al. Surgical treatment of aneurysm and/or dissection of the ascending aorta, transverse aortic arch, and ascending aorta and transverse aortic arch. Factors influencing survival in 717 patients. J Thorac Cardiovasc Surg 1989;98:659–73.

27. Coselli JS, Bueket S, Djukanovic B. Aortic arch surgery: current treatment and results. Ann Thorac Surg 1995;59:19–26.

28. Laas J, Jurmann MJ, Heinemann M, Borst HG. Advances in aortic arch surgery. Ann Thorac Surg 1992;53:227–32.

29. Ueda Y. Retrograde cerebral perfusion with hypothermic circulatory arrest in aortic arch surgery: operative and long-term results. Nagoya J Med Sci 2001;64:93–102.

30. Kawahito K, Adachi H, Yamagucki A, Ino T. Long-term surgical outcomes of aortic arch aneurysm. Kyobu Geka 2002;55:305–8.

CHAPTER 35

STRATEGIES FOR AORTIC ARCH RECONSTRUCTION WITHOUT CIRCULATORY ARREST

SANJIV K. GANDHI, MD, FRANK A. PIGULA, MD

The use of deep hypothermic circulatory arrest (DHCA) has played an important role in developing successful repair techniques for the surgical treatment of both congenital and acquired diseases of the aortic arch. It has the virtue of simplicity, permitting an operative field free of blood and cannulae. It is based on the fundamental concepts that interruption of the cerebral circulation with complete recovery of neurologic function is possible and that brain metabolic rate decreases with temperature. However, in recent years, there has been a trend away from the routine employment of DHCA because of the awareness of potential adverse neurologic outcomes associated with its use.

The search for alternatives has resulted in techniques whereby aortic arch surgery is performed during continuous, or near continuous, circulatory support of the brain. The role of cerebral perfusion techniques is twofold: to avoid the neurologic injury that contributes to morbidity and mortality and to extend the surgeon's capability to treat complex aortic arch pathology.

Although a variety of techniques have been developed, there are only two basic ways to provide circulatory support to the brain during aortic arch surgery: antegrade cerebral perfusion (ACP) and retrograde cerebral perfusion (RCP). This chapter focuses on these techniques and current clinical experience, and reviews the evidence supporting their continued use in both the pediatric and adult cardiac surgical population.

Hypothermia

Hypothermia remains our most effective means of neuroprotection, and, as such, is an essential component to any neuroprotective strategy. By virtue of its ability to reduce ischemic injury, hypothermia has become an indispensable adjunct to the practice of cardiac surgery. Its effectiveness stems from a reduction in the rate of cellular enzymatic reactions, delaying the depletion of energy substrates that lead to a breakdown in cellular homeostasis and organ injury. However, even though hypothermia reduces metabolic activity, it is not abolished, and rewarming occurs as the result of continued metabolic activity. Even with meticulous attention to cooling and warming techniques, in addition to careful monitoring, durations of DHCA exceeding 25 min produce detrimental neurologic outcomes.[1] Various metabolic studies in animals and human beings suggest that cerebral metabolic suppression at clinical levels of deep hypothermia is less complete than had been assumed previously.[2] Thus, a combined strategy of reducing cerebral metabolic demands with hypothermia while providing some degree of cerebral circulatory support is inherently attractive. However, the metabolic needs of the brain during hypothermia remain ill defined and the best technique for providing circulatory support remains unclear.

Antegrade Cerebral Perfusion

Background

Selective ACP has a sound physiologic basis, especially in systems that take advantage of autoregulation of the cerebral blood flow. For the reasons cited above, hypothermia increases the safety margin of the method by reducing the metabolic needs. The combination of selective ACP and hypothermia has been very effective in providing cerebral protection in both laboratory studies and in clinical practice. The supply of nutrients and oxygen at a relatively low flow allows maintenance of appropriate levels of oxygen metabolism at hypothermic temperatures. Crittenden and colleagues exhibited the advantages of ACP over any alternative cerebral protection method, demonstrating the preservation of intracellular pH and energy stores in an experimental model.[3] Sakurada and associates used somatosensory evoked potentials as a monitor of cerebral function and demonstrated ACP at 20°C to be a more protective perfusion modality of the brain than either DHCA or RCP.[4]

The conceptual attractiveness of ACP is not without disadvantage. To perfuse the brain evenly in the face of unknown cerebral vascular anatomy, multiple cannulae are required for multiple arch branches. Multiple cannulations inhibit exposure and may increase the risk of manipulation-related embolization. The potential for hypoperfusion or hyperperfusion exists with any antegrade cerebral perfusion system. At the present time, prevention of perfusion mismatch can be best achieved by continuous monitoring of jugular venous bulb O_2 saturations or use of near-infrared spectroscopy (NIS, see below).

Surgical Techniques and Clinical Experience

With the technique of ACP, some or all of the cerebral vessels are perfused throughout the duration of systemic circulatory arrest. The technique permits numerous variations in implementation. Frist and colleagues, guided by preoperative evaluation of the patency of the circle of Willis, selectively perfused only the innominate artery.[5] Others have employed axillary artery cannulation, either directly or through a graft anastomosed to it.[6] These systems rely on autoregulation of cerebral blood flow. The pump flow rate is determined by the blood pressure in the right radial artery.

Matsuda and associates reported a system of perfusing both the innominate and left carotid arteries via separate pumps and with fixed predetermined flows at 16° to 20°C.[7] Bachet and colleagues employed two pumps and two heat exchangers to perfuse the brain through the innominate and left carotid arteries at 6° to 10°C with low flow and the remainder of the body at 28°C.[8]

Others have described excising the cerebral vessels on an island of native arch, subsequently performing a rapid anastomosis of the arch cap to an appropriately fashioned graft.[9] Flow is re-established via the graft to all three arch branches with the perfusate temperature at 10°C. The flow rate is adjusted to establish a perfusion pressure of 50 mm Hg in the right radial artery. Sites of direct arterial cannulation have also been guided by the use of computed tomography, magnetic resonance imaging, and epiaortic and transesophageal echocardiography to identify potentially embolic material in strategic areas of the aorta.

Optimal implementation demands that all cerebral vessels be perfused with monitoring of pressure and flows. This increases the technical complexity of initiating ACP. In addition, there is the potential disadvantage of manipulation of the cerebral vessels with the attendant risk of dislodging atherosclerotic debris. For operations that require a cerebral protection period of 90 min, ACP is physiologically superior to DHCA and RCP because it supplies sufficient oxygenated blood to the brain in an antegrade direction and can be used to protect the brain for an unlimited period of time.[10]

Several large series exist of patients undergoing aortic reconstructive surgery using ACP. Improved neurologic function and a decrease in mortality rates compared with patients reconstructed with other perfusion techniques have been documented.[11,12] Kazui and colleagues recently reported their experience with ACP in 50 adults undergoing arch replacement for atherosclerotic aneurysms. They reported a perioperative mortality of 2%. Postoperative temporary and permanent neurologic dysfunction was 4% each. The mean ACP time was 78 min. While these authors do not specify ACP pressures or flows, their results compare favorably to other series in which DHCA, with or without RCP, was employed.[1,13]

Antegrade Cerebral Perfusion in the Pediatric Patient: Regional Low-Flow Perfusion

Background

Aortic arch hypoplasia is a common constituent of congenital heart disease. Because of anatomic constraints, repair is most commonly performed during a period of DHCA. Although low-flow cardiopulmonary bypass is a well-described and accepted technique for the repair of many congenital heart defects, it is not routinely applied to neonates requiring aortic arch reconstruction. Anatomically, the diminutive aorta is too small to cannulate and, technically, a bloodless operative field is required for precise anatomic reconstruction. However, evidence of overt brain injury may be found in up to 10% of pediatric patients exposed to DHCA; subtle but detectable neuropsychiatric defects may be identified in up to 50%.[14,15] Thus, the same arguments supporting alternatives to DHCA in adults also apply to the pediatric population. A technique of regional low-flow perfusion (RLFP), an extension of selective antegrade cerebral perfusion as performed during aortic surgery in adults, provides both cerebral and somatic circulatory support of the neonate requiring arch reconstruction while providing the same bloodless exposure enjoyed during DHCA.

Surgical Technique

Several methods of providing cerebral circulatory support in the neonate undergoing arch surgery have been devised. While these procedures may be complicated by the small size of the neonatal vasculature, they are free from the encumbrance of brittle and atherosclerotic vessels found in the adult.

A variety of techniques have been devised and their use can be tailored to the unique anatomic requirements of the case.[16–18] These variations include:

- Direct cannulation of the ascending aorta with advancement of the cannula into the innominate artery (Figure 35-1).

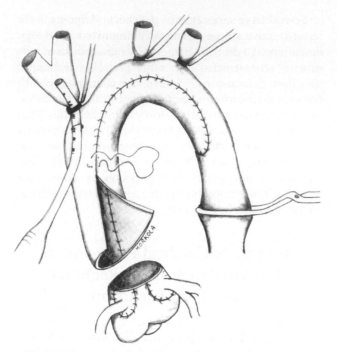

FIGURE 35-1. The right side of the ascending aorta is cannulated 5 mm proximal to the innominate artery. The arterial cannula is advanced into the innominate artery and snared into place. A clamp is placed on the descending thoracic aorta, and the left subclavian and carotid arteries are snared while continuous low-flow cerebral perfusion is maintained through the innominate artery. Reproduced with permission from Tchervenkov CI et al.[18]

- Cannulation of the pulmonary artery confluence perfusing a completed Blalock-Taussig (BT) shunt after division of the main pulmonary artery and obtaining control of the distal pulmonary branches (Figure 35-2).
- Cannulation of the proximal aorta with vascular isolation of the distal arch (Figure 35-3).
- Perfusion of the innominate artery through an arterial cannula attached to the open end of a modified BT shunt following construction of the proximal anastomosis (Figure 35-4).

We employ the last technique, a modification of the technique originally described by Asou and associates.[16] Initially used in single-ventricle palliation in neonates undergoing the Norwood operation for variations of hypoplastic left-heart syndrome, the BT shunt is used as a perfusion conduit such that access to the cerebral circulation is provided via the shunt, innominate, and right common carotid arteries. With control of the brachiocephalic vessels and the descending aorta, RLFP may be delivered during construction of the neoaorta, while exposure and visualization are identical to that achieved during DHCA. RLFP is initiated at 5 mL/kg/min and gradually increased until cerebral blood volume (described below) has reached precirculatory-arrest levels. A small metal-tipped bullet suction device placed through the atrial appendage scavenges venous blood returning to the heart. Systemic temperature is maintained at 18°C during the period of RLFP.

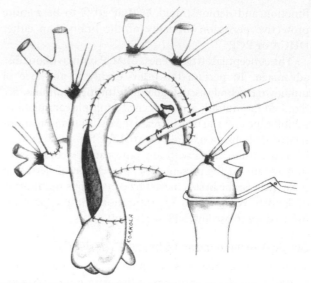

FIGURE 35-2. A modified Blalock-Taussig shunt is fully constructed before cannulation for cardiopulmonary bypass. The arterial cannula is advanced into the pulmonary artery confluence through the patent ductus arteriosus, and low-flow cerebral perfusion is maintained by retrograde flow through the shunt into the innominate artery, with the branch pulmonary arteries snared. Snares on the arch vessels and on the descending thoracic aorta permit reconstruction of the arch. Reproduced with permission from Tchervenkov CI et al.[18]

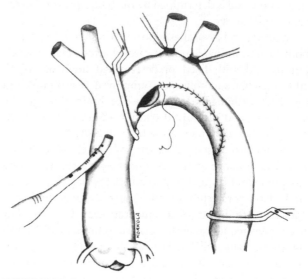

FIGURE 35-3. The distal aortic arch is isolated by applying a clamp just distal to the innominate artery, a second clamp to the descending thoracic aorta, and snaring of the left carotid and left subclavian arteries. While cerebral perfusion is maintained through the ascending aorta into the innominate artery, the aortic arch is reconstructed. Reproduced with permission from Tchervenkov CI et al.[18]

This technique has been modified for use in children with arch pathology undergoing biventricular repair (Figure 35-5).[19] In these situations, the innominate artery, either directly or via a 3.5 mm Gore-Tex graft sewn to it, serves as the sole cannulation site. Upon completion of the repair, the graft, if used, is clipped flush with the innominate artery and oversewn.

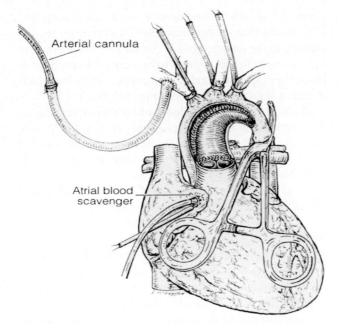

FIGURE 35-4. Arterial inflow is through the cannulated shunt after the anastomosis to the innominate artery is performed. Exposure is maintained by the brachiocephalic snares, a clamp on the descending aorta, and the right atrial blood scavenger. Reproduced with permission from Pigula FA et al.[19]

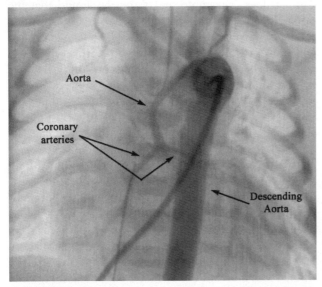

FIGURE 35-5. Hypoplastic ascending aorta in a case of aortic atresia with a normal left ventricle. This patient underwent biventricular repair using RLFP.

Clinical Methodology

NEAR-INFRARED SPECTROSCOPY (NIS)

Control of cerebral circulatory support being a central tenet to any alternative perfusion technique makes a review of the methodology relevant. NIS is a noninvasive method for monitoring the changes of tissue chromophores, namely, oxyhemoglobin and deoxyhemoglobin. NIS exploits unique characteristics of light in the near-infrared spectrum (600 to 1000 nm).[20] Because light of this wavelength can penetrate tissues up to a depth of 6 cm, noninvasive measurements of subsurface tissues, such as the brain and skeletal muscle, is possible.[21,22] Because oxyhemoglobin and deoxyhemoglobin demonstrate well-defined absorption peaks at 929 and 758 nm, respectively, they lend themselves to measurement by using NIS. Summation of these compounds provides an indication of total blood volume. These measurements are, for practical purposes, qualitative. Absolute concentrations of oxyhemoglobin and deoxyhemoglobin are available only if one knows the optical pathlength of the NIS signal within the tissue.[22,23] Because the optical pathlength is dependent upon factors such as skull geometry, interoptode distance, and tissue scatter, absolute concentrations are difficult to obtain. However, for any particular patient, the optical pathlength should remain constant; thus, trend data and relative changes in these compounds should be obtainable and accurate. Monitoring these trends and changes in oxyhemoglobin and deoxyhemoglobin has been found to be clinically useful in a variety of situations.

NIS also has the potential to detect changes in the concentration of oxidized cytochrome aa_3.[24] This compound, representing the last link in the chain of enzymes responsible for cellular aerobic metabolism, is thought to reflect the adequacy of intracellular oxygenation. Although this information is of great interest, measurement of oxidized aa_3 requires complicated algorithms and the use of multiple wavelengths.[25] Because of this, the accuracy of oxidized aa_3 in the clinical setting remains uncertain.[26]

In a recent review, Nollert and associates described the use of NIS in both adult and pediatric cardiovascular surgery patients.[27] In adult patients, brain oxygenation was maintained with mean perfusion pressures of 60 mm Hg.[28] Yao and associates found that cerebral desaturations were associated with prolonged intensive care unit and hospital stay.[29] Furthermore, cerebral saturations less than 40% were associated with frontal lobe dysfunction.

The first description of NIS in pediatric patients was provided by Greeley and associates in 1991.[30] At the Children's Hospital of Pittsburgh, validation studies have been done correlating the jugular bulb saturations with NIS cerebral oxygen saturations, with adjustment of the instrumentation and algorithms appropriate for the pediatric patient. Similar techniques have been used to validate NIS data during hypothermic cardiopulmonary bypass in pediatric patients. To date, no studies establishing safe cerebral saturation criteria have been performed in the pediatric population undergoing cardiac surgery.

NIS has also been applied to measurement of oxygen saturation in human skeletal muscle.[31] Edwards and associates reported a good correlation between NIS and venous occlusion plethysmography in the human forearm.[32] Segal and associates reported the use of NIS on upper extremities to document the effectiveness of sympathectomy on limb blood flow.[33] Others have turned to

NIS as a noninvasive method of assessing the severity of lower-limb ischemia in patients suffering from peripheral vascular disease. Kooijman and associates reported that NIS was an effective noninvasive method for assessing the oxygen debt in the lower extremities of patients suffering from peripheral vascular disease.[34] Komimaya and associates suggested that NIS graded the severity of intermittent claudication in diabetics more accurately than did the ankle:brachial index.[35]

To validate this application of NIS, Tran and associates performed a comparative analysis of nuclear magnetic resonance (NMR) and NIS measurements of intracellular P_{O_2} in human skeletal muscle, and reported that the NIS signals closely match the desaturation kinetics of myoglobin.[36] They concluded that skeletal muscle NIS largely reflects the change in oxyhemoglobin and deoxymyoglobin, rather than hemoglobin. This conclusion would do little to alter the interpretation of limb ischemia. Indeed, an assessment of tissue, rather than hemoglobin oxygenation, would provide a superior assessment of the adequacy of blood flow.

GASTRIC TONOMETRY

The mechanism of gastric tonometry is to measure the partial pressure of CO_2 in the gastrointestinal mucosa via a nasogastric probe tipped with a CO_2-permeable balloon. Because of its physiologic properties, CO_2 is readily diffusible through most tissues.[37,38]

In the standard technique, saline is injected into the balloon and CO_2 is allowed to equilibrate. It is then measured, using a standard blood gas analyzer. Using this technique, Casado-Flores and associates have reported that gastric mucosal pH is of prognostic value in critically ill children.[39] However, saline tonometry is hampered by significant disadvantages, including long equilibration times, contamination of the saline with air, and the stability of CO_2 in saline. Because of this, air has been substituted for saline as the balloon medium, a technique known as gas tonometry. Comparative studies between saline and gas techniques demonstrate shorter equilibration times with less bias using gas tonometry and this has become the preferred technique.[40,41] Automated gas tonometry devices are now commercially available.

Regardless of the technique used, measurement of the gastric mucosal P_{CO_2} allows calculation of the gastric mucosal pH. However, several assumptions are implicit in this calculation and, during low-flow and no-flow states, discrepancies between the indirect measurement of gastric mucosal pH (tonometry) and the direct measurement (pH probe) have been identified.[42] Because of these discrepancies, the difference between the arterial P_{CO_2} and the measured gastric mucosal P_{CO_2}, the P_{CO_2} gap, has also been used as an indicator of gastric mucosal ischemia. An increase in gastric mucosal P_{CO_2}, relative to the arterial P_{CO_2}, may indicate separate but related pathophysiologic processes: CO_2 accumulation as a consequence of impaired blood flow or as a result of increased CO_2 production under anaerobic conditions.[43] Studies examining the linkage between blood flow reduction and P_{CO_2} show that there appears to be a critical lower limit of blood flow (approximately a 60% reduction) below which there is a sudden rise in gastric mucosal P_{CO_2}.[43]

While uncertainty remains about which measurement, P_{CO_2} gap versus calculated mucosal pH, is a more sensitive indicator of mucosal ischemia, experimental evidence supports the use of the P_{CO_2} gap, and this approach is probably more appropriate than the calculation of mucosal pH under conditions of low-flow bypass and circulatory arrest.[44–46]

Experimental Studies

The blood flow requirements of the human brain during hypothermia are unknown. Most of the available data on the physiologic requirements of the brain during hypothermia have been obtained from animal models and extrapolated to the human. Most of this data is consistent between experiments and suggests that brain blood flows somewhere between 10 and 30 mL/kg/min are the minimum requirement. In dogs, Nara and associates reported that flow rates as low as 30 mL/kg/min were able to maintain cerebral oxygenation for up to 120 min.[47] Also in dogs, Miyamoto and associates found that the optimal perfusion rate for the brain at 20°C was 30 mL/kg/min, with oxygen debt and anaerobic metabolism with flow rates below 15 mL/kg/min.[48] In sheep, Swain and associates have shown that flows as low as 10 mL/kg/min may allow the preservation of brain energy substrates.[49] Watanabe and associates found that aerobic metabolism was maintained at flows of 40 mL/kg/min at a pressure of 20 mm Hg.[50]

Besides relatively consistent results, these studies also demonstrated a similar methodology; all examined low-flow perfusion delivered in the ascending aorta via standard cannulation techniques. As such, the distribution of blood flow delivered to a specific organ is variable and related to the relative resistances of the vascular beds. This was also demonstrated by Watanabe and associates, as they reported that, at perfusion rates of 100 mL/kg/min, whole-brain blood flow was 14.2 ± 5.2 mL/kg/min, while kidney flow was 157 ± 114 mL/kg/min and jejunal flow was 63 ± 44 mL/kg/min.[50] Furthermore, these relationships remained stable, except at very low flow rates and perfusion pressures (less than 20 mL/kg/min and systemic blood pressure less than 16 mm Hg).

Thus, not only is the amount of flow delivered important, but the method of delivery is also crucial. Cerebral perfusion requirements during standard cardiopulmonary bypass may differ significantly from those during RLFP, when the brain is perfused in relative isolation. Furthermore, the impact of the least physiologic of all techniques, RCP, remains unclear. For these reasons, cerebral circulatory support remains an active area of clinical investigation.

Clinical Studies

CEREBRAL CIRCULATORY SUPPORT

Because of the sensitivity of the brain to both hypoperfusion and hyperperfusion, a means of evaluating and controlling cerebral blood flow is required. Because of the paucity of information in humans, NIS has been used to regulate flow rates by maintaining cerebral blood volumes at baseline levels (as measured on full-flow bypass). At the present time, most quantitative data have emerged from the pediatric population and are summarized below.

We studied cerebral blood flow requirements in 18 neonates undergoing aortic arch reconstruction by using NIS.[51] Single-ventricle repair was performed in 12 patients and biventricular repair was achieved in 6 patients. Data from these neonates were compared to six other neonates operated on by using DHCA during the same time period.

Operative survival for this cohort of patients was 89% (16/18). Mean duration of RLFP was 49 ± 11 min in the single-ventricle group and 60 ± 52 min in the biventricular group. There were no complications related to RLFP. With RLFP, a short period of DHCA is required for decannulations, recannulations, and atrial septectomy, when necessary. This time, however, is very brief and consistent (9 ± 4 min), and was significantly shorter than that required in control children. Furthermore, children undergoing DHCA demonstrated significantly greater falls in both relative cerebral blood volume (CrBVI) and relative cerebral oxygen saturation (CrSO$_2$) as compared to patients supported with RLFP.

Because cerebral perfusion requirements using RLFP were unknown, we incrementally increased the flow rate until baseline CrBVI (obtained on full-flow hypothermic cardiopulmonary bypass) was obtained. Reacquisition of baseline CrBVI consistently occurred with a RLFP rate of 20 mL/kg/min, and with the reacquisition of CrBVI, CrSO$_2$ was also restored to baseline (measured within 1.3 ± 4.1% and 5.0 ± 8.1%, respectively) (Figure 35-6). This

is in contrast to control children who demonstrated a prompt and predictable decline in both CrBVI and CrSO$_2$ (Figures 35-7 and 35-8).

Blood pressure was routinely measured via a left radial artery line. During the brief period of circulatory arrest required for atrial septectomy and recannulation, radial artery pressure was 0 mm Hg. With RLFP and the reacquisition of baseline CrBVI and CrSO$_2$, the left radial artery catheter measured an average of 22 mm Hg (16 to 28 mm Hg).

Because all flow provided by RLFP enters the innominate artery via the shunt, it is reasonable to assume that higher intracranial blood pressures are attainable with lower flows. In fact, at flow rates of 20 to 30 mL/kg/min, the left radial artery pressure averages 22 mm Hg, a pressure probably unobtainable if this flow were provided into the unrestricted aorta. However, while RLFP focuses circulatory support on the brain, it does not completely isolate the brain. In fact, because of the observation that significant backbleeding occurs from the descending aorta during RLFP, we hypothesized that significant subdiaphragmatic circulatory support was being provided as well.

SOMATIC CIRCULATORY SUPPORT

An unexpected but fortuitous benefit of RLFP in the neonate is its ability to provide subdiaphragmatic circulatory support. We tested this hypothesis in 15 consecutive neonates undergoing arch surgery.[52] Three patients

CIRCULATORY ARREST vs REGIONAL PERFUSION - CrSO$_2$

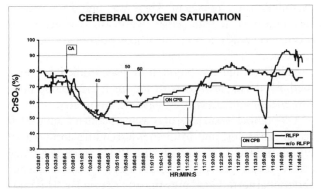

FIGURE 35-7. NIS depicts relative CrSO$_2$ in two infants. The first is a 3.1 kg 5-day-old infant who underwent a Norwood operation for hypoplastic left-heart syndrome (heavy line). The second neonate (thin line) is a 3.0 kg 2-day-old infant who underwent repair of total anomalous pulmonary venous return by using circulatory arrest. Although the rate of desaturation between the two patients is similar, the institution of RLFP restores CrSO$_2$ to baseline levels in patient 1. Sharp declines in CrSO$_2$ in patient 1 on RLFP at circulatory arrest (CA) and cardiopulmonary bypass (CPB) correlate with decannulation and atrial septectomy and with recannulation after reconstruction of the neoaorta. 40 = Initiation of RLFP at 40 mL/min; 50 = 50 mL/min; 60 = 60 mL/min. Reproduced with permission from Pigula FA et al.[19]

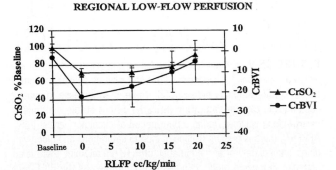

FIGURE 35-6. Relative cerebral blood volume index (CrBVI) and relative cerebral oxygen saturation (CrSO$_2$) as a function of RLFP rate. Reacquisition of baseline CrBVI occurs consistently at approximately 20 mL/kg/min, and is mirrored by return to baseline CrSO$_2$. Reproduced with permission from Pigula FA et al.[19]

CIRCULATORY ARREST vs REGIONAL PERFUSION - CrBVI

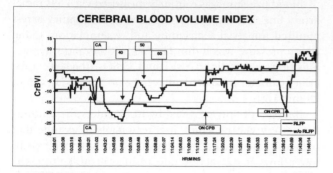

FIGURE 35-8. NIS depicts relative CrBVI in two infants. The first is a 3.1 kg 5-day-old infant who underwent a Norwood operation for hypoplastic left-heart syndrome (heavy line). The second neonate (thin line) is a 3.0 kg 2-day-old infant who underwent repair of total anomalous pulmonary venous return using circulatory arrest. RLFP restores relative CrBVI to near baseline levels in patient 1; CrBVI remains depressed in the neonate who underwent circulatory arrest. Sharp declines in CrBVI in patient 1 on RLFP at circulatory arrest (CA) and cardiopulmonary bypass (CPB) correlate with decannulation and atrial septectomy and with recannulation after reconstruction of the neoaorta. 40 = Initiation of RLFP at 40 mL/min; 50 = 50 mL/min; 60 = 60 mL/min. Reproduced with permission from Pigula FA et al.[19]

underwent biventricular repair and 12 underwent Norwood palliation. The mean circulatory arrest time for these patients was 12 ± 4 min, with a mean duration of RLFP of 53 ± 21 min. There were no observed neurologic sequelae and there were no incidences of renal or hepatic dysfunction in any patient. There was one death, occurring in a neonate with classic hypoplastic left heart syndrome secondary to uncontrollable pulmonary vascular resistance.

Subdiaphragmatic blood flow was studied by three methods during arch reconstruction: arterial blood pressure measurements, NIS, and gastric tonometry.

Differential blood pressures were obtained from the left radial artery line and from the descending aorta via an umbilical artery catheter. During RLFP, when left radial artery blood pressure was 22 mm Hg, simultaneous abdominal aortic blood pressure was 12 mm Hg. This finding explained the backbleeding from the descending aorta and suggested significant subdiaphragmatic perfusion during RLFP. Paired arterial blood gas data (obtained simultaneously from the radial and umbilical artery catheters) were comparable.

NIS quadriceps data were obtained for all 15 patients. Quadriceps blood volume (QrBVI) and quadriceps saturation (QrSO$_2$) were measured on full-flow hypothermic cardiopulmonary bypass, during the brief period of circulatory arrest required for atrial septectomy and shunt cannulation (for those children undergoing Norwood

operations), and during RLFP (Figure 35-9). NIS data showed a significant increase in both QrBVI and QrSO$_2$ in the quadriceps muscle during RLFP as compared to values obtained during the brief period of DHCA, approximating the values obtained on full-flow hypothermic cardiopulmonary bypass.

Because of the role that the gastrointestinal tract plays in the pathogenesis of the systemic inflammatory response, we thought it important to assess the impact of RLFP on splanchnic perfusion. To evaluate the degree of splanchnic flow, gastric tonometry was performed in nine neonates during RLFP and compared to three other infants undergoing ventricular septal defect (VSD) closure during DHCA (mean, 34 min). While the infants under-going VSD closure presented with a slightly negative PCO$_2$ gap (gastric mucosal PCO$_2$ exceeding arterial PCO$_2$), this may reflect their older age and chronic congestive heart failure. Nonetheless, gastric tonometry showed no significant differences in the PCO$_2$ gap before RLFP or DHCA (because arterial blood gases were unobtainable during DHCA, the PCO$_2$ gap was incalculable; thus, comparisons during RLFP and DHCA were impossible). There was, however, a significant gradient observed during rewarming. The children undergoing repair during DHCA demonstrated a PCO$_2$ gap of -3.3 ± 0.3 mm Hg, as compared to 7.8 ± 7.6 mm Hg in the neonates repaired during RLFP. Because CO$_2$ accumulation in the gastric mucosa is thought to result from inadequate blood flow or anaerobic conditions, these data

REGIONAL PERFUSION
QUADRICEPS DATA

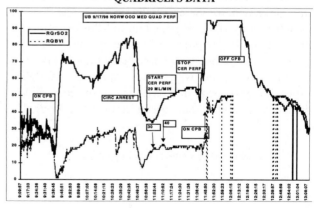

FIGURE 35-9. Quadriceps muscle NIS in a neonate undergoing the Norwood operation for hypoplastic left-heart syndrome. With the initiation of cardiopulmonary bypass (CPB), there is an increase in quadriceps muscle oxygen saturation (RQrSO$_2$) with a stable quadriceps muscle blood volume. During a brief period of circulatory arrest (CIRC ARREST), there is a sharp decline in muscle saturations and blood volumes. Immediately after the initiation of RLFP (20 mL/min), there is an increase in muscle blood volumes that continues as the RLFP rate increases to 30 and then to 40 cc/min. After approximately 5 min, there is a corresponding increase in muscle saturations. With completion of the aortic reconstruction, RLFP is stopped momentarily to allow for central cannulation and standard bypass is resumed. 30 = 30 mL/min; 40 = 40 mL/min. Reproduced with permission from Pigula FA et al.[52]

suggest that children repaired during DHCA experienced ischemia that neonates repaired during RLFP did not. These findings would suggest that the subdiaphragmatic perfusion supplied is physiologically significant.

Summary

Based on our clinical and experimental experience, it is our practice to provide RLFP when the expected circulatory arrest will be in excess of 20 min and when it can be provided without compromise of the surgical repair. To date, we have used RLFP in 40 neonates requiring aortic arch reconstruction. Thirty neonates have received single-ventricle palliation and 10 have received biventricular repairs. One-month and hospital discharge survival has been 73% (22/30) for single-ventricle palliation, predominately the Norwood operation for hypoplastic left-heart syndrome (HLHS), and 90% (9/10) for biventricular repair. These latter patients all had aortic arch hypoplasia or interruption as a component of their pathology. The single death in the biventricular group occurred in a 2 kg neonate with interrupted aortic arch and truncus arteriosus and severe truncal insufficiency. There have been no clinical neurologic complications noted in any patient in either group.

Antegrade cerebral perfusion is an effective means of providing cerebral circulatory support during aortic arch surgery. A variety of techniques have been developed to meet the specific anatomic needs of the patient. Clinical data suggest that this technique is able to provide cerebral and somatic circulatory support to the neonate during the most complex anatomic repairs, without sacrificing exposure. Without the neurologic morbidity related to long periods of DHCA, ACP may extend the capabilities of the surgeon when treating both acquired and congenital diseases of the aortic arch. Further investigation into the optimal deployment of these strategies, such as flow requirements at specific temperatures and the impact of cerebral autoregulatory mechanisms, remains to be pursued.

Retrograde Cerebral Perfusion

Background

The concept of RCP for cerebral protection originated in the treatment of massive air embolism during cardiopulmonary bypass.[53] Retrograde cerebral perfusion is commonly employed in adult thoracic aortic surgery as an adjunct to DHCA to enhance cerebral protection. The mechanisms whereby RCP may accomplish neuroprotection include:

- Delivering oxygen to the brain
- Providing cerebral metabolic support
- Expelling atheromatous and gaseous emboli from the cerebral vasculature
- Maintaining cerebral hypothermia

Surgical Technique

There is no uniformity in the literature regarding the optimal method for implementation of RCP regarding the mode of cannulation, perfusate temperature, and perfusion pressure. The cardiopulmonary bypass technique usually includes bicaval venous cannulation, with the arterial line containing Y-connectors with limbs to the venous line that may be clamped during antegrade cerebral flow (Figure 35-10). At the time of institution of RCP, the superior vena cava is snared, antegrade flow is terminated, the arterial cannula is clamped, and the limb connecting the arterial return line to the superior vena caval cannula is opened. Perfused blood is returned to the oxygenator via cardiotomy suction placed in the open thoracic aorta, the surgical field, and via the inferior vena cava cannula. Retrograde cerebral perfusion may be applied intermittently or continuously. Retrograde cerebral perfusion is generally carried out with monitoring of the venous pressure via either a central venous catheter in the superior vena cava or a jugular bulb catheter. Usually, flow is adjusted to maintain pressure in the range of 15 to 40 mm Hg.[1]

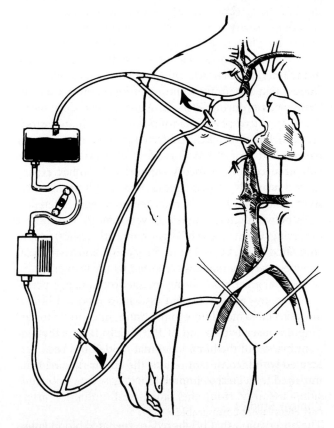

FIGURE 35-10. Retrograde cerebral perfusion circuit. A standard cardiopulmonary bypass circuit is established with bicaval and femoral arterial cannulation, with a bridging circuit established from the femoral arterial inflow arm onto the superior vena caval cannula, through which RCP can be established after the initiation of circulatory arrest. Reproduced with permission from Gardner TJ.[57]

Experimental Studies

The efficacy of cerebral perfusion during RCP has been monitored with a variety of modalities, including NIS, transcranial Doppler assessment of middle cerebral artery blood flow, and central retinal artery flow.[54–56] These and other methodologies suggest that RCP produces cerebral blood flow although they do not provide conclusive evidence that this blood flow is sufficient to support cerebral metabolism.[58–60] Various issues confound the interpretation of human investigations of RCP. The presence and competence of valves in the human internal jugular system are not constant.[61] Variability in cerebral venous anatomy amongst species also confuses the laboratory investigations of RCP. Numerous methods have been employed to assess cerebral blood flow in animals during RCP, including laser Doppler flowmetry and the hydrogen clearance method.[4,62] Capillary flow has also been assessed with the colored microsphere method and with radiolabeled macroaggregated albumin.[63] Overall intracranial flow is approximately 20 to 60% of values achieved during hypothermic cardiopulmonary bypass. Higher flows are limited by the potential for inducing cerebral edema. In a canine study, Oohara and associates reported that RCP, administered at 25 mm Hg, was able to provide about one-third of the cerebral blood flow achieved during full-flow cardiopulmonary bypass.[63] This is in contrast to a recent report by Ehrlich and associates of RCP in a porcine model.[60] They reported that 90% of RCP flow was shunted to the inferior vena cava. Other experimental studies also suggest that significant shunting of blood away from the brain occurs during RCP through venous collaterals.[64] Based on microsphere quantification, Ehrlich and associates concluded that RCP conferred little or no metabolic benefit and that the major effect of RCP was due to enhanced cooling, a theory supported by other experimental work.[60,65] Discrepancies may result from interspecies variation but important methodologic differences exist between these studies. If venovenous shunting is occurring, Oohara's use of larger microspheres (50 μm) as compared to Ehrlich's (15 μm) may contribute to the relatively greater cerebral flows reported by the former.

In a separate study using magnetic resonance perfusion imaging in pigs, Ye and associates reported little if any detectable blood flow to the brain, in contrast to cardiopulmonary bypass and ACP.[66] Finally, histopathologic examination of the brain in animal models has been performed with inconsistent results, the effects ranging from impaired to neutral to improved.[3,67,68]

Clinical Studies

The observation that bright red, oxygenated blood enters the superior vena cava during RCP, with dark, desaturated blood egressing from the brachiocephalic vessels, is undeniable. Exactly which tissues benefit from this support, and for how long, remains controversial. Some investigators suggest that while RCP reduces the risk of embolic stroke and may improve cooling of the brain, little metabolic support of the brain is provided.[69,70]

Despite the lack of convincing evidence that RCP yields a beneficial effect, many centers have adopted it. The relationship between the use of RCP and mortality rates is not entirely clear. RCP is a predictor of death in some investigations and not a predictor of death in others. When comparing RCP and DHCA, the results are also ambiguous. RCP has been found to be associated with comparable mortality rates by some investigators and with reduced mortality rates by other investigators.[13,71–73] In a retrospective review of 109 patients, Ehrlich and associates reported that patients receiving RCP had a lower mortality rate and a lower incidence of permanent neurologic complications than those repaired using DHCA.[74] The incidence of temporary neurologic dysfunction between the two groups was the same. In contrast, Ueda and associates reported the duration of RCP to be a risk factor for death among 249 patients undergoing arch surgery.[73] However, both of these studies suffer from the limitations imposed by the use of historic controls reviewed over many years.

The evidence examining the relationship between RCP and neurologic mortality is also mixed.[75–81] Several analyses of clinical results of RCP demonstrate that long durations of RCP are associated not only with high rates of temporary neurologic dysfunction but, in some studies, with an increased risk of stroke and death after aortic surgery. Safi and associates reported one of the largest series in adults undergoing repair of arch aneurysms.[79] They reported a 9.5% incidence of stroke in patients who did not receive RCP, as compared to a 1.1% incidence of stroke in patients who did ($p < .001$). In contrast, a direct comparison of RCP and DHCA by Usui and associates reported that the duration of DHCA with RCP to be the sole factor predictive of cerebral complications.[82] In the best approximation of a multiarmed trial comparing DHCA versus RCP versus ACP, Hagl and associates retrospectively reviewed 717 patients (588 DHCA, 43 RCP, 86 ACP) undergoing arch surgery.[83] The authors concluded that between cerebral protection times of 40 to 80 min the method of protection did not influence the incidence of stroke. However, ACP did significantly reduce the incidence of temporary neurologic dysfunction.

While even the ability of RCP to provide circulatory support to the brain remains at issue, an interesting report from Ono and associates suggests that RCP does provide support.[58] This group used retinal angiography and fluorescein dye administered via RCP as an indicator of brain perfusion in humans. They demonstrated fluorescein flow into the retinal veins, which progressed through the capillaries and arterioles. While the mean time between administration and retinal appearance of the fluorescein in these five patients was more than 5 min, this report does suggest some perfusion of the human central nervous system during RCP.

An assessment of cerebral metabolism, as approximated by the oxygen extraction ratio (OER), has been measured by several investigators. Cheung and associates found the OER to be increased at the onset of RCP in all patients, an effect that was less pronounced in patients who had sustained previous cerebrovascular events.[84] Cerebral oximetry has been found to be comparable between DHCA and RCP patients in some studies, and others have demonstrated a decrease in cerebral oximetry during the conduct of RCP. Several investigators have compared cerebral oxygen consumption during RCP with that measured during cardiopulmonary bypass.[63] The results of these studies support the notion that there is, in fact, oxygen consumption by tissues perfused during RCP. However, what proportion of the oxygen is consumed by cerebral tissues and whether these values are sufficient to support cellular metabolism remain unclear.

Pediatric Retrograde Cerebral Perfusion

The pediatric experience with RCP is limited to a few case reports. Sung and associates recently reported the use of RCP for the removal of air from the aorta of a 4.9 kg infant following repair of total anomalous pulmonary venous return.[85] To accomplish this, they simply perfused oxygenated pump blood into the right atrium with the pulmonary artery clamped. The authors made no mention, however, about control of the inferior vena cava (IVC) during the 5 min RCP was administered. This child was reportedly neurologically and developmentally normal at 8 months of age. Acikel and associates reported the use of RCP in a 4-year-old suffering from supra-aortic stenosis complicated by endocarditis.[86] Using conventional techniques, these authors also maintained a superior vena cava (SVC) pressure of less than 20 mm Hg for the 26 min cross-clamp time. The authors reported a satisfactory recovery for the child, free from neurologic injury.

While it seems clear that RCP is a useful technique to treat gaseous or embolic contamination of the cerebral vasculature, its role in the perfusion management of pediatric patients requiring arch surgery remains obscure. This is particularly true with the availability of ACP using current techniques.

Summary

A large body of surgical literature is devoted to the use of RCP during aortic arch surgery. Much of this data leads to conflicting conclusions and, based on an analysis of experimental and clinical results, the value of RCP, relative to DHCA alone, should be carefully considered. These variable and discrepant results may stem from the fact that clinicians do not know how to effectively use RCP, do not appreciate whom it should be used on, and do not clearly understand which physiologic or outcome variables to measure as an assessment of its utility. Clearly, the lack of randomized controlled clinical investigations of RCP is a major factor limiting its assessment, and this remains an active area of investigation.

Future Directions

Heart surgeons routinely expose patients to physiologic extremes usually reserved for the animal laboratory. Because of methodologic problems such as interspecies anatomic variation, the relevance of cerebral perfusion techniques is difficult to assess outside of the clinical arena. Emerging technologies, applied appropriately, provide us with spectacular clinical opportunities. Use of these technologies suggests that selective antegrade cerebral perfusion provides significant circulatory support to patients undergoing arch reconstruction, which should be expected to improve survival and neurologic outcome. However, the value of these techniques, and their superiority over alternative perfusion modalities, remain unproven. Cardiac surgical history is a mosaic of techniques and practices adopted on little more than anecdotal evidence. The surgical treatment of congenital heart disease and complex aortic disease in adults is the purview of relatively few intensely focused practitioners treating a defined group of patients in unique ways. As such, we are uniquely positioned to provide insights into human disease and biology through well-organized clinical trials. All forms of cerebral circulatory support would benefit from prospective studies employing recent methodologies, including comprehensive neuropsychiatric evaluations. It is only through such coordinated efforts that the foundation of a truly evidence-based standard of practice can be achieved.

References

1. Ergin MA, Galla JD, Lansman SL, et al. Hypothermic circulatory arrest in operations on the thoracic aorta: determinants of operative mortality and neurologic outcome. J Thorac Cardiovasc Surg 1994;107:788–97.
2. McCullough JN, Zhang N, Reich D, et al. Cerebral metabolic suppression during circulatory arrest in humans. Ann Thorac Surg 1999;67:1895–9.
3. Crittenden MD, Roberts CS, Rosa L, et al. Brain protection during circulatory arrest. Ann Thorac Surg 1991;51:942–7.
4. Sakurada T, Kazai T, Tanaka H, et al. Comparative experimental study of cerebral protection during aortic arch reconstruction. Ann Thorac Surg 1996;61:1348–54.
5. Frist WH, Baldwin JC, Starnes VA, et al. A reconsideration of cerebral perfusion in aortic arch replacement. Ann Thorac Surg 1986;42:273–81.
6. Takahashi T, Shimazaki Y, Watanabe T, et al. Staged perfusion with an axillary artery graft and deep hypothermia during descending aortic replacement. J Thorac Cardiovasc Surg 2001;122:188–9.
7. Matsuda H, Nakano S, Shirakura R, et al. Surgery for aortic arch aneurysm with selective cerebral perfusion and hypothermic cardiopulmonary bypass. Circulation 1989;80:1243–8.

8. Bachet J, Guilmet D, Goudot B, et al. Cold cerebroplegia. A new technique of cerebral protection during operations on the transverse aortic arch. J Thorac Cardiovasc Surg 1991;102:85–94.

9. Galla JD, McCullough JN, Ergin MA, et al. Aortic arch and deep hypothermic circulatory arrest: real-life suspended animation. Cardiol Clin North Am 1999;17:767–78.

10. Griepp RB. Cerebral protection during aortic arch surgery. J Thorac Cardiovasc Surg 2001;121:425–7.

11. Kazui T, Washiyama N, Muhammad BAH, et al. Improved results of atherosclerotic aneurysm surgery using a refined technique. J Thorac Cardiovasc Surg 2000;121:491–9.

12. Okita Y, Minatoya K, Tagusari O, et al. Prospective comparative study of brain protection in total arch replacement: deep hypothermic circulatory arrest with retrograde cerebral perfusion or selective antegrade cerebral perfusion. Ann Thorac Surg 2001;72:72–9.

13. Okita Y, Takamoto S, Ando M, et al. Mortality and cerebral outcome in patients who underwent aortic arch operations using deep hypothermic circulatory arrest with retrograde cerebral perfusion. J Thorac Cardiovasc Surg 1998;115:129–38.

14. Jonas RA, Wernovsky G, Ware J, et al. The Boston Circulatory Arrest Study: perioperative neurologic and developmental outcome after the arterial switch operation. Circulation 1992;86 Suppl:I-360.

15. Hickey PR. Neurologic sequelae associated with deep hypothermic circulatory arrest. Ann Thorac Surg 1998;65: S65–70.

16. Asou T, Kado H, Imoto Y, et al. Selective perfusion technique during aortic arch repair in neonates. Ann Thorac Surg 1996;61:1546–8.

17. Pigula FA, Siewers RD, Nemoto EM. Regional perfusion of the brain during neonatal aortic arch reconstruction. J Thorac Cardiovasc Surg 1999;117:1023–4.

18. Tchervenkov CI, Korkola S, Shum-Tim D, et al. Neonatal aortic arch reconstruction avoiding circulatory arrest and direct arch vessel cannulation. Ann Thorac Surg 2001;72:1615–20.

19. Pigula FA, Nemoto, EM, Griffith BP, Siewers RD. Regional low-flow perfusion provides cerebral circulatory support during neonatal aortic arch reconstruction. J Thorac Cardiovasc Surg 2000;119:331–9.

20. Jobsis FF. Non-invasive infrared monitoring of cerebral and myocardial oxygen sufficiency and circulatory parameters. Science 1977;198:1264–7.

21. VanDerzee P, Cope M, Arridge SR, et al. Experimentally measured optical pathlengths for the adult head, calf and forearm and the head of the newborn infant as a function of interoptode distance. Adv Exp Med Biol 1992; 316:143–53.

22. McCormick PW, Goetting MG, Dujovny M, Ausman JL. Noninvasive cerebral spectroscopy for monitoring cerebral oxygen delivery and hemodynamics. Crit Care Med 1991; 19:89–97.

23. Wyatt JS, Cope M, Delpy DT, et al. Measurement of optical pathlength for cerebral near-infrared spectroscopy in newborn infants. Dev Neurosci 1990;12:140–4.

24. Wray S, Cope M, Delpy DT, et al. Characterization of the near-infrared absorption spectra of cytochrome aa_3 and haemoglobin for the non-invasive monitoring of cerebral oxygenation. Biochem Biophys Acta 1998;933:184–92.

25. Edwards AD, Brown GC, Cope M, et al. Quantification of concentration changes in neonatal human cerebral oxidized cytochrome oxidase. J Appl Physiol 1991;71: 1907–13.

26. Tsuji M. Cerebral monitoring by near-infrared spectroscopy. Intensive Care Med 1996;11:162–72.

27. Nollert G, Shin'oka T, Jonas RA. Near-infrared spectroscopy of the brain in cardiovascular surgery. Thorac Cardiovasc Surg 1998;46:167–75.

28. Tamura M. Noninvasive monitoring of brain oxygen metabolism during cardiopulmonary bypass by near-infrared spectroscopy. Jpn Circ J 1991;55:330–5.

29. Yao FSF, Tseng CC, Boyd MD, et al. Frontal lobe dysfunction following cardiac surgery is associated with cerebral oxygen desaturation. Ann Thorac Surg 1999;68:1458–67.

30. Greeley WJ, Bracey VA, Ungerleider RM, et al. Recovery of cerebral metabolism and mitochondrial oxidation state is delayed after hypothermic circulatory arrest. Circulation 1991;84 Suppl III:400–6.

31. Boushel R, Piantadosi CA. Near-infrared spectroscopy for monitoring muscle oxygenation. Acta Physiol Scand 2000;168:615–22.

32. Edwards AD, Richardson C, VanDerzee P, et al. Measurement of hemoglobin flow and blood flow by near-infrared spectroscopy. J Appl Physiol 1993;75:1884–9.

33. Segal R, Ferson PM, Nemoto EM, Wolfson SK Jr. Flow-monitored transthoracic endoscopic sympathectomy. In: Rengachary SS, Wilkins RH, editors. Neurosurgical operative atlas. Vol. 7. AANS Publications Committee. Baltimore: Williams and Wilkins; 1998. p. 163–71.

34. Kooijman HM, Hopman MTE, Colier NJM, et al. Near-infrared spectroscopy for noninvasive assessment of claudication. J Surg Res 1997;72:1–7.

35. Komimaya T, Shigematsu H, Yasuhara H, Muto T. Near-infrared spectroscopy grades the severity of intermittent claudication in diabetics more accurately than ankle pressure measurement. Br J Surg 2000;87:459–66.

36. Tran TK, Sailasuta N, Kreutzer U, et al. Comparative analysis of NMR and NIRS measurements of intracellular Po_2 in human skeletal muscle. Am J Physiol 1999;276: 1682–90.

37. Bergovsky EH. Determination of tissue Po_2 tensions by hollow visceral tonometers: effect of breathing enriched O_2 mixtures. J Clin Invest 1964;43:192–200.

38. Dawson AM, Trenchard D, Guz A. Small bowel tonometry: assessment of small gut mucosal oxygen tension in dog and man. Nature 1965;206:943–4.

39. Casado-Flores J, Mora E, Perez-Corral F, et al. Prognostic value of gastric intramucosal pH in critically ill children. Crit Care Med 1998;26:1123–7.

40. Temmesfield-Wollbruck B, Szalay A, Olschewski H, et al. Advantage of buffered solutions or automated capnometry in air filled balloons for use in gastric tonometry. Intensive Care Med 1997;23:423–7.

41. Corke CF, Prosco G, Gizycki P, Selvakumaran A. A simple method for frequent monitoring of gastric carbon dioxide. Anaesth Intensive Care 1996;24:590–3.

42. Antonsson JB, Boyle CC, Kruithoff KL, et al. Validation of tonometric measurement of gut intramural pH during endotoxemia and mesenteric occlusion in pigs. Am J Physiol 1990;259:G519–23.

43. Knichwich G, VanAken H, Brussel T. Gastrointestinal monitoring using measurement of intramucosal P_{CO_2}. Anesth Analg 1998;87:134–42.

44. Montgomery A, Hartman M, Jonsson K, et al. Intramucosal pH measurement with tonometers for detecting gastrointestinal ischemia in porcine hemorrhagic shock. Circ Shock 1989;29:319–27.

45. Vallet B, Lund N, Curtis SE, et al. Gut and muscle tissue P_{O_2} in endotoxemic dogs during shock and resuscitation. J Appl Physiol 1994;76:793–800.

46. Tang W, Weil MH, Sun S, et al. Gastric intramural P_{CO_2} as a monitor of perfusion failure during hemorrhagic and anaphylactic shock. J Appl Physiol 1994;76:572–7.

47. Nara M, Yukio C, Niwa H, et al. Experimental determination of the safe minimum perfusion flow rate for low-flow hypothermic cardiopulmonary bypass. Cardiovasc Surg 1999;7:715–22.

48. Miyamoto K, Kawashima Y, Matsuda H, et al. Optimal perfusion flow rate for the brain during deep hypothermic cardiopulmonary bypass at 20°C. J Thorac Cardiovasc Surg 1986;92:1065–70.

49. Swain JA, Anderson RV, Siegman MG. Low-flow cardiopulmonary bypass and cerebral protection: a summary of investigations. Ann Thorac Surg 1993;56:1490–2.

50. Watanabe T, Oshikiri N, Inui K, et al. Optimal blood flow for cooled brain at 20 degrees C. Ann Thorac Surg 1999: 68:864–9.

51. Gandhi SK, Siewers RD, Nemoto EM, et al. Regional low-flow perfusion in complex infant aortic arch reconstruction. Cardiol Young 2001;11 Suppl 1:87.

52. Pigula FA, Gandhi SK, Siewers RD, et al. Regional low-flow perfusion provides somatic circulatory support during neonatal aortic arch surgery. Ann Thorac Surg 2001:72: 401–7.

53. Mills NL, Ochsner JL. Massive air embolism during cardiopulmonary bypass: causes, prevention, and management. J Thorac Cardiovasc Surg 1980;80:708–17.

54. Ganzel BL, Edmonds HL, Pank JR, et al. Neurophysiologic monitoring to assure delivery of retrograde cerebral perfusion. J Thorac Cardiovasc Surg 1997;113:748–57.

55. Tanoue Y, Tominaga R, Ochiai Y, et al. Comparative study of retrograde and selective cerebral perfusion with transcranial Doppler. Ann Thorac Surg 1999;67:672–5.

56. Reich DL, Uysal S, Ergin A, Griepp RB. Retrograde cerebral perfusion as a method of neuroprotection during thoracic aortic surgery. Ann Thorac Surg 2001;72:1774–82.

57. Gardner TJ. Acute aortic dissection. In: Kaiser LR, Kron IL, Spray TL, editors. Mastery of cariothoracic surgery. Philadelphia: Lippincott-Raven; 1998. p. 463.

58. Ono T, Okita Y, Ando M, Kitamura S. Retrograde cerebral perfusion in human brains. Lancet 2000;356:1323.

59. Ye J, Yang L, DelBigio MR, et al. Retrograde cerebral perfusion provides limited distribution of blood to the brain: a study in pigs. J Thorac Cardiovasc Surg 1997;114:660–5.

60. Ehrlich MP, Hagl C, McCullough JN, et al. Retrograde cerebral perfusion provides negligible flow through brain capillaries in the pig. J Thorac Cardiovasc Surg 2001; 122:331–8.

61. Dresser LP, McKinney WM. Anatomic and pathophysiologic studies of the human internal jugular valve. Am J Surg 1987;154:220–4.

62. Fukae K, Nakashima A, Hisahara M, et al. Maldistribution of the cerebral blood flow in retrograde cerebral perfusion. Eur J Cardiothorac Surg 1995;9:496–501.

63. Oohara K, Usui A, Murase M, et al. Regional cerebral tissue blood flow measured by the colored microsphere method during retrograde cerebral perfusion. J Thorac Cardiovasc Surg 1995;109:772–9.

64. Boeckxstans CJ, Flameng WJ. Retrograde cerebral perfusion does not protect the brain in non-human primates. Ann Thorac Surg 1995;60:319–28.

65. Anttila V, Pokela M, Kiviluoma K, et al. Is maintained cranial hypothermia the only factor leading to improved outcome after RCP? An experimental study with a chronic porcine model. J Thorac Cardiovasc Surg 2000;119:1021–9.

66. Ye J, Ryner LN, Kozlowski P, et al. Perfusion imaging to monitor flow distribution in the brain during antegrade and retrograde cerebral perfusion in aortic arch surgery. American Heart Association, 70th session [abstract]. Circulation 1997;96 Suppl:I-185.

67. Imamaki M, Koyanagi H, Hashimoto A, et al. Retrograde cerebral perfusion with hypothermic blood provides efficient protection of the brain: a neuropathological study. J Card Surg 1995;10:325–33.

68. Ye J, Yang L, DelBigio MR, et al. Neuronal damage after hypothermic circulatory arrest and retrograde cerebral perfusion in the pig. Ann Thorac Surg 1996;61:1316–22.

69. Griepp RB, Juvonen T, Griepp E, et al. Is retrograde cerebral perfusion an effective means of neural support during deep hypothermic circulatory arrest? Ann Thorac Surg 1997;64:913–6.

70. Kouchoukos NT. Adjuncts to reduce the incidence of embolic brain injury during operations on the aortic arch. Ann Thorac Surg 1994;57:243–5.

71. Deeb GM, Williams DM, Quint LE, et al. Risk analysis for aortic surgery using hypothermic circulatory arrest with retrograde cerebral perfusion. Ann Thorac Surg 1999; 61:1883–6.

72. Wong CH, Bonser RS. Does retrograde cerebral perfusion affect risk factors for stroke and mortality after hypothermic circulatory arrest. Ann Thorac Surg 1999;67:1900–3.

73. Ueda Y, Okita Y, Aomi S, et al. Retrograde cerebral perfusion for aortic arch surgery: analysis of risk factors. Ann Thorac Surg 1999;67:1879–82.

74. Ehrlich MP, Fang WC, Grabenwoger M, et al. Impact of retrograde cerebral perfusion on aortic arch aneurysm repair. J Thorac Cardiovasc Surg 1999;118(6):1026–32.

75. Ehrlich MP, Fang C, Grabenwoger M, et al. Perioperative risk factors for mortality in patients with acute type A aortic dissection. Circulation 1998;98 Suppl II:294–8.

76. Okita Y, Takamoto S, Ando M, et al. Predictive factors for postoperative cerebral complications in patients with thoracic aortic aneurysm. Eur J Cardiothorac Surg 1996; 10:826–32.

77. Okita Y, Ando M, Minatoya K, et al. Predictive factors for mortality and cerebral complications in arteriosclerotic aneurysm of the aortic arch. Ann Thorac Surg 1999; 67:72–8.

78. Usui A, Yasura K, Watanabe T, et al. Comparative clinical study between retrograde cerebral perfusion and selective cerebral perfusion in surgery for acute type A aortic dissection. Eur J Cardiothorac Surg 1999;15:571–8.

79. Safi HJ, Letsou GV, Iliopoulos DC, et al. Impact of retrograde cerebral perfusion on ascending aortic and arch aneurysm. Ann Thorac Surg 1997;63:1601–7.

80. Coselli JS. Retrograde cerebral perfusion is an effective means of neural support during deep hypothermic circulatory arrest. Ann Thorac Surg 1997;64:908–12.

81. Ehrlich MP, Fang WC, Grabenwoger M, et al. Impact of retrograde cerebral perfusion on aortic arch aneurysm repair. J Thorac Cardiovasc Surg 1999;118:1026–32.

82. Usui A, Abe T, Murase M. Early clinical results of retrograde cerebral perfusion for aortic arch operations. Ann Thorac Surg 1996;62:94–103.

83. Hagl C, Ergin MA, Galla J, et al. Neurologic outcome after ascending aortic and aortic arch operations: effect of brain protection technique in high-risk patients. J Thorac Cardiovasc Surg 2001;121:1107–21.

84. Cheung AT, Bavaria JE, Pochettino A, et al. Oxygen delivery during retrograde cerebral perfusion in humans. Anesth Analg 1999;88:8–15.

85. Sung SC, Jun HJ, Woo JS. Simplified retrograde systemic perfusion for removal of air from the aorta in an infant. Ann Thorac Surg 2001;71:362–4.

86. Acikel U, Ugurlu BS, Karabay O, et al. Retrograde cerebral perfusion with hypothermic circulatory arrest in a child. Ann Thorac Surg 2000;69:1243–4.

CHAPTER 36

AORTIC DISSECTION

G. RANDALL GREEN, MD, IRVING L. KRON, MD

Patients with dissection of the thoracic aorta have challenged physicians for centuries. The precise etiology of thoracic aortic dissection is uncertain but the pathogenesis and clinical sequelae have been fairly well documented over the last 50 years. Disruption of the aortic intima and a variable depth of the media permit the force of aortic blood flow to be redirected from the true lumen into a dissection plane within the media. This is often a lethal event but may result in a chronic condition with aneurysmal dilatation of the dissected aorta and the potential for aortic rupture. Currently, diagnostic algorithms and the subsequent management of thoracic aortic dissection are based primarily on dissection location and on the timing of presentation. Newer imaging modalities, improved medical management, and advances in surgical technique have resulted in improved morbidity and mortality.

The earliest descriptions of aortic dissection appeared in the seventeenth and eighteenth centuries, but Maunoir is credited with first referring to the process as aortic "dissection."[1,2] Early attempts at surgical treatment met with limited clinical success but certain concepts such as fenestration persisted and are still in use today.[3,4] During the era of cardiopulmonary bypass, innovators such as DeBakey and Cooley described surgical correction and altered the natural history of this disease.[5,6] Current surgical procedures for the treatment of aortic dissection have been modified since the pioneering work of these and other earlier investigators, but the concepts introduced continue to guide treatment.

Incidence

Aortic dissection is the most frequently diagnosed lethal condition of the aorta and occurs more frequently than rupture of abdominal aortic aneurysm in the United States.[7] There is an estimated worldwide prevalence of 0.5 to 2.95 of 100,000 persons/yr; the prevalence ranges from 0.2 to 0.8 of 100,000 persons/yr in the United States, resulting in roughly 2,000 new cases per year. These figures are, however, only an estimate. In one autopsy series, the antemortem diagnosis was made in only 15%, revealing that many immediately fatal events go undiagnosed.[8]

Classification

Classification systems for aortic dissection have been critical to design strategies for diagnosis and the subsequent management of individual patients. Although several classification systems exist, the two variables necessary to categorize patients are the location and the timing of dissection. *Acute dissection* has traditionally been used to describe presentation within the first 2 weeks of an event. The more recently added *subacute* designation is used to describe the period between 2 weeks and 2 months, while the term *chronic dissection* is reserved for those presenting at greater than 2 months following the initial event.

The two classification systems most frequently used in clinical practice are the DeBakey and Stanford systems (Figure 36-1). That proposed by DeBakey is a taxonomic system that differentiates between aortic dissection involving only the ascending aorta and those that additionally involve the descending aorta.[9] This system provides the greatest opportunity to segregate like patients for subsequent comparative research. In contrast, the Stanford system proposed by Daily is a functional classification system.[10] All dissections that involve the ascending

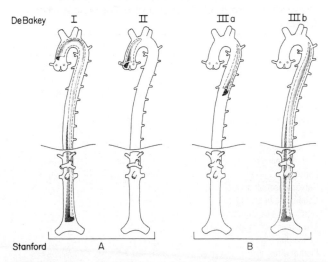

FIGURE 36-1. The DeBakey and Stanford classification systems for thoracic aortic dissection.

aorta are grouped together as type A, regardless of where the primary tear occurs; the clinical behavior of patients with aortic dissection is essentially determined by involvement of the ascending aorta. Critics of the Stanford system suggest that individual patients in the type A classification may be quite different, given the distal extent of dissection. Such a heterogeneous group would not permit rational comparison of similar groups of patients in which the ascending aorta is involved. The descending aortic dissection classifications, DeBakey type III (a and b) and Stanford type B, are equivalent. The Stanford system is used throughout this chapter.

The clinical characteristics of patients suffering acute aortic dissection are somewhat different between the two types (Table 36-1). Type A dissections occur with a greater overall frequency. Both type A and type B dissections occur more frequently in males in the sixth decade of life, while patients with type A dissection are slightly younger. Arterial hypertension is a strong risk factor for type B dissection but less so for type A, whereas the connective tissue disorders are seen more frequently in patients with type A dissection.

Etiology and Pathogenesis

There are several hypotheses regarding the etiology of the intimal disruption (primary tear) that permits aortic blood flow to create a cleavage plane within the media of the aortic wall (false lumen). Originally, this was viewed as a consequence of a biochemical abnormality within the media upon which normal mechanical forces in the aorta acted to create an intimal tear. The link between the abnormal media, termed *cystic medial necrosis* or *degeneration*, and the primary tear has not been scientifically established.

TABLE 36-1. Clinical Characteristics of Patients Presenting with Acute Type A and B Thoracic Aortic Dissection

	Type A	Type B
Frequency	60–75%	25–40%
Sex (M:F)	1.7–2.6:1	2.3–3:1
Age (years)	50–56	60–70
Hypertension	++	+++
Connective tissue disorder	++	+
Pain		
Retrosternal	+++	+,–
Interscapular	+,–	+++
Syncope	++	+,–
Cerebrovascular accident	+	–
Congestive heart failure	+	–
Aortic valve regurgitation	++	+,–
Myocardial infarction	+	–
Pericardial effusion	+++	–
Pleural effusion	+,–	+++
Abdominal pain	+,–	+,–
Peripheral pulse deficit	Upper and lower extremities	Lower extremities

+ and – indicate degree of presence or absence, respectively.

In fact, medial degeneration is found in only a minority of patients with acute aortic dissection and most are children.[11] This theory has lost support over the years. Alternatively, there are data that support a relationship between aortic dissections and intramural hematoma. Advocates of this theory suggest that bleeding from vasa vasorum into the media creates a mass, which results in localized areas of increased stress in the intima during diastole. These areas then permit intimal disruption. In fact, between 10 and 20% of patients thought to have acute aortic dissection are found to have intramural hematoma, suggesting that it may be a precursor to dissection.[12] Penetrating atherosclerotic ulcers have been implicated as the source of intimal disruption in certain cases, yet support for the concept has waned over the years. The pattern of atherosclerotic involvement of the thoracic aorta resulting in penetrating ulcer and the frequency of dissection throughout the aorta do not support this theory.

Once a cleave plane exists in the media, the aortic wall floating within the lumen is termed the *dissection flap* and is composed of the aortic intima and partial thickness media. The primary tear is usually greater than 50% of the circumference of the aorta, but the full circumference is rarely involved. The primary tear in type A dissection is usually located on the right anterior aspect of the ascending aorta and follows a somewhat predictable course spiraling around the arch and into the descending thoracic and abdominal aorta on the left and posteriorly. The dissection may propagate in a retrograde fashion for a variable distance as well, to involve the coronary ostia; this occurs in roughly 11% of all dissections.[13] Myocardial ischemia and aortic rupture into the pericardium are the cause of death in as many as 80% of deaths from acute dissection. Often, the distal false lumen communicates with the true lumen through one or more fenestrations within the dissection flap. The false lumen may also end blindly in as many as 4 to 12% of all dissections, in which case blood in the false lumen thromboses. It may also penetrate the adventitia, causing rupture and death. Regardless of whether the true lumen and false lumen communicate, perfusion of aortic side branches may be compromised by the dissection, causing end-organ ischemia. If these acute complications are avoided, the weakened outer aortic wall, composed of partial media and the adventitia, may dilate, resulting in later aneurysm formation. This long-term complication is the reason for operation in the majority of chronic dissections regardless of type.

Although no single disorder is responsible for aortic dissection, several risk factors have been identified that could damage the aortic wall and lead to dissection (Table 36-2). These include direct mechanical forces on the aortic wall (ie, hypertension, hypervolemia, derangements of aortic flow) and forces that affect the composition of the aortic wall (ie, connective tissue disorders or direct chemical destruction). Hypertension is the mechanical force most often associated with dissection and is found in

TABLE 36-2. Risk Factors for Type A and B Thoracic Aortic Dissection

Hypertension
Connective tissue disorders
   Ehlers-Danlos syndrome
   Marfan's disease
   Turner syndrome
Cystic medial disease of aorta
Aortitis
Iatrogenic
Atherosclerosis
Thoracic aortic aneurysm
Bicuspid aortic valve
Trauma
Pharmacologic
Coarctation of aorta
Hypervolemia (pregnancy)
Congenital aortic stenosis
Polycystic kidney disease
Pheochromocytoma
Sheehan syndrome
Cushing syndrome

greater than 75% of cases. Although increased strain on the aortic wall is intuitive, the mechanism by which hypertension actually leads to dissection is unclear. Similarly, hypervolemia, high cardiac output, and an abnormal hormonal milieu certainly contribute to the increased incidence of dissection in pregnancy, but the mechanism is unclear. Atherosclerosis is not a risk factor for aortic dissection except in pre-existing aneurysms or in the case of atherosclerotic ulceration, which may lead to dissection in the descending thoracic aorta. The fact that distal aortic dissection infrequently accompanies traumatic aortic transection reveals that a primary tear alone is insufficient for subsequent aortic dissection. It should be noted, however, that iatrogenic trauma to the aortic intima may result in dissection. Catheterization procedures, aortic root and femoral artery cannulation for cardiopulmonary bypass, aortic cross-clamping, surgical procedures performed on the aorta (aortic valve replacement and aortocoronary bypass grafting), and placement of intra-aortic balloon pumps have all been reported to result in dissection.

The adventitia provides most of the tensile strength of the aortic wall, with little contribution from the media. The media is composed of concentrically arranged smooth muscle interposed with connective tissue proteins such as collagen, elastin, and fibrillin within the ground substance. Abnormal constituents of the media as in certain connective tissue disorders such as Marfan's disease and Ehlers-Danlos syndrome are associated with aortic dissection. Marfan syndrome is an autosomal dominant inherited disorder in which a point mutation of the fibrillin-1 gene (*FBN1*), located on the long arm of chromosome 15, results in an abnormal media. The incidence of Marfan syndrome is approximately 1 per 5,000 live births. There are, however, many incomplete forms of the disease and as many as 25% of cases may be sporadic, in which no

fibrillin abnormalities are observed. Type IV Ehlers-Danlos syndrome is a connective tissue disorder of the proα1(III) chain of type III. The structurally abnormal media is susceptible to dissection. There are also familial aggregations of dissection without discernible biochemical or genetic abnormalities. Congenital abnormalities of the aortic valve, including bicuspid aortic valve, were found in nearly 10% of fatal dissections in one series. These are usually associated with a pre-existing aortic aneurysm.

Acute Dissection of the Aorta

Clinical Presentation

As many as 40% of patients suffering acute aortic dissection die immediately. Those surviving the initial event may be stabilized with medical management, and it is these patients in whom surgical treatment of aortic dissection has altered the natural history of the disease. The diagnosis of aortic dissection requires a high level of suspicion and should be considered in the setting of severe, unrelenting chest pain that is present in greater than 90% of such patients. Up to 30% of patients ultimately diagnosed with acute dissection are first thought to have another diagnosis. Patients often have no previous episodes of similar pain and are often quite anxious. Pain is located in the midsternum in dissection of the ascending aorta and in the interscapular region for dissection of the descending thoracic aorta (see Table 36-1). It is not unusual for the location of maximum pain to change as the dissection extends in an antegrade or retrograde direction. The character of the pain is often described as "ripping" or "tearing" and is constant with greatest intensity at the onset. Painless dissection has been described and usually occurs in the setting of an existing aneurysm where the pain of a new dissection may not be differentiated from chronic aneurysm pain. Patients may also have signs or symptoms related to malperfusion of the brain, limbs, or visceral organs. These findings may even dominate the presentation following the initial episode of pain. Elements of the past medical history such as primary hypertension, presence of aneurysmal disease of the aorta, or familial connective tissue disorders help to make the diagnosis. Illicit drug use is an increasingly important predisposing factor to dissection that must be investigated.

Patients suffering acute dissection appear ill. Tachycardia may be accompanied by either hypertension in the setting of baseline essential hypertension or hypotension secondary to aortic rupture, pericardial tamponade, acute aortic valve regurgitation, and even acute myocardial ischemia following involvement of the coronary ostia. An abnormal peripheral vascular examination is present in less than 20% of patients with acute aortic dissection, but when present may indicate the type of dissection. Absence of pulses in the upper extremity suggests ascending aortic involvement, whereas pulse deficits in the lower extremities speak to involvement of the distal aorta. These findings are subject to change as the dissection progresses or reentry into the true lumen occurs. Auscultation of the heart may reveal a diastolic murmur or an S3 indicating left-heart volume overload consistent with acute aortic valve insufficiency. Physical exam findings such as jugular venous distension and a pulsus paradoxus are signs of pericardial tamponade that should be identified in any unstable patient to initiate the correct diagnostic and treatment algorithms. Unilateral loss of breath sounds in one thorax, usually the left, may indicate hemothorax as a result of aortic leak or rupture with hemothorax. Alternatively, a pleural effusion may exist secondary to pleural inflammation related to the dissection. This finding requires additional evaluation prior to treatment.

A complete central and peripheral neurologic exam is critical in that abnormalities are present in up to 40% of acute type A dissections. Involvement of the brachiocephalic vessels with loss of brain perfusion may result in transient syncope or stroke. Stroke rarely improves with restoration of blood flow and may even cause hemorrhage and brain death, yet surgery is indicated in such patients. Loss of perfusion to intercostal or lumbar arteries may result in spinal cord ischemia and paraplegia. Peripheral nerve ischemia as a result of malperfusion may yield findings similar to spinal cord malperfusion and should be discerned as these patients often improve with restoration of blood flow. Acute aortic dissection may also cause superior vena cava syndrome, vocal cord paralysis, hematemesis, Horner syndrome, hemoptysis, and airway compression as a result of local compression and mass effects.

Diagnostic Studies

No routine diagnostic study will reliably yield the diagnosis of acute aortic dissection. An electrocardiogram (ECG) is routinely performed and reveals no ischemic changes in most cases. Obvious ischemic changes are present in as many as 20% of acute type A dissections, yet only nonspecific repolarization abnormalities alone are present in up to one-third of patients with coronary ostial involvement. The chest x-ray is abnormal in 60 to 90% of patients with acute dissection (Table 36-3). Although most patients have at least one, if not several, abnormal finding(s), a normal chest x-ray does not rule out the diagnosis. Blood tests obtained at the time of initial obser-

vation are usually unremarkable. There is frequently a mild to moderate leukocytosis. Anemia may result from sequestration of blood or hemolysis. Liver function tests, serum creatinine, myoglobin, and lactic acid may all be abnormal in the setting of certain malperfusion syndromes, depending on duration.

Diagnostic Imaging

The goal of diagnostic imaging is to rapidly demonstrate dissection with minimal distress for the patient. Five advanced imaging modalities are used clinically to diagnose acute aortic dissection: computerized tomography, echocardiography, magnetic resonance imaging, aortography, and intravascular ultrasound. The relative benefits, disadvantages, and diagnostic accuracy of each must be considered in choosing the most appropriate study for a particular clinical situation (Table 36-4). In addition to the essential diagnostic information, certain tests may provide additional important information such as the site of intimal disruption, reentry points, whether there is flow or thrombus in the false lumen, status of the aortic valve, presence and nature of myocardial ischemia, and brachiocephalic and aortic branch vessel involvement.

Aortography was first used to diagnose acute dissection in 1939 and, until recently, was considered the gold standard for diagnosis. It is an invasive test requiring nephrotoxic contrast media in which the aorta is visualized in multiple two-dimensional projections. The diagnosis of dissection depends upon visualization of the intimal flap, two distinct lumen or compression of the true lumen by flow through an adjacent false lumen (Figure 36-2). Indirect signs of dissection include the presence of branch vessel abnormalities and an abnormal intimal contour on injection of the false lumen. The status of the aortic valve may be evaluated, and coronary angiography in the setting of type A dissections is possible only with this diagnostic test. In reality, the coronary ostia are involved in only 10 to 20% of acute type A dissections, and coronary atherosclerosis is present in 25% of all patients with acute aortic dissection. Taking time to perform this test is debatable given that the coronary ostia are easily evaluated at the time of surgery. Aortography is especially useful in type B dissections with evidence of mesenteric ischemia or oliguria, and in type A dissections

TABLE 36-3. Abnormalities Identified on Chest Radiography in Acute Aortic Dissection

Widened mediastinum
Irregular aortic contour
Aortic apical cap
Tracheal displacement
Depression of left mainstem bronchus
Esophageal displacement
Obscure aortic-pulmonary window
Pleural effusion

TABLE 36-4. Sensitivity and Specificity of Various Imaging Modalities Useful for the Diagnosis of Thoracic Aortic Dissection

Imaging Study	Sensitivity (%)	Specificity (%)
Aortography	80–90	88–95
Computerized tomography (CT)	90–100	90–100
Intravascular ultrasonography (IVUS)	94–100	97–100
Echocardiogram		
Transthoracic	60–80	80–96
Transesophageal	90–99	85–98
Magnetic resonance imaging (MRI)	98–100	98–100

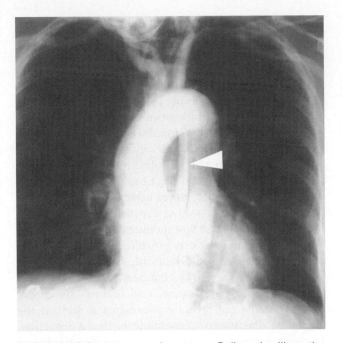

FIGURE 36-2. Aortogram of acute type B dissection illustrating differential contrast enhancement of the true and false lumen in the descending thoracic aorta. The intimal flap (arrowhead) can be seen separating the two lumen.

with signs of malperfusion, because catheter-based intervention may be possible. Aortography may yield false-negative results with thrombosis of one lumen or when contrast equally opacifies each lumen, impairing distinction of a separate true and false lumen. The diagnosis of intramural hematoma is also difficult given the absence of intimal disruption. Aortography requires the presence of skilled personnel whose availability varies with institution. The time required to assemble this team is a detriment when compared to other immediately available diagnostic tests given the high early mortality following acute dissection.

Intravascular ultrasonography (IVUS) is a catheter-based imaging tool that provides dynamic imaging of the aortic wall and a pulsatile intimal flap in patients with aortic dissection. It is particularly useful in delineating the distal extent of dissection and for identifying the true and false lumen in questionable cases during aortography. High-resolution images of the normal three-layered aortic wall are differentiated from the abnormally thin wall adjacent to the false lumen. Because the aortic wall itself is imaged, intramural hematoma and penetrating atherosclerotic ulcers may also be identified. Currently, as an isolated imaging study, it is time-consuming and requires skilled personnel and therefore may not be useful as an initial imaging study. It may be most useful in combination with aortography in the setting of negative imaging studies when a high clinical suspicion remains.

Helical computerized tomography (CT) scanning has become widely available over the last 20 years and is now used most frequently to make the diagnosis of acute aortic dissection. It requires intravenous contrast medium that may limit its use in certain clinical situations but generates images, familiar to most practitioners, that result in a high sensitivity and specificity. This technique can be performed quickly, fulfilling the requirements for use in the early management of acute dissection. Additional structures such as the pleural and pericardial spaces are imaged. The aortic branch vessels are also evaluated with CT scanning; involvement of the brachiocephalic vessels is identified with nearly 96% accuracy. The diagnosis of dissection requires two or more channels separated by a dissection flap (Figure 36-3). Transaxial two-dimensional images can be reconstructed to display three-dimensional reconstructions of the aorta that aid in diagnosis and also are useful for operative planning.

Conventional magnetic resonance imaging (MRI) and the newer contrast-enhanced magnetic resonance angiography generate superior images reliably demonstrating aortic dissection (Figure 36-4). In fact, some consider this the new gold-standard imaging study given the published diagnostic accuracy. Dissection is identified as an intraluminal membrane separating two or more channels. It provides detailed images of the entire aorta, the pericardium, and pleural spaces. Cine imaging may also be used to evaluate left ventricular function, the status of the aortic valve, and flow in aortic branch vessels, as well as flow in the false lumen. It is, however, time-consuming and not widely available, and the presence of ferromagnetic metal contraindicates its use. Another disadvantage of MRI is that artifact is identified in up to 64% of studies, which underscores the need for expert radiologic interpretation of the images. These factors obviously limit its use in the acute setting, but it is a reliable, noninvasive imaging study that is perhaps best used to follow chronic dissections (Figure 36-5).

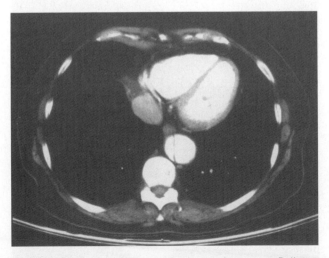

FIGURE 36-3. Axial CT arteriogram image of acute type B dissection. The dissection flap divides the aorta into two distinct lumina within the descending thoracic segment.

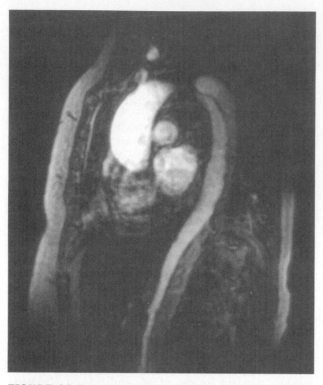

FIGURE 36-4. Sagittal contrast-enhanced magnetic resonance image of acute type B dissection. The dissection extends the entire length of the thoracic and abdominal aorta.

Transesophageal echocardiography (TEE) is currently a preferred method for making the diagnosis of acute aortic dissection. It is widely available, requires no intravenous contrast, and generates dynamic images of the aorta and its branches from which the diagnosis can be made. Criteria for making the diagnosis include visualization of an echogenic surface separating two distinct lumen, repeatedly, in more than one view, and which can be differentiated from normal surrounding cardiac structures (Figure 36-6). The true lumen is identified by expansion during systole and collapse in diastole. Communication between the true lumen and false lumen may be visualized as flow across tears in the dissection flap using color Doppler; similarly the absence of flow indicates false lumen thrombosis. TEE additionally may provide high-quality images of the aortic valve and pericardial space. The coronary ostia and left ventricular function may be assessed to provide information regarding regional wall motion abnormalities to rule out myocardial ischemia as part of the differential diagnosis or as complicating type A dissection. The area surrounding the aorta is also visualized, and therefore, periaortic hematoma indicating leak may be identified. Although the safest setting in which to perform TEE is the operating room under general anesthesia, it can be performed using local anesthesia and minimal sedation in a monitored setting. Relative contraindications to TEE

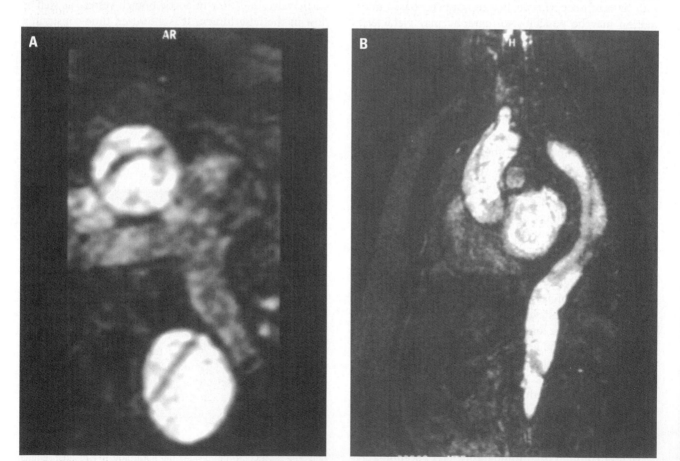

FIGURE 36-5. Axial (A) and sagittal (B) contrast-enhanced magnetic resonance images of a chronic type A dissection.

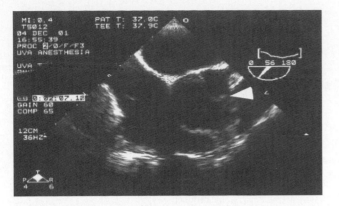

FIGURE 36-6. Transesophageal echocardiographic image of an acute type A dissection. The dissection flap (arrowhead) within the lumen of the aortic root included one aortic valve commissure and freely prolapsed through the aortic valve orifice during diastole.

include esophageal abnormalities and a full stomach, but recognition of these conditions permits safe examination with few complications in the vast majority of patients. Transthoracic echocardiography provides images of the ascending aorta and sections of the aortic arch that may yield the diagnosis but with much less sensitivity than transesophageal imaging (Figure 36-7). As such, transthoracic imaging may prove useful but is generally insufficient to reliably make the diagnosis. Transthoracic evaluation is additionally limited by patient-related factors, including body habitus and emphysema, as well as by operator experience. A negative transthoracic study should be complemented by a transesophageal study that provides greater detail of the entire aorta. To exclude the diagnosis of aortic dissection by TEE, a competent operator must visualize the entire thoracic aorta in a detailed examination.

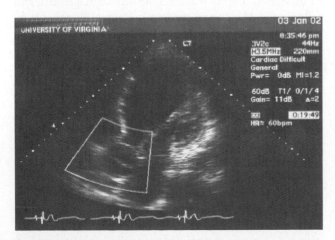

FIGURE 36-7. Transthoracic echocardiographic image of acute type A dissection. Occasionally a dissection flap is identified in the ascending aorta (inset) by using this comparatively insensitive imaging tool. If possible, the diagnosis of aortic dissection should be confirmed by an additional imaging study prior to initiating a particular management algorithm.

Initial Management

Fifty percent of patients suffering acute aortic dissection are dead within 48 hours. A conventional wisdom has evolved that acute aortic dissection carries a "1% per hour" mortality. This demonstrates that patients surviving a dissection must be quickly and aggressively diagnosed and managed.

The initial evaluation of a stable patient suspected of having aortic dissection includes a detailed history and physical examination focusing on those elements likely to rule in the diagnosis. Blood pressure is measured in both arms and immediately treated to achieve a target systolic blood pressure between 90 and 110 mm Hg. During this time, peripheral, and sometimes central, venous and arterial access is obtained; blood is sent for complete blood count, serum electrolytes, creatine kinase with myocardial isoenzymes, and troponin, and a blood type and screen is obtained. The unstable patient may require intubation and mechanical ventilation and possibly placement of a pulmonary artery catheter if necessary. The site of this initial evaluation and resuscitation is determined primarily by the hemodynamic stability of the patient. The unstable patient belongs in the operating room, whereas the stable patient permits a more detailed diagnostic approach from which management follows on an urgent basis. Therefore, the hypotensive patient who may be hypovolemic as a result of blood loss into the thorax or pericardium undergoes the aforementioned evaluation and resuscitation on transfer to the operating room. It is preferable to avoid procedures such as transesophageal echocardiography or central line placement on an awake patient outside the operating room because hypertension resulting from patient discomfort could precipitate aortic rupture or propagation of dissection.

Recognizing the natural history of patients with aortic dissection dictates that management occurs as part of the initial diagnostic evaluation. Blood pressure control in hypertensive patients with pain should first be treated with narcotic analgesics. In general, the goals of hypertension management in acute aortic dissection are twofold.[14] First, aortic wall stress is lowered by decreasing the systolic blood pressure, which reduces the possibility of rupture. Second, shear stress on the aorta is decreased by minimizing the rate of rise of aortic pressure to decrease the likelihood of dissection propagation, so-called anti-impulse therapy. The drugs most commonly used for these purposes are sodium nitroprusside and esmolol. Sodium nitroprusside is a direct arterial vasodilator with a fast onset and short duration of action, which make it ideal to achieve a target systolic blood pressure between 90 and 110 mm Hg. The rate of rise of aortic pressure, however, is increased when sodium nitroprusside is used alone. Esmolol is added to decrease the inotropic state of the myocardium and to decrease the heart rate. This drug is a β_1 selective blocking agent with a short half-life, which can easily be titrated to achieve the target blood pressure.

Loading doses for esmolol and sodium nitroprusside should be avoided to prevent hypotension. Alternative β_1-blocking drugs, such as propranolol or metoprolol, and the combined α- and β-blocker labetalol, are appropriate in the subacute phase. Alternatively, calcium channel blockers may be necessary to reduce systolic blood pressure in those patients with a contraindication to β-blocker use. There are, however, no compelling data supporting their efficacy in acute dissection.

Diagnostic Strategy

The evaluation of suspected acute aortic dissection begins with determination of the likelihood of the diagnosis being correct and the hemodynamic stability of the patient. Unstable patients should undergo ECG and chest x-ray and be transferred to the operating room immediately. These patients should be intubated, mechanically ventilated, and have monitoring lines placed, at which time TEE is performed. Initial medical management is initiated as soon as the diagnosis is suspected prior to transfer to the operating room for subsequent evaluation and management. If TEE fails to yield a diagnosis, then a hemodynamically unstable patient will at that point have a protected airway and invasive monitoring lines placed for subsequent evaluation of alternate diagnoses. If dissection is suspected even in the setting of a negative TEE, CT or aortography (potentially with IVUS) are the next studies of choice.

At the University of Virginia, clinically and hemodynamically stable patients are first evaluated with CT scanning. With a CT scanner in the emergency room, it takes less than 15 min to obtain these data. If that study is negative, yet the diagnosis is still entertained, a transesophageal echocardiogram is obtained. In a recent review, an average of 1.8 imaging studies were used to correctly diagnose acute aortic dissection.[8]

Surgical Indications

The presence of ascending aortic involvement is generally an indication for operative management given that older data indicate a > 90% mortality without surgery in 2 weeks (Table 36-5). The goals are to prevent aortic rupture into the pericardium or pleural space, and to prevent potential coronary ostial or aortic valve involvement. It is important to note that neurologic complications at the time of presentation, including stroke or paraplegia, are not contraindications to surgical correction, as some patients will improve. Thrombosis of either lumen is also not a contraindication to surgery. Although immediate surgical correction of type A dissection is recommended, there are data suggesting that patients who survive type A dissection and who present at greater than 2 weeks may safely undergo elective operation. In fact, poor-risk patients in that same cohort had an acceptable early survival and short-term outcome with medical management alone.[15] In another recent study, type A dissection was

TABLE 36-5. Operative Indications for Types A and B Thoracic Aortic Dissections

Dissection Type	Operative Indication
Acute	
Type A	Presence
Type B	Rupture
	Malperfusion
	Progressive dissection
	Failure of medical management
Chronic	
Type A	Symptoms related to dissection (congestive failure, angina, aortic regurgitation, stroke, pain
	Malperfusion
	Aneurysm
Type B	Symptoms related to dissection
	Malperfusion
	Aneurysm

managed medically in 28% of patients for various reasons, with a 58% in-hospital mortality for that group.[16] Despite this recent recognition that early mortality following type A dissection may be lower than expected, immediate surgical intervention is indicated in the majority of patients.

Aortic rupture and visceral malperfusion are the most frequent causes of death in acute type B dissection. These, however, occur much less frequently when compared with type A dissection, and between 70 and 80% survive the acute and subacute phases with medical management alone. Such success with medical management has traditionally created surgical indications for acute type B dissections, which include complications of medical management or progression of the disease. Specifically included are contained or free aortic rupture, acute aortic expansion, malperfusion syndrome, pain or progression of dissection despite maximal medical management, and failure of medical management to control hypertension. Although medical management of acute type B dissection is the rule in most centers, some centers advocate immediate surgical intervention in selected patients with uncomplicated acute type B dissection. Other factors that may indicate early operation in acute type B dissection are the presence of Marfan syndrome, a large false aneurysm, arch involvement, and presumed medical compliance issues.[17] As in acute type A dissection, acute paralysis does not contraindicate surgery because patients can have remarkable improvement following revascularization.

There is some debate over the treatment of patients diagnosed with intramural hematoma and penetrating atherosclerotic ulcer. The natural history of these so-called dissection variants has made the issue less confusing. Intramural hematoma may lead to acute rupture in up to 35% of patients, whereas regression or no change in the hematoma is seen in the majority of medically managed patients surviving the initial period.[18] Those patients with penetrating ulcer were found to have a rate of acute rupture of 42%. The current recommendations from the Yale group are early operative intervention for intramural hematoma and penetrating ulcer involving the ascending aorta. In the descending aorta, medical management with anti-impulse therapy and a low threshold for operative intervention result in the lowest mortality. These patients require continuous observation and repeat diagnostic imaging after 3 to 5 days in the hospital to monitor the lesion.

Surgical Management

The surgical management of acute aortic dissection must be tailored to the type of dissection and modified by specific patient-related factors, but several general rules apply. In acute type A dissection with involvement of the aortic valve, preservation of the native valve is preferred and accomplished in nearly 85% of cases. Preservation of the aortic valve in patients with connective tissue disorders is performed by some, but long-term data regarding longevity of valve competence lacking. If the valve is preserved in these patients, the sinuses must be replaced or re-created by using various surgical techniques or grafts to prevent aneurysmal dilatation. Preservation of the aortic valve in patients with congenitally bicuspid aortic valves is a matter of debate. Use of an aortic homograft is an alternative surgical strategy for those requiring replacement of the valve and ascending aorta. This is an ideal solution in individuals who have a contraindication to anticoagulation or in young reproductive females.

Management of the aortic arch in patients with type A dissection is determined by whether the intima of the arch is intact or violated. If it is intact, the aortic layers can usually be reunited using either Teflon felt or glue and that site of the arch used for distal anastomosis (Figure 36-8). If the intima is fractured, the brachiocephalic vessels may require reimplantation as a Carrel patch or even individually after reuniting the dissected layers. Isolated dissections involving the aortic arch are rare and are treated as type A dissections with resection of the arch at the site of intimal disruption. Acute type A dissections resulting from retrograde extension into the arch are treated by replacing the arch and reuniting the dissected layers proximally or by going beyond the dissection to normal aorta proximally for the proximal anastomosis. In effect, this converts the dissection to type B.

The goals of surgical management of complicated acute type B dissection are the prevention of free rupture and perfusion of all end organs in the absence of symptoms. The particular operation is based on the specific operative indication and the pattern of dissection. Replacement of the descending thoracic aorta usually begins at the left subclavian artery and the distal anastomosis is ideally made to normal distal thoracic aorta. When dissection involves the entire thoracic aorta, the distal aortic layers are reunited with Teflon felt or glue and that site is used for the distal anastomosis. No more than the proximal third of

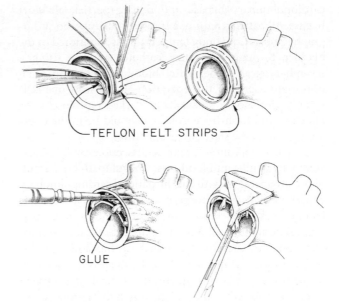

FIGURE 36-8. The intimal flap is reunited with the aortic wall using Teflon felt strips, commercially available glue, or both. Felt strips may be placed on the inside, outside, and/or between the dissected layers of the aorta as the layers are reunited. The specific technique for approximating the layers with glue depends upon the product; fundamentally, glue is applied between the dissected layers, which are then held together manually or with clamps for 3 to 10 min. A seal is formed between the dissected layers that can then be used for primary anastomosis or, if necessary, reinforced with Teflon felt.

the descending thoracic should be replaced if possible. The primary concern when deciding where to place the distal anastomosis in acute type B dissection is preservation of intercostal arteries perfusing the spinal cord. The incidence of paraplegia following surgery for acute type B dissections can be as high as 19%.[19]

Endovascular stent-grafting is currently being tested as a definitive form of management in both acute and chronic forms of type B dissections with acceptable results. Long-term data and prospective comparisons to surgery will be necessary before exclusively percutaneous management can be recommended as an alternative to surgery.

Operative Technique

Anesthesia used during the repair of aortic dissections is often narcotic based, with inhalational agents for maintenance. Single-lumen endotracheal tubes are used for procedures performed through a median sternotomy, while double-lumen endotracheal tubes are useful but rarely mandatory for procedures performed through a left thoracotomy. Monitoring lines often include central venous access with a pulmonary artery catheter and arterial pressure monitoring lines specific to the operation performed. One or two radial arterial lines and at least one femoral line are required to ensure perfusion of the upper and lower body when femoral cannulation is used for cardiopulmonary bypass and during partial left-heart bypass. All patients require a transesophageal echocardiography probe. Core body temperature is monitored in the bladder through the Foley catheter and by using a nasopharyngeal probe. Strict blood conservation is an important aspect of the operation and at least one cell-saver device should be available. Packed red blood cells, platelets, and fresh-frozen plasma should be in the operating room at the start of the operation.

Surgical procedures for aortic dissection can be associated with significant blood loss. Coagulopathy as a result of the preoperative status of the patient, cardiopulmonary bypass, and deep hypothermic circulatory arrest contribute to excessive blood loss. Improvements in vascular graft material have all but eliminated this as a reason for intra- and postoperative blood loss. Antifibrinolytic drugs such as epsilon-aminocaproic acid and aprotinin are useful hemostatic adjuncts. Aprotinin is particularly useful when used in either the full or one-half Hammersmith regimen, and is best administered prior to the operation. In cases in which deep hypothermic circulatory arrest is used, we administer aprotinin only after the period of circulatory arrest. Patients often require transfusion of fresh-frozen plasma, platelets, and possibly cryoprecipitate. Fibrin glues and hemostatic materials such as Surgicel and Gelfoam are useful as systemic coagulopathy is corrected.

There are various options for arterial and venous cannulation sites based upon the type of dissection. Arterial cannulation of the uninvolved aortic arch is preferable in type A dissection. Alternate sites include the right subclavian artery, the innominate artery, or either femoral artery with retrograde aortic perfusion. In any case of retrograde aortic perfusion, it is essential to monitor proximal perfusion with a functioning radial arterial catheter. There is debate over which femoral artery to cannulate in the setting of lower extremity malperfusion with a pulse deficit. Dissection of the abdominal aorta often leaves the left femoral artery originating from the false lumen, and therefore, cannulation of the pulsatile right femoral artery will most often perfuse the true lumen. Potential consequences of false-lumen cannulation are retrograde dissection and malperfusion of aortic branch vessels arising from the true lumen. The solution to this situation begins with prompt recognition of the problem, which requires the appropriate monitoring lines (ie, radial arterial line) and cessation of cardiopulmonary bypass. The goal is then expeditious cannulation of the true lumen and resumption of cardiopulmonary bypass. If the chest has been opened, direct cannulation of the ascending aorta can be successful. An alternative cannulation technique is through the left ventricular apex and aortic valve. The cannula is then held in position with an ascending aortic tourniquet. Venous cannulation is usually through the right atrium by using a two-stage venous cannula while bicaval cannulation is reserved for certain cases in which retrograde cerebral perfusion is used. Because there is often involvement of the aortic valve,

the left ventricle must be vented by a catheter advanced through the right superior pulmonary vein or, rarely, through the left ventricular apex. Cardioplegia is administered retrograde through a coronary sinus catheter.

The formerly popular "clamp-and-sew" technique, which was used for repair of type B dissection, has been supplanted by the use of partial left-heart bypass. Arterial cannulation sites for this technique are either the distal thoracic aorta for limited dissections or the femoral artery for those extending beyond the thorax. Venous drainage of oxygenated blood is from the left inferior pulmonary vein or directly from the left atrium via the appendage. It may be necessary to use deep hypothermic circulatory arrest if a proximal aortic clamp cannot be positioned between the left subclavian and the left common carotid arteries or in the setting of intimal involvement of the distal arch proximal to the clamp. In this case, arterial cannulation of the left femoral artery and vein are recommended and may be complemented by assisted left femoral venous drainage if necessary.

Procedures performed on the dissected aortic arch require disruption of adequate blood flow to the brain. Cerebral protection is achieved by either cessation of electrical activity in the brain through hypothermia or by some form of continued cerebral perfusion. Deep hypothermic circulatory arrest was the first method used to perform operations on the aortic arch and remains an effective method to date for shorter procedures. Generally, periods of circulatory arrest up to 14 min are acceptable at 25°C, and periods up to 31 min appear to result in only transient neurologic sequelae at 15°C in a small number of patients.[20] Some warn that cooling to lower than 15°C may result in a form of nonischemic brain injury. The risk of transient neurologic dysfunction on cognitive testing during circulatory arrest is roughly 10% at less than 30 min, but increases to 15% at 40 min, 30% at 50 min, and 60% at 60 min.[21] It is critical to correctly estimate brain temperature for expected outcome. Nasopharyngeal and tympanic temperature are measured to estimate brain temperature but are imperfect. For that reason, some groups use electroencephalographic silence to determine the appropriate point at which to discontinue cooling and perfusion. This point is reached by slowly cooling on cardiopulmonary bypass maintaining a maximal temperature gradient between perfusate and patient of < 10°C. The head is then packed in ice to maintain a low brain temperature. Methylprednisolone and thiopental administration during cooling are adjunctive measures thought by some to decrease cerebral metabolic requirements during the period of circulatory arrest. Rewarming at the end of the procedure proceeds without exceeding the 10°C temperature gradient to at least 37°C, as core body temperature often falls briefly after cessation of active warming and separation from cardiopulmonary bypass. Furosemide and mannitol are administered to initiate diuresis and as a free radical scavenger following circulatory arrest.

Continued cerebral perfusion during the period of circulatory arrest is a technique used for additional cerebral protection during operations performed on the aortic arch. Flow is delivered in either a retrograde or antegrade fashion. Retrograde cerebral perfusion is useful to flush atherosclerotic material and air from the brachiocephalic vessels. A flow rate to produce a caval pressure of 15 to 25 mm Hg is considered optimal. Recently, selective antegrade cerebral perfusion has become popular. The innominate artery and the left common carotid artery are encircled with vessel occluders and the lumen cannulated with retrograde coronary sinus cannulae. With the left subclavian artery occluded, flow rates are slowly increased to achieve perfusion pressures of 50 to 70 mm Hg at the desired circulatory-arrest temperature.

Aortic arch involvement cannot always be predicted from preoperative studies; consequently, the need for prolonged circulatory arrest is not always known. In that situation, it is useful to systemically cool to 18°C and stop perfusion for a brief period of circulatory arrest. The intima of the aortic arch is then examined. If the intima is intact, the distal anastomosis is performed and the graft cannulated, de-aired, and clamped for resumption of cardiopulmonary bypass with systemic warming. If the intima of the arch is violated, then a hemiarch reconstruction is performed. Only rarely have we done a complete arch resection for an acute dissection.

The exposure for procedures performed on the ascending aorta and the proximal arch is through a median sternotomy. This can be modified with supraclavicular, cervical, or trapdoor incisions to gain exposure to brachiocephalic vessels or the descending thoracic aorta. When dissecting the distal arch, it is important to identify and protect both the left vagus nerve with its recurrent branch and the left phrenic nerve. Replacement of the ascending aorta in type A dissections is best performed by an open distal anastomosis technique if the arch is involved (30%) or if arch involvement is unknown. The open distal anastomotic technique requires clamping the mid-ascending aorta and cardiac arrest via administration of antegrade and/or retrograde cardioplegic solution. The dissected ascending aorta proximal to the clamp is then resected, leaving 5 to 10 mm of normal aorta distal to the sinotubular ridge. The proximal aorta is then reconstructed by reuniting the dissected aortic layers between one or two strips of Teflon felt by using either 3–0 or 4–0 Prolene suture. There has also been a great deal of enthusiasm for reuniting the dissected layers using gelatin-resorcinol-formalin (GRF) glue or the newer BioGlue (Cryolife International Inc., Kennesaw, Georgia). Evaluation and surgical correction of the aortic valve is ideally performed at this time while systemic cooling continues. Once the temperature reaches 20°C, perfusion is discontinued and the aortic clamp is released. The aortic arch is inspected and repaired. If a complex aortic root procedure is required, it is often useful to repair the aortic root with one vascular graft and then to use a separate graft to create the distal aortic anastomosis. The two grafts are then measured, cut, and anastomosed to provide the correct length and orientation for aortic replacement.

If the ascending aorta cannot be cross-clamped, the patient is cooled to 20°C with subsequent circulatory arrest. The distal aortic reconstruction is performed first in this circumstance, at which time the graft is cannulated and proximally clamped with resumption of cardiopulmonary bypass and systemic rewarming. Cannulation of the graft for antegrade systemic perfusion and rewarming is associated with improved neurologic outcome, when compared with retrograde perfusion, and should be performed whenever possible. Newly available vascular grafts include 7 to 8 mm Dacron side-arm grafts for easy cannulation to facilitate this technique. Because a cross-clamp is not applied, the left ventricle must be decompressed once fibrillation starts during systemic cooling (~20°C) to prevent distension and irreversible myocardial injury. Proximal ascending aortic repair is completed during the period of rewarming.

An alternative to the open distal technique is possible when dissection is limited to the ascending aorta or to the proximal arch away from the origin of the brachiocephalic vessels. Arterial perfusion is achieved antegrade, through distal arch cannulation, or retrograde, via cannulation of a femoral artery. An aortic cross-clamp is applied tangentially just proximal to the innominate artery. The ascending aorta is resected to include the inferior aspect of the arch. The layers of the dissected aorta proximal to the clamp are then reunited if necessary, and the aorta is replaced with an appropriately sized, beveled vascular graft. The proximal reconstruction and anastomosis may then be performed without the need for deep hypothermia and circulatory arrest.

When aortic root dissection fails to violate the intima of the coronary artery, repair of the ascending aorta at the sinotubular junction is often sufficient to reunite the aortic root layers and provide unimpeded coronary blood flow. Minimal disruption of the coronary ostial intima may be repaired primarily with 5–0 Prolene suture. If, however, the ostium is circumferentially dissected and an aortic root replacement is necessary, an aortic button should be excised and the layers reunited with either running 5–0 Prolene suture or glue (Figure 36-9). The button may then be reimplanted into a vascular graft or to a separate 8 mm vascular graft as part of a Cabral-type repair. Aortocoronary bypass grafting is performed only when the coronary ostium is not reconstructible and as a last resort.

Aortic regurgitation is present in up to 75% of type A dissections and is often caused by the loss of commissural support of the valve leaflets. Resuspension of the valve commissures using pledgeted 4–0 Prolene sutures passed through the commissure and the reconstructed aortic wall is the simplest and most effective surgical solution (Figure 36-10). The valve commissures may also be resuspended

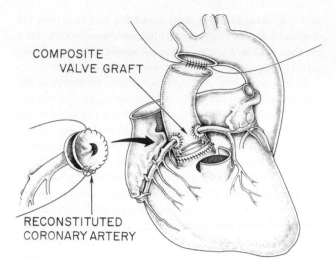

FIGURE 36-9. If the aortic valve cannot be preserved, an aortic root replacement is performed using a composite valve graft. The coronary arteries are excised and the dissected layers repaired with Teflon felt and/or glue as described. The coronary buttons are then reimplanted into a valved conduit as part of a Bentall procedure.

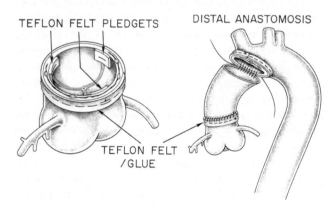

FIGURE 36-10. Reconstruction of the dissected layers of the aortic root is performed using Teflon felt and/or glue. Resuspension of the aortic valve commissures using pledgeted Prolene sutures is often sufficient to achieve aortic valve competence when the intima of the aortic root is intact. The distal ascending aorta is similarly reconstructed and the intervening aorta is replaced with a vascular graft.

into a vascular graft to spare a normal aortic valve in the setting of annuloaortic ectasia.[22] Other surgical techniques exist to recreate the sinuses of Valsalva, which may be more important than previously recognized. If the aortic valve cannot be spared, replacement of the ascending aorta and valve should be performed using a composite valve graft or homograft. The composite valve graft is implanted using horizontal mattress 2–0 Tycron sutures to encircle the annulus and to seat the valved conduit. The previously excised and reconstituted coronary buttons are reimplanted into the vascular graft with running 5–0 Prolene suture. The left button is implanted first, at which time the graft is clamped and placed under pressure to define the proper orientation and position of the right

coronary button. The aortic homograft is similarly implanted using horizontal mattress 2–0 Tycron sutures except that a generous margin of aortic root below the coronary buttons is retained for a second hemostatic suture line of running 4–0 Prolene.

Chronic type A dissection, with or without aneurysmal enlargement, is treated by using many of the same operative techniques described for the acute setting. Treatment of the distal anastomosis is controversial because some surgeons advocate obliteration of flow into the false lumen, whereas other surgeons purposely maintain flow into the true lumen and false lumen through distal resection of the intimal flap. Those surgeons who reunite the chronically dissected aortic layers to perfuse only the true lumen maintain that the false lumen remains perfused through distal reentry tears in more than 50% of patients. Alternatively, there is a theoretical and possibly real concern that important side branches arise exclusively from the false lumen and perfusion may be interrupted with this technique. The practice at the University of Virginia is to resect the distal chronic dissection flap to obviate such concerns. The distal anastomosis is made to the outer wall of the aorta, which has nearly the structural integrity of normal aorta. The rate of aortic valve replacement for aortic regurgitation is much higher in patients with chronic dissection. Morphologic changes in the valvular apparatus appear to occur, which renders the valve irreparable in as many as 50% of cases. Two options exist for aortic valve replacement and repair of the ascending aorta: aortic valve replacement with separate ascending aortic replacement or composite valve replacement. We favor the composite valve graft replacement to remove all potentially abnormal aortic tissue from the root and the potential for aneurysmal dilatation or redissection.

The right lateral decubitus position is optimal for surgical treatment of acute type B dissections requiring operation. The pelvis is canted posteriorly to allow access to both sets of femoral vessels. A posterolateral thoracotomy in the fourth intercostal space provides sufficient access to the aorta; notching the fifth and sixth ribs posteriorly permits visualization of the entire thoracic aorta distally. A thoracoabdominal incision may be required to access the abdominal aorta and is performed either through the abdomen or the retroperitoneum. The left hemidiaphragm is carefully divided in a radial fashion while marking adjacent sites on each side of the division with metal clips. This provides necessary exposure and facilitates subsequent diaphragm approximation.

The operation most frequently performed for acute type B dissection is replacement of the proximal third of the descending thoracic aorta. This includes the site of the primary tear in the majority of cases. After gaining access to the thoracic aorta, the mediastinum between the left subclavian and the left common carotid arteries is dissected and the left subclavian artery encircled with an umbilical tape and Rommel tourniquet. It is essential that the left vagus and recurrent laryngeal nerves are identified and preserved during the course of the dissection. Ultimately, the entire distal arch must be free enough to place an aortic clamp between the left common carotid and the left subclavian arteries. Next, the proximal descending thoracic aorta is circumferentially mobilized, dividing intercostal and bronchial arteries in the segment to be excised. The left inferior pulmonary vein is then dissected and a 4–0 Prolene purse-string suture placed posteriorly. Following the administration of 100 U/kg of intravenous heparin, 14 French cannulae are inserted into the left inferior pulmonary vein and either the descending thoracic aorta or either femoral artery (Figure 36-11). Partial left-heart bypass is then initiated, with flow rates between 1 and 2 L/min. The left subclavian artery is controlled and vascular clamps are placed on the aorta proximally and distally on the midthoracic aorta. Right radial artery pressure is measured to maintain proximal aortic systolic pressure between 100 and 140 mm Hg and mean femoral artery pressure > 60 mm Hg.[23] The aorta is then opened longitudinally and backbleeding intercostal arteries are oversewn. Proximally, the aorta is transected distal to the origin of the left subclavian artery. The size of the vascular graft is based on the diameter of the distal aorta and beveled proximally. The proximal anastomosis is made to undissected aorta using 3–0 Prolene suture and Teflon felt strips if necessary. This anastomosis may include the origin of the left subclavian to deal with dissection in this vessel. A separate 6 to 8 mm Dacron graft can be used if

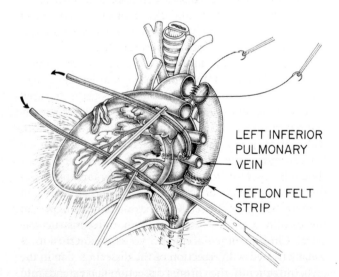

FIGURE 36-11. Partial left-heart bypass is used to repair type B dissections. Cannulation of the normal descending thoracic aorta is possible for limited dissections or aneurysms, but femoral arterial cannulation is sometimes necessary. In the acute setting, repair of the proximal and distal dissected layers with Teflon felt and/or glue and replacement of the proximal third of the descending thoracic aorta are often adequate. Chronic dissections require resection of the intimal flap to maintain perfusion of both lumen and to prevent malperfusion. The chronically thickened outer aortic wall is used in such cases for anastamosis to a vascular graft.

LEFT INFERIOR PULMONARY VEIN

TEFLON FELT STRIP

there is intimal disruption involving the proximal segment of the left subclavian artery. Once the proximal anastomosis is complete, the proximal clamp is released and repositioned on the vascular graft to inspect the anastomosis. Attention is then turned to repairing the distal aorta with Teflon felt or glue for distal anastomosis. The distal anastomosis is completed, the clamps are released, and partial left-heart bypass is terminated. Decannulation and closure are routine. Percutaneously placed femoral artery cannulae that are 15 French or smaller may be removed without direct repair. When cannulae larger than 15 French are required, surgical repair is indicated.

An alternative surgical strategy for acute type B dissection involving the abdominal aorta requires the use of total cardiopulmonary bypass and deep hypothermic circulatory arrest to prevent potential spinal cord and intra-abdominal ischemia.[24] After creation of a thoracoabdominal incision, the thoracic and abdominal aorta is exposed from the left subclavian artery to the aortic bifurcation. The femoral artery and vein are cannulated for cardiopulmonary bypass with systemic cooling and circulatory arrest. Cardiopulmonary bypass is then interrupted and the aorta opened proximally. The arch is repaired if necessary with Teflon felt or glue and the proximal anastomosis created. The graft is clamped distal to the anastomosis and then cannulated for proximal perfusion with resumption of cardiopulmonary bypass. Intercostal arteries to the upper third of the thoracic aorta are divided; larger vessels below T9 are reimplanted into the back of the graft with 4–0 Prolene suture. As vessels are reimplanted, the proximal clamp is moved distally to maintain spinal cord perfusion. Abdominal aortic branch vessels are divided from the wall of the aorta with a 5 mm cuff for reimplantation. Usually the right renal, superior mesenteric, and celiac arteries, as well as several intercostal and lumbar arteries, are removed as a patch and reimplanted into the graft. The left renal artery often originates from a dissected segment of the aorta and is reimplanted after repair. The inferior mesenteric artery and lumbar vessels that bleed are controlled by suture ligation. If the intima of abdominal aortic branch vessels is involved, then repair is carried out with 5–0 Prolene suture. Once all side branches are secured, the distal anastomosis to the aortic bifurcation is performed, reuniting, if necessary, the aortic layers distally. Rewarming should commence as the final aortic branch vessels are being sewn in place.

Two potential situations during repair of acute type B dissection deserve mention. Rupture of the thoracic aorta prior to or during repair often leads to operative death. Successful management requires immediate cannulation of the femoral artery and vein for cardiopulmonary bypass and eventual circulatory arrest, but only if the ruptured area can be locally controlled. While assisted venous drainage through the femoral vein is often adequate, direct cannulation of the right ventricle may also be performed.

Unexpected dissection of the arch extending proximal to the aortic clamp may also require circulatory arrest and performance of an open proximal anastomosis for repair. The techniques for repair of the arch using Teflon felt or glue are identical to those discussed earlier. It is preferable to avoid this situation through preoperative recognition of arch involvement by using high-quality imaging.

Spinal cord ischemia resulting in paraplegia or paraparesis is a catastrophic complication of dissection repair that may now be partially preventable. Spinal cord ischemia occurs in up to 19% of patients following repair of acute dissection; the incidence is much lower, 2.9%, when the indication is aneurysmal disease resulting from chronic dissection.[19] Various strategies to prevent spinal cord ischemia during repair of chronic dissection secondary to aneurysmal dilatation have been devised. Use of partial left-heart bypass appears sufficient for patients with aneurysmal dilatation of the thoracic aorta above the level of T9 and results in paraplegia in fewer than 5% of those patients.[25] Thoracoabdominal aneurysms require additional measures and have a paraplegia rate as high as 10% following surgery. Preoperative identification of the anterior spinal artery origin to preserve its perfusion is one such measure, but its efficacy is controversial. Reimplanting intercostal and lumbar arteries between T9 and L1 while moving the clamp distally has reported benefit in several series.[26] Other methods used for spinal cord protection include measurement of sensory- and motor-evoked potentials, spinal cord cooling, cerebrospinal fluid drainage, and the use of a variety of pharmacologic agents for cellular protection. We presently use left-atrial-to-femoral-artery bypass and reimplant key intercostal arteries.

Malperfusion Syndrome

Malperfusion of aortic branch vessels may occur from the coronary ostia to the aortic bifurcation and may dominate the presentation of certain patients. Although autopsy series yield a greater percentage of patients with evidence of malperfusion, clinical series reveal that dissection is often complicated by malperfusion of at least one organ system (Table 36-6).[13,27] Compression of the true lumen by the false lumen is the mechanism by which aortic branch vessels are occluded in the majority of cases. Branch vessels may also be completely sheared off the true lumen and perfused to various degrees by the false lumen. Malperfusion is treated in a variety of ways, from primary surgical repair of the dissection to catheter-based or open fenestration.

Percutaneous fenestration and stenting are relatively new adjuncts to the surgical management of malperfusion syndromes. Renewed interest in these procedures grew from the recognition that hospital mortality of the various malperfusion syndromes was as high as 60%.[28] Surgical fenestration to treat malperfusion, however, can reduce the mortality to under 20%.[29,30] Indications for percutaneous fenestration and endovascular stent placement were developed to treat malperfusion syndrome in the hope of improving outcome even further. Direct stenting of obstructed branch vessels and percutaneous fenestration with or without placement of a stent in the true lumen are the procedures most commonly performed. In certain situations, stents may be placed across an existing distal reentry tear to maintain patency and perfusion of the true lumen and the branch vessels. Balloon fenestration may be required to create such a communication between the true lumen and false lumen or to prevent thrombosis of the false lumen from which branch vessels may originate. Early results indicate that this procedure is both safe and effective, with restoration of flow in up to 90% of patients with an average 10 to 25% 30-day mortality.[31,32] Given that the majority of postsurgical mortality in this group relates to the duration of concomitant malperfusion in patients with acute dissection, one group advocates percutaneous reperfusion followed by surgical repair.[33] Percutaneous treatment of malperfusion, however, is performed subsequent to surgical repair of the dissection in most reports.

The techniques used for surgical treatment of malperfusion are dependent upon location but are quite similar. Malperfusion of the brachiocephalic vessels is repaired acutely by reuniting the dissected aortic layers proximally and reperfusing the true lumen when the intima is intact. If the intima is violated or the dissection extends into the left common carotid or innominate arteries, the vessel should be resected from the arch, the layers reunited, and the vessel reimplanted into the arch, perhaps with an interposition graft if necessary. Extra-anatomic bypass to the carotid arteries is an option in unreconstructable cases. Chronic brachiocephalic vessel malperfusion is usually treated with resection of the dissection flap in the arch. Infrequently, the chronic dissection flap extends into the branch vessels and may present as transient ischemic attacks or stroke. In such cases, it is often necessary to resect the dissection flap into the branch vessel or to reunite the layers distally prior to reimplantation.

Malperfusion of the intra-abdominal viscera may be apparent at presentation but may also complicate repair of either type A or B dissections. Proximal repair of the dissection is standard treatment, but if this fails, or if malperfusion persists despite repair, an additional procedure is

TABLE 36-6. Frequency and Location of Malperfusion in Acute Type A and B Thoracic Aortic Dissection

Vascular System	Frequency (%)
Renal	23–75
Extremities (upper and lower)	25–60
Mesenteric	10–20
Coronary	5–11
Cerebral	3–13
Spinal	2–9

necessary. The options are either open surgical or percutaneous fenestration of the dissection flap. The percutaneous procedure is performed by pulling an inflated balloon through the dissection flap or by using a fenestration knife. A surgical fenestration procedure is performed through a midline laparotomy with exposure of the infrarenal aorta. Proximal and distal control of the aorta is obtained and a transverse aortotomy created. The dissection flap is resected proximally as far as possible but at least to the level of the renal arteries. The distal dissection flap is reunited with the aortic wall by using Teflon felt or glue, and the aorta closed primarily or by using a short interposition vascular graft. Occasionally, fenestration of intra-abdominal aortic branch vessels is required if the intima is violated beyond the ostia. If the dissection flap cannot be completely excised, the distal vessel layers must be reunited. Consideration should be given to closure of these smaller vessels with patch angioplasty to prevent narrowing. In the event that perfusion is not re-established, extra-anatomic bypass may be required.

Obstruction of the terminal aorta or malperfusion of the lower extremities following operative repair is best treated with percutaneous or open fenestration. The most appropriate surgical option if that fails is femoral–femoral bypass grafting in the setting of unilateral malperfusion, or axillofemoral and femoral–femoral bypass grafting if bilateral lower extremity malperfusion exists.

Postoperative Management

Invasive hemodynamic monitoring is used to ensure adequate end-organ perfusion while maintaining systolic blood pressure between 90 and 110 mm Hg. Early on, blood pressure control is achieved by using narcotics and sedative/hypnotic agents. The patient is allowed to emerge from general anesthesia briefly for a gross neurologic examination. The patient is then sedated for a period to ensure continued hemodynamic stability and to eliminate concerns over bleeding. Coagulopathy is aggressively treated with antifibrinolytic agents and blood products as necessary, and by warming the patient. Hematocrit, platelet count, coagulation studies, and serum electrolytes are obtained and corrected as necessary. An ECG and chest radiograph are obtained to assess for abnormalities and to serve as baseline studies. A full physical exam, including a complete peripheral vascular exam, is performed upon arrival in the intensive care unit. Despite adequate repair of the dissection, perfusion of the false lumen may persist and might cause a malperfusion syndrome. If an abdominal malperfusion syndrome is suspected postoperatively, this should be aggressively evaluated with ultrasound and subsequent angiography if positive. A strong clinical suspicion is enough to warrant this evaluation given the consequences of failed recognition. In the morning, if the patient has been hemodynamically stable without excessive bleeding and has a normal neurologic exam, the patient may be extubated. Management is routine from that point forward.

Long-Term Management

Surviving the operation for acute dissection represents the beginning of a lifelong requirement for meticulous medical management and continued close observation. It has been estimated that replacement of the ascending aorta for type A dissection obliterates flow in the distal false lumen in fewer than 10% of patients. As a result, the natural history of repaired dissection may involve dilatation and potential rupture of the chronically dissected segment of aorta. This occurred and was the reason for late death in nearly 30% of DeBakey's original series in 1982, and is currently the leading cause of late death following surgical repair.[34] Often a multidrug antihypertensive regimen that includes β-blocking agents is required to maintain systolic blood pressure below 120 mm Hg. There are some data indicating that blood pressure control within a narrow range may alter the natural history of chronic dissection by diminishing the rate of aneurysmal dilatation. Follow-up diagnostic imaging is required to monitor aortic size in such patients. The current recommendations for follow-up diagnostic imaging are to obtain a baseline study prior to discharge and at a 6-month interval during the first year. If the aorta remains unchanged, this interval is then prolonged to 1 year. If the aorta is enlarging at a rate greater then 0.5 cm per 6 months or becoming more eccentric on comparison of three-dimensional reconstruction images, then the interval is decreased to 3 months, if surgery is not indicated.

Chronic aortic dissection develops in patients who fail to undergo immediate surgical treatment of type A dissection and in those who are successfully treated medically for type B dissection. The natural history of acute dissection rarely involves spontaneous healing with absence of flow in the false lumen and aortic wall thickening. This phenomenon is observed in 4 to 31% of medically treated patients. As complete thrombosis of the false lumen appears necessary for healing, patients with distal communication of the false lumen may go on to develop aneurysmal dilatation of the aorta. The natural history of this process has been examined and reveals that there is an annual rate of expansion of 2 to 3 mm/year in communicating dissections, and the rate is 1 mm/year in those not communicating. Infrequently, chronic dissection may cause pain and result in paralysis/paraplegia from loss of important intercostal arteries or even distal embolization of thrombus or atheroma from the false lumen. The operative indications for chronic dissection include symptoms, rupture, malperfusion, and aneurysm size.

Spiral CT arteriogram and MRI are the imaging studies of choice to use when following patients with repaired or chronic aortic dissection. MRI and ultrasonography are useful to use with patients with renal insufficiency and for those patients requiring only imaging of the abdominal aorta. Echocardiography is useful for imaging the ascending aorta and provides additional information regarding the aortic valve. It is important to recognize the resolution limitations of each imaging modality and the inherent imprecision of comparing different imaging modalities to evaluate changes. In general, measurements should be made at the same anatomic level with respect to reproducible anatomic structures (ie, the sinotubular ridge, proximal to the innominate or left subclavian arteries or at the diaphragmatic hiatus). It is important to recognize that the false lumen should be included in measurements of aortic diameter whether it is perfused or not. Three-dimensional reconstruction of spiral CT and MRI scans minimize the error introduced by aortic eccentricity when comparing imaging studies and has simplified following this patient population.

The size criteria indicating operative intervention for thoracic aortic aneurysms were recently reviewed by the Yale group and include patients with chronic aortic dissection. These criteria suggest that replacement should be performed for ascending aortic size greater than 5.5 cm, or greater than 5 cm if a connective tissue disorder is present. In the descending thoracic aorta, replacement is indicated at 6.5 cm, or at 6 cm if there is a family history or physical stigmata of a connective tissue disorder.[35] Eccentricity of the aorta was also predictive of rupture as was rapid expansion and continued smoking. Such factors should be considered when deciding whether to operate based on aneurysm size.

Despite appropriate medical management and close follow-up, nearly 23% of patients with chronic dissection require operation for aneurysmal dilatation at 10 years. Reoperation is necessary in 10% at 5 years and in up to 40% at 10 years following type A dissection repair. This number is even higher in patients with Marfan's disease. Nearly 20% of patients require reoperation following valve preservation at the initial operation secondary to progressive aortic regurgitation. These operations carry a higher mortality and morbidity, which is made worse in the emergency setting and when the ascending aorta or arch is involved.

Results

The operative mortality for repair of acute aortic dissection has steadily fallen over the years with development of better vascular graft material, more effective hemostatic agents and improvements in the safety of cardiopulmonary bypass. In the last decade, most centers report an operative mortality for acute type A dissection of between 14 and 27.5%.[36–38] The majority of deaths occur as a result of stroke, myocardial ischemia/heart failure, and malperfusion. The operative mortality of patients suffering acute type B dissection (28 to 65%) is higher than for type A

dissection because the indications for surgery are failure of medical management or complications of dissection, as previously discussed.[39] The most recent data from a multicenter international registry, however, reveal that such a disparity in operative mortality between acute type A and B dissections may be disappearing. The mortality in that study was 27% acute type A and 29% acute type B dissection ($p = $ NS).[16]

The published results for long-term survival for acute type A dissection surgically treated over the last decade are roughly 55 to 75% at 5 years and between 32 and 65% at 10 years.[40, 41] Following operative repair of acute type B dissection, the 5-year survival averages 48%, with 29% alive at 10 years.[41]

The operative mortality for chronic type A dissection is between 4 and 17% and on average is very similar to that reported for chronic type B repair at 10 to 15%.[40,42] The actuarial survival following operation for chronic type A and B dissections is not different at 5 years (59 to 75%) or at 10 years (45%).[41]

References

1. Nicholls F. Observations concerning the body of his late majesty. Philos Trans R Soc Lond 1762;52:265.
2. Laennec R. Traite de l'Ausculattion Mediate. 2nd ed. 1826; T.2:693.
3. Abbott OA. Clinical experiences with application of polythene cellophane upon aneurysms of thoracic vessels. J Thorac Surg 1949;18:435–61.
4. Gurin D. Dissecting aneurysms of the aorta. Diagnosis and operative relief of acute arterial obstruction due to this cause. N Y State J Med 1935;35:1200–2
5. DeBakey ME, Cooley DA, Creech O. Surgical considerations of dissecting aneurysm of the aorta. Ann Surg 1955;142:586–612.
6. Creech O, DeBakey ME, Cooley DA. Surgical treatment of dissecting aneurysm of the aorta. Tex State J Med 1956;52:287–94.
7. Coady MA, Rizzo JA, Goldstein LJ, et al. Natural history, pathogenesis, and etiology of thoracic aortic aneurysms and dissections. Cardiol Clin 1999;17:615–35.
8. Erbel R, Alfonso F, Boileau C, et al. Diagnosis and management of aortic dissection: recommendations of the Task Force on Aortic Dissection, European Society of Cardiology. Eur Heart J 2001;22:1642–81.
9. DeBakey ME, Beall AC Jr, Cooley DA, et al. Dissecting aneurysms of the aorta. Surg Clin North Am 1966;46:1045–55.
10. Daily PO, Trueblood HW, Stinson EB, et al. Management of acute aortic dissections. Ann Thorac Surg 1970;10:237–47.
11. Larson EW, Edwards WD. Risk factors for aortic dissection: a necropsy study of 161 cases. Am J Cardiol 1984;53:849-55.
12. Coady MA, Rizzo JA, Elefteriades JA. Pathologic variants of thoracic aorta dissection: penetrating atherosclerotic ulcers and intramural hematomas. Cardiol Clin 1999;17:637–57.

13. Neri E, Toscono T, Papilia U, et al. Proximal aortic dissection with coronary malperfusion: presentation, management, and outcome. J Thorac Cardiovasc Surg 2001;121:552–60.

14. Wheat MW, Palmer RF, Bartley TD, et al. Treatment of dissecting aneurysms of the aorta without surgery. J Thorac Cardiovasc Surg 1965;50:364–73.

15. Scholl FG, Coady MA, Davies RR, et al. Interval or permanent non-operative management of type A aortic dissection. Arch Surg 1999;134:402–66.

16. Hagan PG, Nienaber CA, Isselbacher EM, et al. The international registry of acute aortic dissection (IRAD): new insights into an old disease. JAMA 2000;283:897–903.

17. Miller DC. The continuing dilemma concerning medical versus surgical management of patients with acute type B dissections. Semin Thorac Cardiovasc Surg 1993;5:33–46.

18. Coady MA, Rizzo JA, Hammond GL, et al. Penetrating ulcer of the thoracic aorta: what is it? How do we recognize it? How do we manage it? J Vasc Surg 1998;27:1006–16.

19. Coselli JS, LeMarie SA, de Figueiredo LP, et al. Paraplegia after thoracoabdominal aneurysm repair: is dissection a risk factor? Ann Thorac Surg 1997;63:28–36.

20. McCullough JN, Zhang N, Reich D, et al. Cerebral metabolic suppression during circulatory arrest in humans. Ann Thorac Surg 1999;67:1895–9.

21. Ergin MA, Griepp EB, Lansman SL, et al. Hypothermic circulatory arrest and other methods of cerebral protection during operations on the thoracic aorta. J Card Surg 1994;9:525–37.

22. David TE, Feindel CM. An aortic valve sparing operation for patients with aortic incompetence and aneurysm of the ascending aorta. J Thorac Cardiovasc Surg 1992;103:617–22.

23. Cunningham JN Jr, Laschinger JC, Spencer FC, et al. Monitoring of somatosensory evoked potentials during surgical procedures on the thoracoabdominal aorta. IV: clinical observations and results. J Thorac Cardiovasc Surg 1987;94:275–85.

24. Kouchoukos NT, Masetti P, Rokkas CK, et al. Safety and efficacy of hypothermic cardiopulmonary bypass and circulatory arrest for operations on the descending thoracic and thoracoabdominal aorta. Ann Thorac Surg 2001;72:699–708.

25. Coselli JS, LeMarie SA. Left heart bypass reduces paraplegia rates following thoracoabdominal aortic aneurysm repair. Ann Thorac Surg 1999;67:1931–4.

26. Safi HJ, Miller CC III, Carr C, et al. Importance of intercostal artery reattachment during thoracoabdominal aortic aneurysm repair. J Vasc Surg 1998;27:58–68.

27. Cambria RP, Brewster DC, Gertler J, et al. Vascular complications associated with spontaneous aortic dissection. J Vasc Surg 1988;7:199–209.

28. Fann JI, Sarris GE, Mitchell RS, et al. Treatment of patients with aortic dissection presenting with peripheral vascular complications. Ann Surg 1990;212:705–13.

29. Lauterbach SR, Cambria RP, Brewster DC, et al. Contemporary management of aortic branch compromise resulting from acute aortic dissection. J Vasc Surg 2001;33:1185–92.

30. Elefteriades JA, Hartleroad J, Gusberg RJ, et al. Long-term experience with descending aortic dissection: the complication-specific approach. Ann Thorac Surg 1992;53:11–20.

31. Slonim SM, Miller DC, Mitchell RS, et al. Percutaneous balloon fenestration and stenting for life-threatening ischemic complications in patients with acute aortic dissection. J Thorac Cardiovasc Surg 1999;117:1118–27.

32. Williams DM, Lee DY, Hamilton BH, et al. The dissected aorta: percutaneous treatment of ischaemic complications-principles and results. J Vasc Interv Radiol 1997;8:605–65.

33. Deeb GM, Williams DM, Bolling SF, et al. Surgical delay for acute type A dissection with malperfusion. Ann Thorac Surg 1997;64:1669–75.

34. DeBakey ME, McCollum CH, Crawford ES, et al. Dissection and dissecting aneurysms of the aorta: twenty-year follow-up of five hundred and twenty-seven patients treated surgically. Surgery 1982;92:1118–34.

35. Coady MA, Rizzo JA, Hammond GL, et al. What is the appropriate size criterion for resection of thoracic aortic aneurysms? J Thorac Cardiovasc Surg 1997;113:476–91.

36. Kirsch M, Soustelle C, Houel R, et al. Risk factor analysis for proximal and distal reoperations after surgery for acute type A aortic dissections. J Thorac Cardiovasc Surg 2002;123:318–25.

37. Ehrlich MP, Ergin MA, McCullough JN, et al. Results of immediate surgical treatment of all acute type A dissections. Circulation 2000;102 Suppl III:III-248–52.

38. Elefteriades JA. What operation for acute type A dissection? J Thorac Cardiovasc Surg 2002;123:201–3.

39. Elefteriades JA, Lovoulos CJ, Coady MA. Management of descending aortic dissection. Ann Thorac Surg 1999;67:2002–5.

40. Sabik JF, Lytle BW, Blackstone EH, et al. Long-term effectiveness of operations for ascending aortic dissections. J Thorac Cardiovasc Surg 2000;119:946–62.

41. Fann JI, Smith JA, Miller DC, et al. Surgical management of aortic dissection during a 30-year period. Circulation 1995;92:II113–21.

42. Safi HJ, Miller CC III, Reardon MJ, et al. Operation for acute and chronic dissection: recent outcome with regard to neurologic deficit and early death. Ann Thorac Surg 1998;66:402–11.

CHAPTER 37

SPINAL CORD PROTECTION DURING OPERATIONS OF THE THORACIC AORTA

LARS G. SVENSSON, MD, PhD

Over the past three decades, much research has focused on the pathophysiology of spinal cord ischemia and methods of protecting the spinal cord during and after surgery. This research, particularly the animal studies, has been reviewed extensively by this author and others. In essence, there are three major events that contribute to spinal cord injury: (1) the degree and duration of spinal cord ischemia during the period of aortic cross-clamping; (2) failure to re-establish spinal cord blood flow during the period of aortic cross-clamping; and (3) postoperative damage to the spinal cord that, at the molecular level, involves complex biochemical cascades of events during the periods of ischemia and reperfusion of the spinal cord. In addition, postoperative events such as hypotension and respiratory problems are important contributing factors to delayed injury.[1-44]

Degree and Duration of Ischemia

Multiple studies show that degree and duration of ischemia are most critical in the development of postoperative spinal cord injury.[1,2,5,7-10,20,24-26,30-32,35,37,40,42,43] There is general agreement that the degree of ischemia is dependent on both the extent of aortic repair and available collateral blood vessels. Indeed, coarctation of the aorta, in which situation there is an extensive network of collateral blood supply, is associated with the lowest risk of postoperative spinal cord injury. In contrast, the extensive Crawford type II thoracoabdominal aneurysm repairs that involve replacement of the aorta from the proximal descending aorta to below the renal arteries are associated with the greatest risk.[9]

Multiple studies show that there is a very strong relationship between aortic cross-clamp time and the risk of neurologic injury, particularly when various protective measures are not used. Thus, performing an expeditious and efficient repair that minimizes the period of aortic cross-clamping continues to be of paramount importance in protecting the spinal cord. As part of this approach, this author and colleagues advocate a method of sequentially and segmentally repairing the aorta that maintains a maximal perfusion of the spinal cord during the period of repair.[1,5,24] Thus, only the proximal part of the descending aorta is clamped off when doing an extensive thoracoabdominal aneurysm repair with distal perfusion of the aorta maintaining intercostal and lumbar artery blood flow up to the proximal descending aorta that is clamped off. After the proximal anastomosis is completed, the clamps are moved further down (typically to above the celiac artery) and the intercostal arteries are then reattached. The proximal descending aorta clamp is then removed and the intercostals reperfused while the segment below the celiac artery clamp is then opened and repaired. This approach effectively maximizes the period of perfusion of the spinal cord during repair. Then, after the visceral segment has been repaired in the type II thoracoabdominal aneurysms, the segment is reperfused and the lower part of the aorta is subsequently repaired. After the distal anastomosis is completed, the patient is rewarmed with distal perfusion. Recently, we reported, in a prospective randomized study based on multivariable analysis, that when using the protective measures and a sequential segmental repair, the intercostal ischemia time was the best predictor of spinal cord injury.

Decreasing the Degree of Ischemia

A useful approach for reducing the degree of ischemia entails maintaining adequate blood flow to the spinal cord as much as possible while simultaneously lowering the metabolic activity of the spinal cord by using hypothermia. The distal perfusion techniques include the use of atriofemoral bypass or perfusion from the left inferior pulmonary vein to the femoral artery with centrifugal pump bypass. Femoral–femoral partial or total cardiopulmonary bypass can also be used, although these are usually reserved for those patients undergoing redo surgery or who have particularly poor pulmonary function from chronic pulmonary disease. Hypothermia can be systemically induced by using atriofemoral bypass or femoral–femoral bypass with a heat exchange in the system, or it can be done locally with epidural cooling, as advocated by Cambria and associates, or by topical cooling of the spinal cord with intrathecal cooling.[15,16,20,43]

Normothermic Distal Perfusion

In a study of 832 descending aorta repairs, in the group of patients who had atriofemoral bypass (247 patients), the incidence of paraplegia/paresis was 6%.[8] The mortality rate was 4%, versus 9% without atriofemoral bypass ($p < .05$). The incidence of acute renal failure was also reduced to 4%, as compared to 8% without atriofemoral bypass ($p < .05$). Furthermore, in a study of 1,509 thoracoabdominal aneurysm repairs, in the 258 patients who had atriofemoral bypass, the incidence of paraplegia was 14%, versus 22% in those patients who did not have atriofemoral bypass ($p = .0025$).[9] For the thoracoabdominal aneurysms, the incidence of acute renal failure was also lowered to 13% in those patients who had atriofemoral bypass, versus 19% in those patients who did not have atriofemoral bypass ($p = .032$). Borst reviewed his experience with 132 patients who underwent atriofemoral bypass with normothermia and reported a 3% mortality rate and a 2.3% paraplegia/paresis rate.[36] Thus, atriofemoral bypass alone appears to have a protective effect, even if done at normothermia.

Hypothermia

Induced hypothermia, typically with deep hypothermia and circulatory arrest, was one of the early techniques used for protecting the spinal cord.[1] This author and colleagues prefer, however, to use active cooling to a moderate hypothermia range of 29° to 32°C based on the method of Swan-Ganz blood temperature monitoring.[1–5] Furthermore, we give patients a lidocaine bolus and put them on a lidocaine drip prior to inducing hypothermia to reduce the risk of any ventricular arrhythmias. In a prospective randomized study of Crawford type I and type II patients, we showed that active cooling with atriofemoral bypass to a moderate hypothermia level was associated with a reduced risk of paraplegia/paresis.[5] In a recent analysis of active cooling with moderate hypothermia and atriofemoral bypass in 72 patients, 3 patients developed a postoperative deficit (1 developed paraplegia; 2 developed paraparesis). Similarly, von Segressor found that active cooling and moderate hypothermia were associated with a reduced negative event rate postoperatively, including paraplegia, death, and surgical revisions.[31]

The use of deep hypothermia with circulatory arrest is usually reserved for complicated cases, such as those patients with distal arch involvement or rupture of the aorta associated with multiple previous descending or thoracoabdominal aorta operations or with intraoperative adverse events. Crawford and colleagues, in their study of deep hypothermia and circulatory arrest through the left chest, reported a 16% mortality rate, a 57% incidence of pulmonary complications, strokes in 9.5%, and paraplegia in 11%.[13] Similarly, Safi and colleagues, using the same technique in high-risk patients, reported a 29% mortality rate and reported that 67% developed pulmonary complications.[32] Of note, encephalopathy was noted in 33% of patients, stroke in 13%, and paraplegia/paresis in 13%.

In contrast, Kouchoukos and colleagues reported excellent results with the more routine use of deep hypothermia with circulatory arrest.[12,33] In a 152-patient series, the 30-day mortality rate was 6.6%, with a 2.7% incidence of paraplegia/paresis; in addition, only 2% developed strokes. Of note in this series, of those patients who underwent emergency operations, the mortality rate was 40%, and for type II thoracoabdominal aneurysms that included emergency surgery, it was 80%. This high mortality rate for emergency thoracoabdominal surgery has been well documented. In one study from Japan, the mortality rate within 3 months of emergency thoracoabdominal aneurysm surgery was 95%. In this author and colleagues' own experience with selective use of profound hypothermic circulatory arrest in 29 patients for aortic arch and/or descending or thoracoabdominal aneurysm repairs, the postoperative mortality rate was 10.3% and the spinal injury rate was 3.6%. Our series included patients who had the entire thoracic or entire aorta replaced in a single operation, extending from the aortic valve down to the celiac artery or to below the bifurcation. By logistic regression analysis we found no significant difference in spinal cord deficits according to the intercostal ischemia time when comparing active cooling with either moderate hypothermia or hypothermic arrest.

The problem following thoracotomy and the use of deep hypothermic circulatory arrest of a high risk of encephalopathy and neurocognitive deficits after surgery was reported in a previous series.[13,32] A possible reason for this could be that air is being trapped in the heart or aortic arch during the repair, which air then embolizes to the brain when reperfusion of the brain recommences with reestablishment of normal cardiac rhythm. Similarly, material in the descending or thoracoabdominal or dissection may embolize during the dissection or femoral perfusion, to cause neurologic injury. A method that this author and colleagues have found useful for establishing cardiopulmonary bypass in these difficult and complex operations is to anastomose an 8 mm tube graft to the right subclavian artery for arterial inflow perfusion.[44] We then place a long venous drainage catheter through the right femoral vein into the right atrium, using transesophageal echocardiography to ensure correct placement of the tip of the drainage cannula. The advantage of this technique is that the arterial inflow of the right subclavian artery can be used for antegrade brain perfusion during a period of circulatory arrest and for flushing out any potential embolic material from the aortic arch. In addition to this method, we routinely flood the field with carbon dioxide at 10 L/min so that any potential air gathering in the heart or aorta is displaced, further reducing the risk of serious air embolization to the brain. Indeed, since we began using this approach, we have been able to reduce the incidence of strokes and neurocognitive deficits.[10]

Cerebrospinal Fluid Drainage with or without Intrathecal Papaverine

The use of cerebrospinal fluid (CSF) drainage was first advocated by Blaisdell and Cooley in the 1960s.[22] Much animal research was performed with varying results as to the effectiveness of CSF drainage.[1–17] In animal studies this author and colleagues did in baboons, we were unable to show that CSF drainage alone during clamping protected the spinal cord, although with the addition of intrathecal papaverine the spinal cord blood flow was improved and paraplegia/paresis was prevented in this group of animals.[17] Also, our measurement of the anterior spinal artery size in these animals showed significant dilation of the vessel, which accounted for improved blood flow to the spinal cord.

In 1991, we performed a prospective randomized study of CSF drainage, although this was limited to a maxium of 50 cc of drainage during a period of aortic cross-clamping and the pressure was kept at 10 mm Hg.[24] Of note, postoperative CSF drainage was not used in this study. This study failed to show any immediate benefit in humans when using CSF drainage with the described protocol, although the incidence of delayed spinal cord injury appeared to be reduced in this group of patients when episodes of hypotension or respiratory failure occurred ($p = .08$). Subsequently, two prospective randomized studies were performed, one by us and one by Coselli and colleagues, that show that for Crawford type I and type II thoracoabdominal aneurysms, CSF drainage significantly reduces the incidence of deficits.[5,35,42] In our study, we also used intrathecal papaverine prior to aortic cross-clamping. During the period of aortic cross-clamping, CSF was allowed to drain freely as long as it was not bloodstained; after aortic clamping, the CSF drainage was stopped until the patient arrived in the intensive care unit. In the intensive care unit, CSF drainage was continued if the CSF pressure exceeded approximately 7 cm of water so that a rate of drainage of approximately 15 to 25 mL an hour was enabled. In that prospective randomized study, the incidence of permanent deficits was 3%. The study by Cosselli documented similar results for type I and type II thoracoabdominal aneurysms. Furthermore, Safi and colleagues advocate the combination of CSF drainage with distal aortic perfusion at normothermia, and in a recent study of descending aortic repairs, the occurence of deficits was 0.9% (1 of 105

patients), and for their thoracoabdominal type I and type II, the incidence was 6% (14 of 239 patients).[7,30,32,39]

Thus, based on our own studies and on the reports by Safi and Coselli, we recommend CSF drainage both during the period of aortic cross-clamping and postoperatively. Indeed, in our study we continued to drain CSF postoperatively for 40 to 48 h after surgery. Of particular note, we and others have found that when delayed paraplegia/paresis occurs, the reinsertion of a catheter for CSF drainage may reverse the incidence of delayed deficits.

For the type I and type II thoracoabdominal aneurysms, the incidence of neurologic deficits was significantly reduced to 3% with CSF drainage and intrathecal preservative papaverine. Although this author and colleagues do not have a prospective randomized study specifically assessing intrathecal papaverine, based on our animal studies, we believe that intrathecal papaverine, has an additive protective effect on the spinal cord, including improving collateral blood flow down the longitudinal vessels on the spinal cord.[1,17] In our first study of intrathecal papaverine in a pilot study of 34 patients, the incidence of deficits was reduced to 2.9%. The one event was related to a delayed deficit. In a more recent evaluation of 61 patients treated with CSF drainage and intrathecal papaverine, 3 patients developed permanent paraplegia/paresis (4.9%). We have also done animal studies using intrathecal perfusion of the spinal cord with cold Ringer lactate and added papaverine to prevent any spinal cord spasm. In the porcine model that we used, the combination significantly reduced postoperative deficits. Cambria and colleagues took a different approach, and in a recent report of 170 patients, they found that using their method of epidural cooling reduced the incidence of spinal cord injury when compared to the historical controls.[20,43]

Finally, in our prospective randomized study showing the relationship of spinal cord injury to the time of aortic cross-clamping, the sigmoid curve shifted to the right with the use of either CSF drainage or intrathecal papaverine. It was shifted even further to the right with active cooling with atriofemoral bypass, and when the two methods were combined, this resulted in the greatest protective effect (Table 37-1).

Reestablishment of Spinal Cord Blood Flow

In 90% of patients the artery of Adamkiewicz arises between T6 and L1, and in 80% of patients the vessel arises from the left segmental intercostal or lumbar arteries.[1,17] While this is the largest of the radicula arteries that supply the spinal cord, the other thoracic radicula arteries are also important to spinal cord blood supply. The reason for this is that the other higher thoracic intercostal arteries that give off the thoracic radicula arteries supply the anterior spinal artery with blood flow up and down the length of anterior spinal artery. This differs from the artery of Adamkiewicz, which is also known as the arteria radicularis magna (ARM), because this artery takes a hairpin bend where it

TABLE 37-1. Techniques that Protect the Spinal Cord

1. Expeditious and efficient repair
   Sequential segmental repair
   Transection of the aorta
   Extensive use of second-stage elephant trunk technique
   Open anastomosis in selected patients

2. Distal perfusion
   Atriofemoral or left inferior pulmonary vein to femoral or partial or total cardiopulmonary bypass

3. Hypothermia
   Systemic
   Local
   Deep hypothermia with circulatory arrest

4. CSF drainage with or without intrathecal papaverine

5. Reattachment of all segmental arteries from intercostal T6 to and including L1

6. Prevention of postoperative hemodynamic instability or deoxygenation or respiratory problems

7. Consideration of pharmacologic agents

8. Consideration of monitoring techniques
   Motor-evoked potentials or spinal cord oxygen saturation

CSF = cerebrospinal fluid.

joins the anterior spinal artery and perfuses the segment of the spinal cord below it, typically the lumbar expansion of the spinal cord. In animal experiments, tying off the ARM has resulted in a 50 to 100% incidence of paraplegia or paresis, particularly in monkey experiments. In the experience of this author and colleagues, however, the ARM may not be quite so critical in spinal cord protection in humans. Rather, in humans, collaterals have developed to the spinal cord because the segmented intercostal or lumbar arteries have been occluded by dissection or clot. We believe that collateral blood flow is an even more important factor in protecting the spinal cord, particularly when dissection or clots within an aneurysm occlude intercostal arteries, especially the artery supplying the ARM. Hence, maintaining blood flow through the other thoracic and lumbar arteries is important, particularly because this can be a vital source of collateral blood flows, as we have documented in some of our studies by using hydrogen mapping of blood-flow patterns to the spinal cord.[4,14,20]

Although preoperative angiography to document the blood supply to the spinal cord has been attempted, there are several problems with this technique.[1] First, patients often require an anesthetic, which procedure has associated risks. Second, the time to do the mapping of the entire potential spinal cord blood supply is lengthy. Third, it is documented that paraplegia or paresis can be induced by the mapping of the spinal cord.[1] Finally, patients have died during the procedure from rupture of the aorta or from complications such as renal failure caused by the large dye load required to perform the mapping.[1] Thus, we do not advocate the use of preoperative angiography for assessment of blood supply for thoracoabdominal aneurysm repairs. Based on our cadaver dissections examining the

spinal cord blood supply in humans, as well as on our studies in primates and the use of hydrogen mapping, we advocate that the critical vessels be reattached during surgery from T6 down to L2. In 98 patients undergoing type I or type II thoracoabdominal aneurysm repairs in whom we carefully examined the patency or occlusion of the segmental arteries, we found that the management of these vessels strongly influenced outcome postoperatively.[10] If patients had patent intercostal or lumbar arteries between the T10 and L1 segments that were not reattached during the time of the aortic repair, the incidence of paraplegia/paresis postoperatively was 63%, in contrast to a 25% incidence rate in patients in whom these vessels were present and reattached ($p = .05$). Similarly, studies by Ross and colleagues and by Safi and colleagues show a higher incidence of paraplegia/paresis when patent intercostal or lumbar arteries were not reattached at the time of surgery in these segments.[38,39]

For patients with descending aortic aneurysm, the importance of these vessels is not quite as clear. The reason for this is as discussed above; the radicula arteries that join the anterior spinal artery can perfuse the spinal cord both upward and downward. Thus, any vessels that are sacrificed during the repair may be compensated for from other radicula arteries and from segments above or below the segment that was repaired. Thus, collateral blood flow may continue to perfuse the anterior spinal artery adequately. This author and colleagues' research in animals, however, shows that if only the ARM is perfused, then the blood flow through this vessel does not protect the lower thoracic spinal cord. In a series of 132 descending aortic repairs, Borst found that all the paraplegia/paresis events that occurred were in those patients in whom the repair was continued to below T8.[36] Similarly, in our study of 832 patients undergoing descending aortic repairs, the patients who had the distal half of the descending aorta replaced had the highest risk of developing paraplegia or paresis.[8] In Estera and colleagues' study of 148 patients undergoing descending aortic repairs in combination with CSF drainage and distal aortic perfusion, the repair of the distal descending aorta was associated with the greatest risk.[30] Similarly, Griepp and colleagues found that clipping most of the descending intercostal arteries was safe, but they did note that the risk of paraplegia was increased with the increasing number of segmental intercostal or lumbar arteries being divided.[40] Based on this research in both animals and humans, we recommend that if the descending aorta is replaced below T8, then these vessels should be preserved.

The results of intraluminal grafting and the incidence of paraplegia/paresis are of interest.[6,41] Because these patients treated by stent grafts do not have significant ischemia during the insertion of the grafts, the incidence of paraplegia/paresis in these patients is largely dependent on the occlusion of intercostal vessels or lumbar arteries or the embolization of these vessels. Thus, just as we showed in 832 patients who underwent aortic repairs, the incidence of paraplegia/paresis increased when the abdominal aorta had been previously repaired.[8] The Stanford studies with intraluminal grafts found similar results.[6,41] In those patients in whom the lower descending aorta was occluded and who had previously undergone abdominal aneurysm repairs, the incidence of paraplegia/paresis was increased.

This author and colleagues have used intraoperative methods in an attempt to determine which vessels need to be reattached at the time of surgery so as to shorten the period of aortic cross-clamping. Our work with hydrogen mapping of the spinal cord showed that this method was accurate and did tend to reduce the period of aortic cross-clamping, although the equipment required is quite cumbersome and it is largely a research method.[4,14,26] Similarly, our research demonstrates that monitoring the spinal cord oxygen saturation with a platinum electrode alongside the spinal cord by using the polargraphic technique was also valuable. The oxygen saturation alongside the spinal cord drops within 30 to 90 s with aortic cross-clamping both in humans and in porcine experiments. With the reestablishment of blood flow to the spinal cord, this is rapidly corrected if the critical intercostal or lumbar arteries have been reattached.[1,4,14,20] This is a method that may have future prospects for monitoring adequate spinal cord blood-flow reestablishment. Our research also shows that, based on using postoperative highly selective angiography in some patients, the reattached intercostal or lumbar arteries clot off in the postoperative period. This is clearly a surgical technique issue that may account for some of the postoperative spinal cord injuries, particularly the delayed deficits associated with hypotension, as we have shown in the porcine model. One operative modification that we have undertaken to reduce this risk is that we no longer use catheters in the individual intercostal or lumbar arteries to prevent backbleeding. This should reduce the risk of injuries and the risk that rupture of these arteries will result in clot formation.

Prevention of Postoperative Hemodynamic Instability and Induced Hypertension

With the increasing success of spinal cord protection during the period of aortic cross-clamping, we have seen a greater proportion of delayed deficits post surgery even though the total number of events has been reduced. To reduce the risk of delayed deficits, we now routinely maintain our patients' postoperative blood pressure at a higher level, typically in a range above 80 mm Hg mean pressure. While this does increase the potential risk of postoperative bleeding, we believe this has contributed to a lower incidence of delayed deficits. In a recent analysis of 132 descending or thoracoabdominal aneurysm repairs, 6 patients developed a delayed deficit (4.5%). In these patients, the deficits were a result of hypotension or pulmonary complications that required the patients to be re-intubated. This further supports the use of CSF drainage for at least the first 2 days post-operation, which is when the patients are most likely to have hypotension or respiratory problems. In addition, extubation is delayed to the second postoperative day.

The Use of Medications

Many animal studies show that specific medications or agents may reduce the incidence of neurologic injury.[1,17] However, there are no successful prospective randomized studies in humans demonstrating that these agents are effective in reducing the incidence of spinal cord injury. Nonetheless, this author and colleagues did notice in one of our prospective randomized studies that patients who received lidocaine for myocardial arrhythmias during surgery tended to have a lowered incidence of postoperative paraplegia or paresis ($p = .1$), albeit not statistically significant.[24] Therefore, we continue to use lidocaine to protect the spinal cord. Animal studies also show that analogs of lidocaine are effective in protecting the spinal cord. In our animal studies, we have examined many agents for spinal cord protection, including superoxide dismutase, allopurinol, steroids, mannitol, flunarizine, naloxone, Selfotel, thiopental, anti-inflammatory agents, white-cell-poor blood transfusions, and angiotensin-converting enzyme blockers. None of these, however, have convincingly reduced the incidence of paraplegia or paresis. Undoubtedly, in the future, agents will be found that are effective in combination with the other documented methods to further reduce the incidence of postoperative paraplegia/paresis.

Conclusion

The incidence of paraplegia/paresis in patients with descending or thoracoabdominal aneurysms has declined significantly in recent years. This is largely a result of extensive research in this area using animal studies and prospective randomized trials in humans. For example, in a recent review of 132 of our patients who underwent descending or thoracoabdominal operations, the incidence of permanent deficits was reduced to 3.8%. This has also contributed to better early and long-term survival rates after surgery for this series of patients, with a mortality rate of 8.3%.

References

1. Svensson LG, Crawford ES. Cardiovascular and vascular disease of the aorta. Philadelphia: WB Saunders; 1997.
2. Crawford ES, Safi HJ, Crawford JL, et al. Thoracoabdominal aortic aneurysms: preoperative and intraoperative factors determining immediate and long-term results of operation in 605 patients. J Vasc Surg 1986;3:389–404.
3. Cooley DA, Baldwin RT. Technique of open distal anastomosis for repair of descending thoracic aortic aneurysms. Ann Thorac Surg 1992;54:932–6.

4. Svensson LG, Patel V, Robinson MF, Crawford ES. Influence of preservation or perfusion of intraoperatively identified spinal cord blood supply on spinal motor evoked potentials and paraplegia after aortic surgery. J Vasc Surg 1991;13:355–65.

5. Svensson LG, Hess KR, D'Agostino RS, et al. Reduction of neurologic injury after high-risk thoracoabdominal aortic operation. Ann Thorac Surg 1998;66:132–8.

6. Dake MD, Miller DC, Semba CP, et al. Transluminal placement of endovascular stent-grafts for the treatment of descending thoracic aortic aneurysms. N Engl J Med 1994;331:1729–34.

7. Safi HJ. Neurologic deficit in patients at high risk with thoracoabdominal aneurysms: the role of cerebrospinal fluid drainage and distal aortic perfusion. J Vasc Surg 1994;20:434–43.

8. Svensson LG, Crawford ES, Hess KR, et al. Variables predictive of outcome in 832 patients undergoing repairs of the descending thoracic aorta. Chest 1993;104:1248–53.

9. Svensson LG, Crawford ES, Hess KR, et al. Experience with 1509 patients undergoing thoracoabdominal aortic operations. J Vasc Surg 1993;17:357–70.

10. Svensson LG, Hess KR, Coselli JS, Safi HJ. Influence of segmental arteries, extent, and atriofemoral bypass on postoperative paraplegia after thoracoabdominal aortic operations. J Vasc Surg 1994;20:255–62.

11. Verdant A, Cosette R, Page A, et al. Aneurysms of the descending thoracic aorta: three hundred sixty-six consecutive cases resected without paraplegia. J Vasc Surg 1995;21:385–91.

12. Kouchoukos NT, Daily BB, Rokkas CK, et al. Hypothermic bypass and circulatory arrest for operations on the descending thoracic and thoracoabdominal aorta. Ann Thorac Surg 1995;60:67–77.

13. Crawford ES, Coselli JS, Safi HJ. Partial cardiopulmonary bypass, hypothermic circulatory arrest, and posterolateral exposure for thoracic aortic aneurysm operation. J Thorac Cardiovasc Surg 1987;94:824–7.

14. Svensson LG, Crawford ES, Patel V, et al. Spinal oxygenation, blood supply localization, cooling, and function with aortic clamping. Ann Thorac Surg 1992;54:74–9.

15. Berguer R, Porto J, Fedoronko B, et al. Selective deep hypothermia of the spinal cord prevents paraplegia after aortic cross-clamping in the dog model. J Vasc Surg 1992;15:62–71.

16. Sun J, Hirsch PD, Svensson LG. Spinal cord protection by papaverine and intrathecal cooling during aortic cross-clamping. J Cardiovasc Surg 1998;39:839–42.

17. Svensson LG, Groenefeldt HT, Von Ritter CM, et al. Cross-clamping of the thoracic aorta: influence of aortic shunts, laminectomy, papaverine, calcium channel blocker, allopurinol, and superoxide dismutase on spinal cord blood flow and paraplegia in baboons. Ann Surg 1986;204:38–47.

18. Kieffer E. Surgical treatment of aneurysms of the thoracoabdominal aorta. Rev Prat 1991;41:1793–7.

19. Maughan RE, Mohan C, Nathan IM, et al. Intrathecal perfusion of an oxygenated perfluorocarbon emulsion prevents paraplegia after extended normothermic aortic cross-clamping. Ann Thorac Surg 1992;54:818–24.

20. Cambria RP, Davidson JK, Zanetti S, et al. Clinical experience with epidural cooling for spinal cord protection during thoracic and thoracoabdominal aneurysm repair. J Vasc Surg 1997;25:234–43.

21. Miyamoto K. A new and simple method of preventing spinal cord damage following temporary occlusion of the thoracic aorta by draining the cerebrospinal fluid. J Cardiovasc Surg 1960;16:188–99.

22. Blaisdell FW, Cooley DA. The mechanism of paraplegia after temporary thoracic aortic occlusion and its relationship to spinal fluid pressure. Surgery 1962;51:351–5.

23. Hollier LH, Money SR, Nashlund TC, et al. Risk of spinal cord dysfunction in patients undergoing thoracoabdominal aortic replacement. Am J Surg 1992;164:210–4.

24. Crawford ES, Svensson LG, Hess KR, et al. A prospective randomized study of cerebrospinal fluid drainage to prevent paraplegia after high-risk surgery on the thoracoabdominal aorta. J Vasc Surg 1991;13:36–46.

25. Acher CW, Wynn MM, Hoch JR, et al. Combined use of spinal fluid drainage and naloxone reduces risk of neurologic deficit in the repair of thoracoabdominal aneurysms. J Vasc Surg 1993;19:236–48.

26. Svensson LG. Intraoperative identification of spinal cord blood supply during repairs of descending aorta and thoracoabdominal aorta. J Thorac Cardiovasc Surg 1996;112:1455–61.

27. Svensson LG. Commentary on De Haan and colleagues: efficacy of transcranial motor evoked myogenic potentials to detect spinal cord ischemia during operations for thoracoabdominal aneurysms. J Thorac Cardiovasc Surg 1997;113:100–1.

28. Williams GM. Treatment of chronic expanding dissecting aneurysms of the descending thoracic and upper abdominal aorta by extended aortotomy, removal of the dissected intima, and closure. J Vasc Surg 1993;18:441–9.

29. Svensson LG. New and future approaches for spinal cord protection. Semin Thorac Cardiovasc Surg 1997;9:206–21.

30. Estera AL, Rubenstein FS, Miller CC, et al. Descending thoracic aortic aneurysm: surgical approach and treatment using the adjuncts cerebrospinal fluid drainage and distal aortic perfusion. Ann Thorac Surg 2001;72(2):481–6.

31. von Segresser LK, Marty B, Mueller X, et al. Active cooling during open repair of thoracoabdominal aortic aneurysms improves outcome. Eur J Cardiothorac Surg 2001;19:411–5.

32. Safi HJ, Miller CC 3rd, Subramaniam MH, et al. Thoracic and thoracoabdominal aortic aneurysm repair using cardiopulmonary bypass, profound hypothermia, and circulatory arrest via left side of the chest incision. J Vasc Surg 1998;28:591–8.

33. Kouchoukos NT, Masetti P, Rokkas CK, et al. Safety and efficacy of hypothermic bypass and circulatory arrest for operations on the descending thoracic and thoracoabdominal aorta. Ann Thorac Surg 2001;72(3):699–707.

34. Nadolny EM, Svensson LG. Carbon dioxide field flooding techniques for open heart surgery: monitoring and minimizing potential adverse effects. Perfusion 2000;15:151–3.

35. Coselli JS, Lemaire SA, Koksoy C, et al. Cerebrospinal fluid drainage reduces paraplegia after thoracoabdominal aortic aneurysm repair: results of a rendomized trial. J Vasc Surg 2002;35(4):631–9.

36. Borst HG, Jurmann M, Buhner B, Laas J. Risk of replacement of descending aorta with a standardized left heart bypass technique. J Thorac Cardiovasc Surg 1994;107:126–32.

37. Huynh TT, Miller CC, Estrera A, Safi HJ. Adjunct (cerebrospinal fluid drainage + distal aortic perfusion) improves outcome following thoracic and thoracoabdominal aortic repair [abstract]. [In press]

38. Ross SD, Kron IL, Parrino PE, et al. Preservation of intercostal arteries during thoracoabdominal aortic aneurysm surgery: a retrospective study. J Thorac Cardiovasc Surg 1999;118:17–25.

39. Safi HJ, Miller CC 3rd, Carr C, et al. Importance of intercostal artery reattachment during thoracoabdominal aortic aneurysm repair. J Vasc Surg 1998;27:58–66.

40. Griepp RB, Ergin MA, Galla JD, et al. Looking for the artery of Adamkiewicz: a quest to minimize paraplegia after operations for aneurysms of the descending thoracic and thoracoabdominal aorta. J Thorac Cardiovasc Surg 1996;112:1202–13.

41. Dake MD, Miller DC, Mitchell RS, et al. The "first generation" of endovascular stent-grafts for patients with aneurysms of the descending thoracic aorta. J Thorac Cardiovasc Surg 1998;116:689–703.

42. Coselli JS, LeMaire SA, Koksoy C, et al. Surgical repair of extent II thoracoabdominal aortic aneurysms: evaluation of morbidity and mortality [abstract]. Ann Thorac Surg 2002;73:1107–15.

43. Cambria RP, Davison JK, Carter C, et al. Epidural cooling for spinal cord protection during thoracoabdominal aneurysm repair: a five-year experience. J Vasc Surg 2000;31:1093–102.

44. Nadolny EM, Svensson LG. Hypothermic arrest for descending aortic rupture in reoperative patients. Ann Thorac Surg 2001;71:2027–30.

CHAPTER 38

THORACOABDOMINAL AORTIC ANEURYSM

HAZIM J. SAFI, MD, TAM T. T. HUYNH, MD, ANTHONY L. ESTRERA, MD,
CHARLES C. MILLER III, PhD, EYAL E. PORAT, MD

Five Decades of Aortic Aneurysm Repair

By devising a method of spinal cord protection, Etheredge, in 1955, launched the modern era of thoracoabdominal aortic aneurysm (TAA) repair.[1] Using a temporary shunt to divert blood flow from the distal thoracic aorta to the distal abdominal aorta, he replaced an aneurysm with a homograft. DeBakey used a similar shunt and homograft technique in the following year.[2] From today's vantage point, early TAA techniques seem cumbersome, and morbidity and mortality rates were admittedly high. Although in the ensuing years, there have been many advances in graft and suture material, anticoagulants, and pump mechanisms, it was the elaborate bypasses and shunts in the lengthy procedures of the 1950s that made surgery a feasible solution for TAA patients.

In 1965, E. Stanley Crawford ushered in a new phase of TAA repair by applying two sound vascular principles: the inclusion technique and routine intercostal artery reimplantation. His technique originated from the early works of Matas and Carrel. In 1888, Rudolph Matas performed an endoaneurysmorrhaphy, or repair of a brachial artery aneurysm within the walls of the aneurysm.[3] Oscar Creech, in 1966, combined the endoaneurysmorrhaphy techniques of Matas with the newest graft replacement developments, which Crawford then applied to TAA repair.[4] In the inclusion technique, the graft is placed inside the aneurysmal sac with visceral branch origins directly reattached to an opening in the graft wall. Alexis Carrel, at the turn of the twentieth century, experimented with different methods for the reattachment of smaller vessels to larger ones, paving the way for the reattachment of intercostal arteries and visceral vessels to a prosthetic graft.[5] The experimental work of Frank Spencer and others further enlightened the surgical community to the significance of intercostal artery reattachment.[6]

In the 1970s, further experimentation in spinal cord protection produced the left-heart bypass with membrane oxygenator, described by Connolly and others.[7] The Gott extracorporeal shunt, placed through proximal and distal ports at the left subclavian and infrarenal abdominal aorta, came into use.[8] In the 1980s, adjuncts continued to be explored. Profound hypothermia and circulatory arrest were less than satisfactory and intraoperative cerebrospinal fluid (CSF) drainage also proved to be a disappointment.[9,10] Distal aortic perfusion and spinal cord monitoring via somatosensory-evoked potential (SSEP) were introduced.[11] SSEPs monitor the status of the spinal cord and can indicate the need for urgent attention if SSEPs change. Accuracy rates were poor. The nonspecificity of the test, that is, the inability to identify ischemia in specific vessels, may have been partially responsible for the conclusion reached by Crawford and associates that there was "... no convincing evidence that one method of operation is likely to be superior to another in preventing neurologic complications."[12] Frustrated by the results, some surgeons for a brief period returned to the simple cross-clamp technique.[13] Sequential clamping of the aorta to reduce periods of ischemia to aortic segments was essential in the cross-clamp technique. Also during this period, thoracoabdominal aortic aneurysm classification was solidified.[13] Our understanding of the pathophysiology of paraplegia and paraparesis expanded and researchers recognized a new entity called *delayed neurologic deficit*.[12]

The 1990s were characterized by further experiments with adjuncts, with different centers focusing on very different techniques. The simple cross-clamp TAA surgery was virtually abandoned.[14–16] This chapter focuses on the techniques that we have found to be most successful in TAA repair and spinal cord protection. We discuss the adjuncts of distal aortic perfusion, CSF drainage, and moderate hypothermia, and explore their impact on neurologic deficits, both immediate and delayed.

Natural History

Ruptured aortic aneurysms remain the thirteenth leading cause of death in the United States, with an increasing prevalence.[17] The increasing prevalence may be attributable to improved imaging techniques, increasing mean age of the population, and overall heightened awareness.[18] The incidence of aortic aneurysms is estimated to be 5.9 cases per 100,000 person-years. The mean age is between 59 and 69 years, with a male predominance of 2:1 to 4:1.[19]

The survival rate for patients with untreated thoracic aortic aneurysms is dismal, estimated to be between 13 and 39% at 5 years.[19–22] The lifetime probability of rupture in untreated thoracic aneurysms and TAA is between 75 and 80%.[19,20] The most common cause of death is rupture.[23] Moreover, the few patients who survive to operation sustain significant morbidity, prolonged hospital course, and, ultimately, a poor quality of life.

The time that elapses between aneurysm formation and rupture is influenced by aneurysm size and growth rate, hypertension, smoking, history of chronic obstructive pulmonary disease, presence of pain, etiology, and age. The size of the aortic aneurysm remains the single most important factor in determining the likelihood of rupture. Rupture is more likely to occur in TAAs exceeding 5 cm in diameter, with the likelihood increasing significantly as the aneurysm enlarges.[20,24–27] Growth rate is a component in formulating the rate of rupture or indication for surgical intervention.[24,28] The rate of growth is exponential, with larger aneurysms growing at greater rates; the rate for aneurysms > 5.2 cm in diameter is 0.12 cm/year.[28,29]

Hypertension and subsequent increased aortic wall tension play a significant role in aneurysm formation. The law of Laplace states that as the diameter of a cylinder increases, the tension applied to the wall also increases. This indicates that the wall tension is directly related to pressure. Although systemic hypertension is widely recognized as a risk factor for aneurysm formation, it is diastolic blood pressure that has been specifically correlated with aneurysm rupture. Multiple reports have noted an association of increased diastolic blood pressure (greater than 100 mm Hg) with rupture of both abdominal and thoracic aortic aneurysms.[24,28,30] As was demonstrated by Wheat in his work on aortic dissections, decreasing the force of myocardial contraction, or *dp/dt*, may decrease the progression of disease and the likelihood of rupture.[31] Consequently, it is recommended that β-adrenergic blocking agents be included in the antihypertensive treatment regimen for patients with known aortic aneurysms.

Although smoking has been implicated as a risk factor for rupture in abdominal aortic aneurysms, a stronger association with chronic obstructive pulmonary disease has been identified.[24,28,32,33] In the study by Cronenwett and associates, chronic obstructive pulmonary disease was defined as a forced expiratory volume in 1 s (FEV1) of less than 50% of predicted.[33] This correlation may be related to increased collagenase activity as seen in smokers.[34] It is theorized that the proteolytic activity may weaken the aortic wall of those patients that are susceptible to aneurysm rupture.[35] An indicator of susceptibility may be seen in patients with chronic obstructive pulmonary disease, in that these patients demonstrate a connective tissue intolerance to smoke-related toxicity.[36] In addition, it has been documented that patients with a history of smoking have a more rapid expansion of thoracic aneurysms.[28,37] This evidence justifies the cessation of smoking in the presence of an aortic aneurysm.

Further implicated in the increased likelihood of aortic rupture are pain, chronic dissection, and age. Vague or uncharacteristic pain in the presence of TAA has been significantly associated with subsequent rupture.[24] Generally, the etiology of TAA is attributed to a degenerative process. It has also been suggested that rupture is associated with chronic dissection, but the evidence is not compelling.[19,38] In a prospective study by Juvonen and associates, aneurysms associated with chronic dissection were observed to be smaller (median diameter of 5.4 cm) than degenerative aneurysms (median diameter of 5.8 cm).[39] Significant alterations in the structure of the aortic wall occur with aging that are distinct from the formation of aneurysms. Age in TAA patients, however, is associated with increased risk of rupture.[40] Furthermore, Juvonen and associates demonstrated that the relative risk for rupture increased by a factor of 2.6 for every decade of age.[39]

The natural course of the majority of aortic aneurysms is rupture and death. Aneurysm size and growth rate, as well as patient age, medical history, and symptoms, must be carefully weighed when considering when to intervene surgically, but elective surgery for TAA repair has been demonstrated to improve long-term survival. Methods have been devised for predicting the risks of surgical repair for TAAs.[24,28] Although these formulas may allow one to preoperatively stratify the risks of surgery for a patient, the decision to operate still remains with the surgeon, the surgeon's clinical evaluation, and the patient's preference.

Preoperative Diagnostic Imaging

Currently, several imaging modalities, revolutionized by computerized hardware and software systems, detect and define TAA.[41] Spiral computed tomography (CT) records data by a 360° rotation of the x-ray beam source around the object being imaged and is replacing conventional CT in most centers. High-quality spiral CT provides faster image acquisition for better image resolution, processing, and reformatting (Figure 38-1). Computed tomographic angiography (CTA) acquires axial images during the arterial phase following a bolus of intravenous contrast.[42–44] The aortic diameter is measured on the CT axial image from the outermost part of the aortic wall on one side to the outermost part of the opposite wall. The scan records

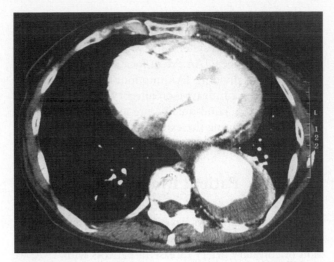

FIGURE 38-1. Computed tomographic angiogram of large TAA.

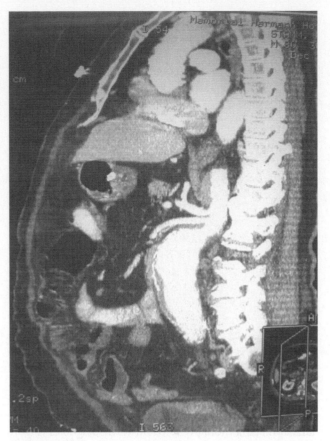

FIGURE 38-2. Sagittal reformatting of computed tomographic angiogram in patient with TAA extent IV.

aortic diameters serially, from the ascending aorta, arch aorta, and thoracoabdominal aorta at various levels to determine the extent of the aneurysms. CTA can define the aortic lumen (such as the distinction between the false and true lumen in aortic dissection), and also shows associated thrombus and/or inflammatory changes in the aortic wall. Also, in cases of acute and chronic aortic dissection, CTA can accurately detect the proximal location of the intimal tear and hence determine the type (DeBakey's I, II, or III; Stanford's A or B) and the mandated management. In patients with small aneurysms and/or chronic aortic dissection, we recommend serial follow-up CT scans every 3 to 12 months to assess possible aneurysm growth.

Coronal reformatting or three-dimensional reconstruction of axial CT images might provide additional views of TAA, but in general is not necessary (Figure 38-2).[45] Thin-slice CTA image acquisition may sometimes show patent intercostal arteries, but this finding has yet to be validated clinically. However, with continued advances in CT technology, thin-slice CTA with three-dimensional reconstruction or reformatting will no doubt become an invaluable tool in TAA assessment for endovascular applications in the near future.

Finally, a general assessment of other intrathoracic, -abdominal, and -pelvic solid organs can be obtained on CT scan, and associated pathology, such as lung or kidney disease, can be detected and evaluated accordingly. Intravenous contrast is not necessary for determining TAA size and extent, and is contraindicated in patients with impaired renal function. However, for patients with normal renal function, we prefer CTA imaging for TAA.

Historically, before CT scan became widely available, conventional aortography was performed in all TAA patients. Today, aortography is limited to patients with suspected aortic branch occlusive disease. In general, because of the magnification, aortography tends to overestimate the TAA size, unless there is an associated thrombus, in which case aortography may underestimate size. Preoperative selective aortography has been reported as a means for identifying patent intercostal arteries and the artery of Adamkiewicz.[46,47] However, these results have not been duplicated in large clinical series. Because of the risk associated with the selective injection of contrast dyes and yet-to-be demonstrated clinical benefits, we do not routinely perform preoperative transesophageal echocardiography (TEE) imaging of intercostal arteries.

Magnetic resonance imaging (MRI) with or without gadolinium (magnetic resonance angiography, or MRA) is a noninvasive imaging modality that has become widely available (Figure 38-3).[41] Its main advantage over CT scan is that it can be performed safely in patients with impaired renal function, because it does not require intravenous radiopaque contrast. However, the image resolution of MRA remains poorer when compared to spiral CT scan. In addition, MRA does not accurately detect calcification and thrombus versus aortic lumen. The time required to acquire images, claustrophobia, internal metallic hardware (such as pacemakers, orthopedic rods, etc), and higher cost are other limiting factors. In general, TAA patients do not require MRA imaging preoperatively.

In patients suspected to have an acute dissection of the ascending aorta associated with hemodynamic instability

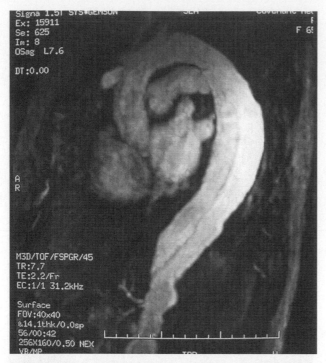

FIGURE 38-3. Magnetic resonance angiogram of TAA extent I with chronic dissection.

or with equivocal CT findings, TEE has emerged as a preferred imaging modality to confirm the diagnosis (Figure 38-4).[48] In addition, TEE provides excellent imaging of the arch and descending thoracic aorta, and accurately detects the presence of aortic dissection in both the acute and chronic phases. However, for technical reasons, TEE visualization is limited to the aortic region above the diaphragm. Usually, for preoperative TAA assessment, TEE is not necessary if good-quality spiral CT scan imaging is available. TEE is invasive and requires an experienced operator for optimal visualization and interpretation.

The CT scan, which came into use in the 1970s, was revolutionary in detecting TAA. It also paved the way to a proper classification system. In 1986, Crawford made the correlation between TAA extent/location and risk of neurologic deficit, dividing TAA into four types, to which we recently added a fifth type or category (Figure 38-5).[13,49] In summary, a good-quality preoperative CT scan is essential for defining the extent of TAA and in the planning operative strategy.

Patient Evaluation

Thoracoabdominal aortic aneurysm patients are usually older and almost always have one or more comorbidities, involving the lungs, kidneys, or heart. In a recent evaluation of coronary artery disease in patients with TAA, we found that ejection fraction was an important predictor of survival. All our patients underwent echocardiography to evaluate their ejection fraction and its impact on immediate and long-term morbidity and mortality rates. Thoracoabdominal aortic aneurysm patients who are asymptomatic, but who show evidence of coronary artery disease, require cardiac catheterization to delineate the coronary anatomy and, if intervention is indicated, undergo either coronary angioplasty and/or stenting. If the coronary anatomy is not amenable to angioplasty, we perform coronary artery bypass. We have learned to use the saphenous vein rather than the internal mammary artery for lesions of the left anterior descending coronary artery. This is because subsequent TAA operations may require aortic clamping proximal to the left subclavian artery, which can cause coronary ischemia. Recovery until TAA surgery is about 4 weeks. If, however, a patient has become symptomatic, TAA is done urgently.

We define chronic obstructive pulmonary disease (COPD) as a history of chronic bronchitis and emphysema,

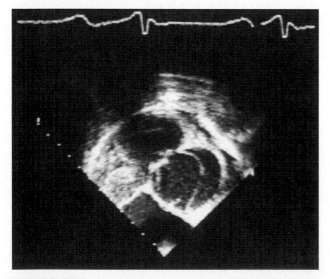

FIGURE 38-4. Transesophageal echocardiogram of type A aortic dissection.

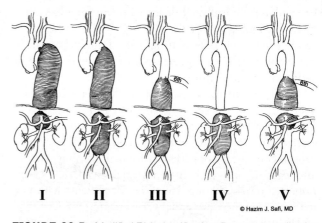

© Hazim J. Safi, MD

FIGURE 38-5. Modified TAA classification. Extent I: from distal to the left subclavian artery to above the renal arteries. Extent II: from distal to the left subclavian artery to the aortic bifurcation. Extent III: from the sixth intercostal space to the aortic bifurcation. Extent IV: from the diaphragm to the aortic bifurcation (total abdominal aorta). Extent V: from the sixth intercostal space to above the renal arteries.

or, while on bronchodilators, < 60% of predicted FEV1. All patients require a pulmonary function test, and then are categorized according to FEV1 and its severity. Patients with severe COPD might require 2 or 3 weeks of intensive pulmonary rehabilitation before we operate. Creatinine levels are measured preoperatively to appraise renal function and, if abnormal, a thorough evaluation of the kidney function by a nephrology team is essential. Renal dysfunction, either preoperatively and/or postoperatively, correlates with high morbidity and mortality rates, both immediate and long-term. Liver function is evaluated, and if a patient has cirrhosis and is not symptomatic, we generally shy away from operating because of the high mortality rate.

Operative Technique: Thoracoabdominal Aorta

After a thorough evaluation of cardiovascular, pulmonary, renal, and general health status, the patient is taken to the operating room. Spinal cord protection is imperative, and critical safeguards are the adjuncts of CSF drainage and distal aortic perfusion, as well as passive (moderate) hypothermia. After being anesthetized and intubated with a double-lumen endotracheal tube, the patient is prepared for surgery. Electrodes attached to the scalp for electroencephalogram (EEG) and along the spinal cord for SSEP assess brain function and spinal cord status. A CSF catheter placed in the third or fourth lumbar space provides CSF drainage and monitoring of CSF pressure (Figure 38-6). The CSF pressure is maintained at less than 10 mm Hg throughout the procedure.

The patient is positioned in the right lateral decubitus position with the hip flexed 45° for accessibility of the left and right groins (Figure 38-7). We tailor the incision to complement the extent of the aneurysm; a modified thoracoabdominal incision for the descending thoracic aorta and extent I TAA, and full thoracoabdominal exploration for TAA extents II, III, IV, and V. The full thoracoabdominal incision begins above the symphysis pubis, goes midline to the umbilicus, and curves straight into the costal cartilage to the bed of the sixth rib. The sixth rib is removed for all except extent IV TAA. The resected rib

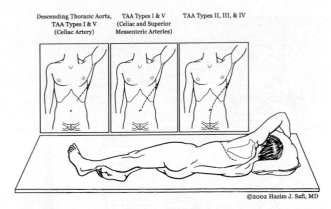

FIGURE 38-7. Illustration of patient in right lateral decubitus position with modified TAA incision and full TAA incisions.

space allows intraoperative identification of the dimension of the aneurysm and the intercostal artery location. The left lung is collapsed. A self-retaining retractor fully exposes the TAA. Taking care to avoid injury to the phrenic nerve, the aortic hiatus and the muscular portion of the diaphragm are cut for passage of the aortic graft.

The pericardium is opened posterior to the phrenic nerve to expose the left atrium. The patient is anticoagulated with 1 mg/kg of heparin. The left atrium is cannulated through the left inferior pulmonary vein. The pericardium is opened to confirm direct cannulation and to prevent postoperative tamponade (Figure 38-8). A Bio-Medicus pump (Minneapolis, Minnesota) with an in-line heat exchanger is attached to this cannula and the arterial inflow is established through the left common femoral artery, or the descending thoracic aorta if the femoral artery is not accessible (Figure 38-9).

The descending thoracic aorta is dissected from the level of the hilum of the lung cephalad to the proximal descending thoracic aorta. We identify the ligamentum arteriosum and transect it, taking care to avoid injury to the left recurrent laryngeal nerve. Distal aortic perfusion is begun as the cross-clamps are applied to the proximal descending thoracic aorta and to the midthoracic aorta

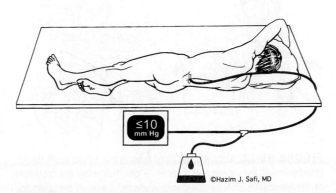

FIGURE 38-6. Cerebrospinal fluid drainage.

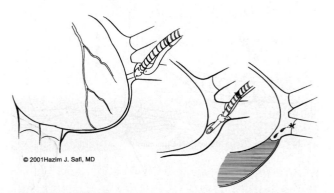

FIGURE 38-8. The pitfalls of cannulating the left pulmonary vein with intact pericardium. Left: Correct cannulation of pulmonary vein. Right: Misplaced cannulation causing cardiac tamponade.

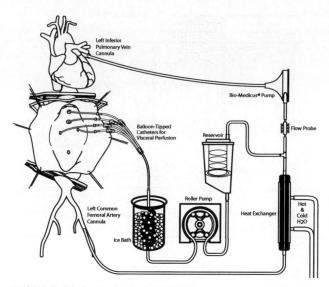

FIGURE 38-9. Illustration of BioMedicus pump and distal aortic perfusion circuit.

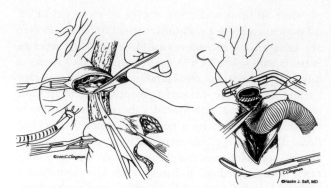

FIGURE 38-11. Illustration of the abandoned inclusion technique and possible esophageal fistula (left) and current method in which the aorta is completely transected (right).

(level of T6) (Figure 38-10). Because of the danger of esophageal fistula, we no longer use the inclusion technique in the proximal anastomosis (Figure 38-11). Instead, we completely transect the aorta to separate it from the underlying esophagus. We prefer a woven Dacron graft for replacement. We suture the graft in end-to-end fashion to the descending thoracic aorta, using a running 3–0 or 2–0 monofilament polypropylene suture. We check the anastomosis for bleeding and use 3–0 pledgeted sutures for reinforcement, if necessary.

For extensive aneurysms, sequential clamping is used and, after completion of the proximal anastomosis, the mid-descending aortic clamp is moved distally onto the abdominal aorta at the celiac axis to accommodate intercostal reattachment. Reattachment of patent, lower intercostal arteries (T8 to T12) is performed routinely, except in cases of occluded arteries, heavily calcified aorta, or when not technically feasible.

With completion of intercostal reattachment, the distal clamp is moved onto the infrarenal aorta, the abdominal aorta is opened, and the visceral vessels are identified (Figure 38-12). The celiac, superior mesenteric, and renal arteries are perfused using No. 9 Pruitt catheters (Cryolife, St. Petersburg, Florida) (Figure 38-13). The cold

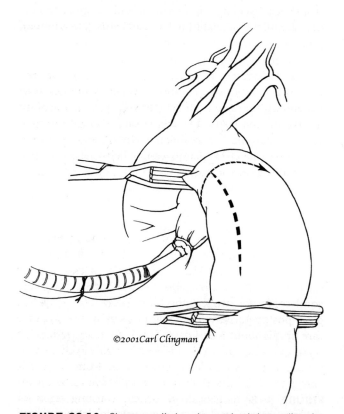

FIGURE 38-10. Clamps applied to the proximal descending thoracic and the midthoracic aorta.

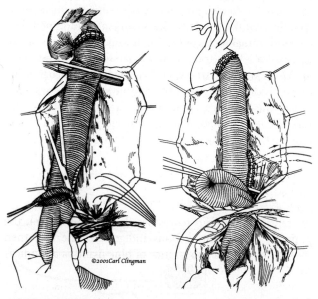

FIGURE 38-12. Left: An elliptical hole is cut in the graft for reattachment of the intercostal arteries. Right: Following reattachment of the intercostal arteries the clamp is moved down on the graft and the graft is tunneled through the diaphragm.

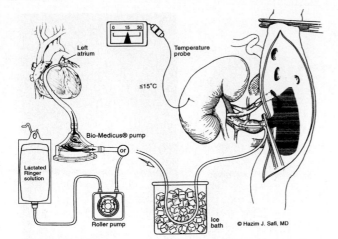

FIGURE 38-13. Illustration of mechanics of visceral artery perfusion.

perfusate (blood at 4°C) delivered to the viscera depends on proximal aortic pressure and is maintained between 300 and 600 mL/min. Renal temperature is directly monitored and kept at approximately 15°C. Because cold visceral perfusion can cause hypothermia, core body temperature is kept between 32° and 33°C by warming the lower circulation, that is, the lower extremities. If we cannot clamp the infrarenal abdominal aorta because of problems such as aortic calcification of an overly large aorta, the patient can be prewarmed to a safe systemic temperature (35°C) and aggressive renal cooling can be achieved. Renal cooling without prewarming could result in a precipitous drop in core temperature below 30°C, leading to serious cardiac dysrhythmias.

The visceral vessels are reattached using the inclusion technique (Figure 38-14). Upon completion of this anastomosis, the perfusion catheters are removed and attention is turned to the distal anastomosis (Figure 38-15). In most cases, an island patch accommodates reattachment of the celiac, superior mesenteric, and both renal arteries. We no longer use a visceral patch for patients with connective tissue disorders such as Marfan syndrome, because of the high incidence of recurrent patch aneurysms in these patients. Instead, we use a specially designed Dacron graft, with side-arm grafts of 10 mm and 12 mm, attached separately to the celiac, superior mesenteric, and the left and right renal arteries. Reattachment of a left renal artery located at too great a distance from other viscera requires an interposition bypass graft. After we release the clamp to restore flow to the viscera, the patient is given intravenous indigo carmine and then monitored for the appearance of blue urine as an indicator of renal function.

Prior to completion of the distal anastomosis, the graft is flushed proximally and the aorta distally. We wean the patient from partial bypass once the rectal temperature reaches 36°C. Protamine is administered and the atrial and femoral cannulae are removed. After hemostasis is

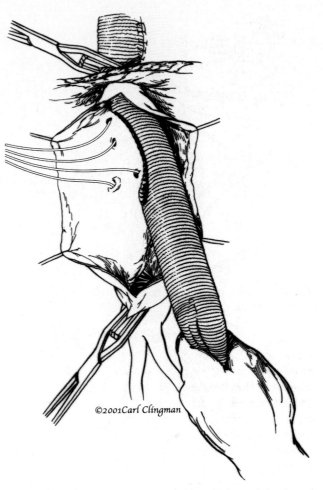

FIGURE 38-14. Illustration of the hole cut in the graft for visceral patch.

achieved, two tubes are placed in the chest for pleural cavity drainage. The pericostal space is approximated using braided absorbable sutures, and the muscular fascia of the chest is closed using monofilament absorbable sutures. The diaphragm and abdominal walls are closed in multiple layers with heavy polypropylene sutures, and the skin is approximated with staples. Figures 38-16 and 38-17 illustrate an extensive TAA before and after surgery.

Postoperative Management

Following surgery, the patient's mean arterial pressure is maintained between 80 and 100 mm Hg. With the patient in a supine position, a single endotracheal tube is exchanged for the bifurcated endotracheal tube. If the vocal cords are swollen, the bifurcation tube is kept in place postoperatively. The length of stay in the intensive care unit is about 3 or 4 days. This is a crucial period. We try to wake the patient as quickly as possible to check neurologic status. After the patient recovers from anesthesia and is moving all extremities, we still have to be on the alert for delayed neurologic deficit. Warning signs for delayed neurologic deficit are unstable arterial blood pressure, hypoxia after extubation, or CSF pressure above

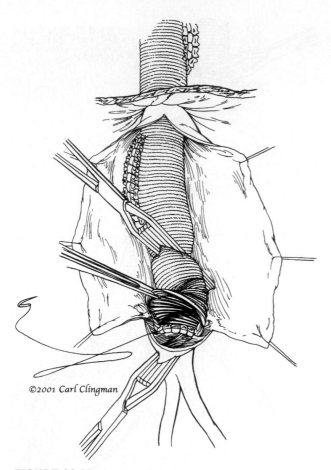

©2001 Carl Clingman

FIGURE 38-15. Distal anastomosis.

10 mm Hg. CSF drainage is discontinued on the third postoperative day, and we transfer the patient to the regular floor. If the patient develops delayed neurologic deficit, the CSF drainage catheter has to be re-inserted and drained freely by gravity for at least 3 days. Usually, the patient will recover his neurologic status if CSF drainage is restored within the first 2 or 3 hours of insult. After the patient is up and about, tolerating a regular diet, afebrile, and has return of normal bowel function, he is discharged, usually in 10 to 12 days following surgery.

Follow-up after TAA repair is essential. The frequency of follow-up visits or CT scans varies somewhat based on TAA etiology, for example, dissection, connective tissue disorders (Marfan syndrome, Ehler-Danlos syndrome), family history, or concurrent aneurysms. For TAA repair, we recommend annual follow-up with CT scan. Regardless of the frequency of CT scans, clinicians must remain on guard for new aneurysm or pseudoaneurysm development.[50]

Operative Technique: Extensive Aortic Aneurysm and the Elephant Trunk Technique

Extensive aortic aneurysms of the ascending aorta, aortic arch, and descending or thoracoabdominal aorta require

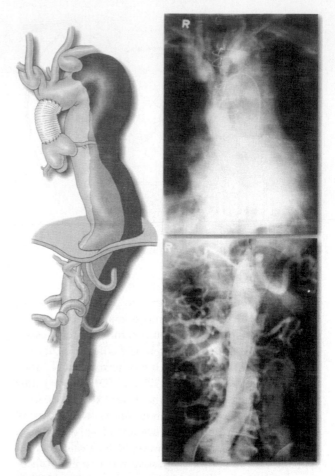

FIGURE 38-16. Illustration and aortogram of extent II TAA with dissection.

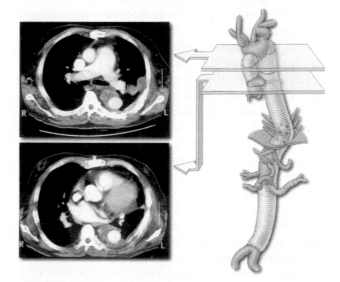

FIGURE 38-17. CT scans and illustration of completed repair of extent II TAA.

innovative surgical techniques. Since 1991, we have routinely used a two-staged approach (Figure 38-18).[51] We perform the first stage, or the elephant trunk technique, in a fashion similar to standard surgery of the ascending

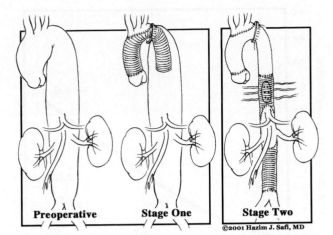

FIGURE 38-18. Illustration of two-staged repair of TAA extent II.

aorta and transverse arch, with the exception that we insert an inverted distal graft. The folded edge of the inverted graft is sutured to the descending thoracic aorta just distal to the left subclavian artery. When the distal anastomosis is completed, the inner portion of the graft is retrieved and the outer portion, or "elephant trunk," is left in the descending aorta. In the first stage, cardiopulmonary bypass, profound hypothermia, circulatory arrest, and retrograde cerebral perfusion provide protection to the brain and guard against stroke.

The second stage of the elephant trunk technique, illustrated earlier in Figure 38-18, is much like standard descending thoracic or thoracoabdominal aortic aneurysm repair. The advantage to this procedure is that by avoiding cross-clamping of the highly vulnerable proximal descending aorta, we avoid dissection between the transverse aortic arch and pulmonary artery, which can lead to catastrophic bleeding from the aorta or pulmonary artery. After induction of anesthesia, a 14-gauge needle is inserted into the third or fourth lumbar space to drain the cerebrospinal fluid. Left-heart bypass is from the left atrial appendage or pulmonary vein to the common femoral artery. With a clamp at the mid-descending thoracic aorta, the proximal third of the descending thoracic aorta is opened. Elimination of the proximal clamp reduces trauma to the aortic wall. The elephant trunk portion of the graft, inserted in the descending thoracic aorta during stage one, is grasped and clamped. A new graft is sutured to the "elephant trunk." Figures 38-19 and 38-20 show an extent II TAA with type A dissection before and after surgery.

Follow-up Results

Mortality

Complex TAA repair potentially exposes the patient to multiorgan ischemic insults and ultimately places the patient at risk for end-organ damage. Mortality rates for TAA repair range between 4 and 21%, depending on the

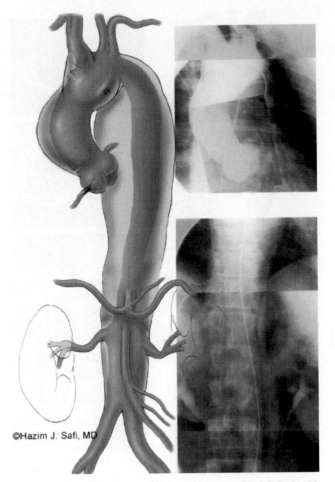

©Hazim J. Safi, MD

FIGURE 38-19. Illustration and aortogram of extent II TAA with type A aortic dissection.

series. In our experience, multivariate risk factors for mortality have been age, renal failure, and paraplegia.[52]

Neurologic Deficit

Although neurologic deficit (paraplegia or paraparesis) continues to have devastating consequences for the patient, the incidence has slowly declined over the past decade. Much of the decline in the incidence of neurologic deficit is attributable to the use of spinal cord protective adjuncts. Many methods have been devised to protect the spinal cord during aortic surgery, including active and passive distal aortic perfusion, total cardiopulmonary bypass, profound hypothermic circulatory arrest, direct spinal cord cooling, cerebrospinal fluid drainage, monitoring of somatosensory- and motor-evoked potentials, and pharmacologic methods that use papaverine, naloxone, or steroids. These adjuncts have had varying degrees of success in preventing neurologic deficit.[12,14,53–57] Despite these advances, neurologic deficit still remains a significant obstacle in the treatment of thoracic and TAA and carries an incidence of between 5 and 10%, depending on the extent of the aneurysm.

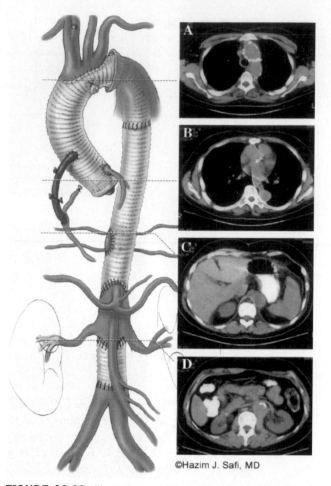

©Hazim J. Safi, MD

FIGURE 38-20. Illustration and CT scans of completed repair of extent II TAA that was performed using the elephant trunk technique.

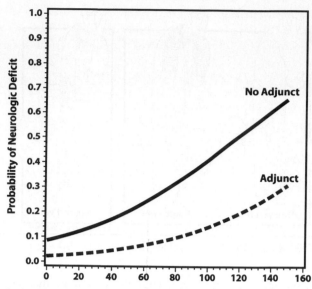

FIGURE 38-21. Logistic regression curve: risk of neurologic deficit during aortic cross-clamp time; simple cross-clamp versus adjunct repair for extent II TAA. Adjunct: distal aortic perfusion and cerebral fluid drainage.

Since 1991, we have used the combination of distal aortic perfusion and CSF drainage for all patients undergoing elective repair of either descending thoracic or TAA aneurysms.[58] We believe that this combination provides significant spinal cord protection. In surgery performed using simple aortic cross-clamping, the incidence of neurologic deficit increases as the length of cross-clamp time increases (Figure 38-21). The aim of the adjuncts is to provide spinal cord protection during the repair to avoid ischemic insult. The pathophysiologic effect of cross-clamping of the descending thoracic aorta is a decreased distal mean arterial pressure and increased CSF pressure, which may lead to a significant reduction in spinal cord perfusion pressure.[59] The adjuncts, by essentially reversing the effects of the cross-clamp—decreasing CSF and increasing distal aortic pressure (DAP)—increase the perfusion pressure of the spinal cord.

Also important in spinal cord protection is intercostal artery reimplantation. We studied the relationship of neurologic deficit to ligation, reimplantation, and pre-existing occlusion of intercostal arteries to determine which arteries and consequent management are most critical to outcome in TAA repair.[60] We concluded that reattachment of the thoracic intercostal arteries is indicated when arteries are patent, and we found the benefit of reattachment to be greater in the lower thoracic regions, specifically T9 to T12.

Neurologic deficit is defined as any paraplegia or paraparesis that occurs upon awakening from anesthesia. If immediate neurologic deficit is observed, then the severity is graded by using the Tarlov scale. If after a period of normal neurologic function, the patient then develops neurologic deficit, this is classified as delayed neurologic deficit. In our experience, this has occurred as early as 2 hours and as late as 2 weeks.[61,62] The incidence was 2.4% in our series of 654 patients, with a median occurrence of 3 days.[61]

Unlike immediate neurologic deficit, which is likely a result of the events that occur during operative repair, delayed neurologic deficit appears to be a result of postoperative factors. Some have hypothesized that all neurologic deficits during aneurysm repair are caused by ischemia that leads to apoptosis or "programmed cell death," and that delayed neurologic deficit is only an extension of the events that occurred during surgery.[63,64] Another theory on the etiology of delayed neurologic deficit is that it may be related to postischemic inflammatory process, possibly causing compartment syndrome.[65]

When we evaluated delayed neurologic deficit, we identified renal insufficiency, presence of acute dissection, and extent II TAA as preoperative factors associated with delayed neurologic deficit.[66] It appears that the postoperative factors that are associated with delayed neurologic deficit are related to the events that affect arterial blood pressure and oxygen delivery, that is, oxygenation, cardiac output, and hemoglobin. Thus, it is our policy to maintain the mean arterial blood pressure at greater than 90 to 100 mm Hg, hemoglobin at greater than 10 mg/dL, and cardiac index at greater than 2.0 L/min. In addition, for 3 days postoperatively, we drain CSF and keep CSF pressure at less than 10 mm Hg. If delayed neurologic deficit occurs while the CSF drain is in place, then the patient is placed supine, and CSF is freely drained until the CSF pressure is less than 10 mm Hg. If the drain has been removed and delayed neurologic deficit occurs, then the CFS drainage catheter is re-inserted and drained for 72 hours. With this protocol, we have observed an improvement in neurologic deficit in greater than 50% of patients, with approximately 40% complete recovery.[61,67]

Renal Protection

The complication of renal failure following TAA repair remains significant.[68] Renal failure increases morbidity, length of stay, and, ultimately, mortality. We have shown that the presence of preoperative renal insufficiency and the development of postoperative renal failure are associated with increased 30-day mortality and neurologic deficit.[68] The incidence of renal failure after TAA repair has ranged from 4 to 29%.[69] In our experiment, the incidence of postoperative renal failure requiring hemodialysis was 15%.[68] Our previous report showed that the risk factors associated with renal failure were increased preoperative creatinine (> 2.0 mg/dL), direct left renal artery reattachment, and the use of simple cross-clamp technique (Table 38-1).

With regard to renal protection, a successful strategy to protect kidney function during surgical TAA repair remains illusive and clinical trials evaluating perioperative renal function are scarce. The goals of perioperative renal protection are to maintain adequate renal oxygen delivery, to reduce renal oxygen utilization, and to reduce direct renal tubular injury. These goals may be addressed by active renal cooling and by directly maintaining renal perfusion, suppressing renal vasoconstriction, preventing micro-occlusion by particulate emboli, and preventing postischemic reperfusion injury.

Our current technique for renal protection involves active visceral cooling with cold blood (4°C) in order to maintain a renal temperature of less than 20°C. We previously used cold lactated Ringer's solution for renal artery perfusion, but discovered that the large amounts of perfusate required to cool the kidneys led to systemic hypothermia, significant hemodilution, and overloading of the heart. Another technique that we have used is retrograde renal vein perfusion, which is under current investigation. Retrograde renal perfusion involves inserting a No. 4 or No. 5 Pruitt balloon catheter into the renal vein and perfusing cold (4°C) lactated Ringer's solution in a retrograde fashion to the kidney. This may have the advantage of flushing of atheromatous debris and can be used in cases of very stenotic renal arteries that would not allow passage of an antegrade perfusion catheter. Despite these techniques, the results of renal protection in our center remain mixed.

Although pharmacologic agents such as dopamine and prostaglandin inhibitors have not been demonstrated to be beneficial for renal protection, we recently found some benefit in the use of fenoldopam. Fenoldopam is a dopaminergic agonist that increases the renal blood flow, sodium excretion, and water excretion, and maintains the glomerular filtration rate (GFR). As an antihypertensive, it causes systemic vasodilation, increased mesenteric vasodilation, and increased coronary vasodilation. Based on animal experiments that are reported to increase the renal blood flow and urine output, with histologic confirmation of renal protection, we have used this as a continuous perioperative infusion.[70] In a randomized placebo-controlled prospective study of 58 patients with elective repair of TAA, we found that fenoldopam decreased the urinary dye clearance time from 17 min to 8 min ($p = .005$). In a study by Gilbert, the use of fenoldopam during TAA repair led to significant improvement in return to baseline renal function for patients with preoperative renal insufficiency.[71]

Visceral Protection

Direct visceral perfusion has been shown to provide protection to the liver.[72] Perfusing the celiac and/or the superior mesenteric artery with either cold or warm blood has the greatest impact on extent II TAA, which is associated with the longest ischemic periods and the highest incidence of postoperative liver dysfunction. In an analysis of TAA patients, we found that acute rupture and emergency presentation were risk factors for hepatic injury following repair.[72] Visceral perfusion during extent II aneurysm repair effectively negated the associated rise in

TABLE 38-1. Factors Associated with Increased Risk of Acute Renal Failure (Model Developed by Stepwise Multiple Logistic Regression Analysis)

Variable	Parameter Estimate	Adjusted Odds Ratio	95% CI	p
Intercept	−3.9355	—	—	.0001
Creatinine > 2.8*	4.2531	70.33	12.01–411.75	.0001
Left renal artery	1.4784	4.39	1.62–11.91	.004
Visceral perfusion	1.2801	3.60	1.18–10.97	.02
Simple clamp	1.2202	3.39	1.07–10.76	.04
TAA type II	0.5569	1.75	0.67–4.52	.25

*Creatinine > 2.8 = preoperative creatinine > 2.8 mg/dL.

We analyzed the factors associated with acute renal failure in 234 patients who underwent TAA or total descending thoracic aneurysm repair, using univariate contingency table and multivariate logistic regression analysis. Acute renal failure, defined as an increase in serum creatinine by 1 mg/dL/d for 2 consecutive days postoperatively, occurred in 41 of 234 patients (17.5%). The univariate odds ratio of death, given acute renal failure, was 6.7 (95% CI 3.2–14.2, $p < .0001$). No significant association was found between the probability of acute renal failure and age, sex, hypertension, right renal artery reattachment, or renal bypass. Factors associated with increased risk of acute renal failure in multivariate analysis were visceral perfusion (OR = 3.6, 95% CI 1.2–11.0, $p < .02$), left renal artery reattachment (OR = 4.4, 95% CI 1.6–1.9, $p < .004$), preoperative creatinine ≥ 2.8 mg/dL (OR = 10.3, 95% CI 12.0–411.8, $p < .0001$), and simple clamp technique (OR = 3.4, 95% CI 1.07–10.76, $p < .04$). There was direct univariate correlation between preoperative creatinine and acute renal failure (OR=3.2 per mg/dL increase, 95% CI 2.7–10.1, $p < .0001$). Reproduced with permission from Safi HJ et al.[68]

postoperative laboratory values for extent II aneurysm repairs done with the simple cross-clamp technique. Intraoperative bleeding was reduced and postoperative liver enzymes more frequently fell within normal range.[72]

Pulmonary Function

Statistically significant predictive risk factors for prolonged postoperative respiratory insufficiency include advanced age, aortic cross-clamp time, number of packed red blood cells transfused, and tobacco use.[73] Since 1994, we cut only the muscular portion of the diaphragm. We found that diaphragm preservation during TAA repair results in a significant improvement in early ventilator weaning (Table 38-2).[73] In addition, this benefit remains present even when the effects of advanced age, tobacco use, extended clamp time, and greater transfusion requirements are accounted for. The preservation of the diaphragm also decreases the length of stay.[74]

Summary

There has been much progress in the field of TAA repair in the last 10 years. The incidence of the major complications—neurologic, renal, respiratory, and hepatic—has fallen. The decline in morbidity and mortality rates can be attributed to improvements in surgical technique, particularly the adoption of adjuncts of distal aortic perfusion and CSF drainage. During the era of the simple cross-clamp technique, routine intercostal artery reimplantation was not feasible because of the necessity to perform surgery quickly. Adjuncts, by providing an ample period of spinal cord protection, permit us to reattach these arteries, providing additional spinal cord protection. Although complications following TAA surgery remain a threat, the current short-term mortality is 5 to 10%, as compared to 20 to 25% 10 years ago.

TABLE 38-2. Intact Diaphragm during TAA Repair Results in a Higher Probability of Early Ventilator Weaning (Multiple Logistic Regression Model)

Variable	Parameter Estimate	Adjusted Odds Ratio	95% CI	p
Intercept	−4.8043	—	—	—
Age	0.0327	1.033	1.008–1.059	.02
Split diaphragm	0.7073	2.029	1.163–3.538	.02
Clamp time	0.0187	1.019	1.005–1.033	.008
Current smoking	0.9459	2.575	1.483–4.472	.0008
Packed red blood cells	0.0538	1.055	1.014–1.098	.008

Two hundred fifty-six TAA patients participated in a study that examined the consequences of diaphragm division. The diaphragm was divided in 150 patients and left intact in 106 patients. Patient demographics, history, physical findings, aneurysm extent, urgency of the procedure, acute dissection, cross-clamp time, homologous and autologous blood product consumption, and adjunctive operative techniques were examined as potential risk factors. FEV1 was also considered in the 197 patients for whom preoperative spirometry was available. Data were analyzed by univariate contingency table and multiple logistic regression methods. Increasing age, current smoking, total cross-clamp time, units of packed red blood cells transfused, and division of the diaphragm were significant, independent predictors of prolonged ventilation. Sixty-seven percent (71/106) of patients whose diaphragms were preserved were extubated in less than 72 hours, as compared to 52% (78/150) of patients who underwent diaphragm division (OR = 0.53, p < .02). Reproduced with permission from Engle J et al.[73]

The neurologic deficit rate for the most troublesome extent II aneurysms has fallen to below 7% from 30 to 40%.[69,75] Future research should focus on extent II TAA.

References

1. Etheredge S, Yee J, Smith J, et al. Successful resection of a large aneurysm of the upper abdominal aorta and replacement with homograft. Surgery 1955;138:1071–81.
2. DeBakey M, Creech O, Morris G. Aneurysm of the thoracoabdominal aorta involving the celiac, mesenteric and renal arteries. Report of four cases treated by resection and homograft replacement. Ann Surg 1956;179:763–72.
3. Matas R. An operation for the radical cure of aneurysm based upon arteriorrhaphy. Ann Surg 1903;37:161–96.
4. Creech O Jr. Endo-aneurysmorrhaphy and treatment of aortic aneurysm. Ann Surg 1966;164:935–46.
5. Carrell A. Results of the transplantation of blood vessels, organs and limbs. JAMA 1908;51:1662–7.
6. Laschinger JC, Cunningham JN Jr, Nathan IM, et al. Intraoperative identification of vessels critical to spinal cord blood supply—use of somatosensory evoked potentials. Curr Surg 1984;41:107–9.
7. Connolly JE, Wakabayashi A, German JC, et al. Clinical experience with pulsatile left heart bypass without anticoagulation for thoracic aneurysms. J Thorac Cardiovasc Surg 1971;62:568–76.
8. Valiathan MS, Weldon CS, Bender HW Jr, et al. Resection of aneurysms of the descending thoracic aorta using a GBH-coated shunt bypass. J Surg Res 1968;8:197–205.
9. Crawford ES, Coselli JS, Safi HJ. Partial cardiopulmonary bypass, hypothermic circulatory arrest, and posterolateral exposure for thoracic aortic aneurysm operation. J Thorac Cardiovasc Surg 1987;94:824–7.
10. Crawford ES, Svensson LG, Hess KR, et al. A prospective randomized study of cerebrospinal fluid drainage to prevent paraplegia after high-risk surgery on the thoracoabdominal aorta. J Vasc Surg 1991;13:36–45; discussion 45–6.
11. Cunningham JN Jr, Laschinger JC, Spencer FC. Monitoring of somatosensory evoked potentials during surgical procedures on the thoracoabdominal aorta. IV. Clinical observations and results. J Thorac Cardiovasc Surg 1987; 94:275–85.
12. Crawford ES, Mizrahi EM, Hess KR, et al. The impact of distal aortic perfusion and somatosensory evoked potential monitoring on prevention of paraplegia after aortic aneurysm operation [published erratum appears in J Thorac Cardiovasc Surg 1989;97(5):665]. J Thorac Cardiovasc Surg 1988;95:357–67.
13. Crawford ES, Crawford JL, Safi HJ, et al. Thoracoabdominal aortic aneurysms: preoperative and intraoperative factors determining immediate and long-term results of operations in 605 patients. J Vasc Surg 1986;3:389–404.
14. Kouchoukos NT, Daily BB, Rokkas CK, et al. Hypothermic bypass and circulatory arrest for operations on the descending thoracic and thoracoabdominal aorta. Ann Thorac Surg 1995;60:67–76;discussion 76–7.
15. Cambria R, Davison J, Zannetti S, et al. Clinical experience with epidural cooling for spinal cord protection during

thoracic and thoracoabdominal aneurysm repair. J Vasc Surg 1997;25:241–3.

16. Safi HJ, Hess KR, Randel M, et al. Cerebrospinal fluid drainage and distal aortic perfusion: reducing neurologic complications in repair of thoracoabdominal aortic aneurysm types I and II. J Vasc Surg 1996;23:223–8; discussion 229.

17. Coady MA, Rizzo JA, Goldstein LJ, Elefteriades JA. Natural history, pathogenesis, and etiology of thoracic aortic aneurysms and dissections. Cardiol Clin 1999;17:615–35; vii.

18. LaRoy LL, Cormier PJ, Matalon TA, et al. Imaging of abdominal aortic aneurysms. AJR Am J Roentgenol 1989;152:785–92.

19. Bickerstaff LK, Pairolero PC, Hollier LH, et al. Thoracic aortic aneurysms: a population-based study. Surgery 1982;92:1103–8.

20. Perko MJ, Norgaard M, Herzog TM, et al. Unoperated aortic aneurysm: a survey of 170 patients. Ann Thorac Surg 1995;59:1204–9.

21. Pressler V, McNamara JJ. Thoracic aortic aneurysm: natural history and treatment. J Thorac Cardiovasc Surg 1980;79:489–98.

22. Crawford ES, DeNatale RW. Thoracoabdominal aortic aneurysm: observations regarding the natural course of the disease. J Vasc Surg 1986;3:578–82.

23. Bonser RS, Pagano D, Lewis ME, et al. Clinical and pathoanatomical factors affecting expansion of thoracic aortic aneurysms. Heart 2000;84:277–83.

24. Juvonen T, Ergin MA, Galla JD, et al. Prospective study of the natural history of thoracic aortic aneurysms. Ann Thorac Surg 1997;63:1533–45.

25. Lobato AC, Puech-Leao P. Predictive factors for rupture of thoracoabdominal aortic aneurysm. J Vasc Surg 1998;27:446–53.

26. Elefteriades JA, Hartleroad J, Gusberg RJ, et al. Long-term experience with descending aortic dissection: the complication-specific approach. Ann Thorac Surg 1992;53:11–20; discussion 20–1.

27. Cambria RA, Gloviczki P, Stanson AW, et al. Outcome and expansion rate of 57 thoracoabdominal aortic aneurysms managed nonoperatively. Am J Surg 1995;170:213–7.

28. Dapunt OE, Galla JD, Sadeghi AM, et al. The natural history of thoracic aortic aneurysms. J Thorac Cardiovasc Surg 1994;107:1323–32; discussion 1332–3.

29. Rizzo JA, Coady MA, Elefteriades JA. Procedures for estimating growth rates in thoracic aortic aneurysms. J Clin Epidemiol 1998;51:747–54.

30. Szilagyi DE, Smith RF, DeRusso FJ, et al. Contribution of abdominal aortic aneurysmectomy to prolongation of life. Ann Surg 1966;164:678–99.

31. Palmer RF, Wheat MW. Management of impending rupture of the aorta with dissection. Adv Intern Med 1971;17:409–23.

32. Strachan DP. Predictors of death from aortic aneurysm among middle-aged men: the Whitehall study. Br J Surg 1991;78:401–4.

33. Cronenwett JL, Murphy TF, Zelenock GB, et al. Actuarial analysis of variables associated with rupture of small abdominal aortic aneurysms. Surgery 1985;98:472–83.

34. Cannon DJ, Read RC. Blood elastolytic activity in patients with aortic aneurysm. Ann Thorac Surg 1982;34:10–5.

35. Busuttil RW, Abou-Zamzam AM, Machleder HI. Collagenase activity of the human aorta. A comparison of patients with and without abdominal aortic aneurysms. Arch Surg 1980;115:1373–8.

36. Ergin MA, Spielvogel D, Apaydin A, et al. Surgical treatment of the dilated ascending aorta: when and how? Ann Thorac Surg 1999;67:1834–9; discussion 1853–6.

37. Lindholt JS, Jorgensen B, Fasting H, Henneberg EW. Plasma levels of plasmin-antiplasmin-complexes are predictive for small abdominal aortic aneurysms expanding to operation-recommendable sizes. J Vasc Surg 2001;34:611–5.

38. Pitt MP, Bonser RS. The natural history of thoracic aortic aneurysm disease: an overview. J Card Surg 1997;12:270–8.

39. Juvonen T, Ergin MA, Galla JD, et al. Risk factors for rupture of chronic type B dissections. J Thorac Cardiovasc Surg 1999;117:776–86.

40. Johansson G, Markstrom U, Swedenborg J. Ruptured thoracic aortic aneurysms: a study of incidence and mortality rates. J Vasc Surg 1995;21:985–8.

41. Fillinger MF. Imaging of the thoracic and thoracoabdominal aorta. Semin Vasc Surg 2000;13:247–63.

42. Balm R, Eikelboom BC, van Leeuwen MS, Noordzij J. Spiral CT-angiography of the aorta. Eur J Vasc Surg 1994;8:544–51.

43. Raptopoulos V, Rosen MP, Kent KC, et al. Sequential helical CT angiography of aortoiliac disease. AJR Am J Roentgenol 1996;166:1347–54.

44. Van Hoe L, Baert AL, Gryspeerdt S, et al. Supra- and juxtarenal aneurysms of the abdominal aorta: preoperative assessment with thin-section spiral CT. Radiology 1996;198:443–8.

45. Bradshaw KA, Pagano D, Bonser RS, et al. Multiplanar reformatting and three-dimensional reconstruction: for preoperative assessment of the thoracic aorta by computed tomography. Clin Radiol 1998;53:198–202.

46. Kieffer E, Richard T, Chiras J, et al. Preoperative spinal cord arteriography in aneurysmal disease of the descending thoracic and thoracoabdominal aorta: preliminary results in 45 patients. Ann Vasc Surg 1989;3:34–46.

47. Williams GM, Perler BA, Burdick JF, et al. Angiographic localization of spinal cord blood supply and its relationship to postoperative paraplegia. J Vasc Surg 1991;13:23–33; discussion 33–5.

48. Sommer T, Fehske W, Holzknecht N, et al. Aortic dissection: a comparative study of diagnosis with spiral CT, multiplanar transesophageal echocardiography, and MR imaging. Radiology 1996;199:347–52.

49. Estrera AL, Rubenstein FS, Miller CC 3rd, et al. Descending thoracic aortic aneurysm: surgical approach and treatment using the adjuncts cerebrospinal fluid drainage and distal aortic perfusion. Ann Thorac Surg 2001;72:481–6.

50. Dardik A, Perler BA, Roseborough GS, Williams GM. Aneurysmal expansion of the visceral patch after thoracoabdominal aortic replacement: an argument for limiting patch size? J Vasc Surg 2001;34:405–9; discussion 410.

51. Safi HJ, Miller CCI, Iliopoulos DC, et al. Staged repair of extensive aortic aneurysm: improved neurologic outcome. Ann Surg 1997;226:559–605.

52. Safi HJ, Campbell MP, Ferreira ML, et al. Spinal cord protection in descending thoracic and thoracoabdominal aortic aneurysm repair. Semin Thorac Cardiovasc Surg 1998;10:41–4.

53. Cambria RP, Davison JK, Carter C, et al. Epidural cooling for spinal cord protection during thoracoabdominal aneurysm repair: a five-year experience. J Vasc Surg 2000;31:1093–102.

54. Dossche KM, Schepens MA, Morshuis WJ, et al. Antegrade selective cerebral perfusion in operations on the proximal thoracic aorta. Ann Thorac Surg 1999;67:1904–10; discussion 1919–21.

55. Ergin MA, Galla JD, Lansman SL, et al. Hypothermic circulatory arrest in operations on the thoracic aorta. Determinants of operative mortality and neurologic outcome. J Thorac Cardiovasc Surg 1994;107:788–97; discussion 797–9.

56. Griepp RB, Ergin MA, Galla JD, et al. Minimizing spinal cord injury during repair of descending thoracic and thoracoabdominal aneurysms: the Mount Sinai approach. Semin Thorac Cardiovasc Surg 1998;10:25–8.

57. Hamilton IN Jr, Hollier LH. Adjunctive therapy for spinal cord protection during thoracoabdominal aortic aneurysm repair. Semin Thorac Cardiovasc Surg 1998; 10:35–9.

58. Safi HJ, Bartoli S, Hess KR, et al. Neurologic deficit in patients at high risk with thoracoabdominal aortic aneurysms: the role of cerebral spinal fluid drainage and distal aortic perfusion. J Vasc Surg 1994;20:434–44; discussion 442–3.

59. Grum D, Svensson L. Changes in cerebrospinal fluid pressure and spinal cord perfusion pressure prior to cross-clamping of the thoracic aorta in humans. J Cardiothoracic Vasc Anesth 1991;5:331–5.

60. Safi H, Miller CI, Carr C, et al. The importance of intercostal artery reattachment during thoracoabdominal aortic aneurysm repair. J Vasc Surg 1998;27:58–68.

61. Huynh TT, Miller CC 3rd, Safi HJ. Delayed onset of neurologic deficit: significance and management. Semin Vasc Surg 2000;13:340–4.

62. Safi HJ, Miller CC 3rd, Azizzadeh A, Iliopoulos DC. Observations on delayed neurologic deficit after thoracoabdominal aortic aneurysm repair. J Vasc Surg 1997;26:616–22.

63. Li GL, Farooque M, Holtz A, Olsson Y. Apoptosis of oligodendrocytes occurs for long distances away from the primary injury after compression trauma to rat spinal cord. Acta Neuropathol (Berl) 1999;98:473–80.

64. Kato H, Kanellopoulos GK, Matsuo S, et al. Neuronal apoptosis and necrosis following spinal cord ischemia in the rat. Exp Neurol 1997;148:464–74.

65. Azizzadeh A, Huynh T, Miller CI, Safi H. Reversal of twice-delayed neurologic deficits with cerebrospinal fluid drainage after thoracoabdominal aneurysm repair: a case report and plea for a national database collection. J Vasc Surg 2000;31:592–8.

66. Estrera AL, Miller CC 3rd, Azizzadeh A, et al. Predictors of delayed neurologic deficit following repair of thoracic and thoracoabdominal aortic aneurysm. AATS abstract, May 2001.

67. Estrera AL, Miller CC 3rd, Huynh TT, et al. Neurologic outcome after thoracic and thoracoabdominal aortic aneurysm repair. Ann Thorac Surg 2001;72:1225–30; discussion 1230–1.

68. Safi HJ, Harlin SA, Miller CC, et al. Predictive factors for acute renal failure in thoracic and thoracoabdominal aortic aneurysm surgery [published erratum appears in J Vasc Surg 1997;25(1):93]. J Vasc Surg 1996;24:338–44; discussion 344–5.

69. Svensson LG, Crawford ES, Hess KR, et al. Experience with 1509 patients undergoing thoracoabdominal aortic operations. J Vasc Surg 1993;17:357–68; discussion 368–70.

70. Halpenny M, Markos F, Snow HM, et al. The effects of fenoldopam on renal blood flow and tubular function during aortic cross-clamping in anaesthetized dogs. Eur J Anaesthesiol 2000;17:491–8.

71. Gilbert TB, Hasnain JU, Flinn WR, et al. Fenoldopam infusion associated with preserving renal function after aortic cross-clamping for aneurysm repair. J Cardiovasc Pharmacol Ther 2001;6:31–6.

72. Safi HJ, Miller CC 3rd, Yawn DH, et al. Impact of distal aortic and visceral perfusion on liver function during thoracoabdominal and descending thoracic aortic repair. J Vasc Surg 1998;27:145–52; discussion 152–3.

73. Engle J, Safi HJ, Miller CC 3rd, et al. The impact of diaphragm management on prolonged ventilator support after thoracoabdominal aortic repair. J Vasc Surg 1999;29:150–6.

74. Huynh TTT, Miller CC 3rd, Estrera AL, et al. Determinants of hospital length of stay after thoracoabdominal aortic aneurysm repair. J Vasc Surg 2002;35:648–53.

75. Safi HJ, Miller CC 3rd, Iliopoulos DC, Griffiths G. Long-term results following thoracoabdominal aortic aneurysm repair. In: Branchereau A, Jacobs MJHM, editors. European vascular course: long-term results of arterial interventions. Armonk, NY: Futura Publishing; 1997. p. 181–93.

CHAPTER 39

Endovascular Stent-Grafts for Thoracic Aneurysms and Dissections

Michael D. Dake, MD

Over the last 10 years, no new cardiovascular interventional technique, with the exception of gene therapy, has had as much unrealized clinical potential as thoracic aortic stent-grafting. Although the theoretical advantages of this less-invasive alternative to open repair are compelling, perhaps even more compelling than the recognized benefits of applying endograft technology to the management of abdominal aortic aneurysms, the potential of this attractive therapy essentially remains an unrealized cliché. It is hard to believe that after more than 10 years of clinical investigation with a variety of thoracic stent-grafts, the medical community interested in treating thoracic aortic diseases still has no access to an Food and Drug Administration approved device for patients with prohibitive operative risks.

Nevertheless, the consensual opinion of surgical and interventional authorities working in this field suggests that in the near future this technology will have an expanded role in the treatment of patients with thoracic aortic diseases and that it will eventually evolve into the primary therapy for selected pathologies in which clear benefits are identified. The traditional standard therapy for descending thoracic aortic aneurysm (TAA) is open operative repair with graft replacement of the diseased aortic segment. Despite important advances in surgical techniques, anesthetic management, and postoperative care over the last 30 years, the mortality and morbidity rates of surgery remain considerable, especially in patients at high risk for thoracotomy because of co-existing severe cardiopulmonary abnormalities or other medical diseases.

The advent of endovascular stent-graft technology provides an alternative to open surgery for selected patients with TAA. Following closely on the heels of early clinical experience with endografts for the treatment of patients with abdominal aortic aneurysms, the application of this new technology was initially focused on the management of descending aortic aneurysms in high-risk surgical candidates.[1–5]

The initial results of these feasibility studies suggest that stent-grafts offer an attractive alternative to open surgical repair that may potentially reduce the operative risk, hospital stay, and procedural cost in selected patients.[5–7] Subsequently, clinical trials of commercially manufactured devices have been initiated to treat patients with descending TAA. Results will be compared with those achieved in an enrolled group of contemporary surgical controls to better determine the effectiveness of stent-graft therapy and quantitate any benefits. Unfortunately, the final results of these studies, including 1-year follow-up data, will not be available until 2002.

Since 1992, when the feasibility and safety of stent-graft therapy for TAA was initially investigated, there has been an increasing number of reports of the application of this technology to treatment of patients with a wide spectrum of thoracic aortic disease, including acute and chronic dissection; intramural hematoma; penetrating ulcer; traumatic injury; Marfan's syndrome; mycotic aneurysm; anastomotic aneurysm; rupture; and emboligenic aortic sources.[5–14] This chapter describes experiences with stent-graft management of specific aortic disease, after a presentation of the currently available devices.

Devices

A detailed discussion of the various first-generation homemade devices is only of modest historical interest. Suffice it to say, most of these prototypical prostheses were self-expanding and based on a combination of polyester graft with a modified type of Gianturco Z stent. Most delivery systems were large (24 to 27 French), relatively rigid, and depending upon the anatomy as well as the length and diameter of the device, difficult to target and deploy due to a marked frictional resistance encountered during withdrawal of the outer device-constraining sheath. Detailed descriptions of individual systems, components, fabrication processes, and deployment techniques are provided elsewhere.[5–14]

Currently, there are two commercially manufactured thoracic stent-grafts that are widely available. The Excluder (W.L. Gore and Associates, Flagstaff, AZ) and the Talent devices (AVE/Medtronic Inc., Santa Rosa, CA) have been each implanted in more than 500 patients with TAA worldwide. Both represent considerable improvements over the prior generation of institutionally fabricated stent-grafts, in terms of ease of use, reliability, and consistency of device manufacturing.

The Gore Excluder (Figure 39-1) is composed of a self-expanding nitinol stent lined with ultrathin wall polytetrafluoroethylene (PTFE) graft material. The PTFE graft has a 30-micron internodal distance similar to the pore size of conventional PTFE grafts used for peripheral vascular reconstructions. The ends of the device have a scalloped contour to enhance graft contact with the aortic wall over a wide range of aortic tortuousities and angulations.

The scalloped projections are covered with PTFE, and their length is directly proportional to the diameter of the graft. The device is very flexible radially and longitudinally.

Two S-shaped stabilization wires anchored 180° apart span the length of the graft to limit longitudinal compression.

The graft is axially compressed onto the end of the delivery catheter and constrained by a PTFE corset that is laced with PTFE suture. The suture runs the length of the catheter and is attached to a deployment knob at the opposite end. Grafts are available in a range of diameters between 26 and 40 mm and in a selection of lengths between 7.5 and 40 cm. The sizes of the delivery system and compatible introducer sheaths vary according to the diameter of the device and scale over a range of 20 to 24 French.

After preliminary arteriographic studies define the preferred proximal and distal stent-graft "landing zones" and these targets are confirmed by transesophageal ultrasonography, the appropriately sized 30-cm-long introducer sheath is advanced over a guidewire to the infrarenal aorta. Alternatively, in certain situations, the catheter delivery system may be introduced over the guidewire without the use of a sheath. In either case, the device catheter is tracked over the wire until it reaches the selected target in a manner that bridges the aneurysm from proximal to distal necks. If more than one device is required because of excessive aneurysm length (> 16 cm) or a mismatch in diameters between proximal and distal necks > 4 mm, the smallest-diameter device is deployed first, irrespective of its location. Subsequently, the larger-diameter device is coaxially placed with at least a 3-cm overlap to enhance the interference seal between the grafts. If the anticipated diameters of multiple grafts are equal, the proximal device is usually deployed first, with additional coaxial devices placed successively distal.

In all cases, there must be sufficiently long proximal and distal aneurysm necks of at least 15 to 20 mm to ensure adequate wall contact for graft fixation and a tight circumferential seal.

After final positioning is completed, the device is deployed by pulling the knob adjacent to the catheter hub. As the knob is smoothly retracted, the attached suture is withdrawn, and opening of the corset occurs initially in the middle and then proceeds toward both ends. An instantaneous release of the underlying self-expanding stent-graft occurs. After deployment, the delivery catheter is removed and a trilobed balloon, designed exclusively to smooth any wrinkles or pleats in the graft without increasing the proximal arterial pressure, is introduced and expanded at the proximal and distal necks, as well as at any device overlap zones. This ensures full graft expansion. The procedure is complete if the desired position of the graft is achieved without arteriographic or transesophageal ultrasound imaging evidence of inadequate sealing and persistent flow within the aneurysm. However, if the device is poorly positioned or not fully expanded and there is a perigraft leak, supplemental maneuvers, including placement of additional stent-graft(s) or balloon expansion over the segment of aneurysm neck where the leak is suspected, may prove beneficial. Additional preprocedural considerations, imaging requirements, procedural techniques, postprocedural patient management, and follow-up issues were detailed earlier.

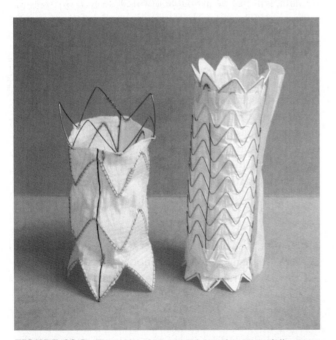

FIGURE 39-1. The two most commonly used commercially manufactured thoracic stent-grafts are the Gore Excluder (left) and the Talent device from AVE/Medtronic.

The second device currently available for treatment of patients with descending TAA is the Talent endoprosthesis (see Figure 39-1). The design of this product has evolved since its clinical introduction.

The current version has a lower profile and more flexible delivery catheter than did the original system. The prosthesis is composed of sinusoidal nitinol stent elements sandwiched between thin layers of polyester graft material. The individual stent forms are secured in place with oversewn sutures to prevent migration; however, they are not connected to one another, and there are segments of unsupported graft interposed between stents.

This design allows independent stent motion and confers a degree of longitudinal flexibility.

Similar to the Excluder device, the Talent uses two longitudinal wires to provide stabilization and prevent longitudinal compression.

A unique aspect of the device is its proximal margin with broad-based nitinol wire scallops. The wide uncovered interstices may be placed across the origin of the left subclavian artery in cases where there is a short proximal neck of between 10 and 20 mm. In this setting, placement of the uncovered stent across the left subclavian artery helps to optimally orient the graft, stabilize its position, and, during deployment, secure precise targeting of the graft material at the distal subclavian margin.

The stent-grafts are available in a wide range of diameters and lengths. In addition, custom fabrication of a prosthesis based upon an individual patient's anatomy is possible within 3 weeks. The delivery profile for Talent is between 22 and 27 French, depending on the diameter and length of the device.

The delivery catheter has a flexible conical tip. Set back from the tip is an integrated balloon that is used for smoothing the graft material and promoting adequate stent expansion following deployment of the self-expanding device. The prosthesis is collapsed over the distal segment of the delivery catheter and maintained in this packed configuration by an overlying transparent sheath. Proximal to the loaded stent-graft is a blunt metal stopper that functions as a brace to maintain the device position as the constraining sheath is withdrawn.

After the stent-graft is properly positioned, usually 1 to 3 cm proximal to the optimal landing zone to mitigate against an inadvertent downstream drift during deployment, the overlying sheath is slowly withdrawn.

As the initial uncovered stent elements cantilever open, gentle retraction of the device is applied until the exact desired position of the proximal graft margin is obtained. After the device is fully deployed, the balloon is withdrawn and expanded within the proximal and distal neck segments to fully expand the prosthesis. Subsequently, the final result is documented angiographically and the arteriotomy repaired surgically.

In an analysis of the relative merits of the devices, it is important to note that both devices have established records of technical and clinical successes. However, in certain cases, the particular disease process and/or anatomy may recommend one over the other. The marked flexibility of the Excluder device and its delivery system, as well as its smaller introduction profile, make it better suited for patients with severely angled aortic anatomy or iliofemoral conduct arteries that are small, calcified, or tortuous.

In TAA cases with short (< 15 mm) proximal necks, or in aortic dissection where the primary entry tear is very close to the left subclavian artery, the Talent device may be preferred because of its leading segment of uncovered stent. In terms of ease of use, the Excluder has some advantages. The maximum graft length available is 20 cm as compared to 13 cm for an individual noncustom Talent device. This, in combination with its simple and straightforward deployment, makes it more efficient to treat patients with long aneurysms. In certain applications, such as aortic dissection, the relative radial force exerted by the prosthesis may be a consideration. In the acute setting, the lower hoop strength of the Excluder may allow adequate coverage of the entry site without causing an iatrogenic secondary tear in the thin fragile dissection flap. On the other hand, the greater radial force of the Talent may be beneficial in cases of chronic dissection to displace a thick and resistant dissection septum and, thus, to enhance the true lumen diameter.

Applications

Currently, the application with the greatest clinical experience remains descending TAA with an estimated 3,000 implementations worldwide (Figure 39-2). Results of controlled studies are not available, long-term data are limited, and comparison of experiences that typically employ a wide variety of prosthetic designs is problematic; however, a consensus pattern of outcomes from centers active in this field is emerging that defines a shared reality.

Irrespective of the device implanted (institutionally crafted first generation or commercially manufactured second generation), in series of more than 40 patients (range, 40 to 260) with nondissection-associated TAA, operative mortalities were between 0 and 4%, technically successful device deployments occurred in 98 to 100% of cases, and immediate aneurysm thrombosis was achieved in 90 to 100%.[15–19] Paraplegia was a complication in 0 to 1.6%, and stroke occurred in a range of 0 to 2.8%. Conversion to open surgical repair occurred in 0 to 4% of cases, and late endoleaks were noted in 2 to 3%.

What have we learned from the experiences accumulated to date? First, it is clear that the ideal endovascular prosthesis for TAA is not yet available. Perhaps, it is unreasonable to expect that one device will be capable of optimally addressing all combinations of TAA etiologies, morphologies, and underlying vascular anatomy. In the end, the individual aspects of each case may dictate

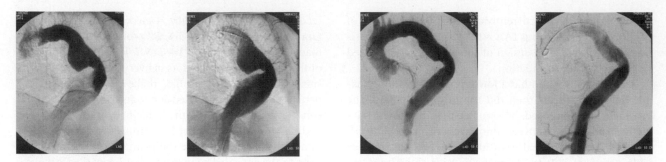

FIGURE 39-2. Aortograms of a 64-year-old man, performed before and immediately after stent-graft placement to isolate a descending thoracic aortic aneurysm.

selection of the best suited prosthesis from a medley of devices.

One factor (eg, short proximal neck, severely angled descending aorta, small or tortuous access arteries) may dominate the decision process. The factors considered in determining which device is preferred for implantation in a 20-year-old with an acute traumatic injury may be different than the factors considered when determining which device is best to deploy in an 80-year-old with a long tortuous degenerative aneurysm.

The reports from the first wave of experiences provide additional insights into the spectrum of results and frequency of complications, some of them unexpected. Indeed, the recorded frequencies for paraplegia are lower than most experienced clinicians would have predicted prior to the initiation of this therapy and are similar to the most favorable results from contemporary series of open surgical repair for TAA. The anticipated potential complication of device migration or kinking has been very rare and observed mostly with the use of "homemade" rigid or semirigid devices and prostheses with unsupported midgraft segments.

The experience with sequelae of stent-graft coverage and occlusion of the left subclavian artery is no longer limited to isolated case reports of inadvertent obstruction due to device misplacement within a short proximal neck segment. The practice of prophylactic left subclavian to left carotid artery transportation or bypass graft placement in patients with an insufficiently long proximal neck in order to avoid possible complications following endograft placement across the subclavian has given way to a trend toward expectant management. If arm, hand, or cerebral symptoms develop after coverage of the branch, then surgical revascularization of the subclavian artery is performed. Early results of this revised algorithm suggest that it is safe in the majority of patients; however, symptomatic malperfusion of the upper extremity requiring interventions occurs with a frequency that is yet to be defined.

In contradiction to the problem of an inadequate proximal neck segment, there are no easy management strategies to deal with a short distal neck above the celiac artery. Intentional coverage of the celiac is not an innocuous tactic despite a coexisting normal superior mesenteric

artery capable of supporting an apparently normal network of collateral flow. There are four known cases of death following intentional stent-graft coverage of the celiac artery during treatment of TAAs with short distal necks. Two of the patients died because of liver failure, and two from sepsis with pancreatic and splenic infarctions, respectively. In all cases, preprocedure catheter maneuvers, including selective arteriographic mapping of possible collateral pathways and hemodynamic pressure recordings, were performed in an effort to predict whether the patients would tolerate occlusion of the celiac artery. Unfortunately, there are no easy operative methods to solve the problem of the short supraceliac neck.

Another concern that still requires attention is the large delivery profile of current devices relative to the iliofemoral arteries. Injuries to conduit arteries and arterial access complications are common, and the clinical sequelae of these complications are often significant. Indeed, the frequency of these events and the more alarming reports of strokes, due in part to manipulations of large, bulky, and semirigid delivery systems within aortic arch, mandate immediate development of smaller, less-traumatic devices.

The issue of endoleaks after stent-graft treatment of patients with TAA is an interesting and important subject. It is now obvious that there are distinct differences between the relative frequencies, various types, and fates of endoleaks identified after stent-graft therapy of TAA and abdominal aortic aneurysm (AAA). There is a clear indication that endoleaks occur less frequently after TAA repair. When they are observed, TAA endoleaks occur more commonly at proximal or distal attachment sites (type 1 endoleak), where there is an incomplete seal between the graft and the proximal or distal aneurysm neck, rather than via retrograde aortic branch vessel flow into the aneurysm from collateral channels (type 2 endoleak). The majority of endoleaks diagnosed early after stent-graft repair of AAA are of the type 2 variety.

Although type 2 endoleaks via intercostal or bronchial arteries have been reported after TAA therapy, the incidence is very low. The reason for this difference is currently unclear.

It is generally accepted that the prognosis for type 1 endoleaks is more serious than the natural history of type

2 endoleaks. The effects from the force of aortic arterial pressure transmitted directly to a TAA after stent-graft placement are potentially lethal, and there are multiple isolated reports of early rupture occurring in this setting. Consequently, aggressive endovascular or surgical intervention is recommended if feasible when type 1 endoleaks are documented more than 2 to 4 weeks after the implantation procedure.

Another thoracic aortic stent-graft application that is receiving increasing attention is the treatment of patients with aortic dissection (Figure 39-3).

There is growing worldwide experience with this procedure in the setting of acute type B dissection and chronic dissection with coexisting descending aortic false lumen aneurysm.[12–14,20,21]

In both pathologies, successful management is predicated on obliteration of the primary entry tear of dissection by placement of the prosthesis within the true lumen across the entry tear. Stent-graft coverage of the entry site closes the primary communication to the false lumen, and its flow is markedly reduced or choked off completely. In acute type B dissection, the true lumen immediately increases in diameter without a corresponding incremental change in the overall aortic diameter. Downstream, any dynamic branch vessel involvement of abdominal aortic true lumen arteries compromised by the dissection process is expeditiously reversed seconds after stent-graft placement.

In both cases of acute and chronic dissection, stagnant blood in the thoracic aortic false lumen clots, and in the majority of patients, progressive thrombosis of the false lumen proceeds from the proximal aspect of the involved thoracic aorta distally, irrespective of the primary tear location. The tempo of this process is variable and presumably based on the size of the false lumen, abdominal branch vessel distribution off the aortic lumens, and the amount of residual thoracic aortic false lumen flow via uncovered additional tears in the thoracic dissection flap, retrograde thoracic aortic false lumen branch vessel flow from collaterals, retrograde perfusion from the abdominal aortic false lumen, and similar considerations.

It is expected that residual isolated patency of the abdominal aortic false lumen will persist via natural fenestration in the dissection flap that exists at levels corresponding to abdominal branches off the false lumen. This phenomenon permits sufficient perfusion of abdominal aortic false lumen branches via true lumen transseptal flow after stent-graft obliteration of the primary thoracic communication to the false lumen. In cases of acute dissection, if thoracic aortic false lumen thrombosis occurs after stent-graft placement, progressive false lumen resolution may occur with a corresponding gradual enlargement of the thoracic true lumen. In this regard, follow-up imaging at 1 year has shown apparent "healing" of the dissection in a number of cases without computed tomography (CT) evidence of a residual thoracic aortic false lumen or dissection flap.[12,13]

Early results from clinical series of stent-graft management in limited numbers of patients with acute type B and acute type A aortic dissection where the primary tear is identified distal to the left subclavian artery are encouraging.[12,16–19,21] Obliteration of flow through the entry tear into the false lumen was achieved in more than 90% of cases, with associated complete thrombosis of the proximal thoracic aortic false lumen segment apparent in 80 to 100% of cases, and distal thoracic segment thrombosis noted less frequently. Progressive thoracic false lumen shrinkage at 1-, 6-, and 12-month follow-up imaging was observed in most cases.

Complications, including paraplegia, rupture, and iatrogenic extension of the dissection into the ascending aorta, were reported anecdotally in early experience with stent-graft placement in acute dissection.[16–19]

In terms of the procedure, there are some technical challenges related to the idiosyncratic morphologic manifestations of aortic dissection that are often discussed when stent-graft therapy is considered. Specifically, the optimal method to select the diameter and length of the prosthesis is a common issue. Because the true lumen is a fraction of the overall transaortic diameter and rarely cylindrical in shape, choosing the "right" device dimension is a unique logistical dilemma. Most practitioners base their selection on more than one measurement. Perhaps, the most compelling measurement is the diameter of the nondissected aorta immediately proximal to the entry tear. This is a good estimate of the original size of the proximal involved segment prior to the dissection. This measurement, plus an oversize factor of 20% to ensure secure anchoring and a tight circumferential seal, is the approximation of device size most frequently used in current practice.

Obviously, if there is retrograde proximal extension of the dissection from the entry site, other planning steps must be taken. These include calculation of the mean true lumen diameter from measurements of the maximum and minimum true lumen dimensions and selection of an arbitrary diameter corresponding to a value larger than the true lumen but smaller than the overall aortic diameter.

In terms of the device length, most investigators implant devices that are clearly longer than the entry tear and usually in the range of 10 to 15 cm long. This added length confers an appearance to the aortic morphology after implantation that is more normal anatomically, especially in the arch, than that observed following placement of a short device focally over the entry tear. In addition, the longer device promotes a more rapid tempo to the formation of thrombus within the proximal thoracic aortic false lumen. Longer extension of the overall device length into the distal one-third of the descending thoracic aorta, however, should be avoided in this setting because of an associated increased risk of spinal cord ischemia.

In cases of aortic dissection with a classic isthmus location of the primary entry site, the tear may be within

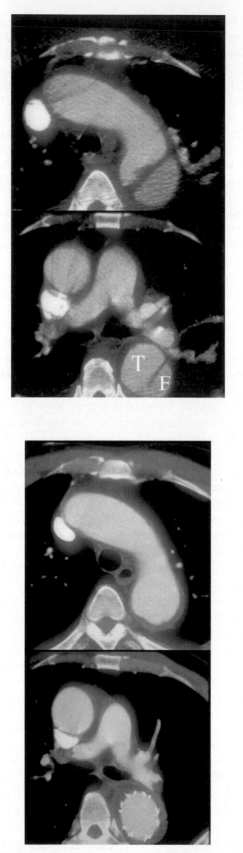

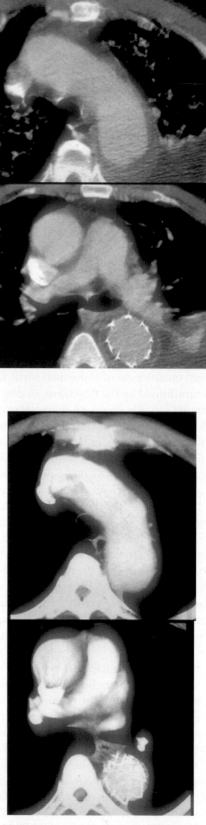

FIGURE 39-3. Series of CT scans performed at the same anatomic levels before and following stent-graft repair of a 53-year-old man with an acute type B aortic dissection complicated by abdominal branch vessel involvement. Immediately after stent-graft placement, there is an increase in the size of the true lumen (T) with resolution of the peripheral ischemia, and subsequently, progressive thrombosis and shrinkage of the false lumen (F).

10 mm of the left subclavian artery. In this situation, a device with a proximal segment consisting of a bare stent can be placed across the left subclavian artery to effectively maximize the length of graft contact with the aortic wall prior to the tear. However, in other settings, where there is retrograde proximal extension of the dissection from the tear to the subclavian artery, it may be necessary to place the graft over the branch, with its leading margin between the left carotid and subclavian arteries. In addition to carefully monitoring the patient post procedure for ischemic symptoms referable to the covered left subclavian, it is important to carefully image the thoracic aorta to exclude persistent perfusion of the false lumen via retrograde subclavian flow around the device into the arch.

Similar to acute type B dissection, experience is mounting with endograft management of chronic aortic dissection as an alternative to open surgical repair in patients with false lumen aneurysm. In this regard, multiple studies report rates of aneurysm, thrombosis, and subsequent false lumen shrinkage that mirror the results recorded in series of acute dissection.[13–20,22] One controlled investigation that compared stent-graft therapy to open surgery in matched groups of patients with chronic type B dissection reported improved survival and decreased neurologic complications with the less-invasive procedure.[13]

Many other applications of stent-grafts for the treatment of patients with a wide variety of thoracic aortic pathologies have been published and are destined to receive increasing attention and clinical study in the future. Most noteworthy are traumatic aortic injury, mycotic aneurysm, aortic rupture, and aneurysms involving arch or abdominal branches.[8–10,22] Details of these experiences are available in earlier publications.

Are there any trends currently evolving? Based on the experience accumulated thus far, and emboldened specifically by the relatively low frequency of paraplegia complicating treatment of TAA, the average stent-graft length appears to be increasing recently. This practice is intended to allow the device to be confidently secured within an ample segment of normal aorta proximal and distal to the aneurysm. It is hoped that this will help to avoid late complications such as endoleak due to degenerative changes within the aortic borders immediately adjacent to the aneurysm.

In conclusion, the recent development of endovascular stent-graft technology and its application as an alternative therapy to open surgical treatment of patients with a variety of thoracic aortic pathologies is an exciting and potentially valuable advance. The next major challenge that interventionists face is the important task of objectively elucidating the "real" benefits, risks, and complications of thoracic stent-grafts through rigorous, prospective, controlled investigations of each possible disease application. This type of controlled experience will no doubt help to better identify the most salutary indications, patients with the best chance for extended benefit, and the frequency of long-term failures. Only after this level of scientific scrutiny is performed can clinicians confidently counsel patients with accurate information regarding their therapeutic options.

References

1. Parodi JC, Palmaz JC, Barone HD. Transfemoral intraluminal graft implantation for abdominal aortic aneurysms. Ann Vasc Surg 1991;5:491–9.
2. Yusuf SW, Baker DM, Chuter TAM, et al. Transfemoral endoluminal repair of abdominal aortic aneurysm with bifurcated graft. Lancet 1994;344:650–1.
3. Moore WS, Vescera CL. Repair of abdominal aortic aneurysm by transfemoral endovascular graft placement. Ann Surg 1994;220:331–41.
4. Blum U, Langer M, Spillner G, et al. Abdominal aortic aneurysms: preliminary technical and clinical results with transfemoral placement of endovascular self-expanding stent-grafts. Radiology 1996;198:25–31.
5. Dake MD, Miller DC, Semba CP, et al. Transluminal placement of endovascular stent-grafts for the treatment of descending thoracic aortic aneurysms. N Engl J Med 1994;331:1729–34.
6. Mitchell RS, Dake MD, Semba CP, et al. Endovascular stent-graft repair of thoracic aortic aneurysms. J Thorac Cardiovasc Surg 1996;111:1054–62.
7. Dake MD, Miller DC, Mitchell RS, et al. The "first generation" of endovascular stent-grafts for patients with aneurysms of the descending thoracic aorta. J Thorac Cardiovasc Surg 1998;116:689–703.
8. Semba CP, Kato N, Kee ST, et al. Acute rupture of the descending thoracic aorta: repair with use of endovascular stent- grafts. J Vasc Interv Radiol 1997;8:337–42.
9. Kato N, Dake MD, Miller DC, et al. Traumatic thoracic aortic aneurysm: treatment with endovascular stent-grafts. Radiology 1997;205:657–62.
10. Semba CP, Sakai T, Slonim SM, et al. Mycotic aneurysm of the thoracic aorta: repair with use of endovascular stent-grafts. J Vasc Interv Radiol 1998;9:41–9.
11. Dake MD, Semba CP, Razavi MK, et al. Endovascular procedures for the treatment of aortic dissection: techniques and results. J Cardiovasc Surg 1998;39:45–52.
12. Dake MD, Kato N, Mitchell RS, et al. Endovascular stent-graft placement for the treatment of acute aortic dissection. N Engl J Med 1999;340:1546–52.
13. Nienaber CA, Fattori R, Lund G, et al. Non-surgical reconstruction of thoracic aortic dissection by stent-graft placement. N Engl J Med 1999;340:1539–45.
14. Sakai T, Dake MD, Semba CP, et al. Descending thoracic aortic aneurysm: thoracic CT findings after endovascular stent-graft placement. Radiology 1999;212:169–74.
15. Dake MD. The advent of thoracic aortic endografting. The First international Summit on Thoracic Aorta Endografting. Tokyo, Japan; 2001.
16. Ehrlich MP. Thoracic aorta endografting: the Australian experience. The First International Summit on Thoracic Aorta Endografting. Tokyo, Japan; 2001.
17. Fattori R. Endovascular treatment of the thoracic aorta. The First International Summit on Thoracic Aorta Endografting. Tokyo, Japan; 2001.

18. Ishimura S. Aorta grafting: the reliable treatment option. The First International Summit on Thoracic Aorta Endografting. Tokyo, Japan; 2001.

19. Lauterjung L. Endovascular stent-grafting for the thoracic aorta. The First International Summit on Thoracic Aorta Endografting. Tokyo, Japan; 2001.

20. Kato N, Hirano T, Shimono T, et al. Treatment of chronic type B aortic dissection with endovascular stent-graft placement. Cardiovasc Intervent Radiol 2000;23:60–2.

21. Czermak BV, Waldenberger P, Fraedrich G, et al. Treatment of Stanford type B aortic dissection with stent-grafts: preliminary results. Radiology 2000;217:544–50.

22. Iwase T. Endovascular repair for chronic aortic dissection by Inoue stent- graft system. The First International Summit on Thoracic Aorta Endografting. Tokyo, Japan; 2001.

CHAPTER 40

INHALED NITRIC OXIDE IN HEART AND LUNG SURGERY

DAVID A. FULLERTON, MD

Hypoxemia and increased pulmonary vascular resistance (PVR) may greatly complicate the management of cardiothoracic surgical patients. They are commonly found in the setting of thoracic organ transplantation, in adult and pediatric cardiac surgical procedures, and in general thoracic surgical procedures. Inhaled nitric oxide (NO) helps in the management of such patients. It improves oxygenation in the setting of acute lung injury and selectively lowers PVR, without producing unwanted systemic vasodilation.

Physiology of Inhaled Nitric Oxide

Inhaled NO is a "selective" pulmonary vasodilator. Once inhaled into the alveolus, it readily diffuses across the alveolocapillary membrane into the subjacent vascular smooth muscle. Within pulmonary vascular smooth muscle, NO stimulates guanylate cyclase to generate cyclic guanosine 3',5'- monophosphate (cGMP). In turn, cGMP activates protein kinase G, which lowers intracellular calcium by ill-defined mechanisms, leading to vascular smooth-muscle relaxation. As NO diffuses through the vascular smooth muscle and into the blood vessel lumen, it is immediately bound to hemoglobin and inactivated; the affinity of hemoglobin for NO is 3,000 times greater than that for oxygen (Figure 40-1). In binding NO, hemoglobin is converted to nitrosyl hemoglobin and then to methemoglobin. Methemoglobin is then converted to nitrates and nitrites by methemoglobin reductase found in erythrocytes. Parenthetically, most of the circulating nitrates and nitrites in human blood are derived from the metabolism of endogenous NO. Thus, by binding to hemoglobin the vasodilating actions of inhaled NO are clinically focused in the pulmonary circulation; unwanted systemic vasorelaxation is avoided. In addition, the vasodilating action of NO is stopped when inhaled NO is withdrawn from the breathing circuit; the half-life of cGMP is less than 1 min. Thus, the pharmacologic effects of inhaled NO are eliminated with cessation of the drug.

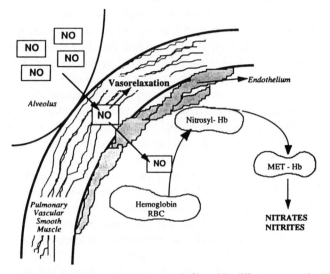

FIGURE 40-1. Inhaled nitric oxide (NO) rapidly diffuses across the alveolocapillary membrane to relax pulmonary vascular smooth muscle. Once it diffuses through the smooth muscle and reaches the blood vessel lumen, it is immediately bound to hemoglobin and inactivated. In this way, the vasodilating actions of NO are focused in the pulmonary circulation. MET-Hb = methemoglobin; Nitrosyl-Hb = nitrosyl hemoglobin; RBC = red blood cell. Reproduced with permission from Fullerton DA et al.[1]

Inhaled NO is potentially toxic to lung tissue. Although early studies suggested that the NO moiety itself is toxic to lung tissue, it now appears the toxicity of inhaled NO is derived from its conversion to NO_2 in the presence of oxygen. In turn, NO_2 may be converted to nitric acid in the presence of water. The rate at which NO is converted to NO_2 is dependent on (1) the square of the concentration of NO and (2) the fraction of inspired oxygen (F_IO_2) to which it is exposed. For example, 10,000 ppm of NO placed in an F_IO_2 of 1.0 will become 50% NO_2 within 24 s. But in a concentration of NO commonly used clinically, such as 10 ppm, and an F_IO_2 of 1.0, 7 h are required to generate 50% NO_2.

Inhaled NO is clinically administered in concentrations of 1 to 80 ppm. To minimize the potential for toxicity during clinical administration, it is necessary to monitor the concentrations of inhaled NO and exhaled NO_2 by chemiluminescence in a continuous fashion, or by frequently checking the concentration of NO delivered and NO_2 exhaled. The lowest possible F_IO_2 should be used to attenuate the conversion of NO to NO_2. The Occupational Safety and Health Administration (OSHA) arbitrarily established a limit for NO, at 25 ppm per 8 h per 24 h interval as the upper limit of safe human exposure. As little as 2 to 3 ppm of NO_2 is extremely cytotoxic in pulmonary histologic studies. The amount of NO_2 to which a patient is exposed may be minimized by placement of a soda lime canister in the inhalational limb of the ventilator circuit (discussed below).

When closely monitored, inhaled NO may be used safely. It may be prudent to "scavenge" the exhaled gas from patients treated with inhaled NO, but recent data suggest that the exposure of hospital personnel to NO or its metabolites from such patients is minimal.

As noted above, once bound to hemoglobin, NO is ultimately converted to methemoglobin. Thus, methemoglobinemia is also a potential toxicity of the use of inhaled NO. Not only is methemoglobin unable to bind oxygen, it shifts the oxygen-hemoglobin dissociation curve to the left, impairing the release of oxygen from hemoglobin. Normal methemoglobin concentrations range from 0 to 3%. Symptoms of hypoxemia result as the concentration of methemoglobin rises. At methemoglobin levels of 0 to 15%, there are typically no symptoms. At levels of 15 to 20%, asymptomatic cyanosis may be noted. Twenty to 25% methemoglobinemia produces weakness, which progresses to acidosis and coma at methemoglobin levels of 50 to 70%. Methemoglobin levels greater than 70% are associated with death. Despite inhalation of high doses of NO (80 ppm) for protracted periods of times, it is uncommon that methemoglobin levels rise significantly. Nonetheless, Curran and colleagues reported methemoglobin levels as high as 7% in children receiving 80 ppm of inhaled NO.[2] In particular, methemoglobin levels must be carefully monitored during the use of inhaled NO in infants, because infants may be deficient in methemoglobin reductase. For example, Roberts and colleagues reported a rise in methemoglobin from 1% to 18.2% on the first day of inhaled NO treatment in a newborn.[3]

Clinical Applications of Inhaled Nitric Oxide

Acute Respiratory Distress Syndrome

Hypoxemia and pulmonary hypertension are universally present in the setting of acute lung injury and acute respiratory distress syndrome (ARDS). Resolution of the acute lung injury is accompanied by improvement in the pulmonary hypertension, whereas progressive pulmonary hypertension produces death from right ventricular failure. Arterial hypoxemia in ARDS is derived from an increase in the intrapulmonary shunt fraction. On the other hand, the pathogenesis of the pulmonary hypertension is multifactorial; it derives from a combination of the injury itself, the inflammatory response to the injury, increased local and circulating levels of vasoconstrictive substances, thromboembolic disease, and iatrogenic factors, including ventilatory support. A less-appreciated component of the pathophysiology of acute lung injury and pulmonary hypertension is impairment of the mechanisms of pulmonary vasorelaxation, which helps the net balance of pulmonary vascular tone in favor of constriction.

Because pulmonary hypertension in acute lung injury appears to play a pivotal role in the pathophysiology, it makes sense that therapy to correct the hypertension would yield beneficial effects. Intravenous vasodilators such as nitroprusside, nitroglycerin, prostaglandin E_1 (PGE_1), and prostacyclin (PGI_2) effectively lower pulmonary artery pressure and vascular resistance. However, their use is limited because their effects are not isolated to the pulmonary circulation; their use leads to systemic hypotension and to an increase in the intrapulmonary shunt, which worsens hypoxemia. Because the pharmacologic actions of inhaled NO are localized to the pulmonary circulation, it is effective in the treatment of ARDS. Inhaled NO is delivered only to ventilated regions of the lung. There it locally vasodilates the pulmonary circulation and "steals" blood from nonventilated regions of the lung. In so doing, intrapulmonary shunt fraction is decreased and arterial oxygenation is improved. At the same time, pulmonary arterial pressure and PVR are lowered without unwanted systemic hemodynamic effects.

Use of inhaled NO in ARDS was first reported by Rossaint and colleagues in 1993.[4] They compared the effects of inhaled NO (18 and 36 ppm) to the effect of intravenous prostacyclin (4 ng/kg/min) in nine patients with ARDS. Inhaled NO produced a reduction of the mean pulmonary artery pressure (MPAP) from 37 ± 3 mm Hg to 30 ± 2 mm Hg and decreased intrapulmonary shunting from $36 \pm 5\%$ to $31 \pm 5\%$. This led to an increase in the partial pressure of oxygen in arterial blood/fraction of inspired oxygen in arterial blood (PaO_2/F_IO_2) ratio from 152 ± 15 mm Hg to 199 ± 23 mm Hg. The mean arterial pressure and cardiac output remained unchanged. Infusion of prostacyclin also reduced pulmonary artery pressure but led to an increase in intrapulmonary shunt, worsening oxygenation, and a decrease in the systemic arterial pressure. The patients were then treated with inhaled NO for 3 to 53 days without evidence of toxicity to lung tissue.

When inhaled NO is used to treat ARDS, the clinical response is usually obvious within 10 min of initiating inhaled NO. There does appear, however, to be a disparity between the effect of NO on oxygenation and pulmonary hypertension in ARDS. Bigatello and colleagues found that the effect of inhaled NO on pulmonary artery pressure was dose-related but that the effects on arterial oxygenation were not.[5] For unclear reasons, inhaled NO at low concentrations (< 10 ppm) was as effective, if not more effective, in increasing arterial oxygenation as higher concentrations. On the other hand, increasing inhaled NO concentrations (5 to 40 ppm) progressively decreased pulmonary artery pressure. Other investigators have confirmed that inhaled NO may be used to lower PVR in patients with ARDS. In turn, right ventricular output and ejection fraction increase, with an associated reduction in right ventricular end-systolic and end-diastolic volumes and a decrease in right atrial pressure. These data suggest that inhaled NO improves right ventricular function in patients with ARDS by reducing the right ventricular afterload.

Unfortunately, not all patients with ARDS respond to inhaled NO. McIntyre and colleagues examined the efficacy of inhaled NO (20 and 40 ppm) in 14 surgical patients with ARDS.[6] All patients had a PaO_2/F_IO_2 ratio < 150 and pulmonary hypertension (MPAP > 30 mm Hg). For the entire group of patients, inhaled NO produced a $43 \pm 9\%$ increase in PaO_2/F_IO_2 ratio at 20 ppm. However, the response was variable; only 69% of patients had a clinically significant improvement in arterial oxygenation (increase in PaO_2/F_IO_2 ratio greater than 20% over baseline). Overall, inhaled NO produced a $15 \pm 4\%$ decrease in the MPAP at 20 ppm NO. Again the response was variable, with only 69% of patients having a significant clinical response (decrease in MPAP of greater than 10% of baseline).

This variable response to inhaled NO in patients with ARDS was confirmed in a large prospective, multicenter, double-blind, placebo-controlled study.[7] In 177 patients with ARDS studied in 30 institutions, only 60% responded to NO (1 to 40 ppm) with > 20% increase in PaO_2. Furthermore, the increase in PaO_2 was not sustained beyond 48 hours. Likewise, the NO had a very modest effect on pulmonary arterial pressure, which was lowered by only 2 mm Hg during the first 24 h of NO administration. The pathophysiologic basis for this variable response to inhaled NO in patients with ARDS is unclear. Improvement in arterial oxygenation and pulmonary hypertension in response to inhaled NO does not seem to correlate well with the baseline pulmonary artery pressure, pulmonary vascular resistance, venous admixture, or etiology of ARDS. Inhaled NO may not cause either a significant reduction in pulmonary artery pressure or an improvement in arterial oxygenation if vascular smooth-muscle–soluble guanylate cyclase is unresponsive to NO.

Results of laboratory animal studies demonstrate that in acute lung injury, cGMP-mediated pulmonary vasorelaxation is significantly impaired.[8] Such findings may offer insight into the variable response to inhaled NO in ARDS by suggesting that the intracellular mechanisms that mediate pulmonary vascular smooth-muscle relaxation may be unable to respond to stimulation by NO in some patients with ARDS.

The mortality rate associated with ARDS remains at approximately 50%. Despite improving oxygenation and right-heart function in the majority of patients with ARDS, use of inhaled NO does not diminish mortality in these patients. An early report by Rossaint and colleagues compared the mortality of 30 patients with ARDS who were treated with inhaled NO with that of matched patients who did not receive inhaled NO.[9] Inhaled NO increased the PaO_2/F_IO_2 ratio by > 10 mm Hg in 83% of patients, decreased the venous admixture by > 10% in 87% of patients, and decreased the MPAP by > 3 mm Hg in 63% of patients. The 30 patients were treated with NO for a mean of 17 ± 2.4 days (range, 2 to 53 days). Despite these effects, the survival in patients treated with NO did not differ from the survival in the matched patients who did not receive NO. Similarly, in the much larger report from Dellinger's multicenter trial, survival was not different between controls and patients treated with NO.[7] Most patients with ARDS die of multiorgan failure, and fewer than 5% die of hypoxemic respiratory failure. Because the actions of NO are clinically focused in the pulmonary circulation yet most deaths in patients with ARDS result from other organ failure, NO may not improve survival in patients with ARDS. Nonetheless, as with other therapeutic modalities available to support respiratory failure, it makes clinical sense to attempt NO therapy in most patients with ARDS.

Adult Cardiac Surgical Patients

Because PVR is the primary clinical determinant of right ventricular afterload, increased PVR may result in right ventricular afterload mismatch, compromising cardiac output. Pharmacologic agents that are currently used as pulmonary vasodilators in cardiac surgical patients include nitroprusside, nitroglycerin, dobutamine, phosphodiesterase inhibitors, and PGE_1. Unfortunately, those intravenous vasodilators produce vasodilation of both the pulmonary and systemic circulations. Such nonselective vasodilation may be hazardous in patients with increased PVR; significant hypotension may result if the degree of systemic vasodilation exceeds that of the pulmonary vasodilation. Such hypotension may impair coronary arterial perfusion pressure to such an extent that right ventricular ischemia and failure are produced.

The pulmonary vasoconstricting effects of cardiopulmonary bypass are well recognized. Increased levels of circulating or local vasoconstricting agonists contribute to increased pulmonary vascular tone following cardiopulmonary bypass. Recent data suggest that pulmonary vascular endothelial cell dysfunction may contribute to pulmonary vasoconstriction following cardiopulmonary bypass; impairment of endothelium-dependent pulmonary vasorelaxation following cardiopulmonary bypass was recently described.[10] Patients with elevated pulmonary artery pressure preoperatively may be particularly susceptible to acute pulmonary hypertension in the postoperative period. Inhaled NO achieves pulmonary vascular smooth relaxation independently of the endothelium and may offer a mechanistic advantage for use as a pulmonary vasodilator following cardiopulmonary bypass.

A recent study of adults undergoing aortocoronary bypass surgery demonstrated that inhaled NO (20 and 40 ppm) produced a consistent reduction in pulmonary arterial pressure and PVR, without change in systemic arterial pressure or systemic vascular resistance (Figure 40-2).[11] Mean pulmonary arterial pressure was lowered from 29 ± 1 to 21 ± 1 mm Hg by inhaled NO; systemic mean arterial pressure remained unchanged during inhalation of NO at 75 ± 3 mm Hg. Pulmonary vascular resistance was lowered from 343 ± 30 to 233 ± 25 dyn·s·cm^{-5} during inhalation of NO, with no change in systemic vascular resistance (SVR). This pulmonary vasodilation produced a significant reduction in transpulmonary gradient as well as right ventricular stroke work index. No greater pulmonary vasodilation was achieved by NO 40 ppm over NO 20 ppm. All hemodynamic variables returned to baseline after cessation of inhaled NO.

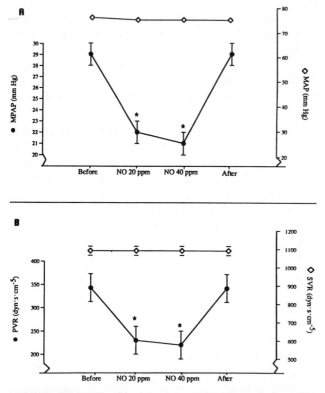

FIGURE 40-2. Hemodynamic effects of inhaled nitric oxide (NO) following coronary artery bypass surgery. As shown in *A*, inhaled NO produced a significant reduction in mean pulmonary artery pressure (MPAP) without change in systemic mean arterial pressure (MAP). As shown in *B*, inhaled NO produced a significant reduction in pulmonary vascular resistance (PVR) without change in systemic vascular resistance (SVR). * *p* < .05. Reproduced with permission from Fullerton DA et al.[11]

Valvular heart disease is the most common reason for pulmonary hypertension among adult cardiac surgical patients. At least three pathophysiologic mechanisms contribute to the pulmonary hypertension seen in long-standing aortic or mitral valvular disease: (1) increased left atrial pressure transmitted retrograde into the arterial circulation; (2) vascular remodeling of the pulmonary vasculature in response to chronic obstruction to pulmonary venous drainage ("fixed component"); and (3) pulmonary arterial vasoconstriction ("reactive component"). Thus, control of PVR in such patients may be a vexing problem. After the elevated left atrial pressure is relieved by valve replacement, increased PVR does not immediately return to normal; several days to weeks may be required. For that reason, perioperative pulmonary vasodilator therapy is most often required in patients undergoing valve surgery, and it is in this group of patients that inhaled NO would theoretically be most useful.

Unfortunately, the efficacy of inhaled NO as a pulmonary vasodilator appears to be less in cardiac surgical patients with pulmonary hypertension from valvular heart disease than in patients undergoing aortocoronary bypass grafting. In six patients studied within 24 h after mitral valve replacement for mitral stenosis, Girard and colleagues reported only a modest reduction in mean pulmonary arterial pressure by inhaled NO (40 ppm).[12] This group of patients had a mean preoperative pulmonary arterial pressure of 49 ± 16 mm Hg. Within 24 h of mitral valve replacement, the mean pulmonary arterial pressure for this group still averaged 41 mm Hg and was modestly lowered to 37 mm Hg by inhaled NO 40 ppm. Although this attenuation of pulmonary arterial pressure was relatively small (9% reduction), it may be a reflection of the structural changes that occur from chronic pulmonary venous outflow pressure brought on by mitral stenosis.

Other investigators have found no response to inhaled NO following valve replacement in patients with pulmonary hypertension secondary to valvular heart disease.[13] Among 20 patients with pulmonary hypertension from valvular heart disease studied in the operating room following mitral valve replacement (alone or in combination with aortic valve replacement), MPAP was 39 ± 3 and PVR was 620 ± 30 before, during, and after NO (40 ppm) (Figure 40-3). In the same study, patients with pulmonary hypertension undergoing aortocoronary bypass served as controls and had a significant response to inhaled NO. In controls, inhaled NO (40 ppm) produced a 24% decrease in MPAP (33 ± 1 to 25 ± 1 mm Hg), a 36% decrease in PVR (375 ± 30 to 250 ± 30 dyn·s·cm^{-5}), and no change in systemic arterial blood pressure. Such data demonstrate the variability of the response to inhaled NO in cardiac surgical patients. Furthermore, the data suggest that inhaled NO may not be an effective pulmonary vasodilator in patients with pulmonary vascular remodeling from left atrial hypertension resultant to valvular heart disease.

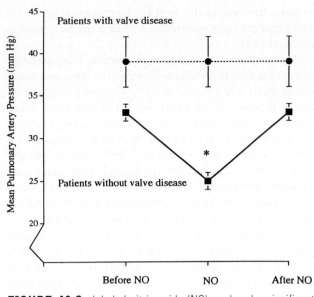

FIGURE 40-3. Inhaled nitric oxide (NO) produced a significant reduction in mean pulmonary artery pressure in patients with pulmonary hypertension without valvular heart disease, but had no effect in patients with valvular heart disease. * $p < 0.05$ versus before and after NO. Reproduced with permission from Fullerton DA et al.[12]

As noted earlier, the intracellular mediator of the vasodilating actions of NO is cGMP. Although the mechanism by which cGMP effects pulmonary vascular smooth-muscle relaxation is unclear, pulmonary vascular tone is assumed to be closely related to intracellular levels of pulmonary vascular smooth-muscle cGMP. In turn, the net concentration of cGMP within pulmonary vascular smooth muscle is determined by the balance of its production by guanylate cyclase and degradation by phosphodiesterase (PDE). In cardiac surgical patients whose pulmonary hypertension failed to respond to

inhaled NO, the effectiveness of inhaled NO was increased by using a two-pronged approach: (1) stimulating cGMP production with inhaled NO plus (2) preventing the breakdown of cGMP by inhibiting PDE (dipyridamole). Such a two-pronged approach may convert cardiac surgical patients with pulmonary hypertension who fail to respond to inhaled NO alone into responders.

In a study of 10 cardiac surgical patients with pulmonary hypertension from aortic and/or mitral valvular disease (MPAP ± 30 mm Hg following cardiopulmonary bypass) studied in the operating room after valve replacement, neither inhaled NO alone (40 ppm) nor dipyridamole (0.2 mg/kg IV) alone lowered PVR or pulmonary artery pressure. However, the combination of inhaled NO *plus* dipyridamole effectively produced significant pulmonary vasodilation, thereby converting nonresponding patients into responders. PVR and MPAP were significantly reduced and cardiac output was increased without change in systemic mean arterial pressure (Figure 40-4).[14] Such combined therapy may be particularly valuable in patients with right-heart dysfunction secondary to pulmonary hypertension by effectively lowering right ventricular afterload.

General Thoracic Surgery

The development of ARDS following pulmonary resection is life-threatening. Although uncommon, it still occurs in 1% of patients following lobectomy and in 2 to 5% of patients following pneumonectomy. The causes are uncertain but are almost certainly multifactorial and include aspiration, interruption of pulmonary lymphatics, and fluid overload. Nonetheless, it is associated with a mortality rate of 30 to 100%. Mathisen and colleagues reported successful use of NO in 10 patients with ARDS following pulmonary resection; 8 patients underwent pneumonectomy.[15] Despite surgical resection of lung tissue, and in

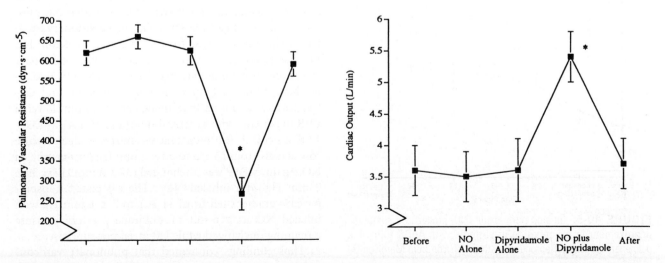

FIGURE 40-4. In patients failing to respond to nitric oxide (NO) alone following cardiac operation, the combination of inhaled NO plus dipyridamole produced a significant reduction in pulmonary vascular resistance and an associated significant increase in cardiac output. Values are mean ± standard error of mean (SEM). * $p = .02$ versus before and after NO. Reproduced with permission from Fullerton DA et al.[14]

most cases a pneumonectomy, NO (10 to 20 ppm) was effective in treating ARDS in these patients. The PaO_2/F_1O_2 ratio rose immediately from 95 ± 13 mm Hg to 128 ± 24 mm Hg. By 96 h of NO therapy, the PaO_2/F_1O_2 ratio had risen to 213 ± 28 mm Hg (Figure 40-5). Three of the 10 patients in this series died, all of sepsis.

Emergency pneumonectomy for trauma is associated with an extremely high mortality rate, which results from acute right ventricular failure secondary to an abrupt rise in PVR. Nurozler and colleagues reported that use of NO following a post-traumatic pneumonectomy was associated with improvement in oxygenation, reduction in pulmonary hypertension and increased cardiac output.[16] Inhaled NO may be of value in the perioperative management of these patients.

Thoracic Organ Transplantation

HEART TRANSPLANTATION

Increased PVR is a risk factor for death following cardiac transplantation. The 30-day mortality rate for cardiac transplantation is more than doubled when the preoperative PVR exceeds 4 Wood units or the transpulmonary gradient exceeds 15 mm Hg; a PVR greater than 6 Wood units is considered a contraindication to heart transplantation. Several factors contribute to this risk. First, the right ventricle of the donor heart is typically accustomed to contracting against normal pulmonary arterial pressure (right ventricular afterload). Second, protection of the unconditioned right ventricle may be compromised during the surgical procedure, because it is more difficult to shield the right ventricle from ambient temperature. Third, the transplanted heart must endure the obligatory injuries of ischemia and reperfusion, which may compromise right ventricular function. For those

reasons, the right ventricle of the transplanted heart is at risk for acute right ventricular failure if the recipient has elevated PVR.

Several contributing factors produce an increased PVR in patients with heart failure. Elevated left atrial pressure is transmitted retrograde, thereby elevating pulmonary artery pressure. In addition, left atrial distension elicits reflex vasoconstriction of the pulmonary arterial circulation, analogous to the situation with mitral stenosis. This "reactive" component of the total PVR is reversible and may be pharmacologically modulated with pulmonary vasodilators. Likewise, left atrial pressure can be expected to normalize following transplantation, thereby eliminating the hydrostatic component. However, long-standing left atrial hypertension may produce architectural remodeling of the pulmonary circulation and a "fixed" component of an increased PVR. Therefore, an essential component of the pre–heart transplant evaluation is an accurate assessment of PVR, and a determination must be made as to whether pulmonary hypertension will be reversible following heart transplantation. In patients found to have increased PVR during the pretransplant evaluation, pharmacologic testing with vasodilators (typically sodium nitroprusside) may be required to determine how much of the PVR is "reactive" and therefore reversible.

Because it is an effective pulmonary vasodilator, inhaled NO has been applied in two roles in cardiac transplantation: (1) to evaluate the "reactive" component of PVR during the pretransplant evaluation of potential cardiac transplant candidates; and (2) as therapy to lower PVR in the early postoperative period following cardiac transplantation. Unfortunately, when given to patients with heart failure pretransplant, inhaled NO may have adverse hemodynamic effects. Loh and colleagues reported that when administered to 19 patients with congestive heart failure, inhaled NO (80 ppm) lowered PVR from 226 $\pm$ 30 to 119 $\pm$ 13 dyn·s·cm^{-5}.[17] This reduction in PVR was associated with a rise in left ventricular end-diastolic pressure from 28 $\pm$ 4 to 34 $\pm$ 5 mm Hg, and pulmonary capillary wedge pressure rose from 25 $\pm$ 3 to 31 $\pm$ 4 mm Hg. Because of the increase in left atrial pressure, pulmonary artery pressure did not change despite a fall in PVR. Others have confirmed these findings. Semigran and colleagues likewise found that inhaled NO (80 ppm) lowered PVR in patients with heart failure from 256 $\pm$ 41 to 139 $\pm$ 14 dyn·s·cm^{-5}.[18] But pulmonary capillary wedge pressure rose acutely from 25 $\pm$ 3 to 32 $\pm$ 2 mm Hg during inhaled NO. Again, MPAP was unchanged (37 $\pm$ 3 mm Hg vs 39 $\pm$ 2 mm Hg with inhaled NO). The calculated transpulmonary gradient fell from 11 $\pm$ 1 to 7 $\pm$ 1 mm Hg with inhaled NO as a result of pulmonary artery pressure remaining unchanged while left atrial pressure rose.

Those findings confirmed that pulmonary vasoconstriction contributes to elevated PVR in patients with heart failure but raised concerns as to whether inhaled NO may somehow depress left ventricular function.

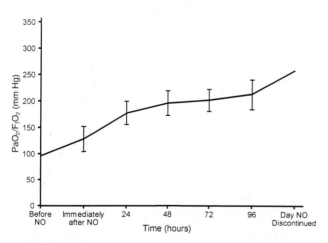

FIGURE 40-5. Inhaled nitric oxide (NO) produced a sustained improvement in oxygenation in patients with ARDS following pulmonary resection. Reproduced with permission from Mathisen DJ et al.[15]

PaO_2 = partial pressure of oxygen in arterial blood

F_1O_2 = fraction of inspired oxygen in arterial blood

Because inhaled NO is immediately bound to hemoglobin and inactivated as it contacts blood, it seems unlikely that NO might reach the myocardium to act as a negative inotrope. In fact, Loh and colleagues found no change in left ventricular contractility (as measured by +dP/dt) during inhalation of NO (80 ppm) in heart failure patients.[17] The rise in left atrial pressure more likely develops because inhaled NO vasodilates the pulmonary circulation, increasing blood flow through the lungs into the left atrium. In heart failure patients, left ventricular dysfunction may preclude accommodation of the increased preload, resulting in increased left atrial pressure. In fact, several cases of pulmonary edema have been reported following administration of inhaled NO to stable patients with heart failure.[19]

Because intravenous vasodilators such as sodium nitroprusside dilate both the pulmonary and systemic circulations, their reduction in left ventricular afterload augments forward flow from the left ventricle, lowers left atrial pressure, and permits the left heart to accommodate the increased blood flow coming through the pulmonary circulation; consequently, left atrial pressure does not rise during infusion of sodium nitroprusside. By lowering left atrial pressure and permitting a determination of pulmonary hemodynamics with a pulmonary venous outflow pressure closer to what the pressure will be following transplantation, nitroprusside offers an advantage over inhaled NO, which raises left atrial pressure. Therefore, inhaled NO should not be used to test for pulmonary vasodilation in the pre–heart transplant evaluation. Instead, an intravenous "nonselective" vasodilator such as nitroprusside is preferable.

On the other hand, inhaled NO may be valuable in the postoperative management of heart transplant recipients. As noted, the right ventricle of the transplanted heart is at risk to fail perioperatively because of a combination of impaired contractility and increased afterload if PVR is elevated. Following cardiac transplantation, such patients may usually be managed with the help of intravenous agents. But if right ventricular output is significantly compromised, intravenous infusion of nonselective vasodilators often produces unwanted systemic hypotension. Successful management of such patients requires effective reduction of PVR without systemic vasodilation.

As a selective pulmonary vasodilator, inhaled NO may be used to optimize right ventricular function by lowering right ventricular afterload. When directly compared to other pulmonary vasodilators following heart transplantation, Kieler-Jensen and colleagues reported that the reduction in pulmonary arterial pressure and PVR produced by inhaled NO was comparable to that produced by intravenous infusions of sodium nitroprusside, PGE_1, and prostacyclin.[20] Unlike intravenous vasodilators, inhaled NO "selectively" lowered PVR without producing systemic vasodilation in heart transplant recipients. Thus, it may be particularly well suited as a pulmonary vasodilator in the postoperative heart transplant patient.

Heart failure patients may require mechanical circulatory support before or after cardiac transplantation. The function of such devices is critically dependent on adequate filling of the mechanical ventricle. Systemic blood flow via a left ventricular assist device (LVAD), which fills by withdrawing blood from the left atrium, may be compromised if increased PVR limits the patient's right ventricle from pumping blood through the pulmonary circulation into the left atrium. The pulmonary vasodilating action of inhaled NO has been effectively used in heart failure to optimize LVAD filling and systemic flow. Hare and colleagues reported that in patients with pulmonary hypertension associated with left ventricular failure supported by an LVAD, inhaled NO (20 and 40 ppm) dilated the pulmonary circulation, lowering PVR by 21.5%.[21] This pulmonary vasorelaxation optimized LVAD filling and increased LVAD flow from $5.3 - 0.3$ to 5.7 ± 0.3 L/min without increasing left atrial pressure.

Those findings were confirmed in patients requiring LVAD support and randomized to receive NO (20 ppm) or placebo (nitrogen gas).[22] In six patients treated with NO, MPAP immediately fell from 35 ± 6 mm Hg to 24 ± 4 mm Hg (Figure 40-6). This reduction in MPAP was associated with an increase in LVAD flow from 1.9 ± 0.2 to 2.7 ± 0.3 L/min/m². In five patients randomized to receive placebo, nitrogen gas had no effect on patients' hemodynamics. These same patients did, however, respond to NO when crossed-over. All patients were successfully weaned

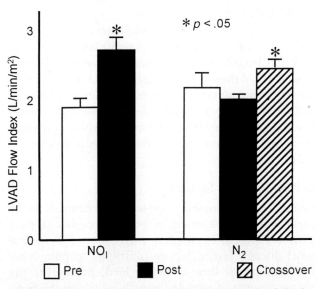

FIGURE 40-6. In patients with pulmonary hypertension following implantation of a left ventricular assist device (LVAD), inhaled nitric oxide (NO) effectively lowered mean pulmonary artery pressure (MPAP). Controls did not respond when given nitrogen gas (N_2) as placebo but did respond to NO. Reduction of MPAP was associated with improved LVAD flow. Reproduced with permission from Argenziano M et al.[22]

from NO within 1 week without complication and were effectively supported with NO until LVAD support alone was sufficient.

LUNG TRANSPLANTATION

The transplanted lung must endure the obligatory injuries of ischemia and reperfusion, each of which produces pulmonary vascular and parenchymal injuries. Cumulatively, these injuries may result in severe lung injury marked by increased pulmonary capillary permeability, pulmonary edema, and increased PVR secondary to pulmonary vasoconstriction. Such allograft lung dysfunction produces hypoxemia secondary to severe intrapulmonary shunting; the clinical picture closely resembles ARDS.

Fortunately, severe allograft lung injury is not common. But when it does occur, the combination of hypoxemia, pulmonary hypertension, and systemic hypotension may quickly become life-threatening; lung transplant recipients typically have little cardiopulmonary reserve. Prompt initiation of inhaled NO therapy has been lifesaving in severe cases of acute allograft lung dysfunction. By producing selective pulmonary vasodilation in the regions of ventilated alveoli, it has decreased intrapulmonary shunting and thereby improved oxygenation. Pulmonary vascular resistance has been lowered by a combination of direct pulmonary vasorelaxation and elimination of hypoxic pulmonary vasoconstriction. In such extreme cases, inhaled NO should be initiated in a concentration of 80 ppm. As the patient stabilizes and begins to improve, the concentration of inhaled NO should be decreased to the lowest level possible to achieve the desired result.

Adatia and colleagues successfully treated six patients (ages 5 to 21 years) with acute allograft lung dysfunction with inhaled NO.[23] Cardiopulmonary bypass had been used in five of the six patients. Inhaled NO (80 ppm) lowered mean pulmonary artery pressure from 38 ± 1.6 to 29 ± 3.1 mm Hg. The mean value for intrapulmonary shunt fraction was lowered from 29% to 21%, which provided a significant improvement in arterial partial pressure of oxygen (Po_2).

Congenital Heart Surgery

Pulmonary hypertension is especially problematic in the perioperative management of pediatric cardiac surgical patients undergoing surgical correction of congenital heart disease. Several factors contribute to pulmonary hypertension in these patients. First, because of the greater amount of vascular smooth muscle in the pediatric pulmonary circulation, children with congenital heart disease are particularly prone to avid pulmonary vasoconstriction. Second, congenital heart lesions that produce excessive pulmonary blood flow or pulmonary venous obstruction might produce hypertrophy and hyperplasia of pulmonary vascular smooth muscle. Over

the long term, such congenital heart lesions may ultimately produce irreversible architectural remodeling of the pulmonary circulation, leading to a fixed increase in PVR. Third, chronic excessive pulmonary blood flow may produce dysfunction of the mechanisms of pulmonary vasorelaxation. Impairment of the mechanisms of relaxation may tip the net balance of pulmonary vascular tone in favor of constriction and lead to an exaggerated vasoconstricting response to pulmonary vasoconstricting agonists. Fourth, following cardiopulmonary bypass, endothelium-dependent pulmonary vasorelaxation is impaired. This postoperative pulmonary endothelial dysfunction exacerbates the tendency of the pulmonary circulation to vasoconstrict. Thus, patients with congenital heart disease may have a particularly "reactive" pulmonary vascular bed superimposed on a "fixed" component of an increased PVR.

Inhaled NO does lower PVR and pulmonary artery pressure when given to patients in the cardiac catheterization laboratory prior to correction of congenital heart defects.

Roberts and colleagues examined the pulmonary vasodilating effects of oxygen (increasing F_IO_2 from 0.21 to 0.90) and inhaled NO (20 to 80 ppm) alone and in combination in 10 children (ages 3 months to 5.5 years) with pulmonary hypertension and congenital heart disease.[24] Both oxygen and inhaled NO alone lowered PVR in these patients, but the combination of inhaled NO (80 ppm) and oxygen (F_IO_2 of 0.90) produced the greatest reduction in PVR and pulmonary arterial pressure. In patients with left-to-right shunts, the reduction in PVR was associated with increased pulmonary artery blood flow. Such data confirm the presence of a reversible component of the PVR and demonstrate that, at least prior to surgical correction, the "reactive" component of the pulmonary hypertension in patients such as these may be attenuated by a combination of oxygen and NO therapy. Such preoperative information may be important in planning the postoperative management in patients with significant pulmonary hypertension.

The surgeon, of course, is primarily concerned with control of the pulmonary circulation in the early postoperative period. Particularly when preoperative pulmonary hypertension reflects excessive pulmonary blood flow from a large left-to-right shunt, pulmonary arterial pressure may fall after surgical repair and may not pose a significant problem in postoperative management.[2] But when significant pulmonary hypertension is present in the early postoperative period, it could compromise right ventricular output and result in systemic hypotension. The first line of therapy to control PVR in such patients should include pharmacologic paralysis, heavy sedation (intravenous fentanyl infusion), respiratory alkalemia with mechanical ventilation (pH 7.50), supplemental oxygen (arterial hemoglobin saturation of 95 to 100%), and intravenous infusion of vasodilating agents. If inotropic support is required, phosphodiesterase inhibitors or dobutamine may be preferable to dopamine or epinephrine because the latter can produce pulmonary vasoconstriction. Unfortunately, these efforts sometimes fail to effectively lower PVR. Furthermore, such patients are prone to experience paroxysmal refractory pulmonary vasoconstriction (pulmonary hypertensive crisis), which is often fatal.

Inhaled NO is lifesaving in postoperative pediatric cardiac surgical patients with pulmonary hypertension refractory to first-line therapy. Curran and colleagues reported a significant reduction in pulmonary artery pressure in 11 of 15 children (ages 1 day to 14 years) who had hemodynamic compromise from pulmonary hypertension refractory to other measures.[2] In 5 of those patients, inhaled NO therapy was initiated emergently to treat a pulmonary hypertensive crisis and was found to successfully lower pulmonary arterial pressure in these patients when other measures had failed. Perhaps most importantly, by providing even a small concentration of inhaled NO (10 to 20 ppm) to these five patients, their clinical course was stabilized and no further episodes of pulmonary hypertensive crisis occurred. These data suggest that providing exogenous NO (inhaled NO) to the pulmonary circulation of infants and children with severe pulmonary hypertension may prevent death from pulmonary hypertension crisis.

Even in patients not in extremis, NO may be useful following certain types of operations.

The postoperative physiology of patients undergoing Fontan-type procedures as well as bidirectional Glenn shunts is somewhat unique in that adequate pulmonary blood flow is critically dependent on very low PVR. Even small increments in PVR, particularly in the early postoperative period, may decrease the transit of blood across the pulmonary vascular bed, thereby impairing oxygenation and left atrial filling. Gamillscheg and colleagues administered NO (1,040 ppm) to nine patients with impaired pulmonary perfusion following total cavopulmonary connection and to four patients following bidirectional Glenn shunts.[25] Administration of NO effectively lowered central venous pressure by 15% to 22% and the transpulmonary pressure gradient by 42% to 55%. Especially following bidirectional Glenn shunts, arterial oxygenation improved (indicative of improved pulmonary blood flow) by 37%.

The postoperative pulmonary physiology of patients undergoing repair of congenital cardiac anomalies is often complex and influenced by a spectrum of variables. This complexity may help to explain why NO has not consistently been shown to improve postoperative pulmonary hypertension or prevent pulmonary hypertensive crises. Day and colleagues randomized 38 patients following biventricular repair or heart transplantation to receive NO (20 ppm) or conventional therapy.[26] Patients were eligible for study with postoperative pulmonary arterial pressures ≥ 50% of systemic arterial pressure. Surprisingly, NO had little if any impact on pulmonary hemodynamics. Furthermore, the use of NO did not prevent pulmonary hypertensive crises; 4 of 19 controls and 3 of 19 NO-treated patients had pulmonary hypertensive crises.

In a much larger study of infants undergoing correction of anomalies known to pose high risk for postoperative pulmonary hypertensive crises, Miller and colleagues found a marked reduction in such with administration of NO.[27] Among infants well-matched for congenital anomalies, 124 were randomized to receive NO (10 ppm) or placebo (nitrogen). Although NO did not completely prevent pulmonary hypertensive crises, the group receiving NO had significantly fewer (median of 4 vs 7). Infants treated with NO were eligible for ventilator weaning 30 h sooner than controls. There was no difference in mortality between the two groups; only one death occurred during study gas administration and resulted from a surgical complication. This study by Miller and colleagues supports the routine postoperative use of NO in infants at risk for pulmonary hypertensive crises undergoing repair of lesions (Figure 40-7).

Children and infants with refractory pulmonary hypertension may require extracorporeal life support (ECLS) to provide systemic perfusion. Because inhaled NO is such an effective pulmonary vasodilator in some such cases, ECLS can be avoided. Goldman and colleagues reported their experience with 10 children (ages 3 days to 10 months) with severe pulmonary hypertension following repair of congenital heart defects.[28] Five of these children could not be separated from cardiopulmonary bypass because of severe pulmonary hypertension, and five had systemic pulmonary arterial pressures causing hemodynamic compromise. Nine of the 10 children responded immediately to inhaled NO (20 ppm). The single child who failed to respond to inhaled NO was placed

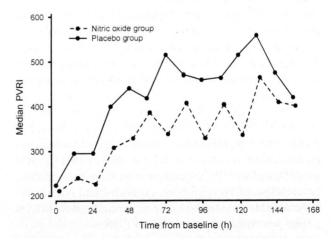

FIGURE 40-7. Inhaled nitric oxide effectively lowered pulmonary vascular resistance index (PVRI) in infants at high risk for pulmonary hypertensive crises following congenital heart surgery. Perioperative morbidity was significantly reduced by nitric oxide, although mortality was not different between the two groups. Reproduced with permission from Miller OI et al.[27]

on ECLS and survived. Six of the nine children who initially responded to inhaled NO survived to be discharged from the hospital. These data suggest that inhaled NO may supplant the need for ECLS in some patients with severe pulmonary hypertension.

Persistent Pulmonary Hypertension of the Newborn

Persistent pulmonary hypertension of the newborn (PPHN) is a syndrome in which pulmonary hypertension secondary to increased PVR produces right-to-left shunting of blood at the levels of the atrium and the patent ductus arteriosus, resulting in profound hypoxemia. The markedly elevated PVR is derived from pulmonary arterial vascular spasm superimposed on smooth-muscle hypertrophy and hyperplasia. Although PPHN is frequently idiopathic, it may be associated with meconium aspiration or sepsis. Survival is possible if the infant can be supported until the pulmonary vasospasm resolves; without improvement in oxygenation, the infant often dies. The role of the cardiothoracic surgeon in the management of these infants is often to provide cardiopulmonary support with ECLS.

As inhaled NO selectively lowers pulmonary rather than systemic vascular resistance, its use may allow blood to preferentially follow the path of least resistance from the pulmonary artery into the lungs rather than through the ductus arteriosus. A prospective multicenter trial examined the effect of inhaled NO in infants with PPHN.[3] Full-term newborn infants without structural cardiac defects with severe systemic hypoxemia (arterial $P_{O_2} < 55$ mm Hg) despite an F_IO_2 of 1.0 were studied. Pulmonary hypertension was determined by echocardiography. Inhaled NO (80 ppm) significantly increased arterial P_{O_2} in 16 of 30 infants (53%), from 41 ± 9 to 89 ± 7 mm Hg. The successful initial response to inhaled NO was maintained in 12 of these 16 infants (75%). In the remaining four infants, oxygenation deteriorated within 12 h, and the infants required ECLS. Infants with a sustained response to inhaled NO were treated for 2 to 8.5 days, during which time the concentration of inhaled NO was progressively lowered. The need for ECLS was significantly lowered by inhaled NO therapy; a well-matched control group required ECLS in 20 of 28 infants (71%), as compared with 12 of 30 infants (40%) in the inhaled NO group. Although inhaled NO successfully improved oxygenation in these infants, it did not improve survival over those treated with ECLS; two patients in each group died. Nonetheless, ECLS is invasive, expensive, and not universally available. Inhaled NO may be used effectively to treat a large percentage of infants with PPHN.

In a similar study of neonates with hypoxic respiratory failure, NO was likewise shown to reduce the need for ECLS.[29] Infants without congenital heart disease were randomized to NO (20 ppm) ($n = 114$ infants) or oxygen (100%) ($n = 121$ infants). Infants treated with NO had much greater improvement in PaO_2 (58 ± 8.5 mm Hg vs

10 ± 5.2 mm Hg). Although no difference in mortality was noted between the two groups, use of NO was associated with a lower need for ECLS (39% vs 55% in controls).

Rebound Pulmonary Hypertension after Withdrawal of NO

In patients responsive to NO, abrupt withdrawal of as little as 1 to 2 ppm NO may result in rebound pulmonary hypertension associated with adverse hemodynamic consequences (Figure 40-8); in fact, it may be life-threatening. Atz and colleagues reported that inhaled NO (80 ppm) lowered MPAP from 36 ± 2 mm Hg to 24 ± 2 mm Hg in five infants following repair of total anomalous pulmonary venous return.[31] After prolonged inhalation of NO (20 ppm), pulmonary artery pressures transiently rose upon cessation of inhaled NO.

In 23 patients receiving NO after correction of a variety of congenital heart defects, Ivy and colleagues found that 7 (30%) demonstrated rebound pulmonary hypertension after withdrawal of NO (see Figure 40-8).[30] In those seven patients demonstrating rebound pulmonary hypertension, pulmonary artery pressure increased by 40%, mixed venous oxygen saturation fell by 17%, and the ratio of MPAP to systemic arterial pressure increased by 46%. Interestingly, administration of dipyridamole (0.6 mg/kg infused over 20 min) effectively attenuated this rebound after NO withdrawal. These data suggest that the intracellular concentration of cGMP within pulmonary vascular smooth-muscle cells is insufficient to maintain pulmonary vascular relaxation after NO withdrawal in some patients. By preventing cGMP metabolism (dipyridamole), its intracellular concentration may be sufficiently maintained to avoid rebound pulmonary hypertension. Although the mechanisms for this rebound phenomenon are unclear, inhaled NO may provide a negative feedback for endogenous endothelial NO production. Regardless, NO should

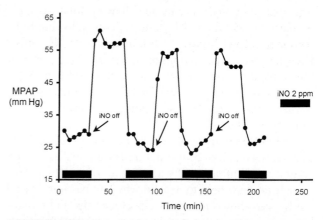

FIGURE 40-8. Abrupt withdrawal of inhaled nitric oxide (iNO) may result in rebound pulmonary hypertension. In this patient, NO was administered for 3 days and withdrawn at a concentration of 2 ppm. Repeatedly, the patient demonstrated rebound pulmonary hypertension. Reproduced with permission from Ivy DD et al.[30]

MPAP = main pulmonary artery pressure

be weaned cautiously when used in patients with critical pulmonary hypertension.

To wean such patients from inhaled NO, this author recommends lowering the concentration of inhaled NO by one-half and carefully observing the patient for any unwanted change in arterial oxygenation or pulmonary arterial pressure. One of the earliest signs of failure to successfully wean from inhaled NO is often a fall in mixed venous oxyhemoglobin saturation. If the patient tolerates the reduction in inhaled NO, the patient should be left in a steady state for approximately 24 h, at which time the concentration of inhaled NO may be cut in half again. The surgeon must be aware that concentrations of inhaled NO as low as 1 to 2 ppm may be critically important to the control of the patient's pulmonary circulation. Consequently, the patient must be closely monitored around the time that inhaled NO is actually stopped.

Summary

Pulmonary hypertension complicates the clinical management of cardiothoracic surgical patients across the disciplines of adult and pediatric cardiac surgery, general thoracic surgery, and thoracic organ transplantation. Among these diverse patient populations, the etiology of the pulmonary hypertension may differ, but inhaled NO is an effective pulmonary vasodilator across the spectrum of cardiothoracic surgical patients. Among these diverse patient populations, the effectiveness of inhaled NO has been variable, although the reasons for this variability are unclear. Inhaled NO need not be considered first-line therapy in the treatment of pulmonary hypertension in heart and lung surgery. Instead, it offers another clinical tool for the surgeon that may in fact be lifesaving in especially difficult cases.

References

1. Fullerton Da, McIntyre RC Jr. Inhaled nitric oxide: therapeutic applications in cardiothoracic surgery. Ann Thorac Surg 1996;61:1856–64.
2. Curran RD, Mavroudis C, Backer CL, et al. Inhaled nitric oxide for children with congenital heart disease and pulmonary hypertension. Ann Thorac Surg 1995;60:1765–71.
3. Roberts JD, Fineman JR, Morin FC III for The Inhaled Nitric Oxide Study Group. Inhaled nitric oxide and persistent pulmonary hypertension of the newborn. N Engl J Med 1997;336:605–10.
4. Rossaint R, Falke KJ, Lopez F, et al. Inhaled nitric oxide for the adult respiratory distress syndrome. N Engl J Med 1993;328:399–405.
5. Bigatello LM, Huford WE, Kacmarek RM, et al. Inhaled nitric oxide is a selective vasodilator in septic patients with severe ARDS. Anesthesiology 1994;80:761–70.
6. McIntyre RC Jr, Moore FA, Moore EE, et al. Inhaled nitric oxide variably improves oxygenation and pulmonary hypertension in patients with acute respiratory distress syndrome. J Trauma 1995;39:418–25.
7. Dellinger RP, Zimmerman JL, Taylor RW, et al. Effects of inhaled nitric oxide in patients with acute respiratory distress syndrome: results of a randomized phase II trial. Crit Care Med 1998;26:15–23.
8. Fullerton DA, McIntyre RC Jr, Hahn AR, et al. Dysfunction of cGMP-mediated pulmonary vasorelaxation in endotoxin-induced acute lung injury. Am J Physiol 1995;268: L1029–35.
9. Rossaint R, Gerlach H, Schmidt-Ruhnke H, et al. Efficacy of inhaled nitric oxide in patients with severe ARDS. Chest 1995;107:1107–15.
10. Wessel DL, Adatia I, Giglia M, et al. Use of inhaled nitric oxide and acetylcholine in the evaluation of pulmonary hypertension and endothelial function after cardiopulmonary bypass. Circulation 1993;88(Pt 1):2128–38.
11. Fullerton DA, Jones SD, Jaggers J, et al. Effective control of pulmonary vascular resistance with inhaled nitric oxide following cardiac operation. J Thorac Cardiovasc Surg 1996; 111:753–63.
12. Girard C, Lehot J-J, Pannetier J-C, et al. Inhaled nitric oxide after mitral valve replacement in patients with chronic pulmonary artery hypertension. Anesthesiology 1992;77: 880–3.
13. Fullerton DA, Jaggers J, Wollmering M, et al. Variable response to inhaled nitric oxide following cardiac surgery. Ann Thorac Surg 1997;63:1251–6.
14. Fullerton DA, Jaggers J, Piedalue F, et al. Effective control of refractory pulmonary hypertension after cardiac surgery. J Thorac Cardiovasc Surg 1997;113:363–8.
15. Mathisen DJ, Kuo E, Hahn C, et al. Inhaled nitric oxide for adult respiratory distress syndrome after pulmonary resection. Ann Thorac Surg 1998;65:1894–902.
16. Nurozler F, Argenziano M, Ginsberg M. Nitric oxide after posttraumatic pneumonectomy. Ann Thorac Surg 2001; 71:364–6.
17. Loh E, Stamler JS, Hare JM, et al. Cardiovascular effects of inhaled nitric oxide in patients with left ventricular dysfunction. Circulation 1994;90:2780–5.
18. Semigran MJ, Cockrill BA, Kacmarek R, et al. Hemodynamic effects of inhaled nitric oxide in heart failure. J Am Coll Cardiol 1994;24:982–8.
19. Bocchi EA, Bacal F, Auler JOC Jr, et al. Inhaled nitric oxide leading to pulmonary edema in stable severe heart failure. Am J Cardiol 1994;74:70–2.
20. Kieler-Jensen N, Lundin S, Ricksten S-E. Vasodilator therapy after heart transplantation: effects of inhaled nitric oxide and intravenous prostacyclin, prostaglandin E_1, and sodium nitroprusside. J Heart Lung Transplant 1995;14:436–43.
21. Hare JM, Shernan SK, Body S, et al. Influence of inhaled NO on systemic flow and ventricular filling pressure in patients receiving mechanical circulatory assistance. Circulation 1997;95:2250–3.
22. Argenziano M, Choudhri AF, Moazami N, et al. Randomized, double-blind trial of inhaled nitric oxide in LVAD recipients with pulmonary hypertension. Ann Thorac Surg 1998;65:340–5.
23. Adatia I, Lillehei C, Arnold JH, et al. Inhaled nitric oxide in the treatment of postoperative graft dysfunction after lung transplantation. Ann Thorac Surg 1994;57:1311–8.
24. Roberts JD, Lang P, Bigatello LM, et al. Inhaled nitric oxide in congenital heart disease. Circulation 1993;87:447–53.

25. Gamillscheg A, Zobel G, Urlesgerger B, et al. Inhaled nitric oxide in patients with critical pulmonary perfusion after Fontan-type procedures and bidirectional Glenn anastomosis. J Thorac Cardiovasc Surg 1997;113:435–42.

26. Day RW, Hawkins JA, McGough EC, et al. Randomized controlled study of inhaled nitric oxide after operation for congenital heart disease. Ann Thorac Surg 2000;69:1907–13.

27. Miller OI, Tang SF, Keech A, et al. Inhaled nitric oxide and prevention of pulmonary hypertension after congenital heart surgery: a randomised double-blind study. Lancet 2001;356:1464–9.

28. Goldman AP, Delius RE, Deanfield JE, et al. Nitric oxide might reduce the need for extracorporeal support in children with critical postoperative pulmonary hypertension. Ann Thorac Surg 1996;62:750–5.

29. The Neonatal Inhaled Nitric Oxide Group. Inhaled nitric oxide in full-term and nearly full-term infants with hypoxic respiratory failure. N Engl J Med 1997;336:597–604.

30. Ivy DD, Kinsella JP, Ziegler JW, Abman SH. Dipyridamole attenuates rebound pulmonary hypertension after inhaled nitric oxide withdrawal in postoperative congenital heart disease. J Thorac Cardiovasc Surg 1998;115:875–82.

31. Atz AM, Adatia I, Wessel DL. Rebound pulmonary hypertension after inhalation of nitric oxide. Ann Thorac Surg 1996;62:1759–64.

CHAPTER 41

EXTRACORPOREAL MEMBRANE OXYGENATION FOR CIRCULATORY SUPPORT

BRIAN W. DUNCAN, MD

The provision of mechanical circulatory support when other forms of treatment fail is increasingly common in the therapeutic approach to patients with cardiac disease. Intraaortic balloon pumps (IABP) and implantable ventricular assist devices (VADs) are standard tools for managing adult patients with advanced left ventricular failure. Extracorporeal membrane oxygenation (ECMO) retains a role in the treatment of adults with circulatory failure because of its ability to expeditiously provide biventricular support. In addition, because of the presence of an oxygenator in the circuit, ECMO provides respiratory support in conditions in which advanced pulmonary disease is also present. ECMO remains the most commonly used form of mechanical circulatory support in children. Isolated left ventricular failure is relatively rare in children, whereas right ventricular failure, pulmonary hypertension, and hypoxia often contribute significantly to circulatory failure in pediatric heart disease. Because of these physiologic differences, support of the left ventricle alone by IABP or left ventricular assist device (LVAD) has more limited application in children. This chapter addresses the current status of ECMO for the provision of circulatory support by examining historical aspects of ECMO development, technical issues related to management of the circuit, clinical features such as indications and contraindications for this treatment, and special situations in which ECMO is especially useful. Because of the prominent role that ECMO occupies in providing mechanical circulatory support for children, much of this chapter discusses topics related to pediatric use; however, ECMO continues to have a place in the treatment of acute circulatory failure in adults, and these applications are covered as well.

The Development of ECMO for Circulatory Support

The use of ECMO as a means of providing circulatory support for cardiac patients arose as a natural extension of work in the 1970s that established the efficacy of ECMO for the treatment of respiratory failure. Baffes and colleagues described an early application of prolonged extracorporeal circulation in congenital heart disease, although the system was used for relatively brief periods of support.[1] However, significant innovations were introduced by these investigators, including the use of the circuit for resuscitation from cardiac arrest and provision of support for perioperative stabilization at the time of palliative cardiac procedures. Soeter was the first to report the use of ECMO for an extended period in a pediatric heart patient; he described the successful use of ECMO to support a 4-year-old girl with severe hypoxia after repair of tetralogy of Fallot.[2] The system described employed a rotary pump with a membrane oxygenator and a heat exchanger. The patient was weaned from support within 48 h, was extubated 2 days later, and was discharged on the thirteenth postoperative day.

Other landmark studies regarding the development of ECMO include those by Hill and Bartlett.[3–5] Although these reports focused on patients with respiratory failure, they also included descriptions of the successful use of ECMO for support after cardiac surgery. Important contributions provided by these early studies included the careful consideration of those aspects of management that make ECMO for cardiac support unique from those required for respiratory failure. Some of the issues addressed by these investigators included how best to handle anticoagulation issues in fresh postoperative cardiac patients. They developed guidelines for indications and contraindications for support and identified the importance of appropriate patient selection for successful outcomes. It is a testimony to the remarkable foresight of these pioneers that the same issues still retain central importance to the success of ECMO used for circulatory support discussed below.

Circuit-Related and other Technical Aspects of ECMO for Circulatory Support

Components of the Circuit

Many of the technical aspects of ECMO used for circulatory support are similar to those of ECMO used for respiratory failure, although with some important additional considerations. ECMO is most often used in a venoarterial mode when used in cardiac patients to provide full cardiopulmonary support. However, several reports describe the successful use of venovenous ECMO for pediatric cardiac patients, which, in addition to providing respiratory support, resulted in improvement in the circulatory status.[6,7] Because a substantial amount of morbidity in congenital heart disease is due to hypoxia, pulmonary hypertension, and right ventricular failure, venovenous ECMO may currently be underused in pediatric cardiac patients. Although not providing cardiac pump support, the use of venovenous ECMO may lead to improved right ventricular function by eliminating hypoxia and decreasing pulmonary vascular resistance. A particularly ingenious approach to venovenous support is the AREC (assistance respiratoire extra-corporelle) system described by Chevalier, which uses a single venous cannula driven by a nonocclusive rotary pump with tidal flow in the circuit provided by alternating clamps.[8] This system has been successfully used in pediatric cardiac patients with hypoxia and pulmonary hypertension as the primary indications for ECMO support.[6]

Most pediatric centers continue to use an ECMO circuit that employs a membrane oxygenator, roller pump, and heat exchanger. The ECMO circuit, however, lends itself to modification, and many pediatric and adult centers currently use systems that incorporate hollow-fiber oxygenators and centrifugal pumps.[9–21] Hollow-fiber oxygenators are highly efficient in terms of gas exchange and are easy to prime, which is especially advantageous when rapid institution of support is necessary, such as in the resuscitation of patients after cardiac arrest.[22,23] In addition, heparin-bonded versions of both the hollow-fiber oxygenators and centrifugal pumps are available, which is a desirable feature in the immediate postoperative state to decrease bleeding. A potential problem of hollow-fiber oxygenators is their limited longevity due to plasma leak requiring frequent replacement with prolonged use.[22] Even though many pediatric centers continue to use roller pumps, centrifugal pumps may also be used; centrifugal pumps maintain venous inflow independent of gravity drainage so that the patient may be at any height relative to the pump. This feature of the centrifugal pump is especially useful in larger patients to maintain adequate venous return at higher flows. An additional advantage of the centrifugal pump is that occlusion of arterial outflow from the pump does not generate excessive arterial line pressure, reducing the risk of "blowout" of the arterial limb of the circuit if distal occlusion occurs. The chief disadvantage of the centrifugal pump is the high negative pressure that may be generated on the venous side of the circuit, potentially leading to hemolysis and cavitation.[24]

Most of the circuits that use roller pumps employ a bladder box, which is a servoregulatory mechanism that turns the pump off if venous inflow is inadvertently interrupted. This device is comprised of an in-line distensible bladder (30-mL volume) that compresses a spring-loaded mechanical switching device. Although widely used, the bladder box is subject to a number of problems related to the sensitivity of the switching device, which may be difficult to adjust. In addition, the bladder forms an area in the circuit with relative stasis of blood flow that may be the site of thrombus propagation. New electronic systems may provide a more accurate approach to pump servoregulation and may be used more widely in the future.[24]

Anticoagulation

The status of each patient's anticoagulation is monitored by the whole-blood activated clotting time (ACT). Achieving an ACT of 180 to 200 s with a continuous heparin infusion maintains the circuit with a minimal risk of important thrombosis.[7,10,13,14,25–27] Platelets are maintained above 100,000 per deciliter, and in patients requiring postoperative support where bleeding is a critical problem, above 150,000 per deciliter. Clotting factors are supplied with infusions of fresh-frozen plasma or cryoprecipitate to maintain fibrinogen levels above 100 mg/dL. For patients who require intraoperative support after cardiopulmonary bypass, we allow the ACT to drift to the 180- to 200-s range as factor levels and platelets are repleted, rather than reversing the heparin effect with protamine.[7] Instituting the heparin infusion may be safely deferred for several hours until the ACT drifts downward in the bleeding postoperative patient.

Heparin-bonded hollow-fiber oxygenators and tubing may be useful for decreasing the amount of systemic heparinization required.[9,17,19] Epsilon-aminocaproic acid (Amicar, Lederle Parenterals, Carolina, Puerto Rico) may also be used to diminish the risk of postoperative hemorrhage.[7,28] Amicar is administered as an intravenous bolus of 100 mg/kg, maintained as a continuous intravenous infusion of 30 mg/kg/h for the initial 48 h of support and then discontinued. Maintaining the infusion for longer periods is usually unnecessary because of abatement of postsurgical bleeding and because of increasing problems with circuit thrombosis resulting from prolonged administration. A recent multicenter trial failed to demonstrate an improvement in the rate of significant intracranial hemorrhage or surgical site bleeding with Amicar infusion for neonates requiring ECMO for respiratory failure; however, the numbers enrolled in the trial were small.[29]

Cannulation and Left Ventricular Decompression

The approach to cannulation should be flexible and based on the setting in which the need for ECMO arises. Transthoracic cannulation of the right atrial appendage and the ascending aorta is most appropriate for cases that require intraoperative support for failure to wean from cardiopulmonary bypass. In the immediate postoperative period, chest cannulation provides the most expeditious route to institute support, especially in patients that suffer cardiac arrest. Excellent venous drainage is assured by chest cannulation; however, significant hemorrhage remains the chief disadvantage making peripheral cannulation sites preferable in most other settings. Cannulation of the right internal jugular vein and the common carotid artery is the preferred peripheral cannulation site in neonates and children who weigh less than approximately 15 kg. Groin cannulation of the femoral vessels provides adequate venous drainage and perfusion for larger children and adults. The addition of a second venous drainage cannula placed in the right internal jugular vein may be employed if venous drainage through the femoral route is inadequate. Lower extremity ischemia can be minimized by placing a perfusion cannula in the distal femoral artery from a side arm brought off of the arterial limb of the circuit.[7,26] Venous congestion of the lower extremity may be prevented by placement of a "saphenous sump" catheter at the time of femoral venous cannulation.[12] The axillary artery and iliac vessels may represent additional cannulation sites in difficult access cases.

Left ventricular distension must be assiduously avoided during ECMO, especially in cases of severe left ventricular dysfunction.[30] We carefully monitor for the development of left-sided distension with echocardiography and direct measurement of left atrial pressure when available. Left-sided distension can often be treated by increasing ECMO flow rates to decrease the volume of pulmonary venous blood returning to the left heart. However, if this is unsuccessful, left atrial venting should be performed to decrease left atrial and left ventricular distension. This can be easily performed in patients who have undergone transthoracic cannulation by cannulating the right pulmonary veins at the atrioventricular groove or by cannulating the left atrial appendage. In patients cannulated by the peripheral route, left-sided decompression may be achieved by

balloon atrial septostomy performed in the cardiac catheterization laboratory or, preferably, at the patient's bedside under echocardiographic guidance.[31,32]

Other Management Points

We maintain ECMO flow rates generally in the range of 80 to 150 cc/kg/min until patients are considered ready for weaning. We usually decrease the doses of inotropes during ECMO, but routinely maintain these patients on low-dose dopamine and vasodilators. This combination hopefully improves peripheral and renal perfusion as well as encourages some degree of ventricular emptying in a further attempt to limit left-sided distension. We feel that it is important to maintain moderate levels of ventilatory support for the cardiac patient who requires ECMO support. Several studies show that coronary perfusion is derived from the left ventricle during ECMO.[33–35] Therefore, blood returning from the pulmonary veins should be fully saturated to maintain adequate myocardial oxygenation and to optimize the chances for ventricular recovery. With the exception of patients that have severe pulmonary parenchymal disease, fully saturated pulmonary venous blood is easily provided by maintaining moderate levels of ventilatory support during ECMO. We maintain the majority of our ECMO-supported cardiac patients with a fractional inspired oxygen of 40%, a respiratory rate of 16, positive end-expiratory pressure of 5 cm H_2O, and a tidal volume of 10 cc/kg.

Weaning from Support

Weaning is performed under echocardiographic guidance to assess ventricular filling and function. We do not routinely place pulmonary arterial catheters for cardiac output and pulmonary capillary wedge pressure determination in most children but would do so in borderline cases. At the time of weaning, flows are gradually turned down over several hours until flows of 25 to 40 cc/kg/min are achieved. Concurrently, ventilatory support and inotrope dosages are increased to appropriate levels. We then clamp the arterial and venous lines, maintaining full anticoagulation, and intermittently flush the cannulas (every 15 to 20 min) until the patient is stable. We routinely perform decannulation at the patient's bedside. We have maintained borderline patients off of ECMO for 1 to 2 h with intermittent flushing of the cannulas until it is clear that support is no longer needed; however, we have not capped the cannulas for periods of 24 h or more as some groups have described for respiratory failure patients. A strategy that we find useful in cases of profound ventricular dysfunction is to lengthen the weaning period over 48 to 72 h, with gradual reduction in flows over that period. It is our observation that especially fragile patients who may have failed with more rapid weaning may benefit from this approach by gradually accommodating to lower flows.

Clinical Aspects of ECMO for Circulatory Support in Children

Cardiac Diagnoses

A recent review of the experience at Children's Hospital, Boston, for pediatric cardiac patients that required mechanical circulatory support with either ECMO or VAD demonstrated that more than half of these cases were patients with complex cyanotic heart disease, possessing either increased pulmonary blood flow (such as transposition of the great arteries) or decreased pulmonary blood flow (such as tetralogy of Fallot).[7] Reviewing reports from other centers reveals this to be a generally representative make-up of patient diagnoses. In Walters' report of a large series of patients requiring postoperative support after cardiac surgery, complete atrioventricular canal (20%), complex single-ventricle anatomy (17%), and tetralogy of Fallot (14%) were the most common diagnoses.[36] In his 1991 review of Extracorporeal Life Support Organization (ELSO) registry data for pediatric cardiac patients, Meliones found patients with left to right shunt (24%), cyanosis with decreased pulmonary blood flow (22%), and cyanosis with increased pulmonary blood flow (17%) to be the most common diagnostic groups.[37] In a comparison of the two modalities, we found ECMO to be superior to VAD for the support of most children with complex cyanotic heart disease where hypoxia, pulmonary hypertension, or biventricular failure contribute significantly to the pathophysiology, necessitating mechanical circulatory support. Because of the presence of an oxygenator in the circuit, ECMO more directly addresses the underlying pathophysiology and provides greater flexibility than VAD.[7]

Indications for Support

Reviewing several large clinical series confirms that indications for support differ according to whether ECMO is required in the preoperative or postoperative period of cardiac surgery. Studies that summarize the preoperative use of ECMO demonstrate that hypoxia and pulmonary hypertension are the most common indications leading to ECMO support.[6,38] Postoperative support is most commonly initiated for failure to wean from cardiopulmonary bypass, cardiogenic shock, or cardiac arrest occurring in the intensive care unit after cardiac surgery.[12–15,25–27,36,39–41]

Our experience, which combined preoperative, postoperative, and cardiac medical patients, demonstrated that hypoxia (36%), cardiac arrest (24%), and failure to wean from cardiopulmonary bypass (14%) were the most common indications for ECMO support.[7] Although hypoxia was the single largest indication in our experience, innovative therapies, such as nitric oxide (NO) administration and high-frequency jet ventilation, may decrease the need for ECMO support in the treatment of pediatric patients with cardiac disease and refractory respiratory failure.[42–44] Kocis reported the use of high-frequency jet ventilation in patients that would have otherwise required ECMO for refractory respiratory failure. Seven of eight patients treated with high-frequency jet ventilation had their respiratory failure reversed, with only a single patient subsequently requiring ECMO.[44] Goldman used NO to treat 10 patients with severe pulmonary hypertension after surgery for congenital heart disease, including 5 who could not be weaned from cardiopulmonary bypass. He was able to avoid ECMO in 8 of these 10 patients, with 80% of the total patients surviving to hospital discharge.[42]

In our experience, the need for ECMO for failure to wean from cardiopulmonary bypass has had a significant negative impact on survival, with only 1 of 11 (9%) of these patients surviving to hospital discharge.[7] Several other studies reported failure to wean from cardiopulmonary bypass as a negative prognostic indicator.[10,15,36] However, a number of studies found inability to wean from bypass was not a risk factor.[26,41] In fact, these latter studies stress the importance of early institution of ECMO before prolonged periods of low cardiac output in the postoperative patient result in end-organ damage. The importance of early institution of ECMO support cannot be overemphasized; however, we have observed that patients who are unable to wean from cardiopulmonary bypass without ECMO fare poorly as a result of excessive mediastinal hemorrhage and often possess less potential for recovery of ventricular function.

Contraindications

As the use of ECMO for cardiac patients has increased, those clinical features defined as contraindications for the institution of support have evolved. There is universal agreement that certain conditions constitute absolute contraindications, including incurable malignancy, advanced multisystem organ failure, extreme prematurity, and severe central nervous system damage.[7,13,36,40] Any patient who is not a transplant candidate should probably be considered ineligible for support in that any patient placed on ECMO may ultimately require cardiac transplantation for recovery.[13]

However, a number of conditions previously thought to be unsalvageable or at risk for further complication with ECMO support may be successfully treated with ECMO and should, at most, represent relative contraindications. Patients with shunted single-ventricle physiology, including patients with hypoplastic left-heart syndrome, were often denied ECMO in the past, because of difficulties in achieving balance between the pulmonary and systemic circulations during support. A number of studies report success with ECMO support of these patients.[7,36,41] Systemic perfusion can usually be maintained by increasing circuit flows; however, blood flow through the shunt may have to be physically limited to insure adequate systemic perfusion and to avoid "flooding" the lungs. We often perform this at the patient's bedside by placing a metallic clip to partially constrict the shunt, which is removed at the time of weaning. Completely occluding the shunt is inadvisable because of the great likelihood of extensive pulmonary infarction.[41] In general, we have not developed rigid contraindications for mechanical support besides those mentioned above; rather, we evaluate each case on its own merits. In addition to shunted single-ventricle patients, we have successfully supported patients with presupport cardiac arrest, patients undergoing palliative cardiac operations, and patients with coexisting congenital diaphragmatic hernia. In our experience, none of these represent absolute contraindications for ECMO support.

Outcome and Risk Factors for Death

Published series report variable survival statistics for pediatric cardiac ECMO. In our experience, two-thirds of all patients placed on ECMO were successfully weaned from support, with 40% of the original patients surviving to hospital discharge.[7] This represents a fairly typical experience, with other studies reporting a weaning rate of 45 to 80% and a hospital survival rate of 22 to 70%.[10,12–15,25–27,36,39–41,45,46]

Reviewing risk factors for death from centers reporting a large experience with ECMO for pediatric cardiac cases reveals a number of unifying concepts. Several studies identified the development of renal failure as a risk factor for hospital death.[7,10,13,36,37] In addition to the development of overt renal failure as a risk factor, we found that survivors had a much greater urine output over the first 24 h of support.[7] Severe hemorrhage, measured directly as the volume of blood lost or the need for excessive transfusion of blood products, was a risk factor for death in a number of studies.[7,15,36,37] In our experience, nonsurvivors had a nearly twofold greater blood loss than did survivors. The presence of residual cardiac lesions after cardiac surgery was a significant risk factor in several reports.[10,12,39] The need for ECMO in cardiac surgical cases that fail to wean from cardiopulmonary bypass represents a risk factor in some reports as discussed above.[10,36] Other risk factors that have been identified in various reports include significant infectious complications, presupport cardiac arrest, and high inotropic dosages while on support.

For postcardiotomy patients, lack of return of ventricular function within 48 to 72 h was an ominous sign in our experience. We compared the rate of return of ventricular function for nontransplanted survivors to that of patients who were unable to be weaned from support (nonsurvivors and survivors who required cardiac transplantation) for both ECMO- and VAD-supported patients.[7] Return of ventricular function was defined as the return of a pulsatile waveform on the peripheral arterial trace on maximal levels of support (80% of normal cardiac output provided by the device). Twenty-four of 25 nontransplanted ECMO survivors (96%) had return of a pulsatile arterial waveform at maximal levels of support by 72 h. All surviving VAD patients had return of a pulsatile arterial waveform within 48 h of the initiation of support, while patients who failed to achieve ejection after this point died or required cardiac transplantation.

We used this data as additional prognostic information for postcardiotomy pediatric cardiac patients. Children who have undergone surgery for congenital heart disease who fail to demonstrate return of ventricular function within 48 to 72 h of ECMO support are currently considered for transplantation or for termination of support if there are contraindications to transplantation. Delaying this decision while awaiting return of ventricular function beyond the first 48 to 72 h of support is not justified based on these results. As a consequence of the scarcity of organ donors in the pediatric population, early consideration for transplantation optimizes the chances of successful organ procurement. It is important to note that these considerations apply to postcardiotomy pediatric cardiac patients; patients who require support for myocarditis may require substantially more time to demonstrate return of ventricular function, which is discussed in the next section.

Special Topics in ECMO Support for Pediatric Cardiac Patients

ECMO for the Treatment of Acute, Fulminant Myocarditis

Indications for the institution of ECMO in patients with myocarditis should be based on the clinical response to intensive care unit management. Most patients who are considered for ECMO support are receiving high-dose inotrope infusions with endotracheal intubation and muscle paralysis. If evidence of a low cardiac output state persists, clinically manifested as oliguria, poor cutaneous perfusion, and hypotension, ECMO should be strongly considered. The need for escalating inotrope doses accompanied by significant ventricular ectopy is an especially lethal combination that should suggest that mechanical circulatory support will be required due to the tendency of these patients to develop sudden and intractable ventricular fibrillation.

The survival rate for children who require mechanical circulatory support for myocarditis is relatively good in most reports.[47–52] The ELSO registry reports that myocarditis has the highest survival of any diagnostic group requiring ECMO, with 58% of these patients being successfully weaned from support.[53] A recent multi-institutional review of 15 patients with viral myocarditis supported by extracorporeal membrane oxygenation (12 patients) or ventricular assist devices (3 patients) demonstrated an overall survival rate of 80%.[54] In this experience, ECMO was thought to be a better choice than VAD for acute support for these children because of the option of peripheral cannulation, maintaining an intact chest cavity. Nine of the 15 patients were weaned from support with 7 survivors (78%), while the remaining 6 patients were successfully bridged to transplantation with 5 survivors (83%). An especially important finding was that all nontransplanted survivors are currently alive with normal ventricular function. Historically, it was believed that a significant percentage of children with acute myocarditis would develop dilated cardiomyopathy with the ultimate need for cardiac transplantation.[55] This study suggests that children with acute, fulminant myocarditis have an overall favorable outcome and a significant degree of disease reversibility if successfully supported during the acute phase of illness.

The reasons for better long-term outcomes and a decreased incidence of progression to dilated cardiomyopathy in patients most severely affected with myocarditis remain unexplained; however, mechanical circulatory support may contribute to the improved long-term outcomes in these children. In patients with dilated cardiomyopathy, prolonged mechanical circulatory support may result in ultimate recovery of ventricular function because of favorable influences on the neurohormonal cardiovascular milieu and unloading of the left ventricle, resulting in normalization of ventricular geometry through "reverse remodeling."[56] The institution of mechanical circulatory support in patients with acute fulminant myocarditis can favorably impact these same factors, resulting in ventricular recovery over a much shorter time course—a process described as "rapid-reverse remodeling."[54] It is compelling to speculate that normalization of ventricular geometry and function by the early institution of support may help to prevent progression to dilated cardiomyopathy.

Based on these results, the optimal approach for children presenting with acute fulminant myocarditis may be to provide mechanical circulatory support, even if required for prolonged periods, in anticipation of eventual ventricular recovery. Previous reports document full return of ventricular function in young adults with myocarditis after weeks or months of mechanical support.[57,58] Pulsatile paracorporeal or implantable VAD systems that allow extended periods of support have been used successfully in pediatric patients in Europe and have demonstrated the feasibility of this approach (see below).[59,60] Prolonged mechanical circulatory support in a larger number of pediatric patients with fulminant myocarditis may reveal that the capability of supporting these children for weeks or months will allow return of native ventricular function, thereby avoiding transplantation in the majority of these children.

Use of Rapid Resuscitation ECMO in the Treatment of Cardiorespiratory Arrest

Cardiac arrest is a common indication for pediatric cardiac ECMO, comprising nearly 25% of all indications

for ECMO in these patients.[7] Several groups have developed systems that allow the expeditious institution of ECMO for children with cardiac disease who suffer cardiac arrest refractory to conventional cardiopulmonary resuscitation.[23,61,62]

One system uses a modified ECMO circuit, an organized team of personnel to perform cannulation, and a streamlined priming process.[61] The "rapid resuscitation" ECMO circuit is maintained vacuum- and CO_2-primed in the intensive care unit and is portable, with a battery power supply enabling it to be quickly used in any location throughout the hospital. If standard cardiopulmonary resuscitation (CPR) is unsuccessful within 10 min of cardiac arrest, the circuit is moved to the patient's bedside and crystalloid priming is initiated while cannulation is proceeding. If cannulation is completed prior to the availability of blood products, ECMO flow is initiated with a crystalloid-primed circuit and blood products are added when available. The excess crystalloid volume is removed as blood is added to the circuit, using exchange transfusions by hand and performing ultrafiltration after the hemodynamics have stabilized. Establishing normal cardiac output with ECMO is the most critical factor for successful resuscitation of these children, even if the hematocrit is low at the time support is instituted due to the use of a crystalloid-primed circuit.

This approach was used for 11 pediatric patients who had suffered cardiac arrest: 9 of these patients were postoperative cardiac surgical patients, 1 child suffered cardiac arrest prior to surgery, and 1 child suffered cardiac arrest in the cardiac catheterization laboratory.[61] All patients were undergoing CPR at the time of ECMO cannulation. The median duration of CPR for these 11 patients was 55 min (range, 15 to 103 min) as compared to a median duration of CPR of 90 min (range, 45 to 200 min) for 7 historical controls resuscitated with conventional means prior to the use of the rapid resuscitation system. All but one of the 11 rapid resuscitation patients were able to be weaned from ECMO, with 7 patients (64%) surviving to hospital discharge, as compared to 2 survivors (29%) of the 7 historical controls.

Jacobs and colleagues reported results for a particularly innovative rapid resuscitation system that uses a hollow-fiber oxygenator to facilitate priming.[23] The circuit employs a centrifugal pump and short lengths of quarter-inch tubing, and is heparin bonded throughout. This system is fully portable and requires a priming volume of 250 mL. The use of the centrifugal pump eliminates the need for gravity drainage, which results in shorter tubing lengths and greater portability. The simplicity of the circuit facilitates priming and minimizes trauma to blood elements, while the heparin bonding results in less blood loss. The authors reported their results with this system in 23 children with cardiac disease, most of whom were status post cardiac surgery. All patients had support instituted with a crystalloid-primed circuit. The simplicity of this system and the avoidance of the blood-priming step enabled set-up time to be as brief as 5 min. The duration of cardiopulmonary resuscitation was only 12 min for the four patients in this series who suffered cardiac arrest prior to cannulation. By using this system, the overall survival in this series was 48%, with all four of the cardiac arrest patients surviving to hospital discharge.

These reports support the concept that pediatric cardiac patients who suffer cardiac arrest are often salvageable and deserve an aggressive approach with prompt institution of ECMO if conventional resuscitative measures fail. Rapid institution of circulatory support with modified ECMO systems can be life-saving, with preservation of end-organ function in these patients.

Clinical Aspects of ECMO for Circulatory Support in Adults

ECMO remains the most commonly used form of mechanical circulatory support in children. Although it has a more limited role in older patients, ECMO has many attributes that make it useful in providing short-term circulatory support in adults.[63] Peripheral cannulation can be performed percutaneously, providing a simple, rapid approach that can be instituted at the bedside. Circuit set-up and priming can be performed quickly, which, in combination with expeditious cannulation, makes ECMO a potential resuscitation tool for patients in cardiac arrest. ECMO provides biventricular cardiac support and pulmonary support for patients who experience right ventricular dysfunction or hypoxia. Unlike implantable VADs, ECMO avoids an apical ventriculotomy in patients who have undergone a recent anteroapical myocardial infarction. Finally, ECMO is relatively less costly than other forms of mechanical circulatory support.

ECMO can provide a period of stabilization and evaluation for patients in cardiogenic shock prior to implantation of more permanent circulatory assist devices or transplantation. Pagani and colleagues compared the outcomes of 32 patients with refractory cardiogenic shock in two groups: group 1 patients were initially stabilized with ECMO and then had LVAD implantation if clinically indicated after evaluation and stabilization; group 2 patients underwent direct LVAD implantation.[63] Seven of the 14 patients initially stabilized with ECMO were subsequently bridged to LVAD, while 1 of these 14 patients was bridged directly to heart transplantation. The remaining 18 patients underwent LVAD implantation without prior ECMO support. Group 1 patients were more critically ill than the group 2 patients, with higher incidences of presupport cardiac arrest, respiratory failure requiring intubation, and renal failure requiring dialysis. Despite the severity of their presupport illness, the patients who survived ECMO support to LVAD implantation had nearly the same 1-year actuarial survival as did the direct LVAD implant group (71% versus 75%, respectively). The authors of this study demonstrated that for patients who are high-risk LVAD candidates, initial treatment with ECMO provides a period during which resuscitation and recovery of end-organ function may occur. In addition, in this experience, approximately 20% of the patients initially supported with ECMO were subsequently found to have contraindications to heart transplantation. Initial ECMO support allowed time for this determination to be made and conserved LVAD and transplantation resources.

Other series have reported the utility of ECMO support for the treatment of postcardiotomy circulatory failure in adults.[16,17,19,20,64] Smedira and associates reported an experience of 202 adult patients who required ECMO support after cardiac surgery.[17] Forty-eight patients were bridged to LVAD ($n = 42$) or directly to transplantation ($n = 6$) with nearly the same 5-year survival (44%) as the 71 patients who were weaned with intent for survival (40%). The remaining 83 patients had ECMO withdrawn for futility. Important factors associated with failure to wean or bridge included renal and hepatic failure and neurologic events on support. In addition, the use of an IABP during support improved the likelihood of weaning or successful bridging. These results corroborated earlier data recommending IABP support for all adult patients requiring ECMO for circulatory support.[65] These authors also reported an analysis of risk factors leading to ECMO support after cardiac surgery.[64] They found the following patient factors to be associated with the ultimate need for ECMO support after cardiac surgery: older age, reoperation, emergency operation, higher creatinine, left main coronary artery disease, greater left ventricular dysfunction, and history of a previous myocardial infarction. Identification of patients with these risk factors allows preoperative management to improve their hemodynamic status and may even suggest the need for preoperative transplant evaluation. For postcardiotomy circulatory failure, these authors advocate ECMO support for 48 to 72 h with conversion to an implantable device if the patient is an acceptable transplant candidate and weaning from ECMO is not possible. Adopting a strategy of ECMO support for initial stabilization with ultimate bridge to transplantation provided by implantable systems may allow continued improvement of results for postcardiotomy cardiac failure.

Other reports have also described the utility of ECMO for postcardiotomy circulatory support in adults.[16,19,20] Magovern found that patients who required ECMO for postcardiotomy circulatory failure after isolated coronary artery bypass grafting had a survival of 56%.[19] This was substantially better than results for patients who required ECMO after valve surgery (13% survival), patients who suffered a postcardiotomy cardiac arrest, or patients who required support for postmyocardial infarction ventricular septal defect (0 survivors in either latter group). ECMO was especially successful in supporting patients during high-risk procedures in the cardiac catheterization laboratory.

In this experience, 85% of cardiac catheterization patients survived with relatively brief support times (mean, 100 ± 11 min). Smith reported the outcome of ECMO for post-cardiotomy circulatory failure in older adults.[16] The mean age of the patients in this group was 69, with a survival to hospital discharge rate of 41%. All of these patients were alive at a median of 21 months after discharge, with 86% reporting satisfactory performance in daily activities.

Summary

The approach to children with increasingly complicated cardiac disease has required the development of innovative measures to help insure successful outcomes. The use of ECMO for cardiac support in children arose naturally in pediatric centers as a result of its widespread and highly successful treatment of respiratory failure in children. The ability to mechanically support the cardiorespiratory system in children is an important component in the development of the field of pediatric cardiac surgery. It would not be overstating its importance to say that reliably successful surgical or medical approaches to many of these cardiac lesions require the availability of ECMO. ECMO retains a role in the treatment of adults with circulatory failure as well. ECMO support can be easily instituted by peripheral cannulation, maintaining an intact chest cavity. This feature, along with rapid circuit set-up, allows the expeditious institution of support in patients whose clinical status is rapidly deteriorating. Perhaps of greatest importance, ECMO provides short-term support for adult patients in refractory cardiogenic shock, allowing a period of resuscitation and evaluation to determine their candidacy for implantable VAD systems or cardiac transplantation.

References

1. Baffes TG, Fridman JL, Bicoff JP, Whitehill JL. Extracorporeal circulation for support of palliative cardiac surgery in infants. Ann Thorac Surg 1970;10:354–63.

2. Soeter JR, Mamiya RT, Sprague AY, McNamara JJ. Prolonged extracorporeal oxygenation for cardiorespiratory failure after tetralogy correction. J Thorac Cardiovasc Surg 1973;66:214–8.

3. Bartlett RH, Gazzaniga AB, Fong SW, Burns NE. Prolonged extracorporeal cardiopulmonary support in man. J Thorac Cardiovasc Surg 1974;68:918–32.

4. Bartlett RH, Gazzaniga AB, Fong SW, et al. Extracorporeal membrane oxygenator support for cardiopulmonary failure. J Thorac Cardiovasc Surg 1977;73:375–86.

5. Hill JD, de Leval MR, Fallat RJ, et al. Acute respiratory insufficiency treatment with prolonged extracorporeal oxygenation. J Thorac Cardiovasc Surg 1972;64:551–62.

6. Trittenwein G, Furst G, Golej J, et al. Preoperative ECMO in congenital cyanotic heart disease using the AREC system. Ann Thorac Surg 1997;63:1298–302.

7. Duncan BW, Hraska V, Jonas RA, et al. Mechanical circulatory support in children with cardiac disease. J Thorac Cardiovasc Surg 1999;117:529–42.

8. Chevalier JY, Couprie C, Larroquet M, et al. Venovenous single lumen cannula extracorporeal lung support in neonates. ASAIO J 1993;39:M654–8.

9. del Nido PJ. Extracorporeal membrane oxygenation for cardiac support in children. Ann Thorac Surg 1996;61:336–9.

10. Langley SM, Sheppard SB, Tsang VT, et al. When is extracorporeal life support worthwhile following repair of congenital heart disease in children? Eur J Cardiothorac Surg 1998;13:520–5.

11. Saito A, Miyamura H, Kanazawa H, et al. Extracorporeal membrane oxygenation for severe heart failure after Fontan operation. Ann Thorac Surg 1993;55:153–5.

12. Black MD, Coles JG, Williams WG, et al. Determinants of success in pediatric cardiac patients undergoing extracorporeal membrane oxygenation. Ann Thorac Surg 1995;60:133–8.

13. Dalton HJ, Siewers RD, Fuhrman BP, et al. Extracorporeal membrane oxygenation for cardiac rescue in children with severe myocardial dysfunction. Crit Care Med 1993;21:1020–8.

14. Kanter KR, Pennington DG, Weber TR, et al. Extracorporeal membrane oxygenation for postoperative cardiac support in children. J Thorac Cardiovasc Surg 1987;93:27–35.

15. Klein MD, Shaheen KW, Whittlesey GC, et al. Extracorporeal membrane oxygenation for the circulatory support of children after repair of congenital heart disease. J Thorac Cardiovasc Surg 1990;100:498–505.

16. Smith C, Bellomo R, Raman JS, et al. An extracorporeal membrane oxygenation-based approach to cardiogenic shock in an older population. Ann Thorac Surg 2001; 71:1421–7.

17. Smedira NG, Moazami N, Golding CM, et al. Clinical experience with 202 adults receiving extracorporeal membrane oxygenation for cardiac failure: survival at five years. J Thorac Cardiovasc Surg 2001;122:92–102.

18. Taghavi S, Ankersmit HJ, Wieselthaler G, et al. Extracorporeal membrane oxygenation for graft failure after heart transplantation: recent Vienna experience. J Thorac Cardiovasc Surg 2001;122:819–20.

19. Magovern GJ Jr, Simpson KA. Extracorporeal membrane oxygenation for adult cardiac support: the Allegheny experience. Ann Thorac Surg 1999;68:655–61.

20. Ko WJ, Lin CY, Chen RJ, et al. Extracorporeal membrane oxygenation support for adult postcardiotomy cardiogenic shock. Ann Thorac Surg 2002;73:538–45.

21. Fiser SM, Tribble CG, Kaza AK, et al. When to discontinue extracorporeal membrane oxygenation for postcardiotomy support. Ann Thorac Surg 2001;71:210–4.

22. Willms DC, Atkins PJ, Dembitsky WP, et al. Analysis of clinical trends in a program of emergent ECLS for cardiovascular collapse. ASAIO J 1997;43:65–8.

23. Jacobs JP, Ojito JW, McConaghey TW, et al. Rapid cardiopulmonary support for children with complex congenital heart disease. Ann Thorac Surg 2000;70:742–50.

24. Hirschl RB. Devices. In: Zwischenberger JB, Bartlett RH, editors. ECMO: extracorporeal cardiopulmonary support in critical care. Ann Arbor, MI: Extracorporeal Life Support Organization; 1995. p. 150–90.

25. Anderson HL, Attori RJ, Custer JR, et al. Extracorporeal membrane oxygenation for pediatric cardiopulmonary failure. J Thorac Cardiovasc Surg 1990;99:1011–21.

26. Delius RE, Bove EL, Meliones JN, et al. Use of extracorporeal life support in patients with congenital heart disease. Crit Care Med 1992;20:1216–22.

27. Raithel RC, Pennington DG, Boegner E, et al. Extracorporeal membrane oxygenation in children after cardiac surgery. Circulation 1992;86 Suppl II:II-305–10.

28. Wilson JM, Bower LK, Fackler JC, et al. Aminocaproic acid decreases the incidence of intracranial hemorrhage and other hemorrhagic complications of ECMO. J Pediatr Surg 1993;28:536–41.

29. Horwitz JR, Cofer BR, Warner BH, et al. A multi-center trial of 6-aminocaproic acid (Amicar) in the prevention of bleeding in infants on ECMO. J Pediatr Surg 1998;33: 1610–3.

30. Shen I, Levy FH, Vocelka CR, et al. Effect of extracorporeal membrane oxygenation on left ventricular function of swine. Ann Thorac Surg 2001;71:862–7.

31. O'Connor TA, Downing GJ, Ewing LL, Gowdamarajan R. Echocardiographically guided balloon atrial septostomy during extracorporeal membrane oxygenation (ECMO). Pediatr Cardiol 1993;14:167–8.

32. Koenig PR, Ralston MA, Kimball TR, et al. Balloon atrial septostomy for left ventricular decompression in patients receiving extracorporeal membrane oxygenation for myocardial failure. J Pediatr 1993;122:S95–9.

33. Shen I, Levy FH, Benak AM, et al. Left ventricular dysfunction during extracorporeal membrane oxygenation in a hypoxemic swine model. Ann Thorac Surg 2001;71: 868–71.

34. Kinsella JP, Gerstmann DR, Rosenberg AA. The effect of extracorporeal membrane oxygenation on coronary perfusion and regional blood flow distribution. Pediatr Res 1992;31:80–4.

35. Secker-Walker JS, Edmonds JF, Spratt EH, Conn AW. The source of coronary perfusion during partial bypass for extracorporeal membrane oxygenation (ECMO). Ann Thorac Surg 1976;21:138–43.

36. Walters HL, Hakimi M, Rice MD, et al. Pediatric cardiac surgical ECMO: multivariate analysis of risk factors for hospital death. Ann Thorac Surg 1995;60:329–37.

37. Meliones JN, Custer JR, Snedecor S, et al. Extracorporeal life support for cardiac assist in pediatric patients. Circulation 1991;84 Suppl III:168–72.

38. Hunkeler NM, Canter CE, Donze A, Spray TL. Extracorporeal life support in cyanotic congenital heart disease before cardiovascular operation. Am J Cardiol 1992; 69:790–3.

39. Rogers AJ, Trento A, Siewers RD, et al. Extracorporeal membrane oxygenation for postcardiotomy cardiogenic shock in children. Ann Thorac Surg 1989;47:903–6.

40. Weinhaus L, Canter C, Noetzel M, et al. Extracorporeal membrane oxygenation for circulatory support after repair of congenital heart defects. Ann Thorac Surg 1989;48:206–12.

41. Ziomek S, Harrell JE, Fasules JW, et al. Extracorporeal membrane oxygenation for cardiac failure after congenital heart operation. Ann Thorac Surg 1992;54:861–8.

42. Goldman AP, Delius RE, Deanfield JE, et al. Nitric oxide might reduce the need for extracorporeal support in children with critical postoperative pulmonary hypertension. Ann Thorac Surg 1996;62:750–5.

43. Journois D, Pouard P, Mauriat P, et al. Inhaled nitric oxide as a therapy for pulmonary hypertension after operations for congenital heart defects. J Thorac Cardiovasc Surg 1994;107:1129–35.

44. Kocis KC, Meliones JN, Dekeon MK, et al. High-frequency jet ventilation for respiratory failure after congenital heart surgery. Circulation 1992;86 Suppl II:II-127–32.

45. Ferrazzi P, Glauber M, DiDomenico A, et al. Assisted circulation for myocardial recovery after repair of congenital heart disease. Eur J Cardiothorac Surg 1991;5:419–24.

46. Trento A, Thompson A, Siewers RD, et al. Extracorporeal membrane oxygenation in children. J Thorac Cardiovasc Surg 1988;96:542–7.

47. Grundl PD, Miller SA, del Nido PJ, et al. Successful treatment of acute myocarditis using extracorporeal membrane oxygenation. Crit Care Med 1993;21:302–4.

48. Frazier EA, Faulkner SC, Seib PM, et al. Prolonged extracorporeal life support for bridging to transplant. Perfusion 1997;12:93–8.

49. Kawahito K, Murata S, Yasu T, et al. Usefulness of extracorporeal membrane oxygenation for treatment of fulminant myocarditis and circulatory collapse. Am J Cardiol 1998;82:910–1.

50. Martin J, Sarai K, Schindler M, et al. Medos HIA-VAD biventricular assist device for bridge to recovery in fulminant myocarditis. Ann Thorac Surg 1997;63:1145–6.

51. del Nido PJ, Armitage JM, Fricker FJ, et al. Extracorporeal membrane oxygenation support as a bridge to pediatric heart transplantation. Circulation 1994;90 Part 2:II-66–9.

52. Cofer BR, Warner BW, Stallion A, Ryckman FC. Extracorporeal membrane oxygenation in the management of cardiac failure secondary to myocarditis. J Pediatr Surg 1993;28:669–72.

53. ECMO registry report. July, 1999. Ann Arbor, MI: Extracorporeal Life Support Organization.

54. Duncan BW, Bohn DJ, Atz AM, et al. Mechanical circulatory support for the treatment of children with acute fulminant myocarditis. J Thorac Cardiovasc Surg 2001; 122:440–8.

55. Greenwood RD, Nadas AS, Fyler DC. The clinical course of primary myocardial disease in infants and children. Am Heart J 1976;5:549–60.

56. Levin GR, Oz MC, Chen JM, et al. Reversal of chronic ventricular dilation in patients with end-stage cardiomyopathy by prolonged mechanical unloading. Circulation 1995;91:2717–20.

57. Holman WL, Bourge RC, Kirklin JK. Circulatory support for seventy days with resolution of acute heart failure. J Thorac Cardiovasc Surg 1991;102:932–4.

58. Levin HR, Oz MC, Catanese KA, et al. Transient normalization of systolic and diastolic function after support with a left ventricular assist device in a patient with dilated cardiomyopathy. J Heart Lung Transplant 1996;15: 840–2.

59. Konertz W, Hotz H, Schneider M, et al. Clinical experience with the MEDOS HIA-VAD system in infants and children. Ann Thorac Surg 1997; 63:1138–44.

60. Stiller B, Dahnert I, Weng Y, et al. Children may survive severe myocarditis with prolonged use of biventricular assist devices. Heart 1999;82:237–40.

61. Duncan BW, Ibrahim AE, Hraska V, et al. Use of rapid-deployment extracorporeal membrane oxygenation for the resuscitation of pediatric patients with heart disease after cardiac arrest. J Thorac Cardiovasc Surg 1998;116:305–11.

62. del Nido PJ, Dalton HJ, Thompson AE, Siewers RD. Extracorporeal membrane oxygenator rescue in children during cardiac arrest after cardiac surgery. Circulation 1992;86 Suppl II:II-300–4.

63. Pagani FD, Lynch W, Swaniker F, et al. Extracorporeal life support to left ventricular assist device bridge to heart transplant: a strategy to optimize survival and resource utilization. Circulation 1999;100 Suppl II:206–10.

64. Smedira NG, Blackstone EH. Postcardiotomy mechanical support: risk factors and outcomes. Ann Thorac Surg 2001;71:S60–6; discussion S82–5.

65. Lazar HL, Treanor P, Yang XM, et al. Enhanced recovery of ischemic myocardium by combining percutaneous bypass with intraaortic balloon pump support. Ann Thorac Surg 1994;57:663–7; discussion 667–8.

CHAPTER 42

LEFT VENTRICULAR VOLUME REDUCTION FOR DILATED CARDIOMYOPATHY

ANTONIO MARIA CALAFIORE, MD, MICHELE DI MAURO, MD,
MARCO CONTINI, MD, GIUSEPPE VITOLLA, MD, PIERO PELINI, MD

In recent years, there has been increasing interest in non-transplant surgical treatment of dilated cardiomyopathy (DCM). The increasing number of patients with heart failure, the shortage of donors for heart transplant and the diffusion of cardiac surgery in countries in which heart transplant, for different reasons, is not available, favored the development of different surgical techniques that could palliate the symptoms of heart failure.

In 1995, Randas V. Batista introduced an unusual approach for treatment of DCM: he proposed the resection of part of the lateral wall to reduce the radius of the left ventricle (LV).[1] The surgical world was shocked by this procedure, and the initial enthusiasm caused a high number of surgeries all over the world. However, early and late results were not proportional to expectations, and the initial interest vanished. Nevertheless, the interest in LV volume reduction did not end, through either a revaluation of the Batista procedure or an extreme application of other techniques, like the Dor or the Guilmet procedure, in patients with large akinetic areas.[2,3]

During the same period another technique became popular: mitral valve surgery to correct the functional mitral regurgitation (FMR) that is always present in DCM in its later stage. Even though Bolling and colleagues proposed this procedure at the beginning of the 1990s, it was the appearance of the Batista procedure (that was in antagonism of Bolling's concept) that stimulated the interest in the pathophysiology of the different aspects of DCM and the search for different surgical possibilities that could fit different aspects of the disease.[4] We acknowledge that without the inspiration and the enthusiasm showed by Batista, and without his dedication to spreading his procedure, his offering to operate on patients everywhere, and his exposing himself to criticism, this fascinating and new chapter of our specialty would have never been written.

First, we define dilated cardiomyopathy, and then we describe briefly Laplace's law, which is often a foundation of surgical procedures of volume reduction.

The chapter discusses *mitral valve surgery,* whose purpose is to stop and possibility to invert left ventricular remodeling, and *left ventricular reshaping,* which includes the procedures that are used to change acutely the left ventricle from a spheroidal to a more elliptical shape.

Definitions

DCM

Some patients with large and hypokinetic hearts cannot be considered as having a DCM. Ejection fraction (EF), by itself, is not a reliable marker of global cardiac function, and low EF can coexist with LV volumes only slightly enlarged (hypokinesia related to severe ischemia). On the other hand, large volumes, by themselves, do not identify DCM, as in patients with large but easily resectable LV aneurysms. Surgical risk and long-term results are completely different in these patients when they are compared to patients with DCM.

We define DCM as LV with EF $\leq$ 35%, with end diastolic volume index (EDVI) higher than 110 mL/m^2, and with functional mitral regurgitation that *has to be corrected.* Dilation of the base of the heart is part of the anatomic aspect. LVs of patients with ischemic disease show the same characteristics; the contractile dysfunction is not explained by the extent of coronary artery disease or ischemic damage. No evidence of residual ischemia has to be demonstrated. Coronary artery bypass graft (CABG) surgery is performed, if necessary, to avoid further coronary occlusions.[5,6]

Laplace's Law

This law estimates myocardial wall stress (MWS) from intraventricular pressure (VIP), radius of curvature (R), and wall thickness (h): MWS = VIP × R/h. According to this law, the increase of the radius of the chronic failing heart exposes the myocytes to a higher wall stress. This leads to chamber and cellular hypertrophy, which, in an adaptive process, renormalizes the wall stress. As the chamber continues to dilate over time, when the limits of hypertrophy are reached, wall stress ultimately increases. As a consequence, a higher part of the cardiac contractile power is used to counteract the wall stress and a minor part is used to eject the blood. Furthermore, a high wall stress is a powerful stimulus for cardiomyocyte apoptosis in the failing heart.[7] A vicious cycle is generated; therefore, reduction of wall stress appears to be a key point in the surgical treatment of DCM.

Mitral Valve Surgery

The appearance of FMR is a negative point in the natural history of DCM, because it increases the degree of heart failure and decreases the rate of survival.[8–10] Mechanisms that lead to FMR are several; however, being the valve normal, they start at the level of subvalvular apparatus. LV enlargement causes displacement of both papillary muscles, which move, according to the specific situation, posterolaterally and apically (Figure 42-1).

As a consequence of geometric distortion of the mitral valve apparatus, there is an increase in the distance over which the mitral leaflets are tethered from the papillary muscles to the anterior annular ring, with a consequent increase of the mitral annular area that must be covered. The leaflets take a tented geometry, their length coaptation is reduced or disappears, and the level where both leaflets meet (mitral valve coaptation depth) is displaced deep in the LV (Figure 42-2). Mitral regurgitation due to postischemic DCM can have, if papillary muscles are involved in the ischemic event, a different start, as restricted motion of leaflets can be the basis of the process. However, when left ventricular dilation starts, the further mechanism of FMR is similar to that described previously.

The increase in mitral valve area causes an increase of the size of the mitral annulus, which causes, by itself, further mitral regurgitation. If papillary muscles are displaced to the same extent, a higher grade of annulus dilation causes a high FMR.

Some authors postulate that the mitral annulus dilates together with the ventricle; as a consequence, it has the same importance as papillary muscle displacement in the determinism of functional mitral regurgitation.[11,12] Even if this hypothesis cannot be completely rejected, mitral leaflets cover an area that exceeds 1.5 to 2.2 times the area subtended by the annulus.[13] Therefore, it needs to be overdilated to cause, by itself, mitral regurgitation. Furthermore, if the annulus were the first (or the only) cause, the amount of regurgitant flow would be fixed and would not change as it does, by definition, in functional mitral regurgitation.

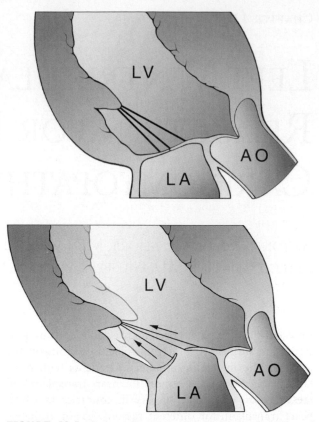

FIGURE 42-1. Both papillary muscles move posterolaterally and apically, as a consequence of left ventricle enlargement. AO = aorta; LA = left atrium; LV = left ventricle.

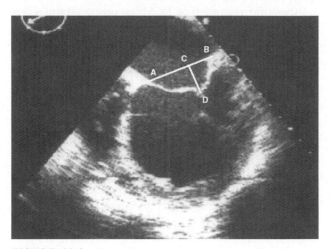

FIGURE 42-2. The leaflets show tented geometry; mitral annulus (A–B = 45 mm) is enlarged and mitral valve coaptation depth (C–D = 13 mm) is increased.

The purpose of surgery is to restore the competence of the mitral valve in order to reduce the symptoms of heart failure. The appearance of FMR increases the end diastolic pressure and, consequently, the wall stress, more than it increases the end diastolic volumes. A characteristic of FMR is its variability from time to time; the LV cannot adapt its shape to continuously changing volumes. Furthermore, LV walls have a different degree of stiffness and are not easily distensible. As a consequence, a sudden change in the degree of FMR is followed by rapid increase in pulmonary pressure with a parallel increase of the level of dyspnea.

Surgical Indications

Being functional, the degree of mitral regurgitation is less important than the abnormalities of mitral valve apparatus. Evaluation of annular dilation, of the motion of both leaflets, of the level of leaflet coaptation, and of LV end diastolic volumes are the key points in surgical indication. Even if high grades of mitral regurgitation (grades 3/4 or 4/4) always need to be corrected, we think that a grade 2/4 mitral regurgitation has to be corrected in the presence of severe abnormalities of mitral valve apparatus. A grade 2/4 mitral regurgitation represents a small part of LV stroke volume in patients with normal EF and volumes; however, if EF is low and the LV is dilated, moderate mitral regurgitation represents a significant portion of LV stroke volume.

Surgical Techniques

The purpose of surgery is to restore mitral valve competence acting on the mitral annulus, which is always dilated. In the great majority of the cases, the mitral valve can be preserved, by applying the technique of the overreduction of the mitral annulus, proposed by Bolling.[4] This can be obtained using a No. 26 ring, a DeVega-like mitral annuloplasty, or a pericardium strip.[14–17] Surgery is addressed to the posterior annulus, whose size can be easily reduced.

We prefer to use a 1 cm wide x 6 cm long pericardial strip, treated for 15 min with a 0.625% glutaraldehyde solution and rinsed for a further 15 min in saline (Figure 42-3). The strip is folded, to avoid any bending during knot tying. When using a pericardial strip, it is necessary to determine its optimal length. We found, based on clinical data, that a 4-cm length is enough to have a correct undersizing of the mitral annulus. The mitral area is approximately 3 cm^2 and the mean gradient is not higher than 2 mm Hg. By using this strategy, the anterior leaflet is able to cover completely the mitral valve area and assures a perfect coaptation with the remaining posterior leaflet, which, functionally, loses its role.

However, even if mitral valve repair can be performed in the great majority of patients, in our experience, there are cases where, due to the severe perturbation of the mitral valve apparatus, the mitral valve has to be replaced. We have found that the distance between the point of the mitral valve leaflet's coaptation and the plane of the mitral valve (mitral valve coaptation depth [MVCD]) is the key determinant of whether the mitral valve is to be repaired or replaced.[5] If this distance is 10 mm or less, the valve can be repaired; if it is 11 mm or greater, the valve has to be replaced. The rationale is that if the papillary muscles are severely displaced, even if the mitral valve annulus is overreduced, the leaflets will not coapt inside the ventricle, leaving the mitral valve incompetent. In these selected

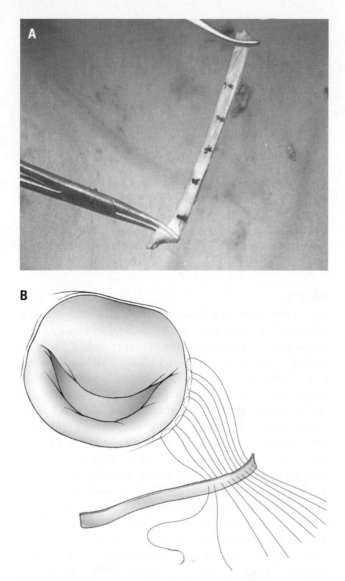

FIGURE 42-3. A pericardial strip is treated for 15 minutes with a 0.625% gluteraldeyde solution and rinsed for a further 15 min in saline (A). The strip is used for posterior annuloplasty (B).

cases, we prefer to insert a prosthesis inside the mitral valve, excising only a small triangle in the anterior leaflet, attracting both papillary muscles toward the annulus (Figure 42-4).

Other authors prefer to always replace the mitral valve.[18] Even if this strategy is acceptable, at least theoretically, we think that mitral valve overreduction provides good midterm results and an improved quality of life to patients, avoiding any possibility of prosthetic dysfunction.

Together with mitral valve surgery, it is often necessary to perform tricuspid annuloplasty. We prefer to use a DeVega-like partial annuloplasty with a 2–0 Ti-Cron suture instead of a polypropylene suture.

Coronary grafting is often necessary, not to reverse ischemia, but to prevent further coronary occlusions that can impair the contractile status.

A **B**

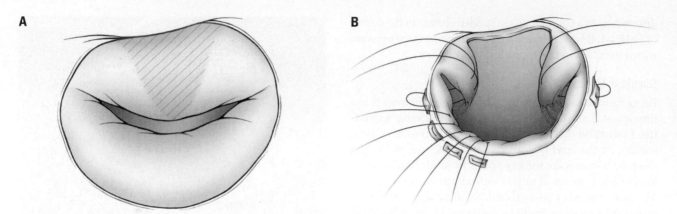

FIGURE 42-4. Mitral valve replacement. Only a small triangle of the anterior leaflets is excised (A). Both papillary muscles are attracted towards the annulus by means of stitches used to insert the prosthesis (B).

Results

The first report of mitral valve repair in patients with dilated cardiomyopathy was by Bolling and colleagues.[4] Subsequently, Bolling updated his experience.[19] Recently, Bolling reported a series of 92 patients who underwent mitral valve repair with an early mortality rate of 5%.[20] Mean preoperative ejection fraction was 14% and end diastolic volumes were 281 ± 86 mL. At mean follow-up of 38 months, 1- and 2-year actuarial survival rates were 80% and 70%, respectively. Radovanovic and colleagues reported a series of 76 patients who underwent mitral and tricuspid valve repair with mean preoperative New York Heart Association (NYHA) class 3.6.[15] Mean echocardiographic end diastolic volumes were 289 ± 87 mL/m² and ejection fraction was 26.6 ± 6.3%. Early mortality rate was 1.3%. Survival rates at 3 and 7 years were 48.7% and 38.1%, respectively. NYHA class decreased from 3.6 to 1.9 during the follow-up. Bishay and colleagues reported 44 patients who had mitral valve surgery with severe left ventricular dysfunction.[21] Mean ejection fraction was 28 ± 6, and mean preoperative end diastolic volume was 183 ± 67 mL/m². Early mortality was 2.3%. 1-, 2-, and 5-year survivals were 89, 86, and 67%, respectively.

PERSONAL EXPERIENCE

From June 1990 to February 2002, 73 patients underwent mitral surgery for DCM at the University of Chieti, Pescara, Italy, of which 23 had mitral valve replacement and 50 had mitral valve repair. Mean ejection fraction was 27 ± 6 % and mean end diastolic volumes were 159 ± 77 mL/m². Three patients (4.1%) died within the first 30 days after surgery. Causes of death were multiorgan failure on the fifth postoperative day, supradiaphragmatic aortic rupture due to an undiagnosed perforating aortic ulcer on the seventh postoperative day, and massive pulmonary bleeding on the eighth postoperative day. All the patients had elective inotropic support for 1 to 141 h (mean, 29.6 ± 32.2 h). Five patients needed an intraaortic balloon pump (IABP) in the operating room and two needed it during their intensive care unit (ICU) stay. Chronic medical treatment included angiotensin-converting enzyme (ACE) inhibitors, diuretics, and beta blockers such as carvedilol. After a mean of 27 ± 29 months, 15 (23.4%) patients died; 7 had had mitral valve repair and 8 had had mitral valve replacement. Causes of death were cardiac in 14 (2 sudden death and 12 heart failure) and noncardiac in 1 (malignancy). Five-year survival was 78.1 ± 4.8%. Patients who had mitral valve repair had better 5-year survival than patients who had mitral valve replacement, even if not statistically significant (84.0 ± 5.2% versus 65.2 ± 9.9%, *p* = not significant [ns]) (Figure 42-5). In the 56 survivors, after a mean follow up of 28 ± 31 months, NYHA class decreased from 3.5 ± 0.6 to 2.2 ± 0.6 (*p* < .001). The probability of being alive with an improvement of at least one NYHA class at 5 years after surgery was 64.4 ± 5.6% and was higher in patients who had repair rather than replacement, even if the values were not statistically significant (70.0 ± 6.5% versus 50.0 ± 10.2%, *p* = ns) (Figure 42-6). Thirty-two of the 56 survivors were carefully followed with serial echocardiographic evaluations. Mitral valve repair gave similar results to mitral valve replacement, even if this latter

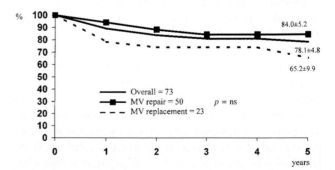

FIGURE 42-5. Mitral valve (MV) surgery. Five-year survival in MV surgery group. Overall (———), MV repair (—■—) and MV replacement (- - - - -). ns = not significant.

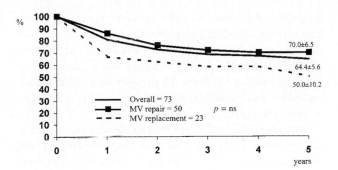

FIGURE 42-6. Mitral valve (MV) surgery. Five-year possibility of being alive with an improvement of at least 1 NYHA class in MV surgery group. Overall (———), MV repair (—■—) and MV replacement (- - - - -). ns = not significant; NYHA = New York Heart Association.

group included the most dilated patients. Volumes, stroke volumes, and ejection fraction did not change, but the postoperative NYHA class was lower than the preoperative class, independent of the surgical procedure on the mitral valve. Residual FMR was present, in different grades, in all but four of the patients who had mitral valve repair (Table 42-1).

Left Ventricle Reshaping

Nonischemic Dilated Cardiomyopathy

Dilation of the left ventricle is a compulsory step in the natural history of nonischemic dilated cardiomyopathy (NIDCM). Although heart transplantation is the best surgical option, there are many practical reasons for not making this procedure the first choice for every patient. Shortage of donors, increased age, pulmonary hypertension, chronic organ failure, or impossibility of using cadaver hearts for religious or legal reasons limit the number of transplanted patients, which reached a plateau in recent years.

Even though mitral valve surgery began in the early 1990s, it wasn't until 1996 that Batista introduced direct surgery on the left ventricle.[1] Batista proposed to resect that portion of lateral wall between the papillary muscles

TABLE 42-1. Postoperative Clinical and Echocardiographic Evolution in 32 Patients (20 Mitral Valve Repair, 12 Mitral Valve Replacement)

	Preoperation (n = 32)	Postoperation (n = 32)	p
NYHA class	3.2 ± 0.6	2.3 ± 0.6	< 0.001
EF (%)	29 ± 6	31 ± 12	ns
EDv (mL/m²)	146 ± 50	133 ± 44	ns
ESv (mL/m²)	101 ± 42	92 ± 38	ns
SV (mL/m²)	45 ± 12	40 ± 16	ns
FMR (20 patients)	3.2 ± 0.7	1.2 ± 0.7	< 0.001
No residual FMR	—	4/20	
Follow up (months)		23.4 ± 17.0	

EDv = end diastolic volume; EF = ejection fraction; ESv = end systolic volume; FMR = functional mitral regurgitation; ns = not significant; NYHA = New York Heart Association; SV = stroke volume.

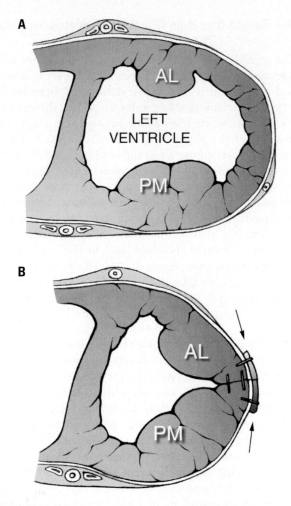

FIGURE 42-7. Batista procedure. The cavity is reduced by excising the lateral wall between the papillary muscles (A, B). AL = anterolateral; PL = posterolateral.

(which could be included in the resection) on the basis of Laplace's law, which postulates the decrease of wall stress if the radius is shortened (Figure 42-7). Early and mid-term results did not fit the expectations, and initial enthusiasm vanished. The main problem was that preoperative patient selection was not clearly defined.

Indeed, there is still a great interest in Batista's concept. Experimental studies show that cardiodepression is caused by increasing the left ventricle radius by using a patch.[22] Patch removal, although not reproducing normality, improves contractility and hemodynamics. Consequently, there is a strong rationale for despherical-ization. On the other hand, a theoretical, but elegant, paper by Artrip and colleagues demonstrated that removing functioning myocardium reduced peak wall stress–pressure relationships but at the expense of increased diastolic wall stiffness, with a net reduction in overall ventricular pump function.[23] Furthermore, in this study, the quality of the remaining myocardium was considered normal.

The Batista Operation (Partial Left Ventriculectomy)

SURGICAL TECHNIQUE

The procedure, as described by Batista, is performed without cardioplegic arrest. The apex of the heart is elevated and an incision is performed, starting 45° from the left anterior descending artery, going up toward the atrioventricular groove. As soon as the left ventricle is open, the position of the papillary muscles is controlled and the incision is carried out along the border of one of the two muscles (Figure 42-8A). The incision is then stopped 1 cm before the groove. Starting from the apex again, a slice of left ventricle is excised, as large as the distance between the two papillary muscles and as long as the first incision (Figure 8B and C). As an alternative, one or both papillary muscles can be resected and eliminated, in this case, together with the mitral valve (Figure 42-9A). The incision is closed with two layers by using Teflon felt. The mitral valve is generally replaced by the ventriculectomy (Figure 42-9B).

CLINICAL RESULTS

Recently, Franco-Cereceda and colleagues reported the Cleveland Clinic midterm results after using the Batista procedure.[24] All the patients were enrolled in the heart transplant program, and all of them had mitral valve surgery. Whereas the 30-day mortality was low (3.2%), 1- and 3-year survival rates were 82% and 64%, respectively. Event-free survival rates (including death, return to NYHA class IV, relisting for heart transplant, implantation of a left ventricular assist device or of a defibrillator) were 49% and 26% at 1 and 3 years, respectively. Independent predictors of higher incidence of adverse events were systolic pulmonary artery pressure beyond 40 mm Hg for survival, reduced maximum exercise oxygen consumption at baseline for rapid return in NYHA class IV, and higher left atrial pressure for lower event-free survival. Modest improvement in ejection fraction was sustained, and redilatation was rare. The authors concluded that the high percentage of failures, which were not predictable from the preoperative clinical studies, makes this procedure a less-than-valuable alternative to heart transplant.

Suma and colleagues reported a different experience in 82 patients.[25] Early mortality was higher (20.7%), but only 8.2% of patients (5 of 61 cases) in elective cases died, and 57.1% of patients in emergency cases died. In elective patients, 1- and 4-year survival rates were 75.5% and 69.3%, whereas no emergency patient survived as long as 3 years.

The high 30-day mortality was confirmed by a survey of Angelini and colleagues that, in a review of the literature that included 12 papers with 506 cases, found an early mortality of 17.4% (88 patients).[24,26–37] Causes of death were low output syndrome in 55 (62.5%), bleeding in 10 (11.3%), malignant arrhythmias in 7 (7.9%), sepsis in 8 (9.1%), and stroke in 5 (5.7%) patients. The cause of death for the remaining 3 patients was heart failure. Long-term results are reported by 10 series (386 patients with a 30-day mortality of 12.7% [49 patients]).[23,25–28,31,32,34–36] Eighty-nine patients died after the first month; causes of death were redilation in 50 (56.2%), malignant arrhythmias in 20 (22.5%), sepsis in 5 (5.6%), and stroke in 2 (2.2%). The cause of death in the remaining 12 patients was unknown. Survival rates after 1 year ranged from 50 to 85%, after 2 years from 45 to 72%, and after 3 years from 33 to 64%. The authors concluded that in spite of a high early mortality, long-term survival seems to be better than expected and that globally, survival data are encouraging.

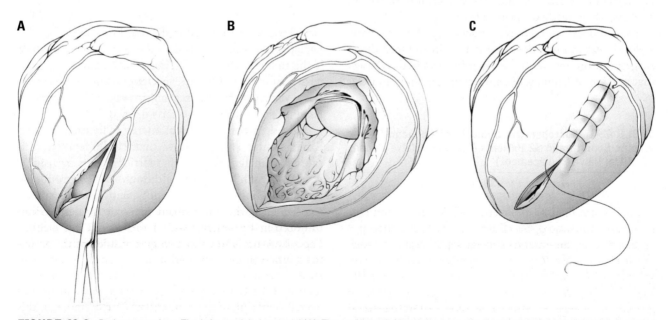

FIGURE 42-8. Batista procedure. The left ventricle is opened (A). The position of the papillary muscles is controlled and the incision is carried out along the border of one of the two. The muscle between the papillaries is excised (B). The incision is then closed (C).

A

B

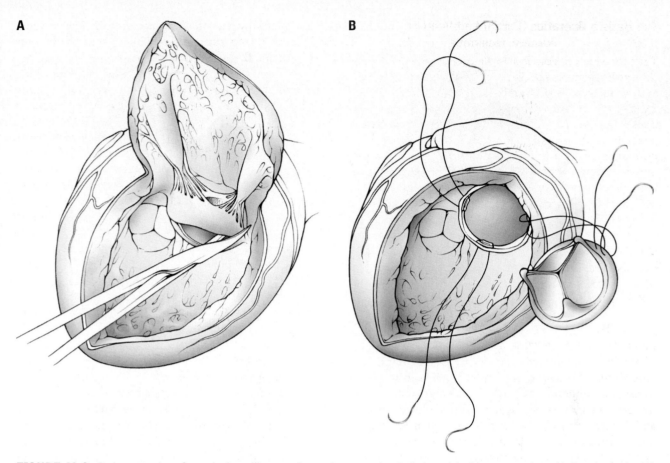

FIGURE 42-9. Batista procedure. One or both papillary muscles can be resected and eliminated, in this case together with the mitral valve (A). The mitral valve is generally replaced from the ventriculectomy (B).

PERSONAL EXPERIENCE

We performed our first Batista operation in January 1996. (We stopped doing Batista operations in June 1998.) Through June 1998, 21 patients had been operated on. In all 21 patients, the mitral valve was replaced. Mean ejection fraction was 21.5 ± 5.0%. Eight patients were dependent on high-dose inotropes and/or IABP. Ten patients showed severe right ventricular failure. Early mortality was 23.1%; the 1-, 3-, and 6-year survival rates were 61.5%, 53.8%, and 53.8%, respectively; and the 1-, 3-, and 6-year event-free survival rates were 61.5%, 46.1%, and 46.1%, respectively (Figure 42-10).

The SAVE Procedure

Some patients with NIDCM have a fibrosis more marked in the septum than in the lateral wall. Yanagida and colleagues demonstrated this clinically; they found that in 8 of 10 patients, the interventricular septal regional work was lower than posteroinferior regional work.[38] In these specific cases, resection of the lateral wall can lead to acute left ventricular failure. Suma and colleagues proposed a procedure that excludes the septum and part of the lateral wall by using a long, oval, longitudinal patch (Figure 42-11) that is fixed to the posterior septum and to the ante-

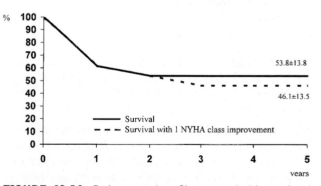

FIGURE 42-10. Batista procedure. Six-year survival (————) and possibility of being alive with an improvement of at least 1 NYHA class (- - - - -).

rior free wall with interrupted sutures.[25] This procedure was used in 12 patients, with 1 early and 1 late death.[39] The follow-up is too short to give an idea of the future developments of this procedure.

Ischemic Cardiomyopathy

If loss of contractile muscle due to myocardial infarction is *transmural*, the area becomes dyskinetic. According to

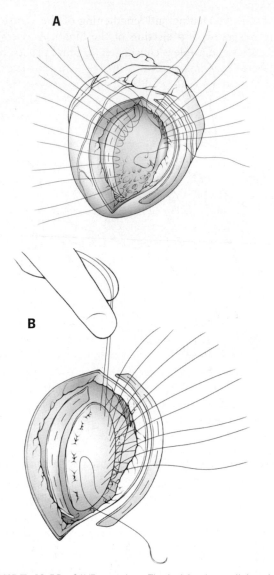

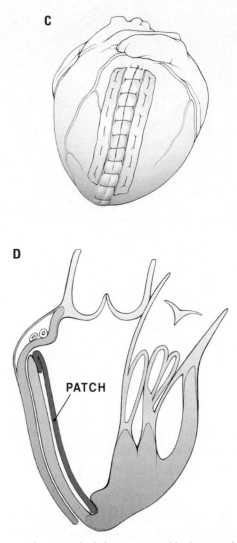

FIGURE 42-11. SAVE procedure. The incision is parallel to the LAD coronary artery. Interrupted stitches are passed in the posterior septum and in the anterior wall (A). A long oval patch is used to reduce the cavity (B). The ventriculotomy is then closed (C). A schematic vision of the procedure (D). LAD = left anterior descending.

the extent of the infarcted area, this situation can cause, by itself, heart failure. Gaudron and colleagues found that 20% of the patients who had myocardial infarction progress toward cardiac decompensation.[40] Over time, the modification in cardiac geometry affects the noninfarcted area (the remote zone), which becomes more hypertrophic and hypercontractile, but later reduces its contractility and dilates. When dilation of the remote zone occurs, the dyskinetic area becomes akinetic.

If myocardial infarction is *not transmural*, as the left anterior descending artery remains open (due to spontaneous fibrinolysis or primary angioplasty), part of the anterior wall and of the septum are replaced by akinetic muscle, which is comprised of roughly two-thirds scar and one-third epicardial muscle salvaged by reperfusion. This anatomic aspect prevents the region from being dyskinetic and collapsing after cardiac decompression in

the operating room; however, these patients present worse hemodynamic parameters, higher volumes, and higher end diastolic pressures with concomitant higher pulmonary pressures.[41] Lack of distensibility increases the endoventricular pressures and affects the remote zones earlier than in patients with dyskinetic areas. Whereas in these latter patients the border between the infarcted and the healthy muscle is clear, with sudden change of contractility, in patients with akinetic scars, the border zone is often hypocontractile and remodeled, and represents an undefined transition zone between scarred and healthy muscle.

In both cases, spatial displacement of the papillary muscles starts the mechanism that leads to functional mitral insufficiency, with rapid progression of heart failure. We consider ischemic cardiomyopathy to be this anatomic situation. Lack of functional mitral insufficiency changes the early and late outcomes, having a lower operative risk and a better late outcome. Even if an inferior myocardial infarction can more easily provide mitral regurgitation, ischemic cardiomyopathy is more often related to anteroseptal myocardial infarction.

The necessity of correcting mitral regurgitation when surgery for left ventricular aneurysms is performed is often underestimated. In 1998, Dor reported the incidence of mitral valve surgery in 100 patients as 10%.[41] Even if the incidence of mitral regurgitation ≥ 2/4 was 45% (86 patients), Mickleborough and colleagues never repaired the valve; postoperative evaluation in 70 of these patients showed an improvement of at least 1 point in the degree of mitral regurgitation in 40 of 70 patients (57%), with 46 of 70 patients (66%) still showing mitral regurgitation ≥ 2.[42] (Some patients showed both conditions.) Conversely, Suma and colleagues performed mitral valve repair in all their patients with mitral regurgitation.[43]

In a recent report, Di Donato and colleagues reported an incidence of late mitral regurgitation in 17 of 44 1-year survivors after the Dor procedure.[44] In 14 of the survivors, preoperative mitral regurgitation was not detectable. The authors found that patients that developed late mitral regurgitation had preoperatively more spherical ventricles and showed an increase of EDVI when compared to early postoperative controls. According to the authors, even if the mechanism of further dilation is not related to the mitral regurgitation itself but is related to a continuous remodeling of the LV, they recommend a more cautious detection of mitral regurgitation before surgery as transesophageal echocardiography. In fact, according to Mickleborough, angiography alone is an insensitive approach to use to evaluate mitral regurgitation.[42] Mickleborough also reported that echocardiograms detected mitral regurgitation in 45% of the patients referred for left ventricular aneurysmectomy who had no evidence of it at the ventriculography.

Surgical Techniques

In the 1980s, because of the work of Jatene and Dor, the concept of restoring the ventricular shape as similarly as possible to the normal shape became widely accepted by the scientific world.[2,45] Myocardial infarction causes loss of viable muscle, but also a change in the spatial orientation of the myocardial fibers. In the normal heart, with normal elliptical shape and oblique fiber orientation, 15% of fiber shortening causes an ejection fraction of 60%. When the shape becomes more spherical, with more transverse fiber orientation, contractile forces in the remote area are reduced and fiber shortening of 15% causes only a 30% ejection fraction.[46] The concept that the cardiac fibers have to be properly oriented was recently emphasized by Torrent-Guasp and colleagues, who proposed that ventricular myocardium, both right and left, exists as a continuous muscle band, oriented spatially as a helix and formed by basal and apical loops.[47] Sequential contraction of this helicoidal band results in

successive shortening and lengthening of the ventricles, causing suction and ejection of the blood. As a consequence, early diastole is considered an active process.[48]

There is general agreement that care must be taken to treat symptoms of heart failure and to reshape the left ventricular chamber to a more normal elliptical rebuilding fiber orientation to obtain an improved contractile function. Recently, Buckberg pointed out that some fundamental aspects of ischemic cardiomyopathy are not normally evaluated by surgeons.[49] Ejection fraction is often considered as the most important aspect of the disease; however, it is not. Other parameters, such as left ventricular end systolic volume index or sphericity indices, are not calculated, even if important for patient selection and as predictors of long-term functional result. Yamaguchi and colleagues reported that a left ventricular end systolic volume index > 100 mL/m^2 with an ejection fraction of less than 30% is related to higher incidences of late deaths and heart failure after isolated myocardial revascularization.[50] Conversely, an ejection fraction higher than 30% and end systolic volumes < 100 mL/m^2 are associated with higher survival and greater freedom from congestive heart failure. Yamaguchi and colleagues' work shows that the choice of surgical strategy must take into account all the variables, not only the ejection fraction. Moreover, their work demonstrates that revascularization alone is unable to reverse symptoms of heart failure in severely dilated hearts.

Because the purpose of surgery is to modify the ventricular shape to reverse the tendency to sphericity, excluding noncontractile areas, and because the septum is a main determinant in the ventricular shape, we describe in more detail the techniques that focus on septoexclusion.

DOR PROCEDURE

The left ventricular cavity is opened in the middle of the aneurysm. If present, clots are removed, and one or more sutures of a 2–0 Prolene monofilament are placed circumferentially, as described by Fontan, approximately 1 cm above the border of the scarred area between normal and diseased muscle to restore the neck of the contracting ventricle and to reestablish a normal oval LV shape.[51] A circular patch (generally 2 cm in diameter) of synthetic tissue (Dacron) is then fixed inside the LV cavity on the border marked by the circular suture, to close the LV cavity (Figure 42-12). To avoid overreduction of the cavity, a balloon inflated with water (50 mL/m^2) is inserted before tying the purse string. The excluded external tissue is then closed.

The technique reported by Jatene has the same objectives that Dor describes.[45] However, the approach is different. Cox recently summarized these differences.[52] Briefly, both Jatene and Dor emphasize the importance of excluding the distal septum. But whereas Jatene imbricates the aneurysmal portion of the distal septum in a posterior-to-anterior direction, stabilizing it and restoring a more physiologic shape, Dor simply excludes this

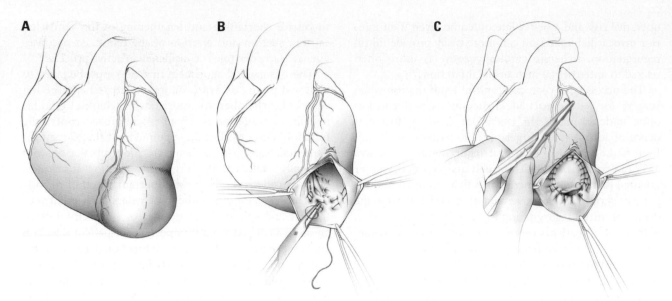

FIGURE 42-12. Dor procedure. The left ventricular cavity is opened in the middle of the aneurysm (A). One or more sutures of a 2–0 Prolene monofilament are placed circumferentially approximately 1 cm above the border of the scarred area between normal and diseased muscle to restore the neck of the contracting ventricle (B). Then a circular patch (generally 2 cm in diameter) in synthetic tissue (Dacron) is fixed inside the left ventricle (LV) cavity on the border marked by the circular suture, to close the LV cavity (C).

septal portion, placing the endocardial patch at the junction of septal scar with normal septum. To restore a conical shape, both Jatene and Dor use a purse string; Jatene places the purse string more proximally on the free wall and more distally on the septum, whereas Dor places it more distally on the free wall and more proximally on the septum (or roughly at the same level). Therefore, whereas the Jatene technique leaves the apex of the left ventricle unchanged in relation to the distal septum, the Dor technique moves the apex in a more lateral position in relation to the ventricular septum.

GUILMET PROCEDURE

This technique is specifically indicated when the septum is more involved than the free wall, as the septal scar starts very high (Figure 42-13). The apex is opened and the greater involvement of the septum in comparison to the free wall is confirmed. An incision is made from the apex upward, 1 cm parallel to the septum (Figure 42-14A). The anterior free wall is sewn obliquely to the septum, starting as high as possible, up to the apical limit of the lateral free wall (Figure 42-14B). About two-thirds of scarred septum is excluded, and the apex is displaced toward the lateral wall. The two edges of the incision, anterior and septal, are sewn together to assure a definitive hemostasis with a running 2–0 Prolene suture (overcoat technique) (Figure 42-14C).

OTHER PROCEDURES

Cooley reported the use of a large endoventricular patch to exclude the scarred tissue without any purse string (endoaneurysmorrhaphy).[53] The goal is to avoid any tension in the sutures placed inside the ventricle (Figure

42-15). Mickleborough reported a modified linear suture, performed on a beating heart, that eliminates the scarred tissue in the anterior wall.[54] Only when the septum is greatly involved is a patch inserted between the septum and the border of the anterior free wall, incorporating this latter part in the closure of the ventriculectomy. This occurred in only 12% of cases reported by Mickleborough and colleagues.

POSTERIOR ANEURYSMS

Aneurysms in the inferior wall of the heart are approached with an incision parallel to the posterior descending artery. Once the anatomy is evaluated, two surgical techniques can be used. A suture with interrupted U stitches can exclude the scarred area from the inside, connecting the healthy lateral muscle to the anterior septum; the suture line is limited by the posteromedial papillary muscle (Figure 42-16A and B). Another option is to insert a triangular or oval patch to obtain the same result (Figure 42-16D).

Clinical Results

Cooley and colleagues reported the results in 136 patients.[55] Among them, 100 (group I) had acute myocardial infarction (AMI) > 30 days before surgery and no previous cardiac operation; 36 (group II) had AMI < 30 days before surgery (18) and previous cardiac operation (18). In group I, operative mortality was low (4%) and the 1-year survival rate was 85.3%. In group II, early mortality was high (30.6%); no survival was reported in this group. Ejection fraction increased in both groups, +10.9% in group I and +13.4% in group II. Mitral valve

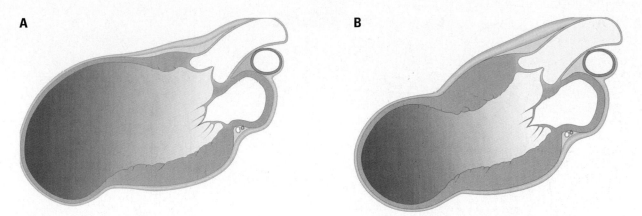

FIGURE 42-13. The Guilmet procedure is indicated when the level of the septal scar is higher in the septum than in the free wall (A). When the level is roughly the same (B), we prefer the Dor technique.

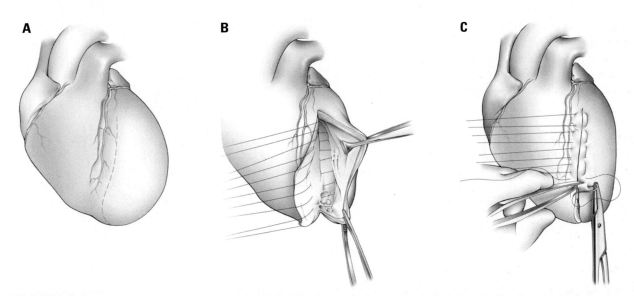

FIGURE 42-14. Guilmet procedure. An incision is made from the apex upward, 1 cm parallel to the septum (A). The anterior free wall is sewn obliquely to the septum, starting as high as possible, up to the apical limit of the lateral free wall (B). The scarred septum is excluded for about two thirds and the apex is displaced toward the lateral wall. The two edges of the incision, anterior and septal, are sewn together to assure a definitive hemostasis with a running 2–0 Prolene suture (overcoat technique) (C).

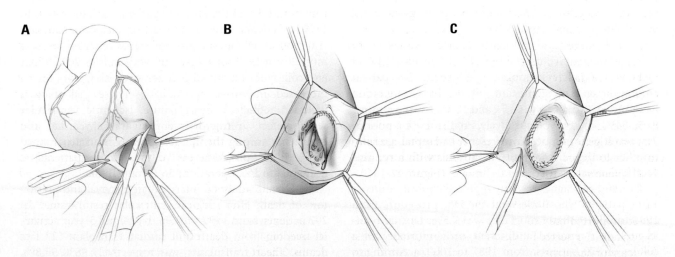

FIGURE 42-15. The aneurysm is opened (A) and a patch is inserted along the border with the healthy muscle (B,C).

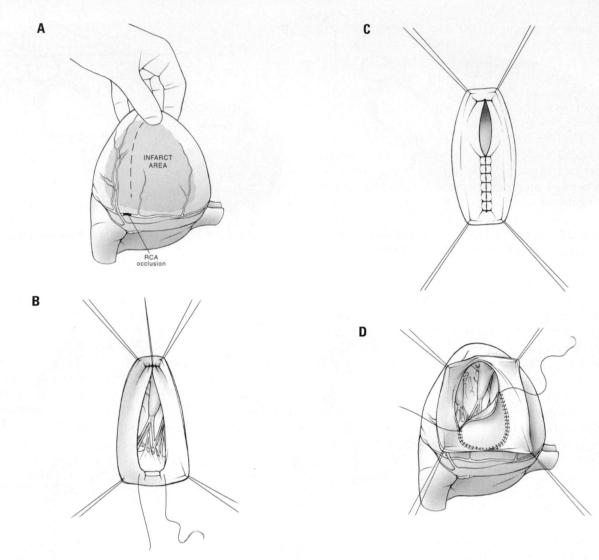

FIGURE 42-16. Posterior aneurysm resection. Incision is parallel to the posterior descending artery (A). Once the anatomy is evaluated, two surgical techniques can be used. A suture with interrupted U stitches can exclude the scarred area from the inside, connecting the healthy lateral muscle to the anterior septum (B,C). The suture line is limited by the posteromedial papillary muscle. Another option is to insert a triangular or oval patch to obtain the same result (D).

surgery was performed in 2% of patients in group I and in 8.3% of patients in group II.

Mickleborough and colleagues reported 196 cases with a very low operative mortality (2.6%).[42] In only 12% of cases was a patch septoplasty performed. No patient among the 86 with significant mitral valve regurgitation had mitral valve surgery; 1-, 5-, and 10-year survivals were 91%, 84%, and 66%, respectively. Predictors of a poor 5-year result were preoperative presence of mitral regurgitation ≥ grades 2/4, symptoms of heart failure, and ventricular tachycardia.

Dor and colleagues recently reported clinical results in 1,011 patients who underwent the Dor procedure from 1984 to 2001.[56] Early mortality was 7.5%. Dor and colleagues also reported a different early mortality of a cohort of 870 patients, from 1987 to 2000, according to different preoperative ejection fraction.[56] Early mortality

rose from 1.3% in the group of patients with EF ≥ 40% to 13% in patients with severely depressed pump function (EF < 30%). Di Donato and colleagues reported an early mortality of 19.3% in 62 patients with an EF ≤ 20%.[57] Dor and colleagues identified preoperative risk factors for an increased operative mortality.[58] These risk factors included refractory heart failure, ischemic ventricular septal defects, refractory ventricular tachycardia, and emergency surgery. In this group, early mortality ranged from 15 to 20%, whereas in the elective patients, it decreased to 5%.

Di Donato analyzed intermediate survival and predictors of death after surgical ventricular restoration.[59] In 207 patients, from 1991 to 1996, 1-, 2-, and 5-year actuarial freedom from death and cardiac transplant (27 late deaths, 3 heart transplants) was, respectively, 98%, 95.8%, and 82.1% (early mortality excluded). Risk factors at Cox analysis were preoperative NYHA class, preoperative and postoperative EF, preoperative end systolic volume index, and remote asynergy. Most late deaths were due to a progressive cardiac decompensation.[59]

Hemodynamic analysis in the postoperative period and at 1 year after the operation showed an increase of the ejection fraction and a decrease of end diastolic volume index. NYHA class decreased significantly from 2.6 ± 0.9 to 1.4 ± 0.6.[60] Mean pulmonary pressure decreased in the early postoperative period but increased 1 year post operation because of progression of left chamber dilatation and functional mitral regurgitation.[59]

Beginning in 1998, two new interventions (balloon sizing and mitral annuloplasty) were introduced in the last 200 cases, reducing the tendency for delayed development of pulmonary hypertension and secondary mitral incompetence to 10%, as compared to a 25% incidence rate before their initiation.[57] According to Dor, surgical repair of mitral insufficiency is needed in more than 25% of patients and can be curative and, sometimes, preventive.

Menicanti and colleagues retrospectively studied 924 patients who underwent surgical ventricular reconstruction that used the Dor procedure during the period 1989 to 2001.[61] Early mortality was 8.2%, increasing from 4.3% in patients who had no mitral valve surgery to 15% in the remaining patients where mitral valve surgery was performed.

Suma and colleagues reported 54 patients who had the Dor procedure.[62] All 54 patients had symptoms of heart failure. Preoperative mean ejection fraction was 23.3%, and 35% of the patients had mitral valve repair. Hospital mortality was 12.9%; 3-year survival was 85.6% in elective patients and 14.8% in emergency patients.

Komeda reported 23 patients who had mitral valve surgery and left ventricular aneurysmectomy.[63] In this selected group of patients, early mortality was 17% and 2-year survival was 71%, cause of late death being mainly congestive heart failure.

PERSONAL EXPERIENCE

Between 1988 and 2001, 93 patients had the Dor operation; 25 patients had concomitant mitral valve surgery. Thirty-day mortality was 8.6%; it was higher when no mitral valve surgery was necessary (4 of 25 [16.0%] vs 4 of 68 [5.9%]). Five- and 10-year survival rates were, respectively, 77.4% and 75.3%, and the possibilities of being alive with one NYHA class improvement at 5 and 10 years were, respectively, 70.0% and 66.7% (Figure 42-17).

We recently reported our results with the Guilmet procedure.[64] Patients were selected for this procedure because the septal involvement was greater than the involvement of the anterior free wall. Twenty-nine patients were operated on between 1998 and 2001. Seven patients had mitral valve surgery. Thirty-day mortality was 6.9%; after surgery, two patients died due to cardiac cause. After a mean follow-up

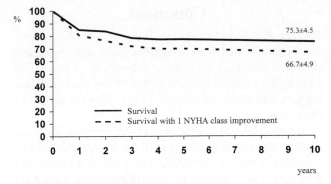

FIGURE 42-17. Dor procedure. Ten-year survival (——) and possibility of being alive with an improvement of at least 1 NYHA class (- - - -).

of 22.5 ± 12.3 months, the NYHA class decreased from 2.9 ± 0.7 to 1.4 ± 0.6 and EDVI decreased from 152 ± 63 to 99 ± 38 mL/m². The possibility of three-year survival with one NYHA class improvement was 82.8% (Figure 42-18).

Globally, from 1997 to 2001, 36 patients had exclusion of anteroseptal scars and mitral valve surgery, 32 had annuloplasty, and 4 had mitral valve replacement. Thirty-day mortality was 16.7%; the 4-year survival rate and the possibility of being alive at 4 years with one NYHA class improvement were 64.0% and 50.0%, respectively (Figure 42-19).

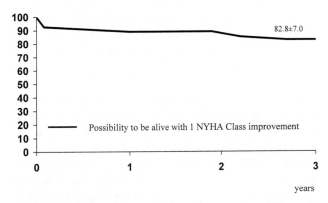

FIGURE 42-18. Guilmet procedure. Three-year possibility to be alive with 1 NYHA Class improvement (——).

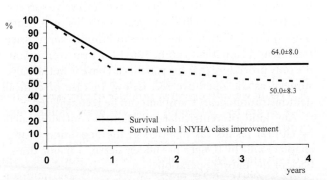

FIGURE 42-19. Exclusion of anteroseptal scars and mitral valve surgery. Four-year survival (——) and possibility to be alive with an improvement of at least 1 NYHA class (- - - -).

Comment

Surgery for dilated cardiomyopathy in selected patients can be performed with acceptable early and reasonable midterm results. Preoperative assessment is crucial in identifying patients who can benefit from nontransplant surgery, and choice of strategy is crucial for the success of the procedure.

It has to be emphasized that, in our opinion, there is a limit to any surgical technique of left ventricular volume reduction in patients with dilated cardiomyopathy, whether it be mitral valve surgery or surgical reshaping. Poor right ventricular function and severe pulmonary hypertension can be considered, in our opinion, a formal contraindication. Surgical experience demonstrates that nothing that can be done, directly or indirectly, on the left ventricle can reverse acutely severe right ventricular failure. Early and late outcomes of these patients are uniformly poor.

In patients with NIDCM, or with IDCM without identifiable and localized scars to be resected, the indication for surgery depends on the presence of a reasonable amount of viable myocardium. We prefer to have a rest myocardial scintigraph to evaluate the extension of the scarred tissue. As a second step, an echo dobutamine stress test is always performed to assess the amount of muscle that thickens under pharmacologic stimulus. These exams give us an idea of the extent of noncontractile tissue, its position, and the quality of the nondiseased myocardium. Lacking standardized guidelines, each case has to be separately evaluated. However, thickening of at least a region of the left ventricle (septum or anterior and lateral or lateral and inferior) allows us to consider the patient for surgery.

Based on our current surgical experience, several key points need to be kept in mind. Early mortality after mitral valve repair is low, and the 3- to 5-year survival rate is reasonable, varying from 70% in reports with ejection fraction around 28%, to 50% in reports with a lower mean ejection fraction. Partial left ventriculectomy has high early mortality and mediocre midterm results. With these points in mind, two common situations can be addressed.

If a patient can be listed for heart transplant, the only procedure that the patient can have is mitral valve surgery. The patient can remain a few years with his own heart, thereby avoiding all the side effects of immunosuppressive treatment. If a patient can be listed for heart transplant, the only procedure that the patient can have is mitral valve surgery, as the operative risk is low. In case of clinical demonstration, heart transplant can be reconsidered.

Any kind of ventricular resection is contraindicated by clinical results (as reported in the beginning of this chapter) and by danger of sudden death, a major drawback of the Batista operation.[65]

Patients with no possibility of heart transplant (because of comorbidities, age, pulmonary hypertension, or lack of availability of heart transplant in their countries), in the presence of mitral regurgitation (from 2+ to 4+), have to undergo mitral valve surgery, because when the clinical status deteriorates, a partial left ventriculectomy can be the next step.

If mitral regurgitation is trivial, partial left ventriculectomy can be scheduled. However, it is necessary to identify, before surgery, the viability of the myocardium, to avoid resection of the only working portion of the heart. Echo dobutamine and myocardial scintigraphy at rest are helpful. Isomura and colleagues suggested identifying the akinetic area in the operating theater before surgery, with the aid of transesophageal echocardiography when the heart is unloaded.[37] The Batista operation or the SAVE operation were chosen by Isomura and colleagues according to the perioperative findings. This strategy was able to reduce early and late mortality significantly.

Whereas results of surgery for NIDCM are easily evaluated, results of surgery for IDCM are difficult to assess because they are included in the results for left ventricular aneurysms. According to the definition we follow, the key reason for identifying postischemic dilated cardiomyopathy is the quality of the remote zone. When it becomes hypokinetic and enlarges, functional mitral valve regurgitation follows and the patient's prognosis is different. This subgroup of patients has a higher 30-day mortality and a lower late survival rate than do patients who undergo left ventricular aneurysmectomy.

There is not yet a general agreement on surgical indications and indications to the specific surgical procedure. However, the number of publications on this topic is increasing, and with time, the better comprehension of pathophysiology of the underlying disease and the more accurate identification of the extent of segmental asynergy will allow surgeons to obtain better and more reproducible results.

References

1. Batista RJV, Santos JLV, Takeshita N, et al. Partial left ventriculectomy to improve left ventricular function for end-stage heart disease. J Card Surg 1996;11:96–7.
2. Dor V, Kreitmann P, Jourdan J, et al. Interest of physiological closure (circumferential plasty on contractile areas) of left ventricle after resection and endocardectomy for aneurysm or akinetic zone. Comparison with classical technique about a series of left ventricular resections [abstract]. J Cardiovasc Surg 1985;26:73.
3. Guilmet D, Popoff G, Dubois C, et al. Nouvelle technique chirurgicale pour la cure des aneurysmes du ventricle gauche. Arch Mal Coeur Vaiss 1984;77:953–8.
4. Bolling SF, Deeb GM, Brunsting LA, Bach DS. Early outcome of mitral valve reconstruction in patients with end-stage cardiomyopathy. J Thorac Cardiovasc Surg 1995;109:676–83.
5. Calafiore AM, Gallina S, Di Mauro M, et al. Mitral valve procedure in dilated cardiomyopathy: repair or replacement? Ann Thorac Surg 2001;71:1146–52.

6. Calafiore AM, Gallina S, Contini M, et al. Surgical treatment of dilated cardiomyopathy with conventional techniques. Eur J Cardiothorac Surg 1999;16 Suppl 1:S73–8.

7. Di Napoli, Taccardi A, Vianale G, et al. Systolic left ventricular wall stress modulates cardiomyocyte apoptosis in patients with severe dilated cardiomyopathy [abstract]. Eur Heart J 2000;21:366.

8. Romeo F, Pelliccia F, Cianfrocca C, et al. Determinants of end-stage idiopathic dilated cardiomyopathy: a multivariate analysis of 104 patients. Clin Cardiol 1989;12: 387–92.

9. Blondheim DS, Jacobs LE, Kotler MN, et al. Dilated cardiomyopathy with mitral regurgitation: decreased survival despite a low frequency of left ventricular thrombus. Am Heart J 1991;122:763–71.

10. Junker A, Thayssen P, Nielsen B, Andersen PE. The hemodynamic and prognostic significance of echo-Doppler-proven mitral regurgitation in patients with dilated cardiomyopathy. Cardiology 1993;83:14–20.

11. Timek TA, Dagum P, Lai TD, et al. Pathogenesis of mitral regurgitation in tachycardia-induced cardiomyopathy. Circulation 2001;104 Suppl I:I47–53.

12. Kono T, Sabbah HN, Rosman H, et al. Left ventricular shape is the primary determinant of functional regurgitation in heart failure. J Am Coll Cardiol 1992;20:1594–8.

13. Brock RC. The surgical pathologic anatomy of mitral valve. Br Heart J 1952;14:489–513.

14. Carpentier A, Deloche A, Dauptain J, et al. A new reconstructive operation for correction of mitral and tricuspid insufficiency. J Thorac Cardiovasc Surg 1971;61: 1–13.

15. Radovanovic N, Mihajlovic B, Selestiansky J, et al. Reductive annuloplasty of double orifices in patients with primary dilated cardiomyopathy. Ann Thorac Surg 2002; 73:751–5.

16. Salati M, Scrofani R, Santoli C. Posterior pericardial annuloplasty: a physiologic correction? Eur J Cardiothorac Surg 1991;5:226–9.

17. Chavaud S, Jebara V, Chachques JC, Carpentier A. Valve extension with glutaraldehyde-preserved autologous pericardium. Results in mitral valve repair. J Thorac Cardiovasc Surg 1991;102:171–8.

18. Buffolo E, de Paula IAM, Palma H, Branco JNR. A new surgical approach for treating dilated cardiomyopathy with mitral regurgitation. Arq Bras Cardiol 2000;74:135–40.

19. Bolling SF, Pagani FD, Deeb GM, Bach DS. Intermediate-term outcome of mitral reconstruction in cardiomyopathy. J Thorac Cardiovasc Surg 1998;115:381–8.

20. Smolens I, Bossone E, Das SA, Bolling SF. Current status of mitral valve reconstruction in patients with dilated cardiomyopathy. Ital Heart J 2000;1:517–20.

21. Bishay ES, McCarthy PM, Cosgrove DM, et al. Mitral valve surgery in patients with severe left ventricular dysfunction. Eur J Cardiothorac Surg 2000;17:213–21.

22. Baretti R, Mizuno A, Buckberg GD, Child JS. Batista procedure: elliptical modeling against spherical distention. Eur J Cardiothorac Surg 2000;17:52–7.

23. Artrip JH, Oz MC, Burkhoff D. Left ventricular volume reduction surgery for heart failure: a physiologic perspective. J Thorac Cardiovasc Surg 2001;122: 775–82.

24. Franco-Cereceda A, McCarthy PM, Blackstone EH, et al. Partial left ventriculectomy for dilated cardiomyopathy: is this an alternative to transplantation? J Thorac Cardiovasc Surg 2001;121:879–93.

25. Suma H, Beyersdorf F, De Oliveira S, et al. Pacopexy—new restoration procedure for non-ischemic dilated cardiomyopathy [abstract]. American Association for Thoracic Surgery 81st Annual Meeting; 2001 May 5–9; San Diego, California.

26. Ascione R, Lim KHH, Chamberlain M, et al. Early and late results of partial left ventriculectomy: single centre experience and review of the literature. International Meeting "Left Ventricular Volume Reduction for Dilated Cardiomyopathy" [abstract]; 2001 September 20–22; Roma, Italy.

27. Gradinac S, Miric M, Popovic Z, et al. Partial left ventriculectomy for idiopathic dilated cardiomyopathy: early results and six-month follow-up. Ann Thorac Surg 1998;66:1963–8.

28. Frazier OH, Gradinac S, Segura AM, et al. Partial left ventriculectomy: which patients can be expected to benefit? Ann Thorac Surg 2000;69:1836–41.

29. Moreira LF, Stolf NA, de Lourdes Higuchi M, et al. Current perspectives of partial left ventriculectomy in the treatment of dilated. cardiomyopathy. Eur J Cardiothorac Surg 2001;19:54–60.

30. Bestetti RB, Moreira-Neto F, Brasil JC, et al. Partial left ventriculectomy: preoperative risk factors for perioperative mortality. Int J Cardiol 1998;67:143–6.

31. Izzat MB, Kabbani SS, Suma H, et al. Early experience with partial left ventriculectomy in the Asia-Pacific region. Ann Thorac Surg 1999;67:1703–7.

32. Konertz W, Khoynezhad A, Sidiropoulos A, et al. Early and intermediate results of left ventricular reduction surgery. Eur J Cardiothorac Surg 1999;15 Suppl 1:S26–30.

33. Vural KM, Tasdemir O. Mid-term results of partial left ventriculectomy in end-stage heart disease. Eur J Cardiothorac Surg 2000;18:550–6.

34. Bhat G, Dowling RD. Evaluation of predictors of clinical outcome after partial left ventriculectomy. Ann Thorac Surg 2001;72:91–5.

35. Lucchese FA, Frota Filho JD, Blacher C, et al. Partial left ventriculectomy: overall and late results in 44 class IV patients with 4-year follow-up. J Card Surg 2000;15: 179–85.

36. Popovic Z, Miric M, Neskovic AN, et al. Functional capacity late after partial left ventriculectomy: relation to ventricular geometry and performance. Eur J Cardiothorac Surg 2001;19:61–7.

37. Isomura T, Suma H, Horii T, et al. Partial left ventriculectomy, ventriculoplasty or valvular surgery for idiopathic dilated cardiomyopathy—the role of intra-operative echocardiography. Eur J Cardiothorac Surg 2000;17: 239–45.

38. Yanagida R, Sugawara M, Kawai A, Koyanagi H. Regional differences in myocardial work of the left ventricle in patients with idiopathic dilated cardiomyopathy: implications for the surgical technique used for left ventriculoplasty J Thorac Cardiovasc Surg 2001;122:600–7.

39. Isomura T, Suma H, Horii T, et al. Left ventricle restoration in patients with non-ischemic dilated cardiomyopathy:

risk factors and predictors of outcome and change of mid-term ventricular function. Eur J Cardiothorac Surg 2001;19:684–9.

40. Gaudron P, Kugler L, Hu K, et al. Effect of quinapril initiated during progressive remodeling in asymptomatic patients with healed myocardial infarction. Am J Cardiol 2000;86:139–44.

41. Dor V, Sabatier M, Di Donato M, et al. Efficacy of endoventricular patch plasty in large postinfarction akinetic scar and severe left ventricular dysfunction: comparison with a series of large dyskinetic scars. J Thorac Cardiovasc Surg 1998;116:50–9.

42. Mickleborough LL, Carson S, Ivanov J. Repair of dyskinetic or akinetic left ventricular aneurysm: results obtained with a modified linear closure J Thorac Cardiovasc Surg 2001;121:675–82.

43. Suma H, Isomura T, Horii T, Hisatomi K. Left ventriculoplasty for ischemic cardiomyopathy. Eur J Cardiothorac Surg 2001;20:319–23.

44. Di Donato M, Sabatier M, Dor V, et al. Effects of the Dor procedure on left ventricular dimension and shape and geometric correlates of mitral regurgitation one year after surgery. J Thorac Cardiovasc Surg 2001;121:91–6.

45. Jatene AD. Left ventricular aneurysmectomy. Resection or reconstruction. J Thorac Cardiovasc Surg 1985;89:321–31.

46. Ingels RB Jr. Myocardial fiber architecture and left ventricular function. Technol Health Care 1997;5:45–52.

47. Torrent-Guasp F, Ballester M, Buckberg GD, et al. Spatial orientation of the ventricular muscle band: physiologic contribution and surgical implications. J Thorac Cardiovasc Surg 2001;122:389–92.

48. Brutssaert DL, Sys SU, Gillebert TC. Diastolic failure: pathophysiology and therapeutic implications. J Am Coll Cardiol 1993;22:318–25.

49. Buckberg GD. Congestive heart failure: treat the disease, not the symptom—return to normalcy. J Thorac Cardiovasc Surg 2001;121:628–37.

50. Yamaguchi A, Ino T, Adachi H, et al. Left ventricular volume predicts postoperative course in patients with ischemic cardiomyopathy. Ann Thorac Surg 1998;65:434–8.

51. Fontan F. Transplantation of knowledge. J Thorac Cardiovasc Surg 1990;99:387–95.

52. Cox JL. Surgical management of left ventricular aneurysms: a clarification of the similarities and differences between the Jatene and Dor techniques. Semin Thorac Cardiovasc Surg 1997;9:131–8.

53. Cooley DA. Ventricular endoaneurysmorrhaphy: a simplified repair for extensive postinfarction aneurysm. J Card Surg 1989;4:200–5.

54. Mickleborough LL. Left ventricular aneurysm: modified linear closure technique. Operative techniques in cardiac and thoracic surgery. Operative Techniques in Thoracic Surgery 1997;2:118–31.

55. Cooley DA, Frazier OH, Duncan JM, et al. Intracavitary repair of ventricular aneurysm and regional dyskinesia. Ann Surg 1992;215:417–24.

56. Dor V, Di Donato M, Sabatier M, et al. Left ventricular reconstruction by endoventricular circular patch plasty repair: a 17-year experience. Semin Thorac Cardiovasc Surg 2001;13:435–47.

57. Di Donato M, Sabatier M, Montiglio F, et al. Outcome of left ventricular aneurysmectomy with patch repair in patients with severely depressed pump function. Am J Cardiol 1995;76:557–61.

58. Dor V. Left ventricular aneurysms: the endoventricular circular patch plasty. Semin Thorac Cardiovasc Surg 1997;9:123–30.

59. Di Donato M, Toso A, Maioli M, et al. Intermediate survival and predictors of death after surgical ventricular restoration. Semin Thorac Cardiovasc Surg 2001;13:468–75.

60. Dor V, Sabatier M, Di Donato M, et al. Late hemodynamic results after left ventricular patch repair associated with coronary grafting in patients with postinfarction akinetic or dyskinetic aneurysm of the left ventricle. J Thorac Cardiovasc Surg 1995;110:1291–9.

61. Menicanti L, Dor V, Buckberg GD, et al. Inferior wall restoration: anatomic and surgical considerations. Semin Thorac Cardiovasc Surg 2001;13:504–13.

62. Suma H, Isomura T, Horii T, Hisatomi K. Left ventriculoplasty for ischemic cardiomyopathy. Eur J Cardiothorac Surg 2001;20:319–23.

63. Komeda M. Left ventricular aneurysm with ischemic mitral regurgitation. In: Buxton B, Fraizer OH, Westaby S, editors. Ischemic heart disease surgical management. St. Louis: Mosby; 1999. p. 313–18.

64. Calafiore AM, Gallina S, Di Mauro M, et al. Left ventricular aneurysmectomy: endoventricular circular patch plasty or septoexclusion. J Card Surg 2002. [In press]

65. Bestetti RB. Sudden cardiac death as a complication of left partial ventriculectomy in patients with end-stage dilated cardiomyopathy. Int J Cardiol 1998;67:183–5.

Chapter 43

Dynamic to Cellular Cardiomyoplasty

Juan Carlos Chachques, MD, PhD, Barbara Cattadori, MD, MS, Alain Carpentier, MD, PhD

Congestive cardiac failure is caused by a decrease in myocardial contractility and elasticity due to mechanical overload or by an initial defect in the myocardial fiber. The alteration in diastolic function is inextricably linked with the pathophysiology of cardiac insufficiency. Despite a widely varying and diverse etiology of congestive cardiac failure, the pathophysiology is, to great extent, constant. The predominant factor is the alteration of myocardial contractility and compliance, resulting in a structural increase in ventricular chamber volume followed by a pathologic remodeling process.

Cardiac Bioassist Procedures

The management of patients with end-stage heart failure is a daily challenge in cardiac surgery. Cardiac transplantation is a limited option for end-stage heart failure because of the shortage of donor organs. Left ventricular assist devices are currently under investigation as permanent therapy for end-stage heart failure, but long-term successful device implantation is limited because of a high rate of infections and the financial cost of the device and the follow-up.

The aim of cardiac bioassist procedures is to restore or enhance the heart pump function by using the patient's electrostimulated muscles, which can be wrapped around the left and right of both ventricles (cardiomyoplasty), the ascending or descending aorta (aortomyoplasty), the right atrium (atriomyoplasty), and around artificial extra-aortic ventricles (skeletal muscle ventricles). A new, emerging approach called *cellular cardiomyoplasty* consists in the use of autologous undifferentiated cells (skeletal or smooth myoblasts, bone marrow cells) that are transplanted into the pathologic myocardium after a 3-week period of in vitro cell expansion. The goal of cellular cardiomyoplasty is the regeneration of the myocardium that potentially may contribute to the improvement of systolic and diastolic ventricular functions. Cardiac bioassist techniques can successfully affect ventricular remodeling and improve cardiac function.[1,2]

Latissimus Dorsi Dynamic Cardiomyoplasty

The biologic support of this operation consists of chronic latissimus dorsi muscle electrostimulation, which induces a physiologic adaptation of skeletal muscle to cardiac work. The metabolism of the rapid glycolytic fatigue-sensitive muscle fibers (type II) are transformed into slow, oxidative fatigue-resistant muscle fibers (type I).

Technically, the cardiomyoplasty (CMP) procedure is a combination of cardiac and plastic surgery with biomedical engineering. Its aim is to prolong and improve the quality of life of patients who suffer from severe chronic cardiac deficiency and who are unresponsive to medical treatment. In CMP, the musculature of the same subject is used, which excludes the risk of rejection and, therefore, no immunosuppressive treatment is necessary.[3–5]

Dynamic cardiomyoplasty has been performed worldwide in more than 1,500 patients; 112 cases were operated in our institution. In addition, 75 patients were operated on by our team abroad, in the scope of an international cooperative program.

Indications

CMP is recommended to patients who suffer from severe chronic cardiac deficiency. The ischemic myocardial deficiency (patients presenting successive infarctions or one largely extended) as well as the dilated cardiomyopathies (generally of unknown origin) are considered to be indications for CMP. Hypertrophic or obstructive cardiomyopathies, however, are excluded for CMP. The time to perform a CMP can be concluded from the postoperative results. The hemodynamic advantage of the CMP is only achieved after a delay of several weeks, corresponding to the adaptation period of the latissimus dorsi muscle (LDM) to its new cardiac assistance function. Consequently, the residual myocardial function has to be taken into account in patient selection (Table 43-1).

TABLE 43-1. Latissimus Dorsi Muscle Cardiomyoplasty: Criteria for Patient Selection

Indications
- Idiopathic dilated or ischemic cardiomyopathies
- Severe heart failure (but not yet end-stage; ie, patient has some cardiac reserve: radioisotopic LV ejection fraction > 15 %; peak VO₂ > 10 mL/kg/min)
- Intact left latissimus dorsi muscle with preserved force
- Adult (fully grown)

Contraindications
- Severe mitral valve regurgitation
- Preoperative dependence on intravenous inotropes or intra-aortic balloon counterpulsation
- Primary hypertrophic or restrictive cardiomyopathy
- Cardiac cachexia

LV = left ventricle
VO₂ = oxygen consumption

Cardiomyoplasty Surgical Technique

This surgical procedure consists of the dissection and the transposition into the chest of the entire latissimus dorsi muscle flap, which will be positioned around both ventricles. Afterward, the LDM will be chronically electrostimulated in synchrony with ventricular systole.[3,6]

Operative Procedure

STAGE ONE: ELEVATION OF THE LATISSIMUS DORSI MUSCLE

The patient is placed in the right thoracotomy position. The left LDM is dissected free with preservation of its axillary pedicle. The largest portion of the LDM is supplied by one common neurovascular bundle, the thoracodorsal artery–vein–nerve complex, which must be carefully

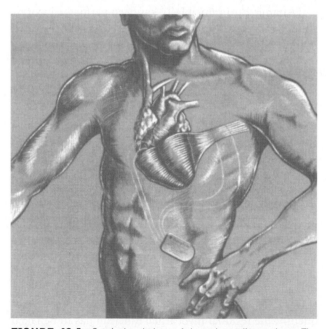

FIGURE 43-1. Surgical technique of dynamic cardiomyoplasty. The left LDM is transposed into the chest and wrapped around the ventricles. Electrodes are inserted for muscle pacing and for heart sensing; afterward, they are connected to an implantable cardiomyostimulator.

isolated and preserved. For chronic muscle pacing, two intramuscular electrodes are implanted. The cathode or proximal electrode is placed near the entrance of the motor nerve branches into the muscle. The second electrode is placed approximately 5 cm distally. The muscle flap and pacing leads are then transferred to the thoracic cavity after segmental resection (6 cm) of the second rib. To avoid left arm motion during electrostimulation and to allow for a bigger LDM surface inside the chest, the LDM humeral tendon is completely divided at its proximal insertion. This tendon is then secured to the third rib in order to prevent traction injury to the neurovascular pedicle.

STAGE TWO: CARDIAC WRAP

The heart is then exposed through median sternotomy and an inverse "C" pericardiotomy overlying the ventricular silhouette. Approximately 20 cc of 1% lidocaine is infused into the pericardial sac to decrease heart excitability and the risk of arrhythmias. Two R-wave sensing electrodes are then implanted into the right ventricular wall. The LDM is wrapped clockwise around both ventricles and fixed with interrupted sutures to the pericardium. The wrapping is then completed by fixing the anterior part of the LDM to the pericardial flap tailored from the right edge of the pericardiotomy. Care is taken to insure that the heart is not subjected to excess tension or compression from the muscle wrapping. Cardiopulmonary bypass is not necessary for this procedure.

STAGE THREE: MUSCLE ELECTROSTIMULATION

Muscle-pacing and heart-sensing electrodes are coupled to an implantable pulse generator (cardiomyostimulator), which includes a heart monitor (sensing chamber), a myostimulator (pacing chamber), and a synchronization circuit processing heart and muscle activities. It enables muscle stimulation synchronized on heart contractions (sensed or paced) using bursts of impulses. Backup cardiac pacing following cardiomyoplasty can be programmed in the sensing channel.

Electrostimulation is started 2 weeks after CMP. This delay is necessary for LDM flap healing and for the development of adhesions between the heart and muscle. The LDM is gradually stimulated by slow increments of burst frequency and number of pulses. To imitate the duration of a systolic contraction, the skeletal muscle should be electrostimulated by using train impulsions with a duration close to the ventricular ejection time span.

Two months after surgery, patients are then stimulated with pulse trains, keeping the heart-to-muscle contraction ratio of 2:1. A programmable synchronization delay enables evoked muscle contractions to be adjusted to the most appropriate period of ventricular contraction. An appropriate synchronization delay between LDM contraction and ventricular systole is achieved, with muscle stimulation starting immediately after closure of the mitral valve evaluated by echocardiography.

The frequency of LDM stimulation is set as a ratio of heart rate, usually 1:2. As the heart rate increases, the muscle will contract more frequently, reducing the relaxation time between successive contractions; this physiologically allows less time for muscle perfusion and for metabolic recovery before the next stimulation. In clinical series using chronically a heart-to-muscle stimulation ratio of 1:1, a deleterious overstimulation muscle pathology was observed. Histologic studies showed LDM fibrosis, atrophy, and fat degeneration.[7]

Cardio-Myostimulator

The contractile power of skeletal muscle is the major component of cardiac bioassist, whether in dynamic cardiomyoplasty, aortomyoplasty, atriomyoplasty, or skeletal muscle ventricles. This power can be elicited by specific devices that sense a cardiac contraction and then electrically stimulate the skeletal muscle with multiple pulses to invoke a contraction that is synchronous with the cardiac contractions. Several pulse generators were manufactured and implanted in patients: Cardio-Myostimulator and Transform System (Medtronic Inc., Minneapolis, MN), Myostim (Telectronics Pacing Systems, Inc., Englewood, CO), Myos (Biotronics, Berlin, Germany), Stiminak and EKS (Moscow Engineering Physics Institute, Moscow, Russia), and, recently, LD-Pace (CCC Uruguay, Montevideo, Uruguay).[8] New devices have been designed to automatically develop a work–rest regimen and a regimen with cessation or slowing down of contractions for several hours each day, in order to avoid LDM pathologic changes as a consequence of muscle overstimulation.

Action Mechanisms of Cardiomyoplasty

The many proposed mechanisms of action of LDM dynamic cardiomyoplasty are (1) systolic assist, (2) limitation of ventricular dilation, (3) reduction of ventricular wall stress (sparing effect), and (4) reverse ventricular remodeling due to the active girdling effect. CMP leads to an increase in ventricular mass by adding a new contractile muscular wall, which, in turn, re-establishes the ratio between the mass and the ventricular diameter in dilated cardiomyopathies.[9–11]

Clinical Experience

PATIENT POPULATION

In our institution, 112 patients aged 15 to 72 years (mean, 51 years) were operated on. All patients presented a severe cardiac deficiency refractory to maximal pharmacologic therapy; 86 were in New York Heart Association (NYHA) class III and 26 were in class IV. Left ventricular (LV) ejection fraction averaged 17% and end-diastolic left ventricular (EDLV) volume was 178 ± 31 mL/m^2. The cause of heart failure was ischemia in 59 patients, dilated cardiomyopathy in 46 patients, and ventricular tumors in 7 patients. Associated pathology (pulmonary hypertension, diabetes, etc) was present in 60% of patients. The technique has evolved from "open fixation" (58 patients), to "nonsuture wrapping" (41 patients), to "mini-invasive technique" (13 patients). Two-stage operations in high-risk patients with mitral valve insufficiency or severe arrhythmia were performed in 6 patients. Associated procedures were performed in 24 patients (coronary artery bypass graft [CABG] = 14, valve = 10).

RESULTS

The postoperative course was often critical (30% low cardiac output syndrome), particularly in ischemic etiology. In 35% of cases, an intra-aortic balloon pump was postoperatively used. Hospital mortality was 53% between 1985 and 1987, 13% between 1988 and 1997, and 8% since the introduction of mini-invasive techniques. Average NYHA class was 3.3 preoperatively and 1.4 post operation. Hemodynamic investigations in the survivors showed significant improvement in ejection fraction (21 to 31%) and cardiac index (1.9 to 2.8 L/min/m^2). Echocardiographic evaluation suggested that dynamic cardiomyoplasty reversed left ventricle (LV) chamber remodeling and improved LV contractility and external work efficiency in 70% of cases. Clinical studies showed an improvement in capacity during exercise, as well as a decrease in patient medication. Furthermore, a decrease was noted in deterioration of their state, which would have required hospitalization.[12–14] Long-term patient survival after cardiomyoplasty was 50% at 8 years (equivalent in our hospital for heart-transplanted patients). Ten patients required heart transplantation in a mean delay of 39 months after cardiomyoplasty, without major technical difficulties. All of these patients survived the operation and were discharged from the hospital.

Comparison of Quality of Life between Cardiomyoplasty and Heart Transplantation

The aim of this specific study was to compare quality of life (QOL) of two groups of patients who received, in our hospital, two types of surgical treatment: cardiomyoplasty ($n = 33$) and heart transplantation ($n = 63$). Quality of life was evaluated by SF-36 questionnaire, 9.7 ± 3 years after the intervention. The two groups did not differ for age and gender.[15,16]

No significant difference was found in QOL subscores or components. Physical component scores were respectively 42.2 ± 10.9 versus 43.5 ± 9.5, and psychic component scores were 49.5 ± 11.9 versus 46.4 ± 11.0 for cardiomyoplasty (CMP) and heart transplantation (HT), very close to standardized scores for the general population (50 ± 10). This result did not change after controlling for the time elapsed since intervention and NYHA stage at the time of evaluation.

These results show that QOL is globally preserved in CMP as well as in HT, several years after surgery. Such data encourage the choice of CMP with contraindications for HT or when the waiting list for transplantation is too long.

Right Ventricular Cardiomyoplasty

Chronically depressed right ventricle (RV) function presents an unsolved therapeutic challenge in cardiac surgery. Despite recent advances in medical and surgical therapies, prognosis remains poor and patient's quality of life and mortality are frequently unacceptable.[17] The RV may fail because of primary diseases or because of delay after left ventricular failure. Congenital anomalies, RV dysplasia, myocarditis, ischemia, and cardiomyopathy are the most frequent etiologies of primary RV failure. Based on the progressive knowledge of patients' selection and management, we applied modifications to the classic cardiomyoplasty procedure by using the left latissimus dorsi muscle to perform a specific RV cardiomyoplasty.[18]

Clinical Experience

Among 187 patients who underwent cardiomyoplasty by our team, 6 consecutive patients underwent cardiomyoplasty for right ventricular failure. Etiology of RV failure was ischemic cardiomyopathy in two cases, and dysplasia, Uhl's disease, congenital cardiomyopathy, and endomyocardial fibrosis, respectively in the remaining four cases. All patients had an advanced stage of heart failure, with five cases in NYHA functional class III and one patient in class III/IV. The preoperative isotopic right ventricle ejection fraction (RVEF) was 20 ± 9.7% and left ventricle ejection fraction (LVEF) was 37 ± 12%.

Surgical Technique

After LDM dissection, implantation of pacing leads, and transposition into the chest, the left LDM flap was placed onto the anterior and diaphragmatic RV free walls. Afterward its distal end was secured to the pericardial sac as far posteriorly as possible at the junction between the diaphragmatic and the posterior parts of the pericardium with interrupted sutures. To synchronize LDM and heart contractions, two sensing epicardial leads were inserted in the LV wall. These leads could not be placed in the RV due to diseased myocardium.

Results

Five patients are alive, with a good quality of life. Three are in NYHA functional class I and two are in class II. One patient died in postoperative year 7 due to stroke, while he was in functional class II. The mean postoperative RVEF is 32 ± 11.3% and LVEF is 51 ± 14.3 %.

Conclusions

The RV myocardial wall and chamber seem to be better adapted than the LV when assisted by an electrostimulated LDM. The hemodynamic characteristics (principally the filling pressures) and the thickness of the RV myocardium are more easily compressed during systole by the paced LDM. Furthermore, anatomically, the RV can be extensively wrapped by the left LDM, which can be positioned in such a manner that the muscular fibers are oriented perpendicularly to the ventricular septum. The results of 10-year follow-up demonstrate hemodynamic and functional improvements following RV cardiomyoplasty, without perioperative mortality and no long-term RV dysfunction–related deaths. We believe that RV cardiomyoplasty, associated with tricuspid valve surgery when it is required, should be an effective treatment for severe RV failure.

Cardiomyoplasty Following Ventricular Tumor Resection

Although cardiac transplantation has been performed for complete removal of ventricular tumors, complete surgical resection with ventricular reconstruction is desirable, insofar as patients with benign tumors would probably be cured, while those with malignant tumors would have a better prognosis. In the following study, extensive and complete surgical resection of ventricular tumors was followed by anatomic ventricular reconstruction using a cardiomyoplasty surgical procedure.

Clinical Experience

Seven patients (four females), mean age of 32.7 years (range of 22 to 55 years) underwent tumor resection and CMP procedure. The most common clinical symptoms were syncopal events, tachyarrhythmias, and heart failure. Cardiac tumors were primary in six patients and metastatic disease was primary in one patient. Distribution of histologic types were fibroma in two patients, and sarcoma, lymphosarcoma, hemangioma, lipoma, and metastatic angiosarcoma, respectively, in the remaining five patients.

Surgical Technique

Surgery consisted of four steps: (1) tumor resection; (2) coronary artery resection, when invaded by the tumor, and CABG; (3) valvular reconstruction, when possible, or replacement; and (4) ventricular wall reconstruction by pericardial patch for closure of the ventricular defect (neoendocardium), covered by the electrostimulated latissimus dorsi muscle flap (neomyocardium).[19]

Results

All patients survived surgery, but two late postoperative deaths are reported. Among the surviving patients, early complications played a major role in their postoperative course and consisted of arrhythmias, atrioventricular block requiring dual-chamber pulse generator, respiratory insufficiency, and heart failure. Two patients were assisted postoperatively with an intra-aortic balloon pump. On postoperative follow-up (mean, 72.4 ± 8.5 months), an improvement in the patients' functional status was observed. Patients moved from NYHA functional class mean 2.8 to a functional class mean 1.2.

Conclusions

The role of CMP in patients with large ventricular tumors is based on the principle that this procedure offers the possibility of reconstructing a contractile ventricular wall, thus preserving an adequate size and shape of the ventricular residual cavities. Moreover, in malignant tumors this technique allows a large resection of the disease without recurrence, avoiding heart transplantation. We believe that CMP is well adapted to reconstruct the ventricular chambers following tumor resection. Historically, it was necessary to adapt this technique for this disease. In this manner, the rationale was to create a new ventricular wall by using autologous pericardium to replace the endocardium, taking advantage of its hemocompatibility. Complementarily, the electrostimulated LDM was used to replace the resected myocardium. Our surgical approach to reconstructing ventricular chambers following tumor resection is to preserve a maximum of the anatomic and functional characteristics of each ventricle, including the valvular apparatus and a compliant ventricular chamber. The excellent long-term evolution without recurrence, ventricular dysfunction and/or thromboembolic complications implies that CMP could be recommended as an alternative to heart transplantation for large-size ventricular tumor therapy.[19]

Electrophysiologic Treatments Associated with Cardiomyoplasty

The patients who have been subjected to a CMP, who are suffering from an ischemic or severe idiopathic cardiomyopathy, present a great risk for ventricular arrhythmias, which are potentially responsible for the occurrence of sudden death. At the same time, electrical and mechanical asynchronisms between the ventricles are frequently observed in these patients. In our institution, CMP was associated with multisite cardiac pacing (for atrioventricular, interventricular, or intraventricular resynchronization) in six cases, and with implantable defibrillators in two cases. The positive results obtained foresee the expansion of this associated technique.

Less-Invasive Techniques for Cardiomyoplasty

Recent clinical experience in cardiovascular surgery demonstrates the interest of using video-assisted mini-invasive and robotic techniques. Fundamentally, the advantage for the patient is aesthetic; however, rehabilitation can be quicker, avoiding the risk of complications of a sternotomy. Thirteen CMPs have been carried out in our department using reduced access and ways with encouraging results.

Discussion

Latissimus dorsi dynamic cardiomyoplasty was indicated for patients presenting with severe left or right ventricular failure, and for ventricular reconstruction following tumor resection. The cardiomyoplasty results improved through experience, through rigorous patient selection, through progress in the operation technique, and through improved postoperative care. Cardiac transplantation is technically feasible after a CMP. Risk factors have been identified, resulting in more precise indications, a lower hospital mortality, and a wider use of this operation. The ventricular function improvement observed after dynamic cardiomyoplasty derived from the direct action of synchronized LDM contraction and from a girdling effect that helps to reverse chamber remodeling and to decrease ventricular wall stress. Technological advances incorporated in the new cardiomyostimulators and electrostimulation protocols will probably improve long-term muscle preservation as well as hemodynamic benefits.[20,21] Clinical improvement has been reported as a consistent finding in cardiomyoplasty follow-up. Clear hemodynamic benefits have been demonstrated in approximately 70% of cardiomyoplasty patients. The mortality after cardiomyoplasty has been significantly higher for patients in persistent NYHA functional class IV, showing that this procedure needs to be indicated earlier than does heart transplantation.[22] Long-term patient survival is equivalent for cardiomyoplasty and for heart transplantation: 50% at 8 years. However, the main problem in cardiac transplantation is the mortality in the waiting list: from 15 to 50%, depending on the country. This is a nonexistent problem in cardiomyoplasty. Worldwide there are thousands of functional class III patients whose quality of life and exercise capacity have worsened despite the use of maximum medical therapy, justifying dynamic cardiomyoplasty indication.[23]

Cellular Cardiomyoplasty

The recent progress in cellular and molecular biology allows the development of new therapies for heart failure. One of the most innovative of the therapies consists of the transplantation of autologous expanded cells into the myocardium for heart muscle regeneration. This approach is called *cellular cardiomyoplasty*. Adult myocardium cannot effectively repair after infarction, due to the limited number of stem cells. Thus, most of the injury is irreversible. For this reason, cell transplantation strategies for heart failure have been designed to replace damaged cells with cells that can perform cardiac work, either in ischemic or idiopathic cardiomyopathies.[24,25] Grafting of healthy cells into the diseased myocardium holds enormous potential as an approach to cardiovascular pathology. Cellular CMP consists of cell implantation to grow new muscle fibers, to develop angiogenesis in the damaged myocardium that potentially may contribute to improve systolic and diastolic ventricular functions, and to reverse the postischemic remodeling process.[26]

Tissue regeneration techniques based on cell transplantation technology have been previously used clinically for the treatment of hemopathies (chronic lymphocytic leukemia, aplastic anemia, immunodeficiencies, myeloma) with excellent results, for diabetes mellitus (transplantation of Langerhans islets), in neurology (Huntington's and Parkinson's diseases, spinal cord regeneration), in hepatology (implantation of hepatocytes as a bridge to liver transplantation), in myology (transplantation of myoblasts in Duchenne's dystrophy), in orthopedics (implantation of chondrocytes for repair of articular defects of the knee), and in dermatology (implantation of cultured epidermal cells).

Current clinical possibilities in cell therapy for heart failure are the transplantation into the damaged myocardium of different types of cells such as autologous myoblasts (originating from skeletal muscle), bone marrow stem cells, peripheral blood stem cells, smooth-muscle cells, angioblasts, and endothelial cells.[27–30]

Indications

ISCHEMIC CARDIOMYOPATHY

Clinical application for cell transplantation should be in patients who present a cardiac dysfunction due to an extensive myocardial infarction, without possibilities of surgical or percutaneous revascularization. The objective of cellular CMP is to limit infarct expansion and cardiac remodeling and to regenerate the myocardium. Patients with right ventricular myocardial infarction and with ischemic mitral valve regurgitation could also be included.

IDIOPATHIC DILATED CARDIOMYOPATHY

Nonischemic cardiomyopathy is also a major cause of heart failure, with high mortality rates. Cell transplantation could offer new hopes in this disease by restoring impaired heart function. Cellular CMP may improve heart function in patients with dilated cardiomyopathy because the grafted cells appear to better survive in the host myocardium because myocardial irrigation in this pathology is not significantly impaired.[25]

Mechanisms of Action

The many proposed mechanisms of action of cellular cardiomyoplasty are reduction of the size of infarct scars, limitation of postischemic ventricular remodeling, improvement of ventricular wall thickening and compliance, and increase of regional myocardial contractility. When skeletal myoblasts are used for cellular CMP, the sequence of actions seems to be that cells transplanted into the myocardium first impact on diastolic dysfunction, and subsequently, when they are sufficiently organized in myotubes and myofibers, systolic performance improves.[31–33]

The technical approach used to implant the cells should influence the efficacy of cellular CMP. Cell mortality after transplantation seems to be important when cells are grafted in the center of high-fibrotic ischemic scars, because there is a great limitation of oxygen and nutrient supply to the chronic ischemic myocardium. Implanting the cells mainly in the peri-infarct areas may improve the

rate of surviving cells; thus, the size of the infarct scars undergo a centripetal reduction.

It is possible that periodically repeated cell injections should be necessary to progressively reduce the infarct scars in ischemic cardiomyopathies or to gradually improve the diseased myocardium in nonischemic cardiomyopathies. This approach should be facilitated by the development of percutaneous catheter-based cell implantation procedures.

Research Protocols

The following experimental studies have been performed in our institution:

1. *Evaluation of segmentary myocardial function.* Autologous myoblasts obtained from skeletal muscles were implanted into the LV wall in an experimental model of partial ventricular akinesia. Chronic cardiac deficiency was developed by local injection of snake cardiotoxin (C 9759, Sigma Chem.) in the LV wall of sheep, through a left minithoracotomy. Echocardiographic studies (Color Kinesis, Hewlett Packard Sonos 5500) were performed after toxin, after cell injections, and at 2 months. Myoblast implantation was associated with the recovery of regional myocardial contractility; regional fraction area change (RFAC) improved and ventricular remodeling partially reversed in the cell-implanted group. Healthy myoblasts organized in multinucleated myotubes were observed in myocardial histologic studies.[34]

2. *Electrostimulation after cellular CMP.* The principles of electrophysiologic conditioning of muscle fibers was applied by our group in cellular cardiomyoplasty. A myocardial infarct model was performed in sheep. Cultured autologous myoblasts were implanted 3 weeks later into and around the infarct areas. Atrial synchronized biventricular pacing was then performed using epicardial electrodes. Evaluation at 2 months showed an increased expression of slow myosin and better organization of transplanted cells in the ventricular wall, as compared with nonstimulated control groups. This histochemical modification seems to be better adapted to perform cardiac work. Simultaneous cardiac resynchronization can also be achieved with this approach.[35]

3. *Endoventricular cell implantation.* We studied the possibilities of endoventricular cell implantation in an experimental sheep model of myocardial infarction. Transcutaneous cell implantation was performed using a specific catheter (NOGA Biosense, Cordis, Johnson and Johnson, Miami Lakes, FL) guided by electroanatomic mapping. The Biosense system allows the precise guidance of the catheter to the infarcted zone. Viable cells were detected in the implantation sites. Periodically repeated cell implantation procedures could be performed with this system.[36]

4. *Association of angiogenic growth factors with cellular CMP.* Locally delivered angiogenic growth factors and cell implantation have been proposed for patients presenting myocardial infarcts without possibility of percutaneous or surgical revascularization. The goal of this study was to compare the effects of these techniques, in an ischemic model in sheep. A myocardial infarction was created by ligation of two coronary branches (distal left anterior descending [LAD] and D2). Three groups were studied: vascular endothelial growth factor (VEGF) group, cell implantation group, and association of cells with locally injected VEGF.[37]

5. *Cell therapy for dilated cardiomyopathy.* A dilated cardiomyopathy model was induced by rapid pacing in sheep. After 4 months of pacing at 200 beats per minute, a definitive heart failure model was achieved. Cellular CMP was performed by using autologous cultured myoblasts injected through multiple injection points performed between the coronary arteries in both ventricles. Hemodynamic and histologic studies were performed.

Clinical Experience

In an attempt to repair damaged heart muscle and to improve cardiac function, we have transplanted a patient's own skeletal muscle cells (autologous myoblasts) directly into infarcted left ventricular areas in two cases.[38,39] Skeletal myoblasts present the advantage of being resistant to ischemia and of expanding rapidly in vitro.

Patients

Procedures were performed in two male patients, aged 66 and 71 years, in NHYA functional class III, presenting impaired LV function (ejection fraction 32% and 28%), LV posterior wall postischemic scars (akinetic and metabolically nonviable), and indications for CABG in remote, viable, and ischemic areas.

Procedure

In December 2001 and February 2002, during an outpatient procedure under local anesthesia, surgical biopsies of 15 and 10 g of a skeletal muscle (the thigh vastus lateralis), were performed. In the cellular biology laboratory, skeletal muscle stem cells (myoblasts) were isolated and expanded in vitro in 17 ± 4 days up to 200 and 300 million. Cells were cultivated in a complete human medium, using the patient's own serum. To obtain a pure myoblast culture, fibroblasts were progressively eliminated from the flasks, using the preplatting technique. At the moment of implantation, the rate of myoblasts was 82 ± 5 % and the rate of viable cells was $95 \pm 3\%$. Afterward, the cells diluted in human albumin were placed in a syringe ready to be injected (Table 43-2). During a surgical procedure, through sternotomy, CABG was performed (to the LAD in the first patient, and to the LAD and D1 in the second case). The muscle cells were then injected (through five

TABLE 43-2. Cellular Cardiomyoplasty

Myoblast implantation protocol:
- Implantation of > 200 million cells
- Cellular density for injection: 50 to 70 million cells per mL
- Time to culture: approximately 21 days
- Myoblast concentration of > 50% myoblasts
- Cell shelf-life at room temperature is 6 h; at 2 to 8°C it is 96 h.

injection points for the first patient, and eight for the second patient) into the posterior wall of the left ventricle, into and around the infarcted areas.

Preliminary Results

Patients had uneventful recovery and were discharged from the intensive care unit 24 and 48 h after surgery. No cardiac arrhythmias were recorded. Echocardiographic studies at 3 months showed improvement of regional myocardial motion (from akinetic scars to hypokinetic ventricular wall); regional fractional shortening improved from $9 \pm 3\%$ to $20 \pm 5\%$. The infarct scar size appears to be significantly reduced, from 18 ± 5 cm² to 7 ± 3 cm² ($p < .05$). The main benefit of the use of autologous human serum for cell cultures is that it can be performed internationally, without any risk of prion, viral, or zoonoses contaminations, unlike traditional cell culture techniques that involve the use of fetal bovine serum for cell growth.

Perspectives

Coronary heart disease is the leading cause of death in the United States, being responsible for approximately 1 of every 5 deaths, or approximately 500,000 deaths each year. Using the patient's skeletal muscle stem cells may eliminate both the ethical and rejection issues that are associated with using fetal stem cells or other types of embryonic cells. Furthermore, autologous bone marrow stromal cells represent an interesting perspective. However, a risk exists that these multipotent mesenchymal stem cells (which can undergo milieu-dependent differentiation) may differentiate into fibroblasts after implantation in a fibrotic scar. Cell transplantation is becoming recognized as a viable strategy to improve myocardial viability and limit infarct growth.[26,34,35] The major challenges for future research programs are the preconditioning for predifferentiation of stem cells before transplantation, the optimization of the rate of surviving cells after myocardial implantation, and the improvement of host-cell interactions (mechanical and electrical coupling).[40]

References

1. Chachques JC, Grandjean PA, Schwartz K, et al. Effect of latissimus dorsi dynamic cardiomyoplasty on ventricular function. Circulation 1988;78 Suppl 3:203–16.
2. Carpentier A, Chachques JC, Grandjean P, editors. Cardiac bioassist. New York: Futura Publishing; 1997. p. 1-632.

3. Chachques JC, Grandjean PA, Carpentier A. Latissimus dorsi dynamic cardiomyoplasty. Ann Thorac Surg 1989;47:600–4.

4. Magovern GJ, Simpson KA. Clinical cardiomyoplasty: review of the ten-year United States experience. Ann Thorac Surg 1996;61:413–9.

5. Moreira LFP, Stolf NAG, Braile DM, Jatene AD. Dynamic cardiomyoplasty in South America. Ann Thorac Surg 1996;61:408–12.

6. Rigatelli G, Carraro U, Barbiero M, et al. New advances in dynamic cardiomyoplasty: Doppler flow wire shows improved cardiac assistance in demand protocol. ASAIO J 2002;48:119–23.

7. Gutierrez PS, Pires WO Jr, Marie SK, et al. Histopathological findings in skeletal muscle used in human dynamic cardiomyoplasty. J Pathol 2001;194:116–21.

8. Chekanov VS, Chachques JC, Brum F, et al. LD-Pace II: a new cardiomyostimulator for cardiac bioassist. ASAIO J 2001;47:50–5.

9. Hwan J, Badhwar V, Chiu RCJ. Mechanisms of dynamic cardiomyoplasty: current concepts. J Card Surg 1996;11:194–9.

10. Schreuder JJ, Van der Veen FH, Ven der Velde ET, et al. Left ventricular pressure-volume relationships before and after cardiomyoplasty in patients with heart failure. Circulation 1997;96:2978–86.

11. Chen FY, deGuzman BJ, Aklog L, et al. Decreased myocardial oxygen consumption indices in dynamic cardiomyoplasty. Circulation 1996;94 Suppl II:239–44.

12. Carpentier A, Chachques JC, Acar C, et al. Dynamic cardiomyoplasty at seven years. J Thorac Cardiovasc Surg 1993;106:42–54.

13. Chachques JC, Berrebi A, Hernigou A, et al. Study of muscular and ventricular function in dynamic cardiomyoplasty: a ten-year follow up. J Heart Lung Transplant 1997;16:854–68.

14. Furnary AP, Chachques JC, Moreira LFP, et al. Long term outcome, survival analysis and risk stratification of dynamic cardiomyoplasty. J Thorac Cardiovasc Surg 1996;112:1640–50.

15. Aaronson NK, Acquadro C, Alonso J, et al. International Quality of Life Assessment (IQOLA) Project. Qual Life Res 1992;1:349–51.

16. Gandek B, Ware JE Jr, Aaronson NK, et al. Tests of data quality, scaling assumptions, and reliability of the SF-36 in eleven countries: results from the IQOLA Project. International Quality of Life Assessment. J Clin Epidemiol 1998;51:1149–58.

17. Juilliere Y, Barbier G, Feldmann L, et al. Additional predictive value of both left and right ventricular ejection fractions on long-term survival in idiopathic dilated cardiomyopathy. Eur Heart J 1997;18:276–80.

18. Fontaine G, Chachques JC, Argyriadis P, et al. Traitement de l'insuffisance ventriculaire droite par cardiomyoplastie. J Chir Thorac Cardiovasc 2001;5:143–8.

19. Chachques JC, Argyriadis P, Latremouille C, et al. Cardiomyoplasty: ventricular reconstruction after tumor resection. J Thorac Cardiovasc Surg 2002;123:889–94.

20. Kashem A, Santamore WP, Chiang B, et al. Vascular delay and intermittent stimulation: keys to successful latissimus dorsi muscle stimulation. Ann Thorac Surg 2001;71:1866–73.

21. Tang ATM, Jarvis JC, Hooper TL, Salmons S. Cardiomyoplasty: the benefits of electrical prestimulation of the latissimus dorsi muscle in situ. Ann Thorac Surg 1999;68:46–51.

22. Herreros JM, Fernandez-Gonzalez AL, Martinez-Monzonis A, et al. Successful dynamic cardiomyoplasty after heart transplantation. J Heart Lung Transplant 1995;14:1218–20.

23. Jessup M. Dynamic cardiomyoplasty: expectations and results. J Heart Lung Transplant 2000;19:68–72.

24. Scorsin M, Hagege A, Vilquin JT, et al. Comparison of the effects of fetal cardiomyocyte and skeletal myoblast transplantation on postinfarction left ventricular function. J Thorac Cardiovasc Surg 2000;119:1169–75.

25. Yoo KJ, Li RK, Weisel RD, et al. Heart cell transplantation improves heart function in dilated cardiomyopathic hamsters. Circulation 2000;102 Suppl 3:204–9.

26. Chachques JC, Hidalgo J, Cattadori B, et al. Cardiomioplastia celular: un nuevo enfoque terapeutico para la disfuncion ventricular. Int Cardiol 2001;10:11–5.

27. Dorfman J, Duong M, Zibaitis A, et al. Myocardial tissue engineering with autologous myoblast implantation. J Thorac Cardiovasc Surg 1998;116:744–51.

28. Atkins BZ, Lewis CW, Kraus WE, et al. Intracardiac transplantation of skeletal myoblasts yields two populations of striated cells in situ. Ann Thorac Surg 1999;67:124–9.

29. Wang JS, Shum-Tim D, Galipeau J, et al. Marrow stromal cells for cellular cardiomyoplasty: feasibility and potential clinical advantages. J Thorac Cardiovasc Surg 2000;120:999–1005.

30. Orlic D, Kajstura J, Chimenti S, et al. Mobilized bone marrow cells repair the infarcted heart, improving function and survival. Proc Natl Acad Sci U S A 2001;98:10344–9.

31. Taylor DA, Atkins BZ, Hungspreugs P, et al. Regenerating functional myocardium: improved performance after skeletal myoblast transplantation. Nat Med 1998;4:929–33.

32. Reinecke H, Zhang M, Bartosek T, Murry CE. Survival, integration, and differentiation of cardiomyocyte grafts. Circulation 1999;100:193–202.

33. Makino S, Fukuda K, Miyoshi S, et al. Cardiomyocytes can be generated from marrow stromal cells in vitro. J Clin Invest 1999;103:697–705.

34. Rajnoch C, Chachques JC, Berrebi A, et al. Cellular therapy reverses myocardial dysfunction. J Thorac Cardiovasc Surg 2001;121:871–8.

35. Chachques JC, Shafy A, Cattadori B, et al. Electrostimulation enhanced fatigue resistant myosin expression in cellular cardiomyoplasty. Circulation 2001;104 Suppl 2:555–6.

36. Chachques JC, Blanchard D, Shafy A, et al. Implantation de myoblastes dans le myocarde par voie endoventriculaire. Arch Mal Coeur 2001;94:1428.

37. Cha JC, Duarte F, Cattadori B, et al. Angiogenic growth factors versus cellular therapy for myocardial infarction. Presented at the American Association for Thoracic Surgery (AATS) 82nd Annual Meeting. Abstracts Book 2002;F17:68.

38. Trainini J, Cichero D, Chachques JC. Cellular cardiomyoplasty at the Avellaneda Hospital, Buenos Aires, Argentina. Personal communication.

39. Herreros J, Prosper F, Chachques JC. Cellular cardiomyoplasty at the University of Navarra, Spain. Personal communication.

40. Chahques JC, Carpentier A. Cellular myoplasty: what are we really trying to achieve? J Thorac Cardiovasc Surg 2002;123:583–4.

CHAPTER 44

CELL THERAPY FOR MYOCARDIAL REPAIR

DAVID W. MARKHAM, MD, DORIS A. TAYLOR, PhD

The last 50 years have seen major advances in our understanding and treatment of acute myocardial infarction (AMI) and congestive heart failure (CHF), two of the most prominent diseases in the Western world. It is a testament to many cardiovascular scientists and physicians that in a short time span we have moved from few therapeutically significant treatments to the current use of a wide array of therapies that prolong life for heart disease victims. These include not only the development of coronary artery bypass surgery, cardiac catheterization, angioplasty, intravascular ultrasonography, and other technologies, but also highly efficacious medical therapy: aspirin, diuretics, thrombolytics, β-adrenergic receptor blockers, and angiotensin-converting enzyme inhibitors, just to mention the most studied and proven drugs now in use.

As AMI therapy has improved, many patients are surviving infarcts but progressing to heart failure. Unfortunately, there are no treatments that reverse or treat the underlying defect in heart failure, the death of cardiomyocytes, resulting in the decompensation of the remainder of the heart. Treatments only delay the progression of heart failure. Therefore, the disease often progresses to an end-stage situation; currently, transplantation is the only lifesaving treatment. Experience with artificial hearts and other mechanical left ventricular assist devices has provided only temporizing measures in the severely ill patient with heart failure, but as these technologies continue to improve, they may provide new therapeutic options. Meanwhile, we are now moving into an exciting new phase of cardiovascular treatment designed to treat the underlying disease process by generating new muscle and vasculature within injured myocardium. Not only could transplanted cells correct cardiovascular anatomic and physiologic disturbances, they may provide "point-of-care" treatment, for instance, at the time of AMI, to aid in the repair of the heart and thus in the prevention of CHF.

The use of cells to repair or regenerate the diseased human body is no longer simply a vision. Instead, it has become an important medical and scientific goal. This work includes a variety of cells, ranging from different populations of stem or progenitor cells to differentiated cells isolated from mature tissue. Significant steps are underway toward using cell therapy in patients with diseases of the central nervous system (CNS), endocrine organs (including novel therapies for diabetes), and the musculoskeletal system. Other treatments have focused on inborn defects of metabolism, and hematopoietic stem cells remain a standard of care in the treatment of particular cancers. The exploitation of stem cells, or other cells capable of *trans*-differentiation, to repair solid organs may be just around the corner. This goal is now especially enticing for the treatment of cardiovascular disease. The impact of advanced and more specific treatment strategies would be enormous not only with regard to the high incidence of coronary disease and congestive heart failure but also for stroke and peripheral vascular disease.

The Heart Is a Nonregenerative Organ

The heart responds to AMI in a complex fashion that involves many processes, including the activation of a variety of molecular signals, recruitment of inflammatory cells, myocyte necrosis, fibrous deposition, scar formation, and remodeling. The end result in CHF is an enlarged, hemodynamically unsuited, scarred heart. This occurs largely because the heart lacks the ability to repair or regenerate functional tissue, unlike many other human tissues such as skeletal muscle or liver. Soon after birth, cardiomyocytes withdraw from the cell cycle and continue to grow via hypertrophy. With cardiac damage, there is little or no effective cardiomyocyte proliferation or regeneration to aid in the healing process. Although there is some debate regarding the level of deoxyribonucleic acid (DNA) synthesis and proliferative capacity of myocardial cells, it is generally accepted that only an exceptionally small population of cells—both histologically and clinically insignificant—is capable of cell division.[1,2]

Interestingly, this debate over cardiac regeneration has recently spilled over into transplant biology. Work has demonstrated Y chromosome–positive cells in female hearts transplanted into male donors—so-called cardiac chimerism.[3–5] Difficulties with immunohistochemistry and proper control groups make chimerism challenging to study. Even though such phenomena are interesting and potentially useful if future technologies allow manipulation, there is almost certainly no significant or physiologic effect on cardiac function.

Much investigational work has addressed both the early stages of cardiomyocyte differentiation and their permanent withdrawal from the cell cycle, in large part to manipulate this process for therapeutic purposes. Yet, this has been frustratingly disappointing. No system has been developed that successfully promotes the survival and integration of differentiated cardiac cells into the infarcted heart. It seems that the intrinsic features of the heart, like the continuous mechanical motion, the highly organized cellular structure, and its efficient capability of scar formation, make terminally differentiated cells unsuited for integration. Certainly, hypoxia and low perfusion make cardiomyocyte integration difficult. Cardiomyocyte cell growth and differentiation are presumably linked, but little is understood regarding the mechanisms. Researchers have engineered cardiac cells to proliferate for potential therapeutic uses, investigated the ability of skeletal muscle to engraft and differentiate in the heart, and studied the pluripotency of various sources of cells to differentiate into cardiomyocytes. All of these approaches have advanced the field, but a definitive treatment strategy to repair diseased human cardiac tissue still does not exist. The goal, at least of our group, is to find a cell capable of engrafting and surviving in the infarcted heart—a cell that can integrate and electrically couple with surrounding cardiomyocytes to increase contractile function. It goes without saying that finding such a cell, especially one that has no negative repercussions on electrical or mechanical conduction, is not an easy task.

Before discussing the state of cardiac cellular transplantation, it is useful to briefly discuss some of the pertinent features of cardiac development and cardiomyocyte differentiation. This is relevant because cardiac engraftment coupled to functional improvement likely relies on the transplantation of cells that have the propensity to differentiate into true molecularly characterized cardiomyocytes.

The heart is the first organ to develop in vertebrates, arising from the migration of precardiac cells. Briefly, these cells converge into a heart tube that begins beating at 20 to 22 days of age in the human. Subsequently, looping, septation, and cushion and outflow tract formation occurs. Thus, in only approximately 8 weeks, the human heart forms from "procardiomyocytes" to become an immature four-chambered organ. It is important to note that myocytes comprise only approximately 30% of the adult heart. Neural crest cells contribute to outflow tract formation,[6,7] and the endothelial mantle contributes to the coronary arteries,[8,9] just to mention examples of how other cell types participate in heart formation. Obviously, this complex developmental process relies on multiple molecular signals controlling polarity, migration, differentiation, and cell–cell coupling, and these features are only partially understood at the present time. The identification of new molecular pathways and cell markers involved in this process could advance our knowledge of heart development and provide insight for developing models for heart regeneration.

Some of the important transcriptional regulators of cardiomyocyte differentiation are known (Figure 44-1). Nkx2.5, a putative homolog of *Drosophila tinman*, is a transcription factor expressed by cardiac progenitors in the early heart field.[10] It is clear from studies of Nkx2.5 that it is an important regulator of genes controlling cardiomyocyte differentiation, including myosin light chains 2 and 3f,[11,12] SM22,[13] and desmin.[14] Other early regulators important for heart formation include GATA-4,[15,16] MEF2C,[17] and dHAND.[18] GATA-4 influences the expression of several proteins, including troponin C, myosin heavy chain (MHC), and atrial and brain natriuretic peptides. The first marker for the ventricular muscle cell lineage, the myosin light chain *MLC2V* gene, encodes a contractile protein important for functional maturation of cardiac muscle.[12]

No single factor has yet been discovered that governs whether a cell will become a cardiomyocyte. For example, expression of Nkx2.5 and Bmp2 do not accurately demarcate the heart-forming region in the developing animal, thus demonstrating a lack of specificity. However, the early markers of cardiac cells are important in allowing us to study which cells form the heart and how they do so. More work is needed to understand how this occurs, and there may be breakthroughs on the horizon from studies of cardiac development and cellular differentiation that

Cardiomyocyte Differentiation

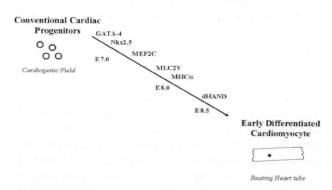

FIGURE 44-1. A simplified schematic of cardiomyocyte differentiation, depicting several transcriptional regulators and contractile proteins that are markers for cells giving rise to functional differentiated cardiomyocytes. Embryonic day (E) indicates number of days following conception in the mouse.

directly impact cellular therapy. A simplified schematic of early cardiomyocyte development appears in Figure 44-1.

Cardiac Cell Therapy

The Goal of Creating a Functional Cardiomyocyte Cell

The lack of postnatal proliferation of cardiomyocytes has led many scientists to attempt to create a readily available source of proliferating cardiac cells. It is well known that cardiac cells transformed with E1A or SV40 T antigen (TAg), two viral oncoproteins, proliferate. E1A binds pocket proteins and drives S-phase entry.[19,20] SV40 TAg interacts with p53 and has been used to derive cell lines using the atrial natriuretic factor (ANF) and α-MHC promoters.[21–25] Although these immortal cell lines proliferate and thus are potentially useful for cardiac repair, the cells lack the ability to completely differentiate or do not retain the capacity for electrical or contractile function.[22] More importantly, as tumor cells, these cardiomyocyte cell lines may potentially be harmful with regard to arrhythmogenesis or outright global heart dysfunction, if transplanted.

AT-1 cells, derived in the laboratory of Dr. Loren Field, express an ANF, the simian virus 40 T antigen fusion gene.[26] These cells proliferate in culture and are detected for as long as 4 months when transplanted into the normal myocardium. Analysis of the transplanted cells show that they are juxtaposed to the host myocardium, and the animals have no evidence of cardiac arrhythmia. Although this individual study shows some promising results, genetically manipulating cells prior to engraftment will involve much more work, especially with regard to differentiation, function, and safety.

Interesting in vitro data demonstrate the possibility of isolating cardiomyocytes from mouse bone marrow stromal cells (BMSCs) immortalized with 5-azacytidine. This finding supports the notion that BMSCs can act as pluripotent stem cells.[27–29] It also offers promise for creating greater accessibility to cultured cardiomyocytes and discovering novel genes regulating their differentiation. In another study, human embryonic stem cells differentiated to cardiomyocytes when plated to form embryoid bodies.[30] These cells may also be useful in future studies, but at present are limited by both technical (ie, tumorigenicity) and ethical concerns.

Another potential source for cardiomyocytes is the fetal or neonatal heart. Some investigators transplanted fetal or neonatal rodent cardiomyocytes into adult myocardium. These cells appear to incorporate following injection and reportedly improve function.[31,32] Similarly, neonatal cardiomyocytes from rats engraft into hearts in which a coronary artery has been ligated; they form cell–cell junctions and align in a parallel fashion with host cardiomyocytes.[33] Although differentiated cardiomyocytes would appear to have increased potential for electromechanical coupling and fatigue resistance, they

have poor tolerance to transplantation in an ischemic environment. There is also the need for immunosuppression for allogeneic cardiac cells. Thus, the transplantation of cardiomyocyte cell lines or primary cardiomyocytes from various sources may prove promising for replacement therapy, but many difficulties still exist. Furthermore, the approach of transplanting fetal or neonatal cells will also be difficult to accomplish in human patients because of ethical concerns.

The perfect cell for cardiomyocyte replacement has not been developed, despite the creation of proliferating cardiomyocyte cell lines. However, these studies have been instructive regarding cardiomyocyte proliferation and differentiation. Although various factors are now known to be important, there is much to be learned. More study is needed to discover the key to maintaining cardiomyocytes that can both proliferate and terminally differentiate. A greater understanding of such progenitor cells may lead to better therapeutic applications.

To summarize, early heart development and cardiomyocyte differentiation are incompletely understood, but we do have growing insight into how gene expression guides these processes. As our understanding increases, many other genes are likely to be implicated in defining a cardiomyocyte. By understanding these processes, we may ultimately be able to induce stem cells, or another plentiful source of noncardiac cells, to differentiate down a cardiomyocyte lineage, but this is presently beyond our current level of understanding.

Stem Cells and the Heart

An alternate approach to using differentiated cells for cardiac repair is to develop novel sources of stem cells. A stem cell is a cell with a high degree of plasticity for multilineage differentiation and the ability to self-renew. Typical examples include hematopoietic stem cells (HSCs), mesenchymal stem cells (MSCs), embryonic stem cells (ESCs), and other tissue-specific cells (such as side population [SP] cells; see "Clinical Cell Transplantation for Cardiac Repair"). The concept of a stem cell is approximately 100 years old.[34] Although much of the history of stem cells has focused on the hematopoietic stem cell, there has been recent attention on other types of these cells that are capable of novel forms of tissue repair. With this has come the idea that stem cells might be used to repair the heart.

Clinical Cell Transplantation for Cardiac Repair

In a recent study, human MSCs isolated from bone marrow were transplanted into the left ventricles of adult mice with severe combined immunodeficiency disease (SCID).[35] The cells survived for greater than 1 week and began to express myogenic markers. In contrast, other investigators have shown that marrow stromal cells injected into scarred myocardium differentiate into nonmyogenic chondrocytes, adipocytes, and osteocytes.

These cells hold great promise if further mechanisms of differentiation and engraftment can be identified and fully understood, but at present their use appears limited. Nonetheless, it was recently shown that bone marrow–derived cells are capable of differentiation to multiple cell types in vitro and in vivo, including to cardiac cells.[27,36–38] These studies focus on two main cell types: BMSCs and SP cells. The BMSC system consists of all nonhematopoietic cells of mesenchymal origin, including macrophages, adipocytes, osteogenic cells, and reticular cells.[39] Orlic and colleagues examined the regeneration ability of lin⁻ c-kit⁺ cells derived from bone marrow.[40] These data showed that these cells can repopulate infarcted mouse hearts. Although exciting, these data need to be reproduced using other species to fully evaluate their differentiation and functional capacity.

Similar studies have used cells known as SP cells, an as yet poorly understood and characterized population of CD34$^{-/low}$ c-kit⁺ sca-1⁺ cells, first identified by their ability to efflux Hoechst dye.[41] These cells homed to the infarcted heart. There they differentiated into cardiomyocytes and endothelial cells in previously lethally irradiated mice, albeit to a low degree (Figure 44-2).[38]

Although the phenomenon of SP cell engraftment in the heart is rare, there is hope in using this information to better identify cells capable of homing to the heart after injury. The full regenerative potential of SP cells is still not known. It is also not known how heterogeneous the SP population is when isolated from various tissues. These studies, combined with the finding that transplanted embryonic dorsal aorta cells can participate in postnatal muscle growth and regeneration, suggest that cell-lineage potential and plasticity of many cell types are more flexible than previously thought.[42] Characterizing these cells and their potential is an important next challenge in the field.

One important issue is what happens to cells once they are transplanted. Do they remain in the heart, do they engraft and become cardiomyocytes, or do they fuse with existing cells and potentially have a negative effect? Two recent studies implicate the role of fusion and spontaneous

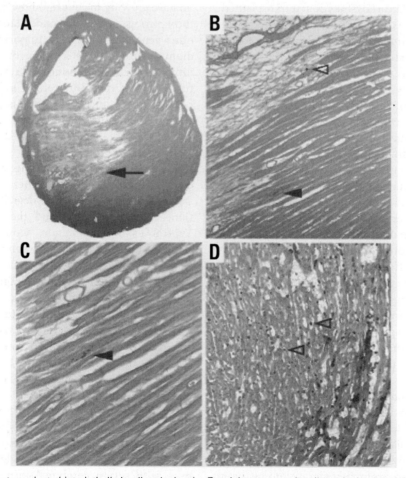

FIGURE 44-2. SP cells transplanted into lethally irradiated mice. LacZ staining occurs primarily at the border of the myocardial infarction. *A,* Lower-power (×10) photograph of mouse myocardial infarction after 4 weeks. The *arrowhead* points to the location of lacZ staining shown in *B* and *C.* The lighter pink tissue to the left and above the arrowhead is primarily fibrotic and results from the infarction. *B,* Higher-power (×20) photograph of the same section, dual-stained for lacZ and antimacrophage Ab F480. The *open arrow* indicates a macrophage; the *closed arrowhead* indicates lacZ-positive cardiomyocytes. *C,* Higher-power photograph of the same section (×40). *D,* Macrophage density of a cardiac section after 1 h of ischemia and 3 h of reperfusion. The *open arrowheads* indicate two of the many macrophages present. The counterstain is eosin.

generation of hybrid cells when cells are grown together.[43,44] These data, especially when applied to in vivo studies, raise the issue of cell fusion. More study is needed to determine whether BMSC or SP cells participate in repair by merely fusing with other cells or by "transdifferentiating" in vivo to become cardiomyocytes. Both processes may actually play a role. At a preclinical level, there will need to be quantitation of fusion events in vivo, and methods will need to be developed to detect the frequency with which fused cells change phenotype and integrate into the heart. These studies will require efficient cell labeling techniques that have little "leakiness" (ie, if a cell is labeled with a particular dye or stain), so that dye transfer can be ruled out. The need to address the issue of fusion comes from the potential that tetraploid fused cells may be tumorigenic or otherwise deleterious.

In summary, there is some debate regarding the mechanism of the multipotency of various sources and populations of stem cells, but there is clearly evidence that warrants further study of stem cells in cardiovascular repair. Stem cells with the capability of differentiating to cardiomyocytes are beginning to be studied in these regards. In fact, several clinical trials have begun, both in Europe and in the United States, where investigators are transplanting bone marrow into infarct to promote either angiogenesis or myogenesis in patients with severe heart disease. Yet, as this technology moves forward, it is critical to understand the phenotype of the cells being transplanted, the purity of the cell population, whether inflammatory cells are present, and how outcomes will be measured. Failure to do so and failure to carefully consider the fate of the cells in vivo could doom an otherwise good treatment paradigm. More information is needed in the fields of heart development and stem cell biology, and both areas would benefit from the discovery of cellular markers for pluripotent cells that can then be isolated and used for muscle reconstitution.

Skeletal Myoblasts As a Source of Cells for Cardiac Repair

The technology of transplanting skeletal muscle grafts onto the myocardium has been used since the mid-1980s. This procedure is called *cardiomyoplasty*, which basically involves wrapping skeletal muscle around the heart. Initial reports in selected patients with CHF demonstrated symptomatic improvement in New York Heart Association (NYHA) class. However, this improvement was not consistently associated with improvement in myocardial performance or survival. Following these results, investigators hypothesized that satellite cells, the cells responsible for skeletal muscle repair, might aid the injured heart if they were transplanted directly into the myocardium. One of the earliest reports of successful injection of satellite cells into injured myocardium was by Chiu and colleagues.[45] Subsequently, the utility of cell transplantation to improve myocardial performance was demonstrated.[46]

Since then, the dramatic increase in understanding of the process of cell differentiation and the therapeutic potential of stem cells has paralleled enthusiasm for myoblast transplantation in the heart—the so-called cellular cardiomyoplasty.

Autologous skeletal myoblasts offer several specific advantages for cardiac repair over other cell types. First, skeletal muscle is abundant and accessible in the body and can be harvested without causing functional disability. Second, skeletal muscle cells can be transplanted in an autologous fashion, and there is no need for immunosuppression to prevent rejection. Also, skeletal muscle is more ischemia resistant than cardiomyocytes and thus more capable of surviving in a heart afflicted by atherosclerotic coronary artery disease. Lastly, by using primary cells rather than immortalized or multipotent cells, there is a decreased likelihood of tumor formation following transplantation.

Transplanting Autologous Skeletal Muscle into Heart

Immature skeletal myoblasts tend to be plastic, as are other undifferentiated stem cells. They are harvested by culturing the cells from a skeletal muscle biopsy specimen. For example, in rabbits, 0.5 mg of soleus muscle is sufficient to begin the process, whereas in pigs, 5 mg is used. To isolate skeletal myoblasts, the tissue is dissected mechanically, then subjected to multiple stages of washing, plating, and growing until enough cells are obtained. At the time of transplantation, myoblast colonies have typically undergone three or four passages. Myoblasts are removed from the culture plates and resuspended in saline or serum albumin–containing solutions prior to injection into the heart.[47]

Cell Delivery

It is useful to discuss the current protocols for cell delivery in more detail and to discuss their limitations. Myoblasts are delivered into areas of myocardial injury by using direct intramyocardial injection. This can be accomplished via myocardial exposure (a surgical approach) or via endocardial injection (a percutaneous approach). The surgical procedure involves anesthetizing the animal (the following details are given for the rabbit) and establishing ventilatory support via intubation. Using a left thoracotomy in the fifth intercostal space, the pericardium is exposed and divided. The myocardial injury is produced by either cryoinjury or coronary artery ligation, depending on the animal model. In the rabbit model, a 1 or 1.5 cm cryoprobe is cooled to −200°C then placed on the heart between the left circumflex artery and the posterior interventricular groove for 3 min. Similar techniques are used in small animals (eg, mice), but much shorter injury times are required (Figure 44-3). During cryoinjury, electrocardiographic leads monitor ST and T wave changes (Figure 44-4).

function, and engraftment. It is unknown how myoblasts integrate into the heart and how they may affect arrhythmogenesis. Also, there is debate whether myoblasts improve function or merely prevent further myocardial deterioration. Preclinical data demonstrate that growth factors, fibroblasts, or other cells may slow the progression of heart failure or even improve diastolic function, but they do not improve systolic function, as do skeletal myoblasts.[58,59,63] The most efficacious means for cell introduction is currently unknown, and safety issues in human trials need to be addressed.

Most studies have used intramuscular injection, but intracoronary devices may be used to deliver cells to the injured area of myocardium by a percutaneous approach. The extent and consequences of the dissemination of skeletal myoblasts to extracardiac organs requires more detailed investigation, especially with regard to potential catheter-based approaches. Essentially, there are many physiologic and molecular questions that need to be answered if skeletal myoblasts, or indeed any cell types, hope to find a place in the clinical armamentarium.

Cell transplantation for cardiac repair moved into the clinic in 1999, when a French group transplanted autologous skeletal myoblasts as an adjunct to coronary artery bypass surgery (CABG). This began an open-label clinical trial in which 10 patients received cells. As indicated in Figure 44-6, even though the cells were injected into an area of the heart remote from the bypass grafts, there was evidence of contraction and viability in the transplanted region.[54] This result is encouraging, in that all patients studied to date have had some improvement in wall thickness or contractility, but we believe that much remains to be studied prior to large-scale clinical trials. As patients have been treated in surgical trials, as an adjunct to CABG and to left ventricular assist device placement and, more recently, in percutaneous trials, a picture has begun to emerge. During a "vulnerable" period that appears to range from 1 to 8 weeks post injection, 10 to 40% of patients in four safety studies appear to develop sustained ventricular tachycardia. Consequently, many of the patients who are now receiving cells are either receiving implantable cardioverter-defibrillators or antiarrhythmic therapy. Interestingly, in the patients who received implantable defibrillators, few of the devices fired.

This unfortunate consequence also appears to hold true in a fraction of patients receiving cells percutaneously. Thus, it is imperative that trials go forward carefully and consider the electrical impact of any transplanted cell. Likewise, it is important to design preclinical studies to elucidate the mechanisms of this outcome. It also points to the importance of going forward clinically only in patients where the greatest opportunity for safety is likely. As such, the introduction of skeletal myoblast transplantation into the clinical arena will most likely take place initially as an adjunct to other cardiac surgical procedures, perhaps in patients with end-stage CHF who require a "bridge" to transplantation, or as an adjunct to CABG. In fact, it appears that a large randomized surgical trial called MAGIC will commence within the year. Lagging, but also underway, is a percutaneous phase II trial in Europe and in the United States. Thus, although skeletal myoblast transplantation is considered a novel therapeutic modality and is being proposed in various clinical settings, like myocardial regeneration, vascular disease, and avascular necrosis of the femoral neck, much needs to be learned before these and other cell trials should be undertaken, since placing patients at undue risk would not be ethically responsible. Moreover, failing to learn from our gene therapy colleagues and moving ahead without careful evaluation of all the forthcoming data could doom a treatment that has been hailed as a paradigm shift in cardiovascular disease.

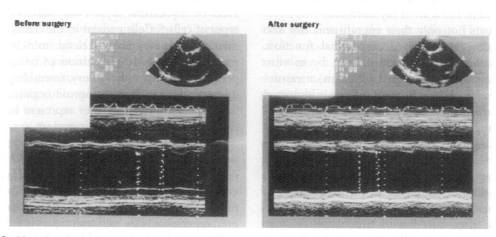

FIGURE 44-6. M-mode echocardiograms before and after surgery in humans. An increase in left ventricular posterior wall contractility occurred after myoblast transplantation. Left ventricular end diastolic dimensions did not change after surgery (70.6 mm [SD, 1.4]) compared with dimensions before surgery (68.6 mm [SD, 3.6]).

The Future of Cell Therapy for Cardiovascular Disease

The cell with optimal characteristics for cardiac engraftment and improvement of function is yet to be identified. Such a cell would have certain characteristics: (1) a high survival rate and long-term engraftment with perhaps a dose effect on improvement in function; (2) minimal associated inflammation or scar formation; (3) optimal electrical and mechanical properties; (4) co-integration with vascular structures; (5) improved cardiac remodeling; and (6) increased patient survival. Contemplating these features has led many investigators to turn toward stem cells because of the potential advantage of using undifferentiated cells that possess the ability to grow, differentiate, and engraft in vivo. However, the molecular signals responsible for controlling differentiation of a stem cell to a functional cardiomyocyte are largely unknown. More investigation is certainly warranted in this area, which may lead to the improved ability to repair the injured heart and possibly the engineering of cells with special features. The most widely studied cell type, the myoblast, shows positive effects clinically, but not without side effects. First characterizing then decreasing its risk benefit ratio are important clinical goals. Doing so may involve altering timing of injections, dosage, location, or even the patient population that receives the cells.

The proper timing of cell delivery is also largely unknown, especially in the human. Promising cell types should be tested for their ability to survive and engraft when transplanted at various times following infarction because the optimal time may vary per cell type. Factors need to be weighed against each other, such as the large amount of inflammation that occurs immediately after infarction and the decreased vascularity of the mature scar. Also in the future, cells may be engineered to produce vascular endothelial growth factor to augment angiogenesis. Other factors may also be used, such as antiapoptotic genes, antioxidants, cell-cycle control genes, or even a combination of cells to give the most efficient engraftment, electromechanical integration, and functional improvement. It must also be remembered that patients are different. We envision tailored therapy for patients with acute myocardial infarction, diffuse native or graft coronary disease, and CHF.

Cell transplantation has the potential to revolutionize the treatment of cardiovascular disease. By combining genomics, tissue engineering, and advanced imaging techniques to more thoroughly study stem cells, tissue-specific stem cells, and muscle-derived cells such as myoblasts, we will gain greater ability to positively affect outcomes in the many patients who suffer from heart disease. Properly designed clinical trials will be an integral part of this process, but much basic science remains to be done before optimal cell therapy exists for the heart.

Acknowledgments

This work was supported in part by NHLBI/NIH awards (R-01 HL-57988, HL-63346, HL-63703) to Doris A. Taylor. The authors gratefully acknowledge the mouse surgical data generated by Tao Wang, MD, Assistant Professor, Duke University Medical Center (DUMC), and also the map data obtained in collaboration with Joe Tranquillo and Craig Henriquez, MD (Biomedical Engineering, DUMC).

References

1. Soonpaa MH, Field LJ. Survey of studies examining mammalian cardiomyocyte DNA synthesis. Circ Res 1998; 83(1):15–26.
2. Anversa P, Kajstura J. Ventricular myocytes are not terminally differentiated in the adult mammalian heart. Circ Res 1998;83(1):1–14.
3. Glaser R, Lu MM, Narula N, Epstein JA. Smooth muscle cells, but not myocytes, of host origin in transplanted human hearts. Circulation 2002;106(1):17–9.
4. Laflamme MA, Myerson D, Saffitz JE, Murry CE. Evidence for cardiomyocyte repopulation by extracardiac progenitors in transplanted human hearts. Circ Res 2002; 90(6):634–40.
5. Hruban RH, Long PP, Perlman EJ, et al. Fluorescence in situ hybridization for the Y-chromosome can be used to detect cells of recipient origin in allografted hearts following cardiac transplantation. Am J Pathol 1993;142(4): 975–80.
6. Kirby M, Waldo K. Neural crest and cardiovascular patterning. Circ Res 1995;77:211–5.
7. Kirby M, Waldo K. Role of neural crest in congenital heart disease. Circulation 1990;82:332–40.
8. Mikawa T, Fischman DA. Retroviral analysis of cardiac morphogenesis: discontinuous formation of coronary vessels. Proc Natl Acad Sci U S A 1992;89:9504–8.
9. Mikawa T, Gourdie R. Pericardial mesoderm generates a population of coronary smooth muscle cells migrating into the heart along with ingrowth of the epicardial organ. Dev Biol 1996;174:221–32.
10. Lints T, Parsons L, Hartley L, et al. Nkx2–5: a novel murine homeobox gene expressed in early heart progenitor cells and their myogenic descendants. Development 1993; 119:969–76.
11. Franco D, Kelly R, Lamers WH, et al. Regionalized transcriptional domains of myosin light chain 3f transgenes in the embryonic mouse heart: morphogenetic implications. Dev Biol 1997;188:17–33.
12. O'Brien TX, Lee KJ, Chien KR. Positional specification of ventricular myosin light chain 2 expression in the primitive murine heart tube. Proc Natl Acad Sci U S A 1993; 90:5157–61.
13. Li L, Miano JM, Mercer B, Olson EN. Expression of the SM22alpha promoter in transgenic mice provides evidence for distinct transcriptional regulatory programs in vascular and visceral smooth muscle cells. J Cell Biol 1996;132:849–59.
14. Kuisk IR, Li H, Tran D, Capetanaki Y. A single MEF2 site governs desmin transcription in both heart and skeletal

muscle during mouse embryogenesis. Dev Biol 1996; 174:1–13.

15. Kuo C, Morrisey E, Anandappa R, et al. GATA4 transcription factor is required for ventral morphogenesis and heart tube formation. Genes Dev 1997;11:1048–60.

16. Molkentin J, Lin Q, Duncan S, Olson E. Requirement of the transcription factor GATA4 for heart tube formation and ventral morphogenesis. Genes Dev 1997;11:1061–72.

17. Lin Q, Schwarz J, Bucana C, Olson EN. Control of mouse cardiac morphogenesis and myogenesis by transcription factor MEF2C. Science 1997;276:1404–7.

18. Srivastava D, Cserjesi P, Olson EN. A subclass of bHLH proteins required for cardiac morphogenesis. Science 1995;270:1995–9.

19. Akli S, Zhan S, Abdellatif M, Schneider MD. E1A can provoke G1 exit that is refractory to p21 and independent of activating cdk2. Circ Res 1999;85(4):319–28.

20. Agah R, Kirshenbaum LA, Abdellatif M, et al. Adenoviral delivery of E2F-1 directs cell cycle reentry and p53-independent apoptosis in postmitotic adult myocardium in vivo. J Clin Invest 1997;100(11):2722–8.

21. Lanson NA Jr, Egeland DB, Royals BA, Claycomb WC. The MRE11-NBS1-RAD50 pathway is perturbed in SV40 large T antigen-immortalized AT-1, AT-2 and HL-1 cardiomyocytes. Nucleic Acids Res 2000;28(15):2882–92.

22. Claycomb WC, Lanson NA Jr, Stallworth BS, et al. HL-1 cells: a cardiac muscle cell line that contracts and retains phenotypic characteristics of the adult cardiomyocyte. Proc Natl Acad Sci U S A 1998;95:2979–84.

23. Daud AI, Lanson NA Jr, Claycomb WC, Field LJ. Identification of SV40 large T-antigen associated proteins in cardiomyocytes from transgenic mice. Am J Physiol 1993; 264(5 Pt 2):H1693–700.

24. Jahn L, Sadoshima J, Greene A, et al. Conditional differentiation of heart- and smooth muscle-derived cells transformed by a temperature-sensitive mutant of SV40 T antigen. J Cell Sci 1996;109 Pt 2:397–407.

25. Sen A, Dunnmon P, Henderson SA, et al. Terminally differentiated neonatal rat myocardial cells proliferate and maintain specific differentiated functions following expression of SV40 large T antigen. J Biol Chem 1988; 263(35):19132–6.

26. Koh GY, Soonpaa MH, Klug MG, Field LJ. Long-term survival of AT-1 cardiomyocyte grafts in syngeneic myocardium. Am J Physiol 1993;264(5 Pt 2):H1727–33.

27. Makino S, Fukuda K, Miyoshi S, et al. Cardiomyocytes can be generated from marrow stromal cells in vitro. J Clin Invest 1999;103:697–705.

28. Pittenger MF, Mackay AM, Beck SC, et al. Multilineage potential of adult human mesenchymal stem cells. Science 1999;284:143–7.

29. Prockop DJ. Marrow stromal cells as stem cells for non-hematopoietic tissues. Science 1997;276:71–4.

30. Kehat I, Kenyagin-Karsenti D, Snir M, et al. Human embryonic stem cells can differentiate into myocytes with structural and functional properties of cardiomyocytes. J Clin Invest 2001;108(3):407–14.

31. Reinecke H, Zhang M, Bartosek T, Murry CE. Survival, integration, and differentiation of cardiomyocyte grafts: a study in normal and injured rat hearts. Circulation 1999;100:193–202.

32. Soonpaa MH, Koh GY, Klug MG, Field LG. Formation of nascent intercalated disks between grafted cardiomyocytes and host myocardium. Science 1994;264:98–101.

33. Matsushita T, Oyamada M, Kurata H, et al. Formation of cell junctions between grafted and host cardiomyocytes at the border zone of rat myocardial infarction. Circulation 1999;100 Suppl 19:II262–8.

34. Regaud C. Etudes sur la structure des tubes seminiferes et sur la spermatogenese chez les mammiferes. Part 1. Archives d'Anatomie microscopiques et de Morphologie experimentale 1901;4:101–56.

35. Toma C, Pittenger MF, Cahill KS, et al. Human mesenchymal stem cells differentiate to a cardiomyocyte phenotype in the adult murine heart. Circulation 2002;105:93–8.

36. Jiang Y, Jahagirdar BN, Reinhardt RL, et al. Pluripotency of mesenchymal stem cells derived from adult marrow. Nature 2002;418(6893):41–9.

37. Mizuno M, Kuboki Y. TGF-beta accelerated the osteogenic differentiation of bone marrow cells induced by collagen matrix. Biochem Biophys Res Commun 1995; 211(3):1091–8.

38. Jackson KA, Majka SM, Wang H, et al. Regeneration of ischemic cardiac muscle and vascular endothelium by adult stem cells. J Clin Invest 2001;107(11):1395–402.

39. Deans RJ, Moseley AB. Mesenchymal stem cells: biology and potential clinical uses. Exp Hematol 2000;28(8):875–84.

40. Orlic D, Kajstura J, Chimenti S, et al. Bone marrow cells regenerate infarcted myocardium. Nature 2001;410: 701–5.

41. Gussoni E, Soneoka Y, Strickland CD, et al. Dystrophin expression in the mdx mouse restored by stem cell transplantation. Nature 1999;401:390–5.

42. De Angelis L, Berghella L, Coletta M, et al. Skeletal myogenic progenitors originating from embryonic dorsal aorta coexpress endothelial and myogenic markers and contribute to postnatal muscle growth and regeneration. J Cell Biol 1999;147:869–78.

43. Terada N, Hamazaki T, Oka M, et al. Bone marrow cells adopt the phenotype of other cells by spontaneous cell fusion. Nature 2002;416:542–5.

44. Ying QL, Nichols J, Evans EP, Smith AG. Changing potency by spontaneous fusion. Nature 2002;416:545–8.

45. Marelli D, Ma F, Chiu RC. Cell transplantation for myocardial repair: an experimental approach. Cell Transplant 1992;1(6):383–90.

46. Atkins BZ, Kraus WE, Glower DD, Taylor DA. Intracardiac transplantation of skeletal myoblasts yields two populations of striated cells in situ. Ann Thorac Surg 1999;67: 124–9.

47. Jain M, DerSimonian H, Brenner DA, et al. Cell therapy attenuates deleterious ventricular remodeling and improves cardiac performance after myocardial infarction. Circulation 2001;103(14):1920–7.

48. Dib N, Diethrich EB, Campbell A, et al. Endoventricular transplantation of allogenic skeletal myoblasts in a porcine model of myocardial infarction. J Endovasc Ther 2002;9(3):313–9.

49. Taylor DA, Atkins BZ, Hungspreugs P, et al. Regenerating functional myocardium: improved performance after skeletal myoblast transplantation. Nat Med 1998;4: 929–33.

50. Atkins BZ, Hueman MT, Meuchel JM, et al. Myogenic cell transplantation improves in vivo regional performance in infarcted rabbit myocardium. J Heart Lung Transplant 1999;18:1173–80.

51. Li RK, Jia ZQ, Weisel RD, et al. Smooth muscle cell transplantation into myocardial scar tissue improves heart function. J Mol Cell Cardiol 1999;31:513–22.

52. Murry CE, Wiseman RW, Schwartz SM, Hauschka SD. Skeletal myoblast transplantation for repair of myocardial necrosis. J Clin Invest 1996;98:2512–23.

53. Reinecke H, MacDonald GH, Hauschka SD, Murry CE. Electromechanical coupling between skeletal and cardiac muscle. Implications for infarct repair. J Cell Biol 2000;149(3):731–40.

54. Menasche P, Hagege AA, Scorsin M, et al. Myoblast transplantation for heart failure. Lancet 2001;357(9252):279–80.

55. Goodell MA, Jackson KA, Majka SM, et al. Stem cell plasticity in muscle and bone marrow. Ann N Y Acad Sci 2001;938:208–18; discussion 218–20.

56. Schlaeger TM, Qin Y, Fujiwara Y, et al. Vascular endothelial cell lineage-specific promoter in transgenic mice. Development 1995;121:1089–98.

57. Atkins BZ, Hueman MT, Meuchel J, et al. Cellular cardiomyoplasty improves diastolic properties of injured heart. J Surg Res 1998;85:234-42.

58. Maher J, Pandolfi PP, Roberts IA. Selection of a highly enriched population of retrovirus-infected human hematopoietic progenitor cells using SNL fibroblasts. Leukemia 1995;9:S29–33.

59. Hutcheson KA, Atkins BZ, Hueman MT, et al. Comparison of benefits on myocardial performance of cellular cardiomyoplasty with skeletal myoblasts and fibroblasts. Cell Transplant 2000;9:359–68.

60. Ogawa E, Saito Y, Harada M. Outside-in signalling of fibronectin stimulates cardiomyocyte hypertrophy in cultured neonatal rat ventricular myocytes. J Mol Cell Cardiol 2000;32:765–76.

61. Van Meter CH Jr, Claycomb WC, Delcarpio JB, et al. Myoblast transplantation in the porcine model: a potential technique for myocardial repair. J Thorac Cardiovasc Surg 1995;110(5):1442–8.

62. Robinson SW, Cho PW, Levitsky HI, et al. Arterial delivery of genetically labeled skeletal myoblasts to the murine heart: long-term survival and phenotypic modification of implanted myoblasts. Cell Transplant 1996;5(1):77–91.

63. Li RK, Jia ZQ, Weisel RD, et al. Survival and function of bioengineered cardiac grafts. Circulation 1999;100 Suppl 19:II63–9.

CHAPTER 45

SKELETAL MUSCLE VENTRICLES

ZULFIKAR A. SHARIF, MD, LARRY W. STEPHENSON, MD

More than a half million people in the United States were diagnosed with heart failure in the year 2002. Of those half million people, nearly 50% will die within 1 year. At present, there are only a few treatment options available for these patients. Medical therapy remains the first line of treatment. However, many patients will continue to deteriorate despite maximum medical therapy. Heart transplantation is limited by high cost and a continued shortage of organs. The remaining option is artificial cardiac assistance. Currently, there are several mechanical pumps being assessed clinically. However, these pumps are limited by the need for continued anticoagulation and a significant risk of stroke and infection.

Energy derived from the contraction of skeletal muscle has been used experimentally and clinically to augment native heart function. Skeletal muscle is capable of efficient transformation of chemical energy into mechanical work. Investigators have shown that it is possible to transform a fatigue-sensitive skeletal muscle into a fatigue-resistant muscle capable of repeated contractions over a sustained period of time. Investigators have used this transformed muscle in an attempt to assist the heart and circulation in a number of novel ways.

Two methods of skeletal muscle cardiac assist—cardiomyoplasty and aortomyoplasty—are currently being used clinically and are discussed elsewhere in this textbook. Cardiomyoplasty involves wrapping the latissimus dorsi muscle around the cardiac ventricles and stimulating the muscle during cardiac systole in an attempt to assist the failing heart. Aortomyoplasty requires that skeletal muscle be wrapped around the aorta and stimulated during diastole to unload the failing ventricle.

This chapter discusses a third approach to skeletal muscle cardiac assistance that uses skeletal muscle ventricles (SMVs), which so far has only been used in laboratory animals. In contrast to the procedures already mentioned, separate pumping chambers are constructed from the muscle and then connected to the circulation in various ways as auxiliary blood pumps.

Early Skeletal Muscle Investigations

Early Functional and Histologic Studies

Rather than using a muscle applied directly to the heart to augment function, our laboratory has focused on the use of pumping chambers constructed from skeletal muscle. These chambers have been constructed from a variety of muscles, including the rectus abdominis, diaphragm, quadriceps femoris, pectoralis major, gluteus maximus, psoas, and latissimus dorsi. We prefer the latissimus dorsi because of its relatively large size, ease in harvesting, single major nerve and blood supply, limited disability associated with mobilization, and anatomic proximity to the heart.

Our current model has evolved over several years after overcoming many obstacles. Cardiac muscle cells are relatively uniform and contract rhythmically over a lifetime without fatiguing. Skeletal muscle, on the other hand, consists of two histologically different types of fibers. Slow-twitch (type I) fibers are relatively fatigue resistant. They contract over a longer duration, develop less tension, and have a longer latency period. The metabolism of these fibers relies primarily on aerobic, oxidative phosphorylation pathways. Fast-twitch (type II) fibers, in contrast, contract over a shorter duration and develop greater peak tension. Their metabolism relies primarily on anaerobic, glycolytic pathways, and they are much more prone to fatigue than type I fibers.

Most muscles are composed of a combination of fiber types, although some muscles have a very high percentage of one type or the other. For example, the postural muscles, such as the soleus and paraspinous muscles, must maintain prolonged contraction and consist of predominantly slow-twitch fibers. In contrast, the extraocular muscles are specialized for sudden, short-term movements and are made up primarily of fast-twitch fibers.

In 1960, Buller, Eccles, and Eccles investigated whether the fiber type was determined by the muscle itself or was influenced by its neural innervation. In their experiments in cats, they switched the motor nerve to the soleus muscle, composed primarily of slow-twitch fibers, with the motor nerve from the flexor digitorum longus muscle, composed predominantly of fast-twitch fibers.[1] After allowing time for nerve regeneration, they found that the slow-twitch soleus muscle was converted to a fast-twitch muscle, whereas the opposite was true of the flexor digitorum muscle.

Salmons and Vrbova discovered, in 1969, that it was the nerve's pattern of electrical stimulation that affected the muscle's functional characteristics.[2] By delivering a continuous low-frequency stimulation to fast-twitch muscle, they were able to show consistent conversion to slow-twitch muscle. Complete transformation required several weeks of stimulation.

Several investigators then studied the functional characteristics of these transformed muscles and found the physiologic, biochemical, and morphologic characteristics of the muscle to be fundamentally changed to those of slow-twitch muscle fibers. The mitochondrial volume density increases, as does the activity of the enzymes involved in aerobic substrate oxidation. The activity of the anaerobic enzymes consequently decreases. There is also a decrease in the cytosolic Ca^{2+} binding, Ca^{2+} sequestration, and a transformation of the sarcoplasmic reticulum membranes. The functional contractile properties of the muscle become transformed as well.[3–5]

Initial Experimental Attempts Using Skeletal Muscle for Cardiac Assistance

In 1959, Kantrowitz attempted to augment the circulation by wrapping the left leaf of the canine diaphragm around the descending aorta.[6,7] The diaphragm was then stimulated via the phrenic nerve to contract in diastole. In these animals, the mean arterial pressure was increased by 26 mm Hg and the mean diastolic pressure was increased by 15 mm Hg. However, the muscle rapidly fatigued over several cardiac cycles.

In 1964, Kusserow was the first to report on the use of skeletal muscle to power a mechanical assist device.[8] He used the rectus femoris muscle to squeeze a bellows-type pump, which was then connected to a hydraulic circuit that allowed the calculation of flow and determination of outflow resistance. These pumps were capable of generating flows of 600 to 720 mL/min against a 20 mm Hg afterload.

In 1975, Vachon and colleagues constructed pumping chambers from denervated pedicle grafts of the diaphragm.[9] They wrapped these around a fluid-filled balloon pressure transducer, which allowed them to vary the outflow resistance while measuring flow, power output, and isovolumic pressure-volume relations. These pedicle grafts were stimulated with electrodes sewn directly into the substance of the muscle. The grafts were able to generate up to 176 mm Hg pressure at a stimulation voltage of 30 volts. They showed that the pressure obtained was proportional to the stimulation voltage and calculated the power output of these grafts to be just over the power output of the right ventricle. However, the muscle fatigued rapidly.

Diaphragmatic pouches were also constructed by Von Recum and co-workers in 1977.[10] These pouches were also stimulated directly. Like the other investigators, they found that the chambers fatigued rapidly within the first several hours. The decline in pressure generation was progressive over the duration of the experiment.

Conditioned Skeletal Muscle Experimentation

In 1982, Macoviak, like Salmons and Vrbova earlier, reported that the continuous stimulation of the canine diaphragm at 10 Hz for 5 weeks resulted in a near complete transformation of the muscle to slow-twitch fatigue-resistant fibers.[11] This was done using an electrode placed directly into the muscle, and the greatest degree of transformation was found close to the electrode. He also showed, however, that a similar degree of transformation could be accomplished with a 2 Hz stimulation frequency. Armenti later showed that by stimulating the phrenic nerve itself, it was possible to transform the entire hemidiaphragm.[12]

The experiments by Macoviak and Armenti were important for three reasons. First, they showed that skeletal muscle could be converted to slow-twitch muscle at only 2 Hz (120 stimuli per min), which would seem much more physiologic than 10 Hz (600 stimuli per min). If chronic stimulation of the muscle is discontinued, the muscle reverts back to its original fiber type over several weeks. Thus, these experiments suggested that a muscle could be transformed and maintain its fatigue resistance while chronically contracting as a cardiac assist device at rates similar to the animal's own heart rate. Second, these experiments indicated that it was more practical to transform skeletal muscle by stimulating its motor nerve as opposed to stimulating the muscle directly. Third, these were the first experiments conducted using fatigue resistant slow-twitch muscle with cardiac assist in mind.

In 1986, Mannion reported that stimulating the latissimus dorsi muscle with either 2 Hz or 10 Hz electrical stimulation resulted in similar increases in fatigue-resistance, but that the 2 Hz stimulation resulted in less decrease in fiber diameter.[13] Clark and Acker then used phosphorous-31 nuclear magnetic resonance (^{31}P-NMR) to show that the conditioned latissimus dorsi muscle has a capacity for oxidative phosphorylation similar to that of the heart.[14]

The effects of burst stimulation have also been investigated. Stimulation of skeletal muscle with a single electrical stimulus results in generation of a single twitch, which by itself is not effective for cardiac assistance. By using an appropriately timed train of stimuli, it is possible to achieve mechanical summation of motor units and generation of a prolonged and significant muscle contraction.

This is referred to as burst stimulation and is typically used to stimulate skeletal muscle for cardiac assist at frequencies of 25 to 35 Hz but sometimes as high as 85 Hz.

The effects of prolonged burst stimulation on the physiologic and histochemical properties of the latissimus dorsi muscle were studied over a 1-year period. Burst cycles causing muscle contractions in the range of 54 to 120 per min were studied. During each contraction cycle, the muscle was typically stimulated in a burst fashion for 25 to 33% of each contraction cycle. In all cases, the burst stimulation frequency was kept at 25 Hz. At 1 year, there was no evidence of muscle fiber damage, no loss of fatigue resistance, and no change in the properties of nerve conduction.[15]

Skeletal Muscle Ventricle Construction

Our laboratory has used the latissimus dorsi muscle of dogs for construction of the SMV. Both the right and left latissimi have been used, depending on the type of assist to be performed. The operation is begun by making an incision from the axilla to the tip of the eleventh rib. The overlying platysma and soft tissue are elevated from the muscle. The attachments to the eleventh and twelfth rib are then incised. The attachment along the posterior spinous processes is then incised, taking care to include a wide margin of thoracodorsal fascia. The underlying collateral blood vessels from the chest wall are then divided. The muscle is fully mobilized up to its humeral attachment, taking care to avoid injury to the neurovascular pedicle.

The thoracodorsal nerve is encircled with a bipolar nerve lead, which is then connected to a nerve stimulator and placed in a subcutaneous pocket over the rectus abdominis muscle. Next, a thoracotomy at the fifth intercostal space is performed to harvest the pericardium, which will line the inner surface of the SMV. The pericardium is then sutured to a Dacron cuff that encircles a plastic mandrel, and the chest is closed. The muscle is wrapped around the mandrel, anchored by the Dacron cuff. Generally, one to two wraps of the muscle are obtained. The thoracodorsal fascia is oriented so that this firm tissue is sewn to the Dacron cuff. Absorbable sutures are then used to secure the layers of the muscle and to close the end of the muscle to form the apex of the pumping chamber. The chamber is then sewn to the surrounding tissue. The SMV has thus been either anchored in the subcutaneous tissue on the chest wall or placed in an intrathoracic position after excision of several ribs.

After mobilization of the muscle, there is relative ischemia in the distal portion. This portion is not able to increase its blood flow in response to the increased demands of stimulation. Mannion and colleagues showed that over the next 3 to 4 weeks, the muscle gradually recovers its ability to increase its blood flow in response to stimulation. We refer to this 3- to 4-week period as the period of vascular delay.[13,16]

The muscle is allowed to recover during this vascular delay period and is then stimulated at 2 Hz continuously over the next 5 to 7 weeks. Following this period of electrical conditioning, the muscle of the SMV has become fatigue resistant and can be used to assist the native heart in a variety of configurations. A second operative procedure is then performed whereby the mandrel is extracted and the SMV is connected to the circulation. A ventricular sensing lead is placed on the myocardium, and the SMV is stimulated to contract synchronously with the heart, using an implantable cardiomyostimulator.

Skeletal Muscle Ventricles as Cardiac Assist Devices

Aortic Diastolic Counterpulsators

The following configuration represents the model most studied in our laboratory. The SMV is connected to the circulation using the bifurcated graft that is anastomosed to the base of the SMV and then to two locations on the descending thoracic aorta. The aorta is ligated between the two limbs of the graft to obligate blood flow through the circuit. A myocardial lead is then used to sense the electrical activity of the native ventricle, and an implantable cardiomyostimulator is used to synchronize contraction to occur in cardiac diastole (Figure 45-1). The contraction of the SMV during cardiac diastole has several useful purposes. First, blood is pumped proximally and distally from

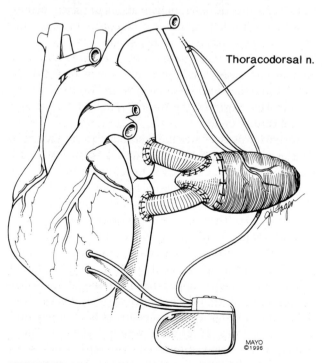

FIGURE 45-1. Skeletal muscle ventricle (SMV) as diastolic counterpulsator. The SMV is connected to the descending aorta by a bifurcated graft. The aorta is ligated between the limbs of the graft to obligate flow through the SMV.

the descending aorta to the periphery. Second, because the coronary arteries are perfused during diastole, there is an increase in coronary artery flow. Finally, relaxation of the SMV chamber at the end of diastole provides a low-pressure system into which the native heart is able to eject, decreasing the energy required for the heart to pump blood, thereby decreasing the heart's oxygen consumption. These hemodynamic improvements are similar to those produced with an intra-aortic balloon pump. Representative figure tracings are shown in Figure 45-2.

Early acute experiments showed that electrically preconditioned SMVs were able to generate a power output of 0.68×10^6 erg, which was approximately half the power output of the native left ventricle and roughly three times the power output of the right ventricle.[17] In 1987, Acker reported on experiments involving five dogs that had SMVs constructed with a modification of the SMV design.[18] These chambers had a cylindrical geometry with inflow and outflow at opposite ends of the chamber. The SMVs were then monitored over time while pumping blood continuously in the circulation. These chambers functioned as diastolic counterpulsators for up to 11 weeks. During periodic measurements of SMV function, the burst frequency was increased from the chronic 25 Hz setting to 43 Hz and then to 85 Hz. These pumps improved aortic flow by 29%, 40%, and 63% at 25, 43, and 85 Hz of thoracodorsal nerve stimulation, respec-

tively. Two-dimensional short-axis echocardiograms of the SMV chambers were obtained; they showed a 70%, 90%, and 100% decrease in the cross-sectional area at the midpoint of the SMV as the burst stimulation frequency increased. The decrease in cross-sectional area was somewhat similar to the ejection function of the SMV. These chambers, however, were prone to thrombus formation, and although all animals had a functional SMV at the time of death, the two longest-surviving animals, 5 and 11 weeks, demonstrated multiple splenic and renal infarctions at the time of autopsy. Neither animal, however, showed evidence of cerebral or coronary embolization.

Over the past decade, modifications in the diastolic counterpulsator model have allowed for improvements in survival. In 1992, Mocek reported on a series of four dogs that survived for more than 6 months with an SMV pumping continuously in circulation.[19] One animal from this series survived for 836 days but showed evidence of some thrombus formation within the chamber at the time of death.

The use of autologous pericardium as a blood-SMV surface lining was then investigated as a possible method of decreasing the incidence of thrombosis. The animal's pericardium was removed at the time of the initial construction of the SMV and wrapped around the mandrel before the muscle wrap was applied. The tissue was oriented so that the inner surface of the pericardium was in

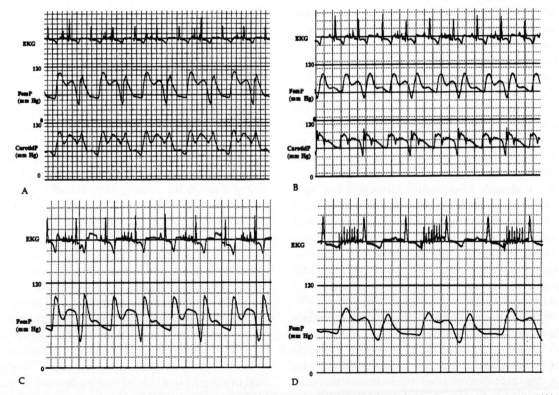

FIGURE 45-2. Pressure and electrocardiographic tracings recorded from the longest surviving animal at the time of connection (A), and after 1 year (B), 2 years (C), and 4 years (D) in the circulation. Stimulation burst frequency is 33 Hz at a 1:2 assist ratio. Carotid P = pressure measured at the carotid artery; Fem P = blood pressure measured at the femoral artery.

contact with the plastic mandrel. When the mandrel was removed several weeks later and the SMV connected to the circulation at the second operation, the blood came in contact with the inner surface of the pericardium. Interestingly, there was no thrombosis noted in either the group with autologous lining or the control group (constructed with the inner layer of the muscle serving as the contact surface for the circulatory blood flow). However, the group with the autologous lining demonstrated a significantly reduced rate of rupture. Sixty-three percent of the SMVs in the control group ruptured over time, as compared to 0% in the group with autologous lining. These investigators concluded that the autologous pericardium improved the structural integrity of the pumping chamber.[20] One animal in the group was electively sacrificed after continuously pumping blood for more than 4 years. To our knowledge, this represents the longest reported survival—clinical or experimental—with a functioning, indwelling cardiac assist device of any type.

Thomas also demonstrated that it is possible to line these chambers with autologous endothelial cells and to retain the endothelial surface while the SMV pumps blood in the arterial circulation. The animal's own jugular vein was used to obtain endothelial cells. After the cells were harvested and grown in culture, the suspended cells were then delivered into the space between the muscle itself and the plastic mandrel at a separate surgical procedure.[21] After allowing several weeks for the endothelial cells to grow and attach, a confluent monolayer of endothelial cells was histologically shown to be present on the inner surface of the pumping chambers. This group also demonstrated that this same result could be obtained by percutaneously injecting the suspended endothelial cells into the space around the mandrel.[22] Finally, they showed that this endothelial cell layer was retained after the SMV had pumped blood in the arterial circulation for 3 h.[23] We believe that this is the first report of the endothelium remaining intact on the surface of a heart assist device while the device pumps blood in the circulation.

The aortic diastolic counterpulsator model has been and continues to be investigated in the setting of heart failure.[24] Because blood supply to the SMV muscle itself may be impaired in the setting of low cardiac output, the possibility of impaired SMV hemodynamic function exists. Propranolol was used to induce heart failure, and it was shown that the percentage improvement in several hemodynamic parameters in this setting was actually better than without propranolol with the SMV functioning. Mean diastolic pressure increased 27.6%, as compared to a 12.9% increase in the same group of SMVs before the induction of heart failure. The endocardial viability ratio, a ratio of myocardial oxygen delivery to myocardial oxygen demand, also increased 28.7% in the setting of heart failure, versus an 11.2% increase before heart failure

induction. However, these studies were performed in an acute setting over 1 h, and the animal's cardiac output promptly returned to normal upon discontinuation of the propranolol.

Currently, our laboratory is using a stable chronic heart failure model that allows evaluation of the function of SMVs in the setting of chronic low cardiac output. We use the rapid ventricular pacing (RVP) technique in conjunction with the aortic diastolic counterpulsator model. Patel examined six dogs with pericardium-lined SMVs created from latissimus dorsi muscles. Each SMV was anastomosed to the descending thoracic aorta with a two-limbed bifurcated polytetrafluoroethylene (PTFE) graft after the usual electrical conditioning period, and the aorta was ligated between the limbs. The SMV was stimulated to contract during diastole at a 1:2 to 1:3 ratio. Chronic heart failure was then induced over the next 7 weeks with the initiation of rapid ventricular pacing at 220 to 230 bpm. SMV contraction resulted in augmentation of the diastolic pressure–time index (DPTI) by 12.1% prior to initiation of RVP and by 33.6% after 7 weeks of RVP.[25] The rapid ventricular pacemaker was turned off temporarily during measurement of left ventricle function, while the SMV was appropriately stimulated with the cardiomyostimulator to again contract synchronously with the heart in a 1:2 or 1:3 ratio. In addition, significant afterload reduction was demonstrated, with increases in peak left ventricular ejection velocity of 22.7% and stroke volume of 6.2%. In three of the six animals, coronary blood flow was measured directly with a coronary artery Doppler flow probe, and flow was shown to be augmented by an average of 47.6%.

Left-Heart Bypass

Hooper and colleagues constructed SMVs and connected the left atrium to the SMV and the SMV to the aorta by using two valved conduits.[26] In this parallel circuit model, the left atrial pressure served as the preload for the SMV. A portion of the systemic cardiac output that would normally have been pumped by the left ventricle (LV) was routed through the parallel SMV circuit and pumped by the contraction of the SMV. Thus, the work required by the native heart was decreased even though the net blood flow produced by the LV and SMV were similar to control. The SMVs in this configuration, as in the aortic diastolic counterpulsator model, are stimulated to contract during diastole because contraction during systole would result in the SMV attempting to eject against an afterload equal to the systolic pressure generated by the LV. Acute experiments over 3 h by Hooper showed that the SMV was able to pump between 21 and 27% of the cardiac output. Although these results showed promise, we have not pursued this model in a chronic setting because of our observation that higher SMV preloads seem to be necessary for optimal SMV performance.

Left Ventricular Apex-to-Aorta Model

In terms of hemodynamic augmentation, the left ventricular apex-to-aorta model is a highly effective experimental model for ventricular assistance, both in vivo and via computer model.[27] This model involves construction of a SMV that is connected in circulation by two valved conduits (Figure 45-3). One conduit is placed from the apex of the left ventricle to the SMV, and the other joins the SMV to the descending thoracic aorta. This model makes use of the higher pressure generated by the left ventricle to serve as preload for the SMV. In addition, when the SMV relaxes and the left ventricle ejects into this low-pressure system, the left ventricle is effectively "unloaded." Figure 45-4 shows representative hemodynamic tracings of this model after 1 year of functioning in circulation.

The blood flow to the muscle layers of the SMV is also likely to be improved in the left ventricular apex-to-aorta configuration when compared to that of the aortic diastolic counterpulsator model. With the left ventricular apex-to-aorta model, there is a substantial period of time during which the pressure inside the SMV itself is much lower than the systemic diastolic pressure. In contrast, with the aortic diastolic counterpulsator model, the walls of the pumping chamber are always exposed to a pressure at least equal to the systemic arterial pressure, which could potentially cause problems with impaired blood flow to the SMV muscle layers.

Initially, acute 3 h experiments were performed; they showed significant improvement in the systolic tension–time index, a measure of myocardial oxygen demand, when the SMV was pumping.[28] The endocardial viability

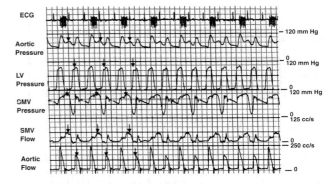

FIGURE 45-4. Hemodynamic recording obtained after 1 year in circulation from a canine with an SMV positioned between the LV apex and the aorta. The SMV is contracting at a 1:2 ratio with the native heart and stimulated at a 33 Hz burst frequency. Arrows indicate effects of SMV contraction in the pressure and flow traces. ECG = electrocardiogram; LV = left ventricle; SMV = skeletal muscle ventricle.

ratio was also significantly improved. At the time of implant and at 1, 2, and 3 h in circulation, the ratio was increased by 68%, 66%, 62%, and 63%, respectively. The SMV circuit in these acute studies pumped 47% of the cardiac output. Stevens and colleagues demonstrated a 31% increase in cardiac output in chronic heart failure in dogs with a left ventricular apex-to-aorta SMV of their own design and constructed from the rectus abdominis muscle.[29]

Subsequently, Thomas documented an SMV in a left ventricular apex-to-aorta configuration that was electively sacrificed after functioning well for 1 year.[30] In a chronic heart failure study, skeletal muscle ventricles were constructed from the latissimus dorsi muscle in 10 dogs. After conditioning, the SMVs were connected to the left ventricle and aorta with two valved conduits, and the SMV was programmed to contract during diastole. At the time of implantation, SMVs stimulated at 33 Hz and in a 1:2 ratio with the heart significantly decreased left ventricular work by 56% at 33 Hz and by 65% at 50 Hz. At a 1:2 ratio, the power output of the SMVs was 59% of left ventricular power output at 33 Hz and 93% at 50 Hz (Figure 45-5). Animals survived 7, 11, 16, 17, 72, 99, 115, 214, and 248 days. Three deaths were directly related to the SMV. In the animal that survived 248 days, SMV power output at 8 months with a 33 Hz stimulation frequency and a 1:2 contraction ratio was 57% of left ventricular power output and 82% at 50 Hz. At a 1:1 contraction ratio, SMV power output was 97% and 173% of the left ventricle, at 33 and 50 Hz, respectively (Figure 45-6).

This study demonstrated that SMVs in a LV apex-to-aorta configuration are able to function effectively in the circulation. Maintenance of significant power output was confirmed in one animal at the 8-month follow-up. Skeletal muscle ventricles significantly unloaded the left ventricle, resulting in decreases in the LV peak pressure, LV

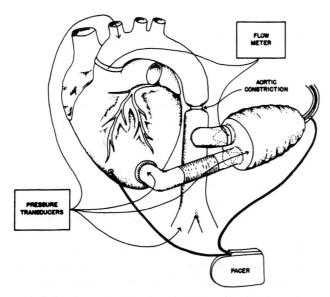

FIGURE 45-3. Skeletal muscle ventricle (SMV) in left ventricular apex-to-aorta configuration. Two valved conduits are connected to the left ventricular apex and the descending thoracic aorta. A 50% aortic constriction was created proximal to the SMV–aortic anastomosis to achieve a slight pressure gradient in the aorta to allow some passive flow through the system, reducing the chances of thrombosis.

CHAPTER 46

MECHANICAL DEVICES FOR TEMPORARY CARDIAC SUPPORT

FRANCIS D. PAGANI, MD, MS, KEITH D. AARONSON, MD, MS

Indications for Device Support and Patient Selection

The goal of temporary mechanical circulatory support (MCS) is to restore normal hemodynamics and oxygen delivery in patients in whom the heart can no longer pump blood to meet oxygen requirements commensurate with the needs of the body. There are no absolute hemodynamic criteria to meet in order to initiate temporary MCS; therefore, appropriate judgment is required to select the proper patients and timing of device intervention. Evidence of cardiogenic shock manifest by a cardiac index < 2.0 L/min/m², systolic blood pressure < 90 mm Hg, pulmonary capillary wedge pressure > 20 mm Hg, with evidence of poor tissue perfusion, reflected by oliguria, rising serum creatinine and liver transaminases, acidosis, mental status changes, and cool extremities, despite the use of optimal pharmacologic therapy, are guidelines to initiate temporary MCS. When patients reach this degree of hemodynamic compromise, the risk of death is substantial. Clinical situations in which temporary MCS is indicated may also include subtle, progressive organ dysfunction despite inotropic therapy in a patient with chronically low cardiac output awaiting heart transplantation, even though hemodynamic parameters may not have significantly changed. Patients with refractory ventricular arrhythmias or life-threatening coronary anatomy with unstable angina not amenable to revascularization, and who are at risk of imminent death (hours, days, or weeks), may be considered for temporary MCS without necessarily meeting hemodynamic criteria.

Patient selection is, perhaps, the single most crucial factor in determining a successful outcome in patients who receive temporary MCS. The patient's history and overall clinical setting are considered in the decision process to initiate MCS. Patients should not be considered for temporary MCS if they have significant contraindications to MCS or if they have significant contraindications to heart transplantation in situations where they are unlikely to wean from temporary MCS after it has been initiated. The presence of irreversible renal, hepatic, or respiratory failure is an absolute contraindication to initiating MCS. Neurologic dysfunction with significant cognitive deficits and the presence of sepsis are additional contraindications to initiating temporary MCS.

Increasing degrees of chronic organ dysfunction also present relative contraindications to initiating MCS. Chronic pulmonary disease associated with significantly impaired pulmonary reserve and systemic oxygenation can contribute to perioperative hypoxia and pulmonary vasoconstriction resulting in right-sided circulatory failure. Patients with severe chronic pulmonary disease may have a fixed (not responsive to pulmonary artery vasodilators) elevation of the pulmonary vascular resistance. A pulmonary vascular resistance > 4 Wood units that is not reversible represents a contraindication to heart transplantation, and thus to temporary MCS, in circumstances where weaning is unlikely. Moderate elevation in pulmonary vascular resistance can be encountered in patients with cardiogenic shock and does not preclude successful use of MCS if reversibility of the pulmonary vascular resistance is documented during initial therapy with inotropes or pulmonary vasodilators. MCS in some instances, however, has been effective in reducing pulmonary vascular resistance in patients previously found to have elevations in their pulmonary vascular resistance not readily responsive to inotropic or vasodilator therapy.

Acute renal failure requiring dialysis is a relative contraindication to initiating MCS. In the setting of cardiogenic shock with acute renal failure, establishing normal hemodynamics with MCS may resolve the renal failure in a relatively short period of time. Thus, the degree and duration of cardiogenic shock, along with the patient's baseline renal function, must be considered in estimating the probability of recovery of renal function. This is important in considering whether the patient will be a transplant candidate or not, in the event that native heart function does not recover while the patient is supported on MCS.[1] Similarly, improvement in hepatic congestion and recovery of synthetic functions of the liver can occur with institution of MCS. The presence of portal hypertension or liver cirrhosis absolute contraindication to initiating MCS, and liver biopsy may be indicated to definitively rule out significant parenchymal fibrosis.

Numerous studies investigating the adverse prognostic factors influencing outcomes following institution of MCS have consistently demonstrated that progressive degrees of organ dysfunction are associated with poor outcome.[2-5] These observations led to the development of risk stratification models.[2] Specifically, the need for mechanical ventilation, oliguria (urine output less than 30 cc/h), preoperative right-sided circulatory failure manifest as an elevated central venous pressure greater than 16 mm Hg, liver dysfunction as measured by a prothrombin time greater than 16 s, and increasing serum creatinine and bilirubin levels are adverse prognostic risk factors for survival following initiation of MCS.[2-5]

In addition to organ dysfunction, other patient factors or clinical settings that have been associated with adverse outcomes include acute myocardial infarction, prior sternotomy, postcardiotomy setting, and advancing age.[3-5] Age may represent an absolute contraindication to initiating temporary MCS if the patient is unlikely to wean and is too old to qualify for heart transplantation. Data from the American Society of Artificial Internal Organs – International Society of Heart and Lung Transplantation registry have demonstrated that although patients older than 70 years of age have a decreased survival on extracorporeal MCS, the probability of weaning from MCS is not affected by age.[6,7] The adverse risk of advancing age is also observed for patients receiving implantable left ventricular assist devices (LVADs).[4]

Timing the initiation of temporary MCS is also crucial to patient outcome. In the setting of postcardiotomy shock, data from the Abiomed BVS 5000 registry demonstrate that delay in initiating temporary MCS for more than 6 h after the initial weaning from cardiopulmonary bypass is associated with a significant decrease in survival (44% versus 14%).[7,8] Early initiation of extracorporeal MCS, based on predictive models for device need that use hemodynamic parameters and degree of intraoperative inotropic support, demonstrates improved rates of weaning and survival to hospital discharge.[9] Delay in instituting MCS also increases the need for biventricular support as opposed to univentricular support alone. Patients requiring biventricular support have a decreased survival.[6,7] As the severity of illness and organ dysfunction increases, patients are more likely to require biventricular support.[10,11] An episode of cardiac arrest prior to the initiation of MCS significantly reduces survival (47% versus 7%).[7,8]

Selection of the appropriate MCS device is also critical to successful outcome and is dependent on a number of factors. These factors include the etiology of the circulatory failure, the duration of expected support, whether biventricular or univentricular support is required, whether combined cardiac and pulmonary failure is present, the size of the patient, the intended use for the device, and current US Food and Drug Administration (FDA) restrictions and regulations for a particular device (Table 46-1). Consideration of all these factors help define the end point of therapy, which may include bridge to recovery or bridge to heart transplantation. There are currently two groups of patients in whom temporary MCS is beneficial and for whom FDA-approved devices exist for those specified indications. The first group consists of those patients who have sustained reversible myocardial injury and for whom there is reasonable expectation that the myocardial function will recover over a short period of support (generally less than 2 weeks). Examples of reversible forms of myocardial injury may include acute myocardial infarction, acute viral myocarditis, and postcardiotomy shock with failure to wean from cardiopulmonary bypass. Under these circumstances there are several types of devices that can be used, including intraaortic balloon pump; extracorporeal ventricular assist devices, either pulsatile or nonpulsatile; and extracorporeal membrane oxygenation (ECMO). The second group of patients are those in whom myocardial function is unlikely to recover (long-standing ischemic, valvular, or idiopathic end-stage heart failure;

TABLE 46-1. Classification and Indications of Mechanical Circulatory Support Devices

Pump Type	Application	Intended Duration of Support*	Flow Characteristics	Pump Location
Intraaortic balloon pump	Left ventricular	Short-term	—	—
ECMO	Biventricular/pulmonary	Short-term	Nonpulsatile, centrifugal	Extracorporeal
Centrifugal pumps and circuit	Biventricular	—	Nonpulsatile, centrifugal	Extracorporeal
TandemHeart pVAD	Left ventricular	Short-term	Nonpulsatile, centrifugal	Extracorporeal
AB-180	Left ventricular	Short-term	Nonpulsatile, centrifugal	Implantable
Thoratec VAS	Biventricular	Short- or long-term	Pulsatile	Extracorporeal
Abiomed BVS 5000	Biventricular	Short-term	Pulsatile	Extracorporeal
HeartMate IP1000 LVAS	Left ventricular	Long-term	Pulsatile	Implantable
HeartMate VE LVAS	Left ventricular	Long-term	Pulsatile	Implantable
HeartMate XVE LVAS	Left ventricular	Long-term	Pulsatile	Implantable
Novacor LVAS	Left ventricular	Long-term	Pulsatile	Implantable
CardioWest	Total artificial heart	Long-term	Pulsatile	Implantable

ECMO = extracorporeel membrane oxygenator; LVAS = left ventricular assist device; VAS = ventricular assist system.
* Short-term (duration of support generally less than 2 weeks).

severe acute myocardial infarction) and who require temporary MCS as a bridge to heart transplantation. Long-term circulatory support devices that are implantable and permit greater patient mobility, rehabilitation, and discharge to home are more appropriate under these circumstances. In the near future, an additional group of patients with the potential for myocardial recovery may be considered for temporary MCS. These patients include those in whom long-term MCS (weeks to months) may be required for ventricular remodeling and recovery from various types of cardiomyopathies.[12] Anecdotal observations from the cumulative experience with long-term temporary MCS for bridge to heart transplantation indication and recent small clinical studies demonstrate that long-term MCS (weeks to months), associated with sustained mechanical unloading of the left ventricle, can improve myocardial function in those patients thought to have irreversible, dilated, end-stage cardiomyopathies.[13,14] In selected patients, device explant with sustained improvement in myocardial function has been observed.[13,14] Several studies demonstrate that long-term MCS can restore ventricular geometry; improve myocyte function, orientation, and size; reduce the prevalence of myocyte apoptosis; and reduce myocardial tumor necrosis factor (TNF)-α gene and protein expression as well as decrease matrix metalloproteinases and associated collagen damage.[15–18] Upregulation of SERCA2a, ryanodine receptor, and sarcolemmal Na^+-Ca^{2+} exchanger also occurs in association with the improvement in the force–frequency relationship of left ventricular trabeculae from patients on long-term MCS.[19] Long-term mechanical unloading reportedly restores β-adrenergic responsiveness and reverses β-receptor downregulation of the failing human heart, in addition to reversing abnormal neurohormonal patterns associated with advanced heart failure, and improving myocardial mitochondrial function.[20,21] These observations have led clinicians to consider MCS, alone or in conjunction with other future possible therapies (gene therapy, myocyte implantation), as a potential modality to reverse end-stage cardiomyopathy. However, to date, only a few patients have successfully been weaned following chronic MCS.[22] Whether this reflects the true potential of recovering chronically dysfunctional hearts or reflects our current level of lack of understanding of markers to predict recovery or how to properly support and wean patients is unknown.

Considerations in Instituting Temporary Mechanical Circulatory Support

Valvular Heart Disease

Abnormalities of the cardiac valves have important adverse consequences in patients being considered for MCS and may require repair or replacement in order to initiate successful MCS or achieve weaning from support.[23] Mild to moderate aortic stenosis in the absence of insufficiency is not a contraindication to placement of a ventricular assist device. However, severe aortic stenosis should be corrected prior to placement of a ventricular assist device, preferably with a bioprosthetic valve, to facilitate future weaning or optimize native heart function in the event of device failure. The presence of even mild to moderate aortic insufficiency can have a significant impact on the effectiveness of ventricular assist devices. In the cases in which left ventricular assistance is initiated with left atrial-to-aortic cannulation, aortic insufficiency will result in left ventricular distension in the presence of significant left ventricular dysfunction. Left ventricular distension adversely affects subendocardial blood flow and can ultimately prevent weaning from MCS. In cases in which left ventricular assistance is initiated with devices that require left ventricular apical-to-aortic cannulation, reductions in left ventricular pressure elicited by mechanical assistance increase the pressure gradient across the aortic valve and increase the degree of aortic insufficiency. Thus, blood pumped into the aortic root by the device will flow backward across the incompetent aortic valve (aortic insufficiency), thereby decreasing net forward flow and compromising end-organ perfusion. Even mild to moderate aortic insufficiency may become severe with initiation of MCS from a left ventricular assist device because the elevated left ventricular end diastolic pressure will be significantly reduced by emptying of the left ventricular cavity by the device, and the aortic root pressure will be elevated above baseline because of device flow. The significance of the regurgitant volume of blood can easily be determined by measuring cardiac output with a thermodilution catheter and comparing it to device flow. In cases in which device flow exceeds the cardiac output, measured by thermodilution technique, by more than 1.5 to 2 L/min, the volume of regurgitation is considered significant. In addition, the presence of significant aortic insufficiency can be confirmed by echocardiography. Patients with a mechanical valve prosthesis in the aortic valve position should have the mechanical valve replaced with a bioprosthetic valve prior to institution of left ventricular assistance. However, bioprosthetic valves in the aortic position are also prone to thrombosis or fusion as a result of complete unloading of the left ventricle with a ventricular assist device that obviates the need for prosthetic valve opening and closing during support. Even fusion of native aortic valve leaflets has been reported with ventricular assist support as a bridge to transplantation.[24] Some surgeons have advocated pericardial patch closure of the aortic valve annulus to prevent thromboembolism from mechanical or bioprosthetic valves in situations of ventricular assist as a bridge to heart transplantation.[23]

Patients with significant preexisting mitral stenosis at the time of initiation of MCS may require correction of the valvular problem before implantation of the device, depending on device selection and site of cannulation. In the setting of significant mitral stenosis, left ventricular filling is impaired. LVADs that use apical ventriculotomy for cannula placement for ventricular drainage may experience limitations in device filling as a consequence of the mitral stenosis. This problem can be circumvented by either choosing a device that can use left atrial drainage or by correcting the underlying valvular pathology (mitral valve repair or replacement with a bioprosthetic valve). In patients with prosthetic valves in the mitral position (either mechanical or bioprosthetic), left ventricular assist should be accomplished with left ventricular apical cannulation to ensure adequate blood flow across the mitral prosthesis to prevent thromboembolism.

Mitral regurgitation does not have an impact on the filling of an LVAD; however, elevations in pulmonary pressures may persist with severe regurgitation, and remodeling of the left ventricle may be adversely affected.[25] In situations where weaning from MCS may be feasible, correction of the mitral pathology, either stenosis or regurgitation, is necessary in order to optimize ventricular function.

Adequate right-heart function is extremely important to maintain LVAD flow in the early postoperative period in patients on univentricular support. Severe tricuspid regurgitation can significantly impair the forward flow of blood on the right side, particularly in situations of high pulmonary vascular resistance. Furthermore, severe tricuspid regurgitation contributes to elevated central venous pressure, hepatic congestion, and renal dysfunction. Severe tricuspid regurgitation may be present preoperatively in the setting of volume overload and biventricular failure or may develop following institution of LVAD support as a consequence of right ventricular dilation from leftward shift of the interventricular septum.[26–28] If severe tricuspid regurgitation is present during the initiation of LVAD support, tricuspid valve repair should be performed to improve right-sided circulatory function.

Coronary Artery Disease

Patients who have significant obstructive coronary artery disease or patients with postcardiotomy shock following failed coronary bypass operations may continue to experience angina during MCS. The presence of obstructive coronary disease with ongoing ischemia may limit the degree of myocardial recovery by significantly impacting the ability to wean from device support or by impacting the ability to wean from cardiopulmonary bypass with left-sided support only in the presence of ischemia of the right ventricle.

Perioperative ischemia of the right ventricle may be of hemodynamic significance during institution of LVAD support. Right ventricular ischemia causing myocardial stunning or infarction that occurs during or soon after implantation of a LVAD can elicit right-sided circulatory failure, resulting in decreased flow to the LVAD. In patients who have had coronary bypass surgery and who are candidates for MCS, patent bypass grafts, particularly to the right coronary artery or left anterior descending coronary artery, should be preserved in order to reduce the risk of perioperative right-sided circulatory failure and arrhythmias. In selected situations, it may be important to perform a coronary artery bypass to the right coronary artery or left anterior descending coronary artery systems to optimize right-heart function in the perioperative period if significant obstructive coronary lesions amenable to bypass are present in the distribution of the these arteries.

Arrhythmias

Atrial and ventricular arrhythmias are common in patients with cardiogenic shock and underlying ischemic heart disease or idiopathic cardiomyopathies. These arrhythmias generally persist in the immediate postoperative period and subsequently resolve with time as the hemodynamic condition of the patient improves and inotropic therapy is weaned. Some patients will have persistence of their arrhythmia, due to their underlying pathology (eg, giant-cell myocarditis). Severe ventricular arrhythmias have traditionally been thought to be a contraindication to univentricular support. However, recent experience reveals that the hemodynamic consequences in patients in whom these arrhythmias develop in the late postoperative period are generally not life-threatening.[29] In the absence of pulmonary hypertension and elevated pulmonary vascular resistance in the postoperative period, patients maintain adequate LVAD flows during ventricular fibrillation. This situation is analogous to a Fontan (systemic vein to pulmonary artery) circulation. In the early perioperative period, some patients with refractory ventricular arrhythmias may require biventricular support indefinitely, or until the pulmonary vasculature resistance drops and a Fontan circulation is tolerated. The addition of right ventricular support for hemodynamic compromise due to refractory ventricular arrhythmia is unusual. In situations where weaning from MCS is feasible or planned, elimination of the ventricular arrhythmias with antiarrhythmic therapy is essential.

Atrial fibrillation and flutter hinders right ventricular filling but is reasonably well tolerated in recipients of ventricular assist devices. Early electrical or pharmacologic cardioversion is indicated to avoid thrombus formation and improve exercise tolerance. Anticoagulation is indicated in patients with persistent atrial or ventricular arrhythmias to prevent thrombus formation (even for those devices for which anticoagulation is otherwise unnecessary).

Intracardiac Shunts

Potential intracardiac shunts such as a patent foramen ovale or atrial septal defect should be closed at the time of initiation of left ventricular assistance to prevent right-to-left shunting. These anomalies should be identified prior to surgery by using transesophageal echocardiography.[30] During the initiation of left ventricular assistance, left atrial pressure is reduced, compared to right atrial pressure. This gradient causes shunting of deoxygenated blood from the right atrium into the left, resulting in significant systemic hypoxemia. In cases where a patent foramen ovale or atrial septal defect has been missed, treatment includes administering pulmonary vasodilators and inotropic agents to decrease the shunt by improving right-heart function and lowering right atrial pressure. If significant hypoxia persists, reoperation or percutaneous interventions to close the anomaly are required.

Adverse Events Associated with Mechanical Circulatory Support

The perioperative morbidity associated with seriously ill patients requiring temporary MCS is significant. In a series of 100 patients undergoing HeartMate LVAD implantation, McCarthy and colleagues[31] reported an incidence of bleeding requiring reoperation of 21%, right-heart failure requiring right ventricular assist device (RVAD) assistance in 11%, bacteremia with positive blood cultures in 59%, and device-related thromboembolic events in approximately 3%. In the clinical evaluation of the HeartMate VE LVAD in 280 patients, Frazier and colleagues reported an incidence of bleeding requiring reoperation in 48%, incidence of right-heart failure requiring RVAD in 11%, infection in 45% of patients, and thromboembolic events occurring in 12%.[4] Catastrophic mechanical failure of the device, which is not amenable to back-up measures, was rare and occurred in 1% of patients. In a randomized trial of LVAD therapy versus medical therapy for severe end-stage heart failure, the risk of adverse events was 2.35 times greater in the LVAD group as compared to the medical group. The risks of bleeding, neurologic dysfunction, sepsis, and renal failure were significantly greater in the LVAD group (odds ratio: 9.47, 4.35, 2.29, and 1.42, respectively).[32] The rate of suspected device malfunction was 0.75 events per patient-year of support.

Bleeding, right-sided circulatory failure, neurologic dysfunction, and progressive multisystem organ failure are the most frequent complications that occur in the early postoperative period following initiation of MCS. Complications that occur most commonly in the late postoperative period include infection, thromboembolism, and device failure.

Bleeding

Bleeding is a frequent, early complication in patients on MCS and generally requires reoperation in the early postoperative period. Risk factors for bleeding include pre-operative hepatic congestion and failure, poor preoperative nutritional status, prolonged cardiopulmonary bypass times, extensive surgical dissection, reoperative surgery, multiple cannulation sites, decreased platelet function, and induction of fibrinolysis as a result of contact with biomaterial surfaces during cardiopulmonary bypass and with MCS devices. The risk of major hemorrhage has decreased substantially with the use of the serine protease inhibitor, aprotinin, and supplemental administration of vitamin K prior to operation.[33,34] In addition, priming the cardiopulmonary bypass circuit with fresh-frozen plasma and blood may reduce significant depletion of clotting factors and prevent the onset of significant coagulopathy at the conclusion of the bypass run. Meticulous surgical technique is also an important factor to reduce hemorrhagic complications.

Right-Sided Circulatory Failure

Right-sided circulatory failure occurs in approximately 10 to 20% of patients supported by left ventricular assistance. The etiology of right-sided circulatory failure is multifactorial and includes primary pathologies within the pulmonary vascular bed and/or right ventricle. Frequently, the occurrence of right-sided circulatory failure is a consequence of both. Factors contributing to right-sided circulatory failure include impaired right ventricular function as a result of intraoperative air embolism, myocardial stunning as a result of poor intraoperative myocardial protection, ischemia and infarction from coronary artery disease, arrhythmias, volume loading, and alteration of right ventricular septal geometry induced by left ventricular unloading. Several studies demonstrate that factors such as elevated central venous pressure, transpulmonary gradient greater than 16 mm Hg, acute decrease in pulmonary artery pressures equal to or greater than 10 mm Hg at the onset of left ventricular assist device support, degree of preoperative pulmonary edema, and increased need for perioperative transfusions, all increase the need for right ventricular mechanical support following LVAD implantation.[2,11,35] Acute unloading of the left ventricle by MCS may cause the septum to shift leftward, increasing right ventricular volume loading and reducing its function.[26,27] The negative consequences of this phenomenon may be offset by the reduction in pulmonary artery pressures and right ventricular afterload caused by device-mediated left ventricular decompression.[26,27] Limiting device flows in the early perioperative period may prevent septal shift and right ventricular overload and thus prevent right-sided circulatory failure in some patients. Hemodynamic stability can be attained with isolated mechanical left ventricular support in approximately 80 to 90% of patients without the need for right ventricular assistance, even in those patients with substantial right ventricular dysfunction, if there is effective replacement of left-sided heart function and aggressive treatment of pulmonary hypertension. More recently, the improved perioperative management of elevated pulmonary vascular resistance, including the use of inhaled nitric oxide, a specific, potent pulmonary vasodilator, in combination with milrinone, isoproterenol, or dobutamine, has significantly reduced the need for placement of a right ventricular assist device.[36] In patients with marked elevation of central venous pressure, multiorgan failure, or severe right ventricular dysfunction with low pulmonary artery pressures, early biventricular or total artificial heart support may be indicated.[10,11,37]

Thromboembolism and Anticoagulation Management

The occurrence of thromboembolic events following MCS is variable and depends on a number of factors, including the type of device, duration of support, location and number of cannulation sites, and the presence of prosthetic valves within the heart. Overall, approximately 10 to 30% of patients receiving MCS will experience a thromboembolic event. Improvement in the rate of thromboembolic events has come from more aggressive antiplatelet therapy in conjunction with warfarin, improved device design, and more frequent use of left ventricular apical as compared to left atrial cannulation. In patients supported for short durations only, anticoagulation is usually achieved with heparin and antiplatelet therapy. Longer-term support usually requires transition to warfarin and antiplatelet therapy for most, but not all, devices.

The single, most significant technological advance in preventing thromboembolic events in patients on long-term left ventricular assistance is attributed to the use of textured blood-contacting surfaces within the devices. This technology was applied in the HeartMate (Thoratec Laboratories, Pleasanton, CA) series of implantable left ventricular assist devices.[38] The interior surfaces of this LVAD were textured by using sintered titanium microspheres on the rigid metallic surfaces and integrally textured polyurethane on the movable diaphragm. This design feature permits a uniform autologous tissue lining to establish on all the blood-contacting surfaces of the pump, minimizing thrombus formation. The tightly adherent fibrin–cellular matrix contains macrophages, mesenchymal cells, endothelial cells, and other blood components. This adherent neointima lining eliminates direct contact between the device and blood elements. In a recent multicenter study, the total thromboembolic event rate for patients supported on the HeartMate device was 0.01 per patient-month of device use among 223 patients supported over a total support time of 531 patient-months.[39] Most thromboembolic events occur either perioperatively due to air or left ventricular thrombus, or occur remotely from the time of device implantation in association with device infection, particularly device fungal infection. Patients supported with the HeartMate LVAD require antiplatelet therapy with aspirin alone, but do not require systemic anticoagulation with heparin or warfarin as with other forms of MCS.

Infection

Infections can be device related (eg, device endocarditis, drive-line or cannula site infection, pocket infection [infection external to an implanted device]) or non-device related (eg, pneumonia, urinary tract infection). The incidence of early nosocomial non–device- or device-related infections in patients undergoing temporary MCS is approximately 30 to 40% in many series and is related to the acuity of illness in this population of patients.[40,41] Patients with persistent or recurrent sepsis and those patients with device-related infections tend to have a higher mortality rate than do patients without these complications. Prolonged hospitalization, immobilization, endotracheal intubation, poor nutritional status, diabetes, obesity, indwelling catheters, intravascular lines, transcutaneous cannulas, and broad-spectrum antibiotic therapy all contribute to the high incidence of nosocomial infections. Device-related infections can sometimes be successfully treated with antibiotic suppression and device exchange or removal. Infections involving the preperitoneal pocket (subfascial space created for device placement) surrounding implantable LVADs require more aggressive treatment, including open drainage, débridement, and rerouting of the drive line through a fresh exit site. However, patients who are device dependent and awaiting transplantation generally cannot tolerate device removal as a therapeutic option to eradicate the infection. In some cases, antibiotic suppression and transplantation are the only chance for cure of device-related infections. Fortunately, these infections do not generally preclude heart transplantation, and transplantation outcomes and survival are generally not significantly affected in this situation. In patients on long-term (more than 2 weeks) MCS, infection remains the single, most significant obstacle to successful outcome. Recent data demonstrate that patients maintained on long-term MCS have significant derangements in their immune system secondary to patient–device interactions. These data suggest that LVAD implantation is accompanied by progressive defects in cellular immunity that seem to be the result of an aberrant state of T-cell activation involving the CD95 (FAS) pathway and activation-induced cell death of CD4 T cells.[42] These defects may predispose recipients of LVADs to fungal infections and other systemic infections as a result of defects in their cellular immunity.[42]

Sensitization to HLA Antigens

The presence of preformed lymphocytotoxic antibodies reactive against donor lymphocytes in recipient serum detected in a routine cross-match is considered a significant obstacle to successful solid organ transplantation. The presence of preformed lymphocytotoxic antibodies is associated with a high incidence of humoral allograft rejection, early graft failure, and poorer patient survival.[43] Recent evidence demonstrates that recipients of MCS support develop prominent B-cell activation, as evidenced by heightened production of anti-HLA (human leukocyte antigen) and antiphospholipid antibodies. The incidence of antibody development to HLA class I or II antibodies may be as high as 80%.[44] This enhanced B-cell reactivity is thought to be secondary to activation-induced cell death of CD4 T cells.[42] However, this high prevalence of anti-HLA class I or II antibodies is not routinely observed, and some investigators report no significant increased risk of cellular or humoral cardiac allograft rejection in the first year following heart transplantation in patients previously supported by an LVAD, nor significant increased risk of death within the first 2 posttransplant years.[45]

Device Malfunction

As with any mechanical device, malfunction is an anticipated occurrence. The types and severity of device malfunctions vary with each of the devices. Many devices have built-in back-up systems that, in the event of catastrophic device failure, provide support to the patient. Also, most patients supported by a LVAD have enough residual left ventricular function to help sustain them until corrective measures can be taken. Device malfunctions in total artificial hearts are more problematic as there is no native heart to provide hemodynamic support in the event of a total device failure. Stringent quality control measures in fabrication and testing and very low mechanical failure rates are, therefore, even more essential with total artificial hearts.

Considerations in Weaning Patients from Mechanical Circulatory Support

A number of factors must be considered when weaning patients from MCS. First and foremost is the consideration of any pathologic abnormalities of the heart, such as valvular disease or severe coronary disease, that has not been addressed and corrected. If the underlying pathology that caused the patient to require MCS is not corrected, then the chances of weaning from MCS are negligible. Cardiac tamponade must also be excluded. Bleeding is a major early complication of MCS, and reoperation for cardiac tamponade and bleeding is frequent. Transesophageal echocardiography may not reliably identify cardiac tamponade in the early postoperative period. Thus, a high index of suspicion and a low threshold for reoperation are critical to rule out tamponade. Volume status, preload and afterload, cardiac rhythm, and degree of inotropic support should be optimized for weaning. Noncardiac causes can contribute to failure to wean from MCS. Pulmonary edema, elevated pulmonary vascular resistance, acute respiratory distress syndrome (ARDS), and pneumonia may hinder right ventricular function.

Once a patient's status has been optimized, weaning from MCS with the use of transesophageal echocardio-graphy is ideal. As device flows are reduced, transesophageal echocardiography provides information on ventricular filling and performance and on valve function. If patients can maintain satisfactory hemodynamics with reduction of pump flow, they can be considered for weaning. In the setting of biventricular support, it is important that device flows on the right side be reduced prior to turning down left-sided device flows to prevent pulmonary edema in the event of inadequate left-sided ventricular function. As device flows are reduced, native heart function will begin to support the circulation, and monitoring of the systemic arterial waveform will demonstrate native heart contractions in synchronization with the electrocardiogram.

If hemodynamics are unsatisfactory during the weaning trial, the patient will require continued support and subsequent weaning trials. In cases in which weaning from temporary MCS is not possible, patients should be evaluated for heart transplantation and bridged to a mechanical device with long-term support capabilities when feasible.

Mechanical Circulatory Support Devices

Intraaortic Balloon Pump

In 1968, Kantrowitz and colleagues reported on the first clinical use of the intraaortic balloon pump (IABP) in three patients suffering from postinfarction cardiogenic shock refractory to medical therapy.[46] Since then, the IABP has become the simplest, most affordable, and most used form of MCS (Figure 46-1). The concept for the IABP was derived from the understanding of the relationship between the area under the arterial pressure trace (time–tension index) and the heart's oxygen consumption. Decreasing the area under the arterial pressure trace during systole by reducing myocardial afterload with an IABP has the effect of reducing myocardial oxygen consumption. Claus and colleagues[47] described a device that lowered the time–tension index by withdrawing blood from the arterial tree just before ventricular systole, returning it to the circulation in diastole. In 1962, a catheter-based balloon was developed that produced hemodynamic effects similar to the pump described by Claus and colleagues.

The major hemodynamic effects of the IABP are a decrease in left ventricular afterload and an increase in coronary artery perfusion pressure. Under ideal circumstances, the IABP may augment cardiac output by as much as 10 to 25%, depending on a number of factors that include balloon size, patient size, degree of aortic compliance, cardiac rhythm, blood pressure, and IABP settings and timing. Patients with ischemic cardiomyopathy generally have the greatest increase in cardiac output as a result of improved cardiac contractility

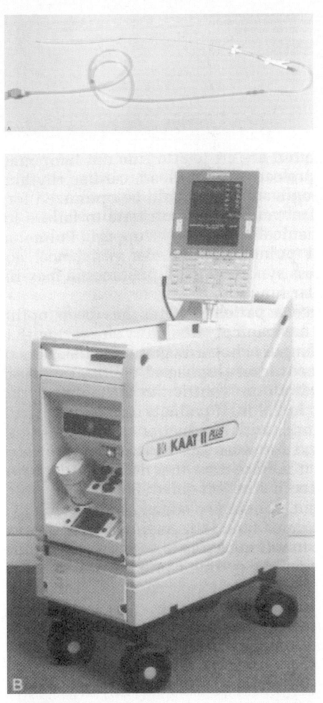

FIGURE 46-1. Intraaortic balloon pump. *A,* Catheter-mounted balloon is typically introduced into the thoracic aorta through a percutaneous insertion in the groin. *B,* Console for the intraaortic balloon pump.

resulting from enhanced coronary perfusion combined with a reduction in systemic afterload.

The IABP is positioned with the tip of the balloon lying just distal to the left subclavian artery. The balloon should fill the aorta so that during the inflation cycle it nearly occludes the vessel. In adults, balloon volumes of 30 to 40 mL are optimal. Inflation should be timed to coincide with closure of the aortic valve, which is obtained by identifying the dicrotic notch of of aortic blood pressure trace (Figure 46-2). Deflation should occur as late as possible to maintain the duration of the augmented diastolic blood pressure but before the aortic valve opens and the ventricle ejects. Deflation is timed to occur with the onset of the electrocardiographic R wave. A regular heart rate with an easily identified R wave or a good arterial pulse tracing with a discrete aortic dicrotic notch optimizes performance of the IABP. Current balloon pumps trigger off the electrocardiographic R wave or from the arterial pressure tracing. During tachycardia, the IABP is usually timed to inflate every other beat. In unstable patients, obtaining a regular rhythm or regularly paced rhythm optimizes proper timing of the IABP.

The IABP can be inserted into the common femoral artery either by the percutaneous technique using a modified Seldinger technique, or by surgical cutdown. A cutdown is generally performed during cardiopulmonary bypass when the arterial pulse is absent due to nonpulsatile flow. During insertion, a guidewire is introduced into the femoral artery, followed by dilating catheters and the balloon. After passage of the flexible guidewire, the soft tissue tract and vessel are progressively dilated until an appropriately sized sheath can be inserted. Sheathless IABP catheters are available. Next, the furled catheter (standard size 9.5 French, with 40-mL balloon) is passed proximally until its tip rests in the thoracic aorta just distal to the left subclavian. In situations where the common femoral or iliac arteries cannot be used because of occlusive disease and an inability to advance the guidewire, the axillary artery, exposed below the middle third of the clavicle, may be used as an alternative entry site. Alternatively, in situations of postcardiotomy failure to wean, the ascending aorta may be used as an insertion site. Fluoroscopy or transesophageal echocardiography should be used to ensure proper positioning of the guidewire. The balloon should be positioned so that during inflation, it does not occlude the left subclavian artery. Heparin is recommended if the IABP will remain in place for more than 24 h. Weaning of the IABP entails observing the clinical response to reducing the ratio of assisted heart beats to total beats from 1:1 to 1:3 or 1:4. At the time of removal of the IABP, every effort should be made to flush out any thrombus as the balloon catheter is removed. Hemostasis should be obtained by application of direct pressure to the entry site for at least 30 to 45 min. Removal of the IABP placed through a cutdown on the femoral artery may require repair of that artery and concomitant embolectomy if there have been signs of ischemia of the lower extremity.

Complications from use of the IABP include leg ischemia; balloon rupture; thrombosis within the balloon; sepsis; infection at the insertion site; bleeding; false aneurysm formation; lymph fistula; femoral neuropathy; vessel perforation with hemorrhage; and aortic dissection

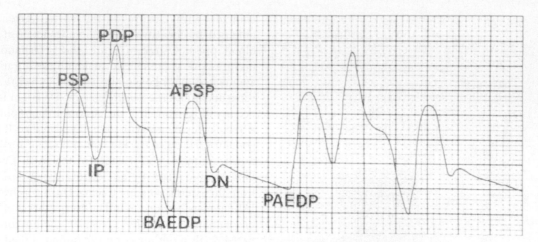

FIGURE 46-2. Aortic pressure tracing during intraaortic balloon pump support. Balloon counterpulsation is occurring after every other heartbeat (1:2 counterpulsation). With correct timing, balloon inflation (IP) begins immediately after aortic valve closure, signaled by the dicrotic notch (DN). When compared with unassisted ejection, the pump augments diastolic blood flow by increasing peak aortic pressure during diastole (PDP). Balloon deflation before systole decreases ventricular afterload, with lower aortic end-diastolic pressure (BAEDP vs PAEDP) and lower peak systolic pressure (APSP vs PSP). (Courtesy of St. Jude Medical, Inc., Cardiac Assist Division, Minneapolis, MN.)

from catheter passage below the intima. Depending on the extent of peripheral vascular disease, balloon position can occlude major branches of the aorta and elicit ischemia of the tissues supplied by these vessels. Examples of this scenario include intestinal "angina" from occlusion of the mesenteric vessels and upper extremity symptoms when the balloon impinges on the left subclavian artery. Female gender, peripheral vascular disease, diabetes, smoking, advanced age, obesity, and cardiogenic shock are risk factors for the development of leg ischemia. Balloon rupture is usually indicated by the appearance of blood within the balloon catheter. Leg ischemia, balloon rupture, and sepsis are an indication for removal of the IABP. If the patient is balloon dependent, a replacement balloon can be inserted in a new site.

The IABP has several disadvantages. In the best of circumstances, cardiac output is augmented by 25% as compared to LVADs that can augment cardiac output by 3 to 5 times baseline flows. The IABP offers no significant support to the right heart. Mobilization and ambulation of the patient is limited while the IABP is being utilized.

Extracorporeal, Nonpulsatile Devices

EXTRACORPOREAL MEMBRANE OXYGENATION (ECMO)

Extracorporeal membrane oxygenation (ECMO; also known as extracorporeal life support [ECLS]) is a temporary form of MCS that uses a modified heart–lung machine to provide circulatory assistance as well as oxygenation and carbon dioxide removal from blood for days to weeks to permit recovery from severe cardiac or pulmonary failure.[48–51] The ECMO circuit is similar in concept to cardiopulmonary bypass, which is routinely used in the operating room; however, safe application of the ECMO circuit for extended periods of time has required certain modifications, particularly the inclusion of membrane

oxygenators. The first successful use of prolonged ECMO was reported by Hill in 1972.[52] Subsequently, ECMO has been used in an increasing number of indications, including neonatal, pediatric, and adult respiratory support; neonatal, pediatric, and adult postcardiotomy support; and as a bridge to an LVAD or to heart and lung transplantation.

ECMO circuits are comprised of a centrifugal pump with either a hollow-fiber or membrane oxygenator, oxygen blender, pump console, heat exchanger, and pump cart. Some centers prefer a roller pump and membrane oxygenator (Figure 46-3).[51] Heparin-bonded circuits are also used. These circuits reduce, but do not eliminate, the need for systemic anticoagulation and may reduce the inflammatory response associated with ECMO. Cannulation for ECMO is extremely variable and depends on the clinical situation and on whether a venoarterial or venovenous circuit is desired. Venovenous circuits are the preferred method for providing respiratory support, while venoarterial circuits can be used for either cardiac and/or respiratory support (Figure 46-4). In emergent situations where institution of MCS is needed within minutes (acute cardiac and/or respiratory arrest), percutaneous cannulation of the femoral vein and artery can be performed (see Figure 46-4). In less urgent situations, cutdown on the internal jugular and carotid artery or respective femoral vessels can be performed. In cases of postcardiotomy failure in the operating room, venous access can be obtained by insertion of a canula in the right atrium, and arterial outflow obtained by cannulation of the ascending aorta (see Figure 46-4).

ECMO provides MCS by draining blood from the venous circulation, oxygenating it, and then returning it to the arterial circulation at physiologic perfusion pressures. ECMO support significantly unloads the right ventricle but does not satisfactorily unload the left ventri-

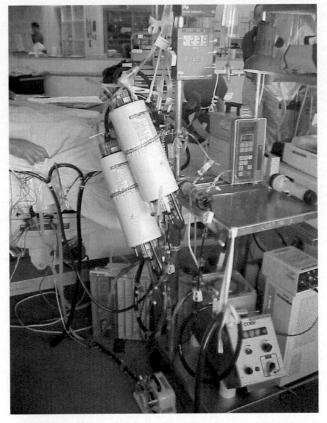

FIGURE 46-3. Photograph of an ECMO circuit used at the University of Michigan. Note the roller pump (bottom center of the photograph) and membrane oxygenator (center of the photograph). (Photograph courtesy of Fresca Swaniker, MD, University of Michigan.)

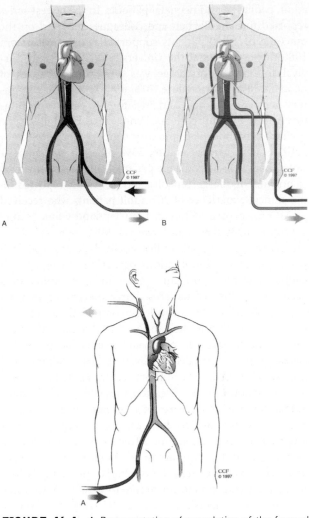

FIGURE 46-4. *A*, Representation of cannulation of the femoral artery and vein for venoarterial ECMO support. Cannulation of the respective femoral artery or vein can be performed by direct surgical cutdown or by percutaneous method. *B*, Representation of cannulation of the ascending aorta and right atrium for venoarterial ECMO support in the postcardiotomy setting. *C*, Representation of cannulation of the femoral vein and internal jugular vein for venovenous ECMO support for respiratory failure.

cle, although left ventricular preload is reduced by decreasing pulmonary venous return. In patients with severe left ventricular dysfunction, left ventricular distension and subsequent development of significant pulmonary hypertension resulting in pulmonary hemorrhage may occur. The use of an IABP may help to reduce left ventricular afterload during systole and improve myocardial contractility. The use of the IABP and inotropic therapy can maintain sufficient cardiac contractility to prevent ventricular distension and thrombus formation. If application of an IABP does not effectively relieve ventricular distension and pulmonary hypertension, an atrial septostomy can be performed to vent pulmonary venous return.[53,54] Alternatively, a left-sided vent can be connected to the venous line of the ECMO circuit to relieve ventricular distension. It is important during ECMO support to maintain some degree of pulmonary blood flow to prevent thrombosis. Venovenous ECMO, unlike venoarterial ECMO, maintains flow through the heart. Additionally, it is important to continue ventilation of the lungs to maintain the oxygen saturation of the blood ejected from the left ventricle above 90%. Poorly oxygenated blood ejected from the left ventricle will perfuse the coronary arteries and the cerebral circulation and may result in hypoxic injury to the heart and brain.

To promote recovery of respiratory function, it is important to manage the patient by using low pressure and oxygen ventilator settings (to avoid ventilator-induced injury), pressure-controlled ventilation, hemofiltration to dry weight, intermittent prone positioning, and nutritional support. Right atrial and left atrial pressures, as well as pump flows, are monitored, and mixed venous saturations are maintained above 75%, which is an accurate reflection of the adequacy of systemic flows. A sudden decrease in venous drainage is usually manifested by chugging of the venous lines, with wide respiratory fluctuations and flow. Causes include hypovolemia, cannula kinking or malposition, pneumothorax, and pericardial tamponade.

Numerous large clinical series have reported successful use of ECMO for cardiac and/or respiratory support in adult, pediatric, and neonatal patients. In the largest series reported to date, Bartlett and colleagues reported on the outcome of 1,000 patients supported with ECMO from 1980 through 1998 at the University of Michigan.[51] Survival to hospital discharge was 88% for 586 cases of neonatal respiratory failure, 70% for 132 cases of respiratory failure in children, and 56% for 146 cases of respiratory failure in adult patients. Venovenous ECMO was the preferred method of respiratory support since 1988. For patients with cardiac failure, 33% of adult patients (31 cases) and 48% of pediatric patients (105 cases) survived to hospital discharge. Smedira and colleagues reported on the clinical experience of 202 adult patients who received ECMO for cardiac failure at the Cleveland Clinic.[55] Survival at 24 h, 30 days, and 1 year was 90%, 38%, and 29%, respectively. For patients alive at 30 days, survival at 5 years was 63%. Complications occurring during ECMO support were significant. Infectious complications occurred in 49% of patients. Forty percent of patients required dialysis, while neurologic complications occurred in 33% and limb complications occurred in 25%. Risk factors for death included older age, thoracic aortic operations, reoperations, decompensated heart failure, and nonuse of an IABP. The authors recommended concomitant IABP support for all patients requiring ECMO support to improve myocardial recovery and improved organ function with pulsatile flow. Magovern and colleagues reported on the outcome of 92 adult patients following institution of ECMO support.[50] Twenty of 55 (36%) patients survived to hospital discharge following ECMO support for postcardiotomy failure to wean. Twenty-three of 27 (85%) patients survived ECMO support following percutaneous interventions in the catheterization laboratory while 2 of 4 (50%) survived ECMO for primary cardiac allograft failure. No patient survived ECMO support for cardiac resuscitation.[56]

EXTRACORPOREAL CENTRIFUGAL PUMPS

Centrifugal pumps are extracorporeal systems that provide short-term MCS.[57,58] The systems are easy to operate, widely available, disposable, and relatively inexpensive when compared to most other forms of mechanical circulatory assist. These systems are most commonly used in cardiopulmonary bypass to support open-heart operations. Thus, there is an extensive knowledge base on the use of these devices. Worldwide, numerous centrifugal pumps are available or are in development for clinical use. However, until recently in the United States, only three centrifugal pumps have been commercially available. All are disposable, cost less than $200.00 (US) per unit, and are relatively simple to operate. The Sarns centrifugal pump (Terumo, Inc., Ann Arbor, MI) uses a spinning impeller system to impart a rotary motion to incoming perfusate. The St. Jude Medical Lifestream centrifugal pump (St. Jude Medical, Inc., Cardiac Assist Division, Chelmsford, MA) employs a curved-vane design and angled-egress blood

flow path that purports to minimize turbulence, decrease hemolysis, and reduce periods of flow stasis. The Bio-Medicus BioPump centrifugal pump head manufactured and marketed by Medtronic BioMedicus, Inc. (Eden Prairie, MN) consists of valveless rotator cones that are made to impart a circular motion to incoming blood by viscous drag and constrained vortex principles, generating pressure and flow. The Carmeda BioMedicus Biopump (Ann Arbor, MI) has heparin covalently bonded to the blood-exposed surfaces. These four disposable pump heads can be magnetically coupled to an electric motor, which is controlled by a computerized console. Control of flow is accomplished by adjusting the revolutions per minute of the spinning pump head. Short-term (generally limited to hours to days) ventricular or pulmonary support can be provided with centrifugal pumps. It can be used for femoral-femoral bypass, conventional cardiopulmonary bypass, left and/or right ventricular assistance, and ECMO.

The most common use of the centrifugal pump, other than for conventional cardiopulmonary bypass operations for open heart procedures, is for patients who have had postcardiotomy failure and cardiogenic shock. Postcardiotomy cardiac failure occurs in 2 to 6% of patients who have cardiac procedures.[57] One percent will require MCS in addition to the IABP for counterpulsation. Results of a voluntary registry reporting the use of the centrifugal pump as right, left, or biventricular assist devices show that approximately 25% of patients were weaned from the device and eventually discharged.[59] The centrifugal pump can be used to provide left, right, or biventricular assistance. Cannulation for left ventricular assistance is most commonly performed through the right superior pulmonary vein into the left atrium, with return into the ascending aorta. Right ventricular assistance is provided by cannulation of the right atrium and pulmonary artery. The pulmonary artery catheter is either placed through the right ventricle and threaded through the pulmonary valve or inserted directly into the pulmonary artery. Cannulas are secured in place with two purse-string pledgeted sutures and tourniquets.

TANDEMHEART pVAD

The TandemHeart pVAD (CardiacAssist, Inc., Pittsburgh, PA) is a percutaneous left atrial-to-femoral artery VAD. The pump is a low-speed, continuous-flow, centrifugal pump that has a very low potential for hemolysis and thromboembolism (Figure 46-5). It is a dual-chamber pump that is comprised of an upper housing and a lower housing assembly. The upper housing provides a conduit for inflow and outflow of blood. The lower housing assembly provides communication with the controller, the means for rotating the impeller of the VAD, and an anticoagulation infusion line integral to the pump, to provide a hydrodynamic bearing, cooling of the bearing, and local anticoagulation. The controller is a microprocessor-based

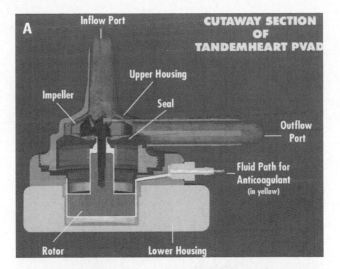

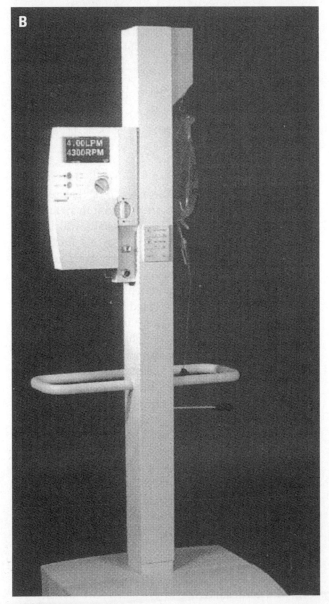

FIGURE 46-5. *A,* TandemHeart pVAD centrifigal pump. *B,* Electrical control console for the TandemHeart pVAD centrifugal pump.

electromechanical drive and infusion system that is designed to operated on AC current or on internal batteries.

Implantation of the device is performed percutaneously through the right femoral vein (Figure 46-6). A standard Brockenbrough catheter is inserted into the superior vena cava. The interatrial septum is punctured in the fossa ovalis by using a Ross needle. The position of the Brockenbrough catheter within the left atrium is documented by manual dye injection. If the position is satisfactory, the Brockenbrough catheter is exchanged for a stiff guidewire with a distal soft wire loop identical to the device used for mitral valvuloplasty when performing the Inoue method. The transseptal puncture site is then dilated to 21 French with a two-stage dilator followed by insertion of a venous inflow cannula, which is sutured to the skin of the thigh. An arterial perfusion catheter of 14 to 19 French is inserted percutaneously into the right femoral artery, or two arterial perfusion catheters of 12 French into both femoral arteries.

Thiele and colleagues reported on the use of the TandemHeart pVAD in 18 patients presenting in cardiogenic shock.[60] Mean duration of support was 4 ± 3 days. Following percutaneous placement of the device, mean cardiac index improved from 1.7 ± 0.3 L/min/m² to 2.4 ± 0.6 L/min/m². Mean device flow during support was 3.2 ± 0.6 L/min. Pulmonary wedge pressure decreased from 31 ± 8 mm Hg to 23 ± 6 mm Hg. Survival at 30 days was 56%.

IMPLANTABLE CENTRIFUGAL PUMPS

The AB-180 (Cardiac Assist Technologies, Inc., Pittsburgh, PA) is an implantable, centrifugal flow LVAD that is identical to the TandemHeart pVAD (Figure 46-7).[61] The intended uses are for treatment of patients with reversible acute forms of cardiogenic shock. The AB-180 weighs approximately 280 g and has a priming volume of 7 mL. The pump is powered by a stationary electromagnetic motor that drives a magnetic rotor and an impeller, which rotates at 2,700 to 4,700 rpm. Pump inflow is provided by a plastic cannula that enters the pump at 180° from the impeller. Outflow leaves the pump at 90° from the inflow. A 10-mm thin-walled polytetrafluoroethylene (PTFE) graft connects to an outflow port and is anastomosed to the aorta. The device can pump up to 6 L/min at a mean arterial pressure of 60 to 90 mm Hg, with inflow pressures > 5 mm Hg. A percutaneous cable connects the pump with the external controller. This cable carries three lines: (1) a DC electric power line, (2) a lubrication line, and (3) a flow occluder. The lubrication line delivers 10 mL/h of heparinized sterile water into the pump, which lubricates the impeller shaft/seal and achieves localized anticoagulation within the pump without the need for systemic anticoagulation. The occluder line consists of a balloon catheter that automatically inflates against the outflow graft if the device fails. There are no valves in the pump, which means that retrograde flow can occur throughout the device, from the aorta to the left atrium, if

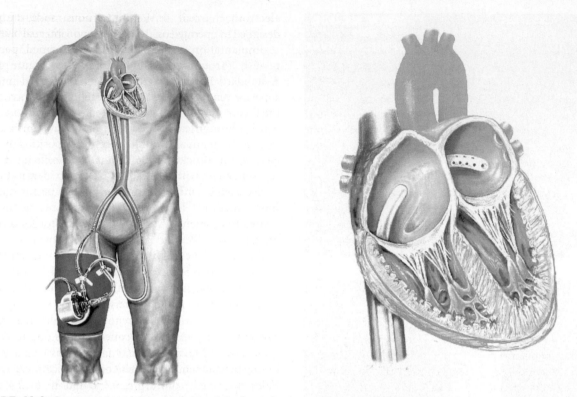

FIGURE 46-6. Representation of the cannulation of the femoral artery and femoral vein with transseptal placement of the inflow catheter within the left atrium from the femoral vein. The TandemHeart pVAD is secured to the patient's right thigh.

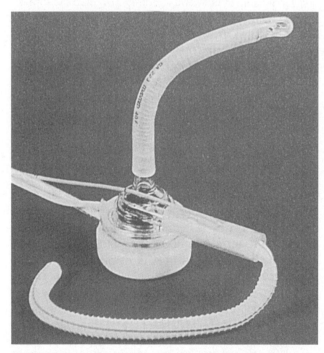

FIGURE 46-7. The AB-180 implantable centrifugal pump.

controller is a microprocessor-based unit that regulates pump speed, alarm function, the lubrication system, and the occluder. It is compact and lightweight, which facilitates patient transport and physical access for nursing care. The device was designed as an implantable pump, and has a single percutaneous line containing power, lubrication, and occluder functions. In postcardiotomy application, the pump is positioned in the right hemithorax on the diaphragm. The pump inflow cannula drains the left atrium by means of the right superior pulmonary vein. Pump outflow is to the ascending aorta by means of a 10-mm PTFE graft. The power cable exits the lower anterolateral thorax through the sixth or seventh interspace. The device has also been used in bridge to transplant situations. In these cases, the pump can be implanted in the left hemithorax by means of a lateral thoracotomy incision, with inflow from the left atrium and outflow to the descending aorta.

In an initial trial of 17 patients from 5 institutions, Magovern and colleagues reported an overall survival to discharge of 29% (5 of 17).[61] The indications for implantation included postcardiotomy failure to wean (12 patients), decompensated cardiomyopathy (2 patients), viral myocarditis (2 patients), and acute myocardial infarction (1 patient). Eight patients weaned from support, with four surviving to discharge; two patients required transplantation, with one surviving to discharge. Mean duration of support was 8.5 days.

the device fails. The occluder system prevents this from occurring. The pump controller is contained in an external console, which is located adjacent to the patient. The

Extracorporeal, Pulsatile Devices

THORATEC VENTRICULAR ASSIST SYSTEM

The Thoratec VAS (Thoratec Laboratories Inc., Pleasanton, CA) is a paracorporeal, pneumatically powered, pulsatile system configured for univentricular or biventricular support that consists of a seamless polyurethane blood sac contained within a rigid polycarbonate housing (Figure 46-8).[62–64] An external drive console sends pressurized air to the pump, which compresses the blood sac and causes blood to be ejected. Bjork-Shiley concavoconvex tilting-disk valves within the inflow and outflow conduits ensure unidirectional blood flow. The device has a stroke volume of approximately 65 mL and a maximum output of 7 L/min. For left ventricular support, the pump inflow cannula can be placed in the left ventricular apex or the left atrium, and the pump outflow conduit is anastomosed to the ascending aorta. For right ventricular support, a large-bore cannula is placed in the right atrium, and the outflow conduit is sewn to the main pulmonary artery. When biventricular support is needed, right pump flow is adjusted so that it is less than left pump flow to prevent excessive pulmonary congestion. After the cannulas have been externalized subcostally, the inflow and outflow cannulas are connected to the pump(s), which resides externally on the anterior surface of the abdomen. During the support period, anticoagulation with dextran, heparin, warfarin, and dipyridamole is required. Patients may be ambulatory but their mobility is limited by the size of the drive console and the paracorporeal position of the pump(s). The Thoratec ventricular assist device can be operated in fixed-rate, volume, or synchronous mode. Volume mode is preferred because it maximizes support of the cardiac output. In the synchronous mode, the pump empties when triggered by the R wave obtained from the patient's electrocardiogram. In this mode, weaning may be achieved by adjusting the device rate to a heart rate ratio in the range of 1:1 to 1:3. Synchronous mode is intended for weaning patients from support. Although the console can function automatically to achieve maximum pump flows, the operator must adjust the systolic driving pressure and diastolic vacuum pressure. The FDA has approved the Thoratec VAS for use as a bridge to recovery and bridge to transplantation. New system designs that are currently being tested include a small, portable drive console that will enhance patient mobility and permit discharge from the hospital and the development of an intracorporeal pump (Figure 46-9).[64,65]

McBride and colleagues reported on the outcomes of 111 patients supported with the Thoratec VAS for acute cardiac failure.[62] Survival at 1 year was approximately 25% for 44 patients treated with the intent to recover. This compared to an approximately 58% 1-year survival for 67 patients treated with the intent to bridge to transplantation. The duration of support ranged from 0.1 to 27 days (mean, 4.5 days) in the recovery group and 0.2 to 184 days (mean, 40.7 days) in the bridge to transplantation group. Complications were significant in both groups. In 104 patients bridged to transplantation with the Thoratec VAS, El-Banayosy and colleagues reported a survival to transplantation of 61%.[63] Approximately 50% of the patients required biventricular support and outcomes were worse for this group. Age, preimplant ventilator use, and higher preimplant total bilirubin were significant predictors of adverse outcome.

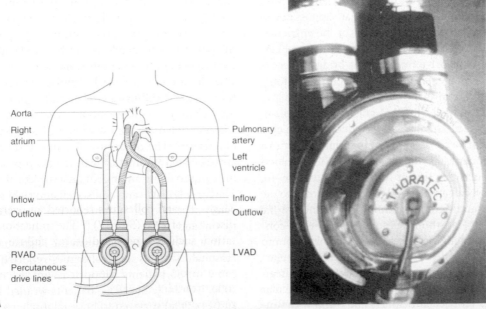

FIGURE 46-8. The Thoratec VAS (Thoratec Laboratories, Inc., Pleasanton, CA). *A,* Representation of the cannulation sites for biventricular support. *B,* Thoratec VAS extracorporeal pneumatic blood pump. LVAD = left ventricular assist device; RVAD = right ventricular assist device.

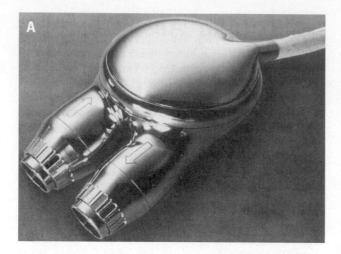

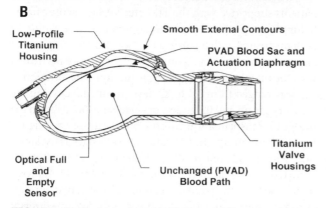

FIGURE 46-9. *A,* Implantable Thoratec VAS pneumatic blood pump. *B,* Representation of the implantable Thoratec VAS pneumatic blood pump. PVAD = pneumatic ventricular assist device.

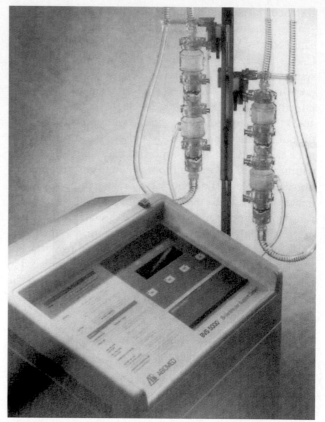

FIGURE 46-10. The pneumatic drive console and blood pumps for the Abiomed BVS 5000 biventricular assist device (Abiomed, Inc., Danvers, MA).

ABIOMED BVS 5000

The Abiomed BVS 5000 (Abiomed Inc., Danvers, MA) support system is an automated ventricular support device intended to provide temporary uni- or biventricular support.[7,8,66,67] The Abiomed BVS 5000 was the first FDA-approved device for short-term MCS as a bridge to recovery in cases of cardiogenic shock due to postcardiotomy failure to wean, acute myocarditis, and myocardial infarction. Positioned externally, this pulsatile system simulates normal physiologic mechanical cardiac function. A microprocessor-based drive console is used to supply power to a disposable, pneumatically driven two-chambered blood pump that supports one side of the heart (Figures 46-10, 46-11, and 46-12). Left atrial blood inflow is returned to the ascending aorta, and right atrial inflow is returned to the pulmonary artery. Transthoracic cannulas are used to connect the external system with the patient. Each blood pump consists of two Angioflex polyurethane atrioventricular-like chambers. Trileaflet polyurethane valves are strategically positioned to separate (1) atrial and ventricular bladders and (2) ventricular bladders and outflow cannulas. One or two disposable blood pumps are operated by a single console, which automatically adjusts beat rate and

systolic/diastolic ratio based on compressed air flow into and out of the external system. The pump is placed at the bedside and blood drains from the patient's left or right atrium by gravity, without the use of vacuum pressure, into the top of the pump and returns to the patient's aorta or pulmonary artery from the bottom of the pump. Filling of the blood pump chambers can be regulated by adjusting the height of the blood pump relative to the patient's heart. The blood pump is a dual-chamber device that incorporates an atrial (filling) chamber and a ventricular (pumping) chamber. Unidirectional flow is ensured by two trileaflet polyurethane valves fabricated from Angioflex, a biomaterial. The durations of pump systole and diastole are calculated automatically by the microprocessor to optimize pump filling and maintain a stroke volume of 83 mL. The console drives and adjusts left and right sides independently of each other. System controls are essentially limited to "on" and "off."

In a 6-year experience from the Hahneman University Hospital, Samuels and colleagues reported on the outcomes of 45 patients supported with the Abiomed BVS 5000.[67] Overall, 22 (49%) patients weaned from support and 14 (31%) survived to hospital discharge. For patients that received optimal timing of insertion by establishing a weaning algorithm, outcomes were improved, with 60%

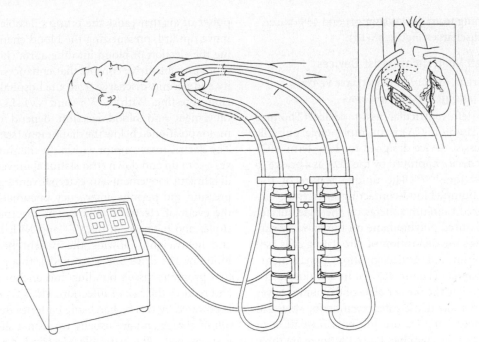

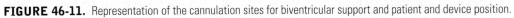

FIGURE 46-11. Representation of the cannulation sites for biventricular support and patient and device position.

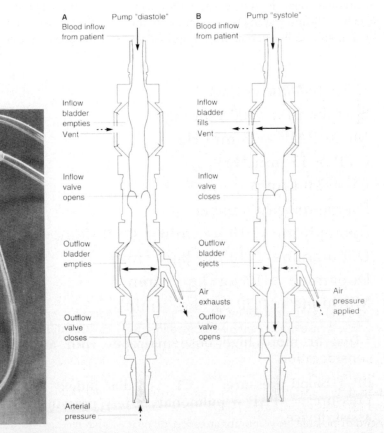

FIGURE 46-12. Photograph and diagram of the Abiomed blood pumps.

of patients weaning from device support and 43% surviving to hospital discharge (Figure 46-13).

Implantable Left Ventricular Assist Devices

HEARTMATE IP 1000 LVAS, HEARTMATE VE LVAS, AND HEARTMATE XVE LVAS

The HeartMate left ventricular assist device (Thoratec Laboratories, Pleasanton, CA) is an implantable, pulsatile left ventricular assist device designed for long-term MCS and was the first device approved by the FDA as a bridge to heart transplantation.[31,68,69] The unique feature of this device is that its pump's blood-contacting surfaces are textured with sintered titanium spheres on the rigid surface and integrally textured polyurethane on the movable surfaces to encourage the deposition of circulating cells (see "Thromboembolism and Anticoagulation Management" earlier in this chapter) (Figure 46-14). In addition to the unique surface design, the pusher plate of the pump moves the diaphragm in a way that creates a wandering vortex in the blood chamber. This feature prevents stagnation of blood in any part of the chamber. Presently, there are three versions of the HeartMate in clinical use—a pneumatic version (IP-1000 LVAS) (Figure 46-15) and two vented electric versions (VE and XVE-LVAS) (Figure 46-16). The HeartMate blood pump consists of a flexible polyurethane diaphragm within a ridged outer titanium alloy housing. The inflow and outflow conduits of the HeartMate device each contain a 25-mm porcine valve within a titanium cage to ensure unidirectional blood flow. The outflow conduit is extended by a 20-mm woven Dacron graft. With the IP-1000 LVAS, a mobile 75-lb external drive console sends pulses of air that cause the pump's flexible diaphragm to move upward, pressurizing the blood chamber and causing the ejection of blood into the aorta (Figure 46-17). A more portable drive console that enhances patient mobility and permits discharge from the hospital is currently in clinical testing. With the VE- and XVE-LVAS, diaphragm movement and blood ejection depend on an electric motor positioned below the diaphragm (see Figure 46-17). The electric rotary motor within the titanium housing drives a cam up and down (translational movement), causing diaphragm movement. An external vent equalizes the air pressure and permits emergency pneumatic actuation in the event of electrical failure. The external system controller and batteries in the VE- and XVE-LVAS are small and lightweight, allowing the patient nearly unlimited mobility. The drive line is covered with a polyester velour that promotes tissue bonding and anchoring to the skin and reduces the risk of infection. The VE- and XVE-LVAS is powered by two rechargeable batteries that provide 4 to 6 h of charge and are usually worn in a shoulder holster, vest, or belt. The wearable electrical devices currently available have external back-up mechanisms to continue support without the need for reoperation in case of failure of the device. If the device should fail, the native heart is able to provide systemic support until the device can be examined. Because the electronic control unit is outside the body, it can easily be repaired should failure of the software, chip, or electronics occur. Finally, if the motor device fails, the single-pusher-plate device can be pneumatically activated with a handheld portable pump or with the 75-lb pneumatic console that operates the IP-1000 model.

Hemodynamic criteria

Systolic BP < 100 mm Hg

Mean PAP > 25 mm Hg

CVP > 15 mm Hg

CI < 2.0 L/min$^{-1} \cdot$ m^{-2}

Pharmacological criteria

Epinephrine ≥ 10 μg $\cdot$ min^{-1} (≥ 0.15 μg $\cdot$ kg$^{-1} \cdot$ min^{-1})

Dobutamine ≥ 10 μg $\cdot$ kg$^{-1} \cdot$ min^{-1}

Dopamine ≥ 10 μg $\cdot$ kg$^{-1} \cdot$ min^{-1}

Milrinone ≥ 0.50 μg $\cdot$ kg^{-1}/min^{-1}

---

[a] Two or more high dose inotropes with low output triggers VAD consideration.

BP = blood pressure; CI = cardiac index; CVP = central venous pressure; PAP = pulmonary artery pressure; VAD = ventricular assist device.

FIGURE 46-13. Algorithm for determining timing of device support. Reproduced with permission from Samuels LE et al.[67]

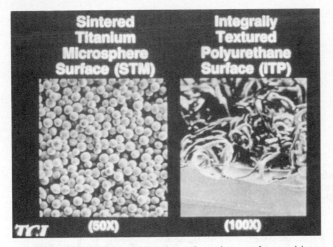

FIGURE 46-14. Sintered titanium microsphere surface and integrally textured polyurethane surface incorporated in the HeartMate left ventricular assist system. (Photograph courtesy of Betty Silverstein Russell, Senior Vice President, Thermo Cardiosystems Inc., Woburn, MA.)

The HeartMate is implanted through an extended median sternotomy incision with the aid of cardiopulmonary bypass. The pump is positioned below the left hemidiaphragm, either within the peritoneal cavity or in a preperitoneal pocket. The inflow tube crosses the diaphragm and is inserted in the apex of the left ventricle. A 20-mm Dacron outflow graft exits from the pocket, crosses the diaphragm, and is anastomosed to the ascending aorta. The drive line is externalized through the right or left abdominal wall and connected to the external power and control unit. The maximum pump flow is 11.6 L/min for the IP-1000 LVAS and 9.6 L/min for the VE- and XVE-LVAS. The HeartMate device can be oper-

ated either in a fixed-rate mode or, more often, in an automatic mode that more closely resembles normal physiologic conditions. In the automatic mode, the device ejects when the pump is 90% full or when it senses a decreased rate of filling. As the patient's activity increases, the pump fills faster and the rate (or stroke volume) automatically increases, resulting in an increase in pump output. With a decrease in activity, pump filling and output decrease. Because the aortic valve rarely opens when the heart is fully supported by a left ventricular assist device, pump output is synonymous with cardiac output. During normal operation, the pump completely unloads the left ventricle and supports cardiac output at physiologic levels. Because of the portability and ease of operation of the HeartMate VE LVAS, patients can be discharged to await heart transplantation outside the hospital.

In a series of 100 patients from the Cleveland Clinic, McCarthy and colleagues reported a survival to transplantation of 76% with the HeartMate LVAD.[31] Of these 100 patients, 64 were bridged with a pneumatic device and 36 were bridged with HeartMate VE. The mean duration of support was 70 ± 41 days. The incidence of perioperative right-sided circulatory failure requiring right ventricular support was 11%. Preoperative risk factors for death included preoperative ventilator support, preoperative ECMO support, low pulmonary artery pressure, and elevated blood urea nitrogen, creatinine, and total bilirubin. In another large series of patients supported with the HeartMate LVAD, Sun and colleagues reported a survival to transplantation of 70% at the Columbia-Presbyterian Hospital.[70] Of 95 patients reported in their series, 62 of 88 eligible patients received transplants, 4 had devices explanted, 2 remained awaiting transplantation, and 3 received devices as destination therapy. In a prospective, multicenter clinical trial of the HeartMate VE LVAD,

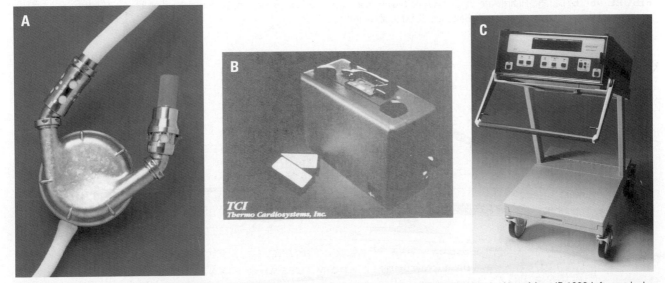

FIGURE 46-15. *A,* The HeartMate IP 1000 left ventricular assist device. *B,* Pneumatic drive console for the HeartMate IP 1000 left ventricular assist device. *C,* Portable pneumatic drive console for the HeartMate IP 1000 left ventricular assist device.

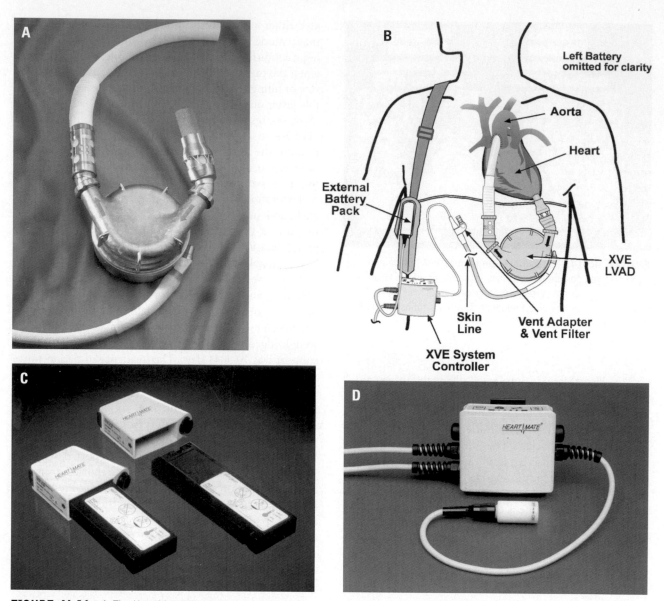

FIGURE 46-16. *A,* The HeartMate VE and XVE left ventricular assist devices. *B,* Representation of location of pump, inflow and outflow cannulas, and percutaneous drive line. *C,* Batteries. *D,* External controller.

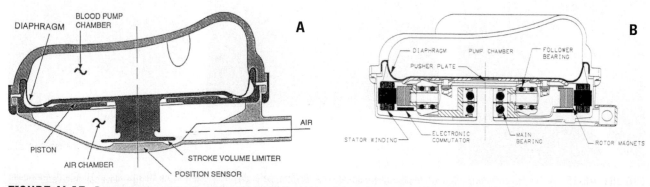

FIGURE 46-17. Representation of the HeartMate IP 1000 (A) and HeartMate VE left ventricular assist devices (B).

Frazier and colleagues reported on 280 patients who received the HeartMate VE device as a bridge to transplantation.[4] Of these patients, 188 (67%) survived to transplantation, while 10 (4%) had the device explanted, and 82 (29%) died awaiting transplantation. When compared to a cohort of historical controls, survival to transplantation was significantly greater for the HeartMate VE group (Figure 46-18). Additionally, 1-year posttransplantation survival was also significantly better in the patients receiving LVAD support (see Figure 46-18). Factors associated with adverse survival to transplantation included age, prior history of cardiac surgery, and elevated total bilirubin and creatinine.

NOVACOR LVAS

The Novacor LVAS (World Heart Corporation, Ottawa, Canada) is a portable, implantable left ventricular assist device designed for long-term circulatory support (Figure 46-19).[71–73] It differs significantly from the HeartMate in its mode of pump actuation and its use of smooth blood-contacting surfaces. During pump systole, two opposing pusher plates compress a seamless polyurethane blood sac, causing ejection of blood (Figure 46-20). Unidirectional flow is ensured by use of 21-mm bioprosthetic valved conduits at the inlet and outlet orifices. The device produces a maximum stroke volume of 70 mL and is monitored by an external drive console. An internal solenoid converts the electric energy from the console to mechanic energy, compressing the pusher plates and pressurizing the pump sac for blood ejection. A percutaneous lead contains the necessary electrical wires and a vent to transfer air. In 1993, the Novacor LVAS was converted from a console-operated system into a wearable system to enhance patient mobility. The wearable system eliminates the need for a bulky console by incorporating a compact controller and rechargeable power packs that are worn on the patient's belt. The wearable system is designed for out-of-hospital use and can be monitored with a bedside monitor. The Novacor is implanted through an extended median sternotomy incision. The pump is positioned in

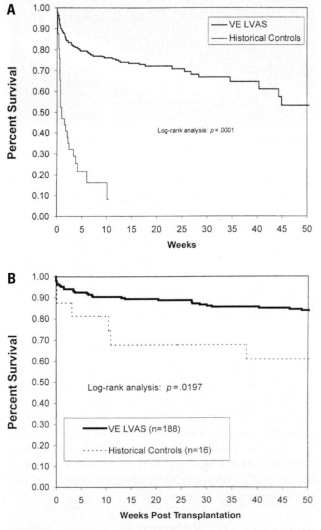

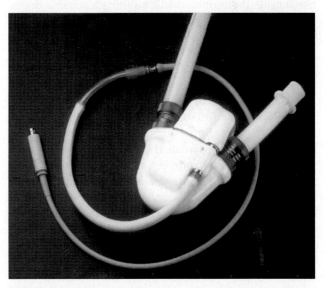

FIGURE 46-19. The Novacor left ventricular assist device (World Heart, Inc., Ottawa, Canada).

FIGURE 46-18. Survival to heart transplantation with LVAD therapy as compared to inotrope therapy (A) and posttransplantation (B). Reproduced with permission from Frazier OH et al.[4] LVAD = left ventricular assist device; VE LVAS = HeartMate VE left ventricular assist system.

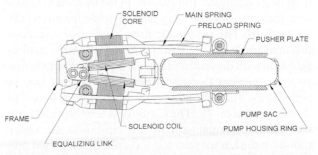

FIGURE 46-20. Representation of the Novacor left ventricular assist device (World Heart, Inc., Ottawa, Canada).

the abdominal wall just anterior to the posterior rectus sheath between the left iliac crest and the costal margin. Cardiopulmonary bypass support is necessary during placement of the left ventricular apical inflow conduit and anastomosis of the outflow graft to the ascending aorta. A percutaneous drive line is brought out through the right lateral abdominal wall and is connected to the cable from the controller. The external controller provides power and allows control and monitoring of the pump. The system can be operated in either a fixed-rate, synchronous, or fill-to-empty mode. The synchronized mode maximizes cardiac unloading. In this mode, an electrocardiographic signal causes pump diastole to correspond with cardiac systole, allowing the heart to fill the pump with little effort. Alternatively, pump output may be maximized by means of the fill-to-empty mode, in which the pumping rate is adjusted automatically, depending on the filling rate of the pump. In addition, the system may be operated in a fixed-rate mode in which the operator sets a constant pumping rate. During device use, anticoagulation with heparin, and later with warfarin and antiplatelet therapy, is necessary to prevent thromboembolism. During long-term support, ambulatory patients can be discharged to live outside the hospital while awaiting a suitable donor heart. The Novacor LVAS is approved by the FDA for use in bridge to heart transplant indication.

Total Artificial Hearts

CARDIOWEST C-70 TOTAL ARTIFICIAL HEART

The CardioWest C-70 total artificial heart (CardioWest Technologies, Inc., Tucson, AZ), formerly called the Jarvik or Symbion total artificial heart, is a pulsatile biventricular cardiac replacement system (Figure 46-21).[37,74] The rigid polyurethane pump contains a smooth, flexible polyurethane diaphragm that separates the blood and air chambers. Two Medtronic-Hall mechanical valves located at the inflow and outflow orifices ensure unidirectional blood flow. Compressed air from the external drive console moves the diaphragm upward, pressurizing the blood chamber and causing ejection of blood. The pump has a maximum stroke volume of 70 mL and a maximum flow rate of 15 L/min, although the average flow rate is < 8 L/min. Pump rate, duration of systole, and driving pressure can be adjusted to achieve optimal flow conditions. The total artificial heart is surgically implanted in the mediastinal space after the ventricles have been excised, while the atrial cuffs are retained. The pneumatic drive lines are externalized percutaneously and attached to the drive console. Anticoagulation with dipyridamole, heparin, and warfarin is necessary to prevent thrombus formation. Patients may be ambulatory, but their mobility is frequently restricted by the large drive console. The CardioWest total artificial heart is currently undergoing clinical investigation at select institutions in the United States. It is currently being used only for a bridge to heart transplant indication. A portable driver is being developed to give the patient greater mobility.

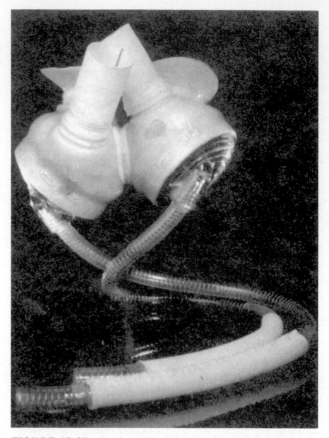

FIGURE 46-21. The CardioWest C-TO total artificial heart.

In a review of clinical outcomes with the CardioWest total artificial heart (TAH) for bridge to transplant indication, Copeland and colleagues reported a 75% survival to transplantation and a survival to discharge of 59%.[74] These outcomes were achieved in 43 patients who represent approximately 11 patient-years of experience. The survival to transplantation and discharge was significantly greater compared to those patients receiving biventricular support with a Thoratec VAS.

Future Directions

Currently, there are several safe and effective options for providing temporary MCS for patients presenting with cardiogenic shock or refractory heart failure. Newer device designs are under development that will increase the options available to patients. Due to technological advances, it will be difficult to predict what ddevices will ultimately prove to be the most efficacious. It is likely that a variety of devices will be necessary, depending on clinical circumstances and patient characteristics.

References

1. Khot UN, Mishra M, Smedira NG, et al. Acute renal failure complicating cardiogenic shock is not a contraindication to mechanical support as a bridge to cardiac transplantation [abstract]. Circulation 2001;104 Suppl II:II-714.

2. Oz MC, Goldstein DJ, Pepino P, et al. Screening scale predicts patients successfully receiving long-term implantable left ventricular assist devices. Circulation 1995;92 Suppl II:II-169–73.

3. Deng MC, Loebe M, El-Banayosy A, et al. Mechanical circulatory support for advanced heart failure: effect of patient selection on outcome. Circulation 2001;103: 231–7.

4. Frazier OH, Rose EA, Oz MC, et al. Multicenter clinical evaluation of the HeartMate vented electric left ventricular assist system in patients awaiting heart transplantation. J Thorac Cardiovasc Surg 2001;122:1186–95.

5. El-Banayosy A, Arusoglu L, Kizner L, et al. Predictors of survival in patients bridged to transplantation with the Thoratec VAD device: a single-center retrospective study on more than 100 patients. J Heart Lung Transplant 2000;19:964–8.

6. Pae WE. Ventricular assist devices and total artificial hearts: a ASAIO-ISHLT registry experience. Ann Thorac Surg 1993;55:295–8.

7. Guyton RA, Schonberger J, Everts P, et al. Postcardiotomy shock: clinical evaluation of the BVS 5000 biventricular support system. Ann Thorac Surg 1993;56:346–56.

8. Jett GK. Postcardiotomy support with ventricular assist devices: selection of recipients. Semin Thorac Cardiovasc Surg 1994;6:136–9.

9. Samuels LE, Kaufman MS, Thomas MP, et al, Wechsler AS. Pharmacologic criteria for ventricular assist device insertion following postcardiotomy shock: experience with the Abiomed BVS system. J Cardiac Surg 1999;14:288–93.

10. Farrar DJ, Hill JD, Pennington DG, et al. Preoperative and postoperative comparison of patients with univentricular and biventricular support with the Thoratec ventricular assist device as a bridge to cardiac transplantation. J Thorac Cardiovasc Surg 1997;113:202–9.

11. Kormos RL, Gasior TA, Kawai A, et al. Transplant candidate's clinical status rather than right ventricular function defines the need for univentricular versus biventricular support. J Thorac Cardiovasc Surgery 1996;111:773–83.

12. Young JB. Healing the heart with ventricular assist device therapy: mechanisms of cardiac recovery. Ann Thorac Surg 2001;71:S210–9.

13. Frazier OH, Myers TJ. Left ventricular assist system as a bridge to myocardial recovery. Ann Thoracic Surg 1999; 68:734–41.

14. Mueller J, Wallukat G, Weng Y-G, et al. Weaning from mechanical cardiac support in patients with idiopathic dilated cardiomyopathy. Circulation 1997;96:542–9.

15. Levin HR, Oz MC, Chen JM, et al. Reversal of chronic ventricular dilation in patients with end-stage cardiomyopathy by prolonged mechanical unloading. Circulation 1995;91:2717–20.

16. Bartling B, Milting H, Schumann H, et al. Myocardial gene expression of regulators of myocyte apoptosis and myocyte calcium homeostasis during hemodynamic unloading by ventricular assist devices in patients with end-stage heart failure. Circulation 1999;100 Suppl II:216–23.

17. Torre-Amione G, Stetson SJ, Youker KA, et al. Decreased expression of tumor necrosis factor-alpha in failing human myocardium after mechanical circulatory support: a potential mechanism for cardiac recovery. Circulation 1999;100:1189–93.

18. Li YY, Feng Y, McTiernan CF, et al. Downregulation of matrix metalloproteinases and reduction in collagen damage in the failing human heart after support with left ventricular assist devices. Circulation 2001;104:1147–52.

19. Ogletree Hughes ML, Stull LB, Sweet WE, et al. Mechanical unloading restores β-adrenergic responsiveness and reverses receptor downregulation in the failing human heart. Circulation 2001;104:881–6.

20. Delgado R 3rd, Radovancevic B, Massin EK, et al. Neurohormonal changes after implantation of a left ventricular assist system. ASAIO J 1998;44:299–302.

21. Lee SH, Doliba N, Osbakken M, et al. Improvement of myocardial mitochondrial function after hemodynamic support with left ventricular assist devices in patients with heart failure. J Thorac Cardiovasc Surgery 1998; 116:344–9.

22. Helman DN, Maybaum SW, Morales DL, et al. Recurrent remodeling after ventricular assistance: is long-term myocardial recovery attainable? Ann Thorac Surg 2000; 70:1255–8.

23. Rao V, Slater JP, Edwards NM, et al. Surgical management of valvular disease in patients requiring left ventricular assist device support. Ann Thorac Surg 2001;71:1448–53.

24. Rose AG, Park SJ, Bank AJ, Miller LW. Partial aortic valve fusion induced by left ventricular assist device. Ann Thorac Surg 2000;70:1270–4.

25. Moazami N, Argenziano M, Kohmoto T, et al. Inflow valve regurgitation during left ventricular assist device support may interfere with reverse ventricular remodeling. Ann Thorac Surg 1998;65:628–31.

26. Santamore WP, Gray LA. Left ventricular contributions to right ventricular systolic function during LVAD support. Ann Thorac Surg 1996;61:350–6.

27. Pavie A, Leger P. Physiology of univentricular versus biventricular support. Ann Thorac Surgery 1996;61:347–9.

28. Mandarino WA, Winowich S, Gorcsan J, et al. Right ventricular performance and left ventricular assist device filling. Ann Thorac Surg 1997;63:1044–9.

29. Aria H, Swartz MT, Pennington DG, et al. Importance of ventricular arrhythmias in bridge patients with ventricular assist devices. ASAIO Trans 1991;37:M427–8.

30. Shapiro GC, Leibowitz DW, Oz MC, et al. Diagnosis of patent foramen ovale with transesophageal echocardiography in a patient supported with a left ventricular assist device. J Heart Lung Transplant 1995;14:594–7.

31. McCarthy PM, Smedira NO, Vargo RL, et al. One hundred patients with the HeartMate left ventricular assist device: evolving concepts and technology. J Thorac Cardiovasc Surg 1998;115:904–12.

32. Rose EC, Gelijns AC, Moskowitz AJ, et al. Long-term use of a left ventricular assist device for end-stage heart failure. N Engl J Med 2001;345:1435–43.

33. Goldstein DJ, Seldomridge JA, Chen JM, et al. Use of aprotinin in LVAD recipients reduces blood loss, blood use, and perioperative mortality. Ann Thorac Surg 1995; 59:1063–8.

34. Kaplon RJ, Gillinov AM, Smedira NG, et al. Vitamin K reduces bleeding in left ventricular assist device recipients. J Heart Lung Transplant 1999;18:346–50.

35. Nakatani S, Thomas JD, Savage RM, et al. Prediction of right ventricular dysfunction after left ventricular assist device implantation. Circulation 1996;94 Suppl 9:II216–21.

36. Argenziano M, Choudhri AF, Moazami N, et al. Randomized, double-blind trial of inhaled nitric oxide in LVAD recipients with pulmonary hypertension. Ann Thorac Surg 1998;65:340–5.

37. Copeland JG, Smith RG, Arabia FA, et al. Comparison of the CardioWest total artificial heart, the Novacor left ventricular assist system, and the Thoratec ventricular assist system in bridge to transplantation. Ann Thorac Surg 2001;71:92S–97S.

38. Rose EA, Levin HR, Oz MC, et al. Artificial circulatory support with textured interior surfaces: a counterintuitive approach to minimizing thromboembolism. Circulation 1994;90 Suppl II:II-87–91.

39. Slater JP, Rose EA, Levin HR, et al. Low thromboembolic risk without anticoagulation using advanced-design left ventricular assist devices. Ann Thorac Surg 1996;62:1321–7.

40. Argenziano M, Catanese KA, Moazami N, et al. The influence of infection on survival and successful transplantation in patients with left ventricular assist devices. J Heart Lung Transplant 1997;16:822–31.

41. Holman EL, Murrah CP, Ferguson ER, et al. Infections during extended circulatory support: University of Alabama at Birmingham experience 1989 to 1994. Ann Thorac Surg 1996;61:366–71.

42. Ankersmit HJ, Tugulea S, Spanier T, et al. Activation-induced T-cell death and immune dysfunction after implantation of left ventricular assist device. Lancet 1999;354:550–5.

43. Itescu S, Tung TC, Burke EM, et al. Preformed IgG antibodies against major histocompatibility complex class II antigens are major risk factors for high-grade cellular rejection in recipients of heart transplantation. Circulation 1998;98:786–93.

44. Nader M, Itescu S, Williams MR, et al. Platelet transfusions are associated with the development of anti-major histocompatibility complex class I antibodies in patients with ventricular assist support. J Heart Lung Transplant 1998;17:876–80.

45. Pagani FD, Dyke DB, Wright S, et al. Development of anti-major histocompatibility complex class I or II antibodies following left ventricular assist device implantation: effects on subsequent allograft rejection and survival. J Heart Lung Transplant 2001;20:646–53.

46. Kantrowitz A, Tjonneland S, Freed PS, et al. Initial clinical experience with intraaortic balloon pumping in cardiogenic shock. JAMA 1968;203:135.

47. Claus RH, Birtwell WC, Albertal G, et al. Assisted circulation, the arterial counterpulsator. J Thorac Cardiovasc Surg 1961;41:447.

48. Muehrcke DD, McCarthy PM, Stewart RW, et al. Extracorporeal membrane oxygenation for postcardiotomy cardiogenic shock. Ann Thorac Surg 1996;61:684–91.

49. Smedira NG, Wudel JH, Hlozek CC, et al. Venovenous extracorporeal life support for patients after cardiotomy. ASAIO J 1997;43:M444–6.

50. Magovern GJ, Magovern JA, Benckart DH, et al. Extracorporeal membrane oxygenation-preliminary results in patients with postcardiotomy cardiogenic shock. Ann Thorac Surgery 1994;57:1462–7.

51. Bartlett RH, Roloff DW, Custer JR, et al. Extracorporeal life support: the University of Michigan experience. JAMA 2000;283:904–8.

52. Hill JD, O'Brien TG, Murray JJ, et al. Extracorporeal oxygenation for acute post-traumatic respiratory failure. N Eng J Med 1972;286:629–34.

53. Pagani FD, Lynch W, Swaniker F, et al. Extracorporeal life support to left ventricular assist device bridge to heart transplant: a strategy to optimize survival and resource utilization. Circulation 1999;100(19):II206–10.

54. Pagani FD, Aaronson KD, Dyke DB, et al. Assessment of an extracorporeal life support to LVAD bridge to heart transplant strategy. Ann Thorac Surg 2000;70:1977–85.

55. Smedira NG, Moazomi N, Golding CM, et al. Clinical experience with 202 adults receiving extracorporeal membrane oxygenation for cardiac failure: survival at five years. J Thorac Cardiovasc Surg 2001;122:92–102.

56. Magovern GJ, Simpson KA. Extracorporeal membrane oxygenation for adult cardiac support: the Allegheny experience. Ann Thorac Surg 1999;68:655–61.

57. Noon GP, Lafuente JA, Irwin S. Acute and temporary ventricular support with BioMedicus centrifugal pump. Ann Thorac Surg 1999;68:650–4.

58. Curtis JJ, Walls JT, Wagner-Mann CC, et al. Centrifugal pumps: description of devices and surgical techniques. Ann Thorac Surgery 1999;68:666–71.

59. Mehta SM, Aufiero TX, Pae WE, et al. Results of mechanical ventricular assistance for the treatment of postcardiotomy cardiogenic shock. ASAIO J 1996;42:211–8.

60. Thiele H, Lauer B, Hambrecht R, et al. Reversal of cardiogenic shock by percutaneous left atrial-to-femoral arterial bypass assistance. Circulation 2001;104:2917–22.

61. Magovern JA, Sussman MJ, Goldstein AH, et al. Clinical results with the AB-180 left ventricular assist device. Ann Thorac Surg 2001; 71:S121–4.

62. McBride LR, Naunheim KS, Fiore AC, et al. Clinical experience with 111 Thoratec ventricular assist devices. Ann Thorac Surg 1999;67:1233–8.

63. El-Banayosy A, Korfer R, Arusoglu L, et al. Bridging to cardiac transplantation with the Thoratec ventricular assist device. Thorac Cardiovasc Surg 1999;47 Suppl 2:307–10.

64. Farrar DJ, Buck KE, Coulter JH, et al. Portable pneumatic biventricular driver for the Thoratec ventricular assist device. ASAIO J 1997;43:M631–4.

65. Reichenbach SH, Farrar DJ, Hill JD. A versatile intracorporeal ventricular assist device based on the Thoratec VAD system. Ann Thorac Surg 2001;71:S171–5.

66. Gray LA, Champsaur GG. The BVS 5000 biventricular assist device. The worldwide registry experience. ASAIO J 1994;40:M460–4.

67. Samuels LE, Holmes EC, Thomas MP, et al. Management of acute cardiac failure with mechanical assist: experience with the Abiomed BVS 5000. Ann Thorac Surg 2001;71:S67–72.

68. Oz MC, Argenziano M, Catanese KA, et al. Bridge experience with long-term implantable left ventricular assist device. Circulation 1997;95:1844–52.

69. Frazier OH, Myers TJ, Radovancevic B. The HeartMate left ventricular assist systems – overview and 12 year experience. Texas Heart Institute Journal 1998;25:265–71.

70. Sun BJ, Catanese KA, Spanier TB, et al. 100 Long-term implantable left ventricular assist devices: the Columbia Presbyterian interim experience. Ann Thorac Surg 1999;68;688–94.

71. Robbins RC, Oyer PE. Bridge to transplant with the Novacor left ventricular assist system. Ann Thorac Surg 1999;68:695–7.

72. El-Banayosy A, Deng M, Loisance DY, et al. The European experience of Novacor left ventricular assist (LVAS) therapy as a bridge to transplant: a retrospective multi-centre study. Eur J Cardiothorac Surg 1999;15:835–41.

73. Murali S. Mechanical circulatory support with the Novacor LVAS: world-wide clinical results. Thorac Cardiovasc Surg 1999;47 Suppl 2:321–5.

74. Copeland JG, Pavie A, Duveau D, et al. Bridge to transplantation with the CardioWest total artificial heart: the international experience 1993–1995. J Heart Lung Transplant 1996;15:94–9.

CHAPTER 47

NEW DEVICES TO SUPPORT THE HEART: PASSIVE VENTRICULAR CONSTRAINT AND DIRECT COMPRESSION

AFTAB R. KHERANI, MD, JOHN H. ARTRIP, MD, MEHMET C. OZ, MD

Since the first left ventricular assist device (LVAD) was successfully used to bridge a patient to transplantation in the late 1980s, technological advances have made these pumps a viable option for a broader spectrum of patients with end-stage heart failure.[1] Devices supporting the heart typically have served as pumps that augment flow in a centrifugal, pulsatile, or axial manner. Recently however, researchers have targeted ventricular geometry in their effort to improve function of the failing heart. Passive ventricular constraint devices favorably mold the heart into a theoretically more efficient pump. Also on the cutting edge of cardiac assist technology are direct compression devices. This concept has been tried in patients in the past, and after a long period of hibernation, companies are again pursuing this niche. Great progress has been made in the areas of direct compression and passive ventricular constraint device technology, and this technology has matured enough to allow comparison to pump devices, which have already established a prominent niche in the surgical management of end-stage heart failure.

Passive Ventricular Constraint Devices

Laplace's law states that wall stress equals the product of intraventricular pressure and radius divided by wall thickness. This is the premise behind the Batista procedure. A partial left ventriculectomy leads to favorable changes in left ventricular geometry, thereby decreasing wall stress and improving function.[2] This, too, is the rationale behind passive ventricular devices. Minimizing dilatation in turn minimizes unfavorable changes in gene expression and neurohormonal stimulation adversely affecting the extracellular matrix. The harmful effects of myocyte stretch are associated with remodeling, an autoinductive process that can lead to heart failure.[3–6] The goal of these devices is to enhance cardiac function by exacting geometric changes that result in augmented ventricular function. The major advantage of these devices lies in their simplicity. Because there is no attached console or power source, they are theoretically easy to maintain once implanted.

Myosplint

The Myosplint (Myocor, Maple Grove, Minnesota) is a 1.4 mm braided polyethylene splint coated with expanded polytetrafluoroethylene. The splint spans the ventricular chamber under tension, attached to thermoplastic polyester-covered epicardial pads at each end (Figure 47-1). To achieve adequate geometric change, three splints are placed, essentially bisecting the failing ventricle. The device is implanted on a beating heart. The needle holes made in the ventricle are occluded by the splint itself, and residual oozing is controlled by the epicardial pads. Once the splints are implanted, the reduction in the effective radius of the chamber translates to decreased wall stress of approximately 20% (derived from left ventricular end-diastolic volume). Typically, a specially designed device is used to place one epicardial pad at the lateral wall and the other at the posterior septum. An obvious emphasis is placed on avoiding the epicardial vessels, papillary muscles, and mitral valve; to this end, two-dimensional echocardiography is used as necessary.

Takagaki and colleagues established that the Myosplint could safely and repeatedly be implanted in dogs, perpendicular to the long axis of the left ventricle, without requiring cardiopulmonary bypass.[7] Another canine study by the Cleveland Clinic Foundation examined the

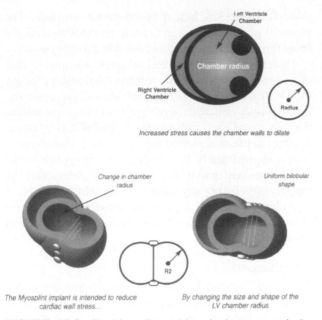

FIGURE 47-1. The Myosplint and how it changes ventricular geometry.

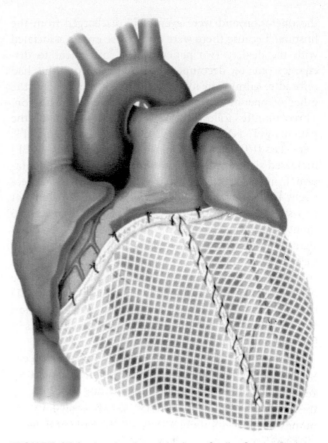

FIGURE 47-2. Anterior view of the Acorn Cardiac Support Device.

effect of the Myosplint on cardiac function. Laplace's law does not exactly apply to the figure-of-eight shape that results from Myosplint placement. Also, wall stress is not uniform around the circumference of the post-Myosplint ventricular chamber. Instead of the calculated 20% decrease in wall tension, animal studies revealed an observed 30% reduction in end-diastolic and a 39% decrease in end-systolic wall stress. Canine studies also demonstrate a significant increase in ejection fraction, from 19% to 36% acutely and 39% at 1 month, and significant decreases in end-systolic and end-diastolic volumes. Cardiac output did not significantly increase by thermodilution, although it did by echocardiography. There was no observed toxic response to the device.[8] Based on early short-term human trials by Klinikum Grosshadern (Munich, Germany) and the Cleveland Clinic Foundation, the Myosplint can be placed safely and effectively in patients.[9]

Acorn Cardiac Support Device

The Acorn Cardiac Support Device (CSD) (Acorn Cardiovascular, St. Paul, Minnesota) is a polyester mesh knit that serves as a jacket around the ventricles (Figure 47-2). It has bi-directional compliance and assists the heart in minimizing the extent of dilation; in addition, it actually reduces the diameter of the ventricle slightly. Six sizes are available, and the surgeon does any minor trimming that may be necessary. Once fitted, the CSD is sewn posteriorly and laterally, just above or below the atrioventricular groove. A final set of anterior stay sutures is placed. CSD implantation can be performed at the time of another cardiac surgical procedure, such as valve repair/replacement or coronary artery bypass grafting.[3]

Power and colleagues published the first large animal study examining the CSD.[10] They paced 12 adult sheep into heart failure. They then implanted the CSD into each animal via a partial lower sternotomy and randomized the animals to device retention (wrap) or removal (sham). Pacing then continued for 28 days, after which time the Australian group observed significant differences in left ventricular fractional shortening, degree of mitral valve regurgitation, and left ventricular long axis area, all favoring the wrap group. A subsequent canine study by the Henry Ford Hospital supported these findings.[11] After 3 months, dogs treated with the CSD demonstrated a significant decrease of almost 20% in left ventricular end-diastolic volume ($p = .04$), as compared to the just over 10% increase experienced by the control group ($p = .002$). The dogs with the device also demonstrated an increase in fractional area of shortening, in contrast to the decrease experienced by the control group. Additionally, CSD-treated animals demonstrated diminished myocyte hypertrophy and interstitial fibrosis, compared to control dogs.

To date, the largest single-center human clinical trial was performed at Charité Universitätsklinikum, Humboldt-Universität zu Berlin, Germany, on 27 patients between April 1999 and March 2000.[12] In 11 cases, CSD placement was the only procedure performed. All patients were New York Heart Association (NYHA) class III or IV at the time of enrollment. All CSD-only patients survived the operation and were eventually discharged from the hospital, because there were no adverse events associated with the device. Two patients died subsequent to discharge: one of decompensated heart failure (he had refused re-admission for medical management) and the other of pneumonia several months after implantation. Three months following CSD placement, 56% of the patients were NYHA class I, 33% were class II, and 11% were class II/III. Left ventricular ejection fraction (LVEF) increased significantly at 3 and 6 months post implantation, from 21.7 ± 1.5 to 27.6 ± 3.2 and 32.8 ± 4.9, respectively. Left ventricular end-diastolic dimension (but not end-systolic dimension) decreased significantly at 3 and 6 months, and the degree of mitral regurgitation decreased significantly at 3 months (there were insufficient data to make a determination at 6 months). Quality of life indices correlated with the objective improvement seen in these patients. This initial clinical safety trial supports CSD implantation as a means of improving cardiac function and symptoms in class III and IV heart failure patients in both the short and intermediate term.

The promise demonstrated by the Berlin experience is supported by the early worldwide experience with 91 patients (Figure 47-3). Mean implant time was 25 minutes, and there were no adverse events related to the device. Additionally, there was no evidence of constrictive disease.[13]

Direct Compression Devices

There are 1.1 million cases of acute myocardial infarction per year; in 7 to 10% of patients, cardiogenic shock follows, carrying an in-hospital mortality rate of 50 to 60%.[14] With these patients, there is demand for a product that can quickly and easily provide temporary mechanical circulatory support without requiring cardiopulmonary bypass. Direct compression devices target this patient population.

In 1965, George Anstadt introduced a mechanical compression device whose purpose was to provide effective, sustained, cardiopulmonary resuscitation.[15] The evolution of the technology pioneered by the original Anstadt cup gave us the CardioSupport System (formerly CTI, Inc., Pine Brook, New Jersey) and the AbioBooster (ABIOMED, Inc., Danvers, Massachusetts). The advances demonstrated by these devices allow for synchronized enhanced compres-

sion. These devices lack a blood-device interface. The potential advantages are significant in terms of theoretically fewer thromboembolic and immunologic complications.[16]

Direct epicardial compression causes an upward shift of the end-systolic pressure-volume relationship, for Pic (V,t) = Ptm (V,t) + PDCC (t), with Pic (V,t) representing intrachamber ventricular pressure, Ptm (V,t) representing the transmural ventricular pressure, and PDCC (t) representing the pressure exerted by the device.[17] The degree of shift is approximately 40% of the pressure applied by the device, so ventricular function must deteriorate by roughly 30% before any substantial benefit is realized. A slight leftward shift is seen in the end-diastolic pressure-volume relationship; this is seen more in the right than left ventricle.[16,18]

CardioSupport

The CardioSupport has been extensively studied in the animal lab and demonstrates promise, particularly in patients suffering acute cardiogenic shock.[16,18] It provides synchronized biventricular cardiac compression and is composed of a rigid outer surface, a vacuum line, polyurethane inflation bladder and inflation line. Implantation was via a thoracotomy, beginning at the apex, and extending up to the atrioventricular groove. In lieu of sutures, vacuum suction (−200 mm Hg) affixed the device to the heart. Lining the CardioSupport were two patch electrodes that enabled electrical synchronization. The device could also operate at a fixed rate, enabling it to serve the same purpose as the original Anstadt cup (CPR).

Animal studies are encouraging. In a canine model of acute heart failure, the CardioSupport doubled both mean arterial pressure and cardiac output in the short term in severely failing hearts. This was accomplished without any increase in myocardial oxygen consumption.[19] Because the device does not appreciably impact the end-diastolic pressure-volume relationship, preload and afterload optimization can maximize the degree of support. CTI, Inc., which developed the CardioSupport, is currently experiencing financial difficulty. The company is likely to be either reorganized or sold, thus ensuring the survival of this promising technology.

AbioBooster

The AbioBooster (Figure 47-4) is a pneumatic device composed of a series of tubular elements. Inflation of the tubes, during systole, helps augment ventricular contraction. The tubes correspondingly deflate in diastole. In vitro studies demonstrate 6.5 L/min of flow generated at an afterload of 115 mm Hg.[20]

Our group studied this device in an ovine model of cardiogenic shock.[21] During ventricular fibrillation, the device was able to increase flow from undetectable levels to 1.5 ± 0.3 L/min (p = .019). Similarly significant increases in flow and stroke volume were seen in sinus rhythm. Additionally, three animals underwent coronary

*p < .05 pre vs follow-up	Pre (n)	6 Mo (n)	12 Mo (n)
LVEDD (mm)	71.1 ± 1.1 (44)	65.2 ± 1.9 (27)	63.1 ± 2.3 (22)
LVEF (%)	22.4 ± 1.3 (44)	29.8 ± 2.2 (28)	31.1 ± 2.3 (23)

FIGURE 47-3. Results from the early global experience with the Acorn Cardiac Support Device. Significant, favorable changes were seen in both left ventricular end-diastolic dimension (LVEDD) and left ventricular ejection fraction (LVEF).

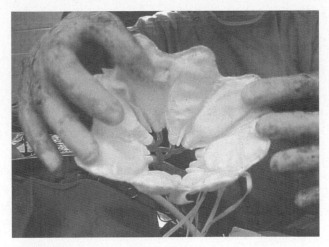

FIGURE 47-4. The AbioBooster device.

artery bypass grafting (CABG). Graft flow was not impeded during 2 h of support. These preliminary animal data show that the AbioBooster can effectively augment cardiac output in cardiogenic shock in the short term and that prior CABG is not a contraindication to device placement.

Conclusion

These devices will not replace traditional ventricular assist devices (VADs), which will continue to occupy a prominent niche in the management of patients who would otherwise suffer multisystem organ failure or die of severe congestive heart failure. In these patients, VADs serve as a bridge to transplantation for many, and can also serve as a bridge to recovery or as long-term outpatient support for patients who are not transplant candidates.[22]

For heart failure patients who are not sick enough for an LVAD, passive constraint devices may prevent end-organ damage and help to inhibit remodeling. Ideally, these devices will prevent heart failure patients from ever requiring a traditional LVAD or transplantation. On the other hand, direct compression devices target patients in postmyocardial infarction or postcardiotomy shock. They can enable a patient to recover from the acute decompensation and can be placed relatively easily and quickly. The advantages of these new devices over traditional LVADs are their relative simplicity and noninvasiveness, with only the Myosplint having any direct interaction with blood. The questions that remain to be answered are concerned with comparisons to medical management and with studies of long-term durability and efficacy. Concerns include reliability, safety, and when, if ever, these devices may be removed. This final point raises ethical and financial issues that will challenge our society. Although early studies of these new devices demonstrate promise, these questions must be answered before their use becomes widespread.

References

1. Argenziano M, Oz MC, Rose EA. The continuing evolution of mechanical ventricular assistance. Curr Probl Surg 1997;34:322–86.
2. Batista RJV, Santos JVL, Takeshita N, et al. Partial left ventriculectomy to improve left ventricular function in end-stage heart disease. J Card Surg 1996;11:96–7.
3. Oz MC. Passive ventricular constraint for the treatment of congestive heart failure. Ann Thorac Surg 2001;71: S185–7.
4. Baig MK, Mahon N, McKenna WJ, et al. The pathophysiology of advanced heart failure. Heart Lung 1999;28:87–101.
5. Pan J, Fukuda K, Saito M, et al. Mechanical stretch activates the JAK/STAT pathway in rat cardiomyocytes. Circ Res 1999;84:1127–36.
6. Minamisawa S, Hoshijima M, Chu G, et al. Chronic phospholamban-sarcoplasmic reticulum calcium ATPase interaction is the critical calcium cycling defect in dilated cardiomyopathy. Cell 1999;99:313–22.
7. Takagaki M, McCarthy PM, Ochiai Y, et al. Novel device to change left ventricular shape for heart failure treatment: device design and implantation procedure. ASAIO J 2001;47:244–8.
8. McCarthy PM, Takagaki M, Ochiai Y, et al. Device-based change in left ventricular shape: a new concept for the treatment of dilated cardiomyopathy. J Thorac Cardiovasc Surg 2001;122:482–90.
9. Schenk S, Reichenspurner H, Groezner JG, et al. Myosplint implantation and ventricular shape change in patients with dilative cardiomyopathy—first clinical experience. J Heart Lung Transplant 2000;20:217.
10. Power JM, Raman J, Dornom A, et al. Passive ventricular constraint amends the course of heart failure: a study in an ovine model of dilated cardiomyopathy. Cardiovasc Res 1999;44:549–55.
11. Chaudhry PA, Mishima T, Sharov VG, et al. Passive epicardial containment prevents ventricular remodeling in heart failure. Ann Thorac Surg 2000;70:1275–80.
12. Konertz WF, Shapland E, Hotz H, et al. Passive containment and reverse remodeling by a novel textile cardiac support device. Circulation 2001;104 Suppl I:I270–5.
13. Oz MC, Konertz WF, Kleber FX, et al. Global surgical experience with the Acorn Cardiac Support Device. [Submitted]
14. Hochman JS, Sleeper LA, Webb JG, et al. Early revascularization in acute myocardial infarction complicated by cardiogenic shock. N Engl J Med 1999;341:625–34.
15. Anstadt GL, Blakemore WS, Baue AE. A new instrument for prolonged mechanical massage. Circulation 1965;31 Suppl II:43.
16. Williams MR, Artrip JH. Direct cardiac compression for cardiogenic shock with the CardioSupport system. Ann Thorac Surg 2001;71 Suppl I:S188–9.
17. Artrip JH, Burkhoff D. Epicardial compression mechanical devices. In: Goldstein DJ, Oz MC, editors. Cardiac assist devices. Armonk, NY: Futura Publishing; 2000. p. 387–402.
18. Artrip JH, Yi G-H, Levin HR, et al. Physiological and hemodynamic evaluation of nonuniform direct cardiac compression. Circulation 1999;100(19 Suppl:II236–43.

19. Artrip JH, Wang J, Leventhal AR, et al. Hemodynamic effects of direct biventricular compression studied in isovolumic and ejected isolated canine hearts. Circulation 1999;99:2177–84.

20. Kung RTV, Rosenberg M. Heart booster: a pericardial support device. Ann Thorac Surg 1999;68:764–7.

21. Kavarana MN, Helman DN, Williams MR, et al. Circulatory support with a direct cardiac compression device: a less invasive approach with the AbioBooster device. J Thorac Cardiovasc Surg 2001;122:786–7.

22. Rose EA, Gelijns AC, Moskowitz AJ, et al, for the Randomized Evaluation of Mechanical Assistance for the Treatment of Congestive Heart Failure (REMATCH) Study Group. Long-term use of a left ventricular assist device for end-stage heart failure. N Engl J Med 2001;345:1435–43.

CHAPTER 48

KANTROWITZ CARDIOVAD: A PERMANENT INTRAAORTIC BALLOON PUMP FOR CONGESTIVE HEART FAILURE

DAVID JAYAKAR, MD, VALLUVAN JEEVANANDAM, MD

Need for Permanent Left Ventricular Assist Device

The treatment of congestive heart failure (CHF) caused by left ventricular dysfunction has evolved dramatically in the last decade.[1,2] Advances in medical treatments have helped patients in all stages of heart failure, even those with New York Heart Association (NYHA) class IV symptoms.[3,4] However, for an expanding group of patients, nonpharmacologic circulatory assistance is the only option. Currently, transplantation is the best option for these patients but is limited by a shortage of donors, leading to a rising mortality for patients on the waiting list. Approximately 16,500 patients are considered to be eligible candidates; only 2,000, however, receive transplants.[5] Furthermore, transplantation is hindered by the complications of immunosuppression and chronic allograft vasculopathy.

These grim statistics have focused attention on mechanical circulatory assist devices for permanent use. Investigators have used mechanical energy in three ways to improve circulation (Table 48-1). The first is direct augmentation of the heart, demonstrated by concepts such as dynamic cardiomyoplasty,[6] the AbioBooster (ABIOMED Inc., Danvers, MA) heart booster,[7] and direct mechanical ventricular actuation (DMVA).[8] Cardiomyoplasty is not effective in advanced stages of heart failure because of operative mortality, the length of time needed to train the latissimus dorsi muscle, chronic muscle fatigue, and only marginal efficacy in improving myocardial function. The AbioBooster and DMVA wrap around and squeeze the heart.[9] These devices are still under development.

Another method of augmenting circulation is pumping blood from the left atria/ventricle to the aorta with enough force to maintain systemic blood pressure. The

TABLE 48-1. Type of Assistance to Heart

Direct mechanical augmentation of heart
 Dynamic cardiomyoplasty
 AbioBooster
 Direct mechanical actuation

Hemodynamic augmentation of left ventricle
 HeartMate
 Novacor
 Thoratec

Hemodynamic augmentation of aorta
 Intraaortic balloon pump
 Kantrowitz CardioVAD

HeartMate/Thoratec[10] (Thoratec Inc., Pleasanton, CA) and Novacor[11] (WorldHeart Corp., Ottawa, Canada) devices follow this principle and are approved by the Food and Drug Administration (FDA) for ventricular assistance as bridges to transplantation. Current devices undergoing trial for permanent implantation include the HeartMate (REMATCH trial),[12] Novacor (INTREPID trial), and the AbioCor total artificial heart (ABIOMED Inc., Danvers, MA).[13] These devices are electrically driven, have valves, and deliver blood in a pulsatile fashion. The console that controls them can be portable, and patients have been successfully placed on these assist devices and discharged home with an excellent quality of life. Another group of devices pump blood in a nonpulsatile fashion using axial flow or centrifugal technology. All these devices are "obligatory," that is, they cannot be stopped even for a short period of time without dire consequences for the patient such as thromboembolic events or ventricular assist device (VAD) regurgitation (Figure 48-1).

The third method of mechanical assistance is to supply energy to portions of the vascular system in order to

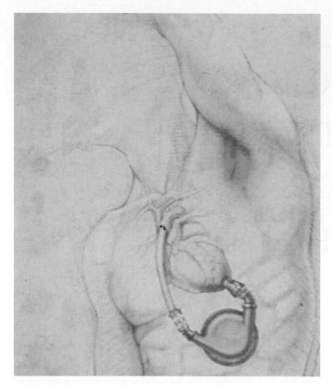

FIGURE 48-1. Devices working in parallel to heart.

decrease the workload of the heart and increase cardiac output. This approach, referred to as *diastolic augmentation*,[14] increases myocardial blood flow, increases diastolic blood pressure, and decreases the systemic resistance applied to the heart during systole. The most common method to augment diastolic pressure is the intraaortic balloon pump (IABP).[15] It is the most frequently used mechanical assist device in the world (> 100,000 uses annually; Datascope Corp., personal communication, March 2002). The most common use has been for treatment of cardiogenic shock,[16] primarily ischemic but also for other causes such as postcardiotomy, myocarditis, and transplantation rejection, and as a bridge to transplantation.[17] Increasing coronary blood flow and decreasing myocardial work give the heart an opportunity to recover. It is even used in chronic heart failure to recover patients from a decompensated state of CHF by decompressing the heart and bringing the myocytes to a better portion of the Starling curve.[18] Once the IABP is removed, the beneficial effects can be long lasting.[17]

Because the temporary IABP can reverse heart failure, development toward a permanent diastolic augmentation device began. The initial attempts used the motor power of the diaphragm to create an auxiliary ventricle.[19] A hemidiaphragm was wrapped around the distal portion of the thoracic aorta and stimulated during diastole, resulting in increased diastolic arterial pressure. Despite the appeal of using skeletal muscle as an auxiliary ventricle, the problem of muscle fatigue could not be overcome.

Next, Dr. Kantrowitz and his colleagues designed a succession of valveless mechanical auxiliary ventricles (MAVs), culminating in a U-shaped unit that spanned the transected aortic arch. In 1966, after a several-year effort in the animal laboratory, this device was implanted in two patients with far-advanced chronic CHF.[20] Both patients succumbed, one on the first postoperative day. The other survived 13 days, during which striking hemodynamic benefits were demonstrated, including prompt and decisive relief of episodes of pulmonary edema. Further clinical use was nonetheless suspended because of the inability to control thromboembolization associated with the U-shaped configuration. The investigators then began exploring the possibilities of implanting a MAV in the aorta or in its wall.

The next-generation MAV initially consisted of an elliptical silicone rubber pumping chamber, covering materials, and a gas conduit. The covering material used for the intravascular surface was Dacron velour backed with a conductive polyurethane. Plain Dacron cloth was used for the outer surface. The prosthesis was implanted on the lateral surface of the descending thoracic aorta between the origin of the left subclavian artery and the diaphragm. Initial clinical implants were encouraging but eventually failed because of thromboembolic episodes and driveline infections. Research then focused on improving the blood interface surface and the transcutaneous exit site.

The Kantrowitz CardioVAD

These changes led to the current-generation device, the Kantrowitz CardioVAD (KCV). The KCV consists of three components: a blood pump, a percutaneous access device (PAD), and drive consoles (Figure 48-2). The blood pump consists of an inflatable bladder mounted on an oblong rigid plastic shell. Valves are not required as backward circulatory flow is inhibited by the native aortic valve. The blood-contacting surface of the bladder is made of a single layer of textured polyurethane and is the only moving part inside the patient. The intravascular surface, similar to that of the HeartMate, fosters formation of a nonthrombogenic pseudointima (Figure 48-3). This obviates the need for long-term anticoagulation. The bladder provides approximately 60 cc of stroke volume, which is designed to approximate that of a normal heart. Displacement of volumes greater than the stroke volume leads to reverse flow of blood in the coronary and cerebral circulations.[17] The pump is designed to displace as much blood as possible during diastole without occluding the aorta. Studies show that occluding the aorta, even transiently, decreases the effectiveness of the pump.[17] This pump is installed in the descending aorta and works in series to the patient's left ventricle (Figure 48-4). It

1. increases the diastolic blood pressure and flow,
2. decreases the afterload for left ventricle,
3. increases the coronary blood flow,
4. increases the mean arterial pressure, and
5. decreases the workload of the left ventricle (Figure 48-5).

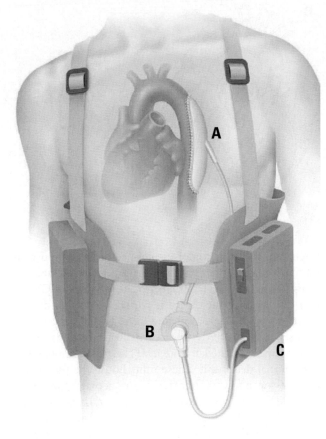

FIGURE 48-2. Components of the Kantrowitz CardioVAD. *A*, Blood pump. *B*, Percutaneous access device. *C*, External drive unit.

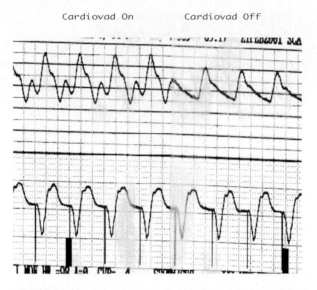

Cardiovad On   Cardiovad Off

FIGURE 48-4. Intraaortic pressure tracing with CardioVAD. The high degree of diastolic augmentation provided by the CardioVAD is because of improved timing and 60 cc balloon displacement volume.

To address potential problems with infection, the PAD was developed to allow for connection of the internal blood pump to the external console. This allows pneumatic and electrical signals to pass between the drive unit and the blood pump (Figure 48-6).

The PAD consists of a Dacron-covered 8 cm diameter disk that rests on the abdominal fascia. A stem made of polycarbonate traverses the epidermal layer. To promote maximal biocompatibility, the polycarbonate is coated with autologous fibroblasts. Fibroblasts are obtained from a skin biopsy 2 weeks prior to implantation. They are cultured and allowed to proliferate. Meanwhile, the polycarbonate stem is exposed to radiation that allows for laser etching of holes measuring 10 microns in depth and 15 microns wide. The fibroblasts adhere to the polycarbonate through growth into the channels. After proper seeding,

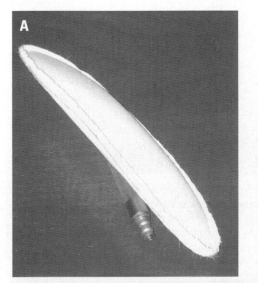

FIGURE 48-3. Balloon pump. *A*, Balloon pump shown without the tube connections. The surface that is in contact with the blood is textured. *B*, Pseudointima formed on the surface of the balloon pump. This is a photograph of the aorta of a calf taken 6 months post operation. The pump surface facing the blood in the aorta is completely endothelialized. The proximal end is to the left. The pseudoneointima is approximately 1 mm thick.

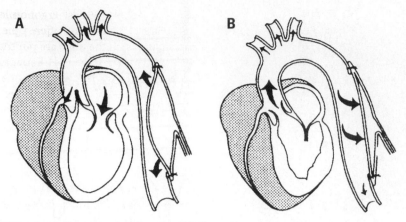

FIGURE 48-5. CardioVAD — descending aorta. *A,* Balloon on. *B,* Balloon off.

these fibroblasts effectively line the surface of the polycarbonate, and healing occurs between the layer of fibroblasts and the patient's granulation tissue (Figure 48-7). This biologic interface prevents downward growth of the epidermal layer, which can lead to marsupialization and creation of infection-prone sinuses.[21] The reliability and infection resistance of the PAD has been demonstrated in long-term experiments using Yucatan or miniature swine

(Figure 48-8).[22] The top of the connector has the port for the pneumatic connection and the electrical tabs for transmitting the electrical electrocardiogram (ECG) signals. The base of the device is connected to the internal blood pump through a silicone tube. Two electrical leads connect from the PAD to epicardial pacing leads placed on the surface of the left ventricle. The final component is the external drive unit. These units house the pneumatic compressor and microprocessor to actuate the blood pump. They are connected to the PAD via a flexible and removal driveline. The microprocessor automatically analyzes the electrical signal from the heart and triggers the KCV during diastole. The KCV can detect alterations in rhythm and trigger the pump accordingly. The compressor shuttles pressurized room air between the console and pump. There is no need for helium because the tube

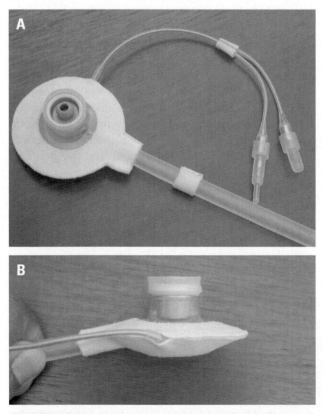

FIGURE 48-6. Percutaneous access device (PAD). This device consists of the necessary electrical and pneumatic connections. The Dacron cuff surrounds the polycarbonate plastic base, the surface of which is coated with the patient's cultured fibroblasts. *A,* Front view. *B,* Lateral view.

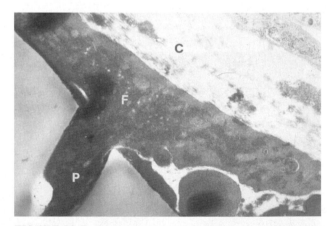

FIGURE 48-7. An electromicrograph of a section through the polycarbonate percutaneous access device (PAD) and the adjacent cultured fibroblasts. One individual fibroblast is seen occupying almost the entire field of the photograph with an arm of its body growing into the 1 μ hole in the polycarbonate body. Above the fibroblast can be seen collagen fibers and portions of other fibroblast bodies. The 1 μ hole is predrilled by exposing the PAD to radiation. The radioactive particles change the chemistry of the polycarbonate. It then can be etched with suitable solvents, leaving a hole in the surface of the polycarbonate about 1 μ in diameter and 15 μ deep.

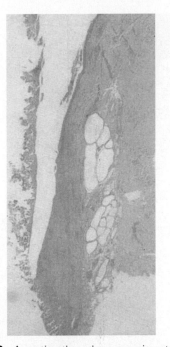

FIGURE 48-8. A section through an experimentally implanted device in a pig without autologous fibroblasts. The blank area is the region where the skin connector was implanted. It was dissolved to allow sectioning. The epidermis keratinocytes are growing down toward the region at the lower end of the slide, adjacent to the skin access device, where the endothelium encounters its own fibroblasts, which are firmly adherent to the skin connector. The normal downward growth of the epithelium is halted upon the recognition of its own fibroblasts. However, there is no adherence to the polycarbonate, leading to free spaces that are potential areas for infection.

that connects the device to the balloon pump is large enough to allow rapid transitions. This drive unit has gone through many modifications to reduce the size and to reduce noise made by the compressor. This unit is available in three configurations (Figure 48-9).

The suitcase model can be powered by alternating current (AC) and has a battery backup. This unit usually resides in the patient's home and is used to power the device through the night while the patient sleeps. It weighs approximately 70 pounds and can be moved with moderate difficulty. This is the quietest console and also has electronic monitoring/telemetry capability.

The other configurations are based around two 2.5-pound rectangular boxes the size of paperback books. One contains rechargeable batteries that are removable and charged through an independent charging unit. The batteries can last from 2 to 4 h, depending on the number of beats required. The other unit contains the microprocessor that senses the ECG from the epicardial electrodes and automatically triggers the pump to inflate during diastole. The units can be separated and carried around as a vest. This configuration is preferred during ambulation. Initially, some patients are too debilitated to be able to carry the extra weight, but after rehabilitation,

the vest offers the best ergonomic design. For limited ambulation, patients are offered the attaché case configuration, in which the units are put together in a case that is well insulated for sound. Patients can use this when ambulating in the house and want a unit that is quiet but not as cumbersome as the suitcase. Most patients use the vest unit except when sleeping.

IMPLANTATION TECHNIQUE

Preoperatively, diagnostic tests are performed to confirm that the device can be implanted into the descending aorta. The initial patients had magnetic resonance imaging (MRI) or computed axial tomography (CAT) scans, but this proved to be limited because of the presence of permanent implantable cardioverter-defibrillators (ICDs) and/or pacemakers. Transthoracic echocardiography (TTE) proved to be more helpful in defining the thoracic aorta and predicting the availability of an area distal to the left subclavian for cross-clamping. The length of the descending aorta is determined by radiography. A minimum of 19 cm is needed from the subclavian to the diaphragm for implantation of the KCV pump.

The first procedure performed after confirming the candidacy of the recipient is a skin biopsy. The skin biopsy is used to culture autologous fibroblasts for coating the polycarbonate component of the PAD. This outpatient procedure is done 2 weeks prior to implantation of the device. This can be done under local anesthesia. A suitable area on the volar aspect of the forearm skin is isolated, and the forearm is prepped. Local anesthesia with 1% Xylocaine is infiltrated around the proposed area. After ensuring adequate anesthesia, a small full-thickness area of skin measuring 1 cm × 5 cm is obtained with a scalpel and is transported to the lab in Krebs tissue culture medium. After adequate hemostasis, the skin defect can be closed with a fine absorbable suture and dressings applied. The patient is discharged home to await maturing of the bladder. Special emphasis is placed on nutritional replenishment and on improving pulmonary function while waiting for the KCV. Patients are instructed concerning the use of incentive spirometers and are given bronchodilator therapy.

After the PAD is adequately prepared (usually 10 days), the patient is admitted to the hospital 10 days later for CardioVAD insertion. A high-thoracic epidural catheter is placed 1 day prior to surgery to aid postthoracotomy pain management. The potential PAD site is also marked on the patient while the patient is wearing his or her customary clothing. The best site is above the belt line in the right upper quadrant.

On the day of surgery, the patient is anesthetized in the supine position with a double-lumen endotracheal tube. Hemodynamics are monitored by using a pulmonary artery catheter and right radial and femoral arterial catheters. Intraoperative transesophageal echocardiography is used to assess the heart function, aortic valve, and

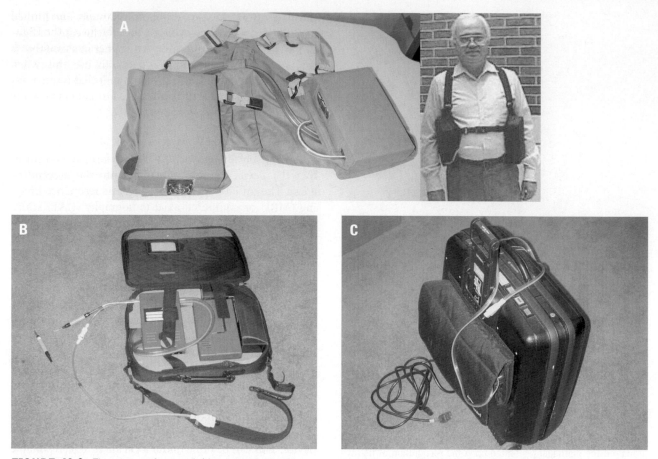

FIGURE 48-9. Three types of external drive units: *A*, portable vest version, 5 lb version; *B*, attaché case version; *C*, suitcase version, which weighs 70 lb.

the pathology in the descending aorta. The patient is secured with a bean bag in true lateral position and the hip rotated laterally to aid exposure to the left groin vessels. The femoral artery and vein are exposed with a vertical skin incision and prepared for cannulation with placement of purse strings.

The left thoracotomy is performed with a lateral skin incision based on the fifth intercostal space. The chest is entered, the left lung is decompressed, and the aorta is isolated. Cardiopulmonary bypass is initiated after activated clotting time (ACT) (> 450 s) – guided heparinization (300 U/kg) using femoral and transverse arch arterial cannulae and a double-stage femoral venous cannula. The heart is allowed to beat, the right lung is ventilated, and the patient is kept normothermic. The aorta is isolated 1 cm distal to the subclavian and at 8 and 16 cm from this area (points A, B, and C, respectively). The aorta is completely encircled at these three points.

The implantation of the balloon pump is done in two stages. During the first stage, the proximal part of the balloon is sewn. The proximal and midaorta are first clamped (points A and B), and the aorta is opened; 3 mm strips of the aorta are removed from the edges. All intercostal vessel bleeders from the aortic wall are controlled with a No. 3 Fogarty balloon catheter. The superior portion of the KCV

is sutured in place with a single layer of 2–0 polypropylene running mattress suture. A felt strip is used on the aortic side as a buttress. The cross-clamp at B (mid) is released and re-applied at point C (distal). The distal portion of the KCV is sewn to the aorta in a similar technique to the proximal end. The point C clamp is removed, and a second layer of running horizontal mattress sutures is used to further secure the KCV (Figure 48-10).

Care is taken to maintain proper spacing of the sutures and to not injure the internal balloon pump. After the KCV pump is implanted, the clamps are released and hemostasis ensured. The pump is connected to the controller with a silastic tube to check for adequate function and for air leaks.

The pericardium is opened, and a suitable area of lateral myocardium is dissected free. Three screw-in surface pacing electrodes (St. Jude Pacesetter, St. Paul, MN) are placed 1 cm apart in a triangular manner. After proper thresholds are checked and confirmed, the pacing leads are tunneled to a left upper quadrant subcutaneous pocket along with the permanent pump driveline. The KCV system is tested and mechanical support initiated. The patient is then weaned off cardiopulmonary bypass (CPB) and heparin-reversed by using protamine. After ensuring proper hemostasis, two chest tubes are placed, and the

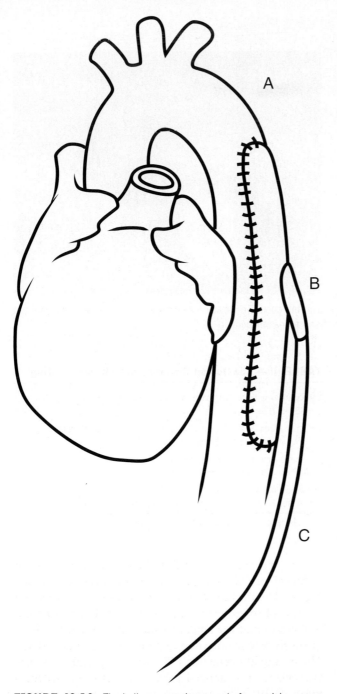

FIGURE 48-10. The balloon pump is secured after excising a part of the aortic wall. Two layers of Prolene 2–0 horizontal mattress sutures are used to secure the pump. The aorta is cross-clamped at point *A*, then sequentially at points *B* and *C*.

company) is centered on the proposed exit site. This punch provides a standardized skin opening for fitting the PAD. The PAD is then carefully inserted. The pacing leads and pneumatic tube from the blood pump that were left in the subcutaneous tunnel are connected to the PAD area. The skin incision above the pad connector is then closed using 2–0 Vicryl and subcuticular 4–0 PDS (Figure 48-11).

The patients are supported with maximum diastolic augmentation, with the device set to inflate immediately after the dicrotic notch. Anticoagulation is not required for the device; patients may receive warfarin (Coumadin) if dictated by the clinical situation.

CLINICAL EXPERIENCE

The initial feasibility trial was designed to test the safety of the device at 1 and 3 months. The enrolled eight patients were nontransplantation candidates who had end-stage cardiomyopathy. All had minimal exercise capacity, and two were bedridden. The hemodynamic criteria for entry into the trial were consistent with other mechanical assist device trials. In addition, the KCV patients received preimplantation IABP as a test to determine whether the KCV would benefit the patient. All patients enrolled in the study benefited from both the IABP and KCV, with the effect of the KCV being superior to the IABP. This is expected because the KCV has a higher stroke volume, has a better timing algorithm, and is permanently fixed to the optimal position in the descending aorta. No patients were rejected from the study as a result of an inadequate response to the IABP. Other entry criteria were similar to that of the REMATCH trial[11]; in fact, four of the patients had either refused entry or were deemed too sick to be candidates for the REMATCH trial.[12] Tables 48-2, 48-3, and 48-4 summarize the inclusion and exclusion criteria.

Three patients had significant plaquing of the aorta (two moderate and one severe), but the KCV could be implanted after cross-clamping and débridement without difficulty. Another surgical consideration is the presence of pleural adhesions. Four patients had previous cardiac surgery and had mild adhesions, which were easily dissected free. One patient had extensive pleural scarring that precluded safe KCV implantation. If a patient has extensive adhesions and the lung cannot be separated from the chest wall without significant pulmonary injury, KCV implantation may have to be aborted because bleeding and air leaks in the presence of prosthetic material could lead to KCV infection.

All patients who had CardioVAD implantation were in severe cardiac failure and had no other treatment options available to them. The seven male and one female patient averaged 70.1 years of age (range, 53 to 74). Of the patients screened, none were excluded because of failure of IABP testing. Six patients had ischemic cardiomyopathy, and five had previous coronary artery bypass graft (CABG) surgery. One patient had valvular cardiomyopathy and had previously received a mechanical aortic valve (St. Jude

chest is closed in routine fashion. The cannulae are removed from the groin and the incision closed.

After the chest and groin incisions are closed, the patient is rotated to the left. The previously marked PAD area is isolated and reprepared for incision. A 10 cm incision is made 6 cm above the proposed center of the PAD and extended down to the fascia. A subcutaneous pocket is developed inferiorly, and the skin punch (provided by the

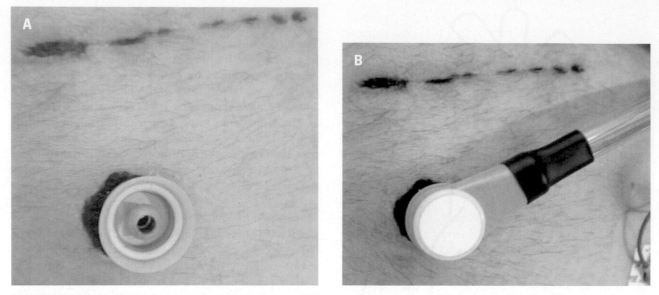

FIGURE 48-11. *A*, Well-healed skin around the connector and the scar of the operative incision used to place the skin pad connector are shown. *B*, PAD with external connector attached. The connector can rotate freely for patient comfort.

TABLE 48-2. General Inclusion Criteria

18 to 80 years of age.

Dilated cardiomyopathy (idiopathic, ischemic, or due to other irreversible cause) not amenable to other invasive/surgical correction.

Limiting CHF symptoms (NYHA class III or IV) refractory to maximal tolerated doses of diuretics, digoxin, angiotensin-converting enzyme inhibitors, β-blockers, and/or intravenous inotropes.

Absence of obstructive valvular disease or aortic regurgitation.

No history of recent myocardial infarction (within 2 weeks).

No irreversible and debilitating renal (chronic dialysis), pulmonary, or hepatic dysfunction.

CHF = congestive heart failure; NYHA = New York Heart Association

TABLE 48-3. Exclusion Criteria from Noninvasive Testing

Leukocytosis indicating an infectious process.

Renal insufficiency not caused by CHF (creatinine > 2.5 mg/dL).

More than three times elevation in liver enzymes and bilirubin level.

Noncorrectable abnormal coagulation parameters.

Uncontrolled atrial or ventricular arrhythmias (heart rate > 120 bpm).

Ejection fraction > 35%.

Severe pulmonary disease (FEV_1 < 1.0 L; FVC < 1.5 L; FEV_1/FVC < 35%; MVV < 50% predicted).

Significant carotid occlusive disease.

Abnormalities of the aorta that would preclude surgery, including aneurysms, coarctation, extreme tortuosity, and inadequate length (< 19 cm).

CHF = congestive heart failure; FCV = forced vital capacity; FEV = forced expiratory volume; MVV = maximal ventilatory volume.

TABLE 48-4. Exclusion Criteria from Invasive Testing

Cardiac index without assistance should be < 2.2 L/min/m² with a PCWP > 15 mm Hg.

During insertion of an IABP, there must be a 15% increase in cardiac output or stroke volume and a 15% reduction in PCWP.

Coagulation and platelet parameters studied prior to and following use of the IABP must be within normal limits.

Irreversible pulmonary hypertension on IABP (transpulmonary gradient > 14 mm Hg and/or pulmonary vascular resistance > 4 Wood units).

IABP = intraaortic balloon pump; PCWP = pulmonary capillary wedge pressure.

Medical Inc., St. Paul, MN). All patients were NYHA class IV and dependent on intravenous inotropic therapy. The ejection fraction (mean ± standard deviation) was 16 ± 5% (range, 9 to 24%). The mean weight loss during the year prior to KCV implantation was 31 ± 12 pounds.

The first patient expired in the operating room from technical problems arising from left atrial to femoral bypass. The implantation was aborted in another patient because of severe pleural adhesions, which did not allow mobilization of the lung. By using partial CPB, all subsequent six patients survived to the first end point (30 days). The mean CPB time was 157 min (range, 120 to 196). A cross-clamp was applied proximally (position A) for a mean of 101 min (range, 69 to 144). The distal cross-clamp was at position B for a mean of 55 min (range, 39 to 77) and at position C for a mean of 46 min (range, 30 to 67). The total cross-clamp time decreased by half from the first to the last patient. For the six patients surviving the operative procedure, there were no reoperations for bleeding and mean chest tube blood loss was only 450 cc (range, 250 to 900). All patients were extubated within 48 h. One patient who was ventilator dependent prior to implantation because of pneumonia required re-intubation 4 days later and received a tracheostomy. The other five patients were ambulatory and dischargeable. One patient stayed in the hospital because of lack of an FDA-approved discharge protocol. All patients were on aspirin, and only one required anticoagulation for his prosthetic aortic valve. Table 48-5 summarizes the hemodynamic and laboratory data before implantation and at 30 days. The reductions in serum creatinine, right atrial (RA) pressure, and pulmonary capillary wedge pressure (PCWP), as well as increase in the cardiac index (CI), were statistically significant when compared with baseline values. Although the quality-of-life (QOL) parameters and the 6 min walk improved, the differences were not significant.

Despite the severity of illness in these patients, the study demonstrated low surgical morbidity and mortality. The first patient done with left atrial to left femoral bypass expired because that amount of support was inadequate for the failing heart. With the use of CPB, all patients have survived and been able to be extubated within 48 h. Bleeding has been minimal, and, subsequently, right-heart failure has not been a problem. Injury to the spinal arteries and potential for paraplegia are potential concerns. However, unlike aneurysm repair, the intercostal arteries are not disrupted. During KCV implantation, they are temporarily occluded with Fogarty catheters to prevent obscuring the surgical field. After KCV implantation, the arteries are allowed to perfuse normally. Additionally, the initial cross-clamp is at the subclavian and

8 cm distal to this area. This arrangement allows sewing the proximal portion of the KCV. The 8 cm clamp is then moved to 16 cm to allow completion of the distal portion of the KCV. This technique limits distal cord ischemia to less than 20 min. When combined with distal arterial perfusion through the femoral artery cannula, this insures adequate cord perfusion.

This study demonstrated the ability to implant the KCV safely. In addition, there is reversal of the heart failure syndrome, with improved hemodynamics. All patients could be weaned off inotropic support while maintaining improved end-organ perfusion. At 1 month, there was reduction in PCWP and RA pressures, with an increase in cardiac index. There also was a significant improvement in renal function with normalization of serum creatinine levels. There was no deleterious effect of the KCV on red blood cells, platelet number, liver function, or coagulation parameters. None of the patients received anticoagulation for the KCV (one patient was placed on Coumadin for a prosthetic mechanical aortic valve), and there were no strokes or thromboembolic events.

The KCV has also shown the capability for intermittent use without any adverse events. Although the patients required KCV assistance for the majority of the time, the device could be disconnected to allow for increased patient comfort. This enables patients to shower or perform other activities of daily life without being tethered to any device. This nonobligatory feature simplifies outpatient management and reduces the impact of device failure in the field. The device is also very easy to use and has only a patient-controlled on/off switch. Table 48-6 lists the advantages of the CardioVAD.

There were two device-related problems that required KCV modifications. The driveline in the earlier patients showed accumulation of small brownish particles, which was discovered to arise from edema fluid that seeped into the PAD and became desiccated by the shunting of compressed air. This problem was corrected by making the PAD connection watertight. The fifth patient had an early leak from the PAD due to a manufacturing defect of the silastic/polycarbonate interface. The connection was reengineered to prevent this problem in the future (LVAD Technology, personal communication, March 2002). Table 48-7 lists the limitations of the CardioVAD.

TABLE 48-5. Results: Hemodynamics and Laboratory Values before and 30 Days after Implantation

	Before KCV Implantation*		30 Days after KCV Implantation†		
	IABP Off	IABP On	KCV Off	KCV On	p Value
Hgb	10.8 ± 1.9		9.9 ± 1.8		NS
Platelets	203 ± 43		187 ± 78		NS
WBC	6.9 ± 1.7		9.7 ± 3.2		NS
Creatinine	2.6 ± 0.5		1.5 ± 0.1		< .05
BUN	58 ± 25		34 ± 4		< .05
LDH	310		220		NS
AST	22 ± 8		32 ± 18		NS
ALT	20 ± 6		18 ± 3		NS
Albumin	3.9 ± 0.3		4.1 ± 0.1		NS
Total protein	7.2 ± 0.3		7.1 ± 0.2		NS
PT (INR)	1.8 ± 0.3		1.3 ± 0.1		NS
APTT (s)	36 ± 11		29 ± 0.5		NS
HR (beats per min)	67	65	68	65	NS
BP systolic (mm Hg)	84 ± 5	100 ± 12	110 ± 13	120 ± 10	NS
BP diastolic (mm Hg)	65 ± 5	55 ± 10	65 ± 5	60 ± 10	NS
RA (mm Hg)	19 ± 1	15 ± 3	17 ± 3	9 ± 2	< .05
PCWP (mm Hg)	32 ± 3	23 ± 7	31 ± 6	14 ± 5	< .05
CI (L/min/m2)	1.7 ± 0.7	2.2 ± 1.0	1.8 ± 0.5	2.6 ± 0.4	< .05
MVO$_2$	45	55	60	70	NS
6 min walk (feet)	375		550		NS

ALT = alanine transaminase; APTT = activated partial prothrombin time; AST = aspartate transaminase; BP = blood pressure; BUN = blood urea nitrogen; CI = cardiac index; Hgb = hemoglobin; HR = heart rate; IABP = intraaortic balloon pump; INR = international normalized ratio; KCV = Kantrowitz CardioVAD; LDH = lactate dehydrogenase; MVO$_2$ = _____; NS = not significant; PCWP = pulmonary capillary wedge pressure; PT = prothrombin time; RA = right atrial pressure; WBC = white blood cell count.

* All patients received inotropes before implantation.

† No patients were on inotropes at 30 days.

TABLE 48-6. Advantages of the CardioVAD

Reverses syndrome of heart failure

Augments cardiac performance by ~ 50%

Implantation less traumatic than with other devices

No hemolysis

No anticoagulation

Nonobligatory, leading to
  Improvement in quality of life
  Reduction in patient anxiety

TABLE 48-7. Limitations of the CardioVAD

Not complete support

Arrhythmias—regular rhythm mandatory for VAD tracking

Aortic valve

Time to adhere cells to PAD

Progression of structural heart abnormalities

Extensive lung adhesions during implant surgery

PAD = percutaneous access device; VAD = ventricular assist device.

Summary

This initial clinical experience with the KCV demonstrates that it can be implanted with very low perioperative morbidity and mortality. It is a novel nonobligatory device that has several advantages over other existing devices. There is no need for anticoagulation, and there are no valves or internal electronics that could fail and force VAD replacement. The control algorithm is simple as the device is triggered "on demand" by the electrical activity of the native heart. Furthermore, it is nonobligatory, so it can be turned on and off at will by the patient without increasing the risk of thromboembolic events. The disadvantages are that it provides only "partial" support. It increases cardiac output by approximately 40%, depending on the afterload condition of the patient. It depends upon native heart activity to function and cannot be placed in patients with severe biventricular function, uncontrolled tachyarrhythmias, or native valvular disease. However, the degree of support obtained seems sufficient to reverse the heart failure syndrome, improve end-organ dysfunction, and remove inotrope dependency.

The KCV is designed for intervention in NYHA class IV patients before there is severe biventricular failure or lack of any myocardial reserve. It is not an acute recovery device. The KCV can be considered equivalent to a mechanical permanent non-energy-depleting inotrope and may have a role in improving the length and quality of life in patients with end-stage heart failure. Perhaps by treating advanced CHF early, the KCV may reduce the number of patients progressing toward cardiac replacement therapy with transplantation or a total artificial heart.

References

1. The RALES Investigators. Effectiveness of spironolactone added to an angiotensin-converting enzyme inhibitor and a loop diuretic for severe chronic congestive heart failure. Am J Cardiol 1996;78:902–7.

2. The SOLVD Investigators. Effect of enalapril on survival in patients with reduced left ventricular ejection fractions and congestive heart failure. N Engl J Med 1991;325: 293–302.

3. The Captopril-Digoxin Multicenter Research Group. Comparative effects of therapy with captopril and digoxin in patients with mild to moderate heart failure. JAMA 1988;259:539–44.

4. Packer M, Bristow MR, Cohn JN, et al. The effect of carvedilol on morbidity and mortality in patients with chronic heart failure. N Engl J Med 1996;334:1349–55.

5. Kottke TE, Pesch DG, Frye RL, et al. The potential contribution of cardiac replacement to the control of cardiovascular diseases. A population-based estimate. Arch Surg 1990;1235:1148–51.

6. Chachques JC, Grandjean PA, Schwartz K, et al. Effect of latissimus dorsi dynamic cardiomyoplasty on ventricular function. Circulation 1988;78 Suppl 3:III-203–16.

7. Kung RTV, Rosenberg M. Heart Booster: a pericardial support device. Ann Thorac Surg 1999;68:764–7.

8. Perez-Tamayo RA, Anstadt MP, Cothran L, et al. Prolonged total circulatory support using direct mechanical ventricular actuation. ASAIO J 1995;41:M512–7.

9. Anstadt MP, Anstadt GL, Lowe JE. Direct mechanical ventricular actuation: a review. Resuscitation 1991;21:7–23.

10. McCarthy PM, Smedira NO, Vargo RL, et al. One hundred patients with the HeartMate left ventricular assist device: evolving concepts and technology. J Thorac Cardiovasc Surg 1998;115:904–12.

11. Murali S. Mechanical circulatory support with the Novacor LVAS: world-wide clinical results. Thorac Cardiovasc Surg 1999;47 Suppl 2:321–5.

12. Rose EA, Eric A, Gelijns AC, et al. Randomized Evaluation of Mechanical Assistance for the Treatment of Congestive Heart Failure (REMATCH) study group, long-term use of a left ventricular assist device for end-stage heart failure. N Engl J Med 2001;345:1435–43.

13. Pennington DG, Swartz MT, Lohmann DP, et al. Cardiac assist devices. Surg Clin North Am 1998;78:691–704.

14. Kantrowitz A. A moment in history: introduction of left ventricular assistance. ASAIO J 1987;10:39–48.

15. Weber KT, Janicki JS. Intraaortic balloon counterpulsation: a review of physiological principles, clinical results and device safety. Ann Thorac Surg 1974;17:602–36.

16. Scheidt S, Wilner G, Muyeller H, et al. Intra-aortic balloon counterpulsation in cardiogenic shock. Report of cooperative clinical trial. N Engl J Med 1973;288:978–84.

17. Kantrowitz A, Cardona RR, Au J, Freed PS. Intraaortic balloon pumping in congestive failure. In: Hosenpud J, Greenberg B, editors. Congestive heart failure: pathophysiology, diagnosis and comprehensive approach to management. New York: Springer-Verlag; 1993. p. 522–47.

18. Dipla KA, Mattiello JA, Jeevanandam V, et al. Myocyte recovery after mechanical circulatory support in humans with end-stage heart failure. Circulation 1998:97;2316–22.

19. Kantrowitz A, McKinnon WMP. The experimental use of the diaphragm as an auxiliary myocardium. Surg Forum 1959;IX:265–7.

20. Kantrowitz A, Akutsu T, Chaptal PA, et al. A clinical experience with an implanted mechanical auxiliary ventricle. JAMA 1966;197:525–9.

21. Freed PS, Wasfie T, Bar-Lev A, et al. Long-term percutaneous access device. ASAIO J 1985;31:230–4.

22. Polinski J, Freed P, Wasfie T, et al. Inhibition of epithelial downgrowth on percutaneous access devices in swine. ASAIO J 1983;29:569–74.

CHAPTER 49

THE NEW ROTARY BLOOD PUMPS: AN ALTERNATIVE TO CARDIAC TRANSPLANTATION?

STEPHEN WESTABY, MD, PhD, FETCS

Heart Failure: the Problem

In the increasingly elderly population, disabling heart failure is a major public health concern. Virtually 5 million people are affected in the United States, accounting for 5% of the health care budget. In 2001, the estimated direct and indirect costs of heart failure were 21 billion dollars (US). In the population older than 65 years of age, the incidence of heart failure approaches 10 per 1,000 population, and despite advances in medical and surgical management, the 5-year mortality rate is around 50%.[1] Between 1979 and 1988, deaths from heart failure increased by 135% while hospitalizations rose by 159%.

Re-admission rates vary from 29 to 47% in the first 6 months after discharge. In the CONSENSUS Study, patients randomized to enalapril spent 15% (30 days) of the mean 6.5-month follow-up time in hospital.[2] Up to one-third of patients gain no symptomatic relief from angiotensin-converting enzyme (ACE) inhibitors, and decompensation through dysrhythmia or pulmonary edema is the trigger for repeated hospital visits.

To date, cardiac transplantation has been the only treatment to provide consistent improvement in quality of life and survival. In 1999, only 2,184 patients in the United States underwent cardiac transplantation, representing less than half of patients on the waiting list. These were carefully selected patients predominantly under the age of 65 years. Seven hundred died while waiting for a donor, and 676 were withdrawn from consideration because of deteriorating end-organ function. In 2001, only 217 cardiac transplantations were undertaken in the United Kingdom. Most heart failure patients cannot be considered because of age limitations, concomitant disease (diabetes, chronic obstructive airways disease, renal impairment, or malignancy), or elevated pulmonary vascular resistance.

Another difficulty is the prediction of outcome for any individual patient without transplantation. Although the degree of left ventricular dysfunction is a prognostic indicator for mortality, many patients with markedly reduced left ventricular ejection faction (LVEF) can survive for years with reasonable functional capacity.[3] From the German transplantation experience (1997), Deng showed that wait-listed patients with ischemic heart disease who did not receive a donor organ had 3- and 4-year survival rates similar to those transplanted.[4] Transplantation listing of more critically ill patients and the use of so-called marginal donor hearts have limited improvement in outcomes after transplantation. In the meantime, the medical and nontransplantation surgical treatment of these patients has improved. Among the surgical options are revascularization of hibernating myocardium, surgical left ventricular remodeling, and the use of left ventricular assist devices.[5,6] In the future, it may be necessary to test the survival benefit of cardiac transplantation over conventional surgical and medical management in a prospective randomized trial. In the meantime, there is a swing away from the practice of transplantation-listing patients with heart failure until alternative methods are considered. This reasoning is in line with the current reassessment of treatment options for patients with end-stage liver, lung, and renal disease.

Lessons Learned with First-Generation Blood Pumps

In the 1970s, the success of cardiac transplantation with cyclosporin immunosuppression was limited by donor organ supply. This, in turn, stimulated the development of implantable circulatory support systems in the 1970s. After 30 years of research and development, mechanical blood pumps are in widespread use for bridge to cardiac transplantation. Two of these first-generation devices, recently licensed by the Food and Drug Administration, are the vented electric HeartMate (Thoratec Laboratories, Inc., Pleasanton, CA) and the Novacor (World Heart Corp., Oakland, CA) left ventricular assist devices (LVADs).[7] Providing stroke volume and pulse pressure, they are implanted in series with, but empty and completely replace, the left ventricle. Unidirectional blood flow is achieved with bioprosthetic valved conduits. A thick percutaneous lead transmits the electrical power line and external vent, which equalizes air pressure behind the pusher plates, through the abdominal wall. Both pumps have portable external power and control systems.

Over the past 15 years, the duration of pretransplantation circulatory support has lengthened considerably as transplant candidates wait longer for a donor heart.[8] This has allowed detailed evaluation of LVAD patients for as long as 4 years. For those patients in a chronic low-output state with multiple organ failure, complete recovery occurs gradually, over months, at a rate that depends on the duration and severity of preexisting heart failure.[9] Most patients return to New York Heart Association (NYHA) class I and are able to wait at home for a suitable donor heart. Hospital discharge improves the patients' psychological state, reduces hospital costs, and decreases the incidence of hospital-based nosocomial infections. Recovery of hemodynamic and nutritional status with a reversal of the metabolic and cellular abnormalities of heart failure has, in turn, improved the success rate of cardiac transplantation.[10]

In the only controlled study of the effects of LVAD support pending transplantation, the control patients met all the device inclusion criteria, but, for logistic problems, no LVAD was available for them.[10] At 90 days after transplantation and despite the surgical risks, the LVAD patients had 71% survival versus 36% for the control patients. The only survivors in the control group received a donor organ within 12 days of entry into the study.

Approximately 75% of LVAD patients undergo successful transplantation, and most are discharged from hospital. Nevertheless, adverse-event complications occur frequently with first-generation blood pumps, and for most patients, the shorter the duration of circulatory support, the better. The most common complications are bleeding, infection, thromboembolism, renal failure, hemolysis, device failure, and stroke.[11,12] Bleeding problems occur in as many as 60% of patients and are caused by hepatic dysfunction and the extensive surgical dissection. Patients who require biventricular assistance with extracorporeal pumps are more susceptible to bleeding than are those patients with LVAD support alone.[13] Pump and driveline infection rates range from 30 to 40% and cause substantial morbidity. Patients who are not rehabilitated fully and who have frequent complications experience stress, major depression, organic mental syndromes, and adjustment disorders.

Are LVADs a Realistic Alternative to Cardiac Transplantation?

As the heart failure population increases in tandem with a global decrease in donor availability, the use of long-term LVAD support seems a logical alternative. The first and only prospective randomized trial of LVAD support versus continued medical therapy began in 1998 and reported in November 2000. The Randomized Evaluation of Mechanical Assistance for the Treatment of Congestive Heart Failure (REMATCH) study employed the vented electric TCI LVAD in NYHA class IV heart failure patients on maximum medical therapy.[14] Entry criteria were left ventricular ejection faction (LVEF) < 25%, peak oxygen consumption of < 12 mL/kg/min, or a continued need for intravenous inotropic therapy for symptomatic hypotension, decreasing renal function, or worsening pulmonary congestion.

The investigating centers had to overcome major ethical, logistic, and economic hurdles in order to recruit 129 patients who were unsuitable for transplantation and willing to be randomized. Mortality from all causes (the primary end point) was 38% lower in the LVAD group. Median survival was 408 days in the device group and only 150 days in the medical therapy group. However, only 23% of LVAD patients survived for 2 years. Anticipated improvement in quality of life was limited by a 28% incidence of device infection by 3 months, a 42% incidence of bleeding by 6 months, and a 35% probability of pump failure by 2 years. Of the 68 patients who received the TCI LVAD, 10 had the device replaced. Nevertheless, the 75% 1-year mortality rate for medically treated patients exceeded that for acquired immunodeficiency syndrome and for breast, lung, and colon cancer. The use of an LVAD was associated with a 48% relative reduction in the risk of death during the follow-up period and a 27% absolute reduction in mortality at 1 year.

These findings suggest that for every 1,000 patients with end-stage heart failure, the use of an LVAD could prevent at least 270 deaths annually. This treatment effect is nearly four times that of β-blockers or ACE inhibitors. Despite the survival benefit, the morbidity and mortality of the TCI LVAD use were considerable. The percutaneous power line was a conduit for bacterial and fungal infection. Immunodeficiency and malnutrition contributed to the infection risk. Immunodeficiency is thought to originate from the lining of the TCI LVAD blood sac, whereas appetite loss occurs through the bulky intraabdominal device pressing on the stomach.

The REMATCH study is a landmark in the evolution of mechanical circulatory support. These findings established mechanical support as an alternative to medical treatment for selected transplantation-ineligible patients or those who prefer not to undergo cardiac transplantation. However, it is clear that long-term mechanical support will only gain widespread acceptance with the use of more user-friendly LVADs.

New Rotary Blood Pumps

In 1994, the Devices and Technology Branch of the National Heart, Lung and Blood Institute invited submissions for the development of innovative new left ventricular support systems. As a result, several new miniaturized implantable LVADs are currently undergoing clinical trials.

The engineering strategy for these second-generation blood pumps features a number of desirable characteristics, including (1) small size and weight that allows the pump to be implanted with closure of the chest; (2) reduced blood–foreign surface interface to decrease contact activation of immune and coagulation proteins; (3) no chronic requirement for anticoagulation with heparin; (4) a simple blood propulsion mechanism that requires few movable parts or prosthetic valves; and (5) a reliable operating system that is easily learned by the patient and safe in the community.

The new axial flow impeller pumps are silent continuous-flow devices that do not provide pulsatility in the circulation. Three models are concurrently undergoing clinical trials in Europe and the United States: the Jarvik 2000 heart, the Micromed-DeBakey LVAD, and the Thermo Cardio Systems II device that was developed at the University of Pittsburgh.

The Jarvik 2000 Heart

The Jarvik 2000 is a silent compact thumb-sized axial-flow pump that it is inserted through an apical cuff into the body of the failing left ventricle (Figure 49-1).[15] An impervious Dacron graft conveys blood to the descending thoracic aorta. The weight is 85 g with a displacement volume of 25 mL. The electromagnetic pumping mechanism consists of a rotor with impeller blades encased in a titanium shell and supported at each end by blood-immersed ceramic bearings < 1 mm in diameter (Figure 49-2). A brushless direct current motor contained within the housing creates the electromagnetic force necessary to rotate the impeller. All the blood-contacting surfaces within the pump are made of smooth titanium. Blood flow is directed through the outflow graft by stator blades located near the pump outlet.

The motor receives power from the external controller through a series of wires. The motor speed is manually adjusted and is regulated by a pulse width–modulated speed control circuit. Lead acid or lithium ion batteries provide a 12-volt power supply (Figure 49-3). The pump's operating range is 8,000 to 12,000 rpm. At speeds set between 9,000 and 12,000 rpm, the pump provides continuous flow of between 3 and 6 L/min, depending on afterload (Figure 49-4). The mean energy consumption remains constant at between 3 and 7 watts.

Two methods of power delivery are available. For bridge to cardiac transplantation, a fine silicone-covered electric cable with Dacron sleeve passes through the abdominal wall. For permanent support, the internal electric wires are

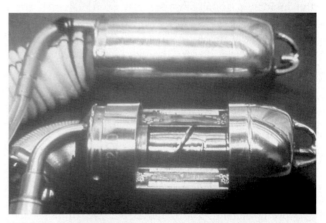

FIGURE 49-2. Jarvik 2000, with cutaway showing the rotor and brushless direct current motor in the titanium housing.

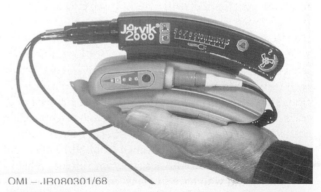

OMI – JB080301/68

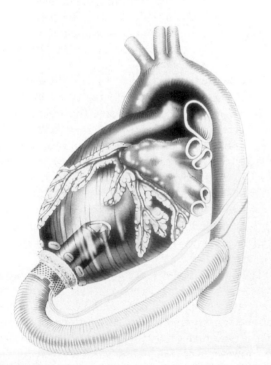

FIGURE 49-1. Diagram showing the intraventricular Jarvik 2000, which offloads the failing heart to the descending thoracic aorta.

FIGURE 49-3. The easily portable external controller (top) and lithium ion battery.

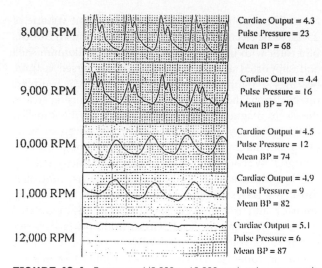

8,000 RPM	Cardiac Output = 4.3 Pulse Pressure = 23 Mean BP = 68
9,000 RPM	Cardiac Output = 4.4 Pulse Pressure = 16 Mean BP = 70
10,000 RPM	Cardiac Output = 4.5 Pulse Pressure = 12 Mean BP = 74
11,000 RPM	Cardiac Output = 4.9 Pulse Pressure = 9 Mean BP = 82
12,000 RPM	Cardiac Output = 5.1 Pulse Pressure = 6 Mean BP = 87

FIGURE 49-4. Pump speed (8,000 to 12,000 rpm), pulse pressure in the systemic circulation, and hemodynamic variables as speed is changed. Device flow is inversely proportional to afterload. Total blood flow is the sum of pump flow plus left ventricular ejection through the aortic valve. The dicrotic notch appears as pump speed is reduced and more blood is ejected via the left ventricular outflow tract. BP = blood pressure.

brought through the left pleural cavity to the apex of the chest and then subcutaneously across the neck to the base of the skull.[16] Here, a rigidly fixed percutaneous titanium pedestal transmits electrical power through the skin of the scalp (Figure 49-5). The combination of immobility and highly vascular scalp skin is known to resist infection in long-standing cochlear implant technology.

The Texas Heart Institute and the Oxford Heart Centre collaborated to evaluate the Jarvik 2000 in bridge-to-transplantation patients (United States) and for permanent treatment of nontransplantation candidates (United Kingdom).[17,18] The implantation technique via left thoracotomy is less complicated than for the larger pulsatile blood pumps. The power cable is first brought out of the chest via the chosen route. The pump outflow graft is then anastomosed to the descending thoracic aorta, using a partial occlusion clamp. The left femoral artery and vein are cannulated for a short period of cardiopulmonary bypass. Ventricular fibrillation is induced, and a circular knife is used to create a device-sized opening in the apex of the left ventricle. A silicone-polyester sewing cuff is sewn to the defect with Teflon-pledgeted mattress sutures. The pump is then inserted within the ventricle and secured with a cotton tape around the cuff and pump housing (Figure 49-6). The heart is defibrillated, and, with native left ventricular ejection, air is removed from the system. As cardiopulmonary bypass is gradually discontinued, the pump is turned on. Pulmonary vasodilators and inotropic agents are used as necessary to support right ventricular function.

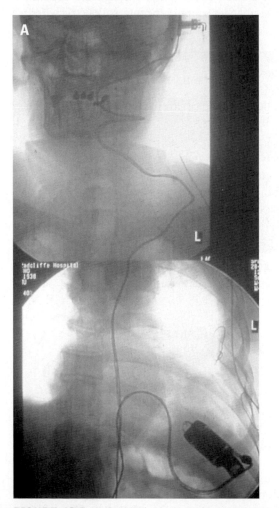

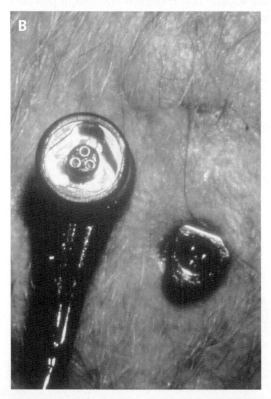

FIGURE 49-5. *A,* Subtraction head, neck, and chest x-ray film showing the permanent power delivery system and the Jarvik 2000 in the intraventricular position. *B,* The percutaneous titanium pedestal and connector.

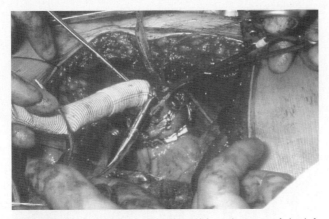

FIGURE 49-6. Jarvik 2000 implanted into the apex of the left ventricle.

Experience suggests that the intraventricular position has important advantages. The device remains well aligned when left ventricular shape changes during unloading (Figure 49-7). In other blood pumps, malalignment of the inflow cannula has caused flow restriction, hemolysis, thrombus formation, and thromboembolism. Avoidance of an external poorly vascularized device pocket reduces infection risk. Only one body cavity is entered, and once implanted, the internal component of the system appears to be imperceptible to the patient.

DEVICE HEMODYNAMICS

Intraoperative hemodynamic assessment is performed with transesophageal echocardiography, a pulmonary artery catheter, an arterial pressure line, and an ultrasonic flow probe on the pump's outflow graft. Flow through the pump can be calculated accurately against varying mean pressures and used to determine optimal impeller speed. The ultrasonic flow probe is removed before the thoracotomy incision is closed.

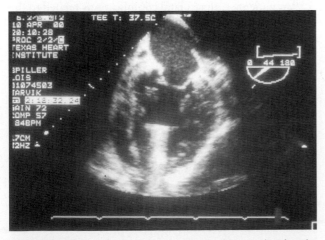

FIGURE 49-7. Two-dimensional echocardiogram showing the device well aligned within the left ventricular cavity.

In the early postoperative period, hemodynamic function is assessed with invasive monitoring and transthoracic echocardiography. The goal is to maintain pump speed at the lowest level compatible with a normal cardiac index and an optimally unloaded left ventricle. Anticoagulation therapy is given to maintain an international normalized ratio (INR) of between 2.0 to 2.5. ACE inhibition and β-blockers are used to reduce afterload and provide a mean blood pressure between 70 to 90 mm Hg.

We doctors use the Jarvik 2000 to partially unload the left ventricle, thereby allowing about 30% stroke volume ejection through the left ventricular outflow tract. In most cases, pump speed is between 9,000 and 10,000 rpm, allowing between 5 and 20 mm Hg pulse pressure in the systemic circulation (see Figure 49-4). This improves coronary blood flow and restores the native left ventricle to a more favorable Frank-Starling relationship.

Compared to preoperative status, the hemodynamic function of all patients improves considerably. Forty-eight hours after device implantation, the average cardiac index has increased by 43%, with a reduction in pulmonary capillary wedge pressure of 52%.

Echocardiographic data confirm the pump's left ventricular unloading effect. Doppler imaging shows continuous flow throughout the entire cycle, with an increase during systolic augmentation when left ventricular contraction boosts preload to the pump. As pump speed increases, ejection flow through the left ventricular outflow tract decreases progressively, as does systemic pulse pressure.

At 12,000 rpm, pulse pressure is usually absent. Pulse pressure increases when pump speed is reduced, and a dicrotic notch appears on the arterial trace when the aortic valve opens. Total system blood flow is the combination of pump output plus left ventricle (LV) ejection through the aortic valve during partial offloading.

When the force of native LV contraction improves, a greater proportion of pump flow occurs during systole. By partially offloading, right ventricular geometry and function are preserved. This is different from pusher plate LVADs that actively empty the native LV and shift the interventricular septum (Figure 49-8). Exercise increases cardiac output through intrinsic mechanisms (elevated heart rate, contractility, and venous return). Flow then increases both through the device and via the LV outflow tract. As a result, activity-responsive electronic mechanisms are unnecessary.

CLINICAL EXPERIENCE

The Jarvik 2000 clinical program began with bridge to transplantation at the Texas Heart Institute and permanent implants for nontransplantation-eligible patients in Oxford.[17,18] To date, 37 implantations have occurred, predominantly in patients with idiopathic dilated cardiomyopathy (61%) and ischemic cardiomyopathy (24%). There have been 30 male and 7 female patients, all NYHA class IV, with ages ranging from 25 to 72 years (mean,

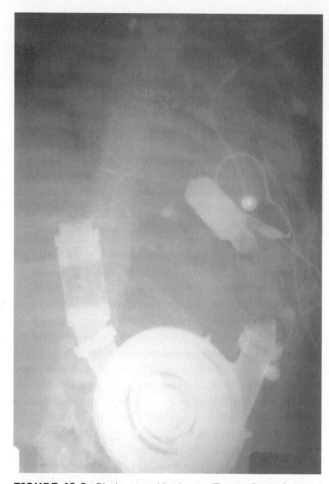

FIGURE 49-8. Displacement blood pump (Thermo Cardio Systems' HeartMate LVAD) and Jarvik 2000 in the same patient. The Jarvik 2000 was used to replace the infected HeartMate LVAD, which was removed the following day. The Jarvik 2000 is roughly the same size as the HeartMate inflow cannula.

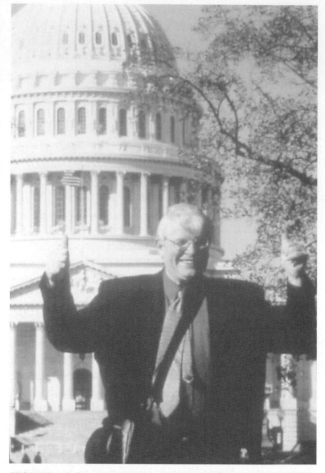

FIGURE 49-9. First permanent Jarvik 2000 patient visits Washington and the Food and Drug Administration to promote long-term mechanical support programs.

53 years). Body surface area ranged from 1.5 to 2.3 m^2 (mean, 1.9 m^2). Preoperative cardiac index ranged from 1.1 to 2.5 L/min/m^2 (mean, 1.7). Left ventricular end-diastolic dimensions ranged from 39 to 97 mm (mean, 68). Peak VO_2 ranged from 5.7 to 11.8 L/min/kg (mean, 8.1), and pulmonary vascular resistance ranged from 0.3 to 8.5 Wood units (mean, 3.0).

Of this population, 10 (27%) are ongoing with a mean support time of 274 days.

The longest surviving Oxford permanent patient is currently NYHA class I 2 years postoperatively (Figure 49-9). Three other permanent implant patients are between 1 and 2 years. Thirteen patients (35%) have been transplanted, including 12 of 25 (48%) in the Houston bridge-to-transplant group. Mean support time for these patients was 95 days. Fourteen patients (39%) have died after a mean support time of 56 days. Cause of death was multiorgan failure in 3, septic shock in 2, right ventricular failure in 2, stroke in 2, acute myocardial infarction in 2, adult respiratory distress syndrome in 2,

and a patient compliance issue in 1. There have been no pump failures in up to 24 months of implantation and in a cumulative support time of 12.6 years. There has been one temporary device-related infection in a bridge-to-transplant patient with an abdominal cable. This was cleared by antibiotics.

Two patients suffered fatal complications related to the skull-mounted pedestal. The first died at 90 days following surgery for intracranial bleeding caused by an implant problem. The second died from left ventricular failure during an attempt to replace a corroded pedestal.

The majority of patients have had very little intraoperative blood loss and were weaned from the ventilator in < 24 h. Left ventricular end diastolic dimensions decreased by 16% during LVAD support (7.1 cm before device implantation and 5.9 cm 48 h postoperatively). There was no significant hemolysis. The average plasma-free hemoglobin level was 14.1 mg/dL as compared to a preimplant value of 7.4 mg/dL.

REHABILITATION AND QUALITY OF LIFE

Operation of the Jarvik 2000 is uncomplicated. The patients and their families are taught to exchange batteries and to identify potential emergency situations. NYHA class I cardiac status was usually achieved within 2 weeks of implantation. Improvement in native ventricular contractility augments pulse pressure while the intravascular volume, pump speed, and vascular tone remain constant. With the pump speed set to the usual submaximal flow rate (9,000 to 10,000 rpm), the aortic valve opens during systole and pulse pressure is detectable in peripheral arteries. Prior to hospital discharge, the patients perform a 5-min "pump off" study to check that cardiac output remains sufficient to cope with an emergency situation. With the pump off, the mean regurgitant flow from descending aorta to the vascular graft was 0.35 L/min/m² (11% of cardiac output). This was well tolerated by all the patients.

The Oxford permanent implant patients left hospital at between 3 and 8 weeks postoperatively with medical management consisting of ACE inhibition, β-blockade and warfarin to maintain INR between 2.5 and 3.5.[18] In each case, left ventricular unloading was accompanied by substantial improvements in both left and right ventricular function and end-organ function. Exercise tolerance increased gradually and was accompanied by a decrease in body weight and a disappearance of peripheral edema and ascites. None of the patients required diuretics after 3 months. As after transplantation, there was a discrepancy between hemodynamic parameters and symptomatic recovery from heart failure. The pump restored cardiac index and left atrial pressure to within normal levels while resolution of breathlessness and fatigue lagged behind hemodynamic improvement. This relates to the skeletal-muscle effects of chronic heart failure. All patients have recorded major improvement in quality of life scores. Activity is unrestricted by the device.

At 2 years postoperation, the first Oxford patient can walk up to 5 miles a day and has completed a long-distance charity walk. He undertakes unaccompanied international air travel and has visited the Food and Drug Administration (FDA) in Washington to discuss his experience. Interruptions of power supply up to 5 h have been well tolerated. On one occasion, the bag containing the control and battery of this patient was stolen by a thief and the external cable was avulsed from the skull pedestal. Power was restored by reattaching the connector, and there was no thromboembolism on restoration of pump flow. For permanent implants, it has been a great advantage to have a completely exchangeable external system.

Survival beyond 2 years is a landmark in continuous-flow pump technology. Demonstration that stroke volume and pulse pressure are not required from an LVAD now facilitates the introduction of less-intrusive continuous-flow devices as a practical alternative to cardiac transplantation for selected patients.

The MicroMed DeBakey VAD

This implantable nonpulsatile extracardiac axial-flow pump was developed in a joint project between the Baylor College of Medicine and the National Aeronautics and Space Administration (NASA)/Johnson Space Center.[19] The titanium device is 3.5 cm in diameter, 7.62 cm in length, and weighs 95 g (Figure 49-10). The inflow cannula is positioned in the apex of the left ventricle. A rigid inflow tube connects to the pump itself situated in an external pocket in the abdominal wall. An outflow vascular graft is directed back through the mediastinum to the ascending aorta and is surrounded by an implanted flow meter. The pump housing contains a brushless direct current (DC) motor stator surrounding the flow path. The pump head consists of a flow straightener that is stationary and that supports the rotor and front ruby sapphire bearing (Figure 49-11). The impeller is the only moving part and features a sophisticated miniature rotor and a stationary diffuser that supports the rotor and rear bearing. The stator on the outside of the flow tube spins in a magnetic field. The impeller contains rare-earth magnets in the blades and acts as the rotor of this brushless motor. Impeller speed ranges from 7,500 to 12,500 rpm. To achieve 5 L/min flow against 100 mm Hg pressure, the rotor spins at 10,000 rpm and requires < 10 watts of input

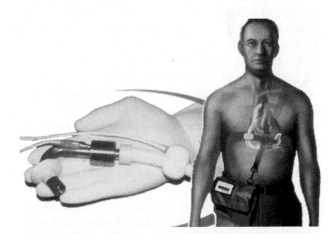

FIGURE 49-10. The MicroMed DeBakey VAD.

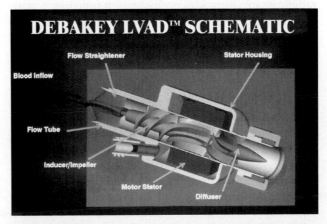

FIGURE 49-11. Diagram showing the blood propulsion mechanism of the DeBakey LVAD.

power. The patient cannot influence the pump speed. As with the Jarvik 2000, there is an inverse relationship between pump speed and pulsatility in the circulation.

CLINICAL EXPERIENCE

The device was introduced in Europe 3 years ago, with CE mark approval for bridge to transplantation in six countries.[20] More recently, it was implanted by the developing team at the Baylor College of Medicine, Houston, TX.[21] At the Second Symposium on Mechanical Circulatory Support at the Berlin Heart Institute, December 2001, Noon described the experience in 110 patients (91 males, 19 females) with the longest implant duration of 441 days. Forty-seven had idiopathic dilated cardiomyopathy, 54 had ischemic cardiomyopathy, and 9 had miscellaneous problems. Average age at implantation was 46 years, which is considerably lower than with other support devices (Novacor patients have an average age of 65 years). The mean duration of support was 63 ± 2 days, during which pump speed was usually set at between 9,000 and 10,500 rpm. The average pump flow in an awake supine patient was 4.8 ± 0.88 L/min.

Noon quoted complication rates similar to those of the Novacor device. Twenty-three percent of patients died postoperatively from multiorgan failure, and approximately 1% died from sepsis. There was a 3% incidence of device failure and a 5.4% incidence of device infection. Indices of hemolysis presented by Turina for Zurich patients showed an average plasma-free hemoglobin of 13 mg/dL and a lactic dehydrogenase (LDH) of 1,776 μ/L. Severe hemolysis has been encountered in some patients, probably related to partial obstruction of the inflow cannula within the left ventricle as the unloaded heart changes shape and the position of the apex remains tethered (Figure 49-12).

With fully ambulatory patients, stress exercise tests show that the pump can practically double the flow rate without adjustment of pump speed. This occurs through increased ventricular filling. Indices of heart failure, including renal, hepatic, and neurologic function, improve rapidly in survivors with normal pump function. A positive nitrogen balance was achieved after 4 to 6 weeks.

So far, no detailed outcome data have been provided for this pump. Heparin coating (Carmeda) was recently applied to the blood interface.

The HeartMate II LVAD

Thermo-Cardio Systems acquired the Nimbus/University of Pittsburgh axial-flow pump, which has been under development since 1992 (Figure 49-13).[22] The device is now being developed by Thoratec.[23] This system consists of three major elements: an integrated pump/rotor, an inflow and outflow cannula set, and an external controller and power supply. The device is manufactured from corrosion-resistant titanium alloy. It has an overall length of 7 cm, an outer diameter of 4 cm, and a displacement volume of

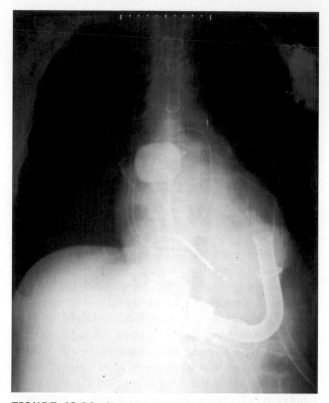

FIGURE 49-12. Plain chest radiograph showing the DeBakey LVAD in situ.

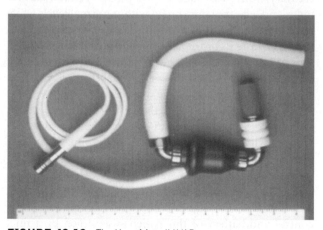

FIGURE 49-13. The HeartMate II LVAD.

62 mL. However, the weight of the device is 370 g, considerably more than the weight of the Jarvik 2000 and DeBakey LVADs. The inflow cannula is made from commercially available 40-French wire-reinforced polyurethane. The outflow cannula is a 14 mm reinforced extended polytetrafluoroethylene vascular graft bonded to a titanium fitting that threads to the pump outflow port with a step-free interface.

The system was designed for univentricular or biventricular support. For left ventricular assist, the inflow and outflow cannulas are configured for connection to the left ventricular apex and the ascending aorta. The pump is then placed under the left costal margin beneath the left rectus abdominus muscle as for the DeBakey VAD.

The inflow cannula leaves the left ventricular apex to cross the diaphragm in the costophrenic angle. It then enters the subrectus pocket to attach to the pump. The outflow cannula is tunneled back under the sternum to the ascending aorta.

The blood-contacting surfaces are textured (as for the TCI pusher-plate LVAD) in an attempt to reduce the incidence of thromboembolic complications and the need for systemic anticoagulation. Pump speed ranges between 3,000 and 15,000 rpm but is normally maintained between 10,000 and 12,000 rpm to produce systemic blood flow > 6 L/min.

In short-term sheep studies, the maximum plasma-free hemoglobin was 27.5 mg/dL but was < 15 mg/dL for animals free from inflow occlusion. Chronic implantations have been performed in six calves for support times between 6 and 181 days (mean, 57 days). Pump speed was maintained at an average of 10,000 rpm with a flow rate of 5 L/min. Maximal flow rates of 8 L/min were possible at the highest pump speed. However, despite anticoagulation with Coumadin, at an INR between 3.0 and 4.0, thrombus was found either in the heart or the device of five of the six animals. This was associated with small renal cortical infarcts.

Further developments with the HeartMate II include a controller system to modulate the pump speed in response to varying physiologic demand and a transcutaneous power system with implantable induction coils.

CLINICAL EXPERIENCE

The first clinical implantation was attempted in Israel in October 2000.[22] Bleeding and hemolysis were said to be problematic, and the patient died soon afterward. Six devices have subsequently been implanted for bridge to transplantation at Bad Oyenhausen, Germany, and Harefield Hospital, United Kingdom. Detailed information on these implants is not yet available. Pump thrombosis is said to have occurred, and the results are currently under review.

The Terumo Magnetically Suspended LVAD

Since 1995, the Terumo Corporation has worked to develop a magnetically suspended centrifugal blood pump without bearings, drive shaft, or seal (Figure 49-14).[24]

The impeller is suspended between the casings, with magnetic forces produced by permanent magnets and electromagnets. The impeller rotates by a magnetic coupling between it and the motor and is suspended by three electromagnets. Three position sensors maintain the free-floating impeller at the center of the pump housing. The blood-contacting surfaces and the inflow and outflow cannula are modified by heparin bonding. Because this is a sealless rotor pump providing contact-free rotation without any material wear, it is expected to be one of the most durable blood pumps, with a theoretical life span of decades. Early prototypes have already operated for more than 2 years in an extracorporeal sheep model with

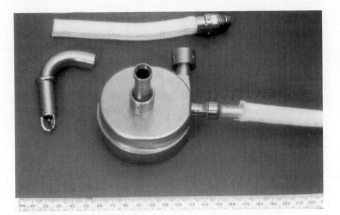

FIGURE 49-14. The Terumo magnetically suspended LVAD.

plasma-free hemoglobin levels remaining within the normal range for all animals up to 864 days. In a sheep model in Oxford, the device produced between 5 and 6 L of blood flow at pump speeds between 2,000 and 3,000 rpm. I have maintained 20 sheep in excellent condition free from hemolyses or thromboembolism without any anticoagulation for > 12 months. All device-related parameters were recorded continuously by computer, and during this time, the systemic circulation was entirely pulseless, with normal end-organ function. The only detectable differences with nonpulsatile circulation were increased plasma renin activity, 5 to 10 mm Hg elevation of mean blood pressure over baseline, and temporary abolition of baroreceptor responses.

Magnetically suspended centrifugal blood pumps are well suited for long-term mechanical circulatory support, and the Terumo LVAD will be introduced clinically in 2003. Similar devices are under development in other laboratories. The INOCOR centrifugal LVAD was recently implanted in two young bridge-to-transplantation patients in Berlin.

Patient Selection and Management of Continuous-Flow LVADs

There are now four well-defined mechanical support strategies for which blood pumps can be used: (1) short-term support for postcardiotomy heart failure, myocardial infarction, or myocarditis; (2) prolonged bridge to myocardial recovery for the limited number of patients with recoverable disease; (3) prolonged bridge to transplantation for those with irrecoverable disease who fit the selection criteria; and (4) permanent circulatory support for nontransplantation candidates with irreversible disease. At present, implantable rotary blood pumps are expensive, and the outcome in postcardiotomy heart failure remains poor. Only 50% of patients are weaned, 35% discharged from hospital, and 25% alive at 1 year. The less-expensive extracorporeal Thoratec Abiomed BVS 5000 or Biomedicus pumps are better suited to limited-duration support in these patients. If recovery is not achieved within 7 days, then the decision may be made to convert to a long-term LVAD for bridge to transplantation.

To date, the implantable axial-flow pumps have performed best when implanted electively into NYHA class IV dilated cardiomyopathy patients before terminal deterioration into cardiogenic shock. In these patients, mechanical unloading promotes functional recovery in the native heart and a symbiotic relationship between the two pumping systems. Absolute end-stage transplantation candidates with ischemic heart disease and high-grade coronary stenoses may suffer coronary thrombosis with nonpulsatile flow and are unlikely to sustain important left ventricular recovery.

Without clinical experience, it was difficult to predict the outcome of circulatory support with nonpulsatile systems. Animal pumping systems, epitomized by the mammalian heart, produce pulse by intermittent contraction and stroke volume ejection with one-way valves. Given this mechanism for blood propulsion, pulse is obligatory, as is a resting phase for the myocyte. There is no evidence that the pulsatility is required for energy exchange at capillary level, where pulse is so dampened as to be virtually continuous.

Until recently, there were no studies of long-term nonpulsatile flow in humans. The closest was with extracorporeal membrane oxygenator (ECMO) in children for several weeks. There is already substantial evidence that the nonpulsatile blood pumps do provide pulsatility in the circulation, particularly when function improves in the unloaded left ventricle.[25] Clinical experience with both the Jarvik 2000 Heart and the DeBakey VAD shows well-preserved hepatic and renal function. Contraction of the unloaded left ventricle provides pressure changes at the pump inlet that provide pulsatile flow in the outflow graft and aorta. Pulsatility even occurs while the native aortic valve remains closed and is not dependent on pump flow, blood pressure, or systemic vascular resistance.[17]

In comparison with the first-generation pusher-plate LVADs, axial-flow pumps are much more sensitive to the differential pressure across the pump (afterload). As a result, continued afterload management with ACE inhibition and β-blockade are required for these patients. If properly applied, axial-flow pumps will continuously unload the failing heart and allow the native ventricle to perform with improved efficacy. In comparison, the larger pusher-plate LVADs empty and capture the whole output of the left ventricle. As such, they are more properly termed left ventricular replacement devices.

Continuous-flow LVADs must be managed differently from pulsatile displacement–type blood pumps. Reduction in preload does not alter the pumping rate of a rotary blood pump. Should continuous flow result in negative pressure throughout the whole native cardiac cycle, then septal shift may occur and produce an hourglass-shaped left ventricle. The left atrium may empty. This impairs right ventricular function and decreases blood flow

through the lungs. Thus, cardiac filling must be balanced with pump speed, a condition that is most challenging in the immediate postoperative period, when blood loss and high pulmonary vascular resistance may further impair blood flow to the left atrium.

Healing the Heart by Mechanical Offloading

Heart failure ensues when myocardial injury produces abnormal mechanical function leading to cardiac remodeling.[26] Precipitating events include a variety of problems such as acute or chronic myocardial ischemia, valve defects with volume or pressure overload, genetic abnormalities, exposure to toxins or infectious agents, and cardiac inflammatory responses in systemic illness. Alterations of myocyte biology in heart failure include attenuation of normal excitation-contraction coupling, reversion to myosin heavy-chain fetal gene expression, and β-adrenergic receptor desensitization.[27] These, together with cytoskeletal protein production, lead to myocyte hypertrophy, myocytolysis, and interstitial fibrosis, which accompany cardiac chamber enlargement and myocardial hypertrophy.[28] Systolic dysfunction is followed by impaired compliance and diastolic dysfunction. Programmed cell death (apoptosis) accelerates the loss of functioning myocytes.[29]

Altered contractility of the left ventricle with remodeling toward a more spherical shape causes mitral regurgitation and diminished stroke volume (see Figure 49-3).[30] The failing circulation causes expression of neurohormonal and inflammatory mediators. Myocyte hypertrophy ensues after the compensatory secretion of growth factors, including catecholamines, endothelin, growth hormone, tumor necrosis factor, angiotensin II, and insulin-dependent growth factor.[31,32] The fibrotic component of remodeling is promoted by activation of the renin-angiotensin-aldosterone axis, as well as through increased endothelin and transforming growth factor-β (TGF-β) responses.[33] Regulation of apoptosis is by changes in the expression of a variety of genes, perhaps adversely influenced by tumor necrosis factor production. Counterregulatory agents are also activated, including atrial- and brain-type natriuretic peptides.[34] Nitric oxide (driven by bradykinin and natriuretic peptides) may also have antigrowth properties, holding uncontrolled cell hypertrophy in check.[35]

Drug treatment in heart failure first focused on symptomatic relief by using diuretics, inotropes, and vasodilators. However, inotropes were soon found to increase mortality. As the importance of remodeling became evident, treatment strategies focused on unloading the heart and arresting disease progression with ACE inhibitors, β-blockers, and new agents, such as angiotensin-receptor blockers, aldosterone antagonists, cytokine inhibitors, neural endopeptidase activators, and endothelin antagonists. These drugs work to lower intracardiac pressures and to improve systemic blood flow. In effect, the beneficial effects of unloading have been apparent since the work of Burch, who advocated prolonged bed rest to ameliorate heart failure.[36]

In the 1990s, transplantation surgeons noted substantial improvement in the native heart of patients bridged to transplantation by LVADs. In 1996, Frazier documented a significant decrease in left ventricular end-diastolic dimensions and a marked rise in ejection fraction (11 to 22%) during chronic offloading.[37] Associated with hemodynamic improvement were dramatic changes in myocardial histology found in samples taken first from the left ventricle during LVAD implantation, and then after cardiac excision during transplantation. Hypertrophied myocytes reverted toward normal size, myocytolysis was reduced, and the sarcoplasmic reticulum handling of calcium flux greatly improved. Other studies confirm these findings and show increased expression of genes involved in calcium metabolism that were downregulated in terminal heart failure (Table 49-1). Levin showed that reversal of the remodeling process was accompanied by normalization of passive pressure-volume relationships and improved contractile response to increased heart rate and β-agonist.[38] Zafeiridis performed detailed histologic studies in 10 patients undergoing LVAD support for a mean of 75 days.[39] Cardiac myocyte volume, length, width, and thickness were determined. In comparison with nonfailing hearts, myocytes taken from failing myocardium exhibited increased volume and length-to-thickness ratio, and there were no differences in any parameter between hearts with ischemic cardiomyopathy or idiopathic dilated cardiomyopathy. However, a consistent finding by several groups has been an increase in interstitial replacement fibrosis.[40]

Milting and colleagues studied the impact of LVAD unloading on apoptosis regulation.[41] This group measured transcription of the apoptosis-associated genes *Fas Exo6 Del*, *Fas receptor*, and *Bel-XL* as markers of recovery. They showed that transcription of apoptosis-inhibiting genes was upregulated in patients supported for more than 6 weeks with an LVAD. Fas receptor messenger

ribonucleic acid (mRNA) remained unaffected by mechanical circulatory support. Their findings of desensitization to apoptotic stimuli suggest reversed molecular remodeling of the heart during LVAD support. Belland also demonstrated both extensive myocyte apoptosis in advanced heart failure and the ability of mechanical unloading to arrest the process.[42]

Left ventricular offloading also has profound effects on the adverse neurohormonal effects of heart failure. In 1995, James demonstrated a profound fall in plasma renin activity, angiotensin II, plasma epinephrine, norepinephrine, and arginine vasopressin.[43] Only atrial natriuretic peptide did not change significantly. These alterations were accompanied by dramatic improvements in cardiac index. Significant attenuation of inflammatory markers also occurs with falling levels of interleukins-6 and -8. Myocardial tumor necrosis factor-alpha (TNF-α) content decreases, particularly in those patients who recover sufficiently to be weaned from the LVAD. This suggests that myocardial expression of genes regulating TNF production are attenuated, which further supports the concept of molecular remodeling in these patients.

Moravec's group showed that mRNA levels for the sarcoplasmic reticulum calcium adenosine triphosphatase (ATPase) enzyme were 1.5 to 4.5 times greater in the left ventricular biopsy specimens removed after LVAD unloading, as compared with the original apical core of myocardium from the same patient.[44] mRNA for atrial natriuretic peptide also decreased, indicating that human heart failure phenotype is reversible and may result in functional recovery of the heart. Takeishi and colleagues studied myocardial regulators of G-protein kinase-C isoforms in paired pre- and post-LVAD samples.[45] They found that LVAD unloading increased the sarcoplasmic reticulum calcium ATPase protein level but left phospholamban concentrations unaffected. Lee and colleagues studied mitochondrial respiratory status and respiratory control index in mitochondria isolated from the myocardium of heart failure patients with and without LVAD support.[46] They found a marked improvement in myocyte mitochondrial function after long-term LVAD use, suggesting that normalization of metabolic function occurs after ventricular unloading. Mutations that lead to disruption of cytoskeletal proteins are found in patients with familial dilated cardiomyopathy. The primary structural functions of dystrophin are to link the cytoskeleton of the cell to the extracellular matrix and to maintain sarcolemmal integrity during mechanical stress. In muscular dystrophies and cardiomyopathic hamsters with S-sarcoglycan deficiency, dystrophin loss is associated with cardiac dysfunction.[47,48] Vatta and colleagues proposed that acquired abnormalities in dystrophin might provide a final common pathway for the progressive dysfunction in heart failure. They recently reported on the expression and integrity of dystrophin in myocardial biopsy samples from ischemic and dilated cardiomyopathy patients

TABLE 49-1. Effects of Left Ventricular Unloading with an LVAD

Reversal of cardiac chamber enlargement
Normalization of diastolic pressure-volume relationships
Reduction in LV global mass
Regression of myocyte hypertrophy
Enhanced inotropic response to β-agonists
Improved cytosolic CA^{2+} transients
Upregulation of apoptosis-inhibiting genes
Improved myocardial mitochondrial function
Attenuation of neurohormonal and cytokine changes
Normalized myocardial phenotype expression (ANP, BNP, SERCA, TNF)
Reversal of degenerative changes in cytoskeletal proteins and dystrophin

ANP = atrial natriuretic peptide; BNP = brain natriuretic peptide; LV = left ventricle; SERCA = _____; TNF = tumor necrosis factor.

bridged to cardiac transplantation.[49] Their findings suggest that decreased contractile function is associated with selective disruption of the amino terminus of dystrophin. Furthermore, the degenerative process was reversed in the myocardium of patients subject to unloading by long-term LVAD support. Alterations in the N terminus of dystrophin in both ischemic and idiopathic cardiomyopathy, suggest that dystrophin-associated lesions occur secondary to heart failure and that relief of mechanical stress may be a future therapeutic option.

Table 49-1 summarizes, collectively, the physical and metabolic responses to LVAD therapy. These findings suggest the potential for mechanical left ventricular unloading as a therapeutic option, particularly for those not eligible for transplantation.

It is now apparent that unloading the heart with an LVAD may improve cardiac function to such an extent that transplantation is no longer necessary. Such improvement results from a better contractile performance of the myocytes, indicating that mechanical unloading affects the expression of genes coding for contractile proteins and metabolic enzymes. Taegtmeyer's group at the University of Texas compared the genetic responses of the heart to unloading with those of hypertrophy and showed that opposite changes in mechanical stress resulted in similar patterns of gene expression.[27] These included the reexpression of growth factors and proto-oncogenes and the isoform-specific shift of transcripts coding for functional proteins from adult to fetal isoforms (see Table 49-1). Taegtmeyer's experiments in rats demonstrated how gene expression in the heart can be exquisitely and acutely turned on or off by variations in mechanical stress. The changes in transcripts were very rapid (preceding the loss of heart weight) and were quickly reversible upon reloading. It was clear that the genetic adaptation of the heart to unloading is a fast and specific process that results from the change in mechanical stress rather than from a loss of cells. The genetic adaptation mostly compromises the preferential expression of fetal isoforms of proteins regulating myocardial energetics in response to changing energy needs of the myocardium.

From the clinical perspective, the work of Taegtmeyer and colleagues supports the concept that functional improvement in the failing heart after left ventricular unloading may have its origin in a reactivation of the fetal gene program. Functional recovery by normalization of left ventricular geometry, improved contractility, and an increased inotropic response in the cardiomyocyte follows changes in the expression of proteins controlling energy production and/or energy consumption. These mechanisms of adaptation to decreased workload are similar to the adaptive mechanisms in cardiac hypertrophy. The heart shifts to a myosin heavy-chain isoform of lower energy consumption and a supply of energy through housekeeping genes, while the genes characterizing heart efficiency are downregulated.[50] With the decreased work during unloading, these mechanisms limiting energy expenditure may allow the failing heart to regain a new cellular homeostasis.

The change in cardiac mass during pressure overload and ventricular unloading is an adaptive mechanism accompanied by the reexpression of fetal genes.[51] However, untreated cardiac hypertrophy can evolve to an uncompensated state of heart failure. In contrast, the process of "atrophy" induced by ventricular unloading rapidly stabilizes and is nonprogressive thereafter.[52] Consequently, cardiac unloading reduces cardiac mass by a self-limited process and limits energy expenditure by preserving the expression of fetal isoforms of proteins regulating myocardial energetics. The plasticity of gene expression by unloading appears to be a specific and reversible phenomenon resulting from an acute decrease in mechanical stress rather than from a nonspecific consequence of atrophy. This therapeutic induction of a fetal gene response may represent the molecular basis for the functional improvement of the failing heart after LVAD treatment and may provide an unexpected alternative to cardiac transplantation or gene therapy in heart failure. The principle of reactivating fetal genes has already been applied to the treatment of muscular dystrophy.

Bridge to Recovery in Clinical Practice

The ability of mechanical left ventricular unloading to alter basic mechanisms of myocyte biology and to arrest heart failure progression points to a new treatment strategy for patients with cardiomyopathy. Consequently, we have taken a step beyond the use of blood pumps solely to sustain life, pending cardiac transplantation. The small continuous-flow devices are suitable for trials of long-term circulatory support as an alternative to transplantation but are also a valuable tool with which to develop the myocardial recovery strategy.[53] Molecular biology and blood pump technology are now advancing in tandem toward a new solution to the heart failure problem.

Some acute pathologic processes leading to cardiogenic shock can be reversed by mechanical support and improved myocardial blood supply. Blood pumps are used routinely to sustain the circulation in postcardiotomy cardiogenic shock when a period of improved myocardial blood supply may limit infarction and result in survival. Equally, short-term mechanical bridge to recovery has been applied successfully in acute viral myocarditis and peripartum cardiomyopathy.[54] Both pulsatile and nonpulsatile blood pumps are effective in this context, and steroids may assist recovery.

To date, the incidence of recovery sufficient to allow LVAD removal in chronic left ventricular dysfunction has been small. Mancini evaluated bridge-to-cardiac transplant patients and prospectively attempted to identify explant candidates by using an exercise testing protocol.[55]

Thirty-nine consecutive patients were studied after insertion of the HeartMate vented electric LVAD. Three months after implantation, a maximal exercise test with hemodynamic monitoring and respiratory gas exchange analysis was performed, with the pump rate reduced by 20 bpm. Hemodynamic measurements were recorded and a repeat exercise test performed if the patient remained stable. In only one patient were the hemodynamics considered adequate to allow device removal. Furthermore, in a retrospective review of 111 consecutive LVAD patients in this program, only 5 explants were identified. However, these studies were performed in end-stage cardiogenic-shock patients with ischemic heart disease or dilated cardiomyopathy and myocardial fibrosis.

Hetzer and colleagues published the largest series of bridge-to-recovery patients. Between 1994 and 1999, 84 patients were supported with either a Novacor or a TCI LVAD with a view to transplantation.[56] Of this group, 65 had idiopathic dilated cardiomyopathy and were studied prospectively with a view to device removal. Twenty-three of the 65 had near-complete reversal of left ventricular failure during an unloading period of between 30 and 794 days. This group underwent elective removal of the LVAD when, during repeated echocardiography, the left ventricular end-diastolic dimension had dropped below 60 mm and the LVEF had risen to > 40%. Device removal was undertaken, leaving the heart as undisturbed as possible. The pump-housing pocket in the left upper abdominal wall was entered, and the inflow and outflow Dacron grafts were transected and oversewn. This left the cannula in the left ventricular apex and the ascending aortic graft in place. Postoperatively, the patients were anticoagulated with warfarin for 6 months in an attempt to avoid thromboembolism from the prosthetic diverticula. β-Blockers, ACE inhibitors, and spironolactone were prescribed indefinitely.

Of the explanted patients, 13 had stable cardiac function without deterioration for between 3 months and 4 years (mean, 23 ± 14 months). Three other patients had echocardiographic decline in cardiac function but without symptomatic deterioration. Seven had recurrent heart failure beginning 4 months to 2 years (mean, 11 ± 7 months) after device removal. These patients were transplanted. Four patients suffered chronic infections within the pump pocket, which caused death in two patients from sepsis and exsanguinations. At the time of LVAD implantation, there were no significant differences between those with sustained recovery and those who relapsed with regard to age, hemodynamics, LVEF, left ventricular end-diastolic dimension (LVEDD), or autoantibody against the β-adrenergic receptor. Those who relapsed had longer duration of heart failure and a more prolonged period of unloading. Patients with sustained recovery demonstrated more rapid improvement in left ventricular function (LVEF and a decrease of LVEDD), and their duration of unloading was shorter. The degree of left ventricular recovery at LVAD explantation was also more complete in these patients. Younger age at the time of LVAD implantation was the only factor to correlate with shorter duration of unloading. The inverse relationship between heart failure recurrence and shorter duration of preoperative left ventricular failure probably reflects the structure of the myocardium. The 42 dilated cardiomyopathy patients who were not explanted improved to a mean LVEF of 25 ± 8% and LVEDD of 59 ± 6 mm, a level deemed insufficient for safe removal of the LVAD.

In summary, younger patients with shorter duration of heart failure have a better chance of recovery and lower probability for recurrence. Lasting recovery correlates with a shorter history and more rapid improvement in cardiac function during unloading. However, no factors were identified that could reliably predict explant candidates before device implantation.

The Berlin experience suggests that 25% of dilated cardiomyopathy patients who require LVAD support can be weaned with stable midterm cardiac function. Frazier has suggested the combination of left ventricular unloading followed by surgical partial left ventriculectomy (PLV) for patients unlikely to receive a transplant.[57] The improvement in left ventricular morphology induced by unloading may improve the likelihood of success after PLV. Frazier's first patient was a 6'6" 240-pound male who was unlikely to receive a donor heart. He was implanted with an electric TCI LVAD and was discharged from hospital after 4 weeks. One year later, he was re-admitted with recurrent heart failure. The left ventricle had redilated after early prosthetic valve failure within the LVAD. It was then decided to remove the LVAD and perform PLV. This resulted in substantial improvement of left ventricular function. At follow-up 1 year later, he remains NYHA class I and has returned to work. A 24-year-old female dilated cardiomyopathy patient underwent 156 days of LVAD support during which she improved from 1.2 to 2.7 L/min/m². Again, the device was removed and PLV performed. One year later, she is NYHA class I. Whether improved myocardial structure and function by LVAD offloading can influence the long-term success of PLV remains to be answered. Another potential surgical maneuver on LVAD removal is passive external support with a polyester-mesh jacket (Acorn device) surgically placed around the ventricles to prevent further dilatation.[58] This method has been employed electively in NYHA class III patients to prevent deterioration.

The Berlin group identified the optimum LVAD weaning time to be 8 to 12 weeks after implantation. This coincides with the disappearance of the autoantibody against the β-adrenergic receptor in dilated cardiomyopathy patients.[59] Histology from patients subjected to much longer duration of support suggested that myocardial atrophy and fibrosis could interfere with weaning although atrophy can be partially reversed by ventricular loading in progressive increments.

To further the therapeutic potential of bridge to recovery, two major challenges must be addressed. First and foremost, better LVADs are necessary. These should be simpler, smaller, safer, more reliable, and easier to insert than the large-displacement blood pumps. The axial-flow pumps, particularly the Jarvik 2000, are well suited because they allow a progressive decrease in support without risk of thromboembolism. Thus, cardiac work can be increased gradually. Second, it is important to clarify the optimal intervention time points as it is likely that success will be related to earlier device implantation. Methods to sustain left ventricular recovery will evolve as the process gains acceptance with time. Given these developments, the mix of mechanical and biologic solutions should provide effective combination therapy and a potential alternative to cardiac transplantation in the advanced heart failure patient.

References

1. Kannel WB, Belanger AJ. Epidemiology of heart failure. Am Heart J 1991;121:951–7.
2. The CONSENSUS Trial Study Group. Effects of enalapril on mortality in severe congestive heart failure. Results of the Co-operative North Scandinavian Enalapril Survival Study (CONSENSUS). N Engl J Med 1987;316:1429–35.
3. Lee KS, Marwick TH, Cook SA, et al. Prognosis of patients with left ventricular dysfunction with and without viable myocardium after myocardial infarction. Relative efficacy of medical therapy and revascularisation. Circulation 1994;90:2687–94.
4. Deng MC, De Meester JMJ, Smits JMA, et al. Effect of receiving a heart transplant: analysis of a national cohort entered onto a waiting list, stratified by heart failure severity. BMJ 2000;321:540–5.
5. Hausmann H, Topp H, Sinaiwski H, et al. Decision making in end-stage coronary artery disease: revascularisation or heart transplant. Ann Thorac Surg 1997;64:1296–301.
6. Westaby S. Nontransplant surgery for heart failure. Heart 2000;803:603–10.
7. Goldstein DJ, Oz MC, Rose EA. Implantable left ventricular assist devices. N Engl J Med 1998;339:1522–33.
8. Frazier OH, Macris MP, Myers TT, et al. Improved survival after extended bridge to cardiac transplantation. Ann Thorac Surg 1996;61:342–6.
9. Hunt SA, Frazier OH, Myers T. Mechanical circulatory support and cardiac transplantation. Circulation 1998; 97:2079–80.
10. Frazier OH, Rose EA, McCarthy P, et al. Improved mortality and rehabilitation of transplant candidates treated with long-term implantable left ventricular assist system. Ann Surg 1995;222:327–36.
11. McCarthy PM, Schmidt SK, Vargo RL, et al. Implantable LVAD infections: implications for permanent use of the device. Ann Thorac Surg 1996;61:359–65.
12. Livingston ER, Fisher CA, Bibidakis J, et al. Increased activation of the coagulation and fibrinolytic systems leads to hemorrhagic complications during left ventricular assist implantation. Circulation 1996;94 Suppl II:II227–34.
13. Farrar DJ, Hill JD, Pennington DG, et al. Preoperative and postoperative comparison of patients with univentricular and biventricular support with the Thoratec ventricular assist device as a bridge to cardiac transplantation. J Thorac Cardiovasc Surg 1997;113:202–9.
14. Rose EA, Gelijns AL, Moskowitz AJ, et al. Long-term use of a left ventricular assist device for end-stage heart failure. N Engl J Med 2001;345:435–43.
15. Westaby S, Katsumata T, Hovel R, et al. Jarvik 2000 heart: potential for bridge to myocardial recovery. Circulation 1998;98:1568–74.
16. Jarvik R, Westaby S, Katsumata T, et al. LVAD power delivery: a percutaneous approach to avoid infection. Ann Thorac Surg 1998;65:470–3.
17. Frazier OH, Myers TJ, Gregoric ID, et al. Initial clinical experience with the Jarvik 2000 implantable axial flow left ventricular assist system. Circulation 2000;105: 2855–60.
18. Westaby S, Banning A, Saito S, et al. Circulatory support as long-term treatment for heart failure. Experience with an intraventricular continuous flow pump. Circulation 2000;105:2588–91.
19. DeBakey ME. A miniature implantable axial flow ventricular assist device. Ann Thorac Surg 1999;68:637–40.
20. Wilhelm MJ, Hammel D, Schmid C, et al. Clinical experience with nine patients supported by the continuous flow DeBakey VAD. J Heart Lung Transplant 2001;20:201.
21. Noon GP, Morley D, Irwin S, Benkowski R. Development and clinical application of the Micromed DeBakey VAD. Curr Opin Cardiol 2000;15;166–71.
22. Griffith BP, Kormos RL, Borovetz HS, et al. HeartMate II left ventricular assist system: from concept to first clinical use. Ann Thorac Surg 2001;71:S116–20.
23. Maher TR, Butler KC, Poirier VL, Gernes DB. HeartMate left ventricular assist devices: a multigeneration of implanted blood pumps. Artif Organs 2001;25:422–6.
24. Saito S, Westaby S, Piggott D, et al. Reliable long-term non-pulsatile circulatory support without anticoagulation. Euro J Cardiothorac Surg 2001;19:678–83.
25. Potopov EV, Loebe M, Nasseri BA, et al. Pulsatile flow in patients with a novel non pulsatile implantable ventricular assist device. Circulation 2000;102 Suppl III:183–7.
26. Braunwald E. Pathophysiology of heart failure. In: Braunwald E, editor. Heart disease: a textbook of cardiovascular medicine. 4th ed. Philadelphia: WB Saunders; 1992. p. 393–418.
27. Depre C, Shipley GL, Chen W, et al. Unloaded heart in vivo replicates fetal gene expression of cardiac hypertrophy. Nat Med 1998;4:1269–75.
28. Towbin JA, Bowles NE. The failing heart. Nature 2002;415: 227–33.
29. Narula J, Haider N, Virmani R, et al. Apoptosis in myocytes in end-stage heart failure. N Engl J Med 1999;335: 1182–9.
30. Swedberg K, Enroth P, Kjekshus J, et al. Hormones regulating cardiovascular function in patients with severe congestive heart failure and their relationship to mortality. Circulation 1990;82:1730–6.
31. Morgan HE, Baker K. Cardiac hypertrophy: mechanical, neural and endocrine dependence. Circulation 1991;83: 13–25.

32. Baker KM, Cherwin MI, Wixson SK, Aceto JF. Renin-angiotensin system involvement in pressure overload cardiac hypertrophy in rats. Am J Physiol 1990;259: H324–32.

33. Weber KT. Extracellular matrix remodelling in heart failure. A note for de novo angiotensin II generation. Circulation 1997;96:4065–82.

34. Troughton RW, Frampton CM, Yandle TG, et al. Treatment of heart failure guided by plasma aminoterminal brain natriuretic peptide (N-BNP) concentrations. Lancet 2000;355:1126–30.

35. Balligard JL, Kelly RA, Margden PA, et al. Control of cardiac muscle cell function by an endogenous nitric oxide signaling system. Proc Natl Acad Sci U S A 1993;90:347–51.

36. Burch GE, De Pasquale NP. On resting the human heart. Am J Med 1968;44:165–7.

37. Frazier OH, Benedict CC, Radovancevich B, et al. Improved left ventricular function after chronic left ventricular unloading. Ann Thorac Surg 1996;62:675–82.

38. Levin HR, Oz MC, Chen JM, et al. Reversal of chronic ventricular dilation in patients with end-stage cardiomyopathy by prolonged mechanical unloading. Circulation 1995;91:2717–20.

39. Zafeiridis A, Jeevanandam V, Houser SR, Margulies KB. Regression of cellular hypertrophy after left ventricular assist device support. Circulation 1998;98:656–62.

40. McCarthy PM, Nakatani S, Vargo R, et al. Structural and left ventricular histologic changes after implantable left ventricular assist device insertion. Ann Thorac Surg 1995;59:609–13.

41. Milting H, Bartling B, Schumann H, et al. Altered levels of mRNA of apoptosis-mediating genes after midterm mechanical ventricular support and dilative cardiomyopathy: first results of the HALLE Assist Induced Recovery study (HAIR). Thorac Cardiovasc Surg 1999;47:48–50.

42. Belland SE, Grunstein R, Jeevanandam V, Eisen HJ. The effect of sustained mechanical support with left ventricular assist devices on myocardial apoptosis in patients with severe dilated cardiomyopathy. J Heart Lung Transplant 1999;17:83–4.

43. James KJ, McCarthy PM, Thomas JD, et al. Effect of the implantable left ventricular assist device on neuroendocrine activation in heart failure. Circulation 1995;92 Suppl II:191–5.

44. Di Tullio M, McCarthy PM, Smedira N, Moravec C. Reversal of the heart failure phenotype by mechanical unloading. Proceddings of the Cleveland Clinic Heart Failure Summit; 1995. p. 65.

45. Takeishi Y, Jalili T, Hoit BD, et al. Alterations in calcium-cycling protein and g-alpha-q signalling after left ventricular assist device supporting failing human hearts. Cardiovasc Res 2000;45:883–8.

46. Lee SH, Doliba N, Osbakken M, et al. Improvement of myocardial mitochondrial function after haemodynamic support with left ventricular assist devices in patients with heart failure. J Thorac Cardiovasc Surg 1998;116:344–9.

47. Danialou G, Comtois A, Dudley R, et al. Dystrophin-deficient cardiomyocytes are abnormally vulnerable to mechanical stress-induced contractile failure and injury. FASEB J 2001;15:1655–7.

48. Ikeda Y, Martone M, Gu Y, et al. Altered membrane proteins and permeability correlate with cardiac dysfunction in cardiomyopathic hamsters. Am J Physiol Heart Circ Physiol 2000;278:H1362–70.

49. Vatta M, Stetson SJ, Perez-Verdia A, et al. Molecular remodelling of dystrophin in patients with end-stage cardiomyopathies and reversal in patients on assistance device therapy. Lancet 2000;359:936–41.

50. Dorn GW, Robbins J, Ball N, Walsh RA. Myosin heavy chain regulation and myocyte contractile depression after LV hypertrophy in aortic banded mice. Am J Physiol 1994;267:H400–5.

51. Sadoshima S, Izumo S. The cellular and molecular response of cardiac myocytes to mechanical stress. Annu Rev Physiol 1997;59:551–71.

52. Soloff LA. Atrophy of myocardium and its myocytes by left ventricular assist device. Circulation 1998;98:1012.

53. Westaby S. New implantable blood pumps for medium and long-term circulatory support. Perfusion 2000;15: 319–25.

54. Westaby S, Katsumata T, Pigott D, et al. Mechanical bridge to recovery in fulminant myocarditis. Ann Thorac Surg 2000;70:278–83.

55. Mancini DM, Beniaminovitz A, Levin H, et al. Low incidence of myocardial recovery after left ventricular assist device implantation in patients with chronic heart failure. Circulation 1998;98:2383–9.

56. Hetzer R, Muller J, Weng Y, et al. Cardiac recovery in dilated cardiomyopathy by unloading with left ventricular assist device. Ann Thorac Surg 1999;68:742–9.

57. Frazier OH. Left ventricular assist device as a bridge to partial left ventriculectomy. Eur J Cardiothorac Surg 1999; 15 Suppl I:520–5.

58. Rahman J, Power JM, Buxton B, et al. Ventricular containment as an adjunctive procedure in ischaemic cardiomyopathy. Early results. Ann Thorac Surg 2000;70: 1124–6.

59. Muller J, Wallukat G, Weng Y, et al. Weaning from mechanical cardiac support in patients with idiopathic dilated cardiomyopathy. Circulation 1997;96:542–9.

CHAPTER 50

CENTRIFUGAL BLOOD PUMPS

NORIYUKI MURAI, MD, PHD, TADASHI MOTOMURA, MD, PHD,
YUKIHIKO NOSÉ, MD, PHD

A centrifugal blood pump is a rotary blood pump. This type of blood pump generates nonpulsatile or continuous blood flow. Such nonpulsatile blood pumps are typically classified into two groups: axial flow blood pumps and centrifugal blood pumps (Table 50-1). An axial flow blood pump is operated like an Archimedes screw, and its size can be reduced to extremely small. The impeller of the axial flow blood pump typically rotates at around 10,000 revolutions per minute (RPM). On the other hand, a centrifugal blood pump propels the blood by using a spinning top inside the chamber. Its typical RPM is approximately one-fifth to one-third that of an axial flow blood pump. Typically, approximately 2,000 to 3,000 RPM is needed to generate clinically needed blood flow of approximately 5 ± 1 L/min against 100 ± 20 mm Hg. Because the impeller of a centrifugal blood pump spins at a much lower speed, its bearing life is expected to be longer than that of an axial flow blood pump. Its endurance life is expected to be longer than 2 years.

Because of the difference in impeller speed, a centrifugal pump is typically larger than an axial flow blood pump. However, when compared with any type of pulsatile blood pump, the centrifugal blood pump is much smaller (see Table 50-1). In this chapter, only centrifugal blood pumps and their physiologic compatibility as a nonpulsatile blood pump are described.

The history of centrifugal pumps is old, especially the concept of centrifugal pumps, which was introduced, in 1968, by Rafferty.[1] Blackshear's group in Minnesota developed the first clinically applicable centrifugal pump for 2 weeks. The early-stage centrifugal pump (first-generation pump) had a shaft that connected directly to an actuator (Figure 50-1). A centrifugal pump, which employed magnetic coupling impeller drive, was later developed (second-generation pump).[2] Most of the currently available centrifugal pumps for cardiopulmonary bypass (CPB) use this impeller-driving method, which eliminates the direct shaft connection between impeller and actuator unit and simplifies the total system. The centrifugal force of the Medtronic pump is generated by the impeller of three cone structures. This cone-type Medtronic centrifugal pump has been used in a variety of clinical applications, particularly for CPB (Figure 50-2A and B). Centrifugal pumps are safe for patients and atraumatic to the blood for CPB and temporary circulatory support. However, using a pump for extracorporeal membrane oxygenation (ECMO) or percutaneous cardiopulmonary support (PCPS) requires long cannulae for blood accesses and circuit tubing. In turn, this requires a higher rotational speed because of the high level of afterload (Figure 50-2C). In this situation, the shear rate and exposure time of the blood impact hemolysis, and often the period of ECMO or PCPS can be more than 2 weeks. Generally, the rate of hemolysis in this cone-type centrifugal blood pump for ECMO application is higher than that of conventional bulky roller pumps. Cone-type centrifugal pumps do not meet such specific extracorporeal circulation with high afterload and low pump flow rate because of high shear-induced hemolysis.[3] A more atraumatic centrifugal pump is needed. Many centrifugal pumps have been developed. The Nikkiso centrifugal pump (HMS-15, Nikkiso Co., Ltd., Tokyo, Japan) demonstrated a low level of hemolysis when compared to a roller pump and a cone-type centrifugal pump, and operated with broad blood flow rate even high afterload (Figure 50-3).[4-7] The key structure of this small centrifugal pump is the impeller vane, which was computer-assisted designed . Vane position and other key structures, such as an angle and length of straight vane, were refined based on the results of computational fluid dynamics (CFD) analysis to provide sufficient blood flow without excessive wall shear stress, which is the primary factor for hemolysis and platelet activation. Another feature of the Nikkiso pump are the washing holes on the impeller base, which aim to prevent stagnant

TABLE 50-1. Comparison of Rotary Blood Pumps and Pulsatile Pumps

Type	RPM of Impeller	Size of Pump (Priming Volume) (mL)
Axial flow pump	$10,000 \pm 2,000$	10 ± 5
Centrifugal pump	$2,500 \pm 500$	25 ± 10
Pulsatile pump	$< 150^*$	$66 (52^{**})$

* Beats per minute (bpm); ** effective stroke volume in revolutions per minute (RPM).

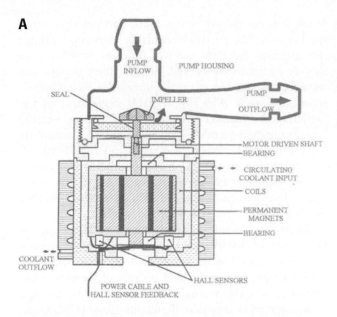

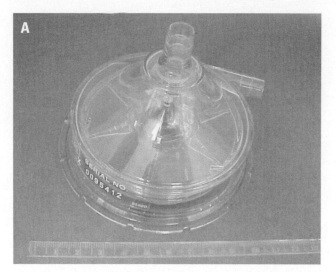

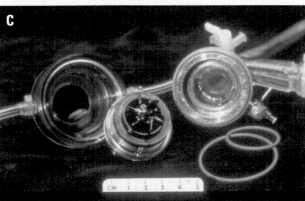

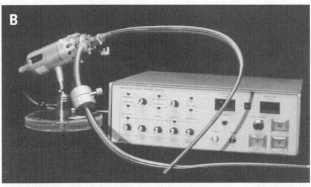

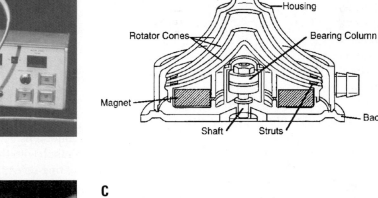

FIGURE 50-1. *A*, Blackshear-Medtronic centrifugal blood pump (cross-sectional drawing). The Blackshear-Medtronic centrifugal blood pump was originally developed by Medtronic USA, Inc., Minneapolis, MN, in the early 1970s. The small impeller inside a pump head was rotated by a DC brushless micromotor with a direct shaft-drive configuration. This pump was different from the current cone-type Bio-Pump, which uses a magnet-coupling drive to rotate the impeller. *B*, Blackshear-Medtronic centrifugal blood pump (pump head and driving console). *C*, Blackshear-Medtronic centrifugal blood pump (impeller and housings).

FIGURE 50-2. *A*, Medtronic Bio-Pump (BP-80X, Medtronic Perfusion Systems, Inc, Minneapolis, MN). *B*, Cross-sectional drawing of Medtronic Bio-Pump. *C*, Hydraulic performance curves of Medtronic Bio-Pump.

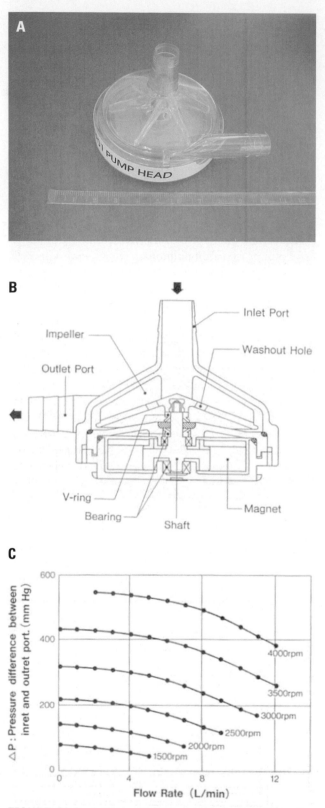

FIGURE 50-3. *A*, Nikkiso HMS-15 centrifugal pump (Nikkiso Co., Ltd., Tokyo, Japan). The HMS-15 is an easy-priming, low priming volume (25 mL), low heat generation, low hemolytic blood pump whose design is based on computational fluid dynamics. Six washout holes are employed on its impeller in order to prevent blood stagnation. *B*, Nikkiso centrifugal pump (cross-sectional drawing). *C*, Hydraulic performance curves of Nikkiso centrifugal pump.

blood flow on the bottom housing, particularly around the bearing. The currently available centrifugal pumps that are used for CPB use two different impeller vane shapes: straight and curved. Several other pumps use washing holes or spaces on the impeller as well. Characteristics of each clinically available centrifugal pump, including the manner of impeller suspension, bearing structure, vane design, washing holes, and inlet design, are summarized in Table 50-2 and Figures 50-2 to 50-10.

Implantable centrifugal blood pumps for long-term left ventricular or biventricular heart assist are currently under development.[8–11] One of such systems employs the floating impeller (described in next section).

The magnet-coupling structure has a sealed bearing at the center of impeller axis, which is disadvantageous because of blood leakage into the bearing itself, because of excessive heat generation, and because of thrombus formation around the bearing shaft during long-term usage.

A centrifugal pump is useful for CPB, ECMO, and PCPS because of easy controllability and high efficiency. This pump can generate high flow without excessive high pressure. Almost all the current centrifugal pumps can generate flow above 5 L/min. Tubing rupture, which frequently occurs with a roller pump, is nonexistent, and the set-up time is very short. In general, a roller-type pump is more traumatic to blood than is a centrifugal pump. Some reports state that a centrifugal pump demonstrates improved blood handling and a reduced risk of emboli production when compared to a roller pump used under standardized conditions, that is, conditions that simulate adult open heart surgery with high flow and low pressure conditions.[12–17] A significant reduction in the number of emboli with the use of a centrifugal pump was at the level of one-seventh of a roller pump.[18,19]

The first clinical data on the use of a centrifugal pump were reported in 1978; the data indicated reduced hemolysis and postoperative chest drainage with the use of a centrifugal pump compared with that of a roller pump.[20] Wheeldon and colleagues found significantly reduced complement activation and better platelet preservation when a centrifugal blood pump was used.[21] Parault and colleagues reported better platelet retention only for higher-risk patients with bypass times greater than 120 min, for patients over 70 years old, and for those patients classified as special case.[22] Jakob and colleagues demonstrated a reduction in plasma hemoglobin, platelet count, β-thromboglobulin, and D-dimers, reaching significance after 90 min of bypass.[23] Berki and colleagues showed that significant differences in platelet count and platelet activation can occur as early as 30 min after initiation of cardiopulmonary bypass.[24] Klein and colleagues reported postoperative chest tube drainage was significantly reduced when a centrifugal pump was used.[19]

Recently, the centrifugal pump was developed as a circulatory assist device. A centrifugal pump as an assist heart device has the advantage of (1) no flexing

TABLE 50-2. Summary of Clinically Available Centrifugal Pumps for Coronary Pulmonary Bypass

Pump	Inlet Port	Bearing	Top Vane‡	Bottom Vane‡	Washing Hole or Window§	Figure Number
Bio-Pump *Medtronics, Inc.*	Straight	Sealed	cone type	No	No	50–2
HMS-15 *Nikkiso Co., Ltd.*	Straight	Sealed	Straight	No	Yes (6 holes)	50–3
Capiox *Terumo Co.*	Straight	Sealed	Straight†	No	No	5U–4
Delphin *Terumo-Sarns 3M*	Straight	Sealed	Curved	No	No	50–5
IsoFlow *St. Jude Medical*	Straight	Sealed	Curved	Yes	Yes	50–6
HiFlow *HIA-Medos AG*	Straight	Sealed	Curved	No	No	50–7
Rota Flow *Jostra AG*	Straight	Seal-less single pivot	Flow channel system	No	No	50–8
Gyro C1E3 *Kyocera Co.*	Angled inlet	Seal-less Peg-top*	Straight	Yes	No	50–9
Revolution *Cobe C.V.*	Angled inlet	Seal-less double pivot	Curved	No	Yes	50 10

* Magnetic-stabilized rotor bearing; † straight blood path; ‡ impeller blade vane; § blood communication channel between the bottom and the top of the impeller.

diaphragm; (2) smaller blood-contacting surfaces; (3) no need for inflow and outflow valves; (4) simpler electronics; (5) fewer moving parts; (6) no requirement for a variable volume chamber; (7) equal or lower energy requirements for the production of continuous flow compared with that of a pusatile flow; (8) good durability; (9) small size; and (10) lower cost (Table 50-3).

Centrifugal blood pumps are widely employed as the blood pumps for cardiopulmonary bypass, with a limited clinical application of up to 6 h. Even though some cases require longer than 6 h of usage, this blood pump is typically classified as a 2-day pump because it operates typically for 48 hours (Table 50-4). Because a centrifugal pump is used for a short length of time and sufficient anticoagulating agents are used, the pump's antithrombogenic features are not a primary design consideration. However, these types of blood pumps should not produce excessive blood trauma. Thus, the major objective is to design an atraumatic blood pump (see Table 50-4). On the other hand, a blood pump applicable for 2 weeks is required in the event of ECMO and PCPS usage. During this period of time, a blood pump has a tendency to produce white thrombosis, particularly at the impeller-supporting shaft areas. Thus, for the development of a 2-week pump, the primary design consideration is an antithrombogenic blood pump.

Other clinical needs for the longer-term blood pumps are for the bridge to transplantation and for the bridge to recovery. Typically, the clinical needs are satisfied if the

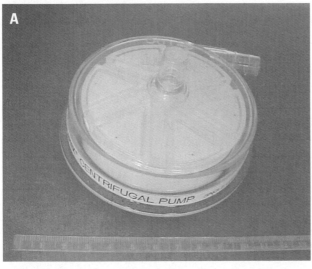

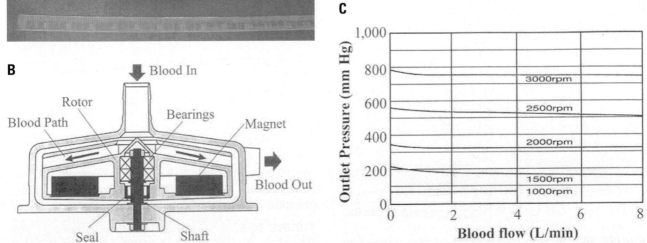

FIGURE 50-4. *A,* Terumo Capiox centrifugal pump (Terumo Cardiovascular, Tokyo, Japan). This pump introduced an impeller with blood passage channels instead of a conventional impeller vane, which reduced priming volume and hemolytic property. Pump flow performance is well maintained against high afterload of greater than 600 mm Hg. Capiox demonstrated significantly less hemolysis than Medtronic Bio-Pump. *B,* Cross-sectional drawing of Capiox centrifugal pump. *C,* Hydraulic performance curves of the Terumo Capiox centrifugal pump.

TABLE 50-3. Blood Pump (Nonpulsatile and Pulsatile)

	Pulsatile	Nonpulsatile
Flexing diaphragm	Yes	No
Valve	Yes	No
Variable volume chamber	Yes	No
Size and weight	Larger and heavier	Smaller and lightweight
Blood contact surface	Larger	Smaller
Electronic control	More complex	Simpler
Moving parts	Lager number	Smaller number
Hemolysis	Higher	Lower

TABLE 50-4. Classification of Pumps

	Clinical Needs	Typical Features
2-Day pump	Cardiopulmonary bypass	Atraumatic pump
2-Week pump	ECMO and PCPS	Antithrombogenic pump
2-Year pump	Bridge to transplantation; Bridge to recovery	Durable pump
5-Year pump	Permanent	Simple pump

ECMO = extracorporeal membrane oxygenator; PCPS = percutaneous cardiopulmonary support.

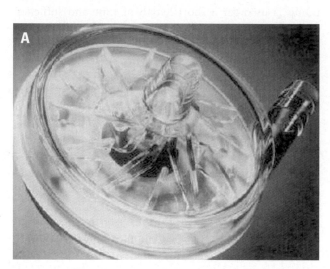

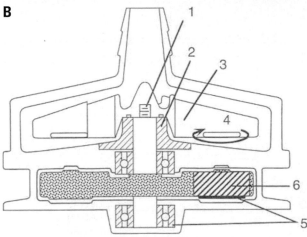

FIGURE 50-5. *A*, Sarns Delphin centrifugal pump (Terumo-Sarns 3M, Ann Arbor, MI). *B*, Cross-sectional drawing of Delphin centrifugal pump (1 = impeller shaft; 2 = sealing part; 3 = vane; 4 = absence of stagnant flow area behind the impeller; 5 = nonsealed ball bearing; 6 = magnet).

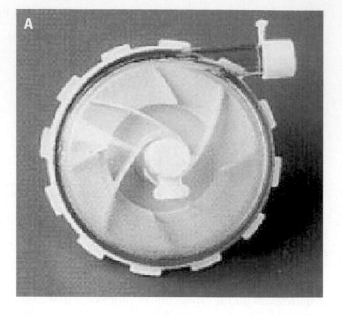

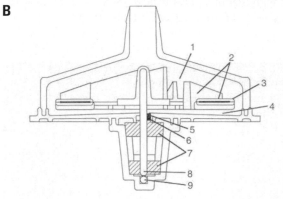

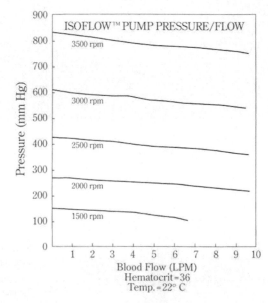

FIGURE 50-6. *A*, St. Jude IsoFlow centrifugal pump (St. Jude Medical, Inc., St. Paul, MN). *B*, Cross-sectional drawing of St. Jude IsoFlow centrifugal pump (1 = blood path; 2 = curved vane; 3 = thin metal drive path; 4 = back side vane; 5 and 6 = quad-ring double seal; 7 = sleeve bearing; 8 = stainless steel shaft; 9 = thrust bearing). *C*, Hydraulic performance curves of St. Jude IsoFlow centrifugal pump.

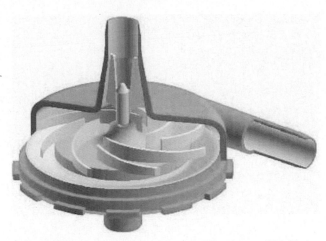

FIGURE 50-7. HIA-Medos HiFlow centrifugal pump (HIA-Medos AG, Stollberg, Germany).

blood pump is implantable with a fail-safe operation of at least 1 year. Thus, this pump's design objective is that it have 2-year durability. The final clinical need is a permanent device. A patient has to be able to live with this device at home for at least 5 years. If the system is complex, there is an increased risk of failure. In addition, the patient or a family member should be able to cope with a system malfunction, should it occur. The system should be as simple as possible (see Table 50-4).

Development of Centrifugal Pumps

Based upon the evolution of impeller activation, a centrifugal blood pump is classified as being within one of four generations (Table 50-5).

The First Generation (Direct Shaft Drive)

The impeller shaft of a centrifugal blood pump is directly connected to an actuator, and almost all of the centrifugal blood pumps initially available for cardiopulmonary bypass fall within this generation (see Figure 50-1). To accommodate this arrangement, the actuator shaft from the outside of the blood pump has to penetrate throughout the pump housing. Thus, a proper water seal is required. At this area, heat generation is very difficult to avoid. In addition, it is also very difficult to avoid thrombus formation near the impeller shaft, eliminating blood stagnation. Based on these limitations, this type of centrifugal blood pump is typically used only for limited periods of time. One exception is the Sun Medical implantable centrifugal Eva Heart pump. Sun Medical incorporated a heat exchange arrangement at the shaft area in order to avoid heat generation and thrombus formation (Figure 50-11).

The Second Generation (Magnetic Coupling)

To avoid a direct impeller shaft connection, a permanent magnet is incorporated inside of the impeller. This magnet is coupled with an electromagnet positioned in a parallel fashion and incorporated in the actuator. Thus, the pump housing could be kept in a completely sealed fashion (see Figures 50-2 to 50-10 and 50-12). The impeller is housed inside the pump. Various types of bearings have been incorporated. Currently, most of the 2-day and the 2-week blood pumps employ this type of impeller arrangement. This type of impeller arrangement has also been incorporated in the longer-term blood pumps.

The Third Generation (Magnet Suspension)

Incorporation of actuation magnets at the bottom of the impeller as well as an additional magnet at the top of the impeller should produce a magnetically suspended impeller when the proper balance is made by the top and the bottom magnets. Once the impeller is suspended, it is possible to eliminate all mechanically produced wear on the impeller (Figure 50-13). This is ideal for long-term implantable blood pumps. Currently, many experimental

TABLE 50-5. Centrifugal Pumps (Past, Present, and Future)

Characteristics	Centrifugal Pump	Uses
Shaft connected to actuator	Ex-type Medtronic Bio-pump	—
	Ex-type Nikkiso pump	—
	Sun Medical Eva Heart	Implantable LVAD
Magnet coupling	Current-type Medtronic Bio-Pump	CPB, ECMO, PCPS
	Current-type Nikkiso pump	CPB, ECMO, PCPS
	Terumo Capiox	CPB, ECMO, PCPS
	Terumo Sarns Centrifugal (Delphin)	CPB, ECMO, PCPS
	St. Jude IsoFlow	CPB, ECMO, PCPS
	Kyocera Gyro C1E3	CPB, ECMO, PCPS
Magnetically suspended (floating impeller)	Thoratec HeartMate III	Implantable LVAD
	Terumo Mag-Lev	Implantable LVAD
	Cleveland Clinic CorAid*	Implantable LVAD
	MedQuest HeartQuest	Implantable LVAD
RPM control dynamic suspension (floating impeller)	Baylor NEDO PI 710	Implantable BVAD

BVAD = biventricular assist device; CPB = cardiopulmonary bypass; ECMO = extracorporeal membrane oxygenation; LVAD = left ventricular assist device; PCPS = percutaneous cardiopulmonary support; RPM = revolutions per minute.

* In stricter sense, this pump is not magnetically suspended; it is a hybrid system with hydrodynamic suspension and magnetic suspension.

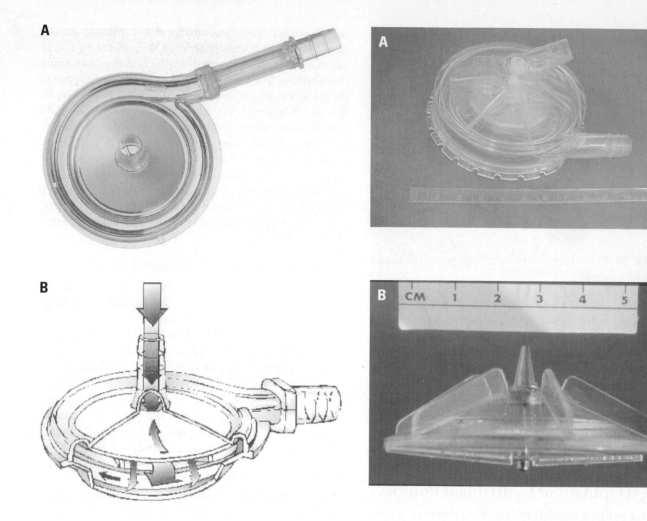

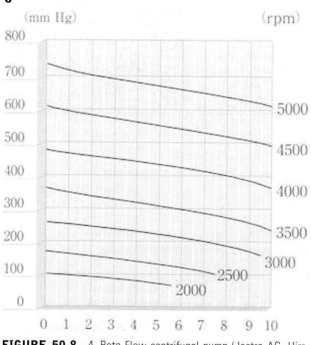

FIGURE 50-8. *A*, Rota Flow centrifugal pump (Jostra AG, Hirrlingen, Germany). *B*, Schematic of Jostra Rota Flow and flow image. *C*, Hydraulic performance curves of Jostra Rota Flow centrifugal pump.

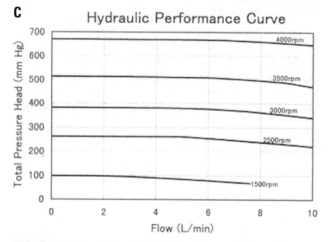

FIGURE 50-9. *A*, Gyro C1E3 centrifugal pump (Kyocera Co., Kyoto, Japan). Gyro C1E3 uses an impeller with two pivot bearings suspended by top and bottom female bearings. The blood inlet port is offset from the center shaft, and angled so-called "eccentric inlet port." (The inlet port is positioned off center.) *B*, Impeller side view of Gyro C1E3 centrifugal pump. Ceramic is used for shaft materials, and this male bearing shaft will last more than 5 years (left ventricular assist device condition) in conjunction with female bearing made of ultrahigh-molecular-weight polyethylene. *C*, Hydraulic performance curves of Gyro C1E3 centrifugal pump.

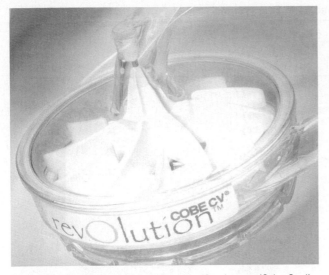

FIGURE 50-10. Cobe Revolution centrifugal pump (Cobe Cardio-vascular, Arvada, CO).

centrifugal blood pumps of this type are under development. They include Thoratec's HeartMate III (Figure 50-14), Terumo's Mag-Lev (Figure 50-15), Cleveland Clinic's CorAid (Figure 50-16), and MedQuest's Heart-Quest (Figure 50-17).

The Fourth Generation (RPM Suspension)

When the impeller is supported by the top and bottom bearings, there is a specific gap between the male and female pivot bearings. It is possible to suspend the impeller at the specific RPMs against a specific pressure head. The current NEDO PI 710 Gyro centrifugal blood pump falls within this category (Figure 50-18).

This pump suspends the impeller when the impeller's RPMs are between 1,700 and 2,000 and when the pressure head is 100 ± 20 mm Hg. Pump flow generated at these conditions is 5 ± 1 L/min. The details are addressed later. With this arrangement, there is no need to have additional hardware or additional power while maintaining the same level of durability. The basic design of this pump is extremely simple. The expected cost of this blood pump is lower than the cost of third-generation blood pumps (Table 50-6). For a permanent blood pump, the design objective is that it be "simple," and this fourth-generation blood pump is ideal for this clinical application.

Another important issue involved in development of a centrifugal blood pump is the design of the impeller, which is a generator of vortex force. The position, the shape, and the size of the impeller blade are extremely important for the optimization of a centrifugal blood pump (see Table 50-2). Also important is the elimination of stagnant blood areas inside the blood pump. Such areas typically reside at the bottom of the impeller. Some blood pumps intend to eliminate this stagnant area at the bottom of the impeller by creating a channel between the bottom and top of the impeller for the blood passage (see Table 50-2).

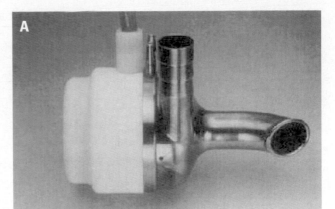

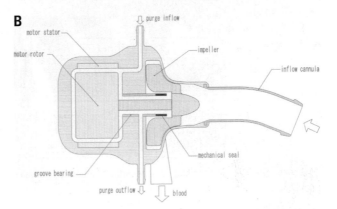

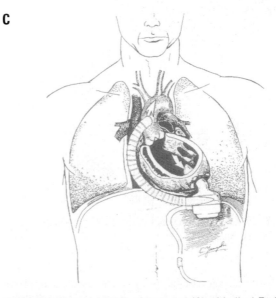

FIGURE 50-11. *A,* Eva Heart pump (Sun Medical Technology Research Corp., Shiga, Japan). *B,* Cross-sectional schematic of the Eva Heart pump. *C,* Anatomic fitting of the Eva Heart.

Current Situation

Cardiopulmonary Bypass and Other Operations

The centrifugal pump is used for cardiopulmonary bypass during heart surgery because it is easy to use and because it prevents excessive outflow high pressure. Because of

TABLE 50-6. Advantages and Disadvantages of Magnetic and RPM Suspension

Centrifugal Pump	Type	Additional Hardware	Additional Power	Construction	Durability	Price of the Device
The third generation	Magnetic suspension	Required	Required	Complex	Yes	Higher
The fourth generation	RPM suspension	Not required	Not required	Simple	Yes	Lower

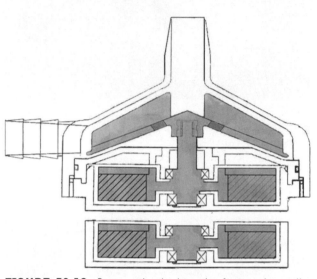

FIGURE 50-12. Cross-sectional schematic of magnetic-coupling impeller drive.

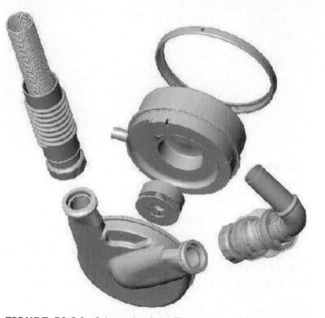

FIGURE 50-14. Schematic of the Thoratec HeartMate III magnet suspension centrifugal pump.

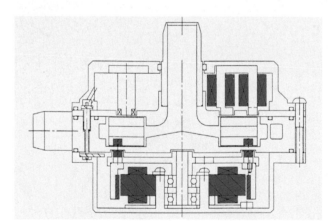

FIGURE 50-13. Cross-sectional schematic of a magnetic suspension centrifugal pump.

these features, centrifugal pumps are used in approximately 50% of adult open heart cases in the United States and Canada. Alamanni reported that using the centrifugal pump reduced device-related complications.[25] Centrifugal pumps can be helpful in reducing the occurrence of some of the most feared neurologic complications of adult cardiac surgery patients. Coselli reported that the centrifugal pump provided excellent pump function and sufficient flow for both distal aortic and selective organ perfusion during thoracoabdominal aortic aneurysm repair. By using the pump, permanent spinal cord injury and distal aortic organ failure was prevented.[26]

Recently, some surgeons have performed cardiac operation by partial sternotomy with a small skin incision. This type of operation is called *minimally invasive cardiac surgery* (MICS). Some authors recommend that a centrifugal pump be used for MICS.[27] Coronary artery bypass graft (CABG) on a beating heart is a MICS application. This approach is often limited to the anterior aspects of the heart because revascularization of the posterior and lateral vessels often requires the heart to be manipulated or contorted. Excessive manipulation can lead to hemodynamic compromise as a result of partially obstructing the pulmonary blood flow. An extracorporeal system with a centrifugal blood pump for right ventricular support is useful for beating-heart coronary anastomoses in the posterior or lateral part without standard CPB.[28]

Often, a centrifugal pump is used in other organ operations. It is useful for a hepatic lobectomy or hepatic vein injury, which may result from trauma suffered in a traffic accident.[29] When a malignant liver tumor invades a hepatic vein, inferior vena cava, or tumor thrombus in the inferior vena cava or right atrium, an extracorporeal bypass using a centrifugal pump is useful.[30,31] When repairing the vena cava affected by Budd-Chiari syndrome, a hepatic vascular exclusion using a centrifugal blood pump is necessary.[32] A centrifugal pump is also useful for maintaining renal

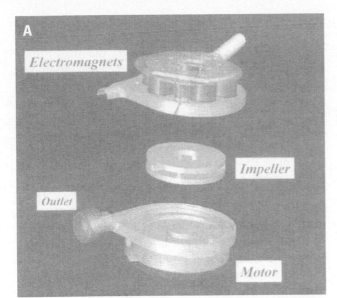

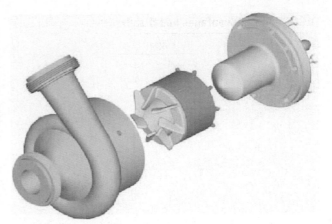

FIGURE 50-16. Cleveland Clinic's CorAid centrifugal pump (Arrow International, Inc., Reading, PA).

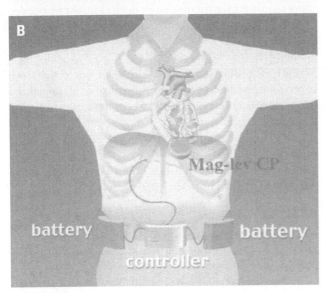

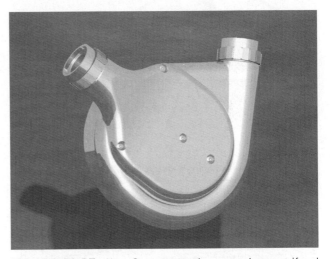

FIGURE 50-17. HeartQuest magnetic suspension centrifugal pump (MedQuest Products, Inc., Salt Lake City, UT).

FIGURE 50-15. *A*, Schematic of the Terumo Mag-Lev centrifugal pump (Terumo Cardiovascular, Tokyo, Japan). *B*, Anatomic fitting of the Terumo Mag-Lev centrifugal pump.

artery blood flow selectively for vascular reconstruction when tumors, such as renal cell carcinoma, invade the inferior vena cava or main renal vascular system.[33]

Extracorporeal Membrane Oxygenation

ECMO is commonly performed in infants and children.[34] Virtually all centers use an ECMO circuit containing an occlusive roller pump, servomechanism, membrane oxygenator, and heat exchanger. The centrifugal pump offers several advantages over the roller pump for ECMO. First, centrifugal pumps are unable to generate high positive pressure that can cause circuit disruption if a line were occluded. They have decreased tendency to suck air emboli when venous return fluctuates, and they are able to trap air emboli while continuing to pump. Second, the pump can be operated at bed level, which decreases the amount of tubing required. Third, the integral battery backup and the ability to operate the pump at bed level make this pump ideally suited for transport. Finally, because of its simple technology, the centrifugal pump enables easy transportation during extracorporeal circulation.[34–36]

The roller pump is often used for long-term ECMO support (about 2 weeks). Almost all oxygenators that use microporous polypropylene hollow-fiber membranes are not durable for the long term. The Kolobow artificial lung, which is made from a silicone gas exchange membrane, is operational for the long-term without serum leakage, but the pressure resistance of the oxygenator is high. This is the reason that centrifugal pumps have not been used for long term ECMO. Recently, a centrifugal pump durable for 1 month was developed.[37] It is expected that a low-pressure–resistant and long-term artificial lung will be developed in the near future.

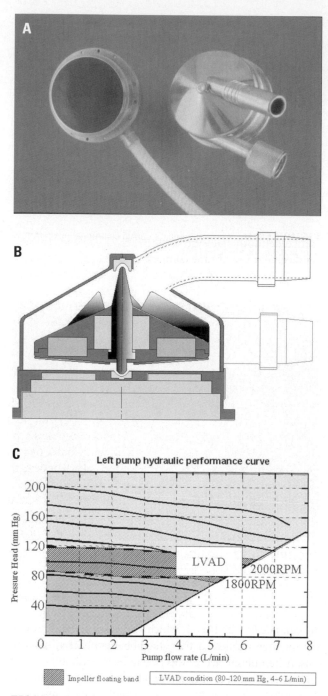

FIGURE 50-18. *A,* Baylor Gyro RPM suspension permanent implantable centrifugal pump (*left,* actuator; *right,* pump head). *B,* Cross-sectional schematic of the Baylor Gyro permanent implantable centrifugal pump. *C,* Hydraulic performance curve of Baylor NEDO PI 710 gyro centrifugal pump and its impeller floating band (oblique line area shows impeller floating band balanced with magnet force and floating force of rotating impeller).

Percutaneous Cardiopulmonary Support

PCPS is a new technique that is used for emergency venoarterial bypass.[38–40] A PCPS device maintains a patient's cardiac and pulmonary function when the patient's cardiac and pulmonary status is failing. This system consists of a centrifugal pump, a control system, a membrane oxygenator, a measuring device for blood flow and pressure, and a heating system to maintain proper blood temperature. A PCPS device is the quickest support available for saving the brain, heart, and other major organs, and a stepwise conversion to advanced circulatory support is important for effective recovery of the failing heart. Rapid priming, rapid insertion, and high flow rate are characteristic of this method. Management or maintenance of PCPS is easy, and it can be used in the operating room as well as in the intensive care unit or ward for patients in a state of profound cardiogenic shock. However, for patients who require mechanical circulatory support, the rates of morbidity and mortality are high. Common complications are bleeding (40%), acute renal failure (30%), and sepsis (30%).[41] Temporary circulatory support for severe cardiac failure showed some improvement of clinical results, but early and proper conversion to more advanced ventricular assist devices might be needed to save patients with intractable biventricular failure.

Temporary Circulatory Support

Recently, the short-term and long-term outcomes from cardiac surgeries have improved because of standardized surgical techniques, sufficient myocardial protection, and the proper management of patients during and after surgery. However, approximately 1% of patients who have open heart surgery still need mechanical circulatory support for severe cardiac dysfunction.[42] Now, the centrifugal pump is used as a short-term assist device.[43]

Bridge to Transplantation

Mechanical circulatory support as a bridge to transplantation is a generally accepted therapeutic option in patients with end-stage heart failure.[43–46]

The devices available are classifiable according to their anatomic position. A centrifugal pump is classified as an extracorporeal device and is applied for short-term support for up to 4 weeks. It is also used in cases of right-heart failure after a left ventricular assist system (LVAS) implantation.[43]

Permanent Ventricular Assist Device versus Cardiac Transplantation: Which Is Better?

Based on the information available from the Institute of Medicine, it is expected that approximately 60,000 patients per year in the United States could be saved by either heart transplantation or cardiac prosthesis implantation. Worldwide, more than 100,000 such patients could be saved every year. Of these 60,000 US patients, approximately 20,000 require heart replacement in the form of a total artificial heart (TAH), biventricular assist device (BVAD), or heart transplantation.[47–49]

Unfortunately, the number of donor hearts available in the United States is approximately 2,000 per year; worldwide the number is approximately 5,000 per year. Under the circumstances, a TAH or BVAD is the only alternative. Unfortunately, a clinically usable long-term BVAD system is not available.

One report recommends permanent ventricular device over transplantation.[50] The reason is as follows. Although the results of a cardiac transplantation are good, the 5-year survival rate is less than 65%, and the 10-year survival rate is less than 45%.[51] It is also important to examine the comorbidity of cardiac transplantation. Data from the International Society of Heart Transplantation define the problems that resulted during the first 2 years in a series of patients transplanted between April 1994 and December 1996. It is anticipated that hypertension, renal dysfunction, hyperlipidemia, diabetes, and malignancy are not risk factors related to LVAS. In the 43% of transplant patients requiring rehospitalization in the first year, 35% were because of rejection, infection, or both. The number of hospitalizations required with LVAS patients is unknown, but there is some indication from the current out-of-hospital ventricular assist device (VAD) patients that repeated hospitalization is not uncommon and occurs in as many as 50% of those who have been out of the hospital over a several-month period.

Consequently, the only way to save these groups of patients is through the use of VADs, rather than not removing the diseased heart and replacing it with a TAH. The life of an artificial heart is limited, and a patient's total dependency on a human-made device is not desirable.

Recently, it is becoming clearer that a cardiomyopathic heart could be recovered if the diseased heart were maintained at the state of a nonfunctioning ventricular unloaded condition.[52–54] Currently, this is only demonstrated with 4% of the approximately 2,000 LVAD patients suffering from cardiomyopathy (from accumulated Novacor and Thermo Cardiosystems, Inc. registry data). However, in Germany, Hetzer's group demonstrated a much higher level of myocardial recovery.[55] It is expected that approximately 30% or more of patients would recover if proper therapeutic measures, including hemodiafiltration for the removal of various types of disease-causing cytokines and plasmapheresis for the removal of antibodies and immunocomplexes, were provided.[56,57]

Even for the ischemic cardiomyopathic patients, removal of low-density lipoprotein (LDL) cholesterol, fibrinogen, and antibodies by plasmapheresis procedures should provide regression of the general atherosclerotic region in 2 years.[58,59] With the improvement of therapeutic procedures and regimen, at least half of the patient population could be saved by treating the basic disease of the natural heart. Thus, it is advantageous to not remove a diseased heart but to keep it to the best of our ability. Currently, approximately 30% of LVAD recipients died because of multiorgan failure secondary to right-heart failure.

Thus, it is increasingly important to provide a BVAD for end-stage heart failure patients. Unfortunately, there is no blood pump available that is small enough so that two can be implanted in a body. We believe that a compact centrifugal pump that has good durability and one that has good antithrombogenicity can be combined to establish a permanently implantable BVAD for longer than 2 years.

Current Problems

Mechanical Destruction of Red Cells: Hemolysis

To develop a 2-day centrifugal pump, it must be developed as an atraumatic blood pump. Under natural physiologic conditions, red cells are destroyed in the reticuloendothelial system and become heme, protein, and cellular membrane components. These cellular membranes, referred to as "ghosts," are metabolized in the body. The human body can clear up to 14 g of free hemoglobin within 24 h, if it has normal renal function; that is, the body can tolerate a continuing hemolysis rate of 0.1 mg hemoglobin/kg/min. This level of hemolysis does not cause any noticeable problems for the body.

However, a blood pump can produce hemolysis. If the pressure decreases below 30% of atmosphere during negative pressure excursion, the pressure has an adverse effect upon the red cells. Thus, negative pressure induces hemolysis. Also, high shear forces induce hemolysis by local turbulence and the velocity gradient. Consequently, wall and surface effects are quite important when designing a pump.[60]

During the past 50 years, many investigators have tried to develop an atraumatic blood pump. They have been faced with controlling mechanically induced hemolysis. Although the body can clear up to 14 g of plasma-free hemoglobin daily, plasma-free hemoglobin of up to 130 mg/dL may be bound to form hemoglobin–haptoglobin complexes in vivo. If the plasma hemoglobin level exceeds this value, hemoglobinuria occurs and, subsequently, organ failure.

In vitro studies have assessed device-induced hemolysis. A hemolysis circuit was primed with 500 mL of fresh human blood and pumped at 6 L/min for 4 h against 110 mm Hg of total pressure head. Plasma-free hemoglobin was sampled at four points in time. Indices of hemolysis were calculated, and their mean value was considered as the final index of hemolysis, defined as the grams of released plasma-free hemoglobin per 100 L of pumped blood. In the literature, three types of formulas are accepted as indices of hemolysis: the traditional index of hemolysis (IH), the normalized index of hemolysis (NIH), and the modified index of hemolysis (Table 50-7).

If the acceptable range of hemoglobin in blood (12 ± 2 g/dL) is limited, the NIH is suitable for comparing results of different hemolysis tests. Fresh human blood should be used in the hemolysis test as part of the final assessment of a developmental device because it is more hemolytic than

TABLE 50-7. Index of Hemolysis (Grams of Hemoglobin Released per 100 L of Pumped Blood)

Index	Equation
1. The traditional index of hemolysis (IH): g/100 L	$IH = \Delta \text{ Free Hb} \times V \times 100/QT$
2. The normalized index of hemolysis (NIH): g/100 L	$NIH = \Delta \text{ Free Hb} \times V \times (100 - Ht)/100 \times 100/QT$
3. The modified index of hemolysis (MIH) (considers both hematocrit and hemoglobin)	$MIH = \Delta \text{ Free Hb} \times V \times (100 - Ht)/100 \times 106/(QT \times Hb)$

From ASTM standard practice for assessment of hemolysis in continuous flow blood pumps. F1841-97.

Δ Free Hb = increase of plasma-free hemoglobin concentration during the sampling period (g/L); Hb = total hemoglobin concentration (g/dL); Ht = hematocrit (%); Q = flow rate (L/min); T = sampling time interval (min); V = the circuit volume (L).

animal blood and because it is analogous to a clinical situation. Of all human blood samples, 93% are in the range of 12 ± 2 mg/dL. Even if hemoglobin is taken into account for calculations using a modified IH, it does not offer better comparability than does the NIH value.

Bovine blood is also recommended for a comparative test among various devices because it is easily available and inexpensive. Varying values of hematocrit and hemoglobin are encountered when using bovine blood. The modified IH has merit as an analysis tool in this situation because it reduces the variation between individual differences.

To establish a basis for comparisons among investigators, the blood donor species, fasting stage, priming volume, flow rate, duration, and pressure must be defined. The hematocrit and hemoglobin values of the blood used are especially important in making comparisons. In addition, the lipid level of the blood substantially influences the rate of hemolysis. The postalimentary lipemic blood is as much as 50 times more fragile than that of canine blood from fasted animals. This information emphasizes fasted blood for the hemolysis test.

The clinically acceptable NIH levels of continuous flow blood pumps should be within the range shown in Table 50-8. It is more convenient to use the NIH that is expressed as milligrams of plasma-free hemoglobin per 100 L of blood pumped (0.001 g/100 L, or 1 mg/100 L).

In recently developed pumps, the impeller design has been modified by changing the diameter and the shape of the vanes to reduce hemolysis.

Thromboembolism and Bleeding

To develop a 2-week centrifugal pump, it is essential that it be an antithrombogenic blood pump. In the development of a 2-day pump, red thrombus formation inside and downstream of the blood pump should be avoided, but the major task of developing a 2-week pump is to avoid white thrombus formation inside and downstream of the blood pump.[44,61] Red thrombosis is generated by the activation of coagulation factors in the blood (Figure 50-19), unlike white thrombosis, which is primarily produced by platelet activation and aggregation, which result from blood exposure to the high shear region inside of the blood pump. Centrifugal pumps are usually used for emergencies or severe cases. The frequency of red thrombosis formation can be decreased if its usage is extended to more than 2 days. Furthermore, red thrombosis formation can be prevented by the administration of proper antithrombotic agents. Even though anticoagulant administration reduces the incidence of thrombus formation at the same time, bleeding complication increases as the side effect. It is obvious that excessive usage of anticoagulant should be avoided. The recently developed centrifugal blood pumps have been generally red thrombosis free because they have been administered with the proper management of anticoagulant. As previously stated, centrifugal blood pumps have a tendency to introduce a high shear environment to the platelets. Immunologic effects accelerate the situation, and the second week of pump usage is the peak time for the formation of white thrombosis.

Neurologic complications after the implantation of blood pumps are a result of blood clotting as well as bleeding.

In a series of patients from St. Louis University who used a pulsatile pump, the thromboembolism rate was

TABLE 50-8. Normalized Index of Hemolysis for VADs and Their Clinical Outcomes

NIH	Clinical Outcomes
> 0.06	Increased level of plasma-free hemoglobin
> 0.04	No increase of plasma-free hemoglobin, but requires blood transfusion
< 0.04	Physiologically acceptable
< 0.02	Clinically acceptable
< 0.01	Design objective of the blood pump

Reproduced with permission from Nosé Y. Design and development strategy for the rotary blood pump. Artif Organs 1998;22(6):438–46.

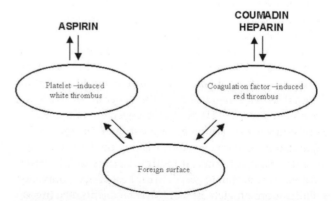

FIGURE 50-19. Blood clot formation on a foreign surface.

14%, whereas the stroke rate was only 9%.[62] In a multi-institutional study of the Thermocardiosystems LVAS (Woburn, MA), the clinical thromboembolic rate was 6% and the stroke rate was approximately 3%. At autopsy, another 3% or 4% incidence of thromboembolic events was identified that had not been apparent clinically.[63] There are no results available documenting long-term use of a centrifugal pump. It is expected that a centrifugal pump's thromboembolic range is smaller than that of a pulsatile pump because a centrifugal pump does not have a mechanical valve and the platelet activation is expected to be less than that of the pulsatile blood pump.

There is considerable difficulty in defining how many of these thromboembolic events are actually related to the device. Other factors are seriously involved. It is likely that if infection can be avoided, the incidence of thromboembolism in assist device patients would be lower.

However, many patients today with mechanical heart valves do very well with chronic anticoagulation. If the total implantable centrifugal pump can be developed, patients will be able to avoid infection and live a comfortable life.

Infection

Infection is a serious complication associated with a device. Risk factors contributing to the development of infection are long-term ventilation after surgery, prolonged hospitalization, and perioperative multiple organ failure, as well as major surgery and extensive blood loss. The effective treatment of patients with an infected device is difficult; therefore, many reports suggest that this complication strongly affects mortality. The infection rate for an extracorporeal assist device is 8.6–50%.[44,61] We are increasingly convinced that the majority of device-centered infections associated with an implanted blood pump are related to the seeding of the pathogenic bacteria during the time of the implant surgery. Thus, it is extremely important to administer high doses of multiple antibiotics prior to surgery and to maintain this regimen for at least 10 to 14 days. A substantial amount of device-centered infections are avoidable by using this aggressive antibiotic regimen prior to, during, and after implant surgery of a blood pump.

Many groups have tried to develop implantable centrifugal assist devices (see Table 50-5). Currently, these devices are in experimental stages; however, we believe that such devices will be available in the very near future.[2,5,6,64]

Hemodynamic Effect of Nonpulsatile Flow

Several authors report that a lower systemic vascular resistance (SVR) exists in pulsatile flow than exists in nonpulsatile flow.[65–67] This issue was further confirmed by earlier papers describing an increase in mean arterial pressure and SVR in the nonpulsatile group.[68–70] During the initial 2 weeks after the implantation of a nonpulsatile blood pump, a patient's autonomic system is in a hyperadrenergic state, which is associated with many hemodynamic abnormalities. However, these hemodynamic abnormalities should become normalized after 2 weeks of implantation. Among the catecholamines, epinephrine and dopamine levels stay constant, whereas the norepinephrine level in the nonpulsatile flow is significantly higher than that in the pulsatile flow. No significant difference was observed in the prostaglandin (PG) level, including 6-keto $PGF_{1\alpha}$ as the end product of PGI_2, PGE_2, and thromboxane B_2 as the end product of thromboxane A_2; or in the levels of antidiuretic hormone, plasma rennin activity, angiotensin-I, angiotensin-II, and atrial natriuretic polypeptide.[71] The findings of higher aortic pressure and norepinephrine levels in the nonpulsatile flow are consistent with the results of recent clinical studies of cardiopulmonary bypass cases.[72,73] There is a possibility that this initial change in SVR and aortic pressure with nonpulsatile flow is correlated with increased circulating catecholamine levels. The presumed higher sympathetic activation in the nonpulsatile flow was in agreement with most of the previous reports showing the increase in afferent nerve activity from carotid sinus and aortic arch baroceptors.[74] But a high SVR condition does not continue for a long time. Yozu reported that at the third postoperative day (POD), the SVR decreased in total in nonpulsatile flow assist animal experiments.[66] Over the following five PODs, although motor speed was not increased, the systemic flow gradually increased from 90 to 130 mL/kg/min and was maintained at this level for the duration of the experiments. This subsequent increase in pump flow correlated with a diminution of the SVR, and this also coincided with the animal being capable of maintaining its own fluid balance.

Mandelbaum and colleagues observed that during a nonpulsatile right-heart bypass preparation, the pulmonary vascular resistance rose to 127% of that seen with pulsatile bypass.[75] Hauge and associates found that there was an improvement in oxygenation under pulsatile flow to abnormal, with edematous lungs having high pulmonary venous pressure, and that this improvement was not observed in normal lungs.[76] In short, pulsatile flow in the pulmonary circuit does not appear to be necessary for normal gas exchange.

In a shock liver model experiment, changes in bile flow and arterial ketone body ratio (AKBR) showed no differences between nonpulsatile and pulsatile groups. Enzyme release was not affected by the pumps; thus, it is concluded that nonpulsatile circulatory assist may not be detrimental to recovery of liver function after profound shock.[77]

Although centrifugal pumps need more flow than pulsatile pumps for organ function maintenance, nonpulsatile blood flow is not a limiting factor for the maintenance of mammalian life.[66,78] In the artificial heart field, nonpulsatile blood pumps have considerable advantages and are promising devices for replacing natural heart function.

Exercise after Centrifugal Pump Implantation

Yozu reported on exercise tests conducted in ventricular-fibrillated-induced models with nonpulsatile centrifugal blood pumps implanted for right ventricular assist device (RVAD) and LVAD in a bypass fashion. Immediately after exercise began, a significant increase in both left arterial pressure (LAP) and right atrial pressure (RAP) and atrial rate were observed. The atrial pressure change appeared to be more pronounced at a higher flow rate, especially LAP. No significant changes in arterial pressure (AP) or pulmonary artery pressure (PAP) were seen, and no significant variation in systemic flow was recognized (less than 3 to 4%). Total oxygen consumption increased significantly after 5 min of exercise (mean increase = 25.0%), corresponding with an increase in the atrioventricular (AV) difference in oxygen content (23.7%). No further increase was observed after 10 min of exercise. After a 15-min rest, all the parameters returned to preexercise levels.[66,79] The comparison tests showed that both nonpulsatile and pulsatile groups tolerate equally moderate exercise tests.[80]

Linneweber reported good results in the exercise tests with nonpulsatile biventricular assist centrifugal blood pumps.[81] Although the pump flows were maintained at a fixed rate, the cardiac output and heart rate increased significantly. It was remarkable to note that the increase in heart rate had no negative effect on the pump performance during this dynamic condition. The decreased ventricle filling time at a higher heart rate did not lead to the "suction phenomenon" frequently observed in rotary blood pumps. In assist devices, the centrifugal pumps provided only a fraction of the increase in cardiac output, while the native heart provided a much larger portion of the cardiac output.

The anaerobic threshold (AT) is defined as the exercise oxygen consumption (VO_2) above which aerobic energy production is supplemented by anaerobic mechanism.[82] At that point, oxygen supply is unable to meet the total oxygen requirements for energy production during heavy exercise; therefore, lactate production is increased as a consequence of energy supplementation produced by activation of the glycolytic pathway. Below the AT, an individual can perform sustained activity. The AT represents an objective measurement of pulmonary and cardiovascular dysfunction and evaluation of a therapeutic response in patients with pulmonary or heart disease.[83,84] The AT has been used as an index to evaluate tolerance to exercise in patients with cardiac diseases.[85,86] Wasserman reported a close relation between oxygen use and the degree of heart failure.[87] In artificial heart research, the AT has been introduced as a possible method for selecting the best artificial heart control scheme.[88]

Yozu and colleagues reported that (1) both nonpulsatile and pulsatile groups show good tolerance to moderate 1.5-miles-per-hour exercise tests without metabolic or hemodynamic deterioration; (2) the increased oxygen demand during exercise is augmented by oxygen extraction for nonpulsatile biventricular bypass and by increased cardiac output and increased oxygen extraction for pulsatile TAH recipients; and (3) the nonpulsatile group has a higher norepinephrine response to exercise tests than does the pulsatile TAH group.[80] Based upon previous studies, the centrifugal blood pump did not increase its output automatically during exercise. Regardless of the same pump flows, the experimental animal could tolerate the same level of exercise imposed on the TAH, which increased cardiac output when the animals were subjected to exercise.

Adaptation Hypothesis of Cardiac Prostheses

For many years, it was believed that a centrifugal blood pump was not physiologically acceptable for long-term use. First, it was not physiologically possible to perfuse the human body with nonpulsatile blood flow, and second, it was difficult to produce a centrifugal blood pump that was clinically applicable that did not produce any blood clots or hemolysis for an extended period of time.

This abnormal physiology was experienced during cardiopulmonary bypass (Table 50-9) because nonpulsatile blood pumps are used during cardiopulmonary bypass. Furthermore, for cardiopulmonary bypass, these pumps are generally used at 20 to 30% below the physiologically required rate of blood flow from the pulsatile natural heart. Consequently, the physiologic abnormalities described in Table 50-9 are not caused by use of a nonpulsatile blood pump; rather, they are primarily caused by blood flow rates lower than the physiologically required level. As a matter of fact, the same nonpulsatile blood pump is physically acceptable when approximately 20% more pulsatile blood flow is maintained (Figure 50-20).

In addition, it has been thought that it is difficult to control a BVAD. However, studies in our laboratory demonstrate that the native heart makes a fine adjustment 2 weeks after implantation of these nonpulsatile assist pumps.[89] In other words, the recipient adjusts to the implanted BVAD 2 weeks after implantation.

TABLE 50-9. Problems Associated with Conventional Cardiopulmonary Bypass

1. Metabolic acidosis
2. Supplemental fluid requirement
3. Alteration and instability of peripheral resistance
4. Interstitial fluid accumulation and edema
5. Postperfusion myocardial dysfunction
6. Reduced urine flow
7. Postoperative bleeding tendency
8. Postoperative neurologic syndrome
9. Postoperative intestinal ischemia
10. "Postperfusion lung" syndrome

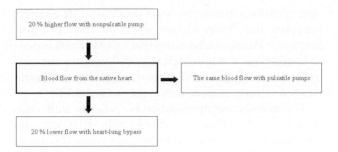

FIGURE 50-20. Different pumps require different blood flow rates.

We base the following hypothesis on our laboratory's 40 years of experience with cardiac prostheses.[37,90]

For many years, it was generally believed that blood pumps with nonpulsatile blood flow are unphysiologic and generate many unphysiologic conditions in patients.

However, patients eventually accept nonpulsatile blood pumps even though the mode of pumping is totally different from that of the natural heart. This type of adaptation or acceptance by the recipient also exists with a pulsatile total artificial heart. After any type of cardiac prosthesis implantation, there is a 6-week adaptation period.

Adaptations to implanted blood pumps by patients are classified in three stages:
- Stage I: Hematologic adaptation–confusion stage (typically, 2 days)
- Stage II: Physiologic adaptation–fighting stage (typically, 2 weeks)
- Stage III: Total adaptation–living together stage (histologic adaptation, typically 6 weeks)[37,90]

Stage I: Confusion Stage

After implantation of a cardiac prosthesis, the recipient experiences the initial 2 days of the confusing stage. This period of time could be termed the "hematologically abnormal stage." Primarily because of surgical impacts, hematologic abnormalities are prominent during this period of time. Actually, the adaptation of the initial blood–material contact should be established within 2 h (typically, 30 min); however, for secondary hematologic adaptation, 2 days are required. Such secondary effect is demonstrated by the surgical implantation of a cardiac prosthesis with a texturized pseudoneointima (PNI)-forming surface. The initial completion of PNI deposition takes 2 days. During this period of time, red thrombosis forms inside and also downstream of the implanted device. To survive this initial hematologic adaptation stage, patients should receive the proper levels of anticoagulation agents. During this period of time, the blood-contacting surface of the device becomes covered with the recipient's plasma protein and establishes proper hematologic adaptation to the device. Also, during this period, the recipient's autonomic nervous system attempts to reestablish its own proper control feedback system with the implanted system. To establish such adaptation, the control system built inside the implant should be as simple as possible and as predictable as possible by the recipient's servo system. To avoid any confusion of the recipient's servo feedback system, it is advisable that any servo control system not be a multiple system. Any challenge of the implant to the recipient's built-in feedback computer should also be avoided. The recipient's computer system would be the loser of such a challenge, and the result would be the death of the recipient.

Stage II: Fighting Stage

During the confusion stage, the local blood material compatibility is established and the recipient's computer system "learns" to understand the human-made machine and its own feedback system. Thus, during the 2 weeks of stage II, the recipient decides whether to live with the implanted device. However, the implanted system is different from the recipient's natural feedback system. So the recipient fights against the foreign system until the implanted system is able to establish the stage II physiologic adaptation to the recipient. During this stage, the recipient is in a hyperadrenergic stage. It is also an immunologically active stage. If a continuous flow blood pump is implanted, it is essential that the blood flow rate be kept 20% higher than that of a pulsatile flow pump.[78] Physiologically, the following circulatory abnormalities are prominent during this stage: higher venous pressure, higher peripheral resistance, and higher circulating blood volume. During this stage, the patient's immunologic response increases. As a result, white thrombus has a tendency to form inside or downstream of the device. Even though such physiologic difficulties are associated with this stage, control of the cardiac prosthesis should be easier during this stage than in the first stage.

Stage III: Living Together Stage

After 2 weeks, the fighting stage is over. All physiologic abnormalities disappear. The general adaptation or the physiologic adaptation of the implanted device is established in 2 weeks. If a continuous flow blood pump is implanted, it is essential to maintain the required blood flow at a rate that is approximately 20% higher than that for a pulsatile pump. During this period of time, tissue reorganization of the recipient's histopathology process begins in order to accept the implanted device more effectively. After 6 weeks of implantation of a nonpulsatile blood pump, an idioperipheral pulsation of 40 beats per minute appears.[64] Although this phenomenon requires an additional study to confirm, we suggest that this type of histologic reorientation inside the recipient's body is occurring effectively.

Stage IV: Accepting Stage (Total Adaptation)

After 6 weeks of implantation, the recipient would accept the implanted cardiac prosthesis not only hematologically and physiologically, but also histopathologically. This is why in vivo studies on cardiac prosthesis implantations (a short-term study of 1 month, which is twice the initial 2 weeks; and a long-term study of 3 months, which is twice the initial 6 weeks) are generally employed to investigate the compatibility with the experimental subjects. Table 50-10 summarizes our adaptation hypothesis after cardiac prosthesis implantation.

In summary, after the final adaptation stage of 6 weeks, normal end-organ function can be maintained with chronic pulsatile or nonpulsatile perfusion. It is important to recognize that the following requirements are necessary to maintain normal physiology.

For a nonpulsatile pump to be acceptable, the blood flow rates need to be cardiac index of the specific patient. In general, pulsatile systems need lower flows than do nonpulsatile devices to maintain the integrity of organ function. However, we should note, that in case of an LVAD, the native heart usually supports the nonpulsatile device with some pulsatility leading to a reduction in necessary flow generated by the pump.

Therefore, mammals seem to be able to adapt to nonpulsatile circulation. Pressure and flow, not pulse, are important to maintain the physiologic function. Chronic nonpulsatile support is not the limiting factor to the maintenance of life.

Bridge to Recovery

Contemporary LVASs afford patients with severe left ventricular dysfunction an improved quality of life and greater mobility than do early-stage devices.[91] Recent studies show that the patients receiving LVAS support experience an improvement in hemodynamic status as well as in their physiologic parameters, such as left ventricular size and the end diastolic pressure–volume relationship.[92,93] In addi-

tion, in patients with severe heart failure who are awaiting transplantation, LVAS support improves renal and liver function.[94] Finally, studies show that some patients experience structural and histologic remodeling of the left ventricle after prolonged LVAS support, suggesting that device removal without transplantation may be possible.[95,96]

The ever-increasing number of patients with end-stage idiopathic dilated cardiomyopathy (IDCM), who are awaiting heart transplantation, has made the use of the VAD a clinical routine to keep patients alive who would otherwise die before they reach the lifesaving transplantation. The time that some of these patients spend on such a mechanical device has now reached several months, and in some cases, even years. Some researchers have observed that during ventricular unloading periods, grossly dilated and failing hearts display an astonishing size reduction and restoration of function.[92,96–101] Mechanical unloading with an LVAS can result in recovery of myocardial function.[101]

There are various reports identifying the cause of these improvements. Normalization of the deranged calcium transport characteristic of advanced heart failure was reported.[102] Heart failure–related changes in gene expression that involve an increase in ventricular expression of atrial natriuretic factor and a decrease in sarcoplasmic reticulum Ca^{2+}-ATPase have also shown improvement after ventricular unloading.[103] Improvements in β-adrenergic density and the contractility of cardiac muscle in response to isoproterenol hydrochloride stimulation likewise have been noted after ventricular unloading.[104]

It is obvious that a mechanical heart assist device and its ventricular unloading effect in fact result in myocardial recovery for a certain number of the patients suffering from untreatable severe cardiomyopathy.

In the case of dilating cardiomyopathic hearts, several pathologic disease-causing macromolecules have been

TABLE 50-10. Summary of Adaptation Hypothesis after Cardiac Prosthesis Implantation

Stage	Term	Adaptation	Typical Phenomenon
I. Confusion	~ 2 days	Hematologic	1. Red thrombosis* 2. High peripheral resistance 3. Difficult to establish proper flows
II. Fighting	~ 2 weeks	Physiologic	1. White thrombosis† 2. High venous pressure High peripheral vascular resistance High circulating blood volume 3. High adrenergic status
III. Living together	~ 6 weeks	Pathologic	1. Interfacial tissue adaptation 2. Near-normal physiology (PA pressure, vascular resistance, etc) 3. System acceptance by tissue reconstruction
IV. Acceptance	~ 6 weeks	Total adaptation	1. Idioperipheral pulsation‡ 2. Normal physiology 3. Total system acceptance

* In the early phase, a thrombus occurring after pump implantation is a red thrombus primarily composed of erythrocytes and fibrin induced by the activation of coagulation cascade.
† White thrombus primarily consisting of rich platelet is formed in this period. Platelet activation and adhesion cause this particular thrombus.
‡ Very-low pulsation appears 6 weeks after establishment of a pulseless condition.
PA = pulmonary artery.

identified. Even though they are not specified as an absolute etiology or disease activator, their normalization might be beneficial for treatment of congestive heart failure. Among them, autoantibodies and tumor necrosis factor have been cited.[105,106] In addition, it is considered that expression and immobilization of other macromolecules are responsible for producing this autoimmunologic disease. Currently, extracorporeal removal systems of such pathologic macromolecules and leukocytes are available.[107–109] Certainly, in cases in which the disease-causing autoantibody is identified, it is possible to effectively remove it by specific immunoadsorption columns or nonspecific membrane systems.[110] Even if pathologic humoral factors are not identified, it is possible to remove all abnormally increased macromolecules.[111] This type of therapy was provided for the treatment of many autoimmunologic diseases in the past, and could be provided to patients together with a bridge to recovery by LVADs.[112,113]

Recently, another approach to bridge to recovery was established. If a patient suffers from hypoperfusion of the heart muscle due to the disseminated atherosclerotic regions of coronary arteries, active and long-term LDL apheresis procedures revealed a therapeutic outcome. Repeated LDL apheresis treatments (preferably twice a month) for longer than 2 years should reverse the atherosclerotic regions of the coronary arteries and reduce the occlusion rate of such vessels.[114,115] Even though these combined therapies have been attempted or provided only experimentally at a few centers in the world, the availability of such active therapeutic artificial organs may provide an additional means of accelerating recovery from heart diseases, as well as provide myocardial rest by mechanical assistance.

Future Prospects

Totally Implantable Nonpulsatile Assist Devices for Long-Term Use

The first group of long-term nonpulsatile blood pumps developed was the axial flow blood pumps.[116–118] The major advantages of these devices over pulsatile are that they are smaller in size, are valve free, eliminate the need for a compliance chamber or external vent tube, have lower power consumption, and cost less. These axial flow blood pumps have a rotor supported by bearings. Because of its high RPM (10,000 ± 2,000), its theoretical life expectancy is less than 2 years. An implantable centrifugal pump's rotational speed is lower than that of an axial flow blood pump. Thus, the centrifugal pump is expected to have a longer useful life span; in addition, it is smaller in size than a pulsatile pump. A centrifugal pump is implantable in small patients, and it is possible to implant two pumps as biventricular assist devices.

The future pump has to be a totally implantable system. A totally implantable system reduces risk of infection and improves quality of life and cosmetic appear-

ance. But some problems remain, including (1) a monitoring tool, (2) an emergency clamp, (3) an energy transmission system, (4) an information transmission system, and (5) an out-of-hospital management system.

It is important to monitor the blood flows of a rotary blood pump. Even though a reliable electromagnetic flow meter is not available, the long-term reliability of an ultrasonic flow meter is acceptable. However, implantation of flow probes and continuous monitoring of the blood flows are not practical. Therefore, the provision for noninvasive pump flow monitoring becomes an important issue. This is also necessary for early detection of a catastrophic failure. If a rotary blood pump is stopped, backflow from the arterial system to the ventricle occurs and is a life-threatening situation. Although most systems are intended to incorporate an emergency clamp on the arterial side of the rotary blood pump, it is imperative to establish a proper occlusion mode. This failure mode addresses not only mechanical and electrical incidents, but also physiologic incidents, including thrombus formation. Transcutaneous energy transmission system (TETS) development began in the 1960s. Now, many researchers have developed TETSs.[119–122] Actually, clinical use of a TETS was applied to the LionHeart (Arrow International, Inc., Reading, PA) ventricular assist system and to the AbioCor total heart (Abiomed Inc., Danvers, MA).[123] But, improvement of energy transmission efficiency and miniaturization are still needed. A system that added information is the transcutaneous energy and information transmission (TEIT) system. Developments in this area are critically needed.

Necessity of Biventricular Assist Device

Right-heart failure, a major complication observed in patients with LVAD support, has an incidence of 11 to 26%, depending on the event.[43,124–126] Therapeutic measures include administration of volume, nitrous oxide by inhalation, inotropic agents, phosphodiesterase type III inhibitors, and prostaglandin. If these measures are unsuccessful, the implantation of a right ventricular assist device is needed.[43] Particularly, severe right-heart failure, which disturbs portal venous return and causes high central venous pressure over 25 mmh, absolutely requires RVAD. RVAD is very effective to recover from impaired venous return and congestive liver failure.[127] Some reports suggest that the percentage of patients needing a BVAD is 50 to 60% of the patient population requiring circulation support.[128] Right-heart failure causes multiorgan failure and sepsis. Currently, some implantable pulsatile LVADs are being used clinically with satisfactory results; however, they cannot be used as an RVAD or BVAD because of their structure and size.[129–132] An axial flow blood pump is the smallest available blood pump due to the high rotational speed of its impeller.[133] As previously stated, the high rotational speed of the impeller imposes greater wear on the bearing system of the pump than on that of the centrifugal blood pump. Thus, its theoretical life expectancy is less than 2 years. The introduction of a centrifugal pump is the only way to develop substantially smaller and durable blood pumps into implantable BVADs.

Baylor Gyro Permanently Implantable Biventricular Assist Device

In 1995, Baylor College of Medicine began development of the Baylor Gyro permanently implantable centrifugal blood pump (Gyro PI pump) (see Figures 50-18 and 50-21). Three long-term in vivo studies were done with an implantable LVAD, with survival up to 284 days.[134] Based on these results, the development of a biventricular assist device system, which requires the implantation of two pumps, is underway. The Gyro PI 700 pump is fabricated from titanium alloy (6% aluminum and 4% vanadium) and has a priming volume of 25 mL, a pump weight of 204 g, a height of 45 mm, and a pump diameter of 65 mm.[135] This pump can provide 5 L/min against 100 mm Hg at 2,000 RPM.[136]

Simple platelet adhesion tests were performed with a smooth surface material of 0.2 μm surface roughness to prove the feasibility of titanium alloy as a pump material.[137] The smooth surface titanium alloy demonstrated minimum platelet adhesion among all the materials subjected to these studies. The normalized index of hemolysis value of the PI 700 was in the range of 0.004 g/100 L.[138] Regarding hemolysis, all in vivo studies showed low levels of plasma-free hemoglobin and no deterioration of the hematocrit level. These results indicate that the Gyro PI 700 pump is suitable as a BVAD system.

The Gyro PI pump was designed to be implanted in the preperitoneal space. After study periods, calves were euthanized and careful inspection was made of the pumps

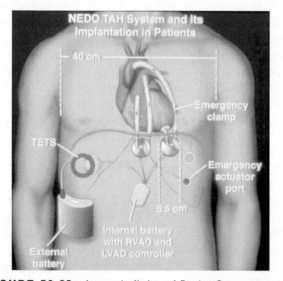

FIGURE 50-21. Anatomic fitting of Baylor Gyro permanent implantable centrifugal pump. LVAD = left ventricular assist device; RVAD = right ventricular assist device; TAH = total artificial heart; TETS = trancutaneous energy transmission system.

and downstream organs for the possible existence of infarct regions or intravascular thrombus formation, except for intracranial tissue. There were no thrombus or infarct regions inside of the pump or in any of the organs studied.[116]

In conclusion, the centrifugal pump is suitable for long-term implantation of 5 years or longer. It is also suitable for the implantation of two pumps, one for right-heart assist and the other for left-heart assist, in a patient having a 40-kg body weight. The energy consumption is low, and the implanted devices do not need a complex control. This simple pump is suitable as a future permanently implantable blood pump (see Table 50-4).

References

1. Rafferty EH, Kletscheka HD, Wynyard M, et al. Artificial heart I, application of nonpulsatile force-vortex principle. Minn Med 1968;51(1):11–6.
2. Dorman F, Bernstein EF, Blackshear PL Jr, et al. Progress in the design of a centrifugal cardiac assist pump with transcutaneous energy transmission by magnetic coupling. Trans Am Soc Artif Intern Organs 1969;15:441–8.
3. Kawahito K, Nosé Y. Hemolysis in different centrifugal pumps. Artif Organs 1997;21(4):323–6.
4. Moon YS, Ohtsubo S, Gomez MR, et al. Comparison of centrifugal and roller pump hemolysis rates at low flow. Artif Organs 1996;20(6):579–81.
5. Orime Y, Takatani S, Sasaki T, et al. Cardiopulmonary bypass with Nikkiso and BioMedicus centrifugal pumps. Artif Organs 1994;18(1):11–6.
6. Shimono T, Makinouchi K, Nosé Y. Total erythrocyte destruction time: the new index for the hemolytic performance of rotary blood pumps. Artif Organs 1995; 19(7):571–5.
7. Ohtsubo S, Naito K, Matsuura M, et al. Initial clinical experience with the Baylor-Nikkiso centrifugal pump. Artif Organs 1995;19(7):769–73.
8. Nonaka K, Linneweber J, Ichikawa S, et al. Development of the Baylor Gyro permanently implantable centrifugal blood pump as a biventricular assist device. Artif Organs 2001;25(9):675–82.
9. Bureque K, Gernes DB, Loree HM, et al. HeartMate III: pump design for a centrifugal LVAD with a magnetically levitated rotor. ASAIO J 2001;47(4):401–5.
10. Nojiri C, Kijima T, Maekawa J, et al. Development status of Terumo implantable left ventricular assist system. Artif Organs 2001;25(5):411–3.
11. Ohciai Y, Golding LAR, Massiello AL, et al. In vivo hemodynamic performance of the Cleveland CorAide blood pump in calves. Ann Thorac Surg 2001;72:747–52.
12. Oku T, Harasaki H, Smith W, et al. Hemolysis. A comparative study of four nonpulsatile pumps. ASAIO Trans 1988;34(3):500–4.
13. Jakob H, Kutshera Y, Palzer B, et al. In vitro assessment of centrifugal pumps for ventricular assist. Artif Organs 1990;14(4):278–83.
14. Moen O, Fosse E, Dregelid E, et al. Centrifugal pump and heparin coating improves cardiopulmonary bypass biocompatibility. Ann Thorac Surg 1996;62:1134–40.

15. Mandl JP. Comparison of emboli production between a constrained force vortex pump and a roller pump. AmSECT Proc 1977:27–31.

16. Uretzky G, Landsburg G, Cohn D, et al. Analysis of microembolic particles originating in extracorporeal circuits. Perfusion 1987;2:9–17.

17. Tamari Y, Lee-Sensiba K, Leonard EF, et al. The effect of pressure and flow on hemolysis caused by Bio-Medicus centrifugal pumps and roller pumps. Guidelines for choosing a blood pump. J Thorac Cardiovasc 1993;106: 997–1007.

18. Triveldi U, Timberlake N, Bennywith O, et al. The impact of centrifugal and roller pump in CABG on microemboli and neuropsychological outcome. Perfusion 1997;12:67.

19. Klein M, Dauben HP, Schulte HD, et al. Centrifugal pumping during routine open heart surgery improves clinical outcome. Artif Organs 1998;22:326–36.

20. Lynch MF, Peterson D, Barker V. Centrifugal blood pumping for open heart surgery. Minn Med 1978;61:536–7.

21. Wheeldon DR, Bethune DW, Gill RD. Vortex pumping for routine cardiac surgery: a comparative study. Perfusion 1990;5:135–43.

22. Parault BG, Conrad SA. The effect of extracorporeal circulation time and patient age on platelet retention during cardiopulmonary bypass. A comparison of roller and centrifugal pumps. J Extra Corpor Technol 1991;23: 34–8.

23. Jakob HG, Hanfner G, Thelemann C, et al. Routine extracorporeal circulation with a centrifugal or roller pump. ASAIO Trans 1991;37(3):M487–9.

24. Berki T, Gürbüz A, Isik Ö, et al. Cardiopulmonary bypass using centrifugal pump. Vasc Surg 1992;26:123–34.

25. Alamanni F, Parolari A, Zanobini M, et al. Centrifugal pump and reduction of neurological risk in adult cardiac surgery. J Extra Corpor Technol 2001;33(1):4–9.

26. Coselli JS, LeMaire SA, Ledesma DF, et al. Initial experience with the Nikkiso centrifugal pump during thoracoabdominal aortic aneurysm repair. J Vasc Surg 1998;27:378 83.

27. Matayoshi T, Yozu R, Morita M, et al. Development of a completely closed circuit using an air filter in drainage circuit for minimally invasive cardiac surgery. Artif Organs 2000;24:454–8.

28. Toomasian JM, Aboul-Hosn W. Coronary artery bypass grafting using a miniature right ventricular support system. Perfusion 2000;15(6):521–6.

29. Taga S, Ezaki T, Yoshida Y, et al. Hepatic venous injury; a case report of atriocaval shunt by a centrifugal pump. Hepatogastroenterology 1997;44:1219–21.

30. Kusano T, Tamai O, Miyazato H, et al. Extracorporeal bypass using a centrifugal pump during resection of malignant liver tumors. Hepatogastroenterology 1999; 46:2483–9.

31. Ohwada S, Kawashima Y, Ogawa T, et al. Extended hepatectomy with ePTFE graft vena caval replacement and hepatic vein reconstruction: a case report. Hepatogastroenterology 1999;46:1151–5.

32. Takano S, Takahashi T, Ohishi H, et al. Radical surgery for Budd-Chiari syndrome. Direct excision and repair for obstruction of the vena cava (Budd-Chiari syndrome) under hepatic vascular exclusion using a centrifugal pump. Eur J Surg 1999;165(7):632–7.

33. Ogawa T, Ohwada T, Ohtaki A, et al. Successful resection of renal cell carcinoma with tumor thrombi extending into right atrium: a case report. Hepatogastroenterology 1999;46:2535–9.

34. Trittenwein G, Golej J, Burda G, et al. Neonatal and pediatric extracorporeal membrane oxygenation using nonocclusive blood pumps: the Vienna experience. Artif Organs 2001;25(12):994–9.

35. Kress DC, Cohen DJ, Swanson DK, et al. Pump-induced hemolysis in a rabbit model of neonatal ECMO. ASAIO Trans 1987;33(3):446–52.

36. McDonald JV, Green TP, Steinhorn RH. The role of the centrifugal pump in hemolysis during neonatal extracorporeal support. ASAIO J 1997;43(1):35–8.

37. Nosé Y. Design and development strategy for the rotary blood pump. Artif Organs 1998;22(6):438–46.

38. Phillips SJ, Ballentine B, Slonine D, et al. Percutaneous initiation of cardiopulmonary bypass. Ann Thorac Surg 1983;36:223–5.

39. Philips SJ, Zeff RH, Kongtahworn C, et al. Percutaneous cardiopulmonary bypass: application and indication for use. Ann Thorac Surg 1989;47:121–3.

40. Urbanek P, Bock H, Vicol C. Percutaneous cardiopulmonary support (PCPS). Cardiology 1994;84: 216–21.

41. Paolini G, Triggiani M, Di Credico G, et al. Assist circulation in postcardiotomy heart failure: experience with the Bio-Medicus centrifugal pump in ten patients. Cardiovasc Surg 1994;2:630–3.

42. Kitamura M, Aomi S, Hachida M, et al. Current strategy of temporary circulatory support for severe cardiac failure after operation. Ann Thorac Surg 1999;68:662–5.

43. El-Banayosy A, Körfer R, Arusoglu L, et al. Device and patient management in a bridge-to-transplant setting. Ann Thorac Surg 2001;71:S98–102.

44. Körfer R, El-Banayosy A, Posival H, et al. Mechanical circulatory support: the Bad Oeyhausen experience. Ann Thorac Surg 1995;59:S56–63.

45. Körfer R, El-Banayosy A, Arusoglu H, et al. Single-center experience with Thoratec ventricular assist device. J Thorac Cardiovasc Surg 2000;119:596–600.

46. El-Banayosy A, Arusoglu L, Kizner L, et al. Complication of circulatory assist. Perfusion 2000;15:327–31.

47. Hogness JR, VanAntwerp M. Executive summary. In: Hogness JR, VanAntwerp M, editors. The artificial heart: prototypes, policies, and patients: committee to evaluate the artificial heart program of the National Heart, Lung, and Blood Institute. Washington, DC: National Academy Press; 1991. p. 1–13.

48. Funk D. Epidemiology of end-stage heart disease. In: Hogness JR, VanAntwerp M, editors. The artificial heart: prototypes, policies, and patients: committee to evaluate the artificial heart program of the National Heart, Lung, and Blood Institute. Washington, DC: National Academy Press; 1991. p. 251–61.

49. Oz MC, Rose EA, Levin HR. Selection criteria for placement of left ventricular assist devices. Am Heart J 1995; 129:173–7.

50. Pennington DG, Oaks TE, Lohmann DP. Permanent ventricular assist device support versus cardiac transplantation. Ann Thorac Surg 1999;68:729–33.

51. Hosenpud JD, Bennett LE, Keck BM, et al. The registry of the International Society of Heart and Lung Transplantation: Fourteenth Official Report—1997. J Heart Lung Transplant 1997;16:691–712.

52. Mueller J, Wallukat G, Weng Y, et al. Weaning from mechanical cardiac support in patients with idiopathic dilated cardiomyopathy. Circulation 1997;96:542–9.

53. McCarthy PM, Nakatani S, Vargo R, et al. Structural and left ventricular histolic changes after implantable LVAD insertion. Ann Thorac Surg 1995;59:609–13.

54. Levin HR, Chen JM, Oz M, et al. Potential of left ventricular assist devices as outpatient therapy while awaiting heart transplantation. Ann Thorac Surg 1994;58:1515–20.

55. Loebe M, Mueller J, Hetzer R. Ventricular assistance for recovery of heart failure. Curr Opin Cardiol 1999;14:234–48.

56. Dipla K, Mattiello JA, Jeevanandam V, et al. Myocyte recovery after mechanical circulatory support in humans with end-stage heart failure. Circulation 1998;97:2316–22.

57. Furukawa Y, Kobuke K, Matsumori A. Role of cytokines in autoimmune myocarditis and cardiomyopathy. Autoimmunity 2001;34(3):165–8.

58. Matsuda Y, Nosé Y. The next generation extracorporeal method for the management of atherosclerosis. Artif Organs 1995;19(9):877–9.

59. Kajinami K, Mabuchi H. Therapeutic effects of LDL apheresis in the prevention of atherosclerosis. Curr Opin Lipidol 1999;10(5):401–6.

60. Kawahito K, Nosé Y. Hemolysis in different centrifugal pumps. Artif Organs 1997;21:323–6.

61. Karl TR, Sano S, Horton S, et al. Centrifugal pump left heart assist in pediatric cardiac operations. Indication, technique, and results. J Thorac Cardiovasc Surg 1991;102:624–30.

62. Pennington DG, McBride LR, Peigh PS, et al. Eight years' experience with bridge to cardiac transplantation. J Thorac Cardiovasc Surg 1994;107:472–81.

63. Slater JP, Rose EA, Levin HR, et al. Low thromboembolic risk without anticoagulation using advanced-design left ventricular assist device. Ann Thorac Surg 1996;62:1321–8.

64. Nosé Y, Tsutsui T, Butler KC, et al. Rotary pumps: new developments and future perspective. ASAIO J 1998;44:234–8.

65. Nakayama K, Tamiya T, Yamamoto K, et al. High-amplitude pulsatile pump in extracorporeal circulation with particular reference to hemodynamics. Surgery 1963;54:798–809.

66. Yozu R, Golding LAR, Jacobs G, et al. Experimental results and future prospects for a nonpulsatile cardiac prosthesis. World J Surg 1985;9:116–27.

67. Giron F, Birtwell WC, Soroff HS, et al. Hemodynamic effects of pulsatile and nonpulsatile flow. Arch Surg 1966;93:802–10.

68. Trinkle JK, Helton NE, Wood RE, et al. Metabolic comparison of a new pulsatile pump and a roller pump for cardiopulmonary bypass. J Thorac Cardiovasc Surg 1969;58:562–9.

69. Jacobs LA, Klopp EH, Seamone W, et al. Improved organ function during cardiac bypass with a roller pump to deliver pulsatile flow. J Thorac Cardiovasc 1969;58:703–12.

70. Dunn J, Kirsh MM, Harness J, et al. Hemodynamic, metabolic, and hematologic effects of pulsatile cardiopulmonary bypass. J Thorac Cardiovasc Surg 1974;68:138–47.

71. Tatsumi E, Toda K, Taenaka Y, et al. Acute phase response of vasoactive hormones to non pulsatile systemic circulation. ASAIO J 1995;41:M460–5.

72. Minami K, Vyska K, Körfer R. Role of the carotid sinus in the response of integrated venous system to pulsatile and nonpulsatile perfusion. J Thorac Cardiovasc Surg 1992;104:1639–46.

73. Minami K, Körner MM, Vyska K, et al. Effects of pulsatile perfusion on plasma catecholamine levels and hemodynamics during and after cardiac operations with cardiopulmonary bypass. J Thorac Cardiovasc Surg 1990;99:82–91.

74. Chapleau MW, Abboud FM. Determination of sensitization of carotid baroreceptors by pulsatile pressure in dogs. Cir Res 1989;65:566–77.

75. Mandelbaum I, Burns WH. Pulsatile and nonpulsatile blood flow. JAMA 1965;191:657–60.

76. Hauge A, Nicolaysen G. Pulmonary O_2 transfer during pulsatile and non-pulsatile perfusion. Acta Physiol Scand 1980;109:325–32.

77. Satoh H, Miyamoto Y, Shimazaki Y, et al. Comparison between pulsatile and nonpulsatile circulatory assist for the recovery of shock liver. ASAIO J 1995;41:M596–600.

78. Sugita Y, Golding L, Jacobs G, et al. Comparison of osmotic and body fluid balance in chronic nonpulsatile biventricular bypass (NPBVB) and total artificial heart (TAH) experiments. Trans Am Soc Artif Intern Organs 1984;30:148–54.

79. Valdés F, Golding LR, Harasaki H, et al. Hemodynamic response to exercise during chronic ventricular fibrillation and nonpulsatile biventricular bypass. Trans Am Soc Artif Intern Organs 1981;27:449–53.

80. Yozu R, Golding LAR, Shimomitsu T, et al. Exercise response in chronic nonpulsatile and pulsatile TAH animals. Trans Am Soc Artif Intern Organ 1985;31:22–7.

81. Linneweber J, Nonaka K, Takano T, et al. Hemodynamic exercise response in calves with an implantable biventricular centrifugal blood pump. Artif Organs 2001;25:1018–21.

82. Wasserman K. The anaerobic threshold measure measurement to evaluate exercise performance. Am Rev Respir Dis 1984;129 Suppl:S35–40.

83. Matsumura N, Nishijima H, Kojima S, et al. Determination of anaerobic threshold for assessment of functional state in patients with chronic heart failure. Circulation 1983;68:360–7.

84. Fortini A, Bonechi F, Taddei T, et al. Anaerobic threshold in patients with exercise-induced myocardial ischemia. Circulation 1991;83 Suppl III:III-50–3.

85. Itoh H, Taniguchi K, Koike A, et al. Evaluation of severity of heart failure using ventilatory gas analysis. Circulation 1990;81 Suppl II:II-31–7.

86. Sullivan MJ, Cobb FR. The anaerobic threshold in chronic heart failure: relation to blood lactate, ventilatory basis, reproducibility, and response to exercise training. Circulation 1990;81 Suppl II:II-47–58.

87. Wasserman K. Overview and future direction. Circulation 1990;81 Suppl II:II-59–64.

88. Yozu R, Shimomitsu T, Jacobs G, et al. Use of the anaerobic threshold for evaluating various total artificial heart control algorithms in calves. Artif Organs 1985;9:279–83.

89. Yoshikawa M, Nakata KI, Nonaka K, et al. Right ventricular assist system feedback flow control parameter for rotary blood pump. Artif Organs 2000;24:659–66.

90. Nosé Y, Linneweber J, Ishitoya H, et al. The ICMT publication on artificial organs. Vol III. Artificial heart, past, present, and future. Houston: ICMT Press; 2002.

91. Frazier OH. First use of an untethered, vented electric left ventricular assist device for long-term support. Circulation 1994;89:2908–14.

92. Levin HR, Oz MC, Chen JM, et al. Reversal of chronic ventricular dilation in patients with end-stage cardiomyopathy by prolonged mechanical unloading. Circulation 1995;91:2717–20.

93. McCarthy PM, Savage RM, Fraser CD, et al. Hemodynamic and physiologic changes during support with an implantable left ventricular assist device. J Thorac Cardiovasc Surg 1995;109:409–18.

94. Frazier OH, Macris MP, Myers TJ, et al. Improved survival after extended bridge to cardiac transplantation. Ann Thorac Surg 1994;57:1416–22.

95. McCarthy PM, Nakatani S, Vargo R, et al. Structural and left ventricular histologic changes after implantable LVAD insertion. Ann Thorac Surg 1995;59:609–13.

96. Frazier OH, Benedict CR, Radovancevic B, et al. Improved left ventricular function after chronic left ventricular unloading. Ann Thorac Surg 1996;62:675–82.

97. Hetzer R, Müller J, Weng Y, et al. Cardiac recovery in dilated cardiomyopathy by unloading with a left ventricular assist device. Ann Thorac Surg 1999;68:742–9.

98. Holman WL, Bourge RC, Kirklin JK. Case report: circulatory support for seventy days with resolution of acute heart failure. J Thorac Cardiovasc Surg 1991;102:932–4.

99. Nakatani T, Sasako Y, Kumon K, et al. Long-term circulatory support to promote recovery from profound heart failure. ASAIO J 1995;41:M526–30.

100. Levin HR, Oz MC, Catanese KA, et al. Transient normalization of systolic and diastolic function after support with a left ventricular assist device in a patient with dilated cardiomyopathy. J Heart Lung Transplant 1996;15:840–2.

101. Frazier OH, Myers TJ. Left ventricular assist system as a bridge to myocardial recovery. Ann Thorac Surg 1999;68:734–41.

102. Bick RJ, Poindexter BJ, Buja LM, et al. Improved sarcoplasmic reticulum function after mechanical left ventricular unloading. Cardiovasc Pathobiol 1998;2:159–66.

103. Dilulio NA, DiPaola NR, Smedira NG, et al. Reversal of the heart failure phenotype by mechanical unloading [abstract]. J Heart Lung Transplant 1999;18:89–90.

104. Ogletree-Hughes ML, Barrett-Stull L, Smedira NG, et al. Mechanical unloading restores beta-adrenergic responsiveness in the failing human heart [abstract]. J Heart Lung Transplant 1999;18:63.

105. Magnusson Y, Hjalmarson Å, Hoebeke J. Beta 1-adrenoceptor autoimmunity in cardiomyopathy. Int J Cardiol 1996;54(2):137–41.

106. Blum A, Miller H. Role of cytokines in heart failure. Am Heart J 1998;135:181–6.

107. Sueoka A. Present status of apheresis technologies: part 2. Membrane plasma fractionator. Ther Apher 1997;1(2):135–46.

108. Sueoka A. Present status of apheresis technologies, part 3: adsorbent. Ther Apher 1997;1(3):271–83.

109. Sueoka A. Present status of apheresis technologies: part 4. Leukocyte filter. Ther Apher 1998;2(1):78–86.

110. Wallukat G, Reinke P, Dörffel WV, et al. Removal of autoantibodies in dilated cardiomyopathy by immunoadsorption. Int J Cardiol 1996;54(2):191–5.

111. Matsuda Y, Malchesky PS, Nosé Y. Low-density lipoprotein removal methods by membranes and future perspectives. Artif Organs 1996;20(4):346–54.

112. Matsumari A, Yamada T, Suzuki H, et al. Increased circulating cytokines in patients with myocarditis and cardiomyopathy. Br. Heart J 1994;72:561–6.

113. Tayama E, Nose Y. Can we treat dilated cardiomyopathy using a left ventricular assist device? Artif Organs 1996;20:197–201.

114. Kroon AA, Aengevaeren WRM, Werf TVD, et al. LDL-apheresis atherosclerosis regression study (LAARS): effect of aggressive versus conventional lipid lowering treatment on coronary atherosclerosis. Circulation 1996;93:1826–35.

115. Matsuda Y, Malchesky PS, Nosé Y. Low-density lipoprotein removal methods by membranes and future perspectives. Artif Organs 1996;20:346–55.

116. Butler KC, Dow JJ, Litwak P, et al. Development of Nimbus/University of Pittsburgh innovative ventricular assist system. Ann Thorac Surg 1999;68:790–4.

117. Macris MP, Parnis SM, Frazier OH, et al. Development of an implantable assist system. Ann Thorac Surg 1997;63:367–70.

118. DeBakey ME. A miniature implantable axial flow ventricular assist device. Ann Thorac Surg 1999;68:637–40.

119. Takatani S, Orime Y, Tasai K, et al. Totally implantable total artificial heart and ventricular assist device with multipurpose miniature electromechanical energy system. Artif Organs 1994;18:80–92.

120. Marlinski E, Jacobs G, Deirmengian C, et al. Durability testing of components for the Jarvik 2000 completely implantable axial flow left ventricular assist device. ASAIO J 1998;44:M741–4.

121. Thomas DC, Butler KC, Taylor LP, et al. Progress on development of the Nimbus-University of Pittsburgh axial flow left ventricular assist system. ASAIO J 1998;44:M521–4.

122. Burke DJ, Burke E, Parsaie F, et al. The HeartMate II: design and development of fully sealed axial flow left ventricular assist system. Artif Organs 2001;25:380–5.

123. Snyder A, Pae W, Boehmer J, et al. First clinical trials of totally implantable destination therapy ventricular assist system. J Congest Heart Fail Circulatory Supp 2001;1:185–92.

124. McCarthy PM, Smedira NO, Vargo RL, et al. One hundred patients with the HeartMate left ventricular assist device: enveloping concepts and technology. J Thorac Cardiovasc Surg 1998;115:904–12.

125. El-Banayosy A, Arusoglu L, Kizner L, et al. Novacor left ventricular system versus HeartMate vented electric left ventricular system as a long-term mechanical circulatory support device in bridging patients. A prospective study. J Thorac Cardiovasc Surg 2000;119:581–7.

126. Poirier VL. The HeartMate left ventricular assist system: wordwide clinical results. Eur J Cardiothorac Surg 1997;11Suppl:S39–44.

127. Nose Y, Ohtsubo S, Tayama E. Therapeutic and physiological artificial heart: future prospects. Artif Organs 1997;21:592–6.

128. Farrar DJ, Hill JD, Pennington DG, et al. Preoperative and postoperative comparison of patients with univentricular and biventricular support with the Thoratec ventricular assist device as a bridge to cardiac transplantation. J Thorac Cardiovasc Surg 1997;113:202–9.

129. Dohmen PM, Laube H, de Jonge K, et al. Mechanical circulatory support for one thousand days or more with the Novacor N100 left ventricular assist device. J Thorac Cardiovasc Surg 1999;117:1029–30.

130. Koul B, Solem JO, Steen S, et al. HeartMate left ventricular assist device as a bridge to heart transplantation. Ann Thorac Surg 1998;65:1625–30.

131. Frazier OH, Rose EA, Macmanus Q, et al. Multicenter clinical evaluation of the HeartMate 1000 IP left ventricular assist device. Ann Thorac Surg 1992;53:1080–90.

132. Arabia FA, Smith RG, Jaffe C, et al. Cost analysis of the Novacor left ventricular assist system as an outpatient bridge to heart transplantation. ASAIO J 1996;42:M546–9.

133. Kawahito K, Damm G, Benkowski R, et al. Ex vivo phase I evaluation of the DeBakey/NASA axial flow ventricular assist device. Artif Organs 1996;20:47–52.

134. Ohtsuka G, Nakata K, Yoshikawa M, et al. Long-term in vivo left ventricular assist device study for 284 days with Gyro pump. Artif Organs 1999;23:504–7.

135. Yoshikawa M, Nonaka K, Linneweber J, et al. Development of NEDO implantable ventricular assist device with Gyro centrifugal pump. Artif Organs 2000;24:459–67.

136. Nosé Y, Nakata K, Yoshikawa M, et al. Development of totally implantable biventricular bypass centrifugal blood pump system. Ann Thorac Surg 1999;68:775–9.

137. Groth T, Campbell EJ, Hermann K, et al. Application of enzyme immunoassays for testing haemocompatibility of biomedical polymers. Biomaterial 1995;16:1009–15.

138. Takami Y, Makinouchi K, Nakazawa T, et al. Hemolytic characteristics of a pivot bearing supported gyro centrifugal pump (C1E3) simulating various clinical applications. Artif Organs 1996;20:1042–9.

CHAPTER 51

NEW IMPLANTABLE PULSATILE BLOOD PUMPS

KENNETH L. FRANCO, MD

The National Heart, Lung and Blood Institute and the American Heart Association state that there are approximately 5 million people in the United States who have congestive heart failure. This number has doubled in the last 10 years and there are about 500,000 new cases diagnosed each year. The acceleration comes from the improved treatment of acute heart failure, patients living longer, and the success of treating other conditions that previously were fatal at an earlier age. Many of these patients survive for many years, dying of congestive heart failure later in life (the largest group is those persons who are older than 65 years of age). The mortality rate for congestive heart failure at 5 years from the initial diagnosis is 50%.[1] The incidence of congestive heart failure is closely related to advancing age, and with the generalized aging of our growing population, it insures the magnitude of this public health problem will grow even larger in the future. Congestive heart failure is a debilitating and costly disease. Patients with advanced heart failure are extensive users of health care services, especially hospital services. Of those persons who are older than 65 years of age, congestive heart failure is the most frequently listed hospital discharge diagnosis (DRG 127), primary for nearly 1 million hospital stays and secondary in more than 2 million hospital stays. In 1998, total direct expenditures for the treatment of congestive heart failure were estimated at $20 billion (US).

For people with intractable congestive heart failure who no longer respond to medical management and for whom all other options have been exhausted, the only available standard treatment is heart transplantation. In 1999, 2,500 heart transplants were performed in the United States, with many patients dying while on the waiting list. The number of people with end-stage congestive heart failure who could benefit with chronic ventricular support with a mechanical device has been estimated at 35,000 to 100,000 a year in the United States. New pulsatile and nonpulsatile cardiac assist devices are being developed to provide chronic support for patients with congestive heart failure (Table 51-1). The lack of a suitable number of human donor organs and the success of several pulsatile devices used as a bridge to transplantation have created a significant need for devices that can provide chronic support. For these devices to be effective, they must provide sufficient cardiac output to allow the patient to perform their usual daily activities, have a low risk of thromboemboli, be fully implantable (thereby reducing the risk of infection by removing the drive line), and have a low incidence of device malfunction that requires part or all of the device to be replaced.

Throughout the history of mechanical device development, we have been trying to mimic the native heart and have built several pulsatile devices that are currently used clinically to support the circulation of end-stage cardiac patients. Although they have been used successfully to support the circulation of end-stage cardiac patients for a prolonged duration, they tend to be large, inefficient, and costly, requiring expensive valves in the inflow and outflow positions. On the other hand, continuous flow devices offer several advantages over the pulsatile system, including being smaller, less expensive, using less energy, and not requiring valves. The only limitation of continuous flow pumps is nonpulsatility, which may be unphysiologic. However, earlier chronic animal studies and current clinical trials demonstrate that mammals, including humans, can tolerate nonpulsatile flow for a prolonged duration. Synthetic continuous flow pumps, although unphysiologic in nature, could maintain the circulation of humans for a prolonged period of time. Recovery of heart function was also reported even with nonpulsatile flow by the appearance of the pulses. Patients could tolerate even mild exercise in the rehabilitation process. This evidence supports that mammals could adapt to nonpulsatile blood flow. Pulse may not be necessary from the perspective of peripheral organ perfusion, but flow and pressure are more important than the presence of a pulse. However, when recovery of heart function is concerned, pulse may be a necessity. The heart continues to provide oxygen and nutrients by means of pumping blood every minute; it contracts using energy, then rests to supply itself with the energy for survival. Biologically it was not possible to

TABLE 51-1. Pulsatile Mechanical Assist Devices

	Arrow LionHeart LVAS	HeartSaver VAD	Thoratec IVAD
Pump Type	Intracorporeal	Intracorporeal	Intracorporeal
Pump actuation	Electrohydraulic	Electrohydraulic	Electromechanical
Valves	Delrin monostrut	Bioprosthetic	Delrin monostrut
Blood chamber material	Titanium	Proprietary polyurethane	Thoralon polyurethane
Flow type	Pulsatile	Pulsatile	Pulsatile
VAD configuration	LVAD	LVAD	LVAD, RVAD, BiVAD
Intended indication	Long-term—alternative to transplantation or medical therapy	Long-term—alternative to transplantation or medical therapy	Bridge to transplantation and to recovery
LVAD implant site	Within abdominal wall and within chest wall	Intrathoracic	Within abdominal wall
Totally implantable device	Yes	Yes	No
Power transmission	TETS	TETS	Percutaneous lead
Remote communication	No	Yes	No
Power source	Batteries	Batteries	Battery or external portable power console
SV (stroke volume)	64 mL	70 mL	65 mL
Pump output	8 L/min	7.5 L/min	7.2 L/min
Total volume displacement	250 mL	560 mL	252 mL
Pump weight	680 g	900 g	339 g
Clinical implants	23	—	—

BiVAD = biventricular assist device; IVAD = implantable ventricular assist device; LVAD = left ventricular assist device; LVAS = left ventricular assist system; RVAD = right ventricular assist device; TETS = transcutaneous energy transfer system; VAD = ventricular assist device.

create a continuous working system, so when recovery of the heart function is desired, the usual approach may be use of a pulsatile device to augment the diastolic pressure so that perfusion pressure through the coronary arteries is increased and maintained.[2] The cost for a device implant or a heart transplant are about the same, but there is still a huge gap between the supply and demand for donor hearts, and after the first year of recovery, transplant patients will have to bear the cost of rejection drugs for the rest of their lives, which drugs are expensive. This author suspects that the costs of mechanical devices will continue to decrease as less complex, implantable, and more efficient devices are developed.

A study was recently published comparing the long-term use of left ventricular assist devices (LVADs) to medical therapy in patients with end-stage heart failure who were not candidates for heart transplantation (Rematch study).[3] The study followed 129 patients with end-stage heart failure who were not eligible for cardiac transplantation and who were randomly assigned to receive an LVAD or optimal medical management. All patients had symptoms of heart failure and were in New York Heart Association class IV. Kaplan-Meier estimates of survival at 1 year were 52% in the device group and 25% in the medical therapy group, and at 2 years were 23% and 8%, respectively. The frequency of serious adverse events in the device group was 2.5 times that in the medical group, with the predominance being infection, bleeding, and malfunction of the device. The quality of life was significantly improved

at 1 year in the device group. Within 3 months after implantation, the probability of infection of the LVAD was 28%. Although most of the infections were in the driveline tract and pocket, which were treated with local measures and antibiotics, fatal sepsis was common. Within 6 months after implantation of the LVAD, the frequency of bleeding was 42%. No system had failed by 12 months but the probability of device failure was 35% at 24 months. The device was replaced in 10 patients. Terminal heart failure caused the majority of deaths in the medical therapy group, whereas the most common cause of death in the device group was sepsis and failure of the device. The study demonstrates that long-term support with an LVAD resulted in substantial improvement in survival in patients with serious heart failure who were not candidates for heart transplantation, and the findings also establish LVADs and heart transplantation as treatment options for patients with end-stage heart failure.

The Arrow LionHeart Left Ventricular Assist System

The Arrow LionHeart left ventricular assist system (LVAS) is manufactured by Arrow International, Inc. (Reading, PA), and is designed for use as destination therapy for patients with progressive, irreversible end-stage class IV congestive heart failure for which heart transplantation is not an option. It is not intended as a bridge to transplant or as a bridge to recovery of ventricular function. In other words, it is a long-term therapeutic option for patients who are considered ineligible for heart transplantation.[4] The LVAS has several unique features, including being the first fully implantable LVAS in clinical use with no lines or cables exiting the skin to power the device, which should reduce the incidence of infections. In addition, it uses a transcutaneous energy system to charge the internal batteries and to power the device, and it uses a compliance chamber, eliminating the need for a vent tube (Figure 51-1). The LionHeart LVAS is the result of a 7-year collaboration with the Department of Surgery's Section of Artificial Organs at Pennsylvania State University (Hershey, PA). Essential research in the area of sustained mechanical circulatory support that helped to define the LionHeart LVAS has been ongoing at Penn State for more than 30 years. The first human implant occurred on October 26, 1999, at the Heart and Diabetes center in Bad Oeynhausen, Germany. As of December 1, 2001, 17 patients have had the device implanted in Europe. A 30-patient European clinic trial sponsored by Arrow International is being conducted to demonstrate the safety and performance of the LionHeart LVAS. The additional European centers involved include Hospital La Pitie, the University of Vienna Medical Center, and the Berlin Heart Institute. A Food and Drug Administration (FDA)–sponsored Investigational Device Exemption (IDE) clinical trial in the United States began in 2001; to date, seven patients have been implanted with the LionHeart LVAS.

The key features of the LionHeart LVAS include fully implantable components, transcutaneous energy transfer, fully automated control algorithm, and modular design. The fully implantable components eliminate drive and vent lines exiting the skin, which allows for reduction in the risk of infection, improved mobility, and a better quality of life. The current percutaneous drivelines are eliminated by the use of the transcutaneous energy transfer to batteries, which allows patients to be untethered for 20 to 30 min. The fully automated control algorithm responds to changes in the patient's condition, and the LVAS will pump as much blood as the patient requires. The modular design will allow for exchange of discreet subsystems that will require replacement over time due to wear or infection.

The implanted subsystem components include the blood pump, the motor controller, the internal coil, the compliance chamber, and the access port (Figure 51-2). The combined weight of the implanted components is 1.5 kg. The blood pump is electrically powered and is implanted in the preperitoneal space beneath the left costal margin. The apex of the left ventricle is cored with a coring punch, and a sewing cuff is sutured in place. The inlet cannula is positioned as desired and locked in place with a clamping mechanism. The outlet cannula is routed to the ascending aorta where the coated vascular graft section of the cannula is trimmed to length and sewn in place via an end-to-side anastomosis. The cannulas are connected to the blood pump with self-locking collet-type connectors. The blood pump features a motor, a pusher-plate mechanism, a smooth polyurethane sac, and two tilting-disc valves for unidirectional flow. The blood pump is connected to the native circulation via inlet and outlet cannulas. The Arrow LionHeart blood pump assembly uses a brushless direct current (DC) motor to drive a roller screw mechanism. The roller screw is connected to a

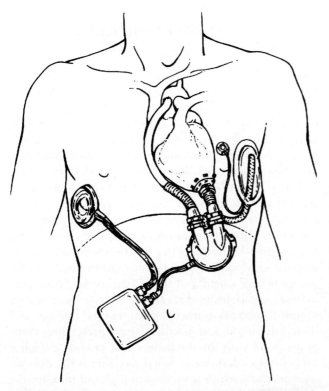

FIGURE 51-1. The totally implantable Arrow LionHeart LVAS. Drawing courtesy of Arrow International, Inc. (Reading, PA).

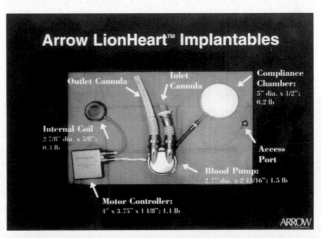

FIGURE 51-2. The Arrow LionHeart implantables, which include the inlet and outlet cannulae, the internal coil, the motor controller, the blood pump, the compliance chamber, and the access port. Photograph courtesy of Arrow International, Inc. (Reading, PA).

pusher plate. As the rotor spins in clockwise and counter-clockwise directions, the pusher plate is driven back and forth within the blood pump housing to compress and empty a blood sac that has been passively filled with blood from the left ventricle through a one-way tilting-disc valve. The blood pump works continuously in a fill-to-empty mode to pump blood. In other words, whenever the sac is full, the pump empties it. In this context the blood pump functions asynchronously with respect to the heart. The motor controller and internal coil control the operation of the blood pump. The blood pump and electronic motor controller are powered by either external sources or rechargeable batteries located in the motor controller. External power is received transcutaneously by the internal coil and sent to the motor controller and blood pump for continuous operation. Internal power is delivered by the motor controller's rechargeable batteries and allows the LVAS recipient to function totally free of the external power source for approximately 20 to 30 min. The motor controller is placed under the anterior abdominal wall in the preperitoneal space beneath the right costal margin. The internal coil is placed in the subcutaneous tissue of the chest wall. The compliance chamber and access port serve as a gas volume accumulator. The compliance chamber provides gas to evacuated chambers of the blood pump during its operation. This compliance chamber is periodically charged, via the access port, with room air every 4 to 5 weeks. The compliance chamber is placed in the left pleural space. The access port is passed through the intercostal space located in the subcutaneous tissue over the left anterior chest wall.

The external subsystem components include the power transmitter (PT) coil, power pack with batteries, and the charger. The PT transfers power across the intact skin. The PT is connected to the power pack in normal operation and is likely to be worn on the belt or in a pack. The power pack with the battery packs provides power to the LionHeart LVAS. The power pack weighs approximately 3.6 kg when loaded with two battery packs. The rechargeable battery packs each provide approximately 2 to 3 h of power for mobile operation. The power pack is worn either with a shoulder harness or in a backpack or is pulled on a hand cart. The charger is floor based and recharges depleted battery packs, tests the battery packs, and provides alternating current (AC) power to the system when it is connected between an AC power source and the power pack. This is the normal configuration when the LVAS recipient is sleeping. In addition to the system components above, other accessories have been developed. These accessories include wearable accessories to facilitate mobility, surgical implant tools, alternate power supplies, and a system monitor. The system monitor is intended to provide the clinician with the ability to interrogate the LVAS for its functional status and operating condition during follow-up appointments or remotely, if indicated (Figure 51-3).

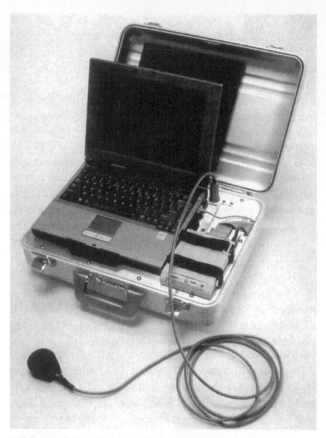

FIGURE 51-3. The Arrow LionHeart LVAS system monitor. Photograph courtesy of Arrow International, Inc. (Reading, PA).

HeartSaver Ventricular Assist Device

The HeartSaver VAD is manufactured by World Heart Corporation and was developed for long-term use in patients with end-stage congestive heart failure (Figure 51-4). The HeartSaver VAD consists of these implantable components: the implanted VAD unit (which consists of the blood chamber, volume displacement chamber, electrohydraulic axial flow pump, and electronic controller) (Figure 51-5); the internal transcutaneous energy transfer and biotelemetry coil; the internal battery pack; and the inflow and outflow conduits with integrated tissue valves. These components are capable of providing the required blood pumping function without needing external components for periods determined by the energy storage capacity of the internal battery pack. The external components include the remote biotelemetry monitor, external transcutaneous energy transfer and biotelemetry coil, and external battery pack. These components are worn by the patient and provide complete mobility. An additional external accessory is the clinical-user interface, which is used to control and monitor the device during implantation, to monitor device function in the early perioperative period, and for remote monitoring

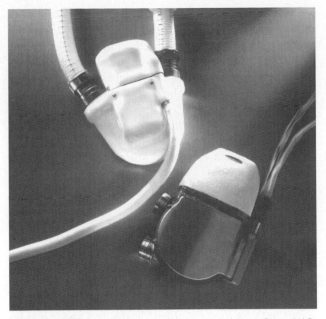

FIGURE 51-4. The Novacor LVAS and the HeartSaver VAD. Photograph courtesy of World Heart Corporation (Ottawa, Canada).

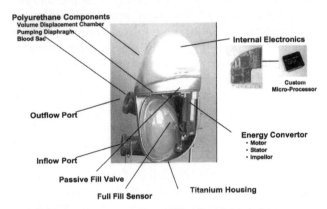

FIGURE 51-5. The HeartSaver VAD unit with labeled components. Photograph courtesy of World Heart Corporation (Ottawa, Canada).

control of the implanted device in the outpatient setting. The HeartSaver VAD has these advantages: it can be implanted in the thoracic position, which eliminates the need for body openings for venting and reduces the length of connections to the heart; it has a sleek and compact design; it uses a design that should minimize the risk of thromboembolic complications; it is completely implantable, which should minimize the risk of postoperative infections; it is much easier to implant than other systems that require perforation of the diaphragm and major abdominal interventions to permit implantation in the abdomen; and it allows the patient to be remotely monitored. The ability to monitor patients remotely and to make adjustments to the VAD for optimal performance is a tremendous advantage in monitoring patients in the outpatient setting.

The HeartSaver VAD system is an implantable, pulsatile electrohydraulically actuated ventricular assist device that combines the blood chamber, the volume displacement chamber, electrohydraulic axial flow pump, and control electronics into a single unit with an overall volume of approximately 500 mL.[5] The unit is designed for implantation in the left hemithorax and the geometry is based on cadaveric and intraoperative anatomic fit studies, as well as fluid dynamics optimization. An integrated volume displacement chamber (VDC) adjacent to the lung allows the pressure of the system to equalize with atmospheric pressure, thus eliminating the requirement for external venting. The unit is powered by a transcutaneous energy transfer (TET) system to eliminate the need for percutaneous power cables. The TET system provides power to operate the unit from a wearable external battery and/or other power source (eg, automobile cigarette lighter and household AC outlet). The TET system also charges an internal implantable rechargeable battery, which allows the recipient to bathe, shower, and perform other activities without the need for an external power source. Control and monitoring of the implanted unit is accomplished using an infrared biotelemetry system integrated with the TET system. A wearable external controller provides device system displays and warning alarms. The controller also offers the clinician the capability to perform routine device monitoring from a remote location by using phone lines or other public telecommunications infrastructure (eg, satellites, Internet, and asynchronous transfer mode systems), which enables a patient to leave the hospital and reduces the number of return visits for routine device assessment. Selection of the intrathoracic implant site for the device was based on several factors. First, the inflow cannula length may be shortened compared to intra-abdominal devices (Figure 51-6). It is speculated that the short inflow cannula may improve inflow characteristics. Second, the rib cage provides a secure anchoring site to eliminate device migration. Finally, the incision does not have to extend into the abdomen, thereby improving patient comfort and postoperative mobility while avoiding the necessity of perforating the diaphragm for passage of the inlet cannula.

To design the implantable unit for intrathoracic placement, the overall size, weight and geometry of the unit had to be optimized to fit within the available space in the left hemithorax.[6] To assess the available space a series of cadaveric and intraoperative fit trials were conducted. Based on these studies the overall geometric constraints of the device were determined and the unit's configuration was adapted to meet these demands. The implantable unit has a total volume displacement of about 500 mL and a weight of 680 g. It consists of a 70 mL blood chamber with a flexible polyurethane diaphragm within a rigid housing. The silicone-based hydraulic fluid is pumped during systole through the energy converter that consists of a bidirectional brushless DC motor, a bladed impeller, and a bladed

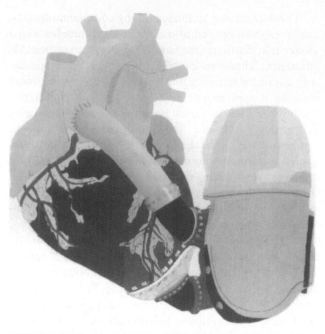

FIGURE 51-6. The HeartSaver VAD connected to the heart by a small inlet cannula attached to the apex and a longer outlet cannula attached to the ascending aorta. Photograph courtesy of World Heart Corporation (Ottawa, Canada).

housing. The hydraulic fluid actuates the flexible blood chamber diaphragm that ejects the blood from the chamber. The blood chamber fills passively during diastole, with the hydraulic fluid returning to the volume displacement chamber through a one-way valve. The diastolic filling may be augmented with reversal of the motor in the active filling mode. Filling and ejection of blood is monitored by using Hall effect sensors and a magnet embedded in the blood pumping diaphragm, which allows the position of the flexing diaphragm to be dynamically determined throughout the pumping cycle by internal electronic module. The bioprosthetic valves are mounted in the inflow and outflow cannulas, which should reduce anticoagulation requirements. To eliminate the need for percutaneous venting, a VDC was integrated into the implantable unit. The VDC allows for the displacement of the actuating hydraulic fluid during device diastole and consists of an integrated hydraulic fluid chamber with a flexible diaphragm. The flexible diaphragm is in contact with the lung tissue, which, in turn, is in contact with atmospheric pressure, thus eliminating the need for a percutaneous vent tube. In the case of the HeartSaver VAD, the VDC also performs a secondary function, namely, heat dissipation from the internal electronic module. The internal electronic module is mounted within the VDC surrounded by the actuating hydraulic fluid, which allows excess heat generation to be transferred over the entire surface area of the implanted unit. Heat transfer to the body is accomplished across the blood diaphragm into the blood stream, across the VDC diaphragm to the lung tissue, and across the

housing to the surrounding tissue. By allowing large areas of heat transfer potential, local hot spots are eliminated and operating temperatures well within the physiologic limits can be obtained. In addition to not requiring external venting, total implantability would only be possible if power for the device was internal and could be delivered transcutaneously.

To provide power to the device without percutaneous lines, a TET system was developed. The TET system transfers power from an external source across the intact skin and tissue to the device using electromagnetic induction. This is accomplished by using a pair of wire coils, one implanted subcutaneously and one located directly over the implanted coil on the skin surface. By selecting an appropriate operating frequency from the coil geometry, a coupling coefficient suitable for power transfer across intact skin and tissue can be obtained. The TET system provides two major functions: it provides operating power from an external battery source (battery, wall socket, etc) to the implanted device and also provides power to recharge the implanted battery, which is used as a backup power supply. The implanted battery also provides the patient with the ability to bathe, shower, swim, and perform other activities, unencumbered by any external components. To monitor and control the device without the need for percutaneous connections, a biotelemetry system was developed. This system uses infrared data communications to transfer control and monitoring information across the intact skin and tissue. Electronic modules consisting of multiple infrared receivers and the transmitter components are mounted in both the energy transfer coils, establishing a bidirectional communications path between the implanted device and the outside of the body. The infrared method was selected based primarily on its immunity to electronic noise, which insures a high level of accuracy for this life-critical application. A remote biotelemetry capability has been added to the HeartSaver VAD, which allows health care providers at a remote site to control and monitor the device by using public communications infrastructure (telephone lines, asynchronous transfer mode, satellites, internet, etc) (Figure 51-7). This feature is expected to offer patients improved convenience and quality of life by reducing the number of visits to the hospital or clinic for routine device or patient checkups. Basically, patients can connect the wearable external controller to a telephone line or cellular phone at their home or other location and a health care provider at the hospital or clinic can have access to control and monitor functions of the implanted device. This remote communications capability should also help to alleviate fears that some patients have exhibited related to leaving the hospital with a complex implantable medical device. In addition, because a patient will no longer be required to return as frequently to the hospital for routine device or patient checkups, the cost of follow-up of patient care will also be reduced. The Heart-

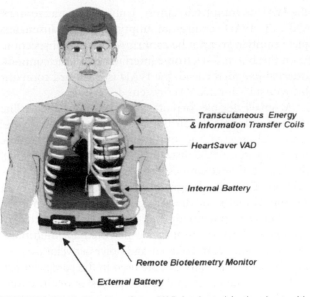

FIGURE 51-7. The HeartSaver VAD implanted in the chest with the remote biotelemetry monitor and external battery attached to the waist. Drawing courtesy of World Heart Corporation (Ottawa, Canada).

Labels in figure:
Transcutaneous Energy & Information Transfer Coils
HeartSaver VAD
Internal Battery
Remote Biotelemetry Monitor
External Battery

Saver VAD is expected to deliver enhanced quality of life to the device recipient in both the short and long terms. The intrathoracic position should reduce incision length and abdominal manipulation, thereby reducing postoperative pain and minimizing associated complications. Total implantability will offer improved patient mobility and, it is hoped, early patient discharge. Finally, the remote biotelemetry capability will allow for ease of follow-up with patients living away from hospital-based resources.

The entire HeartSaver VAD, including the TET biotelemetry subsystems, were assessed in vivo in a series of bovine experiments. During these experiments, the animals were supported for periods as long as 5 days to assess the system design, implantability, and overall function. To allow further development of the TET biotelemetry system (independent of the implantable unit), it was tested with a percutaneous power and information cable. Testing focused on performance of inflow and outflow cannulas, device positioning in the calf model in preperation[7] for chronic testing of the final design, and team preparation. Thirteen experiments were performed in animals with a mean weight of 102 kg. Duration of implantation ranged from 14 h to 30 days. Modifications resulting from these tests included abandoning cardiopulmonary bypass support during cannula implantation to reduce pulmonary complications, use of a stainless steel wire-reinforced cannula to prevent kinking, use of a Dacron coating to prevent abrasion of adjacent tissue, changes in the control software, and improvements to monitoring systems for blood chamber filling and ejection. There were no infection-related complications during the series of experiments and there was only one case of thrombosis in the blood chamber that was later determined to be caused by

breakage of the polyurethane housing component, which has since been resolved by using a cast titanium housing. There were also two cases of cannula clotting related to cannula kinking, which has been resolved through cannula reinforcement and straightening. Six studies were electively terminated because various goals were achieved; three studies were terminated because of insufficient inflow to the device; three were terminated because of pulmonary dysfunction, three because of bleeding tamponade, two because of respiratory insufficiency, and two because of faulty electrical connections; two were terminated because of housing defects resulting in hydraulic fluid loss; one was terminated because of thromboembolic complications related to the anticoagulation protocol, one because of ventricular fibrillation during implantation, one because of an air embolism during device implantation, and one because of a power failure in the facility. Most of the study terminations were due to the medical/surgical complications experienced during the development of a suitable implantation protocol in the animal model. These issues have now been specifically addressed and satisfactorily resolved. Long-term studies out to 90 days are in progress and it is expected that early clinical trials will begin in Canada in the fall of 2002.

Thoratec IVAD

Thoratec's (Pleasanton, CA) paracorporeal VAD offers clinicians the advantages of an externally worn device, which is especially important for a wide range of body sizes and for ease of device removal. However, Thoratec recognizes that some clinicians prefer implantable pumps if prolonged VAD support is anticipated because of the patient's size, blood type, or elevated antibodies. In light of this, and based on extensive experience with the paracorporeal device implanted up to 550 days, Thoratec has developed an implantable VAD (IVAD). The IVAD has the same blood flow path and Thoralon polyurethane blood pumping sac as the paracorporeal VAD but the housing is a smooth, contoured polished titanium alloy (Figure 51-8). The IVAD has a new sensor to detect when the

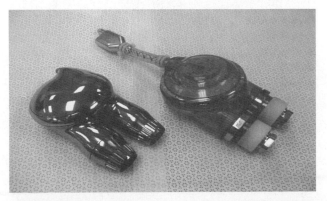

FIGURE 51-8. Thoratec's paracorporeal LVAD and the implantable VAD. Photograph courtesy of Thoratec Corporation (Pleasanton, CA).

pump is full and empty, and is controlled with the Thoratec TLC-II portable VAD driver, which is a small, briefcase-size, battery-powered pneumatic control unit.[8] A small, flexible percutaneous pneumatic drive line for each VAD is tunneled out of the body from the LVAD or right ventricular assist device (RVAD) in the preperitoneal position. Small size and simplicity are the major advantages of the IVAD. The IVAD weighs 339 g and has an implanted volume of 250 mL, which is approximately 50% that of current implantable pulsatile electromechanical LVADs available today (Figure 51-9).

The overall size and shape of the IVAD facilitates implantation in a diverse patient population.[9] A low-profile housing is fabricated from a titanium alloy known to have good tissue biocompatibility properties. The smooth external contours are designed to minimize dead space in the preperitoneal pocket and to reduce the risk of infection. In addition, the surface of the device is polished to take advantage of the potential bacterial colonization resistance associated with smooth metallic surfaces. The IVAD contains an optical infrared sensor to detect when the blood sac is full or empty. The small 2.2 mm–thick sensor allows for substantial reduction in the overall size of the housing. The optical sensor replaces a Hall effect switch in the paracorporeal VAD and does not require the associated switch diaphragm and magnet, which further simplifies the implanted components contained in the IVAD. An external microprocessor-based circuit analyzes the sensor's signal and provides the driver with a full signal equivalent to the paracorporeal VAD Hall switch output. This external electronic interface, contained in the electric lead, also has an indicator lamp that flashes when

the IVAD is completely empty. Unlike the paracorporeal VAD, the IVAD requires an empty signal, because complete emptying cannot be confirmed by visual inspection. With the external electronic interfacing and the common external pneumatic lead, the IVAD is backward compatible with all Thoratec VAD system drivers.

A small flexible percutaneous pneumatic driveline delivers and vents the air that activates the 9 mm–diameter velour-covered line and also carries an electric cable for the sensor.[9] At the distal end of the line, a special small diameter fitting combines electrical and pneumatic connections. Extensive design efforts were made to achieve an 11 mm diameter for the fitting that is tunneled through the skin. The pneumatic line tubing is constructed of Thoralon, Thoratec's proprietary polyurethane multipolymer, with wire reinforcement and polyester velour covering, the same materials that are used in the paracorporeal VAD percutaneous cannulas. The polyester velour covering promotes tissue ingrowth, providing an effective barrier to infection and anchoring the VAD within the body. The geometry of the blood path is identical between the clinically proven paracorporeal VAD and the IVAD. The IVAD uses the same blood sac, actuation diaphragm, and unidirectional blood valves as the paracorporeal VAD without modifications. Both the paracorporeal VAD and the IVAD have a smooth, seamless, flexible pumping chamber or blood sac made of Thoralon. For both VADs, two monostrut valves with Delrin occluder disks maintain unidirectional flow through the blood pump. The pumping chamber is separated from the air chamber by a polyurethane actuation diaphragm. The diaphragm serves as both a volume limiter and safety chamber. To prevent abrasion, silicone oil lubricates the surfaces where the diaphragm and VAD case contact the blood sac. The blood-contacting geometry of the valve housing, and the components that connect the cannula to the VAD, are identical for the two pumps. The only difference is that the paracorporeal valve housings are constructed of stainless steel whereas the IVAD valve housings are constructed of a more damage-resistant titanium alloy. The effective stroke volume is the same for both pumps, at 65 mL.

The cannulas for the IVAD have the same internal dimensions and blood-contacting material as the cannulas used for the paracorporeal VAD. The lengths of the cannulas are reduced to accommodate the intracorporeal placement of the IVAD. The cannulas are secured to the valve housing of the IVAD by means of a collet nut that contains a captured collet. The IVAD is designed for left ventricular apical cannulation with return to the ascending aorta. For RVAD application, either right ventricular or right atrial cannulation can be used with return blood flow to the pulmonary artery. Right ventricular cannulation has the advantage of providing greater RVAD flow rather than right atrial cannulation. The IVAD is designed for implantation in a preperitoneal or intraperitoneal position by using standard surgical techniques. Curved

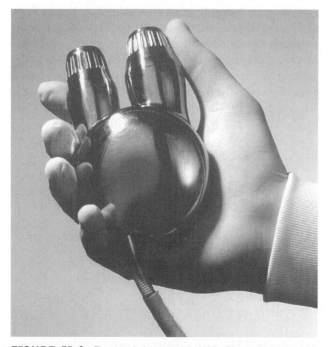

FIGURE 51-9. Thoratec's implantable VAD. Photograph courtesy of Thoratec Corporation (Pleasanton, CA).

12.7 mm–diameter tunnelers have been designed to creat a tunnel to allow passage of the pneumatic lines from the pocket to the exit site. It is anticipated that an FDA-sponsored clinical trial of the IVAD will begin in the United States in 2002.

References

1. O'Connell J, Bristow M. Economic impact of heart failure in the United States: time for a different approach. J Heart Lung Transplant 1994;13:5107–22.

2. Takatani S. Can rotary blood pumps replace pulsatile devices. ASAIO J 2001;25:671–4.

3. Rose E, Gelijus A, Moskowitz A, et al. Long-term use of left ventricular assist devices for end-stage heart failure. N Engl J Med 2001;345:1435–43.

4. Weiss WJ, Rosenburg G, Snyder AJ, et al. A completely implanted left ventricular assist device—chronic in vivo testing. ASAIO J 1993;39(3):M427–32.

5. Mussivand TV, Masters RG, Itendry PJ, et al. Totally implantable intrathoracic ventricular assist device. Ann Thorac Surg 1996;61:444–7.

6. Mussivand TV, Hendry PJ, Masters RG, et al. Development of a ventricular assist device for out-of-hospital use. J Heart Lung Transplant 1999;18:166–71.

7. Mussivand TV, Hendry PJ, Masters RG, et al. Progress with the HeartSaver ventricular assist device. Ann of Thorac Surg 1999;68:785–9.

8. Farrar D, Reichenbach S, Rossi S, et al. Development of an intracorporeal Thoratec ventricular assist device for univentricular and biventricular support. ASAIO J 2000; 46:351–3.

9. Reichenbach S, Farrar D, Hill J. A versatile intracorporeal ventricular assist device based on the Thoratec VAD system. Ann Thorac Surg 2001;71:S171–5.

CHAPTER 52

IMPLANTABLE LEFT VENTRICULAR ASSIST DEVICE INFECTIONS

STEVEN M. GORDON, MD, PATRICK M. MCCARTHY, MD

Reflecting on the recent death of Dr. Christiaan N. Barnard on September 2, 2001, it is remarkable to note that cardiac transplantation has been performed an estimated 100,000 times around the world since the world's first human heart transplant in 1967. Today, heart transplantation is carried out in 160 hospitals in the United States with an overall 1-year survival rate of 85 to 90%. However, as the prevalence of patients with heart failure increases each year, the number of patients that could benefit from heart transplantation (approximately 20,000 patients in the United States) outstrips the limited supply (about 2,000 hearts annually) despite efforts to increase the availability of human allografts. Although numerous therapeutic approaches are under investigation, at present, mechanical support by means of ventricular assist devices is the most promising alternative to transplantation.[1]

Currently, there are three types of Food and Drug Administration (FDA)–approved implantable left ventricular assist devices (LVADs) for bridge to transplantation—two HeartMate devices (Thoratec, Pleasanton, CA) and the Novacor device (Worldheart, Ottawa, Canada). Two devices are electrical pulsatile devices, one is pneumatic, and all are implanted through a median sternotomy with an inflow cannula in the apex of the left ventricle and an outflow tube anastomosed to the ascending aorta. Within the device are two trileaflet porcine valves to maintain unidirectional flow and a woven Dacron outflow graft anastomosed to the ascending aorta. A single drive line containing the electrical cable and the atmospheric air vent leads transcutaneously from the implanted pump to the power pack outside.

Complications associated with ventricular assist devices, including infection, bleeding, and thromboembolism, occur frequently in these patients. Infections occur in approximately 50% of patients with ventricular assist devices (VADs) and might be life-threatening or might prevent consideration of transplantation. Patients with implantable pumps are at high risk for infections because of a variety of reasons, including the design of the pumps and host-immune factors. In particular, the extra corporeal drive lines (13.5 to 15 mm in diameter) breach the normal cutaneous defenses against infection, providing a portal of entry for potential pathogens.[2–4] This chapter reviews the epidemiology, diagnosis, and management of, and strategies for, treatment and prevention of infections in patients with implantable LVADs.

Definition and Classification of Infection

In addition to being at risk for postimplantation infections (including device-associated infections), patients with implantable LVADs may also have preexisting nosocomial infections at the time of implantation. The Centers for Disease Control and Prevention have developed standard definitions for nosocomial infections, including ventilator-associated, bloodstream, and surgical site infections.[5] In contrast, there are no standard definitions of VAD-associated infections; consequently, studies reporting infections in patients with ventricular devices may be hard to compare. For example, the HeartMate left ventricular assist system multicenter clinical trial defined the presence of infection by (1) a white blood cell count > 12,500/µL, (2) a temperature > 38°C, and (3) a need for antibiotic therapy. Although sensitive (perhaps too sensitive), these criteria for infection are not specific. Holman and colleagues at the University of Alabama define infections as an antemortem positive culture and classifies infections into four categories based upon site (bloodstream vs nonbloodstream), source (VAD related or not), and severity (mediastinitis or endovascular components of VAD) (Table 52-1).[6] At our institution, we have used Centers for Disease Control and Prevention definitions for nosocomial infections and adapted definitions for implantable devices to characterize LVAD-associated infections (Table 52-2).[4,7]

TABLE 52-1. University of Alabama Classification of Infection

Class I
Patient-related nonblood infections that involve urine, wounds, sputum, chapter tips from indwelling lines (mediastinal infections excluded).

Class II
Infections that entail bloodborne organisms detected by blood culture.

Class III
Ventricular assist system–related infections that affect percutaneous guidelines or cannula insertion sites.

Class IV
Ventricular assist system–related infections that involve blood-contacting surfaces or device intracorporeal components (mediastinitis included).

TABLE 52-2. Cleveland Clinic Classifications of Ventricular Assist Device Infections

Class I
1. Culture or histologic evidence of infection
   a. Drive line
   b. Pump pocket
   c. Inflow/outflow conduits
2. Bloodstream infection with same organism cultured from the device
3. No other obvious source for the bloodstream infection

Class II
1. Culture or histologic evidence of infection
   a. Drive line
   b. Pump pocket
   c. Inflow/outflow conduits
2. Local or systemic signs of infection
   a. Local: purulent exudate, warmth, erythema, tenderness, induration
   b. Systemic: temperature > 38°C, white blood cell count 15,000/mL
3. No bloodstream infection
4. No other obvious source of infection

Class III
1. Local or systemic signs of infection
2. Clinical response to antimicrobials, device removal, or both
3. No culture or histologic evidence of device or bloodstream infection
4. No other obvious source of infection

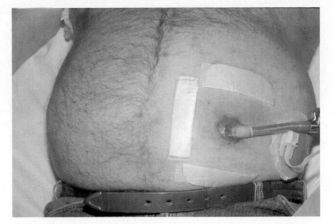

FIGURE 52-1. Drive line infection with associated erythema, edema, and purulent drainage.

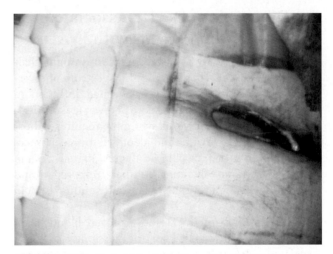

FIGURE 52-2. Pocket infection with subsequent erosion of drive line through skin.

Case Definitions for Ventricular Assist Device–Associated Infections

A drive line–associated infection is defined by purulent drainage around the drive line with or without positive cultures (Figure 52-1). Pump pocket infection is defined as purulent drainage around the LVAD pocket from percutaneous aspiration or erosion through skin (Figure 52-2).

A nosocomial bloodstream infection (BSI) is defined by using criteria from the Centers for Disease Control and Prevention.[5] An LVAD-associated BSI is defined as one in which the same pathogen is cultured from purulent drainage around any portion of the device, including drive lines, and the blood, with no other obvious source. LVAD endocarditis is defined by culture and/or histopathologic evidence of infection from the inflow/outflow conduits or from the porcine valves at the time of transplantation or autopsy (Figures 52-3 and 52-4).

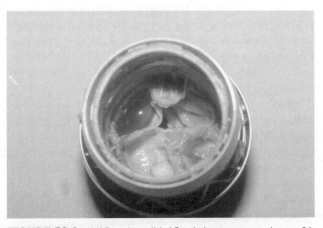

FIGURE 52-3. LVAD endocarditis (*Staphylococcus aureus*), case 24, Table 52-6.

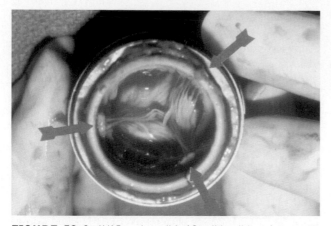

FIGURE 52-4. LVAD endocarditis (*Candida albicans*), case 19, Table 52-6.

Diagnosis of Device-Associated Infections in Patients with LVADs

The diagnosis of LVAD-associated infections can be challenging for the clinician and ranges in spectrum of severity from a localized drive line–associated infection to infective endocarditis. The presence of fever, leukocytosis, increased flow rates, or sepsis syndrome requires a thorough evaluation to exclude and identify a source of infection. Inspection of indwelling catheters, drive line, and pump pocket, and obtaining cultures from blood and other sites when appropriate (urine and sputum) should be performed.

A patient with an LVAD and a proven bloodstream infection must be assessed for the possibility of VAD-associated endocarditis. Unfortunately, current imaging studies are limited in their ability to provide data for the clinician. Echocardiography remains sensitive and specific for imaging of native valves, but not helpful in VAD-associated endocarditis. Visualization of inflow- and outflow conduits by transthoracic or transesophageal echocardiography are often impossible or difficult. Catheter-based ultrasound may allow imaging the interior pump components or surfaces. Cardiac catheterization can identify severe incompetence of the valves. Computed tomography (CT) scans and ultrasound can determine presence of collections around the device and guide aspiration of these collections for culture and cell counts. Magnetic resonance imaging (MRI) scans are precluded in these patients. Although there has been at least one report of immunoscintigraphy of ^{99m}Tc-labeled granulocytes being helpful in the diagnosis of a case of LVAD endocarditis, current nuclear imaging techniques are not considered robust in this regard, with problems of sensitivity and specificity, and remain impractical for the intensive care unit (ICU) patient.[8]

Epidemiology of Infections in Patients with LVADs

Despite a lack of accepted consensus criteria for standardization of LVAD-associated infections, the incidence of types of infection (device associated vs other) and the spectrum of device-associated infections (drive line to endocarditis) can be estimated from published studies to date, especially from registry reports or high-volume transplantation centers.

The likelihood of a patient developing an infection during support with a VAD is approximately 50%. Registries of patients with LVADs reporting infections provide a meaningful number of patients despite a lack of a standard definition for infection. Table 52-3 shows the infection rates from the FDA Premarket, Safety, and Effectiveness Summaries for the Novacor and HeartMate VE and IP VADs in 358 patients in bridge-to-transplantation studies.[9,10] The average infection rate was 54% (range, 44 to 66%). In two other registry reports involving 842 patients, the average infection rate was 30%. The data include an international registry of 584 bridge-to-transplantation patients with VADs or total artificial hearts and 258 European patients supported by a variety of devices for myocardial recovery (Table 52-3).[11–14]

Drive Line–Associated Infections

Drive line–associated infections, as defined by purulent drainage around the drive line with or without positive cultures, are the most common device-associated infections occurring in patients with LVADs (Table 52-4). The

TABLE 52-3. Infection in Patients with Ventricular Assist Systems (VAS)

Reference	Ventricular Assist Systems (VAS)	Number of Patients	Infection Rate (%)
FDA 9	Novacor	156	103 (66)
FDA 10	HeartMate (pneumatic)	86	38 (44)
FDA 10	HeartMate (vented electric)	116	53 (46)
13	Novacor	25	12 (48)
14	HeartMate	60	29 (48)
11	Total artificial heart and VAS	584	166 (29)
12	Total artificial heart and VAS	258	82 (32)
TOTAL		1,285	483 (38)

TABLE 52-4. Drive line and Pump Pocket Infections in Patients with Ventricular Assist Systems (VAS)

Reference	VAS	Number	Drive Line Infection (%)	Pump Pocket Infections (%)
15	HeartMate/ Novacor/Thoratec	162	54 (33)	—
2	HeartMate	150	35 (23)	15 (10)
2	Novacor	55	10 (18)	4 (7)

incidence of drive line infections was 33% among 162 patients who had a mechanical bridge to transplant with at least 60 days of support, and increased significantly with duration of support (49% vs 25%, $p < .002$) after 100 days.[15] At our institution, drive line infections occurred in 35 patients (23% of 150 patients) with HeartMate devices and in 10 patients (18% of 55 patients) with Novacor devices.[2]

Pocket-Associated Infections

Pocket-associated infections often present with fever, localized pain, tenderness, erythema, and, eventually, erosion of the device through the skin or with purulent drainage from the drive line or other incisions. The incidence of pocket-associated infections among LVAD patients at our institution is approximately 10% (see Table 52-4).[2,15]

Nosocomial Bloodstream Infections in Patients with LVADs

Patients with implantable ventricular assist devices have a high incidence of nosocomial BSI (approximately 8 per 1,000 device days). We identified 140 BSIs among 214 patients with LVADs for an attack rate of 49% (104 of 214 patients with BSIs), of which 38% (of the 140 BSIs) were determined to be device associated.[16] A review of published reports of infections in patients with implantable LVADs with an emphasis on bloodstream infections are comparable to our findings (Table 52-5).[6,13–23] The overall attack rate for BSI was 38% (162 episodes in 425 patients; range, 16 to 53%) with an incidence of 5 per 1,000 device days (range, 1.8 to 7.9).

Approximately 50% of the pathogens causing BSI are gram-positive cocci (coagulase-negative staphylococci,

Staphylococcus aureus, and enterococci); approximately 10% are *Candida* species; and approximately 30% are gram-negative bacilli (*Pseudomonas aeruginosa, Enterobacter* sp, and *Klebsiella*).[16] The mean interval from implantation of device to onset of BSI was 23 days, with a difference in interval to bloodstream infections when stratified by pathogen group (fungi > gram-positive cocci > gram-negative rods).

Importantly, there appears to be a significant association between increased mortality while on device support for patients with BSIs. When stratified by pathogen groups, fungemia had the highest hazard ratio (10.9) for death on device, followed by gram-negative bacilli bacteremias (5.1), and then bacteremias due to gram-positive cocci (2.2). In addition, survival after cardiac transplantation in our series was not affected by an antecedent nosocomial BSI during LVAD support.

The most dramatic and, fortunately, least-common type of VAD-associated infections involves infection of the LVAD endovascular surface or valves, associated with fungemia or bacteremia (often relapsing). Diagnosis can be difficult, as extracardiac and device sources are often possible (eg, indwelling intravascular catheters). Direct visualization of inflow and outflow conduits by transthoracic or transesophageal echocardiography are difficult, but indirect measurements of flow may indicate a high degree of suspicion of conduit valve insufficiency. Cardiac catheterization theoretically can identify severe incompetence of the valve.

We identified 24 cases of LVAD endocarditis reported in the English literature, including 6 cases at our institution (Table 52-6).[3,8,14,24–27] Patients usually present with persistent or relapsing bloodstream infections and/or stroke. The most prevalent pathogens associated with LVAD endocarditis are *Candida* sp (33%), *Enterococcus* sp (21%), and *Pseudomonas aeruginosa* and coagulase-nega-

TABLE 52-5. Infections in Patients with Left Ventricular Assist Devices with an Emphasis on Bloodstream Infections (BSI)

Reference	Location	Study Time	N	Mean Onset to LVAD Infection (range)	LVAD Infection Attack Rate	LVAD BSI Attack Rate	LVAD (days)	LVAD BSI Incidence Rate*
13	Germany	1993–1996 Novocor	25	85 d (56–114)	48% (12/25)	16% (4/25)	—	—
17	Chicago	1994–1995 HeartMate	20	39 d (4–115)	30% (6/20)	20% (4/20)	—	8.4
18	Kansas City	1991–1995 HeartMate	18	37 d (3–77)	44.4% (8/18)	—	679	1.8
19	Ann Arbor	1996–1999 HeartMate	35	73 (13–133)	51.5% (18/25)	—	2,565	7
14	Columbia	1990–1995 HeartMate	60	93 (0–566)	—	27% (16/60)	—	—
20	Texas Heart Center	1986–1996 HeartMate	56	92.5 (0–504)	45% (25/56)	18% (10/56)	5,179	4.8
21	Sweden	1993–1999 HeartMate	10	241 (56–873)	40% (4/10)	—	2,410	—
22	Germany	1993–1999 HeartMate/Novocor	66	126 (18–244)	4.5% (3/66)	—	—	—
23	Germany	1993–1999 HeartMate	9	113.8 (23–205)	—	22% (2/9)	1,026	1.9
6	Alabama	1988–1997 HeartMate and Thoratec	41	74 ∀ 94 d	—	53% (22/41)	3,274	6.7
15	Pittsburgh (registry)	HeartMate/Novocor	162	—	33% (54/162)	—	—	—
16	Cleveland Clinic	1991–2000 HeartMate/Novocor	214	23 d	—	49% (104/214)	17,831	7.9
TOTAL			718		34% (130/382)	38% (162/425)	32,964	5

* Per 1,000 LVAD days.

TABLE 52-6. Clinical Presentation, Management, and Outcome in 24 Cases of LVAD Endocarditis

Reference	Patient	Clinical Presentation	Device	Onset (days)	Therapy/ Intervention	Outcome	Pathogen	Histopathology
14	1	Bacteremia/fever	HeartMate	225	Antibiotics	Survival/trx	Enterococcus faecalis	
14	2	Bacteremia/fever	HeartMate	80	Transplantation	Death	Staphylococcus epidermidis	
14	3	Fungemia/fever	HeartMate	77	LVAD replaced	Survival/trx	Candida parapsilosis	
14	4	Cachexia/failure to thrive	HeartMate	198	Antibiotics	Death	Escherichia coli	
14	5	Inflow obstruction	HeartMate	101		Survival	Pseudomonas aeruginosa	
14	6	Outflow graft rapture	HeartMate	26	Graft repair	Death	Staphylococcus aureus	
14	7	Cerebral embolization	HeartMate	23	Antibiotics	Death	Staphylococcus epidermidis	
14	8	Cerebral embolization	HeartMate	169	Transplantation	Survival/trx	Candida albicans	
24	9	Persistent fever/leukocytosis	HeartMate	77	Transplantation	Survival/trx	Candida albicans	Diaphragm of device
24	10	Cerebral embolization	HeartMate	50	Transplantation	Survival/trx	Candida albicans	Outflow graft and valve
24	11	LVAD outflow obstruction	HeartMate	17	LVAD explanted	Death	Syncephalastrum racemosum	Outflow graft
25	12	Fungemia/fever	HeartMate	210	Transplantation	Survival/trx	Candida albicans	Vegetations
25	13	Bacteremia/cerebral embolization	HeartMate	165	Exchange of device	Death	Vancomycin-resistant enterococcus	
21	14	Sepsis syndrome	HeartMate	78	Antibiotics	Death	—	Vegetations (autopsy)
8	15	Bacteremia	Novacor	100	Exchange of valves on VAD	Survival	Staphylococcus aureus	
26	16	Fungemia	Thoratec	—	Removal of VAD	Death	Candida albicans	
27	17	Relapsing bacteremia/ cerebral embolization	Novacor	416	Antibiotics	Death	Enterococcus faecium	
27	18	Relapsing bacteremia	Novacor	172	Exchange of device and transplantation	Survival/trx	Pseudomonas aeruginosa	
3	19	LVAD pocket infection	HeartMate	101	Transplantation	Survival/trx	Candida albicans	Inflow and outflow vegetations
3	20	Sepsis and relapsing fungemia	HeartMate	32	Replacement of device	Death	Candida albicans	Autopsy showed infection of new LVAD
Present report	21	Relapsing fungemia with embolic lesions (skin)	HeartMate	67	Transplantation	Survival/trx	Candida albicans	Vegetations
Present report	22	Cerebral embolization/sepsis	HeartMate	150	Antibiotics	Death	Staphylococcus aureus	Vegetations
Present report	23	Relapsing bacteremia	HeartMate	60	Antibiotics	Death	Vancomycin-resistant enterococci	Vegetation on autopsy
Present report	24	Relapsing bacteremia	HeartMate	75	Transplantation	Survival/trx	Staphylococcus aureus	Vegetations on inflow valve at explantation

trx = transplanted

tive staphylococci (8.3% each). The associated mortality with LVAD-associated endocarditis is 50%; however, 11 of 12 patients with LVAD-associated endocarditis who underwent transplantation survived.

The incidence of LVAD-associated endocarditis is difficult to ascertain, partly because investigators may use differing definitions. Investigators at Columbia reported a 13% incidence of endocarditis in patients with HeartMate LVADs (8 of 60 LVADs).[14] Notably, explanted HeartMate LVADs are immediately disassembled during surgery, allowing visual inspection and culturing of all blood-contacting LVAD surfaces (diaphragm, inflow-outflow valves, and inflow-outflow grafts). Disassembly of the Novacor inflow and outflow grafts in the operative theater is more difficult and limited compared to the HeartMate device. The incidence of LVAD-associated endocarditis among our 225 patients with LVADs (through 1999) was 3% (6 cases).

Management of LVAD-Associated Infections

Treatment of infected left ventricular assist devices includes both nonsurgical (antimicrobials) and surgical procedures such as débridement, device exchange, explantation, or flap coverage. Serious infections can be successfully managed with appropriate antimicrobial therapy and adjuvant surgical treatment, including tissue débridement, localized antimicrobial irrigation, drainage of infected fluids, and device exchange or device removal at the time of cardiac transplantation or following cardiac recovery.[6] At Columbia Presbyterian, almost 25% of the first 88 LVAD implantations developed device-associated infections. Forty percent (8 of 20) of these patients underwent surgical interventions with 63% survival, including three patients who were successfully transplanted.[28] Treatment plans should be tailored to the extent of infection and clinical situation of the patient, but first and foremost, one should always consider device explantation (with or without infection) if the patient can tolerate it hemodynamically.

Drive line exit-site infections unresponsive to conservative therapy may require surgical revision of the site, as described by McCarthy.[3] These infections are often associated with skin breakdown and are often caused by Staphylococcus sp (coagulase negative or positive).

Deep wound infections of either the mediastinum or abdominal pocket may require surgical exploration. Successful treatment of a preperitoneal pocket infection with S. epidermidis with in situ slow-release antibiotic-impregnated beads (vancomycin and tobramycin and polymethylmethacrylate), open irrigation, and drainage of the pocket has been reported.[29] This innovative approach has the advantage of high local concentrations of antimicrobials while avoiding systemic toxicities.

Mediastinitis complicating an LVAD has been successfully treated with a prolonged course of mediastinal and parenteral antibiotics, but most require surgical intervention.[30] Providing well-vascularized tissue has been well established in treatment of infections, and muscle flaps can accelerate the time to functional recovery. Omental transfer and muscle flaps in the posttransplant period have been used successfully in managing LVAD-associated mediastinitis. A rectus muscle flap is located adjacent to the site of device implantation, is often available for harvest, and provides sufficient bulk to cover the device. One must ensure the vascularity of the rectus has not been compromised (patients may have had coronary artery bypass graft with internal mammary artery graft) and determine whether the rectus abdominis muscle was previously transected by the drive line. If additional vascularized tissue is required, one may be able to raise an omental flap as well.

Externally exposed ventricular assist devices are associated with underlying infections of the preperitoneal pocket causing mediastinitis and high mortality rates. The options for surgical intervention are challenging at best. Device removal is usually not possible and device exchange may result in catastrophic complications.[3] Successful salvage often requires frequent and creative reconstructive procedures, often combining use of the omentum, musculocutaneous flaps, and systemic antimicrobial agents.[25]

Treatment of suspected or proven LVAD endocarditis is most challenging and associated with high rates of morbidity and mortality. Patients with relapsing bloodstream infections (episodes of positive blood cultures with the same organism) or persistent bloodstream infections without an extracardiac or device focus should be considered to have endovascular infection until proven otherwise. Endovascular infection in the setting of LVAD implantation is difficult to eradicate with antimicrobial agents. Reported surgical options include orthotopic heart transplantation, device exchange, or exploration with in situ valve exchange of the inflow and outflow graft valves in the Novacor devices without cardiopulmonary bypass.[8,31]

Morbidity and Mortality Associated with Device Infections

It is often difficult to distinguish between patients who die with infections from those in whom infection is directly attributed to the cause of death. Mortality rates attributed to infections (device and nondevice) during ventricular support range from 15 to 44%. Mortality from LVAD endocarditis has been reported at a single center to be almost 50%.[14,32]

The results of the Randomized Evaluation of Mechanical Assistance for the Treatment of Congestive Heart Failure (REMATCH) study underscores the significance of infections with long-term use of LVADs. A total of 129 patients with end-stage heart failure who were ineligible for cardiac transplantation were randomly assigned to receive either an LVAD (HeartMate) or optimal medical management.[33] Median survival was significantly longer in the device group (408 days vs 150 days) and mortality from all causes was 48% lower in the device group. However, late survival was similar at 24 months, with 41% (17 of 41) of deaths in the LVAD group attributed to sepsis.

Posttransplantation Outcomes: Impact of LVAD-Associated Infections

An area of controversy has been the transplantation of LVAD patients with active infections. Sihna and colleagues reported on 11 patients with active infections at the time of transplantation (6 device-associated).[34] Although two of these patients succumbed to infections within 30 days of transplantation, there was no significant difference in 6-month mortality between patients with and without infections while on LVAD support (18% noninfected vs 11% infection). The persistence of bloodstream infections or device-related infections with multidrug-resistant pathogens can serve as a basis to increase the urgency of transplantation. At the time of transplantation, the device and all foreign material are removed with the recipient's heart. The mediastinum, pump pocket, and pericardium are all carefully débrided, and then the donor heart is placed with meticulous hemostasis.

Infections persisting through the posttransplantation period require therapy, often 4 to 6 weeks, depending on pathogen, site, and clinical course.

Risk and Prevention of Infections in Patients with LVADS

The term *risk factor* has a particular meaning in epidemiology, and in the context of surgical site infection pathophysiology and prevention, it strictly refers to a variable that has a significant, independent association within the development of a surgical site infection after a specific operation.[7] Risk factors can be identified by epidemiologic studies by using both univariate and multivariate analyses. Knowledge of risk factors may allow for risk stratification of procedures (high vs low) and may identify targeted prevention measures. A surgical site prevention measure can be identified as an action or set of actions taken to reduce the risk of surgical site infections.

For VADs to reach their full potential, it will be necessary to better understand the pathogenesis of device-associated infections and to devise strategies for prevention. Although elimination of the drive lines with totally implantable systems remains a desirable goal, it will not eliminate all infectious complications (eg, pacemakers, prosthetic valve endocarditis). Basic research into the mechanism of biofilm production may identify surface interactions that can be manipulated to deter microbial colonization. Optimization of antimicrobial therapy (targeted to the results of cultures and the least-broad spectrum) is important to reduce selective pressure for antibiotic-resistant pathogens.[35]

There is increased interest in the immunologic effects of patients with implantable ventricular assist devices and associated infections with progressive defects in cellular immunity that may be the result of T-cell activation. These defects are associated with increased risk of candidal and other systemic infections.[36] Targeted approaches to downregulating abnormal immune reactivation in LVAD recipients may reduce the infection risk in patients on long-term support.

Patients who are receiving ventilatory support and those who are immobile are at risk for atelectasis and postoperative pneumonia. We make it a policy to mobilize patients and to wean them from ventilator support as soon as possible.

Malnourishment may lead to increased susceptibility to infection, and we try to provide enteral nutritional support as soon as possible, which may also prevent bacterial translocation from the gut. Parenteral nutrition is considered for patients with ileus.

Antimicrobial Prophylaxis in Patients with Ventricular Assist Devices

With the high rates of infections associated with patients with implantable assist devices there have been strategies to prevent infections with prophylactic use of antimicrobial agents. In particular, *Candida* sp has been identified as a pathogen of serious infection in patients with ventricular assist devices (up to 10% of bloodstream infections and 50% of endocarditis; see Table 52-6).[16] Skinner and colleagues recently reported on the burden of fungal infection or colonization (44% of 36 patients with LVADs).[26] Extended antifungal prophylaxis (use of azole or nystatin until all patients were extubated or all antibiotics were discontinued) was no more effective than use of antifungal agents for documented fungal colonization or infections.

Our approach to antimicrobial use in patients with implantable ventricular assist devices is to try to reduce or target antimicrobial therapy whenever possible and to avoid prophylaxis. We also employ oral antimicrobial agents (if the gut is functional) for treatment of nonendovascular infections (without sepsis syndrome) whenever possible. Patients who report questionable penicillin allergies (without anaphylaxis) should undergo skin testing to reduce unnecessary use of broad-spectrum antimicrobials.[37]

Preoperative nares colonization with *S. aureus* (carried in 20 to 30% of healthy humans) may be an independent risk factor for surgical site infections following cardiothoracic operations. Mupirocin ointment is effective as a topical agent for eradicating *S. aureus* from the nares of colonized patients or health care workers. Two studies associated intranasal mupirocin prophylaxis with a 60% reduction in wound infections following cardiac surgery when compared to historical controls.[38,39] However, approximately four patients would need to be exposed to drug for every patient colonized, resulting in overuse, increased cost, and problems with antimicrobial resistance. There are no studies of eradication of nasal carriage of *S. aureus* as an effective surgical wound infection prevention method in LVAD recipients.

We are currently looking into DNA sequence–based identification of *S. aureus* from nasal swabs among patients scheduled for cardiac surgery, which would permit timely targeted prophylaxis, using intranasal mupirocin for those patients colonized with *S. aureus*.

Prevention of Device-Associated Infections

We recommend early complete immobilization of the drive line site in the postoperative period to promote tissue in-growth to occur. An abdominal binder may be used for patient comfort and drive line immobilization if the pump has been placed in the preperitoneal position.

All wound care must be performed with sterile technique, including mask and gloves. We routinely use a silver-impregnated dressing (Arglaes, Medline Industries, Inc., Mundelein, IL) for the drive line exit site for all patients with VADs. The dressing is designed to slowly release ionic silver at the application site in response to contact with water vapor. The transparent dressing allows for inspection of the wound without disturbing the tissue or healing process. For uncomplicated wounds, the dressing may be left intact for a period of 7 days.

An antimicrobial-impregnated drive line may be another strategy to prevent infections. Successful animal models employed drive lines impregnated with chlorhexidine, triclosan, and silver sulfadiazine, and plans for human trials are underway.[40]

Surgical Considerations: Pump Placement

The pump can be placed in most patients within the abdomen or within the preperitoneal space or rectus sheath.[41,42] In one study, device-associated LVAD infections were significantly lower in intraperitoneal HeartMate-supported patients (intraperitoneal, 14% [5 of 37], vs extraperitoneal, 46% [5 of 11]).[41] However, intraabdominal implantation may cause adhesions to the viscera, with increased risk of obstruction or colonic perforation. At the Cleveland Clinic, preperitoneal placement of ventricular assist devices is preferred, and intraabdominal sites for selected patients expected to have long-term implants (eg, permanent implants or those who are highly sensitized to human leukocyte antigens).

Vaccinations in Patients on Ventricular Assist Devices

All patients with VAD should be assessed for vaccine-preventable illness, including pneumococcal infection, influenza, and hepatitis B. The adult pneumococcal vaccine contains the capsular polysaccharides of 23 pneumococcal types and should be given as a single intramuscular dose (0.5 mL). Revaccination is recommended for patients who received their first immunization more than 6 years earlier.

Influenza vaccine contains two type A strains and one type B strain, which represent the most recent influenza viruses circulating in the world. The vaccine is inactivated and cannot cause infection. All patients with VADs should undergo vaccination (unless a patient has a true egg allergy) as a primary prevention for influenza. We have had several documented cases of nosocomial influenza infections in patients with VADs, and in one patient, influenza caused the postponement of heart transplantation.

We also recommend immunization of all nonimmune patients with implantable assist devices to reduce the risk of transmission of hepatitis B from the donor at the time of transplantation.

Devices for the Future

Infectious complications associated with our current ventricular assist systems are the major limitations to long-term use of LVAD support in patients who are not transplant candidates.[33,43] Control of infection in these devices may be improved with new designs, antibiotic-impregnated drive lines, and innovative therapies. For example, the Jarvik 2000 system consists of a small (90 g) intraventricular axial flow pump that transmits power and data via internal electronics through a thin power line attached to a skill-based pedestal. It does not have valves (therefore no risk of device-associated endocarditis) and is currently being investigated as a bridge to transplantation.

The next generation of ventricular assist systems should be inherently less susceptible to infections because of smaller size, reduced thrombogenicity, and transcutaneous energy transmission systems.[44]

References

1. Goldstein DJ, Oz MC, Rose EA. Implantable left ventricular assist devices. N Engl J Med 1998;339:1522–33.
2. Kasirajan V, McCarthy PM, Hoercher K, et al. Clinical experience with long-term use of implantable left ventricular assist devices: indications, implantation, and outcomes. Semin Thorac Cardiothorac Surg 2000;12:229–37.
3. McCarthy PM, Schmitt SK, Vargo RL, et al. Implantable LVAD infections: implications for permanent use of the device. Ann Thorac Surg 1996;61:359–65.
4. McCarthy PM, Sabik JF. Implantable circulatory support devices as a bridge to heart transplantation. Semin Thorac Surg 1994;6:174–80.
5. Garner JS, Jarvis WR, Emori TG, et al. CDC definitions for nosocomial infections. Am J Infect Control 1988;16:128–40.
6. Holman, WL, Skinner JL, Waiter KB, et al. Infection during circulatory support with ventricular assist devices. Ann Thorac Surg 1999;68:711–6.
7. Mangram AJ, Horan TC, Pearson ML, et al. Guideline for prevention of surgical site infection, 1999. Infect Control Hosp Epidemiol 1999;20:250–78.
8. de Jonge KC, Laube HR, Dohmen PM, et al. Diagnosis and management of left ventricular device valve endocarditis: LVAD valve replacement. Ann Thorac Surg 2000;70:1404–5.
9. United States Food and Drug Administration. Summary of safety and effectiveness data for the Novacor left ventricular assist system. http://www.fda.gov.cdrh/pdf/p980012b.pdf.
10. United States Food and Drug Administration: Summary of safety and effectiveness data for supplemental application. HeartMate vented electric left ventricular assist system (VE LVAS). http://www.fda.gov.cdrh/pdf/p920014s007b.pdf.
11. Mehta SM, Aufiero TX, Pae WE Jr, et al. Combined registry for the clinical use of mechanical ventricular assist pumps and the total artificial heart in conjunction with heart transplantation: sixth official report—1994. J Heart Lung Transplant 1995;14:585–93.
12. Quania E, Pavie A, Chieco S, Mambrito B. The Concerted Action (Heart) European registry on clinical application of mechanical circulatory support systems: bridge to transplant. The Registry Scientific Committee. Eur J Cardiothorac Surg 1997;11:182–8.
13. Herrmann M, Weyand M, Greshake B, et al. Left ventricular assist device infection is associated with increased mortality but is not a contraindication to transplantation. Circulation 1997;95:814–7.
14. Argenziano M, Catanese KA, Moazami N, et al. The influence of infection on survival and successful transplantation in patients with left ventricular assist devices. J Heart Lung Transplant 1997;16:822–31.
15. Griffith BP, Kormos RL, Mastala CJ, et al. Results of extended bridge to transplantation: window into the future of permanent ventricular assist devices. Ann Thorac Surg 1996;61:396–8.
16. Gordon SM, Schmitt SK, Jacobs M, et al. Nosocomial bloodstream infections in patients with implantable left ventricular assist devices. Ann Thorac Surg 2001;72:725–30.
17. Fischer SA, Trenholme GM, Costanzo MR, Piccone W. Infectious complications in left ventricular device assist device recipients. Clin Infect Dis 1997;24:18–23.
18. Prendergast TW, Todd BA, Beyer AJ, et al. Management of left ventricular assist device infection with heart transplantation. Ann Thorac Surg 1997;64:142–7.
19. Malani PN, Dyke DB, Chenoweth CE. Nosocomial infections in left ventricular assist devices [abstract]. 38th Annual meeting of Infectious Disease Society of America; 2000 September 7–10. New Orleans.
20. Springer WE, Wasler A, Radovancevic B, et al. Retrospective analysis of infection in patients undergoing support with left ventricular assist systems. ASAIO J 1996;42:M763–5.

21. Peterzen B, Granfeldt H, Lonn D, et al. Management of patients with end-stage heart disease treated with an implantable left ventricular assist device in a nontransplanting center. J Cardiothorac Vasc Anesth 2000;14: 438–43.

22. Tjan TDT, Asfour B, Hammel D, et al. Wound complications after left ventricular assist device implantation. Ann Thorac Surg 2000;70:538–41.

23. Arusoglu L, Koerfer R, Tenderich G, et al. A novel method to reduce device-related infections in patients supported with the HeartMate device. Ann Thorac Surg 1999;68: 1875–7.

24. Nurozler F, Argenziano M, Oz MC, Naka Y. Fungal left ventricular assist device endocarditis. Ann Thorac Surg 2001;71:614–8.

25. Turowski GA, Orgill DP, Pribaz JJ, et al. Salvage of externally exposed assist devices. Plast Reconstr Surg 1998;102: 2425–9.

26. Skinner JL, Harris C, Aaron MF, et al. Cost-benefit analysis of extended antifungal prophylaxis in ventricular assist devices. ASAIO J 2000;45:587–9.

27. Vilchez R, McEllistrem MC, Harrison LH, et al. Relapsing bacteremia in patients with ventricular assist device: an emergent complication of extended circulatory support. Ann Thorac Surg 2001;72:96–101.

28. Hutchinson OZ, Oz MC, Ascherman JA. The use of muscle flaps to treat left ventricular assist device infections. Plast Reconstr Surg 2001;107:364–73.

29. McKellar SH, Allred BD, Marks JD, et al. Treatment of infected ventricular assist device using antibiotic-impregnated beads. Ann Thorac Surg 1999;67:554–5.

30. Rooks JR, Burton NA, Lefrak EA, Macmanus Q. Mediastinitis complicating successful mechanical bridge to heart transplantation. J Heart Lung Transplant 1992;11: 261–4.

31. Schmitz C, Roell W, Dewald O, et al. Replacement of the valves of a Novacor LVAS without cardiopulmonary bypass. Thorac Cardiovasc Surg 2000;48:380–1.

32. Oz MC, Argenziano M, Cantanese KA, et al. Bridge experience with long-term implantable left ventricular assist devices: are they an alternative to transplantation? Circulation 1997;95:1844–52.

33. Rose EA, Gelijns AC, Moskwitz AJ, et al. Long-term use of a left ventricular assist device for end-stage heart failure. N Engl J Med 2001:345:1435–43.

34. Sinha P, Chen JM, Flannery M, et al. Infections during left ventricular assist device support does not affect post-transplant outcomes. Circulation 2000;102 Suppl III: III-194–9.

35. Burns GL. Infections associated with implanted blood pumps. Int J Artif Organs 1993;16:771–6.

36. Ankersmit HS, Tugulea S, Spanier T, et al. Activation of T-cell death and immune dysfunction after implantation of left ventricular device. Lancet 1999;354:550–5.

37. Arroliga ME, Wagner W, Bobek MB, et al. A pilot study of penicillin skin testing in patients with a history of penicillin allergy admitted to a medical intensive care unit. Chest 2000;118:1106–8.

38. Cimochowski GE, Harostock MD, Brown R, et al. Intranasal mupirocin reduces sternal wound infection after open heart surgery in diabetics and nondiabetics. Ann Thorac Surg 2001;71:1572–9.

39. Kluytmans JAJW, Mouton JW, VandenBergh MFQ, et al. Reduction of surgical-site infections in cardiothoracic surgery by elimination of nasal carriage of Staphylococcus aureus. Infect Control Hosp Epidemiol 1996;17: 780–5.

40. Choi L, Choudhri AF, Pillarisetty VG, et al. Development of an infection-resistant LVAD drive line: a novel approach to the prevention of device-related infections. J Heart Lung Transplant 1999;18:1103–10.

41. Wasler A, Springer WE, Radovancevic B, et al. A comparison between intraperitoneal and extraperitoneal left ventricular assist system placement. ASAIO J 1996;42: M573–6.

42. Oz MC, Goldstein DJ, Rose EA. Preperitoneal placement of ventricular assist devices: an illustrated stepwise approach. J Card Surg 1995;10:288–94.

43. Meyers TJ, Khan T, Frazier OH. Infectious complications associated with ventricular assist systems. ASAIO J 2000; 46:S28–36.

44. McCarthy PM, Smith WA. Mechanical and circulatory support: a long and winding road. Science 2002;295: 998–9.

CHAPTER 53

CURRENT STATUS OF TOTAL ARTIFICIAL HEARTS

ROBERT D. DOWLING, MD, LAMAN A. GRAY JR, MD

The prevalence of congestive heart failure continues to increase, and current estimates are that heart failure affects 4.7 million people in the United States alone, with 500,000 new cases diagnosed annually. Despite improvements in medical management, 5-year survival remains below 50% for all patients with heart failure, and for those patients with advanced disease, 1-year survival is quite poor. A significant portion of these patients could benefit from some type of cardiac replacement therapy. Currently, heart transplantation is the only approved method for replacing the failing heart. However, there is a severe shortage of donor organs, with only 2,198 heart transplants being performed in the United States in the year 2000. Furthermore, in 3 of the last 4 years, there has been a decrease in the number of heart transplants performed in the United States.[1] Transplantation is also limited by strict medical, psychosocial, and financial criteria. The need for chronic immunosuppression and aggressive surveillance also place severe limitations on the potential impact of heart transplantation. Long-term survival has also been limited, primarily by the development of allograft coronary artery disease. Clearly, there is a significant need for alternative approaches to replace the failing heart.

The first use of a total artificial heart was as a bridge to transplantation in 1969. This initial patient was sustained for 62 hours until a donor heart could be transplanted.[2] In 1982, the Jarvik 7 was implanted into Dr. Barney Clark.[3] This device was intended as a permanent replacement for the natural heart. The Jarvik 7 device was pneumatically actuated and required large percutaneous lines with the patient being tethered to large control consoles. Due to complications associated with the device, clinical implants as destination therapy were halted in 1990. The Jarvik heart was used successfully in 1985 as a bridge to transplantation. This system is currently known as the CardioWest Total Artificial Heart and has been used since 1993 by the group at the University of Arizona as a bridge to transplantation, with an 80% survival rate.[4] After initiation of clinical trials of the Jarvik 7 heart, the National Heart, Lung and Blood Institute initiated funding for a total arti-

ficial heart with the potential of improved quality of life by allowing for patient discharge and improved ability to perform the activities of daily living. Initially, six centers were funded, with this number eventually being decreased to two—the Penn State Total Electrical Artificial Heart, which was developed in conjunction with the 3M company, and the AbioCor Implantable Replacement Heart.[5] Recently, ABIOMED Inc. (Danvers, MA) acquired the Penn State Total Artificial Heart, making this the only system that will be undergoing clinical trials in the near future.

Device Description

The AbioCor Implantable Replacement Heart consists of both internal and external components.[6,7] The internal components are the AbioCor thoracic unit, internal battery, controller, and transcutaneous energy transfer (TET) coil (Figure 53-1). The internal battery is lithium ion based and is able to power the thoracic unit for brief periods of time (up to 30 min). The internal controller regulates the thoracic unit and transmits device performance data to a bedside console via radiofrequency telemetry. The internal TET coil receives energy transmitted across

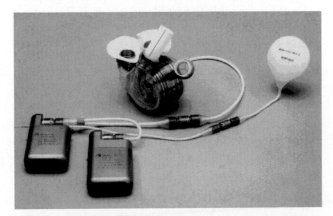

FIGURE 53-1. Internal components of the AbioCor Implantable Replacement Heart system include the thoracic unit, controller, battery, and TET coil.

the skin from the external TET coil and transmits it to the thoracic unit and to the internal battery. The AbioCor thoracic unit itself consists of two pumping chambers that function as the left and right ventricles. An energy converter is situated between the right and left ventricles, which contains an electrically driven centrifugal pump which provides continuous unidirectional hydraulic fluid motion. Hydraulic fluid flow reversal is achieved by a two-position switching valve that alternates the direction of hydraulic flow between the left and right pumping chamber; this results in alternate left and right systole. The beat rate of the thoracic unit is determined by the frequency ("the rate") of the switching valve. The pump motor impeller and the switching valve are essentially the only moving parts of the energy converter. All blood-contacting surfaces of the AbioCor thoracic unit, including the trileaflet valves (24 mm internal diameter), are polyurethane (Angioflex). This results in a smooth, continuous blood-contacting surface from the inflow cuffs to the outflow grafts. The beat rate of the device can be varied between 60 and 150 beats per minute. Stroke volume is 60 to 65 cc, and the device is therefore capable of providing a flow rate of 4 to 10 L/min. An atrial balance chamber is present and allows for decreased right-sided stroke volume to maintain right and left fluid balance.[3] Essentially, a portion of hydraulic fluid is shunted into the balance chamber rather than to the right pumping chamber. The balance chamber has effectively provided for left-to right-balance in all of the preclinical implants and all of the clinical implants to date.

External components consist of an external TET coil, external batteries, and external patient-carried electronics (Figure 53-2). The external TET coil transfers energy from batteries or a standard wall outlet across the skin to the internal TET coil. An adhesive alginate hydrocolloid dressing (Kendall Co., Mansfield, MA) with Velcro attachments is placed directly over the internal TET coil. The external TET coil is then connected to the dressing via the Velcro attachments. This has resulted in excellent patient comfort and minimal episodes of TET coil dislodgment. The external batteries are able to provide up to 1 h of support per pound of battery. The external batteries can either be carried in a vest or a handbag, or attached to a Velcro belt. The patient-carried electronics contains basic alarm systems similar to current-generation LVADs. When the patient is not mobile, device performance data are transmitted to a bedside console via radiofrequency telemetry. This is done on a beat-by-beat basis and includes parameters such as left and right motor speed, energy requirements, right and left hydraulic fluid pressures, and beat rate.

Preclinical Experience

Preclinical experience with the AbioCor device was initiated at the Texas Heart Institute under the direction of O.H. Frazier, MD. Initial experience allowed for refine-

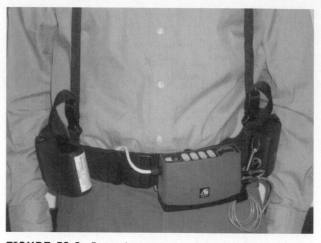

FIGURE 53-2. External components of the AbioCor Implantable Replacement Heart system include the batteries and a portable TET module, which contains basic alarms.

ment of the operating technique, which rapidly allowed for the long-term in vivo implants. In 1994, Parnis and colleagues reported on the Texas Heart Institute experience with chronic in vivo implants.[8] They demonstrated excellent performance of the device for more than 2 months in calves with weights in excess of 100 kg. The device was able to adequately maintain normal end-organ function and did not result in elevated plasma-free hemoglobin. The balance chamber was effective in maintaining left–right balance as evidenced by normal left and right atrial pressures over a range of cardiac outputs. These initial studies, which involved placement of the AbioCor thoracic unit alone, were followed by further animal studies that eventually incorporated all the internal components as described above. Further in vivo experiments were performed by our group at the University of Louisville. Working with the Texas Heart Institute team, we were rapidly able to become proficient with the implant procedure. We began a series of 30-day implants, culminating in 29 implants performed under Good Laboratory Practice guidelines and submitted to the US Food and Drug Administration for review. All animals that underwent operation had implantation of pressure catheters in the superior vena cava (SVC), inferior vena cava (IVC), pulmonary artery, and carotid arteries. A side port on the atrial cuffs allowed for continuous monitoring of the right and left atrial pressures. We were also able to demonstrate that animals maintained normal kidney and liver function without evidence of significant hemolysis. The presence of a catheter in the pulmonary artery allowed for daily measurements of mixed venous saturations, which demonstrated adequate tissue perfusion with hematocrits in the mid to low twenties. All animals demonstrated normal systemic pressures as well as normal pulmonary artery pressures. There was excellent function of the atrial balance chamber as evidenced by normal left and right atrial pressures. These animals demonstrated normal neurologic activity and were ambulated at least three times a week, either on a large animal treadmill or in the halls. Serial measurements of serum lactate levels demonstrated that animals with the AbioCor device were able to maintain aerobic metabolism not only at rest but also with low levels of exercise. The AbioCor thoracic units did not have any device malfunctions, and there was also excellent function of the internal battery, internal controller, and TET coil. We did not see any evidence of thermal injury related to the transcutaneous energy transfer system.

Clinical Trials

Because the AbioCor Implantable Replacement Heart is designed as destination therapy, patients selected for the initial clinical trials cannot be candidates for other types of therapy, including heart transplantation. Because of the nature of the clinical trial, it was thought best to select patients with a high predicted mortality. All patients who were considered as candidates had a 30-day predicted mortality of greater than 70% based on the AbioScore prognostic model or acute myocardial infarction (AMI) shock scores. The AbioScore mortality prediction model was developed by the team at ABIOMED and was based on previous prognostic models; parameters were selected that were appropriate for patients with end-stage heart failure. Initial retrospective studies were followed by prospective studies to verify that this was an accurate prediction model. Potential candidates must be adult patients with biventricular failure who are dependent on inotropes or unable to tolerate inotropes due to severe arrhythmias. Patients are excluded from the study if they are felt to be candidates for other conventional therapies or if they have a predicted survival of greater than 70% at 30 days. Patients are also excluded if they have end-organ dysfunction that is thought not to be reversible. A complete psychosocial evaluation is performed on all potential recipients, similar to that performed in patients being considered for transplantation. We feel that an adequate support system is crucial to help the patient in the recovery period. Patients meeting the appropriate inclusion criteria undergo computerized tomography scan of the chest, followed by an AbioFit virtual fit evaluation. The AbioFit evaluation is a three-dimensional computerized image of the AbioCor thoracic unit superimposed upon the imagery of the patient's mediastinal and chest wall structures. This computer simulation allows us to view the position of the AbioCor in the potential recipient's chest from every possible angle. This virtual surgery allows us to determine whether we can position the AbioCor thoracic unit in the chest without impinging on vital structures such as the left pulmonary veins and the left lower-lobe bronchus. The surgical implant team must believe that the AbioFit program does predict that the thoracic unit will fit in the chest prior to proceeding with operative therapy.

During this extensive evaluation, the patient and the patient's family receive intensive education on the device, including the results of reliability studies, preclinical trials, and the results of previous human implants.

For every patient that enters or considers entering the AbioCor clinical trial, an independent patient advocate is made available to them and their families to assist in the understanding of the potential risks and benefits of entering the clinical trial. This represents an unprecedented innovation in the protection of human subjects in clinical research projects that was introduced by ABIOMED. The patient advocate is able to help the patient and the patient's family to interpret the contents of the informed consent document. After the implant procedure, the patient advocate continues to be available to the patient and family for assistance in making other important medical decisions. All patient advocates have background in clinical medicine and all function completely independently of both the sponsoring company and the medical teams.[6]

Operative Approach

The operative approach for the AbioCor system was initially developed in a bovine model. This operative approach consisted of placement of the thoracic unit and other internal components through a left thoracotomy. As we approached clinical trials, we performed a number of implants in the cadaver lab in an attempt to finalize the details of the operative approach in humans prior to beginning the human clinical trials. We also began implanting the AbioCor device in a pig model through a median sternotomy, again to re-create as closely as possible a model similar to what would be used in the clinical studies.

At operation, an infraclavicular incision is made and a pocket is created above the pectoral muscle fascia for placement of the internal TET coil. A median sternotomy incision is then made, and the TET coil is placed in its pocket with the cable being passed to the lower part of the sternotomy incision. The incision over the TET coil is then closed in two layers with running suture. The pocket for the TET coil is made first so that this can be completed before the patient is given heparin, in the hope that this will decrease the likelihood of a pocket wound hematoma. A sternal retractor is placed and a pericardial cradle is created. Dissection for the internal battery and controller is made. This can be performed either in the preperitoneal space or deep to the rectus abduminus muscle (ie, on top of the posterior rectus sheath). The patient is heparinized and cannulas are placed. Cannulation of the aorta or femoral artery is performed, depending on the length of aorta available, as most of these patients will have had previous cardiac surgery. An SVC cannula is placed and a venous cannula is placed through the femoral vein and guided up into position just below the junction of the IVC and the right atrium. Cardiopulmonary bypass is initiated, the caval tapes are snared down, and the aorta is cross-clamped. The right and left ventricles are excised just above the AV groove. The mitral and tricuspid valves are excised. The left atrial cuff is trimmed to appropriate diameter and sewn to the native left atrium at the level of the annulus, using two layers of running 4–0 Prolene reinforced with felt strips. Leak testing is performed after the creation of each anastomosis to decrease the likelihood of suture line bleeding after placement of the device. Anastomosis of the right atrial cuff to the native right atrium is then performed in similar fashion, followed by leak testing to insure that the suture line is likely to be hemostatic. A dummy model of the AbioCor device is positioned in the chest to determine the appropriate length and orientation of the outflow grafts to the aorta and pulmonary artery. These outflow grafts are then sewn end-to-end to the great vessels with running 4–0 Prolene suture. The AbioCor thoracic unit is then brought up to the operative field and appropriate electrical connections are made. The AbioCor is placed in the pericardial space and attached to the atrial cuffs via screw-lock quick-connects. The device is completely de-aired by allowing air to be ejected through side ports arising from the outflow grafts. Once the right side of the heart has been de-aired, the side port of the pulmonary artery outflow graft is occluded and the left side of the heart is de-aired through the side port that arises from the aortic outflow graft. After the device is adequately de-aired, the cross-clamp is removed and the patient is rapidly weaned from cardiopulmonary bypass onto full AbioCor support. The left and right filling pressures are used to determine adjustment of the beat rate and to adjust the balance chamber. The anesthetic management for these patients has been previously described.[9]

Clinical implants of the AbioCor Implantable Replacement Heart were initiated on July 2, 2001. The first recipient was a 59-year-old African American male with a history of ischemic cardiomyopathy and end-stage heart failure. He had a history of emergency coronary artery bypass surgery after acute anterior wall myocardial infarction. He had developed progressive worsening of symptoms and had been evaluated by a number of excellent transplant centers and felt not to be a candidate due to severe malnutrition, pulmonary artery hypertension, and chronic renal insufficiency. He was placed on maximal medical therapy including three inotropes. This patient had seen a description of the AbioCor device in the lay press and approached his cardiologist, who was familiar with the preclinical work. When initially seen by our group he was noted to be severely malnourished and on three inotropes, with systolic blood pressures in the seventies. Placement of a pulmonary artery catheter demonstrated a maximum cardiac index of 1.4 with pulmonary artery pressures in the 60 to 70 mm Hg range. His admission serum creatinine of 3.4 improved after placement of an intraaortic balloon pump. The patient was found to

meet all inclusion criteria, and the AbioFit predicted an excellent fit of the device in the chest. The patient's intraoperative course was unremarkable despite the presence of severe adhesions from a previous surgery. His initial postoperative course was remarkable for gastrointestinal (GI) bleeding each time he was placed on appropriate anticoagulation. He did have a history of remote GI bleeding, and because of this history, he underwent upper endoscopy as part of his preoperative evaluation. There were no abnormalities found on a complete upper endoscopy, and the preoperative assessment was that he would be unlikely to have significant problems with upper GI bleeding. However, when he was placed on heparin, he consistently developed punctate bleeding from multiple sites in his stomach. During his first 2 postoperative months, he was managed solely on antiplatelet therapy for 80% of the time. By the third month, as his nutritional status improved, he was able to tolerate therapeutic Coumadin in addition to his antiplatelet therapy. He continued to gain strength, and plans were being made for his discharge from the hospital. On postoperative day 130, he suffered a large stroke. His anticoagulation was therefore increased and he subsequently developed a psoas muscle bleed, which resulted in multisystem organ failure. He expired on postoperative day 151 following his implant.

The second AbioCor recipient was a 70-year-old male with ischemic cardiomyopathy. He had refractory heart failure despite the multiple inotropes and placement of an intraaortic balloon pump. He has had no previous surgery, which facilitated placement of the AbioCor device. His postoperative course has been complicated by aspiration pneumonitis and malignant neuroleptic syndrome with peak temperature of 41.7°C. Fortunately, this central fever responded dramatically to initiation of therapy with dantrolene. Currently, he is more than 6 months from his surgery and has continued to improve. He is doing well after being discharged to home 4 months ago. He has had no thromboembolic events.

Summary

Clinical trials with the AbioCor Implantable Replacement Heart recently began after decades of development. The key design feature is the absence of percutaneous lines, which is achieved by energy transfer across the skin, using inductive coupling. An atrial balance chamber is also present in the thoracic unit, which has allowed for left-to-right balance in all the preclinical implants and in all the clinical implants to date. The initial cohort of patients demonstrates that this system is well tolerated and allows for excellent patient mobility. Continuations of the clinical trials are needed to define the roles of this technology in the treatment of patients with severe end-stage heart failure.

References

1. UNOS Critical Data. U.S. Facts about Transplantation (n.d.). http://www.unos.org/newsroom/critdata_main.htm (accessed April 23, 2002).

2. Cooley DA, Liotta D, Hallman GL, et al. Orthotopic cardiac prosthesis for two-staged cardiac replacement. Am J Cardiol 1969;24:723–30.

3. Devries WC. The permanent artificial heart: four case reports. JAMA 1988;259:849–59.

4. Copeland JG 3rd, Smith RG, Arabia FA, et al. Comparison of the CardioWest Total Artificial Heart, the Novacor left ventricular assist system and the Thoratec ventricular assist system in bridge to transplantation. Ann Thorac Surg 2001;71:S92–7.

5. Frazier OH. Mechanical cardiac assistance: historical perspectives. Semin Thorac Cardiovasc Surg 2000;12(3):207–20.

6. Dowling RD, Etoch SW, Stevens KA, et al. Current status of the AbioCor implantable replacement heart. Ann Thorac Surg 2001;71:S147–9.

7. Dowling RD, Etoch SW, Stevens K, et al. Initial experience with the totally implantable AbioCor replacement heart at the University of Louisville. ASAIO J 2000;46:579–81.

8. Parnis SM, Yu LS, Ochs BD, et al. Chronic in vivo evaluation of an electrohydraulic total artificial heart. ASAIO J 1994;40(3):M489–93.

9. Theilmeier KA, Pank JR, Dowling RD, Gray LA. Anesthetic and perioperative considerations in patients undergoing placement of totally implantable replacement hearts. Semin Cardiothorac Vasc Anesth 2001;5:335–44.

CHAPTER 54

HEART PRESERVATION

JOHN V. CONTE, MD

Successful cardiac transplantation is dependent on the safe procurement and preservation of the donor heart. Current techniques of heart preservation allow a 4- to 6-h period of safe ischemic storage in most cases. The limited donor supply and growing recipient waiting lists make it imperative that every available organ is used, regardless of the distance between the donor hospital and the recipient institution. By the very nature of its function, cardiac transplantation is different from other types of solid-organ transplantation—immediate function of the donor organ is necessary for recipient survival. This limits the ability to use marginal donors and makes optimal preservation mandatory.

While the optimal method for heart preservation has yet to be identified, many of the mechanisms involved in cell injury and death during organ preservation are known. An understanding of these mechanisms can help with understanding the current approaches to cardiac preservation and the goals of current research efforts. This chapter provides the reader with an appreciation of the historical highlights of cardiac preservation and an understanding of the current state of the art of clinical cardiac preservation and laboratory studies, which may impact on the future of solid-organ preservation.

Historical Highlights

Lower and Shumway studied heart preservation, using immersion in hypothermic saline more than four decades ago, and hypothermia has subsequently proved to be the most important unifying concept in organ preservation.[1,2] Hypothermia reportedly reduces the tissues' metabolic rate by as much as 99%, and cooling produces a twofold decrease in the activity of most cellular enzymes for every 10°C decrease in temperature.[3,4] Even today, despite a dramatically advanced understanding of cellular metabolism and organ preservation, hypothermia remains the time-proven central component of organ preservation of all solid organs.

As the finite limits of hypothermic organ preservation became apparent, Robicsek, in 1969, in an attempt to prolong the acceptable periods of cardiac preservation, introduced ex vivo continuous perfusion of organs with normothermic blood to mimic the native condition.[5]

Later, clinical experience was obtained at the University of Pittsburgh by using an autoperfusion apparatus for heart–lung preservation.[6,7] This technique was abandoned because of the logistical problems, the cumbersome nature of these systems, and the general impression that the beneficial effects of continuous oxygen delivery, substrate enhancement, and the washout of metabolic byproducts were offset by the increased tissue edema caused by the perfusion apparatus and sequestration of white blood cells. However, recent success with ex vivo preservation and resuscitation of renal allografts has led to renewed interest in cardiac perfusion techniques for organ preservation. Investigations of perfusion preservation techniques that use both blood-based and asanguinous solutions are currently underway.[8,9]

Donor core cooling on cardiopulmonary bypass was introduced initially for combined heart–lung transplantation, to uniformly cool the donor. It carries with it the beneficial properties afforded by using blood as a perfusate in that it is a colloid; contains free radical scavengers, natural buffers, oxygen, and metabolic substrates; and avoids unequal distribution of the flush solution and organ cooling which can occur with single-flush techniques.[10] At least one center's report showed no advantage over hypothermic single-flush techniques and that center has abandoned its use.[11] Although this technique is cumbersome and expensive because of the additional personnel and equipment required, it is still the preferred technique at some centers.[12]

The single-flush technique emerged in the 1970s, coincident with the explosion of coronary artery surgery. The essential components of this technique consists of clamping the aorta and perfusing the heart with a K^+-containing solution to arrest the heart and render it asanguinous and hypothermic before it is excised and stored in a hypothermic crystalloid solution. The combination of electromechanical silence and organ cooling was felt to reduce the metabolic rate to allow an extended period of ischemic tolerance and enable successful distal procurement. A variety of cardioplegic solutions have evolved, which were successfully employed in laboratory, and later in clinical, transplantation.[13–15] The development of new solutions or modifications of known solutions, has remained a central focus of organ preservation researchers for much of the last two decades. In a 1992 report of a survey of cardiac transplantation programs by researchers at Papworth Hospital, 92% of programs employed a single-flush technique.[16] Despite the near universal use of a single-flush technique, the techniques used at different institutions are rendered unique by manipulation of the many variables discussed throughout this chapter.

Donor Organ Injury

Some degree of tissue injury is inevitable with organ preservation. Donor injury can occur at many points in the donor procurement process. This injury can be exacerbated by multiple factors prior to harvest, during preservation, and following implantation. Brain death itself is incompletely understood and may initiate pathologic processes that negatively impact on the ability of a given organ to tolerate ischemia during organ preservation. Increased intracranial pressures lead to the development of neurohormonal axis abnormalities of thyroid hormone, antidiuretic hormone, and cortisol regulation in brain-dead patients. These abnormalities likely play an important role in donor management and, ultimately, in the suitability of an organ for transplantation.

Hypoxia at the time of the initial event leading to brain death can be the initial insult to the donor organ. This hypoxic injury can be compounded during resuscitative efforts and through attempts to achieve hemodynamic stability. This can include mechanical injury due to cardiopulmonary resuscitation, cardiac distension due to fluid overload secondary to volume resuscitation, and prolonged use of high-dose inotropes and vasoconstricting agents. Hemodynamic instability, loss of thermal regulation, massive fluid shifts, and metabolic derangements are all common problems following brain death. Hemodynamic instability can lead to microinfarctions caused by hypo- and hypertensive episodes. Metabolic and electrolyte imbalances and fluid shifts can result in tissue edema and cellular dysfunction. The net effect of these events may be cardiac injury and functional derangements occurring even before the donor organ is inspected and its suitability for transplantation determined.

Further damage may occur during the procurement process, due to mechanical trauma and cardioplegia, and during the period of hypothermic storage. Hypothermia, despite being the cornerstone of organ preservation, can have deleterious effects resulting in cytoplasmic and nuclear swelling as well as mitochondrial injury.[1] Hypothermic inactivation of membrane-bound enzymes alters the permeability of lipid bilayers of the cell wall, resulting in edema formation. Cell volume regulation is lost as the Na^+-K^+–adenosine triphosphatase (ATPase) pump is inhibited, permitting the entry of sodium. Water passively enters the cell to equalize the osmotic and ionic gradients. Further alterations of the internal milieu occurs when the Ca^{2+}–ATPase pump is inactivated, resulting in

the intracellular sequestration of calcium. Despite the reduction of cellular metabolism during hypothermic storage, high-energy phosphate stores are eventually depleted, resulting in the need for alternate pathways for adenosine triphosphate (ATP) to power vital cellular functions.

Finally, implantation can result in additional injury due to mechanical trauma, inadvertent warming during implantation, ischemic reperfusion injury, excessive demands placed on the implanted organs to assume life-sustaining functions, and high-dose inotropic agents.

The pathophysiology of ischemia reperfusion injury is complex, multifactorial, and still incompletely understood. The generation of oxygen-derived free radicals is thought to play a significant role in ischemia reperfusion injury. As ATP is catabolized to produce energy for cellular metabolism, hypoxanthine accumulates in ischemic tissue. The free radical molecules are produced via the endothelial xanthine oxidase pathway when hypoxanthine is reduced to xanthine, releasing oxygen-derived free radicals. Newly generated free radicals overcome the natural intracellular free radical scavengers (superoxide dismutase, catalase, and peroxidase), resulting in widespread oxidation of membrane lipids and denaturation of proteins. This leads to disruption of myocyte and endothelial cell homeostatic mechanisms. Intracellular calcium metabolism is affected by damage to the sarcoplasmic reticulum, and oxidative phosphorylation is impaired by mitochondrial damage. Leukocyte chemotactic factors released during this process lead to sequestration of white blood cells in the ischemic tissues. Accumulated leukocytes in ischemic tissue play a significant role in reperfusion injury. The expression of neutrophil adhesion molecules on endothelial cells following ischemic damage leads to leukocyte binding during reperfusion. Leukocytes, in turn, release cytotoxic molecules, including oxygen and halide radicals, granule proteases, and arachidonic acid metabolites mediating direct tissue injury and vasoconstriction, as well as initiating the activation of complement and other blood components. Ischemic injury in the heart is manifested as myocardial edema and ischemic band contracture histologically. Physiologically, it is reflected as reduced ventricular compliance, reduced fractional shortening, decreased stroke volume, and diminished cardiac output. This overall decreased function results in a need for an increased heart rate to maintain the cardiac output, increasing the oxygen demand and exacerbating the ischemic injury.

Single-Flush Technique

Surgical Technique

The heart is visually inspected and palpated to identify areas of hypokinesis, contusion, palpable coronary artery disease, or the unexpected thrill of a valvular lesion or congenital abnormality. The aorta, superior vena cava

(SVC), and inferior vena cava (IVC) are encircled with vessel loops. The donor is systemically heparinized (30 mL/kg). Inflow occlusion is then accomplished by ligating the SVC and clamping the IVC at the diaphragm. The heart is allowed to beat empty, and the aorta is then cross-clamped. The flush solution is infused in the ascending aorta. The IVC proximal to the clamp and the left atrial appendage, or a pulmonary vein, are incised to allow egress of blood and flush solutions. Several liters of cold saline are poured over the heart to initiate topical cooling. Once the flush solution is delivered, the heart is excised and packaged for storage in a sterile container containing the storage solution. If the lungs are to be simultaneously harvested, intravenous prostaglandin E_1 (PGE_1) is infused prior to the cross-clamping, at rates varying from 20 to 50 ng/kg/min, until there is a significant (ie, 20%) drop in systemic blood pressure. At that point, inflow occlusion is initiated and the aorta is clamped. Additional PGE_1 (ie, 500 µg), can be injected into the main pulmonary artery, or the entire dose can be delivered via that route, prior to initiating the pulmonary flush. The lungs are flushed with a solution through a catheter in the main pulmonary artery, simultaneous to the cardiac flush.

Maintenance of hypothermia during implantation is an extension of organ preservation. To achieve this, moderate hypothermia to a temperature of 28°C in the recipient is used while on cardiopulmonary bypass to decrease the degree of organ rewarming due to the recipient's ambient body temperature. Bronchial artery blood return to the left atrium is drained to prevent allograft warming from blood in the recipient's circulation. Finally, the heart is continuously bathed with cold saline or covered with saline slush during the implantation until reperfusion is initiated, to prevent inadvertent warming during implantation.

FLUSH AND STORAGE SOLUTIONS

Variables in the single-flush technique begin with the flush (cardioplegia) and storage solutions. A clear distinction should be made between the two. The primary goal of the flush solution is to arrest the heart and to begin cooling the tissue to decrease energy use. Additional goals are to create a milieu in which cellular damage is minimized, to provide glucose and other substrates as a source of energy, and to render the heart asanguinous. The goals of the storage solution are to achieve and maintain hypothermia, provide insulation between the cold source (ice) and the organ, provide a noninjurious milieu for storage, and to provide glucose and other substrates for energy. The effect of using different solutions for flush and storage is unknown and has not been extensively studied.

Flush Solution

The ideal solution remains unknown. Two main categories of crystalloid solutions have emerged, based on their electrolyte composition. Intracellular solutions are generally characterized by moderate to high concentra-

tions of potassium (> 100 µmol/L) with little to no calcium and low concentrations of sodium.[17] Extracellular solutions are characterized by high sodium and low to moderate potassium concentrations. Various additives are added to the electrolyte solution to give each solution its unique composition. Table 54-1 lists the composition of commonly used solutions.

The goal of intracellular solutions is to reduce the electrochemical gradient across the cell membrane and prevent cellular edema. Sodium influx and the obligatory passive entry of water into the cell to achieve osmotic equilibrium is minimized. Energy conservation is achieved by limiting the activity of the Na^+-K^+-ATPase pump to reestablish the normal cellular ionic gradient. Examples include the University of Wisconsin (Viaspan), Collins, Euro-Collins, and Cardiosol solutions. The term *intracellular* is sometimes applied to solutions with low sodium concentrations, such as the Stanford and Bretschneider (HTK) solutions, without taking into account their potassium concentrations. The optimal concentrations of potassium and calcium are unknown and have generated the most controversy. The primary concern in the use of intracellular-type solutions is the K^+-induced (Ca^{2+} influx) vasoconstriction. The concern is that hyperkalemia may cause endothelial cell injury and coronary vascular dysfunction leading to an early impaired reperfusion and possibly post-transplant vasculopathy. Conclusive evidence of significant damage to the hypothermic allograft by hyperkalemic intracellular solutions is lacking. Proponents of intracellular solutions feel that the K^+-induced spasm is short-lived because hypothermia inactivates membrane activity and the K^+-induced Ca^{2+} influx.[17] Some solutions are supplemented with pharmacologic agents to counteract the calcium-induced spasm, such as verapamil, butanedione, 2-monoxine, and nisoldipine; agents that are nitric oxide donors, such as nitroglycerin and sodium nitroprusside; or agents that bind calcium, such as lactobionate and phosphate.[17–21] It should be kept in mind that just as cellular enzymatic systems are affected by ischemia and various degrees of hypothermia, so are the pharmacologic activities of additives to the various preservation solutions.

Extracellular solutions avoid the theoretical cellular damage and increased vascular resistance associated with hyperkalemic solutions; however, there is concern over sodium influx and cellular swelling as well as an intracellular accumulation of calcium because of impaired exchange mechanisms. Calcium accumulation can result in myocardial contracture and impaired performance. Celsior, St. Thomas' Hospital, Perfadex (LPD) solutions are representative examples of extracellular solutions.

While the Papworth survey did not find the type of cardioplegic solution used to be a predictor of mortality by multivariate analysis, it is noteworthy that several solutions used today (eg, Viaspan, Celsior, and Perfadex) were not included in that study.[15] A similar, more recent,

TABLE 54-1. Commonly Used Donor Preservation Solutions: Composition of Lung Preservation Solutions

Class	I	I	I	I	I	I	E	E	E	E
Components	Stanford	HTK	Collins	EC	UW	Cardiosol	St. Thomas'	Plegisol	LPD	Celsior
Sodium	15	15	10	10	35	40	140	120	138	100
Potassium	17	10	115	115	125	125	16	16	6	15
Chloride	17	50	50	10	—	—	139	160	142	42
Bicarbonate	15	—	10	10	—	—	10	10*	1*	—
Mg	—	4	30	8	5	4	16	32	0.8	13
Calcium	—	—	—	—	—	—	1.2	2.4	—	0.25
Phosphate	—	—	58	100	25	25	—	—	0.8	—
SO$_4$	—	—	—	8	5	—	—	—	0.8	—
Glucose	250	—	—	120	—	—	—	—	5	—
Raffinose	—	—	—	—	30	30	—	—	—	—
HES	—	—	—	—	50	—	—	—	—	—
Dextran (g/L)	—	—	—	—	—	—	—	—	50	—
PEG	—	—	—	—	—	50	—	—	—	—
Mannitol	72	—	—	—	—	—	30	—	—	50
Lactobionate	—	—	—	—	100	100	—	—	—	80
Glutathione	—	—	—	—	3	—	—	—	—	3
Adenosine	—	—	—	—	5	—	—	—	—	—
Histidine	—	180	—	—	—	—	—	—	—	30
Histidine HCl	—	18	—	—	—	—	—	—	—	—
Tryptophan	—	2	—	—	—	—	—	—	—	—
Ketoglutarate	—	1	—	—	—	—	—	—	—	—
Glutamate	—	—	—	—	—	—	—	—	—	20
Insulin (U/L)	—	—	—	—	100	—	—	—	—	—
Decadron (mg/L)	—	—	—	—	8	—	—	—	—	—
Penicillin (mg/L)	—	—	—	—	133	—	—	—	—	—
Allopurinol	—	—	—	—	1	—	—	—	—	—
Desferal	—	—	—	—	—	7.1	—	—	—	—
Nitroglycerin	—	—	—	—	—	2.5	—	—	—	—
THAM/TRIS	—	—	—	—	—	—	—	—	1*	—
pH (4°C)	7.8	7.1	7.4	7.4	7.4	7.8	7.8	7.8	7.4	7.3
Osmolarity	440	310	320	360	320	325	290	304	290	320

Adapted from Wheeldon D et al;[16] Conte JV et al.[25]

All values expressed in mmol/L unless specified.

E = extracellular solution; EC = Euro-Collins solution; HES = hydroxy ethyl starch; HTK = Bretschneider's solution; I = intracellular solution; LDP = low potassium dextran (Perfadex) solution; PEG = polyethylene glycol; UW = University of Wisconsin (Viaspan) solution; THAM/TRIS = tromethamine/tris (hydroxymethyl) aminomethane.

* Added to solution prior to use to achieve final composition.

survey-type study reviewed the use of preservation solutions at US transplantation centers and had some interesting findings.[22] Solutions were classified as intra- or extracellular; based on Na$^+$ content (> 70 mEq/L). Only 55% of the solutions used were "standard" formulations; the remainder were somehow modified by the center. This study did show a small survival advantage at 1 month and 1 year with intracellular solutions. However, given the nature of this uncontrolled retrospective review, a case for a true advantage of one class of preservation solution over the other cannot be made.

Storage Solution

It would appear intuitive that the same solution be used to flush and store the donor heart if there is a definite benefit to a particular preservation solution. However, only 12% of programs in the Papworth survey used the same solution for both flush and storage. Saline was the most common storage solution and was used in 47% of centers. Additionally, the use of high-potassium cardioplegic solutions for storage was associated with increased mortality.

It is unclear whether using different solutions for flush and storage has any real effect on preservation or whether it detracts from the expected beneficial effects of a specific flush solution. Presently, there is no evidence to clearly support the use of any flush or storage solution, given the current ischemic periods of 4 to 6 h for heart preservation. However, specific studies to investigate this issue have not been carried out, and the issue remains open to debate.

Temperature

The ideal temperature of the preservation solution for flushing and storage is unknown, and the literature on the subject is confusing and often contradictory. Very few programs actually measure the temperature of the flush or storage solutions. Only 3% of the programs in the Papworth survey measured the temperature, but 73% reported their storage temperature to be 40°C.[15] It is generally believed that the optimal temperature is around 10°C for heart preservation. The ideal temperature will sufficiently decrease cellular metabolism but will allow critical cellular processes to continue. Although myocardial temperatures lower than 100°C impair vasomotor function and affect calcium homeostasis and other cellular transport mechanisms by impairing membrane-bound enzymes, temperatures above 100°C impair the effect of some preservation solutions and provide inferior preservation.[23] Excessive cooling to temperatures below 100°C can result in significant injury and should be carefully avoided. Unmonitored, it can happen in as quickly as 60 min in standard saline solution storage on ice.[24]

Volume

The optimal volume of flush solution is unknown. A single dose of antegrade flushing is standard. The methodology used to determine the volume delivered varies greatly. Some methods deliver a set volume or a set volume per body weight; other methods choose continuous flushing until the coronary sinus or left atrial effluent appears clear. For heart transplantation, volumes of 500 cc to 2 L or 10 to 20 mL/kg have been given. Although antegrade delivery is most commonly used, retrograde coronary sinus flushing is used by some. Multiple doses of cardioplegia or blood can easily be delivered during implantation through the same catheter to maintain hypothermia.

The ideal pressure at which to flush the donor organs is unknown for heart preservation. While most programs agree there is an optimal pressure at which to infuse the flush solution, most programs do not monitor pressure. Many different techniques have been reported and are used clinically. Some centers deliver the flush through a pump apparatus at a given pressure; most centers, however, hang the bag of flush solution at a prescribed height (eg, 30 to 80 cm) or in a pressure bag inflated to infuse the solution at a prescribed pressure. Pressure bags inflated to a pressure of 150 to 250 mm Hg, which reflect the pressure used to infuse cardioplegia solutions for coronary artery surgery, are commonly employed for hearts.

PRESERVATION SOLUTION ADDITIVES

A wide variety of substances have been added to the flush and storage solutions to take advantage of their biologic, chemical, or physiologic properties. The main categories of solution additives are discussed.

Impermeants

These agents are employed to reduce cellular swelling. They counteract the movement of fluid into cells driven by the higher intracellular osmotic pressure through cell membranes impaired by hypoxia and hypothermia. In the literature, these agents are variously referred to as impermeants, osmotic agents, and colloids. They are large molecules to which cell membranes are impermeable. They remain in the intravascular space, increasing the intravascular oncotic pressure, and, in some cases, adding other beneficial effects, such as decreasing the generation of oxygen-derived free radicals via the Haber-Weiss pathway

by binding Fe^{2+}. Dextran, mannitol, lactobionate, gluconate, raffinose, histidine and hydroxy ethyl starch are examples of impermeants.[25]

Substrate Enhancement

The goal of substrate enhancement is to prevent the depletion of high-energy phosphates and to encourage their replenishment during ischemia. Although cell metabolism is decreased during preservation, it does continue, requiring energy in the form of high-energy phosphates. As components of the biologic systems that generate ATP via the purine salvage pathway and Krebs citric acid cycle, amino acids such as adenosine, L-glutamate, L-arginine, and L-pyruvate are believed to prevent ischemic contracture due to energy depletion. Experimental models show that amino acid supplementation maintains energy stores and improves functional recovery.[26] Although the literature supports substrate-enhanced cardioplegia in the form of sugars and amino acids for cardiac surgery, its use in organ preservation is unproven. The length of the ischemic period and the duration and degree of hypothermia are greatly different in these two scenarios. It is unknown whether profoundly hypothermic cells with depressed metabolic processes can use exogenously supplied substrates and incorporate them into useful compounds to make a significant difference.

Antioxidants

The recognition that oxygen-derived free radicals play a significant role in ischemia reperfusion injury has led to investigations into methods to mitigate their effects. Pharmacologic interventions have been employed to supplement the naturally occurring antioxidants catalase, superoxide dismutase, and glutathione. Exogenously delivered compounds aim to prevent the formation of or bind the reactive oxygen molecules before they can bind to and injure cell membranes. The delivery of antioxidant agents concomitant with reperfusion aims to bind or prevent the generation of toxic free radical moieties. Free radical scavengers that have been employed experimentally and clinically include superoxide dismutase, catalase, glutathione, allopurinol, mannitol, and histidine.[25] In addition to free radical scavengers and impermeants, compounds that bind the transition metals iron and copper, such as desferrioxamine and neocuproine, have been employed to inhibit the generation of oxygen-derived free radicals by removing these metals necessary for the production of free radicals via the Haber-Weiss and Fenton reactions. Conflicting experimental and clinical results make the utility of these drugs unknown.

DONOR PRETREATMENT

Attempts have been made to improve donor organ function by treatment prior to procurement. The goal is to treat the donor with pharmacologic agents in an attempt to improve function, increase the tolerance to ischemia, and prevent ischemia reperfusion injury. The list of agents that have been used for donor pretreatment is extensive. They generally have a well-grounded scientific basis for their use and are effective in laboratory studies; however, none have been shown to be superior to standard donor management in the few controlled clinical trials performed to date (Table 54-2).[27–43]

The use of triiodothyronine (T_3) and thyroxine (T_4) to treat cardiac donors is controversial. Acting via the influx of Ca^{2+} and an efflux of K^+, thyroid hormones have been reported to improve donor hemodynamics and graft survival of donor hearts. The use of these agents is controversial because of the inconsistent results reported in clinical studies despite the findings that many brain-dead donors are hypothyroid.[42,43]

STRATEGIES TO REDUCE RECIPIENT REPERFUSION INJURY

Reperfusion injury is a complex multifactorial injury that occurs during the initial reperfusion of ischemic tissues. The maximum release of oxygen-derived free radicals occurs during reperfusion, a period in which the organ is susceptible to significant injury. A wide variety of strategies and pharmacologic interventions have been employed clinically and experimentally to reduce reperfusion injury. Strategies include controlled reperfusion of ischemic tissues at low pressures, leukocyte depletion via chemical and mechanical means, pharmacologic addition to flush solutions, donor and recipient pretreatment, and enhancement of natural protective mechanisms via ischemic preconditioning.

Controlled Reperfusion

Controlled reperfusion at a low pressure is felt to be beneficial in cardiac surgery by minimizing the hydrostatic pressure faced by hypothermic ischemic tissues with dysfunctional capillaries and cell membranes. By keeping the hydrostatic pressure portion of the Starling equation low until after the high energy stores are repleted, tissue edema will form. Controlled reperfusion of the transplanted heart with blood or blood cardioplegia decreases the amount of inotropic support, decreases postoperative

TABLE 54-2. Agents Used for Donor Preconditioning in Clinical and Laboratory Studies on Cardiac Preservation

Lidocaine	Methylprednisolone
Nicorandil	Halothane
Propanolol	T_3/T_4
Chlorpromazine	Insulin
Verapamil	Glucose
Nicardipine	Allopurinol
Dipyridamole	Antidiuretic hormone
Adenosine	L-Arginine

Adapted from Schaub R et al;[27] Sugimoto S et al;[28] Portnoy VF et al;[29] Thomas GE et al;[30] Walpoth B et al;[31] Guffin AV et al;[32] Brown PS et al;[33] Mechant FJ et al;[34] Fremes SE et al;[35] Busuttil RW et al;[36] Bretschneider HJ et al;[37] Stow DF et al;[38] Du ZY et al;[39] Ferrero ME et al;[40] Novitsky D et al;[41] Orlowsky JP et al;[42] Randell TT et al.[43]

arrhythmias, increases spontaneous recovery of sinus rhythm, lessens ICU and hospital stays, and reduces ischemic damage on endomyocardial biopsies. The combination of oxygen delivery, substrate enhancement, energy repletion, low reperfusion pressure, and buffering capacity is thought to reduce reperfusion injury and to improve function.[44–49]

Leukocyte Depletion Strategies

Leukocyte sequestration in donor organs is known to play a significant role in ischemia reperfusion injury. Leukocyte reduction during reperfusion may reduce free radical–mediated tissue injury, and various pharmacologic and mechanical strategies, such as leukocyte filters in the cardiopulmonary bypass circuit, have been employed.[49]

Adhesion to myocytes and endothelial cells is critical for the release of free radicals and proteases by activated neutrophils. Pharmacologic interventions attempt to block adhesion and activation by direct and indirect mechanisms. Monoclonal antibodies to the integrin and selectin adhesion molecules directly block this critical step in neutrophil-mediated injury and reduce the degree of reperfusion injury in pulmonary and cardiac models, respectively.[50,51] Several commonly used drugs, including pentoxifylline, lidocaine, nitroprusside, and mycophenolate mofetil, have been shown experimentally to prevent neutrophil adhesion and to decrease reperfusion injury but have yet to find widespread clinical use.[52–55]

Nitric Oxide Donors

Of all the pharmacologic interventions, the use of nitric oxide donors is particularly promising. Nitric oxide is synthesized by endothelial cells from L-arginine by nitric oxide synthetase. Nitric oxide plays a major role in vascular homeostasis by relaxation of vascular smooth muscle and the inhibition of leukocyte and platelet adhesion. Reperfusion injury is thought to be partly mediated by disruption of vascular homeostasis, manifested by "leaky capillary membranes," resulting in tissue edema, leukocyte infiltration, and platelet adherence. Nitric oxide levels are decreased in the transplanted tissue following reperfusion.[56] L-Arginine is an example of one of many different types of nitric oxide donors that have improved the recovery of endothelial cell and overall cardiac function in models of myocardial ischemia.[56–59]

Phosphodiesterase Inhibitors

Phosphodiesterase inhibitors block the degradation of cyclic adenosine monophosphate (cAMP) by blocking the enzyme phosphodiesterase. Numerous studies suggest that increased levels of cAMP can attenuate the increased microvascular permeability associated with ischemia reperfusion injury by maintaining tight intracellular junctions through effects on actinomycin myofibrils within endothelial cells, by decreasing the release and effects of various cytokines, tumor necrosis factor, and thrombomodulin, and by reducing the expression of adhesion molecules. Clinically used phosphodiesterase inhibitors such as theophylline reduce reperfusion injury in animal models, and because of their familiarity to clinicians, may be more readily employed than other agents.[60]

NEW AND FUTURE TECHNIQUES

Ischemic Preconditioning

The general hypothesis of ischemic preconditioning is that a brief period of ischemia will activate protective mechanisms and increase ischemic tolerance. Animal studies show preservation of high-energy phosphates, decreased creatine kinase leakage, and improved contractile function after global hypothermic ischemia in cardiac models, and reduced reperfusion injury in lung models.[61,62] Activation of ATP-sensitive potassium channels has been postulated as providing endogenous protection against myocardial ischemia and is thought to play a pivotal role in the cardioprotective effects of ischemic preconditioning.[63] A number of potassium channel–opening drugs exist that are cardioprotective in the setting of myocardial ischemia.[63] While ischemic preconditioning is impractical in the setting of multiorgan procurement, pharmacologic preconditioning is not and may be particularly relevant in the use of non–beating-heart donors.

Continuous Perfusion

The concept of continuous mechanical perfusion was recently re-introduced experimentally with the hope that low-pressure perfusion with a high colloid osmotic pressure perfusate would prevent the tissue edema seen with earlier systems. Perfusion systems have been successful in resuscitating and preserving renal allografts.[8] Although encouraging laboratory data on perfusion preservation of cardiac allografts using donor blood and preservation solutions have been reported, clinical data have not been reported to date.[64–68]

Gene Therapy

Gene therapy has many potential applications in transplantation. Gene transfer has been accomplished during hypothermic storage in both hearts and lungs.[69,70] In a model of murine cardiac ischemia reperfusion, transgenic overexpression of superoxide dismutase conferred significant functional benefit over control animals.[71] In another study, the gene that codes for heat shock protein was successfully transferred to donor lungs and decreased ischemic reperfusion injury.[72] These studies validated the potential use of gene therapy to modify the donor organ to protect it against injury during preservation. The implications of this technology are great.

Novel and New Compounds

A number of new compounds have been investigated that have demonstrated beneficial effects in animal models of ischemic reperfusion injury and heart and lung preservation. Some medications have beneficial effects in limited clinical experiences; however, the questions regarding the ultimate utility of any compound will only be determined following human clinical trials. Among these compounds are a variety of different prostaglandins, lazaroids, platelet-activating factor antagonists, heat shock protein agonists, vasoactive intestinal peptide, calcium channel blockers, tumor necrosis factor antagonists, interleukin antagonists, and perfluorochemicals.[73–83]

Conclusion

The current acceptable period of cardiac preservation is 4 to 6 h when using the single-flush technique and hypothermic storage. The ideal method and the ideal solution for cardiac preservation have yet to be identified. This chapter summarized common practices in cardiac preservation and identified those areas of current investigation that may lead to significant future contributions to the field.

References

1. Lower RR, Stofer RC, Hurley EJ, et al. Successful homotransplantation of the canine heart after experimental models of anoxic preservation for seven hours. Am J Surg 1962;104:302.
2. Hendry PJ, Walley VM, Koshal A, et al. Are temperatures attained by donor hearts during transport too cold? J Thorac Cardiovasc Surg 1989;98:517–22.
3. Bigelow WG, Mustard WT, Evans JG. Some physiological concepts of hypothermia and their application to cardiac surgery. J Thorac Surg 1954;28:463.
4. Belzer FO, Southard JH. Principles of solid organ preservation by cold storage. Transplantation 1988;45:673–6.
5. Robicsek F, Tam W, Daugherty HK. Survival of heart grafts. Arch Surg 1969;99:750–2.
6. Hardesty RL, Griffith BP. Autoperfusion of the heart and lungs for preservation during distant procurement. J Thorac Cardiovasc Surg 1987;93:11–8.
7. Ladowksi JS, Kapelanski DP, Teodori MF, et al. Use of autoperfusion for distant procurement of heart-lung allografts. J Heart Transplant 1985;4:300–33.
8. Xenos ES. Perfusion storage versus static storage in kidney transplantation: is one superior to the other? Nephrol Dial Transplant 1997;12(2):253–4.
9. Oshima K, Morishita Y, Yamagishi T, et al. Long-term heart preservation using a new portable hypothermic perfusion apparatus. J Heart Lung Transplant 1999;18:852–61.
10. Baumgartner WA, Williams GM, Fraser CD, et al. Cardiopulmonary bypass with profound hypothermia. An optimal preservation method for multiorgan procurement. Transplantation 1989;47:123–7.
11. Haverich A, Wahlers T, Schafers HJ, et al. Distant organ procurement in clinical lung and heart–lung transplantation. Cooling by extracorporeal circulation or hypothermic flush. Eur J Cardiothorac Surg 1990;4:245–9.

12. Yacoub MH, Khaghani A, Banner N, et al. Distant organ procurement for heart and lung transplantation. Transplant Proc 1989;21:2548–50.

13. Reitz BA, Brody WR, Hickey PR, Michaelis LL. Protection of the heart for 24 hours with intracellular (high K$^+$) solution and hypothermia. Surg Forum 1974:25:149–51.

14. Baumgartner WA, Reitz BA, Stinson EB. Cardioplegia in human heart transplantation. In: Engleman RN, Levitsky S, editors. A textbook of clinical cardioplegia. Mount Kisco [NY]: Futura Publishing; 1982. p. 373.

15. Vega JD, Oschner JL, Jeevanandam V, et al. A multicenter randomized, controlled trial of Celsior for flush and hypothermic storage of cardiac allografts. Ann Thorac Surg 2001;71:1442–7.

16. Wheeldon D, Sharples L, Wallwork J, et al. Donor heart preservation survey. J Heart Lung Transplant 1992;11:986–93.

17. Wicomb WN, Portnoy VF, Collins GM. Advances in heart storage: In: Cooper JDK, Miller LW, Patterson GA, editors. The transplantation and replacement of thoracic organs. Boston [MA]: Kluwer; 1997. p. 675–87.

18. Bolotina VM, Najib S, Palacino JJ, et al. Nitric oxide directly activates calcium dependent potassium channels in vascular smooth muscle. Nature 1994;368:850–3.

19. Coulombe A, Lefevre IA, Deroubaix E, et al. Effect of 2,3,-butanedione 2-monoxime on slow inward and transient outward currents in rat ventricular myocytes. J Mol Cell Cardiol 1990;22:921–2.

20. Herbaczynska-Cedro K, Gordon-Majszak W. Nisoldipine inhibits lipid peroxidation induced by coronary occlusion in pig myocardium. Cardiovasc Res 1990;24:683–7.

21. Stringham JC, Southard JH, Fields BL. Improved myocardial preservation with 2,3-butanedione monoxime, calcium and the UW solution. Transplant Proc 1993;25:1625–6.

22. Demmy TL, Biddle JS, Bennett LE, et al. Organ preservation solutions in heart transplantations. Patterns of usage and related survival. Transplant 1997;63:262–9.

23. Keon WJ, Hendry, Taichman GE, Mainwood GW. Cardiac transplantation: the ideal myocardial temperature for graft transport. Ann Thorac Surg 1988;46:337–41.

24. Amrani M, Ledingham S, Jayakumar J, et al. Detrimental effects of temperature on the efficacy of the University of Wisconsin solution when used for cardioplegia at moderate hypothermia. Comparison with St. Thomas Hospital solution at 4 degrees and 20 degrees C. Circulation 1992;86 Suppl 5:II 280–8.

25. Conte JV, Baumgartner WA. Overview and future practice patterns in cardiac and pulmonary preservation. J Card Surg 2000;15:91–107.

26. Lasley RD, Mentzer RM. The role of adenosine in extended myocardial preservation with the University of Wisconsin solution. J Thorac Cardiovasc Surg 1994;107:1356–63.

27. Schaub R, Lemole G, Pinder G. Effects of lidocaine and epinephrine on myocardial preservation following cardiopulmonary bypass in the dog. J Thorac Cardiovasc Surg 1977;74:571–5.

28. Sugimoto S, Puddu PE, Monti F, et al. Pretreatment with the adenosine triphosphate-sensitive potassium channel opener nicorandil and improved myocardial protection during high potassium cardioplegic hypoxia. J Thorac Cardiovasc Surg 1994;108:455–66.

29. Portnoy VF, Dvortsin GF, Shargorodskaya AY, et al. The effect of increasing propanolol doses on cardiac function and myocardial pH during total ischemia. J Surg Res 1981;3:6.

30. Thomas GE, Levitsky S, Feinberg H. Chlorpromazine inhibits loss of contractile function, compliance, and ATP in ischemic rabbit hearts. J Mol Cell Cardiol 1983;15:621–6–12.

31. Walpoth B, Bleese N, Zhao H, et al. Assessment of rabbit hearts during reperfusion after hypothermic long-term storage: the role of verapamil and effect on myocardial calcium. Surg Forum 1984;35:288–91.

32. Guffin AV, Kates RA, Holbrook GW, et al. Verapamil and myocardial preservation in patients undergoing coronary artery bypass surgery. Ann Thorac Surg 1986;41:587–91.

33. Brown PS, Parenten GL, Holland FW, et al. Pretreatment with nicardipine preserves ventricular function after hypothermic ischemic arrest. Ann Thorac Surg 1991;51:739–43.

34. Mechant FJ, Feinberg H, Levitsky S. Reversal of myocardial depression by dipyridamole following aortic cross clamping. Surg Forum 1972;23:162–4.

35. Fremes SE, Zhang J, Furukawa RD, et al. Adenosine pretreatment for prolonged cardiac storage. An evaluation with St. Thomas' Hospital and University of Wisconsin solutions. J Thorac Cardiovasc Surg 1995;110:293–9.

36. Busuttil RW, George WJ, Hewitt RL. Effect of methylprednisolone on the heart during ischemic arrest. J Thorac Cardiovasc Surg 1975;70:955–61.

37. Bretschneider IIJ, Hubner G, Knoll D, et al. Myocardial resistance and tolerance to ischemia: physiological and biochemical basis. J Cardiovasc Surg 1975;16:241–6.

38. Stowe DF, Habazett H, Graf BM, et al. One-day hypothermic preservation of isolated hearts with halothane improves cardiac function better than low calcium. Anesthesiology 1995;83:1065–77.

39. Du ZY, Hicks M, Spratt P, et al. Cardioprotective effects of pinacidil pretreatment and lazaroid (U74500A) preservation in isolated rat hearts after 12-hour hypothermic storage. Transplantation 1998;66:158–63.

40. Ferrero ME, Marni A, Parise M, et al. Protection of rat heart from damage due to ischemia reperfusion during procurement and grafting by defibrotide. Transplantation 1991;52:611–5.

41. Novitsky D, Cooper DKC, Reichart B. Hemodynamic and metabolic responses to hormonal therapy in brain dead potential organ donors. Transplantation 1987;43:852–8.

42. Orlowsky JP, Spees EK. Improved cardiac transplant survival with thyroxine treatment in hemodynamically unstable donors. Transplant Proc 1993;25:1535–8.

43. Randell TT, Hockerstedt KAV. Triiodothyronine treatment is not indicated in brain dead multiorgan donors: a controlled study. Transplant Proc 1993;25:1552–8.

44. Pradas G, Cuenca J, Juffa A. Continuous warm reperfusion during heart transplantation. J Thorac Cardiovasc Surg 1996;111:784–90.

45. Carrier M, Leung TK, Solymoss BC, et al. Clinical trial of retrograde warm blood reperfusion versus standard cold topical irrigation of transplanted hearts. Ann Thorac Surg 1996;61:1310–4.

46. Richens D, Junius F, Hill A, et al. Clinical study of crystalloid cardioplegia vs aspartate-enriched cardioplegia plus warm reperfusion for donor heart preservation. Transplant Proc 1993;25:1608–10.

47. Nataf P, Pavie A, Bracamontes L, et al. Myocardial protection by blood cardioplegia and warm reperfusion of the heart. Ann Thorac Surg 1992;53:525–6.

48. Soots G, Crepin F, Prat A, et al. Cold blood cardioplegia and warm cardioplegic reperfusion in heart transplantation. Eur J Cardiothorac Surg 1991;5:400–4.

49. Pearl JM, Drinkwater DC, Laks H, et al. Leukocyte-depleted reperfusion of transplanted human hearts: a randomized double blind clinical trial. J Heart Lung Transplant 1992;11:1082–92.

50. Byrne JG, Smith WJ, Murphy MP, et al. Complete prevention of myocardial stunning, contracture, low reflow, and edema after heart transplantation by blocking neutrophil adhesion molecules during reperfusion. J Thorac Cardiovasc Surg 1992;104:1589–96.

51. Lefer DJ, Flynn DM, Phillips L, et al. A novel sialyl-Lewis x analog attenuates neutrophil accumulation and myocardial necrosis after ischemia and reperfusion. Circulation 1994;90:2390–401.

52. Schmid RA, Yamashita M, Ando K, et al. Lidocaine reduces reperfusion injury and neutrophil migration in canine lung allografts. Ann Thorac Surg 1996;61:949–55.

53. Yamashita M, Schmid RA, Ando K, et al. Nitroprusside reduces lung allograft reperfusion injury. Ann Thorac Surg 1996;62:791–6.

54. Paul LC, Valentin JF, Brujin JA, Zhang S. Donor treatment with mycophenolate mofetil protects against ischemia reperfusion injury. Transplant Proc 1999;31;1026.

55. Chapelier A, Reigner J, Mazmanian M, et al. Amelioration of reperfusion injury by pentoxifylline after lung transplantation. J Heart Lung Transplant 1995;14:676–83.

56. Katori M, Tamaki T, Tanaka M, et al. Nitric oxide donor induces upregulation of stress proteins in cold ischemic rat hearts. Transplant Proc 1999;31:1022–3.

57. Nakanishi K, Vinten-Johansen J, Lefer J, et al. Intracoronary L-arginine during reperfusion improves endothelial function and reduces infarct size. Am J Physiol 1992; 263:H1650–8.

58. Keefer LK, Nims RW, Davies KM, Wink DA. NONOates (1-substituted Diazen-1-ium-1,2diolates) as nitric oxide donors: convenient nitric oxide dosage forms. Methods Enzymol 1996;268:281–93.

59. Du ZY, Hicks M, Jansz P, et al. The nitric oxide donor diethylamine nonoate enhances preservation of the donor rat heart. J Heart Lung Transplant 1998;17: 1113–20.

60. Adkins WK, Barnard JW, May S, et al. Compounds that increase cAMP prevent ischemia reperfusion injury. J Appl Physiol 1992;72:492–7.

61. Karck M, Rahmanian P, Haverich A. Ischemic preconditioning enhances donor heart preservation. Transplantation 1996;62:17–22.

62. Grover GJ. The role of ATP-sensitive potassium channels in myocardial ischemia: pharmacology and implications for the future. In: Kamazyn M, editor. Myocardial ischemia: mechanisms, reperfusion, protection. Basel: Birkhauser-Verlag; 1996. p. 313–20.

63. Hearse DJ. Activation of ATP sensitive potassium channels: a novel pharmacological approach to myocardial protection? Cardiovasc Res 1995;30:1–10.

64. Rao V, Feindel CM, Weisel RD, et al. Donor blood perfusion improves myocardial recovery after heart transplantation. J Heart Lung Transplant 1997;16:667–73.

65. Ferrera R, Marscek P, Larese A, et al. Comparison of continuous microperfusion and cold storage for pig heart preservation. J Heart Lung Transplant 1993;12:463–9.

66. Ferrera R, Hadour G. A reliable method for long-term (24-hour) hypothermic transport of cardiac grafts. Transplant Proc 1998;30:4320–43.

67. Oshima K, Morishita Y, Yamagishi T, et al. A new portable hypothermic perfusion apparatus for long-term heart preservation in canine models. Transplant Proc 1999;31: 1072–3.

68. Chien S, Maley R, Oeltgen PR, et al. Canine lung transplantation after more than 24 hours of normothermic preservation. J Heart Lung Transplant 1997;16:340–51.

69. Gojo S, Niwaya K, Taniguchi S, et al. Gene transfer into the donor heart during cold preservation for heart transplantation. Ann Thorac Surg 1998;65:647–52.

70. Boasquevisque CH, Mora BN, Schmid RA, et al. Ex vivo adenoviral-mediated gene transfer to lung isografts during cold preservation. Ann Thorac Surg 1997;63: 1556–61.

71. Chen EP, Bittner HB, Davis RD, et al. Physiologic effects of extracellular superoxide dismutase transgene overexpression on myocardial function after ischemia and reperfusion injury. J Thorac Cardiovasc Surg 1998;115:450–9.

72. Yano M, Mora BN, Ritter JM, et al. Gene transfer of heat shock protein 70 protects the lung from ischemia reperfusion injury. Ann Thorac Surg 1999;67:1421–7.

73. Hendry PJ, Anstdt MP, Plunkett MD, et al. Improved donor myocardial recovery with a new lazaroid lipid antiperoxidant in the isolated canine heart. J Heart Lung Transplant 1992;11:636–45.

74. Sasaki S, Alessandrini F, Lodi R, et al. Improvement of pulmonary graft after storage for 24 hours by in vivo administration of lazaroid U74389G: functional and morphologic analysis. J Heart Lung Transplant 1996;15: 35–42.

75. Novick RJ, Menkis AH, McKenzie FN. New trends in lung preservation: a collective review. J Heart Lung Transplant 1992;11:377–92.

76. Qayumi AK, English JE, Duncan S, et al. Extended lung preservation with platelet activating factor antagonist TCV-309 in combination with prostaglandin E1. J Heart Lung Transplant 1997;16:946–55.

77. Gowda A, Yang C, Asimakis GK, et al. Heat shock improves recovery and provides protection against global ischemia after hypothermic storage. Ann Thorac Surg 1998;66:1991–7.

78. Kojima R, Tamaki T, Kawamura A, et al. Expression of heat shock proteins induced by L-glutamine injection and survival of hypothermically stored heart grafts. Transplant Proc 1998;30:3746–7.

79. Alessandrini F, Sasaki S, Said SI, et al. Enhancement of extended lung preservation with a vasoactive intestinal peptide enriched University of Wisconsin solution. Transplantation 1995;59:1253–8.

80. Kuroda Y, Kawamura T, Tanioka Y, et al. Heart preservation using a cavitary two-layer (University of Wisconsin solution perfluorochemical) cold storage method. Transplantation 1995;59:699–705.

81. Chen RH. The scientific basis for hypocalcemic cardioplegia and reperfusion in cardiac surgery. Ann Thorac Surg 1996;62:910–4.

82. Hachida M, Lu H, Kaneko N, et al. Protective effects of JTV519 on prolonged myocardial protection. Transplant Proc 1999;31:1094–8.

83. Koyano T, Takeyoshi I, Takahashi T, et al. Effects of FR167653 on ischemia reperfusion injury: evaluation through preservation and transplantation in canine hearts. J Heart Lung Transplant 1998;17:1247–54.

CHAPTER 55

ADVANCES IN IMMUNOSUPPRESSION

JACOB JOSEPH, MD, SANJEEV TREHAN, MD, DAVID O. TAYLOR, MD

The evolution of organ transplantation into a viable long-term option in end-stage cardiac and pulmonary disease has its underpinnings in the rapid strides made in our knowledge of the immune response to a grafted organ. This expansion of knowledge has resulted in multiple new avenues directed toward achieving more specific and controlled immunosuppression. Although reasonable success has been achieved with present modalities, the quest for optimal immunosuppressive strategies is far from over. This chapter briefly presents the immunologic principles behind, and potential clinical relevance of, select new modalities that are currently in use or making the transition from bench to bedside.

Immunobiology of Transplant Rejection

Rejection of a transplanted organ by preformed antibodies (hyperacute rejection) has been greatly reduced by preoperative screening for alloreactive antibodies and prospective, donor-specific crossmatching in sensitized recipients and nowadays is an extremely rare event. However, acute cellular rejection remains a significant problem in solid organ transplantation, and its basis in T lymphocyte–mediated immune responses is the main focus of our discussion. Allograft vasculopathy, or "chronic rejection," is a complex process that involves immunologic injury and vascular proliferative responses; it is discussed in detail in a separate chapter. The T lymphocyte plays a major role in supporting antibody production by B cells and in the immune response of allograft vasculopathy; hence, understanding the T cell response to immune encounters may be important in modulating hyperacute rejection as well as allograft vasculopathy.[1-4] Figure 55-1 shows a simplified schema of the immune response of the recipient to an allograft.

Various immune cells, including T lymphocytes and antigen-presenting cells (APCs), adhere to the endothelium because of the interaction of adhesion molecules with ligands on the endothelial cell surface as part of the initial inflammatory response.[1-4] Quiescent endothelial cells are induced to express adhesion molecules by ischemia, surgical manipulation, or cytokines, resulting in leukocyte adhesion and transmigration. Figure 55-1 and its inset show this crucial reaction and some of the major adhesion molecules involved. The adhesion molecule–ligand interaction plays a major role in the immune response and offers potential targets for attenuating the T cell response. In view of the fact that most transplanted organs undergo damage from anoxia or surgical manipulation and consequent upregulation of endothelial adhesion molecules, prophylactic blockade employing antibodies against one or more of these components may attenuate initial T cell responses during engraftment. The major adhesion molecule–ligand pairs involved are CD2:LFA3 (leukocyte function associated antigen [LFA]-3) and ICAM-1 (intercellular adhesion molecule-1):LFA-1, which enhance the interaction of T cells with both endothelium and APCs. Blockade of these interactions attenuates immune response in animal models, and the initial clinical experience is encouraging, as is discussed below.

The T cells may be activated against alloantigen by (1) "direct" interaction with foreign antigens presented by endothelial cells, myocytes, or passenger dendritic cells in association with donor major histocompatibility complex (MHC) antigens, and by (2) "indirect" interaction with foreign peptides processed and presented by recipient APCs. The T cell activation leads to a series of intracellular events resulting in an "activated" T cell, which secretes various cytokines, including interleukin-2 (IL-2). A positive feedback ensues, resulting in amplification of the T cell response by expression of IL-2 receptor, occupancy by IL-2, and stimulation of T cell proliferation (see below). Other cytokines secreted (interferon-gamma [IFN-γ], tumor necrosis factor-alpha [TNF-α], IL-4, IL-5, and IL-6) stimulate the activation and proliferation of macrophages, B cells, and other cells involved in the inflammatory response. The immune cascade, involving helper T cells, cytotoxic T cells, natural killer (NK) cells,

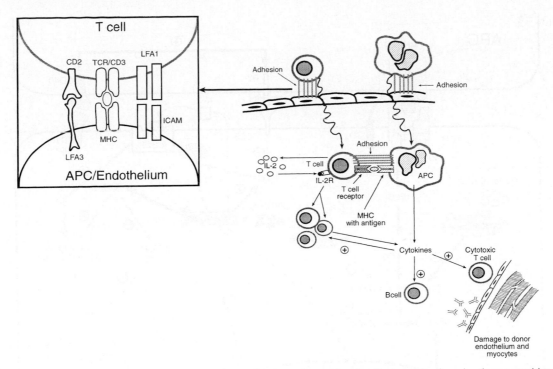

FIGURE 55-1. Overview of the donor–recipient immune interaction. Inset shows relevant adhesion molecule and antigen recognition receptors. APC = antigen-presenting cell; CD2 and CD3 = clusters of differentiation markers; ICAM = intercellular adhesion molecule-1; IL-2R = interleukin-2 (receptor); LFA1 and LFA3 = leukocyte function associated antigen 1 and 3; MHC = major histocompatibility antigens; TCR = T cell receptor.

B cells, antibodies, and complement, culminates in damage to donor endothelium and myocytes, manifesting as rejection.

The crucial reactions involved in activation of a T cell after it encounters an antigen are shown in Figure 55-2, along with putative sites of action of immunosuppression modalities discussed here.[1–4] The initiation point for the T cell response is the direct or indirect presentation of the alloantigen and binding to the T cell receptor/CD3 complex. This leads to activation of several tyrosine kinases such as $p56^{lck}$, $p59^{fyn}$, and ZAP-70. The ensuing phosphorylation activation of phospholipase C (PLC) leads ultimately to a rise in intracellular calcium. Calcium, along with calmodulin, activates the serine threonine phosphatase calcineurin. Calcineurin dephosphorylates the cytoplasmic subunit of nuclear factor of activated T cells (NFAT-c), enabling its translocation to the nucleus, where it complexes with the nuclear subunit (NFAT-n). This complex binds to the promoter regions of various cytokine genes, especially the IL-2 promoter, upregulating transcription. IL-2 enables the proliferative response of activated cells as well as other immune cells in both an autocrine and paracrine fashion. Cyclosporine and tacrolimus (FK506), in complex with their cytoplasmic binding proteins, cyclophilins and FK-binding proteins (FKBPs), respectively, inhibit the function of calcineurin and thus downregulate expression of IL-2 and other cytokines. The CD4 molecule is closely associated with the T cell receptor of helper T cells and plays a major role in immune amplification. Blocking the function of the CD4 molecule can selectively block the response of a helper T cell to MHC class II–alloantigen complex.

IL-2 binds to its receptor on the T cell and elicits a series of intracellular events ultimately resulting in the activation of various cyclin kinases. These kinases are important cell cycle regulatory proteins. The consequent progression of the activated T cell through the cell cycle is critical for effective cellular proliferation and subsequent immune amplification. The cell passes through G1 to the synthetic (S) phase, which is dependent on nucleic acid synthesis in preparation for mitosis. The lymphocyte is primarily dependent on the de novo pathway of purine and pyrimidine synthesis unlike other cells capable of rapid division, where the "salvage" pathways can contribute to a significant extent. Mycophenolate mofetil, by inhibiting a key enzyme of the de novo pathway, inosine monophosphate dehydrogenase (IMPDH), blocks the proliferative response of T cells. Sirolimus (rapamycin) acts to block several events downstream of the IL-2 receptor. This drug binds to the same binding proteins as tacrolimus (primarily FKBP-12), but rather than inhibiting calcineurin, it inhibits cytoplasmic proteins collectively termed target of rapamycin (TOR) proteins. These proteins are required for cell-cycle progression in response to IL-2 stimulation, and hence sirolimus is able to block the proliferative response of T cells after immune stimulation. Sirolimus inhibits 70 kD S6 kinase (p70s6k),

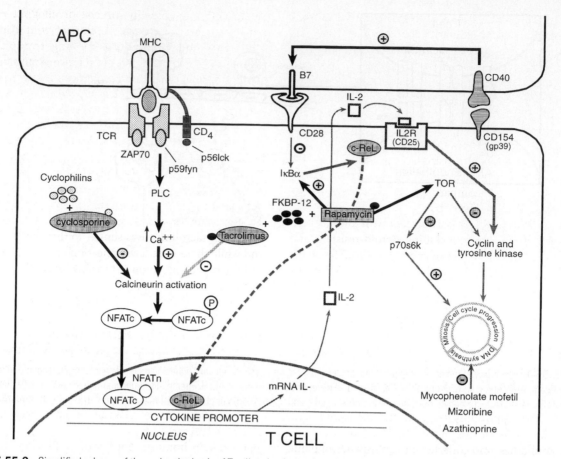

FIGURE 55-2. Simplified schema of the molecular basis of T cell activation and mechanisms of action for the newer immunosuppressive agents. APC = antigen-presenting cell; CD = clusters of differentiation markers; c-Rel = CD28 response element; FKBP-12 = FK-506 binding protein 12; IκBα = I kappa B alpha; IL-2R = interleukin-2 (receptor); MHC = major histocompatibility antigens; NFATc = nuclear factor of activated T cells, cytoplasmic component; NFATn = nuclear factor of activated T cells, nuclear component; PLC = phospholipase C; p56fyn = tyroine kinase FYN; p56lck = tyrosine kinase LCK; p70s6k = phosphoprotein 70 ribosomal protein S6 kinase; TCR = T cell receptor; TOR = target of rapamycin.

preventing the phosphorylation of S6 ribosomal protein, which is thought to be involved in the translation of cell-cycle regulatory proteins. Another very promising approach is blockade of the IL-2 receptor by monoclonal antibodies directed against specific components of the receptor complex.

We have already mentioned the importance of adhesion molecules in enhancing the T cell response to antigen, independent of the antigen–receptor interaction. Another critical interaction involves the "co-stimulatory" signals, which are antigen-independent pathways that significantly enhance the T cell responses. In fact, co-stimulatory signals are necessary for full activation as T cell receptor (TCR) stimulation, without a co-stimulatory signal, leads to programmed cell death or anergy.[5] The CD28 and CD40 molecules and their ligand interactions are the two signals best studied to date. The CD28 molecule, found on T cells, interacts with its ligand (B7-1 [CD80], B7-2 [CD86], and B7-3) on activated APCs. This interaction amplifies the T cell response by downregulating IκBα; this leads to enhanced translocation of a CD28 response element (c-Rel) to the nucleus, where it up-

regulates IL-2 gene expression. The second co-stimulatory signal involves the interaction between CD40 on the APC with its ligand on activated T cells, CD154 (gp 39), a member of the TNF family. This interaction has effects on both T and B cells. In the B cell, this signal leads to direct activation. In B cells and other APCs, the signal causes upregulation of the expression of B7-1, B7-2, and B7-3. Upregulation of B7 molecules will lead to an increased CD28/B7 signal, amplifying the immune response as noted above. In several small and large animal models, antibody-mediated blockade of these co-stimulatory pathways markedly attenuates the immune response to the transplanted organ. Sirolimus is also thought to interfere with this pathway by inhibiting the downregulation of IκBα.

Tacrolimus

Tacrolimus (FK506) is a macrolide antibiotic isolated from the fungus *Streptomyces tsukubaensis*. As shown in Figure 55-2, it binds to cytosolic proteins collectively termed FK-binding proteins and inhibits the function of calcineurin, thus blocking the upregulation of IL-2 transcription, in a manner similar to cyclosporine (CsA). The major therapeutic effect of tacrolimus is preventing IL-2 production and activation of the T cell. Tacrolimus is 10 to 100 times more potent than CsA and can be expected to have differences in the side-effect profile as compared to CsA, which binds to a different set of cytoplasmic proteins before converging on calcineurin.

Extensive clinical experience has been reported in liver and kidney transplantation, commencing with a favorable effect on rejection refractory to conventional immunosuppression.[6] Trials comparing CsA- and tacrolimus-based regimens in liver transplantation show that tacrolimus-based therapy is associated with a lower incidence of acute rejection, including steroid-resistant and refractory rejection.[7,8] Several trials suggest a favorable profile for tacrolimus in thoracic transplantation. Investigators at the University of Pittsburgh first reported clinical experience in heart recipients, which was later summarized by Pham and colleagues in a retrospective report comparing tacrolimus and CsA-based regimens.[9] Patients in the CsA group ($n = 121$) were further classified into two subgroups based on whether or not they received lympholytic induction (LI) therapy. Although patient survival rates did not differ, tacrolimus-treated patients ($n = 122$) had significantly lower linearized rejection rates as compared to both CsA groups (0.09 episodes per 100 patient days for tacrolimus group vs 0.13 episodes per 100 patient days and 0.26 episodes per 100 patient days for the CsA group with and without LI, respectively). The requirement for pulse steroid treatment of rejection was lower in the tacrolimus group, and all cases of refractory rejection in the CsA group were successfully managed by tacrolimus rescue. There was no significant difference in actuarial freedom from allograft coronary disease for up to 5 years of follow-up. The tacrolimus group demonstrated a lower risk of hypertension, lower requirement for steroids, and similar serum creatinine at 2 years. The incidences of bacterial, viral, and fungal infections were not significantly different between the two groups.

Two prospective, multicenter, randomized, controlled trials were recently completed. The US Tacrolimus in Heart Transplant Multicenter Study compared open-label tacrolimus- and cyclosporine-based immunosuppression in 85 primary heart transplant recipients.[10] There were no significant differences in survival, probability, and overall incidence of each grade of rejection or types of treatment required. However, lower incidences of treated hyperlipidemia (41% vs 71%, $p = .01$) and hypertension (48% vs 71%, $p = .05$) were observed in the tacrolimus group, and the incidences of renal dysfunction, hyperglycemia, hypomagnesemia, and hyperkalemia were similar in the two groups. The European Tacrolimus Multicentre Heart Study compared open-labeled tacrolimus- and cyclosporine-based immunosuppression in 82 primary heart transplant recipients.[11] As in the US trial, there were no

significant differences in survival or allograft rejection between the two groups. A clinical trial comparing tacrolimus and cyclosporine in lung transplantation showed similar survival rates in the two groups but fewer acute rejection episodes and a significantly lower incidence of obliterative bronchiolitis in the tacrolimus group.[12] The overall incidence of infection was the same in both groups (although bacterial infections were more common in the CsA group); however, the tacrolimus group had a higher incidence of fungal infections. Groetzner and co-workers recently reported their experience with 73 patients who were undergoing primary heart transplantation and who were randomized to cyclosporine or tacrolimus.[13] During a 3-year follow-up period it was noted that the long-term toxicity of tacrolimus was similar to that of cyclosporine, and while there were fewer rejection episodes, tacrolimus had no impact on survival. Tacrolimus has also been used effectively as rescue immunosuppressant in heart transplant recipients who had refractory rejection or who were intolerent to cyclosporine.[14] A study by Mehra and co-workers raises the intriguing possibility of better outcomes in black heart transplant recipients with tacrolimus-based regimens.[15] In a small, prospective, randomized trial ($n = 42$), they showed that tacrolimus combined with adjunctive mycophenolate therapy, when compared with cyclosporine, reduced allograft rejection with a similar side-effect profile.

Mycophenolate Mofetil

Mycophenolate mofetil (MMF) is a derivative of mycophenolic acid (MPA); MPA reversibly inhibits the enzyme IMPDH, which is the rate-limiting step in the de novo pathway of purine synthesis. In contrast to most other replicating cells, lymphocytes rely primarily on the de novo pathway. In addition, the type II isoform of IMPDH, which is the major isoform in lymphocytes, is about four times more sensitive to the drug effect than the type I isoform found in most other cells. Thus, MPA confers a relatively lymphocyte-specific antiproliferative effect.[3]

Clinical efficacy and toxicity have been well studied in kidney transplant recipients. Halloran and associates recently reported a pooled analysis of the three large, randomized, multicenter, double-blind clinical trials that had enrolled nearly 1,500 patients.[16] Comparisons were made between MMF doses of 2 and 3 g/d and azathioprine (AZA) or placebo. Graft survival rates were not significantly different. Mycophenolate mofetil significantly reduced the incidence of rejection (40.8% in the AZA/placebo groups vs 19.8% and 16.5% for the 2 g and 3 g MMF groups, respectively). This translated into better renal function in both MMF groups at 3, 6, and 9 months.

Promising results from small pilot studies in heart transplant recipients led to the large, international, multicenter, randomized, double-blind trial that compared the efficacy of MMF to AZA in cardiac transplantation.[17–20] Target doses chosen were 1.5 g bid for MMF and 1.5 to 3 mg/kg/d for AZA in addition to cyclosporine and corticosteroids. Data analysis, on an intention-to-treat basis, revealed slightly lower incidences of death, retransplantation, and biopsy-proven rejection, which did not reach statistical significance. A major limitation of the study was that 11% of randomized patients withdrew from the study prior to receiving the study drug and subsequently received open-label AZA, likely affecting the intention-to-treat results. In the 578 patients who received at least one dose of the study drug, 1-year mortality was lower in the MMF group (6.2% vs 11.4%, $p = .03$). Cumulative biopsy-proven rejection episodes were not significantly reduced by MMF; yet, interestingly, biopsy-proven rejection with severe hemodynamic compromise was associated with 12 deaths in the AZA group as opposed to no such deaths in the MMF group. There were no significant differences in allograft vasculopathy at 1 year as assessed by angiography and intravascular ultrasonography. Mycophenolate mofetil patients had a greater incidence of diarrhea (45% vs 34%, $p = .008$) and esophagitis (7% vs 3%, $p = .02$), while AZA patients had a greater incidence of leukopenia (39% vs 30%, $p = .04$). The incidence of malignancy was similar in the two groups. Opportunistic infections, especially with the herpes viruses, were more prevalent in the MMF group (53% vs 44%, $p = .025$). Overall, this study demonstrates the safety of MMF in cardiac transplant recipients, with a possible trend toward reducing severe rejection, albeit at the expense of increased susceptibility to opportunistic infections. Further data regarding the long-term effects of MMF on allograft vasculopathy are forthcoming. Interestingly, Taylor and co-workers demonstrated an increased incidence of rejection when stable heart transplant recipients ($n = 43$) were converted from MMF to azothioprine.[21] These patients were on MMF therapy for an average of 41 months as part of an open-label safety study prior to conversion to either MMF or AZA. There was a significant increase in treated allograft rejection episodes in the AZA conversion group, accompanied by an increase in the mean biopsy score.

Although MMF drug levels are not often monitored, recent data suggest the value of monitoring. A retrospective analysis of 215 heart transplant recipients who had routine monitoring of MMF trough levels showed that MMF trough levels of 2 microgram/mL (µg/L) or greater was associated with a decreased incidence of rejection.[22] Another retrospective analysis of a tacrolimus-based regimen suggested that mycophenolic acid (MPA) plasma levels of greater that 3 µg/mL was associated with freedom from rejection.[23] However, a definite therapeutic window has still not been established, as shown by Hesse and co-workers, who did not find a significant correlation between MPA trough levels and acute rejection.[24] These authors did note, however, a significant increase in MPA trough levels in patients converted from cyclosporine to tacrolimus, which indicates a need for monitoring drug levels during changes in therapy.

Augmentation of immunosuppression with MMF may allow a decrease in cyclosporine dose and recovery of renal function in cyclosporine-induced nephropathy. In a prospective pilot study, heart transplant patients (mean of 8.6 years post-transpant) with deteriorating renal function were changed from AZA to MMF, allowing decrease in cyclosporine dosage and improvement in renal function, without acute rejection episodes over a 4- to 12-month follow-up period.[25] Other small studies also document a similar benefit, indicating that a switch to MMF may be appropriate in cyclosporine-induced nephropathy to enable recovery of renal function without jeopardizing graft survival.[26,27] However, long-term follow-up studies are required before such a procedure can be advised in stable heart transplant patients with cyclosporine-induced nephropathy.

Sirolimus (Rapamycin)

Sirolimus (rapamycin) is a macrocyclic antibiotic isolated from *Streptomyces hygroscopicus,* having powerful immunosuppressive properties. Although it is structurally similar to tacrolimus and complexes with the FKBP family of proteins, it interacts with different intracellular activation pathways. As was shown earlier in Figure 55-2, there are several potential targets. The sirolimus–FKBP complex inhibits a set of protein kinases termed mTOR (mammalian target of rapamycin), which appear to be required for cell-cycle progression. Sirolimus–FKBP inhibits activation of 70 kD S6 kinase, thereby interfering with the function of the S6 ribosomal protein and preventing translation of cell-cycle regulatory proteins. Also, as described earlier, it may inhibit CD28-mediated downregulation of IκBα, preventing the enhancement of cytokine transcription. Thus, sirolimus acts at several sites and, unlike tacrolimus and cyclosporine, can inhibit already activated T cells. This unique action makes it an attractive candidate in multidrug protocols with calcineurin inhibitors (tacrolimus and cyclosporine) and antimetabolites (azathioprine and mycophenolate mofetil).

An exciting feature of the potential of rapamycin lies in its ability to interfere with growth-factor–mediated cell proliferation. This combined effect on immune response and cell proliferation may be beneficial in the prevention of allograft vasculopathy. In a rat model of cardiac transplantation, administration of high doses of rapamycin early in the transplant course with continued maintenance led to a significant decrease in infiltration by leukocytes and macrophages and to subsequent intimal proliferation.[28] Efficacy in preventing allograft vasculopathy in humans would completely alter the long-term survival of solid-organ transplantation.

The clinical profile of this drug has only been tested in a few small trials so far. A phase I study in quiescent renal transplant patients receiving a CsA/steroid–based regimen tested sirolimus in three ascending doses against placebo.[29] Oral sirolimus or placebo was administered for 14 days. The main side effect was a reversible decrease in platelet and white blood cell counts. Sirolimus did not significantly alter the CsA concentrations. The drug was also not associated with increased incidences of hypertension, renal insufficiency, or hepatic dysfunction in combination with CsA, thus offering great promise in enhancing CsA-based therapy without increasing toxicity. A similar study testing ascending doses of sirolimus up to 15 mg/m² in stable renal transplant recipients also showed no serious adverse events, the only event attributed to sirolimus being a single case of thrombocytopenia.[30] Kahan and colleagues recently presented their results in renal transplant patients on a sirolimus–CsA maintenance regimen.[31] Steroid withdrawal was attempted in 32 human leuco antigen–mismatched living-donor recipients, and in 35 cadaveric-donor kidney recipients free of acute rejection or renal dysfunction, beginning 1 month after transplantation. Successful steroid withdrawal was accomplished in 77% of patients (78% in living-related and 77% in cadaveric-donor kidney recipients). Of note, patients on sirolimus-cyclosporine had lower levels of cholesterol, triglycerides, creatinine, and white blood cell counts than did patients remaining on sirolimus-cyclosporine-prednisone or cyclosporine-prednisone. Snell and co-workers[32] recently published results of sirolimus use in 23 lung transplant and 13 heart transplant recipients. Of the 56 indications for use, the commonest reason was renal dysfunction (30 of 56). Other indications were acute rejection prophylaxis, refractory acute rejection, myopathy, refractory chronic rejection, and cyclosporine-induced neurotoxicity. A 10 mg loading dose followed by a 5 mg daily maintenance dose was used prior to November 1999 to achieve a whole-blood level of 10 to 40 µg/L. After preliminary analysis and review of literature showed excess infections at this dose, the dose was reduced to a 5 mg loading dose followed by a 3 mg daily maintenance dose to achieve a blood level of 5 to 13 µg/L. As a result, there was improvement or stabilization of 35 of 56 indications. However, 37 infectious complications were seen in 21 patients, highlighting the need for carefully balancing the augmented immunosuppression with risk of infection. Several multiorgan phase III trials of sirolimus and a rapamycin derivative, SDZ RAD, are currently either underway or planned.

Methotrexate

Methotrexate inhibits the enzyme dihydrofolate reductase, thereby interfering with the pathway supplying the methyl groups for synthesis of thymidylate. By virtue of its antiproliferative effects, it interferes with both T and B cell–mediated immune responses. The predominant role explored for methotrexate has been in recalcitrant rejection.[33,34] The addition of weekly methotrexate courses (generally 2.5 to 25 mg/week) for 8 to 12 weeks is generally associated with decreased rejection episodes, decreased corticosteroid use, and acceptable toxicity.[33,34] A retrospective analysis of the use of methotrexate and total lymphoid irradiation in 57 patients with recalcitrant rejection showed comparable efficacy.[35] When methotrexate was used for rejection prophylaxis early after heart transplantation along with quadruple therapy with CsA, steroids, AZA, and OKT3, no significant effect on preventing rejection was seen.[36]

Monoclonal Antibodies and Fusion Proteins

Monoclonal antibodies directed against a specific molecular interaction offer great potential in achieving controlled and specific immunosuppression. The clinical success of OKT3 has led to the development of a variety of monoclonal antibodies. As was shown earlier in Figures 55–1 and 55–2, a number of cellular and subcellular interactions offer themselves to controlled inhibition.

Adhesion molecules and their ligands are expressed by various cells recruited into the immune cascade. Blockade of adhesion molecule function may inhibit perpetuation of endothelial injury at the time of transplantation as well as interfere with various steps of the immune encounter with foreign antigen (see Figure 55-1). Adhesion molecule blockade results in prolonged allograft survival in a variety of animal models.[4] Briscoe and associates demonstrated, in human heart transplant biopsies, that increased expression of the adhesion molecules ICAM-1, VCAM-1 (vascular cell adhesion molecule-1), and E-selectin was seen to correlate with CD3+ T cell infiltrates and the degree of rejection.[37] Antibodies to the adhesion molecule LFA-1, which binds to ICAM-1, has been compared to rabbit antithymocyte globulin (ATG) in 101 patients receiving their first kidney transplant.[38] Anti–LFA-1 antibody was better tolerated, although rejection rates at 15 days and at 3 months were not significantly different in the two treatment groups. The percentage of functioning grafts was similar at 1 year, as was the incidence and severity of infections. Interestingly, fewer patients required post-transplantation dialysis in the anti–LFA-1 group (19% vs 35%, a difference that did not reach statistical significance). This suggests a potential role for adhesion molecule blockade in preventing early renal allograft dysfunction. Another adhesion molecule–ligand pair tested is the LFA-3/CD2 interaction. A soluble human LFA-3 construct, which binds CD2 on the T cells and inhibits responses of T cells in vitro, was studied in a primate cardiac allograft model.[39] In baboon heart recipients, injections of LFA-3 for 12 consecutive days, starting 2 days before transplantation, significantly delayed graft rejection as compared to control (human IgG). Grafts from treated animals also showed markedly diminished endothelialitis. Despite persistent blood levels up to 1 to 2 weeks after the last injection, circulating antibodies to the LFA-3 construct were not detected in serum.

The CD4 recognition of the major histocompatibility complex of the APC is an important event in the immune response, and its inhibition has been successfully shown to prolong allograft survival in animal models. A phase I study of anti–CD4 antibody (OKT4A) was undertaken in cadaveric renal allograft recipients.[40] Thirty patients were given OKT4A for 12 consecutive days in ascending doses along with standard triple-drug therapy. The drug was well tolerated without the cytokine release side effects associated with OKT3, achieved a high percentage of saturation of CD4 receptors in all groups, and was devoid of significant side effects. A low 3-month rejection rate (37%) and an excellent 2-year graft survival rate were seen in this study.

The establishment of the critical role of co-stimulation in the complete immune response has been an exciting development, and two major pathways have been studied in detail. As can be seen from Figure 55-2, the close interrelation between the actions of CD40/ligand and CD28/B-7 protein suggest the potential for dual inhibition to achieve a powerful inhibition of the immune response. In biopsy samples from human cardiac allografts manifesting rejection, CD40 and its ligand CD154 (gp39/CD40 ligand) are expressed at high levels.[41] Kirk and associates studied the effects of blocking both pathways in a primate model of renal transplantation.[42] In this preclinical model, the fusion protein CTLA4-Ig (B-7 specific) and the monoclonal antibody 5C8 (CD40-ligand specific) were tested singly and in combination without any other background immunosuppression. Both drugs inhibited the mixed lymphocyte reaction, with the combination being 100 times more effective. Renal allografts were rejected in control animals in 5 to 8 days, while brief therapy with either drug prolonged rejection-free survival for 20 to 98 days. The most exciting aspect of this trial was that the agents were only administered briefly during the immediate perioperative period without any other immunosuppressive drugs, suggesting the possibility that this regimen was associated with immunologic tolerance. Surprisingly, for such a powerful modality, there were no significant side effects during treatment. This opens up the possibility of inducing acceptance of the allograft with a safe short-term therapy as opposed to the aggressive, chronic strategies employed at present.

Inhibition of function of the activated T cell can also be achieved by blockage of the interleukin-2 receptor (IL-2R). Genetically engineered human IgG_1 monoclonal antibody to the α chain of IL-2R (daclizumab) was tested in a randomized, placebo-controlled trial of 55 primary heart transplant recipients.[43] The drug or placebo was administered within 24 hours after transplantation and subsequently once every other week, for a total of 5 doses, while standard triple-drug immunosuppressive therapy was continued. The mean frequency of acute rejection episodes decreased from 0.64 per patient in the control group to 0.19 per patient in the daclizumab group ($p = .02$). The incidence of acute rejection was decreased from 63% in the control group to 18% in the daclizumab group. However, the frequency of rejection episodes after the 3-month induction period was similar between the two groups. There was no increased incidence of infections or maglignancies in the daclizumab group. No major adverse effects were reported with the drug. The absence of significant immunogenicity and side effects, coupled with demonstrable efficacy, offers promise for this drug in thoracic transplantation. The same authors reported a benefit of induction with daclizumab in decreasing incidence of graft athoerosclerosis at 1 year post transplant.[44] However, long-term studies in a larger number of patients are required to determine long-term survival benefits and optimal dosing schedules.

Basiliximab, a chimeric (human and mouse) antibody also against the IL-2R α subunit, has also shown great promise. Nashan and associates conducted a randomized, placebo-controlled trial of basiliximab in 380 renal allograft recipients receiving CsA and steroid therapy.[45] Two doses of basiliximab or placebo were given on days 0 and 4, providing IL-2R suppression for 4 to 6 weeks. The intention-to-treat analysis revealed a 32% reduction in biopsy-proven acute rejection episodes and a 13% reduction in steroid-resistant first rejection episodes in the basiliximab group. The mean daily dose of steroids was significantly higher in the placebo group, at 2 and 4 weeks. The incidence of graft loss and adverse events, including infections, was similar in the two groups. Basiliximab was well tolerated acutely, without cytokine-release phenomena. Another trial in kidney recipients by Kahan and colleagues showed similar results, with a significant 31% reduction in the incidence of acute rejection during the first 12 months after transplantation in patients given basiliximab, with a similar adverse effect profile compared to placebo.[46]

Photopheresis

Photopheresis involves the treatment of lymphocytes extracorporeally with long-wavelength ultraviolet light after exposure to the photosensitive drug 8-methoxypsoralen. Photoactivated 8-methoxypsoralen binds to the DNA and other cellular components of the treated lymphocytes, resulting in cell death. Re-infusion of these photoactivated, dying cells leads presumably to an "autoimmune" response against them as well as the larger pool of untreated clones.[47] In four patients at very high risk for rejection after cardiac transplantation (two with high panel reactive antibody [PRA] and two multiparous women), the addition of photopheresis to standard immunosuppression was associated with a surprisingly low incidence of rejection.[47] In a small pilot study, Meiser and associates reported that the early postoperative application of this therapy in addition to standard triple-drug therapy was associated with a reduction in cardiac rejection episodes without an increase in infections.[48] These encouraging early results led to a larger, prospective, multicenter, randomized trial of 60 primary heart recipients who were assigned to receive standard triple-drug therapy with or without photopheresis.[49] The treatment group received 12 two-day cycles during the first 6 months post transplant. Patient survival was similar during 6 months of follow-up. The photopheresis group had a 2.13 times greater likelihood of being rejection-free than did the control group, while the control group had 2.64 times greater relative risk of multiple rejection episodes.[49] This was accomplished without an increase in the incidence of infections; in fact, the detection of *Cytomegalovirus* deoxyribonucleic acid by polymerase chain reaction was significantly less frequent in the photopheresis group in a study by Barr and colleagues (unpublished). Barr and co-workers also reported a decreased coronary artery intimal thickness at 1 year post transplant in cardiac transplant patients treated with prophylactic photopheresis.[50]

Total Lymphoid Irradiation

In situ irradiation of lymphocytes is another method of achieving profound depression of the immune response. Currently, it is only used as rescue therapy in thoracic transplantation. In a small study of 19 heart transplant recipients with recurrent or early severe rejection, total lymphoid irradiation (TLI) was associated with a significant decrease in rejection rates.[51] However, the total dose of 800 rad resulted in an increased incidence of infections and depressed white blood cell (WBC) and platelet counts.[51] Similar doses have been used successfully in treating drug-resistant cardiac transplant rejection and rejection in heart-lung and lung allografts.[52,53] Hence, the current role of TLI may be in treating resistant rejection, and it is generally well tolerated in the short term with close surveillance of WBC and platelet counts and adjustment of doses and intervals as required. However, the effects of TLI appear to be permanent, and a report of the late development of acute leukemias in patients causes concern.[54]

Donor Bone Marrow Transfusion

Donor bone marrow infusion has been successfully used to modulate the immune response and to induce tolerance to allografts in a variety of animal models. Potential mechanisms are many and include donor cell microchimerism due to implantation of host tissues with graft cells, induction of anergy, clonal deletion, suppressor cell activity, and regulation of cytokines.[55] Zeevi and associates recently reported the presence of microchimerism in the majority of allograft recipients at the University of Pittsburgh who received donor bone marrow–augmented transplants.[56]

There was a trend toward a lower incidence of rejection in the first 100 days after transplantation in the heart recipients as compared to historic controls. The incidence of bronchiolitis obliterans was decreased in lung recipients during 18 months of follow-up as compared to historic controls. Another study from the same institution showed a 73% incidence of microchimerism in heart and lung recipients treated with donor marrow infusion at time of transplantation.[57] In a larger cohort of 24 heart and 20 lung recipients, the same investigators later reported that unmodified donor bone marrow infusion was associated with similar survival and overall rejection rates; however, 38% of the bone marrow–augmented patients were rejection-free during the first 6 months, as compared to only 11% of the control patients.[58] There were no apparent complications related to the bone marrow infusion itself. There are currently several studies of bone marrow or stem cell–augmented cardiac, hepatic, and renal transplantation underway.

Conclusion

Transplantation immunosuppression is moving rapidly away from broad, nonspecific therapies and toward specific, molecular targets. The number of potential therapeutic agents is expanding rapidly as the molecular basis of allograft rejection becomes clearer. The ultimate transplant immunotherapy, namely, complete allograft acceptance, is likely only a few developments away.

References

1. Lodish H, Baltimore D, Berk A, et al. Immunity. In: Molecular cell biology. New York: Scientific American Books; 1995. p. 1295–340.
2. Parham P. Immunobiology of transplantation. In: Haber E, editor. Molecular cardiovascular medicine. New York: Scientific American Books; 1995. p. 289–310.
3. Trehan S, Taylor DO, Renlund DG. New pharmacologic immunosuppressive agents. In: Cooper DKC, Miller LW, Patterson GA, editors. The transplantation and replacement of thoracic organs. Lancaster: Kluwer Academic Publishers; 1997. p. 635–60.
4. Perico N, Renuzzi G. Prevention of transplant rejection. Current treatment guidelines and future developments. Drugs 1997;54(4):533–70.
5. Sayegh MH, Turka LA. The role of T cell costimulatory activation pathways in transplant rejection. N Engl J Med 1998;338:1813–21.
6. US Multicenter FK506 Liver Study Group. Comparison of tacrolimus (FK506) and CsA for immunosuppression in liver transplantation. N Engl J Med 1994;331:1110–5.
7. European FK506 Multicenter Liver Study Group. Randomized trial comparing tacrolimus and CsA in prevention of liver allograft rejection. Lancet 1994;344:423–8.
8. Fung JJ, Todo S, Abu Elmagd K, et al. Randomized trial in primary liver transplantation under immunosuppression with FK506 or cyclosporin. Transplant Proc 1993;25:1130.

9. Pham SM, Kormos RL, Hattler BG, et al. A prospective trial of tacrolimus (FK506). In: Clinical heart transplantation. J Thorac Cardiovasc Surg 1996;111:764–72.

10. Taylor DO, Barr ML, Radovancevic B, et al. A comparison of tacrolimus- and cyclosporine-based immunosuppression in cardiac transplantation. J Heart Lung Transplant 1997;16(1):72.

11. Reichart B, Meiser B, Vigano M, et al. Tacrolimus (FK506) vs. cyclosporin in heart transplantation: results from a randomized European, multicentre pilot study. J Heart Lung Transplant 1997;16:43.

12. Keenan RJ, Konishi H, Kawai A, et al. Clinical trial of tacrolimus versus cyclosporine in lung transplantation. Ann Thorac Surg 1995;60:580–5.

13. Groetzner J, Meiser BM, Schirmer J, et al. Tacrolimus or cyclosporine for immunosuppression after cardiac transplantation: which treatment reveals more side effects during long-term follow-up. Transplant Proc 2001;33:1461–4.

14. De Bonis M, Reynolds L, Barros J, Madden P. Tacrolimus as a rescue immunosuppressant after heart transplantation. Eur J Cardiothorac Surg 2001;19(5):690–5.

15. Mehra MR, Uber PA, Scott RL, et al. Racial differences in clinical outcome using tacrolimus and mycophenolate mofetil immunosuppression in heart transplantation. Transplant Proc 2001;33:1613–4.

16. Halloran P, Mathew S, Tomlanovich S, et al. Mycophenolate mofetil in renal allograft recipients. Transplantation 1997;63:39–47.

17. Taylor DO, Ensley DR, Olsen SL, et al. Mycophenolate mofetil (RS-61443): preclinical, clinical, and three-year experience in heart transplantation. J Heart Lung Transplant 1994;13:571–82.

18. Kirklin JK, Bourge RC, Naftel DC, et al. Treatment of recurrent heart rejection with mycophenolate mofetil (RS-61443): initial clinical experience. J Heart Lung Transplant 1994;13:444–50.

19. Renlund DG, Gopinathan SK, Kfoury AG, et al. Mycophenolate mofetil (MMF) in heart transplantation: rejection prevention and treatment. Clin Transplant 1996;10:136–9.

20. Kobashigawa J, Miller L, Renlund D, et al. A randomized active-controlled trial of mycophenolate mofetil in heart transplant recipients. Transplantation 1998;66:507–15.

21. Taylor DO, Sharma RC, Kfoury AG, Renlund DG. Increased incidence of allograft rejection in stable heart transplant recipients after late conversion from mycophenolate mofetil to azathioprine. Clin Transplant 1999;13(4):296–9.

22. Yamani MH, Starling RC, Goormastic M, et al. The impact of routine mycophenolate mofetil drug monitoring on the treatment of cardiac allograft rejection. Transplantation 2000;69(11):2326–30.

23. Meiser BM, Pfeiffer M, Schmidt D, et al. Combination therapy with tacrolimus and mycophenolate mofetil following cardiac transplantation: importance of mycophenolic acid therapeutic drug monitoring. J Heart Lung Transplant 1999;18(2):143–9.

24. Hesse CJ, Vantrimpotn IC, van Reimsdijk-van Overbeeke T, et al. the value of routine monitoring of mycophenolic acid plasma levels after clinical heart transplantation. Transplant Proc 2001;33:2163–4.

25. Dureau G, Obadia JF, Chizel M, Boissonnat P. Introduction of mycophenolate mofetil and cyclosporine withdrawal in heart transplant patients with progressive deteriorating renal fundtion. Transplant Proc 2000;32:461–2.

26. Aleksic I, Baryalei M, Busch T, et al. Improvement of impaired renal function in heart transplant recipients treated with mycophenolate mofetil and low-dose cyclosporine. Transplantation 200;69(8):1586–90.

27. Sanchez V, Delgado JF, Blasco R, et al. Benefits of mycophenolate mofetil in cardiac transplant recipients with cyclosporine-induced nephropathy. Transplant Proc 1999;31:2515–6.

28. Schmid C, Heeman U, Azuma H, et al. Rapamycin inhibits transplant vasculopathy in long-surviving rat heart allografts. Transplantation 1995;60:729–33.

29. Murgia MG, Jordan S, Kahan BD. The side-effect profile of sirolimus: a phase I study in quiescent cyclosporine-prednisone-treated renal transplant patients. Kidney Int 1996;49:209–16.

30. Brattstrom C, Tyden G, Sawe J, et al. A randomized, double-blind, placebo-controlled study to determine safety, tolerance, and preliminary pharmacokinetics of ascending single doses of orally administered sirolimus (rapamycin) in stable renal transplant recipients. Transplant Proc 1996;28:985–6.

31. Kahan BD, Pescovitz M, Chan G, et al. One-year outcome after steroid withdrawal from a sirolimus–cyclosporine–prednisone regimen in cadaver- and living-donor recipients. Transplantation 1998;65:S167.

32. Snell GI, Levvey BJ, Chin W, et al. Rescue therapy: a role for sirolimus in lung and heart transplant recipients. Transplant Proc 2001;33:1084–5.

33. Costanzo-Nordin MR, Grusk BB, Silver MA, et al. Reversal of recalcitrant cardiac allograft rejection with methotrexate. Circulation 1998;78 Suppl III:III-47–57.

34. Olsen SL, O'Connell JB, Bristow MR, Renlund DG. Methotrexate as an adjunct in the treatment of persistent mild cardiac allograft rejection. Transplantation 1990;50:773–5.

35. Ross HJ, Gullestad L, Pak J, et al. Methotrexate or total lymphoid radiation for treatment of persistent or recurrent allograft cellular rejection: a comparative study. J Heart Lung Transplant 1997;16:179–89.

36. Taylor DO, Olsen SL, Ensley RD, et al. Methotrexate for rejection prophylaxis after heart transplantation. J Heart Lung Transplant 1995;14:950–4.

37. Briscoe DM, Yeung AC, Schoen EL, et al. Predictive value of inducible endothelial cell adhesion molecule expression for acute rejection of human cardiac allografts. Transplantation 1995;59:204–11.

38. Hourmant M, Bedrossian J, Durand D, et al. A randomized multicenter trial comparing leukocyte function-associated antigen-1 monoclonal antibody with rabbit antithymocyte globulin as induction treatment in first kidney transplantations. Transplantation 1996;62:1565–70.

39. Kaplon RJ, Hochman PS, Michler RE, et al. Short-course single-agent therapy with an LFA-3-IgG1 fusion protein prolongs primate cardiac allograft survival. Transplantation 1996;61:356–63.

40. Cooperative Clinical Trials in Transplantation Research Group. Murine OKT4A immunosuppression in cadaver

donor renal allograft recipients. Transplantation 1997; 63:1087–95.

41. Reul RM, Fang JC, Denton MD, et al. CD40 and CD40 ligand (CD 154) are coexpressed on microvessels in vivo in human cardiac allograft rejection. Transplantation 1997;64:1765–74.

42. Kirk AL, Harlan DM, Armstrong NN, et al. CTLA4-Ig and anti-CD40 ligand prevent renal allograft rejection in primates. Proc Natl Acad Sci U S A 1997;94:8789–94.

43. Beniaminovitz A, Itescu S, Lietz K, et al. Prevention of rejection in cardiac transplantation by blockade of the interleukin-2 receptor with a monoclonal antibody. N Engl J Med 2000;342:613–9.

44. Mancini D, Beniaminovitz A, Edwards N, et al. Effect of daclizumab induction therapy on the development of cardiac transplant vasculopathy. J Heart Lung Transplant 2001;20(2):194.

45. Nashan B, Moore R, Amlot P, et al. Randomised trial of basiliximab versus placebo for control of acute cellular rejection in renal allograft recipients. Lancet 1997;350: 1193–8.

46. Kahan BD, Rajagopalan PR, Hall ML, et al. Basiliximab (Simulect) is efficacious in reducing the incidence of acute rejection episodes in renal allograft patients: results at 12 months. Transplantation 1998;65:S189.

47. Rose EA, Barr ML, Xu He, et al. Photochemotherapy in human heart transplant recipients at high risk for fatal rejection. J Heart Lung Transplant 1992;11:746–50.

48. Meiser BM, Kur F, Reichenspurner H, et al. Reduction of the incidence of rejection by adjunct immunosuppression with photochemotherapy after heart transplantation. Transplantation 1994;57:563–8.

49. Barr ML, Eisen HJ, Meiser BM, et al. Immunomodulation with photopheresis: clinical results of the multi-center cardiac transplantation study. Fifteenth Annual Meeting ASTP, Chicago 1996; (Program and Abstracts):170.

50. Barr ML, Baker CJ, Schenkel FA, et al. Prophylactic photopheresis and chronic rejection: effects on graft intimal hyperplasia in cardiac transplantation. Clin Transplant 2000;14(2):162–6.

51. Salter MM, Kirklin JK, Bourge RC, et al. Total lymphoid irradiation in the treatment of early or recurrent heart rejection. J Heart Lung Transplant 1992;11.902–12.

52. Evans MA, Schomberg PJ, Rodeheffer RJ, et al. Total lymphoid irradiation: a novel and successful therapy for resistant cardiac allograft rejection. Mayo Clin Proc 1992;67:785–90.

53. Valentine VG, Robbins RC, Wehner JH, et al. Total lymphoid irradiation for refractory acute rejection in heart-lung and lung allografts. Chest 1996;109:1184–9.

54. Bourge RC, Kirklin JK, Giffin DC, et al. Total lymphoid irradiation after cardiac transplantation: is there a risk of late leukemia? J Heart Lung Transplant 1998;17:75.

55. Brennan DC, Mohanakumar T, Flye MW. Donor-specific transfusion and donor bone marrow infusion in renal transplantation tolerance: a review of efficacy and mechanisms. Am J Kidney Dis 1995;26(5):701–15.

56. Zeevi A, Pavlick M, Banas R, et al. Three years of follow-up of bone marrow-augmented organ transplant recipients: the impact on donor-specific immune modulation. Transplant Proc 1997;29:1205–6.

57. Pham SM, Keenan RJ, Rao AS, et al. Perioperative donor bone marrow infusion augments chimerism in heart and lung transplant recipients. Ann Thoracic Surg 1995; 60:1015–20.

58. Pham SM, Zeevi A, Rao A, et al. Three-year experience on combined donor bone marrow infusion and thoracic organ transplantation. J Heart Lung Transplant 1997; 16:69.

CHAPTER 56

ALLOGRAFT CORONARY ARTERY DISEASE

JIGNESH K. PATEL, MD, PhD, JON A. KOBASHIGAWA, MD

Transplant coronary artery disease (TCAD) was first noted during the 1960s in experimental animal models of heart transplants. These studies demonstrated a time-dependent prevalence of atherosclerosis in the donor heart that appeared unrelated to allograft rejection. TCAD was noted clinically in the 1970s, when histologic studies of coronary artery lesions in transplant hearts revealed extensive disease in vessels that had appeared to be normal angiographically at the time of transplantation. Although the introduction of cyclosporine-based immunosuppression in the early 1980s was followed by improved survival rates among transplant recipients, no corresponding decrease in the prevalence of TCAD was observed.[1]

TCAD is the principal determinant limiting the long-term survival of cardiac allografts. According to the registry of the International Society of Heart and Lung Transplantation, the overall half-life of allograft survival is only 8.7 years, and following the first year, there is a constant annual mortality rate of 4%. This is despite significant improvements in therapy to prevent allograft rejection in recent years. After the first year of transplantation, coronary artery disease accounts for a significant number of all deaths.

Incidence and Prognosis

Despite its limited sensitivity, coronary angiography remains the preferred method of the clinical detection of TCAD.[2] More recent studies suggest promising potential for noninvasive methods such as the detection of coronary calcification by electron beam computerized tomography.[3,4] The reported incidence of TCAD has varied widely due to differences in definition of disease and patient populations. In one of the largest cohorts studied, angiographically significant TCAD was noted in 42% of the patients at 5 years with 7% developing severe disease leading to death or retransplantation.[5] TCAD may occur as early as 1 year after transplantation, and disease that appears early following transplantation is more aggressive and associated with a worse prognosis, with two-thirds of patients developing coronary events 5 years following

detection of TCAD in one study.[6] In one study, those patients with angiographic disease had a relative risk of any cardiac event of 3.4 and of death of 4.6 when compared to those without disease.[7]

Pathologic Characteristics of TCAD

Conventional atherosclerosis is a manifestation of chronic inflammation affecting the vessel wall with ingress of inflammatory cells including macrophages, T cells, and smooth-muscle cells. This process is thought to be a "response to injury" of the endothelium, as first hypothesized by Ross.[8] A number of factors have been implicated in causing the initial insult to the endothelium, including cholesterol, hypertension, oxidative stress, and even possibly infections such as *Chlamydia pneumoniae* and *Cytomegalovirus* (CMV). Similarly, transplant vasculopathy is thought to result from an initial injury to the allograft endothelium. Principal determinants (Figure 56-1) include preservation injury, alloimmune response, and possibly chronic *Cytomegalovirus* infection, in addition to the conventional risk factors for atherosclerosis. The general distinguishing feature of transplant vasculopathy (Figure 56-2), when compared to conventional atherosclerosis, is its more diffuse nature, with frequent involvement of large- and medium-sized vessels as well as the microvasculature (Table 56-1). Lesions also tend to be concentric, limiting detection by conventional angiography.[9] Many transplant recipients with TCAD also have lesions typical of more conventional atherosclerosis, but for the most part, lesions tend to be lipid poor and calcification seems to occur relatively late. A wide spectrum of lesion type is therefore apparent (Figure 56-3). The disease not only affects the intima but the media and adventitia frequently undergo fibrous infiltration. As a consequence, compensatory remodeling of the artery is inhibited (the Glagov phenomenon), and the artery may even undergo constriction.[10] In some cases, subepicardial inflammatory infiltrates are noted even in the absence of myocardial interstitial inflammatory infiltrates. Intravas-

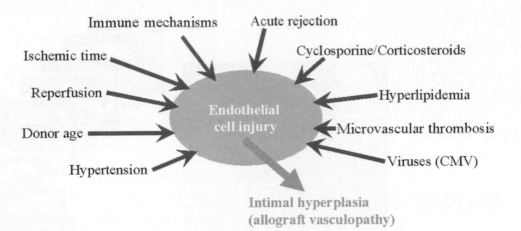

FIGURE 56-1. Proposed mechanisms contributing to endothelial injury in the development of transplant coronary artery disease. Endothelial cell injury has been proposed as the event that initially triggers proliferation of smooth-muscle cells and macrophages.

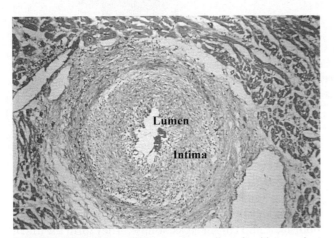

FIGURE 56-2. Myocardial artery in an allograft with transplant vasculopathy showing concentric intimal hyperplasia and compromise in luminal area (hematoxylin and eosin ×40 original magnification).

TABLE 56-1. Typical Features of Nontransplant Atherosclerosis and Transplant Coronary Artery Disease

Nontransplant Atherosclerosis	Transplant Coronary Artery Disease
Affects mostly epicardial vessels	All arteries affected, including microvasculature
Slow progression	Rapid progression
Lesions eccentric	Lesions concentric
Generally lipid rich	Generally lipid poor
Calcification seen early	Calcification occurs late
Compensatory remodeling (Glagov phenomenon)	Arteries constrict

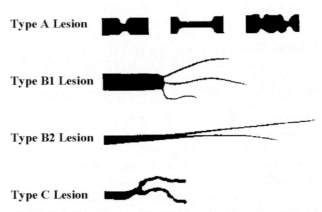

FIGURE 56-3. Diagrammatic representation of types of lesions seen angiographically in heart transplant recipients. Type A lesion: discrete tubular or multiple stenoses. Type B1 lesion: abrupt transition from a normal proximal vessel, with distal diffuse concentric narrowing and obliterated vessel. Type B2 lesion: gradual concentric tapering, with distal portion having residual channel. Type C lesion: narrowed, irregular vessel that terminates abruptly.

imaging techniques allow direct imaging of the vessel wall (Figure 56-4). This has been useful in determining characteristics of donor-related lesions (conventional atherosclerosis) by examination early following transplantation and comparing transplant-acquired lesions later on in the same regions.[11,12] Furthermore, as TCAD often presents as diffuse concentric disease not easily appreciated angiographically, intravascular ultrasonography provides more detailed assessment with increased sensitivity.[13]

Clinical Presentation

Because of the denervated state of the transplanted heart, cardiac ischemia or infarction does not typically present with chest pain.[14] Many patients do, however, develop evidence for cardiac reinnervation, and cases of chest pain due to ischemia and infarction have been documented.[15–17]

cular thrombus is also a frequent finding at autopsy or following explant for retransplantation.[9]

Angiographic lesions have been classified to describe the spectrum of lesions seen in TCAD. Type A lesions have features of conventional coronary atherosclerotic disease. Type B and C lesions represent more typical transplant-related disease (see Figure 56-3). Intravascular

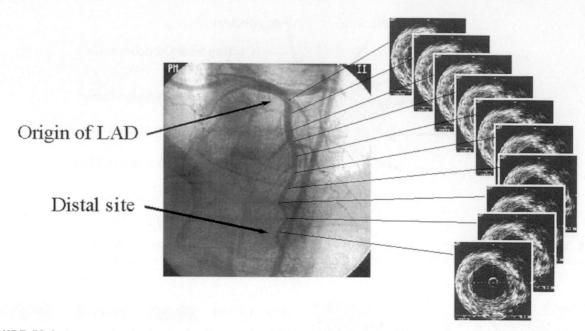

FIGURE 56-4. Intravascular ultrasonography allows sequential cross-sectional analysis of epicardial vessels. Coronary angiography (left) reveals a seemingly normal left anterior descending (LAD) artery with no identifiable disease; however, the intravascular ultrasound images of the same artery (right panels) reveal an eccentric noncalcified plaque. The central circle represents catheter artifact. For the detection and quantification of intramural atherosclerosis, intravascular ultrasonography is superior to coronary angiography.

Patients with myocardial infarction frequently do not have typical electrocardiogram (ECG) changes to baseline abnormalities nor do they have changes as a consequence of heterogenous disease resulting from diffuse vasculopathy.[18] In general, the lack of symptoms and electrocardiographic findings often lead to less frequent use of revascularization therapies, which results in worse outcomes, presenting as heart failure, arrhythmia, or sudden death.[7,18]

Immune Mechanisms Contributing to TCAD

The transplanted heart is a major stimulus to the recipient immune system. The principal determinant of the recipient immune response is the recognition of foreign antigens encoded by the major histocompatibility complex (MHC). Both class I (HLA A, B, C) and class II (HLA DR, DP, DQ) antigens are highly polymorphic glycoproteins encoded on chromosome 6 in humans. A substantial portion of circulating donor T lymphocytes are able to recognize these antigens and hence mount a robust immune response which leads to production of a variety of cytokines (interleukins, interferon-γ, and tumor necrosis factor-α). These cytokines subsequently allow development of effector mechanisms, including cytotoxic T cells, infiltrating macrophages, and antibody production.

Although much of this immune response is responsible for the allograft dysfunction seen in acute rejection, there is evidence to suggest that it also plays an important contributory role in the development of TCAD. This phenomenon is, therefore, also frequently termed *chronic*

rejection, a process not only seen in the transplanted heart, but also in renal, lung, and liver allografts. In transplanted lungs, chronic rejection presents as obliterative bronchiolitis, and in liver allografts, the equivalent process is known as vanishing bile duct syndrome.

Endothelial cells likely play a pivotal role in mediating both acute and chronic rejection.[19,20] They form the initial interface between donor and the host circulating lymphocytes and maintain a barrier to the egress of inflammatory cells into the interstitium. They are also highly responsive to cytokines and are able to express class II antigens, particularly in the microvasculature and coronary arteries (Figure 56-5).[21–23] They also act as antigen-presenting cells (APCs).[24,25] In vitro, endothelial cells from human coronary arteries are able to stimulate allogeneic T cells.[26]

Although T-cell injury to the myocardium in acute cellular rejection is limited by immunosuppressive agents, it appears that these agents have a limited effect on the development of TCAD. One reason may be that these agents are more effective at suppressing interleukin (IL)-2 production and less effective at suppressing the production of cytokines that lead to antibody production.[27] The majority of patients following solid-organ transplantation continue to make antibodies to the allograft. Anti-HLA antibody production in recipients has been associated with a higher mortality.[28] More specifically, production of antiendothelial antibodies correlates with the development of TCAD.[29] The majority of patients with TCAD seemed to have developed antibodies to the intermediate filament vimentin, a protein characteristic that is not restricted to endothelial cells. Vimentin is diffusely

Graft Vascular Endothelium

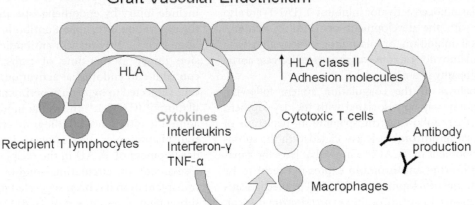

FIGURE 56-5. Endothelial cells play a central role in rejection. Recipient T cells may be activated due to HLA alloantigen recognition leading to cytokine production. In a simplified scheme, this leads to both further endothelial activation and recruitment of supplemental mediators of endothelial injury. These include macrophages, cytotoxic T cells, and the production of antiendothelial antibodies (for example, antivimentin antibodies). (TNF = tumor necrosis factor.)

expressed in the intima and media of normal and diseased coronary arteries. Therefore, injury early following transplantation, for example, by ischemia and reperfusion, may lead to release of vimentin into the circulation. The protein may be taken up by APCs and presented as an autoantigen as it is not normally exposed to the immune system. Interestingly, these antibodies do not seem to mediate complement-mediated cytotoxicity to endothelial cells in vitro, a process associated with hyperacute rejection. Consequently, antivimentin antibodies may exert a more subtle form of low-grade damage in a process in keeping with the chronic progressive course of TCAD development. One possible mechanism may be the upregulation of endothelial cell adhesion molecules, which, over a period of time, would allow adherence and transmigration of inflammatory cells into the intima.[30]

Hemostatic Factors

A distinguishing feature of TCAD is the diffuse nature of the disease; it affects both the arterial network as well as the capillary network and the venous system, suggesting that this is truly a panvascular disease.[31] The normal cardiac microvasculature is highly resistant to thrombosis. However, as early as 1 month following cardiac transplantation, endomyocardial biopsy specimens begin to show evidence of microvascular fibrin deposition, which subsequently significantly correlates with the development of TCAD.[32] Microvascular thrombosis also results in acute myocardial cell damage from ischemia. Labarrere recently demonstrated that troponins, sensitive markers for myocardial damage, are indeed elevated in transplant patients with evidence of microvascular fibrin deposition on endomyocardial biopsy specimens.[33] Furthermore, patients with persistently elevated troponins in the first year had a significantly higher likelihood of developing

graft failure or severe TCAD. Elevated troponins in the first month following cardiac transplantation are very common, presumably related to the ischemia/reperfusion injury that occurs at the time of transplantation. The persistent elevation in the following months, which occurs in some patients and which also correlates with ongoing microvascular thrombosis, presumably relates to a more persistent thrombogenic insult. One possibility is that this relates to cellular rejection. Certainly, severe acute allograft rejection is frequently associated with microvascular thrombosis. However, patients with myocardial fibrin deposits and elevated troponins do not show more cellular rejection episodes than those without.[32] Other possibilities include the development of antiendothelial cell antibodies, including those against vimentin. Multiple time-dependent factors may be involved, with ischemia/reperfusion injury being important early following transplantation, and development of antibodies or cytokine-dependent endothelial cell activation being more important later on. The early events may serve to release endothelial cell antigens, such as vimentin, to which a humoral response is subsequently mounted.

The propensity for vascular thrombosis depends upon the balance between procoagulant status and endogenous fibrinolytic activity. Decreased fibrinolytic activity would prevent removal of fibrin, and in a prothrombotic microvasculature, would facilitate further production of thrombin and fibrin. Both increased plasma fibrinogen concentration and decreased plasma fibrinolytic activity are associated with increased arterial intimal thickening in cardiac transplant patients.[34,35] Labarrere noted a significantly increased incidence of angiographic coronary artery disease in transplant patients with lower levels of tissue plasminogen activator (t-PA) on endomyocardial biopsies.[35] These patients developed earlier and more aggressive disease than did those patients with normal t-PA levels within the arteriolar microvasculature. Circulating levels of t-PA and plasminogen activator inhibitor-1 (PAI-1) are also associated with the development of TCAD.[36] Recently, experimental inhibition of plasminogen activators with viral antiinflammatory serpin was shown to decrease aortic graft vasculopathy in a rat model.[37]

Abnormalities of the coagulation system following transplantation may be associated with the development of TCAD. Early following transplantation, depletion of microvascular antithrombin is associated with the subsequent development of TCAD.[38] Grafts that have the capability of recovering antithrombin expression seem to be less prone to the development of TCAD. The mechanisms leading to change in antithrombin expression are unclear. Release of cytokines following episodes of cellular rejection or other factors related to the process of transplantation may lead to alteration in the expression or availability of molecules which bind antithrombin, such as heparan sulfate proteoglycan molecules.[39] Ischemia and reperfusion may be particularly important due to release of enzymes from recruited neutrophils, including neutrophil elastase and heparinase. Lack of antithrombin binding because of subsequent loss of heparin sulfate leads to generation of thrombin, a process that leads to further loss of heparin sulfate proteoglycan, thereby sustaining a prothrombogenic milieu within the microvasculature.

Endothelial Activation

Allograft vascular endothelial cells express HLA class II antigens and adhesion molecules such as intercellular adhesion molecule-1 (ICAM-1) and vascular cell adhesion molecule (VCAM).[35,40] These molecules are not usually expressed on endothelium of normal hearts. The expression of these molecules on endothelium is a phenomenon referred to as *endothelial activation*. Although expression of adhesion molecules on endothelium is a feature of nontransplant atherosclerosis, the expression of HLA antigens seems to be unique to the transplant endothelium. Furthermore, coculture of these cells in vitro with CD4+ T cells results in their proliferation and production of IL-2.[40] This implies that donor endothelium may provide a sustained stimulus to recipient lymphocytes to maintain a chronic immunologic response. Allografts with expression of ICAM-1 and HLA-DR on arterial and arteriolar endothelium develop transplant vasculopathy.[41] A recent study has also suggested that a certain ICAM-1 polymorphism detected in the donor heart may be protective from the development of TCAD, which may relate to an allelic change that renders decreased ICAM-1 binding to B cells.[42]

A number of factors may lead to endothelial activation (see Figure 56-5). Cytokines released from inflammatory cells following an episode of acute rejection may lead to this process, and an increased incidence of TCAD correlates with the frequency of acute allograft rejection

episodes.[43] Other possibilities of endothelial activation include injury by endothelial-specific T lymphocytes or the generation of recipient antibodies to donor endothelium such as antivimentin antibodies. Ischemia/reperfusion injury at the time of transplantation may also contribute to endothelial activation. Human endothelial cells subjected to hypoxia experimentally do show upregulation of ICAM-1.[44] In animal models, the induction of adhesion molecules on allograft endothelium prior to transplantation is also associated with the subsequent development of TCAD in the recipient.[45] In humans, the assessment of circulating soluble ICAM-1 following transplantation has been suggested to be a marker for the subsequent development of TCAD.[46]

Integrins and Chemokines

Integrins and chemokines may also contribute to transplant vasculopathy. Recent studies imply a correlation between sustained expression of the vitronectin receptor (integrin α-V,β-3) and progression of TCAD by intravascular ultrasonography (IVUS).[47] The chemokine RANTES (regulated on activation, normal T cell expressed and secreted), a chemokine that selectively chemoattracts T lymphocytes, natural killer (NK) cells, monocytes, and eosinophils, is expressed in human TCAD.[48] In an animal model, sustained RANTES production was required for both monocyte recruitment and the development of intimal thickening, and this required the presence of CD4+ cells.[49]

Nonimmune Factors in the Development of TCAD

Insight into the role of nonimmunologic factors in the development of chronic rejection is provided by studies on renal allografts. Donor kidneys and hearts that are well matched for HLA antigens clearly have longer graft survival.[50] On the other hand, grafts from living unrelated donors have survival comparable to grafts from related donors and consistently superior to matched grafts from cadaveric donors.[51] Nonimmune factors must therefore play a significant role in the development of chronic graft dysfunction. It is also possible that immune factors may be important in the development of early graft vasculopathy whereas nonimmune factors may determine the propensity to develop TCAD late following transplantation.[52]

Cadaveric organs are procured often under profound physiologic derangements. Donors frequently have sustained massive central nervous system injuries, often with periods of labile blood pressure requiring prolonged inotropic support. Organ harvesting may take place under less-than-ideal conditions before being perfused with subphysiologic electrolyte preservation solutions. Organs are then stored in the cold for several hours prior to final engraftment. Further changes during reperfusion then take place.

To determine specific risk factors for fatal donor allograft vasculopathy, a multi-institutional analysis of more than 7,000 cardiac transplants over a period of 10 years was recently performed.[53] By multivariable analysis, risk factors for fatal allograft vasculopathy included older donor age, male donor, younger recipient age, earlier date of transplant, ischemic etiology, history of recipient cigarette use, history of gouty arthritis, black recipient, and positive donor CMV serology (Table 56-2). Allografts from donors older than 50 years of age had a 50% chance of developing moderate to severe TCAD at 5 years. This presumably relates to the extent of preexisting atherosclerosis in the older donor. In contrast, however, programs that actively pursue the use of older grafts have not seen a significant difference in overall survival or in the development of TCAD when compared to recipients with younger allografts.[54] Furthermore, the presence of preexisting coronary artery disease does not seem to accelerate the progression of TCAD.[55]

A number of important changes that may impact upon the performance of the donor heart occur following brain death. Circulating neuroendocrine hormonal levels may be increased while levels of other hormones may decrease.[56] Inflammatory markers, including cytokines and adhesion molecules, may be upregulated, leading to apoptosis and cardiac dysfunction.[57] Interestingly, however, the use of adrenergic agents in optimizing donors prior to transplantation has been associated with improved renal allograft survival but impaired cardiac allograft function following transplantation.[58]

Ischemia occurring during organ procurement and storage and subsequent reperfusion following engraftment may produce endothelial changes that may be central to the subsequent development of TCAD over the ensuing years.[59] Acutely, changes include desquamation and retraction of endothelial cells, increasing their permeability. A number of endothelial genes can be induced by hypoxia, including vascular endothelial growth factor (VEGF), basic fibroblast growth factor (bFGF), and platelet-derived growth factor (PDGF).[60–62] Both bFGF and PDGF may induce intimal smooth-muscle migration and proliferation whereas VEGF stimulates endothelial proliferation and enhances vascular permeability.[63]

TABLE 56-2. Risk Factors for the Development of Transplant Coronary Artery Disease

Older age
Male donor
Young recipient
Ischemic etiology for transplantation
Recipient history of smoking
History of gouty arthritis
Black recipient
Donor positive CMV status
Hyperlipidemia in recipient
Hypertension in recipient

CMV = *Cytomegalovirus*.

Angiotensin II is also a potent mitogen for smooth-muscle cell proliferation and, experimentally, its inhibition is effective in inhibiting the development of TCAD.[64,65] Similarly, inhibition of angiotensin-converting enzyme (ACE), whose expression is increased in injured vessels, is also effective experimentally in ameliorating transplant vasculopathy, and ACE inhibitors could be potentially of some value as preventive agents.[64]

Ischemia may also lead to increased expression of CD11/CD18 adhesion molecules on circulating leukocytes and corresponding increase in expression of ICAM-1 and MHC molecules on endothelial cells. As a result, avidity of CD11/CD18 for ICAM-1 is promoted and leukocytes are activated, which leads to release of proinflammatory mediators. Experimentally, anti-ICAM-1 antibodies limit myocardial damage following ischemia/reperfusion injury.[66]

Hyperlipidemia

Approximately half of all cardiac transplantations are performed on patients with ischemic cardiomyopathy. A substantial portion of these patients have a history of hyperlipidemia as a major contributor to their disease. Lipid levels are also widely elevated following cardiac transplantation.[67] A number of factors are thought to contribute to post-transplant hyperlipidemia. Steroids contribute to increased apolipoprotein B production and also contribute to post-transplant obesity. Cyclosporine may enhance this effect and may also independently increase hepatic lipase activity and decrease lipoprotein lipase activity.[68] The effect would be impaired very-low-density lipoprotein (VLDL) and low-density lipoprotein (LDL) clearance.

Hyperlipidemia is a well-established risk factor for nontransplant atherosclerosis. Both clinical and experimental observations suggest that it may be important in the development of transplant vasculopathy.[69–71] In a small retrospective study, elevated lipid values 6 months following transplantation had a strong predictive value for the development of TCAD at 3 years.[70] In a more recent study, post-transplant elevation of LDL at 1 year was the only predictor for the development or progression of TCAD by IVUS.[72] Experimentally, rabbits fed a high-cholesterol diet following cardiac transplantation develop accelerated graft atherosclerosis.[73] The allogeneic state of the transplanted heart which also leads to endothelial activation may further augment the vascular response to hyperlipidemia. In this respect, greater intimal thickening, more intimal angiogenesis, and a greater accumulation of T cells are seen in transplanted vasculature when compared to native vessels in animals exposed to the same level of hyperlipidemia.[74,75] Interestingly, treatment initiated within 2 weeks of transplantation with an inhibitor of the rate-limiting enzyme in the cholesterol biosynthetic pathway, hydroxymethylglutaryl coenzyme A (HMG

CoA) reductase, is associated with decreased development of coronary intimal thickening as well as a lower frequency of hemodynamically compromising rejection episodes and improved survival.[76] These agents likely have an immunosuppressive effect in addition to their lipid-lowering activity. As hyperlipidemia is so common following transplantation, these findings suggest that all cardiac transplant recipients should receive HMG CoA reductase inhibitors where tolerated.

Hypertension

There is a clear link between hypertension and conventional coronary atherosclerosis. Hypertension is a common problem following cardiac transplantation, related in part to the use of corticosteroids, frequent associated weight gain, and use of calcineurin inhibitors. Although no studies have specifically addressed the issue of whether hypertension is a risk factor for the development of TCAD, it seems likely that it is.

There is evidence that use of calcium channel blockers may attenuate the development of TCAD. In one study, patients randomized to diltiazem demonstrated a significant decrease in coronary artery luminal diameter by quantitative coronary angiography (QCA) when compared with baseline at 1 and 5 years.[77] At 5 years there was also a significant difference in freedom from both death and TCAD. In a rat heterotopic transplant model, amlodipine significantly decreased the development of allograft vasculopathy.[78] In vitro, calcium channel blockers stabilize endothelial cell function, inhibit platelet aggregation, and decrease the release of platelet-derived growth factors.[79]

Drugs and TCAD

The impact of immunosuppressive agents on transplant vasculopathy is not well defined. The indirect effects of long-term steroid therapy on lipid metabolism have already been described. This effect is enhanced with the use of cyclosporin although there is some evidence that substitution of cyclosporin for the newer calcineurin inhibitor tacrolimus may abrogate the rise in serum lipids.[80] The number and severity of episodes of acute rejection may contribute to the subsequent development of TCAD.[43,52] Thus, more effective immunosuppressive regimens may have a beneficial impact on the development of allograft vasculopathy.

Tacrolimus, a calcineurin inhibitor with actions similar to cyclosporine, has been studied extensively in liver transplantation and shown to be superior to cyclosporine in preventing chronic rejection (Williams, 1996 No. 1198).[81] Although it causes less hypertension and hyperlipidemia than cyclosporine in cardiac transplantation, data on preventing TCAD are less conclusive.[80] In one study, treatment with tacrolimus was associated with the lower incidence of antiendothelial antibodies.[82] In a more recent study, there was a trend toward more TCAD by intravascular ultrasonography in patients treated with tacrolimus when compared to cyclosporine.[83]

Mycophenolate mofetil (MMF), an inhibitor of the de novo pathway for purine biosynthesis, is more effective at reducing cardiac allograft rejection and post-transplant mortality.[84] More recent studies suggest that it may also be more effective at reducing allograft vasculopathy.[85] This effect may be related at least in part to the ability of mycophenolate to reduce B-cell responses, as patients treated with this agent developed lower antivimentin titers, which was correlated with the lower incidence of TCAD by IVUS.

Sirolimus (rapamycin), a macrolide antibiotic with potent immunosuppressive effects, has antiproliferative effects on smooth-muscle cells in vitro and in experimental animal models of vascular injury. It was also recently shown to reduce the process of in-stent restenosis following angioplasty and stent placement in native coronary artery disease in a small-scale human trial.[86] It clearly holds great potential as a primary immunosuppressive agent in cardiac transplantation with the promise of preventing TCAD, a process in which intimal smooth-muscle proliferation is the hallmark. Clinical trials are currently pending. Another agent not yet available for clinical use and currently undergoing trials, FTY720, experimentally reduces the development of TCAD in mice.[87]

Leflunomide is a new immunosuppressive agent that is effective in both allo- and xenotransplantation in animal models. In vitro, it is able to inhibit smooth-muscle cell proliferation. In animal models, it prevents allograft vasculopathy.[88] In one study, leflunomide was even able to reverse transplant vasculopathy when the agent was started late, and this correlated with a decrease in antibody formation.[88]

Cytomegalovirus

Among the many possible etiologic factors implicated in the development of TCAD, *Cytomegalovirus* infection has held a prominent position over the years. Human CMV has a wide global distribution, and exposure to it increases with age, so much so that by age 60 years, up to 90% of humans have evidence of prior exposure. Fortunately, CMV poses little threat to the vast majority of humans who have a well-developed competent immune system, with most infections resulting in mild subclinical disease. However, in patients with acquired immunodeficiency syndrome (AIDS), cancer patients undergoing chemotherapy, and organ transplant recipients, CMV infection can be life-threatening, leading to systemic viremia, hepatitis, pneumonitis, retinitis, colitis, and other manifestations. In cardiac transplantation, CMV infection is associated with accelerated allograft vasculopathy. Both clinical and experimental studies suggest that CMV infection may play an important role in the development of

TCAD. In one of the earlier studies of 102 transplant recipients, 16% developed transplant vasculopathy, of whom 62% had evidence of CMV infection as compared to only 25% of patients without TCAD.[89] Similar findings were confirmed by Loebe and colleagues.[90] In animal studies, rat aortic allografts develop neointimal proliferation when the recipients are infected with CMV at the time of transplantation.[91]

The mechanisms by which CMV infection may contribute to transplant vasculopathy are unclear. CMV infection of human endothelial cells does not seem to result in induction of HLA class II antigens, and infected cells are refractory to induction of these antigens by interferon-γ due to interruption of the signal transduction pathway.[92] The induction of class I molecules by interferon-γ is also similarly blocked by CMV.[93] Endothelial cell infection, however, does lead to upregulation of adhesion molecules on both infected and noninfected cells. Production of IL-1β is implicated in this paracrine effect.[94] Coculture experiments suggest that CMV infection of T cells results in production of interferon-γ and tumor necrosis factor-α, which are then able to induce expression of class I and class II antigens, VCAM-1, and ICAM-1. CMV infection of smooth-muscle cells may also contribute to neointimal proliferation by inhibition of apoptosis.[95]

Detecting Transplant Coronary Artery Disease

Transplant coronary disease is usually very advanced and beyond therapeutic intervention by the time symptoms develop. Surveillance is therefore the major approach to monitoring the development of TCAD. Both noninvasive and invasive approaches have been used for diagnosis. In general, noninvasive methods are unable to detect early disease as these techniques depend upon the presence of hemodynamically significant lesions. Ultrafast CT has been used to detect coronary calcification and may be useful in the detection of TCAD but still does not provide detailed information about the vessel lumen or wall.[96] Consequently, invasive methods are the mainstay of TCAD detection.

Coronary angiography relies upon the ability to compare normal segments of the vessel with diseased segments. The diffuse nature of TCAD often results in underestimation of disease because there is no reference segment in which the normal diameter of the vessel can be assessed. Minimal luminal irregularities may suggest the presence of early disease and is therefore often commented upon. Comparison with prior studies may help to determine development of disease but requires the use of the same angiographic protocol at each study for precise evaluation to avoid confounding by technical factors such as angiographic projections and magnification. Moreover, this allows use of computer-assisted QCA, which improves sensitivity of detection of TCAD. However, QCA also has its limitations because it does not allow evaluation of the vessel wall and may miss early disease where compensatory dilatation of the vessel may occur to preserve luminal area.

IVUS is currently the only technique that allows evaluation of the vessel wall. Cross-sectional images of the coronary vessel wall comparable to histologic sections are obtained. Intimal area can be quantitatively planimetered to accurately assess even early plaque burden (Figure 56-6). Sequential images are usually obtained as the catheter is pulled back to determine the extent of disease along a vessel wall (see Figure 56-4). Several studies show that IVUS is more sensitive than angiography in detecting TCAD.[11,97,98] The technique, however, has several limitations: it is highly invasive, it requires anticoagulation, it uses expensive single-use catheters, and evaluation is mainly limited to the major epicardial vessels.

Determination of coronary flow reserve with intracoronary Doppler flow measurement may be useful in assessing TCAD although the clinical importance of this information has yet to be determined. Intracoronary flow velocities are determined using a Doppler transducer mounted on a guidewire. Pharmacologic interventions such as intracoronary adenosine can be used to measure maximal coronary flow and to calculate flow reserve. Coronary flow reserve is reduced in patients with TCAD and deteriorates with increasing time after transplantation.[99] Measurement of coronary flow reserve reflects changes in the microvasculature as well as the epicardial vessels.

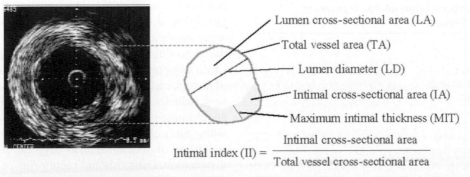

FIGURE 56-6. Intravascular ultrasonography enables quantitative analysis of coronary lesions to determine both extent and progression of disease when lesions are studied sequentially over a time period.

Production of vasodilatory mediators by the endothelium plays a major role in the regulation of vascular tone. Endothelial dysfunction is not only an early feature in the development of atherosclerosis but likely also plays a fundamental role in the development of TCAD. Nitroglycerin is a direct vasodilator acting on vascular smooth muscle. Acetylcholine works indirectly through its action on the endothelium. Its vasodilatory property is dependent upon an intact functional endothelium. The loss or attenuation of endothelium-dependent vasodilatation can be used to determine endothelial cell dysfunction. Both QCA and IVUS can be used to assess changes in vessel diameter in response to pharmacologic challenge. Abnormal responses to acetylcholine have been reported after transplantation.[100]

Treatment of TCAD

Clinically apparent disease is associated with a poor prognosis, and therefore prevention is an important strategy in addressing transplant vasculopathy. Agents used in the treatment and prevention of conventional atherosclerosis are also used for TCAD (Table 56-3). Aspirin is widely used, given its widely established use in nontransplant coronary disease. Control of hypertension and hyperlipidemia was already discussed. The use of HMG CoA reductase inhibitors is particularly important because they also help to prevent allograft rejection. Newer immunosuppressive agents such as mycophenolate mofetil and rapamycin may have additional benefits in preventing TCAD, but further studies are needed.

Once clinically apparent TCAD is apparent, a number of approaches are available to relieve ischemia. For focal disease, percutaneous coronary intervention (PCI) with balloon angioplasty has been successful although restenosis is particularly common in the transplant setting.[101] Stenting has helped to address this problem. The use of intracoronary radiation to prevent restenosis in TCAD is currently undergoing evaluation. In the near future, the availability of rapamycin-coated stents offers further hope for optimism. The use of atherectomy techniques and laser therapy has been reported in a small number of patients.[102–104] No studies are available to show whether

TABLE 56-3. Treatment Options for Transplant Coronary Artery Disease

Prevention
    Aspirin
    Control of hypertension
    HMG CoA reductase inhibitors
    Mycophenolate mofetil
    ?Rapamycin
Treatment
    Balloon angioplasty/stenting
    ?Intracoronary radiation
    Coronary artery bypass surgery
    Retransplantation

HMG CoA = hydroxymethylglutaryl coenzyme A.

percutaneous coronary intervention alters the prognosis of TCAD, and because many patients with significant disease are asymptomatic, intervention often presents a dilemma.

Patients with multivessel focal disease with adequate distal target vessels may be candidates for coronary artery bypass surgery (CABG). Efficacy is difficult to determine because relatively small numbers have been reported, reflecting the many patients who do not have adequate targets and the preferential use of PCI.

Retransplantation may be a consideration for many patients with advanced TCAD that is not amenable to PCI or CABG. Survival rates reported after retransplantation are consistently lower than those after primary transplantation. Retransplantations within the first 6 months after original transplantation have the worst outcomes, with a 1-year survival rate of only 38%.[105] These were, however, most commonly performed for treatment of refractory rejection. In a Stanford study, the 1-year actuarial survival of those patients who underwent retransplantation specifically for TCAD was 69 ± 10%, which approaches the 1-year survival rate following primary transplantation.[106] This study also showed that patients having a second heart transplant do not have an increased risk for developing TCAD in the second donor heart. The actuarial freedom from TCAD in the entire heart retransplantation population at 5 years was 89 ± 7%, and, in patients who underwent retransplantation for TCAD, the actuarial freedom from this disease process in the retransplanted heart at 5 years was 91 ± 9%. Such data suggest that heart transplant patients who develop severe TCAD may be suitable candidates for retransplantation. The scarcity of donor hearts, however, creates an ethical dilemma. Some authors argue that it is better to use organs to give more patients the opportunity of a first transplant rather than allocate two organs to the same individual. Other authors believe that patients needing a second transplant should be considered on the same basis as those being evaluated for first transplants.

Conclusion

Transplant vasculopathy is an important and major complication that limits the long-term survival of cardiac allografts. The disease has many features that are similar to nontransplant atherosclerosis, but there also important differences in both pathology and distribution of the disease. Development of TCAD is dependent upon a number of factors, including conventional atherosclerosis risk factors, ischemic injury at the time of organ harvest, host alloimmune response, hemostatic factors, and the modulating effect of post-transplant medications. Clinical presentation of TCAD is also atypical due to surgical denervation. Diagnosis and monitoring of disease depend mostly on invasive techniques. Given the relatively poor prognosis of TCAD, prevention remains an important strategy. Greater understanding of its pathology will offer more promising immunosuppressive regimens and improved methods of organ preservation in the near future, which, it is hoped, will have a significant impact upon the development of this disease in the transplant population. In the meantime, those with established disease have conventional revascularization techniques available to them for palliation, and retransplantation may be a consideration for a few.

References

1. Gao SZ, Schroeder JS, Alderman EL, et al. Prevalence of accelerated coronary artery disease in heart transplant survivors. Comparison of cyclosporine and azathioprine regimens. Circulation 1989;80:III100–5.

2. Gao SZ, Hunt SA, Schroeder JS. Accelerated transplant coronary artery disease. Semin Thorac Cardiovasc Surg 1990;2:241–9.

3. Lazem F, Barbir M, Banner N, et al. Coronary calcification detected by ultrafast computed tomography is a predictor of cardiac events in heart transplant recipients. Transplant Proc 1997;29:572–5.

4. Barbir M, Lazem F, Bowker T, et al. Determinants of transplant-related coronary calcium detected by ultrafast computed tomography scanning. Am J Cardiol 1997;79: 1606–9.

5. Costanzo MR, Naftel DC, Pritzker MR, et al. Heart transplant coronary artery disease detected by coronary angiography: a multi-institutional study of preoperative donor and recipient risk factors. Cardiac Transplant Research Database. J Heart Lung Transplant 1998;17:744–53.

6. Gao SZ, Hunt SA, Schroeder JS, et al. Early development of accelerated graft coronary artery disease: risk factors and course. J Am Coll Cardiol 1996;28:673–9.

7. Uretsky BF, Kormos RL, Zerbe TR, et al. Cardiac events after heart transplantation: incidence and predictive value of coronary arteriography. J Heart Lung Transplant 1992;11:S45–51.

8. Ross R, Glomset J, Harker L. Response to injury and atherogenesis. Am J Pathol 1977;86:675–84.

9. Arbustini E, Roberts WC. Morphological observations in the epicardial coronary arteries and their surroundings late after cardiac transplantation (allograft vascular disease). Am J Cardiol 1996;78:814–20.

10. Kobashigawa J, Wener L, Johnson J, et al. Longitudinal study of vascular remodeling in coronary arteries after heart transplantation. J Heart Lung Transplant 2000;19: 546–50.

11. Kapadia SR, Nissen SE, Ziada KM, et al. Development of transplantation vasculopathy and progression of donor-transmitted atherosclerosis: comparison by serial intravascular ultrasound imaging. Circulation 1998;98:2672–8.

12. Kapadia SR, Nissen SE, Tuzcu EM. Impact of intravascular ultrasound in understanding transplant coronary artery disease. Curr Opin Cardiol 1999;14:140–50.

13. St Goar FG, Pinto FJ, Alderman EL, et al. Intracoronary ultrasound in cardiac transplant recipients. In vivo evidence of "angiographically silent" intimal thickening. Circulation 1992;85:979–87.

14. Aranda JM Jr, Hill J. Cardiac transplant vasculopathy. Chest 2000;118:1792–800.

15. Stark RP, McGinn AL, Wilson RF. Chest pain in cardiac-transplant recipients. Evidence of sensory reinnervation after cardiac transplantation. N Engl J Med 1991;324: 1791–4.

16. Ramsdale DB, Bellamy CM. Angina and threatened acute myocardial infarction after cardiac transplantation. Am Heart J 1990;119:1195–7.

17. Schroeder JS, Hunt SA. Chest pain in heart-transplant recipients. N Engl J Med 1991;324:1805–7.

18. Gao SZ, Schroeder JS, Hunt SA, et al. Acute myocardial infarction in cardiac transplant recipients. Am J Cardiol 1989;64:1093–7.

19. Rose ML. Role of endothelial cells in allograft rejection. Vasc Med 1997;2:105–14.

20. Bishop DK, Shelby J, Eichwald EJ. Mobilization of T lymphocytes following cardiac transplantation. Evidence that CD4-positive cells are required for cytotoxic T lymphocyte activation, inflammatory endothelial development, graft infiltration, and acute allograft rejection. Transplantation 1992;53:849–57.

21. Shirwan H. Chronic allograft rejection. Do the Th2 cells preferentially induced by indirect alloantigen recognition play a dominant role? Transplantation 1999;68:715–26.

22. Daar AS, Fuggle SV, Fabre JW, et al. The detailed distribution of MHC Class II antigens in normal human organs. Transplantation 1984;38:293–8.

23. Page C, Rose M, Yacoub M, Pigott R. Antigenic heterogeneity of vascular endothelium. Am J Pathol 1992; 141: 673–83.

24. Rose ML, Page C, Hengstenberg C, Yacoub MH. Identification of antigen presenting cells in normal and transplanted human heart: importance of endothelial cells. Hum Immunol 1990;28:179–85.

25. Rose ML. Endothelial cells as antigen-presenting cells: role in human transplant rejection. Cell Mol Life Sci 1998; 54:965–78.

26. McDouall RM, Page CS, Hafizi S, et al. Alloproliferation of purified CD4+ T cells to adult human heart endothelial cells, and study of second-signal requirements. Immunology 1996;89:220–6.

27. Han CW, Imamura M, Hashino S, et al. Differential effects of the immunosuppressants cyclosporin A, FK506 and KM2210 on cytokine gene expression. Bone Marrow Transplant 1995;15:733–9.

28. Suciu-Foca N, Reed E, Marboe C, et al. The role of anti-HLA antibodies in heart transplantation. Transplantation 1991;51:716–24.

29. Dunn MJ, Crisp SJ, Rose ML, et al. Anti-endothelial antibodies and coronary artery disease after cardiac transplantation. Lancet 1992;339:1566–70.

30. Pidwell DJ, Heller MJ, Gabler D, Orosz CG. In vitro stimulation of human endothelial cells by sera from a subpopulation of high-percentage panel-reactive antibody patients. Transplantation 1995;60:563–9.

31. Oni AA, Ray J, Hosenpud JD. Coronary venous intimal thickening in explanted cardiac allografts. Evidence demonstrating that transplant coronary artery disease is a manifestation of a diffuse allograft vasculopathy. Transplantation 1992;53:1247–51.

32. Labarrere CA, Nelson DR, Faulk WP. Myocardial fibrin deposits in the first month after transplantation predict subsequent coronary artery disease and graft failure in cardiac allograft recipients. Am J Med 1998;105:207–13.

33. Labarrere CA, Nelson DR, Cox CJ, et al. Cardiac-specific troponin I levels and risk of coronary artery disease and graft failure following heart transplantation. JAMA 2000;284:457–64.

34. Meckel CR, Anderson TJ, Mudge GH, et al. Hemostatic/fibrinolytic predictors of allograft coronary artery disease after cardiac transplantation. Vasc Med 1997;2:306–12.

35. Labarrere CA, Pitts D, Nelson DR, Faulk WP. Vascular tissue plasminogen activator and the development of coronary artery disease in heart-transplant recipients. N Engl J Med 1995;333:1111–6.

36. Warshofsky MK, Wasserman HS, Wang W, et al. Plasma levels of tissue plasminogen activator and plasminogen activator inhibitor-1 are correlated with the presence of transplant coronary artery disease in cardiac transplant recipients. Am J Cardiol 1997;80:145–9.

37. Lucas A, Dai E, Liu L, et al. Transplant vasculopathy: viral anti-inflammatory serpin regulation of atherogenesis. J Heart Lung Transplant 2000;19:1029–38.

38. Labarrere CA, Torry RJ, Nelson DR, et al. Vascular antithrombin and clinical outcome in heart transplant patients. Am J Cardiol 2001;87:425–31.

39. Labarrere CA. Anticoagulation factors as predictors of transplant-associated coronary artery disease. J Heart Lung Transplant 2000;19:623–33.

40. Salomon RN, Hughes CC, Schoen FJ, et al. Human coronary transplantation-associated arteriosclerosis. Evidence for a chronic immune reaction to activated graft endothelial cells. Am J Pathol 1991;138:791–8.

41. Labarrere CA, Nelson DR, Faulk WP. Endothelial activation and development of coronary artery disease in transplanted human hearts. JAMA 1997;278:1169–75.

42. Borozdenkova S, Smith J, Marshall S, et al. Identification of ICAM-1 polymorphism that is associated with protection from transplant associated vasculopathy after cardiac transplantation. Hum Immunol 2001;62:247–55.

43. Kobashigawa JA, Miller L, Yeung A, et al. Does acute rejection correlate with the development of transplant coronary artery disease? A multicenter study using intravascular ultrasound. Sandoz/CVIS Investigators. J Heart Lung Transplant 1995;14:S221–6.

44. Zund G, Uezono S, Stahl GL, et al. Hypoxia enhances induction of endothelial ICAM-1: role for metabolic acidosis and proteasomes. Am J Physiol 1997;273:C1571–80.

45. Poston RS Jr, Billingham ME, Pollard J, et al. Effects of increased ICAM-1 on reperfusion injury and chronic graft vascular disease. Ann Thorac Surg 1997;64:1004–12.

46. Labarrere CA, Nelson DR, Miller SJ, et al. Value of serum-soluble intercellular adhesion molecule-1 for the noninvasive risk assessment of transplant coronary artery disease, posttransplant ischemic events, and cardiac graft failure. Circulation 2000;102:1549–55.

47. Yamani MH, Masri S, Ratliff NB, et al. The role of vitronectin receptor and tissue factor in the pathogenesis of transplant coronary vasculopathy [abstract]. J Heart Lung Transplant 2001;20:185.

48. Pattison JM, Nelson PJ, Huie P, et al. RANTES chemokine expression in transplant-associated accelerated atherosclerosis [abstract]. J Heart Lung Transplant 1996;15:1194–9.

49. Yun JJ, Fischbein MP, Laks H, et al. RANTES production during development of cardiac allograft vasculopathy. Transplantation 2001;71:1649–56.

50. Opelz G, Wujciak T, Dohler B, et al. HLA compatibility and organ transplant survival. Collaborative Transplant Study. Rev Immunogenet 1999;1:334–42.

51. Gjertson DW, Cecka JM. Living unrelated donor kidney transplantation. Kidney Int 2000;58:491–9.

52. Hornick P, Smith J, Pomerance A, et al. Influence of acute rejection episodes, HLA matching, and donor/recipient phenotype on the development of "early" transplant-associated coronary artery disease. Circulation 1997;96:II-148–53.

53. Costanzo MR, Eisen HJ, Brown RN, et al. Are there specific risk factors for fatal allograft vasculopathy? An analysis of over 7,000 cardiac transplant patients [abstract]. J Heart Lung Transplant 2001;20:152.

54. Drinkwater DC, Laks H, Blitz A, et al. Outcomes of patients undergoing transplantation with older donor hearts. J Heart Lung Transplant 1996;15:684–91.

55. Botas J, Pinto FJ, Chenzbraun A, et al. Influence of pre-existent donor coronary artery disease on the progression of transplant vasculopathy. An intravascular ultrasound study. Circulation 1995;92:1126–32.

56. Arita K, Uozumi T, Oki S, et al. The function of the hypothalamo-pituitary axis in brain dead patients. Acta Neurochir (Wien) 1993;123:64–75.

57. Birks EJ, Yacoub MH, Burton PS, et al. Activation of apoptotic and inflammatory pathways in dysfunctional donor hearts. Transplantation 2000;70:1498–506.

58. Schnuelle P, Berger S, de Boer J, et al. Effects of catecholamine application to brain-dead donors on graft survival in solid organ transplantation. Transplantation 2001;72:455–63.

59. Day JD, Rayburn BK, Gaudin PB, et al. Cardiac allograft vasculopathy: the central pathogenetic role of ischemia-induced endothelial cell injury. J Heart Lung Transplant 1995;14:S142–9.

60. Kourembanas S, Hannan RL, Faller DV. Oxygen tension regulates the expression of the platelet-derived growth factor-B chain gene in human endothelial cells. J Clin Invest 1990;86:670–4.

61. Levy AP, Levy NS, Wegner S, Goldberg MA. Transcriptional regulation of the rat vascular endothelial growth factor gene by hypoxia. J Biol Chem 1995;270:13333–40.

62. Lindner V, Reidy MA. Proliferation of smooth muscle cells after vascular injury is inhibited by an antibody against basic fibroblast growth factor. Proc Natl Acad Sci U S A 1991;88:3739–43.

63. Dvorak HF, Brown LF, Detmar M, Dvorak AM. Vascular permeability factor/vascular endothelial growth factor, microvascular hyperpermeability, and angiogenesis. Am J Pathol 1995;146:1029–39.

64. Furukawa Y, Matsumori A, Hirozane T, Sasayama S. Angiotensin II receptor antagonist TCV-116 reduces graft coronary artery disease and preserves graft status in a murine model. A comparative study with captopril. Circulation 1996;93:333–9.

65. Richter M, Skupin M, Grabs R, et al. New approach in the therapy of chronic rejection? ACE- and AT1-blocker reduce the development of chronic rejection after cardiac transplantation in a rat model. J Heart Lung Transplant 2000;19:1047–55.

66. Yamazaki T, Seko Y, Tamatani T, et al. Expression of intercellular adhesion molecule-1 in rat heart with ischemia/reperfusion and limitation of infarct size by treatment with antibodies against cell adhesion molecules. Am J Pathol 1993;143:410–8.

67. Stamler JS, Vaughan DE, Rudd MA, et al. Frequency of hypercholesterolemia after cardiac transplantation. Am J Cardiol 1988;62:1268–72.

68. Superko HR, Haskell WL, Di Ricco CD. Lipoprotein and hepatic lipase activity and high-density lipoprotein subclasses after cardiac transplantation. Am J Cardiol 1990;66:1131–4.

69. Kobashigawa JA, Kasiske BL. Hyperlipidemia in solid organ transplantation. Transplantation 1997;63:331–8.

70. Eich D, Thompson JA, Ko DJ, et al. Hypercholesterolemia in long-term survivors of heart transplantation: an early marker of accelerated coronary artery disease. J Heart Lung Transplant 1991;10:45–9.

71. Esper E, Glagov S, Karp RB, et al. Role of hypercholesterolemia in accelerated transplant coronary vasculopathy: results of surgical therapy with partial ileal bypass in rabbits undergoing heterotopic heart transplantation. J Heart Lung Transplant 1997;16:420–35.

72. Kapadia SR, Nissen SE, Ziada KM, et al. Impact of lipid abnormalities in development and progression of transplant coronary disease: a serial intravascular ultrasound study. J Am Coll Cardiol 2001;38:206–13.

73. Alonso DR, Starek PK, Minick CR. Studies on the pathogenesis of atheroarteriosclerosis induced in rabbit cardiac allografts by the synergy of graft rejection and hypercholesterolemia. Am J Pathol 1977;87:415–42.

74. Tanaka H, Sukhova GK, Libby P. Interaction of the allogeneic state and hypercholesterolemia in arterial lesion formation in experimental cardiac allografts. Arterioscler Thromb 1994;14:734–45.

75. Raisanen-Sokolowski A, Tilly-Kiesi M, Ustinov J, et al. Hyperlipidemia accelerates allograft arteriosclerosis (chronic rejection) in the rat. Arterioscler Thromb 1994;14:2032–42.

76. Kobashigawa JA, Katznelson S, Laks H, et al. Effect of pravastatin on outcomes after cardiac transplantation. N Engl J Med 1995;333:621–7.

77. Schroeder JS, Gao SZ, Alderman EL, et al. A preliminary study of diltiazem in the prevention of coronary artery disease in heart-transplant recipients. N Engl J Med 1993;328:164–70.

78. Atkinson JB, Wudel JH, Hoff SJ, et al. Amlodipine reduces graft coronary artery disease in rat heterotopic cardiac allografts. J Heart Lung Transplant 1993;12:1036–43.

79. Betz E, Weiss HD, Heinle H, Fotev Z. Calcium antagonists and atherosclerosis. J Cardiovasc Pharmacol 1991;18:S71–5.

80. Taylor DO, Barr ML, Radovancevic B, et al. A randomized, multicenter comparison of tacrolimus and cyclosporine immunosuppressive regimens in cardiac transplantation: decreased hyperlipidemia and hypertension with tacrolimus. J Heart Lung Transplant 1999;18:336–45.

81. Williams R, Neuhaus P, Bismuth H, et al. Two-year data from the European multicentre tacrolimus (Fk506) liver study. Transplant Int 1996;9 Suppl 1:S144–50.

82. Jurcevic S, Dunn MJ, Crisp S, et al. A new enzyme-linked immunosorbent assay to measure anti-endothelial antibodies after cardiac transplantation demonstrates greater inhibition of antibody formation by tacrolimus compared with cyclosporine. Transplantation 1998;65:1197–202.

83. Klauss V, Konig A, Spes C, et al. Cyclosporine versus tacrolimus (FK506) for prevention of cardiac allograft vasculopathy. Am J Cardiol 2000;85:266–9.

84. Kobashigawa J, Miller L, Renlund D, et al. A randomized active-controlled trial of mycophenolate mofetil in heart transplant recipients. Mycophenolate Mofetil Investigators. Transplantation 1998;66:507–15.

85. Rose MLD, Smith JD, Keogh AM, et al. Mycophenolate mofetil (MMF) depresses antibody production after cardiac transplantation [abstract]. Circulation 2000;102:II.490.

86. Rensing BV, Smits P, Foley D, et al. Coronary restenosis prevention with a rapamycin coated stent [abstract]. J Am Coll Cardiol 2001;37:47A.

87. Hwang MW, Matsumori A, Furukawa Y, et al. FTY720, a new immunosuppressant, promotes long-term graft survival and inhibits the progression of graft coronary artery disease in a murine model of cardiac transplantation. Circulation 1999;100:1322–9.

88. MacDonald AS, Sabr K, MacAuley MA, et al. Effects of leflunomide and cyclosporine on aortic allograft chronic rejection in the rat. Transplant Proc 1994;26:3244–5.

89. McDonald K, Rector TS, Braulin EA, et al. Association of coronary artery disease in cardiac transplant recipients with cytomegalovirus infection. Am J Cardiol 1989;64:359–62.

90. Loebe M, Schuler S, Zais O, et al. Role of cytomegalovirus infection in the development of coronary artery disease in the transplanted heart. J Heart Transplant 1990;9:707–11.

91. Lemstrom KB, Bruning JH, Bruggeman CA, et al. Cytomegalovirus infection enhances smooth muscle cell proliferation and intimal thickening of rat aortic allografts. J Clin Invest 1993;92:549–58.

92. Scholz M, Hamann A, Blaheta RA, et al. Cytomegalovirus- and interferon-related effects on human endothelial cells. Cytomegalovirus infection reduces upregulation of HLA class II antigen expression after treatment with interferon-gamma. Hum Immunol 1992;35:230–8.

93. Miller DM, Zhang Y, Rahill BM, et al. Human cytomegalovirus blocks interferon-gamma stimulated up-regulation of major histocompatibility complex class I expression and the class I antigen processing machinery. Transplantation 2000;69:687–90.

94. Dengler TJ, Raftery MJ, Werle M, et al. Cytomegalovirus infection of vascular cells induces expression of pro- inflammatory adhesion molecules by paracrine action of secreted interleukin-1beta. Transplantation 2000;69:1160–8.

95. Zhu H, Shen Y, Shenk T. Human cytomegalovirus IE1 and IE2 proteins block apoptosis. J Virol 1995;69:7960–70.

96. Farzaneh-Far A. Electron-beam computed tomography in the assessment of coronary artery disease after heart transplantation [abstract]. Circulation 2001;103:E60.

97. Rickenbacher PR, Kemna MS, Pinto FJ, et al. Coronary artery intimal thickening in the transplanted heart. An in vivo intracoronary ultrasound study of immunologic and metabolic risk factors. Transplantation 1996;61:46–53.

98. Konig A, Theisen K, Klauss V. Intravascular ultrasound for assessment of coronary allograft vasculopathy. Z Kardiol 2000;89:IX/45–9.

99. Mullins PA, Chauhan A, Sharples L, et al. Impairment of coronary flow reserve in orthotopic cardiac transplant recipients with minor coronary occlusive disease. Br Heart J 1992;68:266–71.

100. Hartmann A, Mazzilli N, Weis M, et al. Time course of endothelial function in epicardial conduit coronary arteries and in the microcirculation in the long-term follow-up after cardiac transplantation. Int J Cardiol 1996; 53:127–36.

101. Sharifi M, Siraj Y, O'Donnell J, Pompili VJ. Coronary angioplasty and stenting in orthotopic heart transplants: a fruitful act or a futile attempt? Angiology 2000; 51:809–15.

102. Strikwerda S, Umans V, van der Linden MM, et al. Percutaneous directional atherectomy for discrete coronary lesions in cardiac transplant patients. Am Heart J 1992; 123:1686–90.

103. Patel VS, Radovancevic B, Springer W, et al. Revascularization procedures in patients with transplant coronary artery disease. Eur J Cardiothorac Surg 1997;11:895–901.

104. Topaz O, Bailey NT, Mohanty PK. Application of solid-state pulsed-wave, mid-infrared laser for percutaneous revascularization in heart transplant recipients. J Heart Lung Transplant 1998;17:505–10.

105. Hosenpud JD, Novick RJ, Breen TJ, et al. The registry of the International Society for Heart and Lung Transplantation: twelfth official report—1995. J Heart Lung Transplant 1995;14:805–15.

106. Smith JA, Ribakove GH, Hunt SA, et al. Heart retransplantation: the 25-year experience at a single institution. J Heart Lung Transplant 1995;14:832–9.

CHAPTER 57

ADVANCES IN CARDIAC TRANSPLANTATION

NILOO M. EDWARDS, MD, MAURICIO GARRIDO, MD

Cardiac transplantation continues to evolve as a treatment for patients with end-stage heart failure. Advances in immune suppression, surgical technique, and perioperative patient management have all contributed to improved survival in the current era of transplantation. But as outcomes improve and eligibility criteria expand, there is a simultaneous decrease in the availability of "suitable" donors. Consequently, the current era of heart transplantation is marked by a balance of these advances in medical and surgical management against declining numbers of traditionally "suitable" donors.

Recipient Selection

Transplantation is the treatment of choice for patients with end-stage heart disease who have a life expectancy of less than 1 year. Risk of dying in these patients can be estimated by symptoms (New York Heart Assoication functional class), left ventricular ejection fraction, and maximal exercise VO_2. Of these, the single best predictor of outcomes of medical treatment is peak VO_2, even though it may be influenced by deconditioning, motivation, or body composition.[1] However, pretransplant risk stratification for ambulatory patients can be improved by considering other independent predictors of death. Using seven variables (Table 57-1)—presence of coronary artery disease; resting heart rate; left ventricular ejection fraction; mean arterial blood pressure; presence of an intraventricular conduction delay; peak VO_2; and serum sodium—Aaronson developed a mathematical model that is a better predictor of outcome with medical management.[2] On this scale, patients with scores greater than 8.1 had excellent survival with medical management when compared to those patients with scores less than 7.2. At Columbia-Presbyterian Medical Center, we have incorporated this heart failure survival score (HFSS) into our preoperative assessment of suitability for transplantation.

Currently we will consider patients for transplantation if they are New York Heart Association (NYHA) functional class III or IV despite maximal medical management and have a peak VO_2 greater than 14 or a heart failure score less than 8.1. If the candidates meet these criteria, they proceed to a full transplantation evaluation, which includes right-heart catheterization and studies to exclude significant comorbidities (Figure 57-1).

TABLE 57-1. Heart Failure Survival Score = Sum of Variable × Beta Coefficient

Variable	Beta Coefficient
Ischemic cardiomyopathy (yes = 1; no = 0)	+0.6931
Resting heart rate (bpm)	+0.0216
Left ventricular ejection fraction (%)	−0.0464
Mean arterial blood pressure (mm Hg)	−0.0255
Intraventricular conduction delay (yes = 1; no = 0)	+0.6083
Peak VO_2 (mL/kg/min)	−0.0546
Serum sodium (μmol/L)	−0.047

Exclusion Criteria

Exclusion criteria fall into three broad categories (Table 57-2): (1) factors that limit long-term survival (eg, age, cancer, diffuse arteriosclerosis, end-organ dysfunction); (2) factors that increase perioperative mortality (eg, pulmonary hypertension, recent pulmonary infarction, active infection, active peptic ulcer disease); and (3) factors that affect the patients' ability to care for themselves (eg, untreated psychiatric illness, recent substance abuse). Experience demonstrates, however, that excellent outcomes may be achieved in patients with many of these exclusion criteria; consequently we are reevaluating and modifying many of our exclusion criteria. Additionally, experience with "high-risk" donors has allowed programs such as ours to offer these donors to recipients with limited life expectancy (eg, older age, human immunodeficiency virus [HIV]), further blurring the borders of exclusion and inclusion.

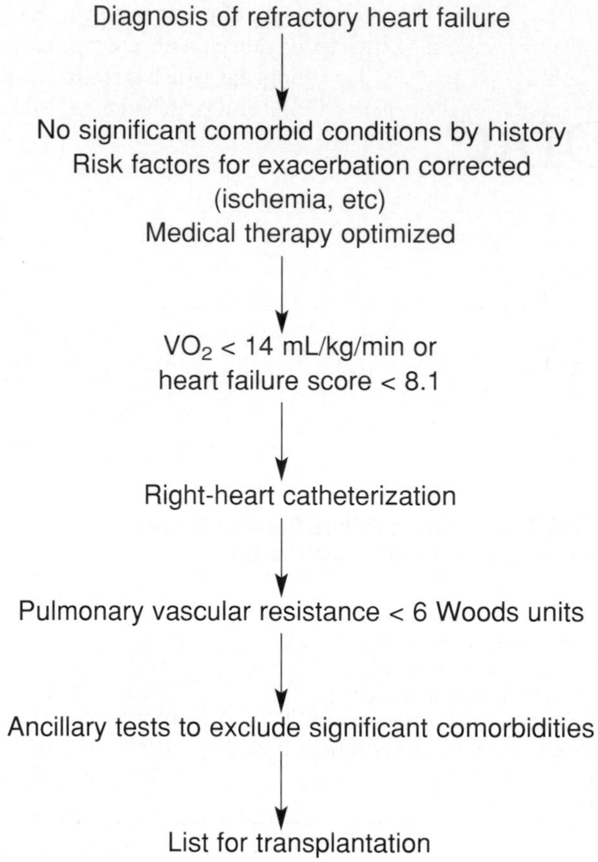

Diagnosis of refractory heart failure

↓

No significant comorbid conditions by history
Risk factors for exacerbation corrected
(ischemia, etc)
Medical therapy optimized

↓

VO$_2$ < 14 mL/kg/min or
heart failure score < 8.1

↓

Right-heart catheterization

↓

Pulmonary vascular resistance < 6 Woods units

↓

Ancillary tests to exclude significant comorbidities

↓

List for transplantation

FIGURE 57-1. Cardiac transplantation candidate selection.

TABLE 57-2. Exclusion Criteria

Factors that decrease long-term survival
___ Age > 65 yr
___ Significant end-organ damage (renal: creatinine > 2.5, or creatinine clearance < 25 mL/min; hepatic: bilirubin > 2.5, ALT/AST > twice normal; pulmonary: moderate to severe chronic bronchitis, COPD; hematologic: significant coagulation disorder)
___ Brittle diabetes
___ Chronic illness impairing survival
___ Severe peripheral vascular disease
___ Poorly controlled hypertension despite multiple medications
___ Active or recent malignancy
___ Human immunodeficiency virus (HIV) seroconversion

Factors that increase perioperative risk
___ Pulmonary hypertension
___ Recent peptic ulcer disease
___ Pulmonary infarction within 6 to 8 weeks
___ Active infection
___ Severe obesity (> 130% ideal body weight)
___ Cachexia (< 80% ideal body weight)

Factors that affect ability to care for oneself
___ Chronic illness affecting function
___ Drug, tobacco, or alcohol abuse within 6 months
___ Untreated psychiatric illness
___ Psychosocial instability

ALT = alanine aminotransferase; AST = aspartate aminotransferase; COPD = chronic obstructive pulmonary disease.

From 1983 to 1994, pretransplantation pulmonary hypertension (PHTN) greater than 6 Woods units correlated with 30-day mortality in our institutional experience; a more recent examination of 229 patients transplanted between 1994 and 1999 suggests that neither pulmonary vascular resistance nor pulmonary vascular resistance index in this era are predictive of 30-day mortality.[3,4] This probably reflects a number of programmatic changes during the current era, which include increased use of perioperative phosphodiesterase inhibitors, earlier implantation of left ventricular assist devices, adoption of the bicaval anastomotic technique, and liberal administration of postoperative nitric oxide.

Similarly, favorable outcomes in assist device patients with active infections and in patients who are either obese or cachexic have forced us to consider these as relative rather than absolute exclusion criteria. Not infrequently, patients actively using tobacco will undergo postcardiotomy assist device placement and consideration for transplantation. Despite the fact that these patients do not meet criteria, we tend to err on the side of the patient, hoping that this life-threatening event will induce a change in habits without requiring a formal 6-month proof of abstinence.

Clearly recipient exclusion criteria are changing as clinical outcomes predict better survival in patients once thought to be at too high a risk. We advocate an annual reexamination of program exclusion criteria based on national and program results.

Donor Acceptance Criteria

The ideal donor is one who is ABO blood type compatible, size matched to within 20% of the recipient's body weight; male younger than 40 or female younger than 45 years of age; normal heart function by echocardiogram; on minimal pressors; has an anticipated ischemic time of less than 4 h; and has no evidence of infection, HIV, hepatitis B or C, or malignancy. Unfortunately, the probability of finding a donor who meets even two of these criteria is becoming increasingly remote, but there are increasing data to support transgression of all these criteria with good results—including ABO mismatching in the pediatric transplant population.[5,6]

To determine the impact of the "extended donor" variables on early and intermediate post-transplant survival, we performed a retrospective review of the consecutive donors used in 161 patients who were transplanted between 1995 and 1997. Thirty donors (19%) were identified as marginal, based on accepted criteria (age > 50 years, echocardiographic evidence for wall motion abnormality, ischemic time > 240 min), but no impact of use of "marginal donors" was demonstrable with respect to 45-day or 1-year mortality. In this study, only donor-recipient size mismatch of greater than 20% body weight was found to be a significant predictor of 45-day mortality ($p = .03$) but not 1-year mortality.[7]

Our approach to donor selection is not to decline donors based on any fixed criteria but to consider the acuity of the recipient because, ultimately, donor selection is a function of the medical condition of the recipient. Additionally, the creation of a "high-risk recipient program" has allowed us to use turned-down hearts for recipients who would not otherwise be candidates for transplantation, based on their comorbidities.

Surgical Technique

In the 1960s, Lower and Shumway introduced what has become the standard technique for orthotopic heart transplantation. This method of implantation involves the anastomosis of donor to recipient at the level of a mid-atrial cuff. Although this is still the procedure of choice in many programs, we prefer the bicaval anastomotic technique, in which the left atrial anastomosis is at the level of a midatrial cuff, but the right-sided connections are at the level of the inferior and superior venae cavae. This technique has been associated with improved right ventricular function, improved atrial geometry, less tricuspid valve regurgitation, less sinus node dysfunction, decreased need for pacemaker placement, and overall improved survival.[8]

In a nonrandomized trial, Milano compared 65 consecutive standard atrial cuff implantation procedures with 75 consecutive bicaval transplants.[8] Despite similar immunosuppression regimens, donor and recipient selection criteria, and postoperative management, the cardiac index at 24 h after transplantation was significantly higher in the bicaval group, and inotrope requirements and tricuspid regurgitation were significantly less. Although mortality was similar for both groups, the average postoperative length of stay was significantly longer in the standard group (20.4 vs 12.1 days). In a larger study by Aziz, which compared bicaval to standard implantation technique, a significantly improved actuarial survival was demonstrated at 5 years (81% vs 62%, respectively) in the bicaval cohort.[9] Additionally, other retrospective studies have demonstrated a lower incidence of atrial flutter and atrial fibrillation in the bicaval groups (4% vs 40%), which may be due to improved right atrial geometry with the bicaval technique.[10]

Immunosuppression

Most transplantation centers use a triple immunosuppression regimen consisting of prednisone, cyclosporine, and azathioprine. The maintenance immunosuppression protocol at Columbia-Presbyterian Medical Center consists of cyclosporine adjusted to maintain serum levels of 300 to 350 ng/mL in the first 3 months, 200 to 300 ng/mL for months 4 to 12, and then a level of 100 to 150 ng/mL; steroids, which are started before cardiopulmonary bypass and then rapidly tapered to 5 mg of prednisone per day by the third month (a quarter of our patients are weaned off steroids by 1 year); and azathioprine, which is started in the immediate postoperative period and switched to mycophenolate mofetil (MMF) when the patient is able to eat.

Twenty percent of centers prefer to use tacrolimus instead of cyclosporine. Tacrolimus has a similar mechanism of action to cyclosporine and is effective in cardiac transplantation although there are no clear data to demonstrate any superiority over cyclosporine. Both agents have comparable incidences of nephrotoxicity and neurotoxicity, and although the incidence of hypertension and hyperlipidemia is lower with tacrolimus, the frequency of glucose intolerance is higher.[11] Additionally, tacrolimus may play a role in the treatment of refractory rejection in patients on a cyclosporine-based regimen; a study by Armitage demonstrated a reversal of allograft rejection in 90% of patients when tacrolimus was substituted for cyclosporine.[12] It may also be a more appealing drug for female recipients who have developed hirsutism and gingival hyperplasia from cyclosporine.

More recent additions to the immunosuppression armamentarium are rapamycin and interleukin (IL)-2 receptor–specific antibodies. Rapamycin is structurally similar to FK506 (tacrolimus) and binds to the FK-binding protein. The combination of this drug and cyclosporine or tacrolimus is synergistic and allows reduced doses of both agents; however, side effects include thrombocytopenia, leukopenia, anemia, and hyperlipidemia. Equally tantalizing is the possible role for rapamycin in patients with transplant coronary artery disease. Our experience with 35 patients with angiographically documented transplant coronary artery disease, who were randomized to either rapamycin or continued current immunosuppression, has demonstrated a slower progression of transplant coronary artery disease in the rapamycin group.

Antibodies to the activated IL-2 receptor are available in a chimeric form (basiliximab) or a humanized form (daclizumab). These agents are designed to prevent IL-2–induced clonal expansion of activated T cells, by selectively blocking the IL-2 receptor, thereby preventing rejection. We randomized 55 nonsensitized recipients, within 24 h of cardiac transplantation, to either daclizumab (28 patients) or placebo (27 patients) in combination with the standard immunosuppression protocol of cyclosporine, mycophenolate mofetil, and corticosteroids. The daclizumab-treated group had significantly fewer rejection episodes over a 1-year period, had a longer time to first rejection, and did not require rescue therapy, despite similar infection rates in both groups.[13]

The Sensitized Patient

Some patients have high panel-reactive antibody (PRA) levels and are considered "sensitized" if these levels are in excess of 20%; often, this is the result of repeat transplantation, blood transfusions, or multiple pregnancies. The presence of lymphocytotoxic (immunoglobulin G [IgG]) donor-specific antibodies can cause early graft failure and is associated with an increased frequency of, and shorter time to, acute cellular rejection, as well as earlier onset of transplant coronary artery disease.[14,15] Because sensitized candidates must undergo donor-specific T-cell crossmatch, they have longer waiting times and increased waitlist mortality, but the waiting time to transplantation and mortality for these patients can be decreased to that of nonsensitized recipients by the pretransplant administration of cyclophosphamide and intravenous immunoglobulin.[16,17]

Survival

The expected 1-year survival for heart transplantation is 80%, with a linear attrition of 4% per year, and the patient half-life is 9.1 years or 11.6 years for patients who survive their first post-transplant year.[18] Outcomes continue to improve with time. In a retrospective analysis of 1,137 consecutive transplants performed at Columbia-Presbyterian Medical Center from 1977 to 1999, patients were divided into three cohorts based on the immunosuppression protocol and the era of transplantation: Group I = steroids + azathioprine ($n = 25$; 1977 to April 1983); Group II = cyclosporine + steroids ($n = 40$; April 1983 to April 1985); and Group III = cyclosporine + azathioprine + steroids ($n = 1,027$; April 1985 to August 1999). With each era of transplantation, survival odds increased and the incidences of malignancy, transplant coronary artery disease, and infection decreased.[19] One- and 5-year survival was, respectively, 44% and 18% for Group I, 63% and 55% for Group II, and 81% and 68% for Group III.

In a separate study of 65 recipients surviving longer than 10 years, a multivariable analysis of donor and recipient factors found that only a pretransplantation diagnosis of ischemic cardiomyopathy was independently predictive of an adverse long-term outcome.[20] Further analysis of 507 consecutive heart transplant recipients at Columbia-Presbyterian Medical Center from 1993 to 1998 was performed to identify risk factors that might affect early and late survival in the current era. In this study, neither pulmonary vascular resistance (PVR) nor sensitization adversely impacted on early mortality. Early mortality (< 30 days) was associated with older donors (> 50 years of age), donor–recipient gender mismatch, and pretransplantation diagnosis of congenital cardiomyopathy. Additionally there was a significant decrease in early mortality, from 16% in 1993 to 5% in 1999, confirming the trend to improved outcomes with more recent era of transplantation.[21]

The International Society for Heart and Lung Transplantation data further substantiate these improvements in survival with more recent era of transplantation.[18] Interestingly, this survival improvement coincides with a quadrupling in the use of donors older than age 50 years, which highlights the contrast between our increasing ability to transplant sicker patients with better results, against a shrinking donor pool. It can only be hoped that the next era of heart transplantation will be marked by innovation in heart replacement options for the greater numbers of patients with end-stage heart disease waiting to be transplanted, in addition to the improved outcomes for the diminishing numbers of patients who are transplanted.

References

1. Mancini D, Eisen H, Kussmaul Y, et al. Value of peak exercise consumption for optimal timing of cardiac transplantation in ambulatory patients with heart failure. Circulation 1991;82:778–86.
2. Aaronson K, Schwartz J, Chen T, Mancini D. Development and prospective validation of a clinical index to predict survival in ambulatory patients referred for cardiac transplantation evaluation. Circulation 1997;95:2660–7.
3. Chen J, Levin H, Michler R, et al. Reevaluating the significance of pulmonary hypertension prior to cardiac transplantation, determining optimal thresholds, and quantification of the effect of reversibility on perioperative mortality. J Thorac Cardiovasc Surg 1997;114: 627–34.
4. Chen JM, Sinha P, Rajasinghe HA, et al. The diminishing impact of pretransplant pulmonary hypertension on perioperative mortality after cardiac transplantation. J Heart Lung Transplant 2001;2:235–6.
5. Sweeney ML, Lammermeier DE, Frazier OH, et al. Extension of donor criteria in cardiac transplantation: surgical risk versus supply side economics. Ann Thorac Surg 1990;50:7–10.
6. John R, Rajasinghe H, Chen JM, et al. Impact of current management practices on early and late death in more than 500 consecutive cardiac transplant recipients. Ann Surg 2000;232:302–11.
7. Chen JM, Sinha P, Rajasinghe HA, et al. Short and long-term impact of donor characteristics on recipient survival, 1995–1999. Heart Lung Transplant 2002;21:608–10.
8. Milano CA, Shah AS, Trigt PV, et al. Evaluation of early postoperative results after bicaval versus standard cardiac transplantation and review of the literature. Am Heart J 2000;140:717–21.
9. Aziz T, Yonan N, Burgess M, et al. Bicaval and standard techniques in orthotopic heart transplantation: medium-term experience in cardiac performance and survival. J Thorac Cardiovasc Surg 1999;118:115–22.
10. Brandt M, Harringer W, Hirt S, et al. Influence of bicaval anastomosis on late occurrence of atrial arrhythmia after heart transplantation. Ann Thorac Surg 1997;64:70–2.
11. Pham SD, Kormos RL, Hattler BG, et al. A prospective trial of tacrolimus (FK506) in clinical heart transplantation: immediate-term results. J Thorac Cardiovasc Surg 1996;111:764–72.
12. Armitage JM, Kormos RL, Griffith BP, et al. A clinical trial of FK506 as primary and rescue immunosuppression in cardiac transplantation. Transplant Proc 1991;23: 1140–52.

13. Beniaminovitz A, Itescu S, Lietz K, et al. Prevention of rejection in cardiac transplantation by blockade of the interleukin-2 receptor with a monoclonal antibody. N Engl J Med 2000;42:613–9.

14. Smith JD, Danskine AJ, Laylor RM, et al. The effect of panel reactive antibodies and the donor-specific crossmatch on graft survival after heart and heart-lung transplantation. Transplant Immunol 1993;1:60–5.

15. Itescu S, Tung T, Burke E, et al. Preformed IgG antibodies against major histocompatibility class II antigens are major risk factors for high-grade cellular rejection in recipients of heart transplantation. Circulation 1998;98: 786–93.

16. John R, Leitz K, Burke E, et al. Intravenous immunoglobulin reduces anti-HLA alloreactivity and shortens waiting time to cardiac transplantation in highly sensitized left ventricular assist device recipients. Circulation 1999;100 Suppl 19:II229–35.

17. Itescu S, Burke E, Lietz K, et al. Intravenous pulse administration of cyclophosphamide is an effective and safe treatment for sensitized cardiac allograft recipients. Circulation 2002;105:1214–9.

18. Hosenpud JD, Bennett L, Keck BM, et al. The Registry of the International Society for Heart and Lung Transplantation: eighteenth official report—2001. J Heart Lung Transplant 2001;20:805–15.

19. Edwards NM, Rajasinghe HA, John R, et al. Cardiac transplantation in over 1000 patients: a single institution experience from Columbia University. Clin Transpl 1999;15:249–61.

20. John R, Rajasinghe HA, Itescu S, et al. Long-term survival (> 10 years) after cardiac transplantation in the cyclosporine era: evaluation of risk factors and graft function. J Am Coll Cardiol 2000;37(1):189–94.

21. John R, Rajasinghe HA, Chen JM, et al. Impact of current management practices on early and late mortality in 500 cardiac transplant recipients. Ann Surg 2000;232: 302–11.

CHAPTER 58

HEART-LUNG TRANSPLANTATION

SOON J. PARK, MD

Human beings have long been fascinated with the concept of organ transplantation. In the early twentieth century, attempts were made in animal models by Alexis Carrel and Charles Guthrie, who described the technical feasibility of vascular anastomoses in solid organ transplantation.[1] In 1950, extensive experimental work on thoracic organ transplantation was presented by Vladimir Petrovich Demikhov.[2] Some of his models involved combined heart and left lung transplants in 20 dogs, 4 of which lived 3 to 8 days post transplantation. Over the next 30 years, many other investigators continued to work on various animal models of heart-lung transplantation. In 1972, Aldo Castañeda demonstrated the technical feasibility of autologous heart-lung transplants in baboons, with good functional outcome as late as 24 months post transplant.[3,4] In an allograft animal model, success in heart-lung transplantation came with the discovery of cyclosporine.[5] It was remarkably efficacious in suppressing the immune system and preventing rejection, yet it was devoid of serious side effects.[6] In 1980, Bruce Reitz reported on three long-term survivors in a monkey allograft heart-lung transplant model.[7]

This experimental success set the stage for Reitz to usher in the clinical era of heart-lung transplantation, beginning in 1981. That year, more than a decade after the first clinical attempt by Cooley in 1968, a 45-year-old woman with primary pulmonary hypertension underwent a successful heart-lung transplant, the fourth human patient to undergo such a transplant.[8] She became the first long-term survivor; at 20 months post transplant, her exercise tolerance test results were normal.[9] Although Reitz's experimental surgical technique required minor modifications, it is still widely accepted in clinical practice today. A key component remains cyclosporine.

From 1982 to 1989, the number of heart-lung transplants reported to the International Society for Heart and Lung Transplantation (ISHLT) registry expanded rapidly, peaking at 240 in 1989. Since 1989, the number has been decreasing. In 2000, only 104 patients worldwide underwent a heart-lung transplant, according to the registry.[10] Indications and therapeutic options have changed over the years. Lung transplants have become more successful, especially after the difficulty of bronchial dehiscence (frequently seen in the early clinical experience) was over-

come. More patients with primary pulmonary hypertension (PPH) or cystic fibrosis (CF) are now treated with a bilateral single-lung transplant, rather than with a heart-lung transplant.

Indications

The major indications for a heart-lung transplant are reported, by underlying disease, by the ISHLT registry.[10]

Patients with combined end-stage cardiac and pulmonary disease should be considered for a heart-lung transplant. Eisenmenger's syndrome, which is caused by congential heart disease, accounts for 32% of the cases in the registry; PPH accounts for 25%. In the 1980s, a heart-lung transplant was the only option for PPH patients. Now, most are treated with a bilateral single-lung transplant; a heart-lung transplant is reserved only for those with advanced right ventricular failure secondary to PPH.

CF, the third most common diagnosis requiring a heart-lung transplant, accounts for 16% of the cases in the registry. The transplant communities in North America and Europe seem to differ in philosophy regarding the best option for CF patients. In 2000, of all heart-lung transplants, only 2% were performed for CF patients in North America, as compared with 29% in Europe. The European centers that have had good success with heart-lung transplants for cystic fibrosis patients continue to advocate this practice with a concomitant "domino" heart transplant.[11–13] Most of the North American centers prefer bilateral single-lung transplants.[14–15]

Other diagnoses (such as α_1-antitrysin deficiencies, idiopathic pulmonary fibrosis, and chronic obstructive pulmonary disease) as well as retransplants account for 27% of the registry.

Recipient Selection Criteria

In North America, patients with Eisenmenger's syndrome or with PPH and advanced right-heart failure are typically referred for a heart-lung transplant. Most transplant centers have an upper age limit of 50 years. Transplant candidates must not have other irreversible organ failure that would compromise their long-term survival or quality of life post transplant. Candidates often have concomitant hepatic or renal dysfunction because of their underlying cardiopulmonary disease, but such dysfunction usually improves post transplant. The expected survival time and quality of life with the underlying disease, if left untreated, must be worse than those expected post transplant. According to the ISHLT registry, the current survival rate for heart-lung recipients is 60% at 1 year and 40% at 5 years post transplant.[10]

Patients with cyanotic heart disease often develop extensive systemic to pulmonary collateral vessels. Prior thoracic surgery in such patients could mean significant technical challenges at the time of the transplant, so it is a relative contraindication to a heart-lung transplant.[16]

Thorough evaluation and proper selection of heart-lung recipients is mandatory to ensure optimal outcome posttransplant. Tables 58-1 and 58-2 show the current workup and eligibility guidelines used at the University of Minnesota.

Donor Selection Criteria

The cadaver heart-lung donor must meet all donor eligibility criteria for both the heart and the lungs separately. The donor heart must have near-normal right and left ventricular function, without significant hypertrophy, valvular disease, or coronary artery disease. Electrocardiographic and echocardiographic evaluations are essential. Coronary angiography is recommended for donors who are older than 40 years of age.

The donor lungs must demonstrate satisfactory oxygenation and ventilation parameters on a reasonable tidal volume of 10 to 15 mL/kg. Oxygen partial pressure (Po_2) must be greater than 100 on 40% fraction of inspired oxygen (F_IO_2) and greater than 250 on 100% F_IO_2. Lung compliance must be normal. Chest roentgenography must not demonstrate any significant infiltrate consistent with either pulmonary contusion or pneumonia. Minimal or no smoking history is preferred, but smoking history, per se, is not an absolute contraindication to lung donation. The donor's lifestyle and level of physical activity tolerated before brain death could provide important insights into the cardiopulmonary reserve of the donor organs.

At the time of organ procurement, intraoperative inspection of the heart and lungs is an important part of the donor organ evaluation. Visual inspection of the heart's size and right ventricular function is helpful. Palpation for atherosclerotic plaques in the coronary arteries and for thrills at the valves is also useful. Palpation and visualization of the lungs for nodules or contusion, as well as bronchoscopic inspection for trauma, purulent secretion, or aspiration pneumonia, should be done routinely. Once the organs are found to be acceptable for transplantation, communication and coordination between the donor and recipient surgical teams are vital to minimize ischemic time. The simple system now in use allows preservation and storage of heart-lung organs for up to 4 h.[17]

Procurement

A median sternotomy and midline abdominal incision are commonly used for multiple organ procurement. The pericardium and both pleura are opened to enable inspection of thoracic organs (as described above). The superior vena cava is freed up and encircled with a suture, well away from the sinus node. The ascending aorta is encircled with an umbilical tape distally, near the innominate artery. The posterior pericardium is incised between the superior vena cava and the ascending aorta, to expose the trachea. The membranous portion of the trachea should be approached with care, to avoid tearing it. The trachea is encircled with an umbilical tape proximally, away from the carina.

When other organ procurement teams are ready to proceed with the actual removal of organs, the donor is given intravenous heparin at 3 mg/kg. A cardioplegia catheter is placed in the ascending aorta, and a sump catheter (14-French) is inserted in the main pulmonary artery to deliver preservation solution. The superior vena cava is ligated away from the sinus node, and the inferior vena cava is partially transected, right at the diaphragm, to bleed out the donor. Once the heart empties itself out within 2 to 3 beats, the ascending aorta is cross-clamped distal to the cardioplegia catheter.

Preservation solutions are delivered to the heart and lungs. High-potassium-based crystalloid cardioplegia, such as Stanford solution, is commonly used for heart preservation. Both Euro-Collins and University of Wisconsin (UW) solutions have been successfully used for heart or lung preservation.[18] Lower-potassium-based solutions, such as Celsior and low-potassium dextran, are now being tested for heart and lung preservation; early results are promising.[19,20]

The left atrial appendage is partially amputated to let out the lung effusate, thereby helping to prevent left ventricular distension and pulmonary venous congestion during preservation. During the period of preservation solution infusion, the heart and lungs are covered in cold saline solution mixed with ice slush. One liter of high-potassium crystalloid cardioplegia, infused under pressure, is adequate to induce a prompt arrest of the heart. Four liters (60 cc/kg body weight) of lung preservation solution is infused under either partial pressure or gravity drainage. During the infusion period, the lungs are ventilated with room air at 4 to 6 breaths per minute, to promote even distribution of the preservation solution. The lungs should turn asanguinous; the effusate out of the left atrial appendage should turn clear as well.

Excision of the heart-lung block is next. The superior vena cava and inferior vena cava are transected. The aorta is transected distal to the nominate artery, to ensure adequate length of the ascending aorta. The pericardium is incised on both sides and extended posteriorly at the level of the diaphragm. The inferior pulmonary ligaments are

TABLE 58-1. University of Minnesota Potential Heart-Lung/Lung Recipient Evaluation

A. Admit to transplant center, Dx_____ Eval Date: _____

B. Pulmonary medicine attending physician: Dr._____ Pager: _____

Appointment: _____

C. Consults
1. Thoracic transplant surgeon consult
2. Social-work consult
3. Precatheterization appointment (scheduled with cardiovascular center)
4. Transplant coordinator teaching: Coordinator: _____ Pager: _____
5. Dietitian
6. ENT (cystic fibrosis patients only)
7. Respiratory therapy teaching
8. Cardiopulmonary evaluation (except PPH patients)
9. Chaplain
10. Pretransplant home monitoring consult

D. Laboratories
1. Chemistry
a. GNEC, PO4, Amylase, AST, Total bilirubin, AP, TSH, Total protein, Albumin, Transferrin, 24-h Urine for Creatinine Clearance
b. Fasting labs: Chol, Trig, HDL, LDL
2. Hematology
a. CBC with differential
3. Coagulation Studies
a. PT/INR, PTT
4. Immunology
a. ABO typing and screen
b. HLA, A, B, C, DR Typing, Panel Reactive Antibody (PRA)
Lung transplant recipient must be marked on immunology sheet.
c. Quantitative immunoglobulins with G subclasses I, II, III, IV.
5. PSA (for men over age 55)
6. UA/UC, urine cotinine
7. Microbiology
a. Sputum for routine culture and fungus
8. Virology
a. Titers for CMV, EBV, VZV, HSV, Toxoplasmosis
b. Hepatitis profile (all A, B, C), HIV
9. Stool guaiacs ×3

E. Tests
1. Chest x-ray (PA & lateral, and AP supine at 40" height)
2. 12-lead ECG
3. CT of chest without contrast. Include high resolution cuts
4. MUGA scan (first pass right and left ejection fractions)
5. DEXA scan of spine and hips
6. CT before of sinuses prior to ENT consult if cystic fibrosis
7. Lung scan, perfusion only
8. Bilateral mammogram for female patients (women 35 & older) if not done in the past year
9. Echocardiogram (with estimate of RV pressures) w/bubble study, if no known shunt
10. Cardiac cath. Must include pulmonary artery pressures and resistance. Left ventricular gram and coronaries if > 40 years old. R heart cath if < 40 years old. Double-check with coordinator if CF dx. Modified vasodilator studies if PA pressure > 40 systolic .
11. Full medicine pulmonary function tests
12. 6-min walk tolerance test (respiratory therapy)
13. Skeletal x-rays
a. Spine (thoracic and lumbar)
b. Hip, bilateral
14. PPD (5 test units), mumps & candida (adults only) skin tests for patients with no prior history of positive PPD or verified TB.
15. Pneumovax (pneumococcal vaccine) 0.5 mL IM. Give only if patient has not received.
16. Hepatitis A vaccine. If Hep A screen is negative, give first dose and instruct patient to obtain second dose in 6 months.
17. Hepatitis B vaccine. If Hep B screen is negative, give first dose and instruct patient to obtain second dose in 1 month, and third dose in 6 months. Use standard dosing.

*MUST BE COMPLETED BEFORE CARDIAC CATHETERIZATION

F. Patient to attend Heart-Lung Transplant Clinic Support Group, Monday 11:00 am, Hegman Conference Room. The first Monday of the month, the support group meets at 7 pm in the Hegman Conference Room.

G. Patient to have complete dental exam by their local dentist prior to activation on transplant list and complete current OB/GYN exam.

TABLE 58-2. University of Minnesota Thoracic Transplant Program· Patient Care Protocols

Recipient Selection Criteria

A. Age 50 years or younger for heart-lung transplants (determined by the patient's age on first contact with our program).

B. Absence of conditions likely to limit survival or rehabilitation potential.
   Depending on disease severity and individual circumstances, the following may represent absolute or relative contraindications:
   - Significantly impaired hepatic function, with persistent marked elevation of LFT (eg, > 2× normal AST or bilirubin). Patients with suspected liver dysfunction should undergo ultrasound and Doppler study to assess for cirrhosis, portal hypertension, or reversal of portal blood flow.
   - Active peptic ulcer disease.
   - Bleeding diathesis.
   - Complicated or uncontrolled diabetes.
   - History of malignancy with appreciable risk of recurrence.
   - Present abuse of alcohol or recreational drugs (for present or past problems, chemical dependency consultation is required).
   - Inability to understand procedure and risks involved or to comply with follow-up care.
   - Infection outside the lungs and upper respiratory tract.
   - Obesity: body weight > 140% ideal body weight before activation on list.
   - Cachexia: body weight < 80% predicted before activation on list.
   - History of major (eg, psychotic) psychiatric illness with appreciable risk of recurrence.
   - Inadequate financial or insurance resources.
   - Cigarette smoking within 4 months before activation on list (for recent smokers, a smoking cessation program is required).
   - Inadequate support system to assist in pretransplant and post-transplant care.
   - Chronic systemic corticosteroid medication pretransplant. However, low doses of corticosteroids (ie, ~ 20 mg prednisone or equivalent per day) and intermittent short courses of higher steroid doses (3 to 4 days) are NOT contraindications.
   - Pleural disease (chest CT scan Required). Previous thoracotomy and sternotomy are NOT absolute contraindications. Extensive pleural scanning and previous pneumonectomy are relative contraindications.

C. Absence of surgically remediable chronic thromboembolic disease.

AST = Aspartate aminotransferase   CT = computed tomography   LFT = Liver Function Test

---

divided, and a pre-esophageal plane is developed for mediastinal dissection. The posterior pleural reflections, including azygos vein, are divided. The lungs are kept partially inflated with room air. A TA 30 stapler with 3.5 mm staples is placed at the proximal trachea, well away from the carina, as the endotracheal tube is pulled back. The tissues between the anterior chest wall and the trachea on either thorax are divided away from the hilum on each side. The heart-lung block is placed in a sterile container filled with cold saline, then packaged and transported to the transplant center.

The Transplant

After the intraoperative inspection at the donor hospital finds the donor organs to be acceptable, the recipient is brought to the operating room, well in advance of the expected arrival of the donor organs, to minimize ischemic time. Either a bilateral submammary or a median sternotomy incision can be done; the latter is our incision of choice. Recipients often have significant systemic to pulmonary collateral vessels, so meticulous hemostasis is critical during all phases of the operation. The superior vena cava is cannulated directly. The inferior vena cava is cannulated through the right atrial wall, near the caval atrial juncture, for venous drainage. The ascending aorta is cannulated distally near the innominate artery.

Cardiopulmonary bypass is initiated, and the recipient is cooled to systemic hypothermia of about 28° to 30°C. Both venae cavae are snared with umbilical tapes, and the ascending aorta is cross-clamped. The recipient cardiectomy is performed first, followed by bilateral pneumectomy. The cardiectomy should be tailored for either right atrial or bicaval anastomosis. The right atrium is transected, leaving atrial cuffs around the superior vena cava and inferior vena cava for the bicaval anastomosis.[3,7] The right atrium and interatrial septum are retained for atrial anastomosis (Figure 58-1).[21,22] The ascending aorta and the main pulmonary artery are transected. The pulmonary veins or the left atrium is transected to complete the recipient cardiectomy. Some modifications in cardiectomy technique are required if the heart is to be used as a donor heart in a "domino" heart transplant.

The cardiectomy improves visualization for the recipient pneumonectomy. The phrenic nerves are identified on both sides, and a strip of pericardium is preserved around the phrenic nerves to protect them from injury. The inferior pulmonary ligaments are divided, and the lungs are removed one at a time. Surgical dissection around the ligamentum arteriosum must be conducted carefully, to minimize the risk of injuring the recurrent laryngeal nerve. A segment of the pulmonary artery should be left behind, around the ligamentum, during the left pneumonectomy (Figure 58-2).[22] The vagus nerves are also protected from injury during the dissection: injury might result in delayed gastric emptying posttransplant. The remnants of the pulmonary arteries and pulmonary veins are freed from their pericardial attachments. The remnants of mainstem bronchi are freed up and traced to the distal trachea. The posterior pericardium is incised, to expose the carina and bronchial stumps. The distal trachea is transected, just above the carina, to remove the

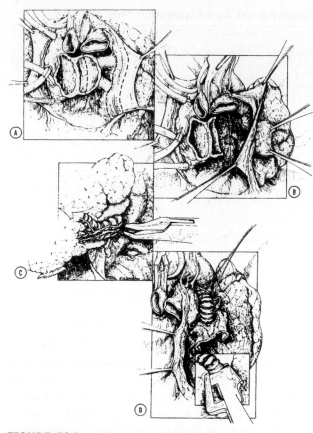

FIGURE 58-1. *A*, The recipient atria after removal of the heart. Incisions are made so as to preserve the phrenic nerve in a "ribbon" of pericardium. The left and right pulmonary veins are separated by a longitudinal incision in the posterior left atrial wall and thus into the oblique sinus. *B*, The left pulmonary veins are withdrawn beneath the phrenic nerve. The vagus nerve is immediately posterior. *C*, The left lung is progressively mobilized, and the bronchial arteries are secured. *D*, The left pulmonary artery is divided, and the bronchus is stapled and cut. Reproduced by permission from Mosby.

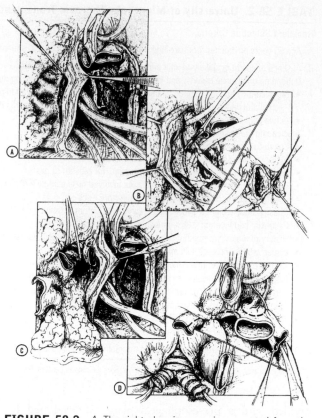

FIGURE 58-2. *A*, The right phrenic nerve is separated from the hilum. *B*, The right pulmonary veins are separated from the right atrium. *C*, The right pulmonary ligament is divided, the lung is mobilized, and the pulmonary artery and bronchus are cut. *D*, The remnants of the pulmonary artery are removed, leaving the area around the ductus ligament and recurrent nerve. The trachea and bronchial remnants are exposed to the right of the aorta. The trachea is cut just above the carina. Reproduced by permission from Mosby.

carina and bronchial stumps. The bronchial vessels are then controlled for hemostasis. Before sewing the organs in, satisfactory hemostasis must be achieved in the posterior mediastinum. Bleeding there could be very difficult to control, given the heart-lung block's anatomic position after implantation.

The donor organs are examined and fashioned for implantation. The trachea is divided about one to two rings above the carina. Any type of dissection that could potentially devascularize the tracheobronchial tree must be avoided. The incision in the left atrial appendage is closed. The heart is examined for any patent foramen ovale or atrial septal defect; if either of the latter is found, the defect is closed primarily. Before implantation, excess donor tissue, such as pericardium, fat, or lymphatics, is removed. The heart-lung block is brought into the recipient chest cavity. The right and left lungs are placed in the corresponding pleural spaces, through the opening, posterior to the phrenic nerve pericardial strip. It is impor-

tant to inspect the lungs, to avoid unintended torsion at the hilum.

The tracheal anastomosis is constructed first. Running 3–0 Prolene sutures are used to approximate the trachea in an end-to-end fashion. Next, the aortic anastomosis is completed in an end-to-end fashion. Two layers of Prolene suture lines are often used to achieve satisfactory hemostasis. The first layer is approximated with horizontal mattress sutures, followed by a second layer of running 4–0 Prolene sutures. The superior vena cava and inferior vena cava are anastomosed next, using 4–0 Prolene sutures in an end-to-end fashion. We prefer bicaval anastomoses, although a single right atrial anastomosis can be utilized (Figure 58-3).[22] A meticulous de-airing maneuver is essential to prevent air embolus to the right coronary system.

The aortic cross-clamp is released, and caval snares are released. The recipient is fully rewarmed to normothermia. The lungs are ventilated and inspected to confirm absence of atelectatic segments, and an appropriate tidal volume is delivered to ventilate the lungs. The heart should

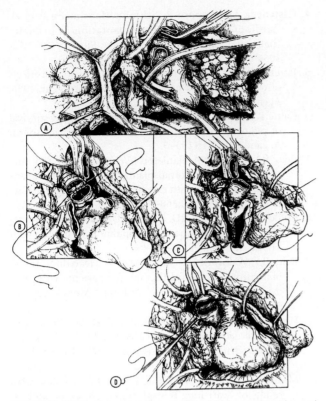

FIGURE 58-3. Reimplantation. *A,* The right lung passes beneath the right atrial remnant and the phrenic nerve. *B,* The tracheal anastomosis is performed first, commencing with the posterior wall. *C,* The right atrial anastomosis. *D,* The aortic anastomosis. Reproduced with permission from Mosby.

be supported with isoproterenol or epinephrine (or both) for chronotropic and inotropic aid. The recipient is weaned off cardiopulmonary bypass; cardiac and pulmonary functions are monitored closely. Satisfactory oxygenation and ventilation are confirmed with arterial blood gas. Pulmonary artery pressure, mixed venous oxygen saturation (SVO$_2$), and cardiac output are monitored to ensure the recipient's cardiopulmonary stability off cardiopulmonary bypass. Protamine is given to reverse heparin. The cardiopulmonary bypass cannulas are removed. Both pleural spaces and the mediastinum are drained with chest tubes, and the sternum is closed.

If the recipient develops cardiac or pulmonary dysfunction when being weaned from cardiopulmonary bypass support, extracorporeal membrane oxygenator (ECMO) support may be helpful, especially in dealing with reversible allograft dysfunction (such as ischemia-reperfusion injury). A high success rate has been reported for weaning patients off ECMO support for acute lung injury after heart-lung transplants.[23]

Post-transplantation Care

Allograft dysfunction may develop hours post transplant. Clinical deterioration may continue, despite aggressive measures (such as more inotropes and significantly increased ventilator support). Early institution of ECMO support may need to be considered. Acute allograft dysfunction within 24 h post transplantation seems to be mostly related to ischemia-reperfusion injury; such dysfunction often reverses within 2 to 4 days of ECMO support.[23–25] Early ECMO support may avert additional injury often associated with excessive ventilatory trauma or with other organ dysfunction related to a low-flow state. Postoperative bleeding can complicate the patient's care. At the time of transplantation, surgical technique must be meticulous, to minimize surgical bleeding. Recipients often have pre-existing coagulopathy due to hepatic congestion; such coagulopathy worsens with prolonged cardiopulmonary bypass support (eg, during a difficult transplant operation). To correct coagulopathy, aggressive blood product replacement with platelets, fresh-frozen plasma, and cryoprecipitates is important.

With heart-lung transplants, right ventricular dysfunction with an elevated central venous pressure must be aggressively managed. Respiratory acidosis, hypoxemia, and atelectasis—all strong stimuli for pulmonary vasoconstriction—must be avoided to minimize an undue increase in afterload for the right ventricle. Nitroglycerin or nitric oxide (or both) may help lower pulmonary hypertension.

If a recipient develops inadequate urine output because of renal dysfunction, either ultrafiltration or hemodialysis is indicated; fluid must be removed to lower central venous pressure to a more physiologic level of less than 15 mm H$_2$O. Recipients with persistent postoperative bleeding in the face of corrected coagulopathy, or those who develop hemodynamic instability from bleeding, must return to the operating room promptly.

Immunosuppression

Immunosuppressive protocols may vary from one transplant center to another. The most common therapy involves three drugs: cyclosporine or FK506; azathioprine or mycophenolate mofetil (MMF); and steroids. Our typical protocol includes Solu-Medrol (1g before the allograft is reperfused, then 125 mg intravenously every 8 h over the next 24 h), cyclosporine, MMF, and prednisone.

Post-transplant care of heart-lung recipients is similar to that of lung recipients. The incidence of rejection is much more frequent in the lungs than in the heart. In heart-lung recipients (in contrast to heart recipients), surveillance right ventricular endomyocardial biopsies are not recommended unless specifically indicated.[26,27] Instead, heart-lung recipients undergo routine postoperative surveillance bronchoscopy lung biopsies to monitor for rejection episodes that may be clinically silent. During the first week post transplant, the tracheal anastomosis is inspected and bronchial lavage is done. At 4 weeks post transplant, a follow-up bronchoscopy and transbronchial biopsy are done (unless indicated earlier on clinical grounds). Then, routine surveillance bronchoscopy and lung biopsies are done every 2 months for the first year, and every 6 months thereafter.[28]

Infection

Broad-spectrum antibiotics are used perioperatively as prophylaxis against bacterial infection. At the time of transplant, the donor lungs are cultured for bacterial pathogens and the post transplant antibiotics are modified according to the bacterial pathogens found. Invasive or disseminated fungal infection needs aggressive treatment with intravenous amphotericin B. Asymptomatic recipients with positive fungal culture results in their transplanted lungs are also treated with itraconazole or amphotericin B. *Cytomegalovirus* (CMV) infection, either a primary infection or reactivation of latent virus, can occur within the first few weeks to months post transplant. Prophylactic intravenous ganciclovir three times weekly is as effective as daily administration.[29] We are currently evaluating the efficacy of an oral form of ganciclovir called valganciclovir, which is administered orally from day 8 to day 90 post transplant as CMV prophylaxis (except in CMV-negative recipients of CMV-negative organs). *Pneumocystis carinii* pneumonia (PCP) can occur in lung recipients unless they receive preventive therapy. Our standard prophylaxis against PCP is trimethoprim-sulfamethoxazole (TMP-SMX): adult heart-lung recipients take 1 single-strength tablet twice weekly indefinitely. If they cannot tolerate TMP-SMX, inhaled pentamidine or oral dapsone can be substituted.

Long-Term Care

Infection and rejection are the two most common causes of death within the first year after a heart-lung transplant. Subsequently, bronchiolitis obliterans syndrome (BOS) is the leading cause of death and of loss of pulmonary function.[10] Monitoring the forced expiratory volume in 1 s post transplant is important because a worsening BOS grade may warrant different or additional immunosuppression. Recipients are also at risk for hypertension, kidney dysfunction, hyperlipidemia, post-transplant lymphoproliferative disorder, and other nonlymphomatous malignant neoplasms.

References

1. Carrel A, Guthrie CC. The transplantation of veins and organs. Am Med 1905;10:1101–2.
2. Demikhov VP. Experimental transplantation of an additional heart in the dog. Bull Exp Biol Med (Russia) 1950;1:241–52.
3. Castañeda AR, Arnar O, Schmidt-Habelman P, et al. Cardiopulmonary autotransplantation in primates. J Cardiovasc Surg 1972;37:523–31.
4. Castañeda AR, Zamora R, Schmidt-Habelmann P, et al. Cardiopulmonary autotransplantation in primates (baboons): late functional results. Surgery 1972;72:1064–70.
5. Borel JF, Feurer C, Gubler HU, Stahelin H. Biological effects of cyclosporin A: a new anti-lymphocytic agent. 1976. Agents Actions 1994;43(3-4):179–86.
6. Calne RY, White DJG, Rolles K, et al. Prolonged survival of pig orthotopic heart grafts treated with cyclosporin A. Lancet 1978;1:1183–5.
7. Reitz BA, Burton NA, Jamieson SW, et al. Heart and lung transplantation: autotransplantation and allotransplantation in primates with extended survival. J Thorac Cardiovasc Surg 1980;80:360–72.
8. Cooley DA, Bloodwell RD, Hallman DG, et al. Organ transplantation for advanced cardiopulmonary disease. Ann Thorac Surg 1969;8:30–46.
9. Reitz BA, Wallwork JL, Hunt SA, et al. Heart-lung transplantation: successful therapy for patients with pulmonary vascular disease. N Engl J Med 1982;306:557–64.
10. Hosenpud JD, Bennett LE, Keck BM, et al. The Registry of the International Society for Heart and Lung Transplantation: eighteenth Official Report—2001. J Heart Lung Transplant 2001;20(8):805–16.
11. Madden BP, Hodson ME, Tsang V, et al. Intermediate-term results of heart-lung transplantation for cystic fibrosis. Lancet 1992;339(8809):1583–7.
12. Yacoub MH, Banner NR, Khaghani A, et al. Heart-lung transplantation for cystic fibrosis and subsequent domino heart transplantation. J Heart Transplant 1990;9(5):459–66; discussion 466–7.
13. Smith JA, Roberts M, McNeil K, et al. Excellent outcome of cardiac transplantation using domino donor hearts. Eur J Cardiothorac Surg 1996;10(8):628–33.
14. Mendeloff EN. Lung transplantation for cystic fibrosis. Semin Thorac Cardiovasc Surg 1998;10(3):202–12.
15. Barlow CW, Robbins RC, Moon MR, et al. Heart-lung versus double-lung transplantation for suppurative lung disease. J Thorac Cardiovasc Surg 2000;119(3):466–76.
16. Burke CM, Baldwin JC, Morris AJ, et al. Twenty-eight cases of human heart-lung transplantation. Lancet 1986;1:517–9.
17. Baldwin JC, Frist WH, Starkey TD, et al. Distant graft procurement for combined heart and lung transplantation using pulmonary artery flush and simple topical hypothermia for graft preservation. Ann Thorac Surg 1987;43:670–3.
18. Stringham JC, Love RB, Welter D, et al. Impact of University of Wisconsin solution on clinical heart transplantation. A comparison with Stanford solution for extended preservation. Circulation 1998;98 Suppl 19:II-157–61; discussion II-162.
19. Muller C, Furst H, Reichenspurner H, et al. Lung procurement by low-potassium dextran and the effect on preservation injury. Munich Lung Transplant Group. Transplantation 1999;68(8):1139–43.
20. Wildhirt SM, Weis M, Schulze C, et al. Effects of Celsior and University of Wisconsin preservation solutions on hemodynamics and endothelial function after cardiac transplantation in humans: a single-center, prospective, randomized trial. Transpl Int 2000;13 Suppl 1:S203–11.

21. Reitz BA, Pennock JL, Shumway NE. Simplified operative method of heart and lung transplantation. J Surg Res 1981;31:1–5.

22. Jamieson SW, Stinson EB, Oyer PE, et al. Operative technique for heart-lung transplantation. J Thorac Cardiovasc Surg 1984;87:930–5.

23. Nguyen DQ, Kulick DM, Bolman RM III, Park SJ. Temporary ECMO support following lung and heart-lung transplantation. J Heart Lung Transplant 2000;19(3):313–6.

24. Glassman LR, Keenan RJ, Fabrizio MC, et al. Extracorporeal membrane oxygenation as an adjunct treatment for primary graft failure in adult lung transplant recipients. J Thorac Cardiovasc Surg 1995;110(3):723–6; discussion 726–7.

25. Meyers BF, Sundt TM 3rd, Henry S, et al. Selective use of extracorporeal membrane oxygenation is warranted after lung transplantation. J Thorac Cardiovasc Surg 2000;120(1):20–6.

26. Glanville AR, Imoto E, Baldwin JC, et al. The role of right ventricular endomyocardial biopsy in the long-term management of heart-lung transplant recipients. J Heart Transplant 1987;6:357–61.

27. Hutter JA, Higenbottam T, Stewart S, Wallwork J. Routine endomyocardial biopsy is redundant in heart-lung recipients. J Heart Transplant 1988;7:48.

28. Hertz MI, editor. Manual of lung transplant medical care. 2nd ed. Minneapolis, MN: Fairview Publications; 2001.

29. Hertz MI, Jordan C, Savik SK, et al. Randomized trial of daily versus three-times-weekly prophylactic ganciclovir after lung and heart-lung transplantation. J Heart Lung Transplant 1998;17(9):913–20.

CARDIAC XENOTRANSPLANTATION

William E. Beschorner, MD

Heart transplantation is certainly a success story of modern medicine. To illustrate, adult heart transplant candidates with a United Network of Organ Sharing (UNOS) priority code of 1A ("Urgent") have a life expectancy of less than 7 days. Those who receive a transplant have a 5-year survival of almost 70%,[1] with survival for more than 10 years being typical.

The problem is that human donors will provide only a small portion of the heart grafts needed. In the United States, 4 to 5 million people have heart failure, with approximately 750,000 dying annually.[2] The number of patients younger than age 65 years who could benefit from a heart transplant is estimated at 50,000 or more per year.[3] In year 2000, 2,286 heart allograft transplantations were performed in the United States for end-stage heart failure.[4] If a lifeline can be offered to only 5% of those in need, then the actual success rate is limited.

Understandably, intense efforts are directed at fulfilling this large unmet need. In addition to improved medical treatment, investigators have been pursuing implantable ventricular assist devices and mechanical hearts, tissue engineering using myocardial cells derived from stem cells, and xenotransplantation.

Presently, none of these approaches is satisfactory. Mechanical hearts continue to improve, but outcomes are limited by coagulation problems, thromboembolism, infections, and device failure. Tissue engineering is at a very early and naive stage of development. Besides the problems of developing complex organs in three dimensions with multiple cell lines, there are questions about reliability and reproducibility of stem cell lines, immune rejection, the risk of teratomas, and ethical concerns. Xenotransplantation is currently limited by severe rejection events involving many antigens and multiple immune reactions. The immune suppression that would be currently required would be prohibitive. Until there is a successful technology that can be offered to those in need, the rational response is to pursue all reasonable technologies.

Optimism for xenotransplantation was initially very high. Many believed that when hyperacute rejection by preformed antibodies to alphaGal (alpha-1,3-galactose) was prevented, pig heart xenografts would be commonplace. As the field matured, however, the initial optimism was not realized. Instead, the barriers to xenotransplantation, the antigens and immune reactions, became better defined. Comprehensive strategies of tissue accommodation and immune tolerance will need to complement the piecemeal strategies of antigen resolution and immune suppression. Compared with allotransplantation, xenotransplantation provides the opportunity to accomplish these goals within the donor, prior to transplantation, sparing the recipient much of the risk of transplantation. It is regrettable that as the promise of xenotransplantation approaches reality, institutional and corporate support is limited. They must be encouraged to continue and extend their participation and support.

This brief review describes the potential benefits of cardiac xenotransplantation, the problems as currently understood, promising solutions for these problems, and the steps needed to take the technology into clinical trials.

The Potential for Cardiac Xenotransplantation

While the cardiac allotransplant story is certainly a technical success, the individual transplants are usually an adventure. Many factors that substantially affect the outcome of the transplant are largely beyond the control of the transplantation team. Nothing can be done with a potential donor until the patient is declared brain-dead. Medical decisions and interventions are made for the benefit of the patient, not the organ donation. The transplantation must be performed within hours of death, including obtaining permission, performing tests, procuring the donor organs, identifying the appropriate recipient, transportation to the recipient, and preparation of the recipient and the heart transplant. The donor may have significant problems that preclude transplantation, such as advanced age, cardiovascular disease, infections, and the like. Drugs administered during the final moments of life often adversely affect the quality of the transplant. Organ procurement may be adversely affected by local conditions. Rather than defining the optimal donor for a recipient, the optimal recipient is selected for a donor organ. The transplantation is performed as an emergency procedure, necessitating the potential recipients and transplantation personnel to be on constant alert. The condition of potential recipients typically deteriorates while waiting for a donor organ, leading to a prolonged and complicated postoperative recovery or premature death.

In contrast, with xenotransplantation the process would be totally controlled by the xenotransplant program. The donor pigs and the procurement of organs would be produced using procedures and facilities that satisfy requirements established by the US Food and Drug Administration. The donor pigs would be young, healthy, and free of infections. Quality assurance tests would be performed before procurement of the organ. The most appropriate donor, based on size, age, and other factors, would be produced for the recipient. The transplant organ would be obtained by a full-time xenograft procurement team. For patients with chronic heart failure, the transplantation procedure would be scheduled ahead of time and performed on an elective basis. By preventing a prolonged waiting period, the recipient would be in better condition at the time of transplantation, reducing the cost and length of postoperative recovery.

With human organ transplants, the goals of transplantation, prolonged graft acceptance and maintenance of immune competence, must be achieved within the recipient. There is little that can be done with the donor. Xenotransplantation presents the opportunity to achieve these goals within the donor. To the extent that they are accomplished within the donor pig, the risk to the recipient is reduced. For example, while inducing accommodation of the graft within the patient, the graft may be lost to rejection. If induced within the donor pig, prior to transplantation, accommodation of the graft is confirmed prior to transplantation. In the patient, measures to reduce antigraft antibodies are necessary. If accomplished in the donor, those measures are not needed in the recipient. Xenografts can be modified in many ways, including inbreeding, transgenic pigs with complement inhibitors or knockout of antigens, and cellular chimerism.

The Challenge of Xenotransplantation

With so many potential advantages, why, then, are xenotransplantations not performed routinely? The overriding issue is xenograft rejection. Protocols and drugs that are effective in preventing or reversing rejection of human allografts are ineffective with xenograft rejection. Allografts are rarely transplanted into recipients with preformed antibodies. Recipients of pig xenografts, however, typically have high titers of preformed antibodies. Allograft rejection involves relatively few histocompatibility antigens. Xenografts have many recognized antigens. Allograft rejection is primarily T cell rejection, so drugs that selectively inhibit these reactions can be used without a global immune deficiency. Xenograft rejection involves multiple reactions, including antibody-mediated rejection, T cell–mediated rejection, and natural killer (NK) cell rejection. There are currently no agents that are effective in suppressing B cell reactions. If the drugs were available, however, suppressing all of the potential reactions would leave the recipient severely immune deficient.

The challenge for xenotransplantation, therefore, is to prevent multiple rejection reactions to multiple antigens while preserving the immune competence of the recipient.

The Xenograft Antigens

Intuitively, two disparate species like humans and pigs would be expected to express many disparate antigens. Therefore, one would expect that pig tissues would express many antigens not present in humans, stimulating multiple immune reactions.

Most of the focus of pig antigens has been directed at alphaGal, an oligosaccharide produced in most mammals, including pigs. However, humans, apes, and Old World monkeys have a deficiency in the enzyme alpha-1,3-galactosyltransferase and therefore do not constitutively produce this epitope. The oligosaccharide is generally expressed on intestinal bacteria, which most likely sensitizes hosts that do not constitutively produce it. Consequently, humans, apes, and Old World monkeys develop natural antibodies to alphaGal.[5] The natural preformed antibodies are primarily directed at an epitope on the endothelial membrane, a glycoprotein with a terminal galactose alphaGal residue.

Although alphaGal is the most prevalent antigen expressed on pig endothelial cells, other antigens certainly contribute to rejection. When the antibodies to alphaGal were depleted, pig lungs were still lost to hyperacute rejection (HAR).[6] In transgenic knockout mice lacking the alphaGal antigen, pancreatic islets were rejected by antibodies to unrelated antigens.[7] Pig hearts transplanted into dogs were rejected by HAR within minutes although dogs produce alphaGal constitutively and do not have alphaGal antibodies.[8]

Multiple antigens other than alphaGal have been identified on pig red cells that are recognized by natural antibodies and bind complement.[9] Thirty-four non-alphaGal antigens from pig endothelial cells were recently identified in cynomolgus monkeys that rejected human decay-accelerating factor (hDAF) transgenic pig hearts by acute vascular rejection.[10]

The Rejection Reactions

HYPERACUTE REJECTION

When a pig heart is transplanted into a primate with pre-formed natural antibodies, the heart xenograft typically becomes dark and stops beating within minutes to hours of restoring circulation as a consequence of HAR. Antibody binds to the endothelial cells throughout the graft, and complement is activated, leading to adhesion of platelets, thrombosis, and ischemic necrosis of the tissue.

HAR of pig xenografts by Old World monkeys involves the immediate binding of circulating preformed antibodies to the endothelium and the classic pathway of complement fixation.[11–15] The binding of complement to the endothelial cells can then lead to loss of heparin sulfate, activation with change in shape, cell death and coagulation, and adhesion of neutrophils.[16] The widespread thrombosis of the vessels causes ischemic destruction of the xenograft.

In contrast to HAR of allografts caused by sensitization, the responsible xenophyllic antibodies involves primarily immunoglobulin (Ig) M rather than IgG.

ACUTE VASCULAR REJECTION

Initially it was thought that if HAR was resolved, the immune reaction to xenografts would be relatively weak and the grafts accepted with only modest immune suppression. However, that hope was not realized, and xenografts were vigorously and irreversibly rejected in 2 to 8 days.

The histology of the rejected grafts shows vascular thrombosis and swelling of endothelial cells. There is an infiltrate of large mononuclear cells, including macrophages and NK cells. Lymphocytes represent a minor population.[17] IgG is typically deposited on the endothelial cells, and complement may be detectable.

Acute vascular rejection appears to be identical to an entity previously called delayed xenograft rejection.[18] The antibody specificity observed in acute vascular rejection differs from the IgM natural antibodies seen in HAR. The antibodies include IgG and are directed against the alpha-Gal antigen, as well as against other antigens.[19] The binding of IgG suggests that the reaction is a secondary response to antigens. A study of sera from patients treated with extracorporeal perfusion of pig livers showed an early rise in IgG1 following the perfusion.[20]

The contribution of T cells to acute vascular rejection is unclear. In the guinea pig-to-rat model, acute vascular rejection does not appear to require T cells because the reaction is also observed in nude rats.[21] Immunohistochemistry of the rejected graft showed a dense infiltrate of macrophages and NK cells but no B cells or T cells (α/β T cell receptor).

Other models support the participation of T cells. For example, chemotherapy agents effective against T cells (eg, cyclosporine, cyclophosphamide) can delay pig xenograft rejection in primates.[22,23] Furthermore, it is possible that the few residual T cells remaining in the nude rats contribute to the rejection process.[24,25]

CELLULAR REJECTION BY T LYMPHOCYTES AND NATURAL KILLER CELLS

As seen previously, the prevention of one major xenograft rejection reaction may not lead to prolonged survival but may simply unmask a subsequent rejection reaction. Quite possibly, therefore, the prevention of acute vascular rejection may simply reveal acute cellular rejection. If acute cellular rejection is similar to that seen with allografts, it could be prevented with currently available drugs. The data suggest, however, that cellular xenograft rejection differs in at least two respects from acute allograft rejection: antigen recognition and the nature of the effector cells.

Antigen-presenting cells (APCs) in the recipient of a xenograft may be defective in presenting the antigens to the recipient T cells. However, porcine endothelial antigens are able to stimulate human T cells directly, bypassing the need for APCs.[26]

In immunopathology descriptions, the T cell infiltrates typically constitute a minor population, as compared to a major component with allograft rejection. The major components consist of bound immunoglobulins, natural killer cells, and macrophages.

Nonetheless, studies support a significant function for T cells in xenograft rejection. When human blood is perfused through a porcine kidney, the T cells and NK cells are removed from the blood. These cells were later identified attached to the vascular endothelial cells of the perfused graft.[27]

In vitro cell-mediated cell lysis assays suggest that T cells and NK cells collaborate in the destruction of pig endothelial cells. Lymphocytes from humans, as well as from newborn baboon xenograft recipients, spontaneously lysed labeled pig endothelial cells.[28,29] The lysis was enhanced by interleukin-2 and inhibited by antibodies to CD2. Cell-mediated lysis correlates with acute rejection.

CD4+ T cells are particularly important for acute cellular xenograft rejection. With the depletion of CD4+ cells by using monoclonal antibodies, fetal pig islets enjoyed prolonged survival.[30] The recipients were unable to mount antibody responses to pig cells. These studies indicated that CD4+ cells were important in at least the afferent limb of the immune response, particularly regarding the antibody response.[31] Although the studies emphasize CD4+ T cells, it is assumed that the antibodies also depleted CD4+ monocytes and macrophages as well.

Although the CD4+ cells certainly would contribute to the humoral response,[32] the CD4+ cells can destroy the target cells directly. Adoptive transfer studies of cell populations to severe combined immunodeficiency disease (SCID) mice showed that the transfer of CD4+ cells without B cells led to rapid rejection of pig skin grafts.[33,34]

With allograft rejection, CD8+ cells are the effector cells that lead to tissue injury. With xenografts, however, the CD8+ cells are less important.[35]

Pig endothelial cells stimulate the proliferation of both purified CD4+ and CD8+ human lymphocytes.[36,37] Cytokine analysis of the mouse versus rat mixed lymphocyte reaction (MLR) indicates that the CD4+ helper cells are those of TH2 subtype, as compared with the usual TH1 subtype seen with allogeneic reactions.[32] Whereas TH1 cells participate in delayed-type hypersensitivity reactions, TH2 cells typically contribute to the humoral response.

CHRONIC REJECTION

Chronic rejection is a major problem with allografts, leading to loss of grafts months or years post transplantation. The grafts undergo accelerated atherosclerosis, with diffuse intimal thickening and proliferation of the fibroblasts.

Currently, there is relatively little experience with long-term xenografts and therefore little experience with chronic rejection. Graft atherosclerosis has been observed in two baboon recipients of monkey hearts.[38] The recipients died at 74 and 502 days post transplanttion. The findings resembled accelerated arteriosclerosis seen with chronic allograft rejection. In the hamster-to-rat heart and aorta transplant models, chronic vascular rejection has been described, also resembling chronic allograft rejection.[40–42]

In a systematic and quantitative study of hamster aorta xenografts, Scheringa demonstrated thickening and infiltration of the adventitia during the acute rejection (14 days).[39] This subsided and was followed during chronic rejection by a progressive thickening of the intima (at 56 days). Localized IgM deposits are seen in the arterial lesions.

Chronic xenograft rejection might prove to be more resistant to chemotherapy than allografts.[42] Continuous cyclosporine or mycophenolate mofetil is effective in reducing the intimal thickening seen in chronic xenograft rejection.[39,40,43]

Other Potential Issues

Zoonotic Infections

The immune-deficient recipient is at significant risk for contracting infectious diseases from the organ donor. This has been demonstrated for allografts with the transmission of herpes viruses (including *Cytomegalovirus* and Epstein-Barr), human immunodeficiency virus, hepatitis, *Toxoplasma gondii*, and other viruses. Precautions are now taken to minimize that risk. The risk of a human opportunistic infection would be minimized with animal donors. For example, even primates such as baboons are resistant to hepatitis B and human immunodeficiency virus.[44]

On the other hand, there is a potential risk for transmission of an infectious agent harbored by the animal donor. The zoonotic agents include exogenous infections as well as endogenous agents such as retroviruses. While the exogenous agents can potentially be eliminated from the herd, endogenous retroviruses are coded within the genome.

In comparing the potential use of swine and primate organs, the greatest concern has been expressed for the use of nonhuman primates as xenograft donors.[15,16] Whereas swine can be bred rapidly and can be raised under controlled conditions, the conditions for primates cannot be as well controlled. There are several examples of viruses that are relatively benign in primates but have produced catastrophic results when they infect humans, such as the Marburg virus and the Ebola virus.[47,48] Although these viruses have a high mortality rate in humans, human hosts are unable to sustain the amplification for prolonged periods of time.[49] Proviral deoxyribonucleic acid for endogenous retroviruses is found in baboons and monkeys. When human cells are cocultured with baboon cells, the virus can be detected.[50]

Swine also pose a small risk for zoonotic infections, although most consider the risk to be much less than with nonhuman primates.[51] Multiple agents can potentially be passed from humans to pigs, which in turn could infect xenograft recipients. These include bacterial infections (such as *Salmonella*, *Campylobacter*, and *Yersinia*), parasites such as *Schistosoma*, and viruses such as influenza virus. Swine may also carry herpes viruses, including a swine *Cytomegalovirus* and circoviruses.[52]

High standards of animal husbandry have made these entities more theoretical than real. A thorough necropsy examination of 10 pigs was performed, including 150 tests. The stool contained some parasites considered to be commensals. No agents pathogenic for humans were identified.[53]

Transformed porcine cell lines produce C type endogenous retroviruses. When two such cell lines, PK-15 and MPK, were cocultured with human cell lines, porcine virus could be identified within the human cells.[54] The study raised the possibility that porcine retroviruses might infect humans. That, in turn, raises the risk that the virus may behave more aggressively in humans or transform into a more aggressive virus.

At this time, the concern is more theoretical than real. When severely immune-suppressed baboons were transplanted with porcine endothelial cells, there was no evidence of porcine endogenous retrovirus (PERV) in the blood or multiple tissues.[55] Human recipients of porcine pancreatic islets were followed for up to 7 years post transplantation. No evidence of PERV was found in the blood.[56] Neither PERV nor antibodies to PERV could be detected in patients after perfusion of their blood through porcine kidneys.[57]

An extensive retrospective study of 160 patients exposed to viable pig tissues up to 12 years previously suggests that the risk is minimal at worst.[58] The specimens were analyzed in multiple laboratories, including the

Centers for Disease Control and Prevention in Atlanta, Georgia. The analyses used a highly sensitive polymerase chain reaction assay for PERV.[59] Because PERV is present in most pig cells, the analysis distinguished between the presence of PERV because of chimerism and true PERV infection. The patients included those treated with extracorporeal splenic perfusion, extracorporeal perfusion of whole liver and whole kidney, skin grafts, islet transplants, and treatment with artificial liver devices incorporating porcine hepatocytes. There was no evidence of PERV infection in any of the subjects, even though some demonstrated microchimerism up to 8.5 years after exposure. The failure to detect PERV infection after prolonged chimerism with porcine cells suggests that the lack of infection is more likely related to an unfavorable environment than to the absence of an immune response.

The hypothetical risk to the public posed by PERV is a theoretical concern without supporting data. Extensive ongoing research has failed to demonstrate that PERV is either contagious or pathogenic. Indeed, it may be impossible to prove unequivocally the safety of xenotransplants, in that negative data can never prove safety. What would have happened if virologists had raised a similar concern about human endogenous retroviruses? Would that have prevented the widespread use of blood transfusions and human organ transplants?

Perhaps a more productive line of investigation would be to define the factors responsible for the strong resistance of human cells to PERV in vivo. Then the factors in the pigs could be monitored as quality control and the human factors monitored preclinically and in clinical follow-up. If the factors were absent, the transplantation would not be done. Strains of swine have been discovered, in which PERV does not pass to human cells in culture, no matter what is done. This may be helpful, although the coculture test proved to be totally unreliable for predicting PERV infection in vivo.

Not all porcine cells can transmit PERV in culture. For example, cells from miniature swine cocultured with human cells did not lead to transmission.[60] PERV from islets of swine grown in New Zealand also could not be transmitted to nude or nonobese diabetic mice.[61] The frequency of swine that cannot transmit PERV in culture is not known.

Before PERV can become a public health problem, it theoretically needs to undergo multiple transformations before becoming contagious and pathologic. It would be valuable to define those transformations and how they can be detected.

The Food and Drug Administration has held hearings and issued suggested guidelines as related to infectious diseases from xenotransplantation.[46,62,63] The suggestions include the formation of a registry for xenotransplantation, formation of institutional xenotransplant committees including experts in infectious diseases, the surveillance of both animal donors and human recipients, the archiving of blood and tissues from donors and recipients, and husbandry measures designed to provide pathogen-free animal donors.

Xenograft Function

The anatomy and physiology of the pig heart closely resembles the human heart, making the pig very attractive as the donor species.[64] There are some minor differences, including a lower electrical threshold for pacing pig hearts and the presence of the left azygous vein draining the intercostal blood.[65,66] Overall, however, the ventricles, atria, and coronary arteries are very close between the two species. Organ dysfunction has not been a problem in pig-to-primate transplantations when rejection is prevented.[67]

Pigs grow rapidly and can become quite large. If the heart grew at the same rate, it could soon be too large for the recipient. Within the pig, however, the heart does not keep pace with the growth of the body. The heart weight/body weight is approximately 0.8% at birth, 0.5% at sexual maturity, and 0.3% at maturity. One suggestion is to use miniature pigs. However, the relative size of hearts in miniature pigs is larger than in commercial pigs, so there is limited advantage to using smaller pigs.[67] Following transplantation, studies indicate that the growth of pig organs is very limited in the new host if rejection is prevented.[68] Consequently, host growth factors rather than organ transplant factors may define the post transplantation size of the xenograft.

Prevention of Rejection

The two primary goals of transplantation are long-term acceptance of a functional graft and maintenance of immune competence of the recipient. In the broadest terms, these goals can be accomplished with either a piecemeal strategy or a comprehensive strategy. In the piecemeal strategy, individual antigen differences are identified between the donor and recipient and resolved as much as possible. Individual immune reactions responsible for rejection are identified and suppressed. The comprehensive strategy resolves multiple immune problems in a manner that leaves the recipient immune competent. Accommodation conditions the graft to resist injury by antigraft antibodies, regardless of the individual antigens. Immune tolerance reprograms the recipient's immune response to selectively ignore the graft while remaining reactive to other antigens.

The goals of transplantation can potentially be accomplished within the recipient or within the donor. To the extent that they are accomplished within the donor, the risk to the recipient is reduced. The goals are accomplished and confirmed before transplantation. The optimal conditions can be defined and controlled better within the donor than the recipient.

With human allografts, the strategy has been primarily a piecemeal strategy, with tissue typing and selective suppression of the immune reactions. The goals were pursued within the recipient by default, since there is little that can be done with a human donor.

With xenotransplantation, the transplantation goals can potentially be accomplished within the recipient or within the donor. These efforts would need to block preformed antibodies, complement fixation, NK cell reactions, T cell responses, and B cell responses.

Individual strategies have been developed for each of the specific xenograft rejection reactions. Antibodies can be removed from the recipient by absorption.[69,70] Antibodies to alphaGal antigen can be neutralized with soluble oligosaccharides.[71,72] Complement fixation can be blocked with soluble complement receptor.[73,74] T cell responses can be inhibited with drugs such as cyclophosphamide, cyclosporine, tacrolimus, leflunomide, rapamycin, and mycophenolate mofetil, among other drugs.[23,75-79] Currently, good drugs are not available to block B cell or NK cell reactions. If agents were available for all of the immune responses, the combination would leave the recipient severely immune deficient, with a high risk for infectious diseases and toxicity. The piecemeal strategy, by itself, will not prevent xenograft rejection while maintaining immune competence.

The donor pigs can be modified to address individual immune reactions or antigen disparities. To block complement fixation after preformed antibodies bound to the graft, transgenic pigs were produced with high levels of human complement inhibitors. Pig heart xenografts transplanted into baboons were not lost to hyperacute rejection. The complement inhibitors, however, had little effect in preventing acute vascular rejection.

Heart xenografts from transgenic pigs with hDAF were transplanted heterotopically or orthotopically into baboons.[80] The heterotopic hearts survived an average of 23.5 days (range, 2 to 99) while the orthotopic grafts survived an average of 11.7 (range, 1 to 39) days. Post transplantation, the recipients received four-drug immune suppression, a protocol associated with leukopenia.[81] The predominant pathology observed in the grafts not lost to either HAR or technical failure was acute vascular rejection, with areas of myocardial infarcts and thrombosis, IgM and IgG, complement, macrophages, and variable numbers of NK and T cells.

Transgenic pigs have been produced to reduce or eliminate expression of the alphaGal antigen. The expression of fucosyl transferase produces the O antigen with a concomitant reduction in alphaGal.[82,83] Transgenic pig grafts carrying the enzyme and complement inhibitor did not, however, survive longer than grafts with complement inhibitors alone in large animal studies.

The direct way to eliminate the alphaGal gene would be to disrupt it with homologous recombination, leading to a knockout of the gene. Fetal pig fibroblasts were so treated and cloned into pigs.[84,85] Being hemizygous, the founder pigs still produced alphaGal. Recently, homozygous pigs were produced by treating fibroblasts from the transgenic pigs to knock out the second gene. After selection, those fibroblasts were cloned into pigs, producing homozygous double-knockout pigs.[86] Transplantation of vascular xenografts into baboons will be performed shortly. It has been noted that there is a second galactosyl transferase allele that produces alphaGal in pigs. The organs from the double-knockout pigs have not yet been transplanted into primate recipients.

The comprehensive strategies of accommodation and tolerance would substantially reduce the need for immune suppression. However, they can be difficult to achieve within the recipient. Furthermore, there is some risk to the recipient during the induction phase.

If graft rejection by antibodies can be prevented for several weeks, the graft eventually may become accommodated or resistant to injury. For example, if antidonor antibodies are reduced in recipients of incompatible kidney allografts, after several weeks the graft survives in spite of persistent antibodies.[87] The molecular basis for accommodation has been studied and some protective proteins identified.[88,89] Accommodation has been proposed as a pathway to prolonged xenograft acceptance and prevention of acute vascular rejection.[90-92] During the induction phase the risk is substantial that the graft, will be lost to antigraft antibodies. Antibody-mediated rejection can be prevented by removing the antibodies with plasmapheresis or inhibition of complement. With these steps, however, the recipient is at increased risk for infection.

Specific immune tolerance potentially could eliminate the need for immune suppression by reprogramming the immune system to selectively ignore the xenograft. The recipient would become specifically hyporesponsive to the antigens on the pig tissues but would be appropriately responsive to unrelated antigens on infectious agents.

Several methods of immune tolerance have been proposed for xenotransplantation. Mixed chimerism in the recipient can be achieved by ablating the recipient's immunity and reconstituting the recipient with a mixture of donor pig and recipient hematopoietic cells. Efforts have focused on minimizing the period of severe immune deficiency and on enhancing chimerism.[93,94] In large animal studies, prolonged chimerism with pig cells was achieved in recipients with restored immune competence. However, organ xenografts, which express antigens not present on hematopoietic cells, are typically rejected.

The thymus produces T lymphocytes that are self-tolerant. In addition to maturation of the T cells, self-reactive T cell clones are deleted. Suppressor T cells are produced, which help to control autoreactive processes. Specific tolerance to foreign grafts could potentially be achieved by reprogramming the thymus, involving depletion and recruitment of new dendritic cells or injection of cells into the thymus. Another approach involves transplantation of fetal thymus tissue from the donor pig. Reprogramming has not yet been shown to lead to long-term survival of xenografts in large animal models. The tolerance would be limited to T cells, and if the main effect is reprogramming clonal deletion, the recipient would be subjected to a period of severe immune deficiency.

Blocking the co-stimulation process of T cells has the potential advantage of inducing immune tolerance without a period of severe immune deficiency. For effective sensitization of T cells, both the T cell receptor and a second receptor, such as CD28, must interact with the corresponding ligands of the antigen-presenting cells, such as B7-1. If the second interaction is blocked, as with CTLA-4, an antibody to B7-1, the T cell becomes anergic. Co-stimulation blockade has prolonged heart xenograft survival in small animal models with T cell depletion.[95] While large animal models of heart transplants have not yet been tested, antibody to CD40 ligand, combined with T cell depletion, irradiation, and chemotherapy, prevented an antibody response to non-alphaGal antigens when pig hematopoietic cells were infused into baboons.[96]

The comprehensive strategies of accommodation and tolerance are being pursued within the donor pig. By inducing cellular chimerism within the donor pig, accommodation of the pig tissues and immune tolerance to the pig tissue antigens can be induced. Because the heart xenograft is accommodated outside the recipient, before transplantation, it is not necessary to remove the antibodies or complement from the recipient. By producing and transferring specific suppressor cells to the recipient, immune tolerance can be conveyed to the recipient without a period of severe immune deficiency. Pursuing these strategies provides an added opportunity of defining the conditions that are optimal for induction of accommodation and tolerance. Fetal pigs offer an environment conducive to the growth of foreign cells, the induction of accommodation through low levels of antipig antibodies, and the development of specific suppressor cells that suppress the reactions to pig antigens. The fetal environment is naturally sterile, providing a low-cost bioreactor for accomplishing the goals.

A large animal model of chimeric donor pigs demonstrates the feasibility of this approach.[97] Bone marrow from the recipient sheep was infused into fetal pigs. After delivery, the pigs were assessed for chimerism. Tolerant splenocytes were infused into the recipient sheep, and the heart xenograft was transplanted heterotopically into the neck of the recipient. Modest suppression consisting of cyclosporine and tapered steroids was administered post transplantation. All 12 of the control xenografts (no or minimal chimerism) were lost to acute vascular rejection. In contrast, only 1 of 13 experimental xenografts (with more than 1% chimerism) developed acute vascular rejection. The antipig antibody response decreased by 10-fold in the experimental group. Most importantly, the white cell, lymphocyte, and platelet counts were normal throughout the course. The IgG and IgM levels were normal. Minimal complications or infections were experienced. Prolonged xenograft survival was achieved without severe immune suppression.

As a large animal model of pig heart xenotransplantation, it is valuable and supports the feasibility of xenotransplantation. No animal model is perfect, however, and there are some remaining issues relevant to translation to clinical trials. Sheep do not produce preformed or induced antibodies to alphaGal, a major pig antigen. Will the accommodation of the pig heart provide protection against these antibodies? Will the alphaGal disparity lead to severe graft-versus-host disease when human cells are infused into fetal pigs? Will the human cells produce specific suppressor cells?

Accommodation of pig hearts provides protection against high titers of antipig antibody in sensitized sheep. Heart explants function for a prolonged period during ex vivo perfusion with sensitized sheep plasma.[98] Chimeric pig hearts transplanted into sensitized sheep functioned well, even when the titer of cytotoxic antipig antibodies exceeded 1,000.[99] Assays have been developed to assess pig tissue accommodation before procuring the organ.[100] Ex vivo perfusion of a heart explant from a pig chimeric with sheep cells functioned for 4 h when perfused with whole human blood, while the nonchimeric control heart stopped in 20 min.[101]

Human marrow and cord blood cells have been grown within fetal pigs. With partial depletion of T cells, high levels of chimerism are achieved without graft-versus-host disease. Large numbers of suppressor cells are generated, capable of specifically suppressing the reaction of human lymphocytes to pig cells.[102]

The transplantation of pig hearts into baboons or monkeys would be a more stringent test of xenotransplantation than pig-to-sheep transplantations. If human hematopoietic cells can be grown in fetal pigs, then most likely non-human primate cells will grow in fetal pigs. If human chimerism leads to antigen-specific suppressor cells and accommodation, then most likely nonhuman primate cells will also lead to accommodation and tolerance.

The Near Future of Cardiac Xenotransplantation

Once the technology is proven feasible, the transplantation of pig hearts into human recipients should be implemented. Orthotopic transplantations of pig hearts into baboons demonstrated appropriate function as long as followed. The Food and Drug Administration has issued guidelines for assuring the safety of xenotransplantation and for monitoring recipients and close contacts. The main remaining issue is whether immune modulation can provide for prolonged heart xenograft survival while maintaining immune competence in the recipient. As discussed earlier, progress on this challenge is promising.

The Food and Drug Administration Center for Biologics Evaluation and Research has sponsored hearings and workshops that have helped formulate their issued guidelines for xenotransplantation. These proceedings were a combined effort with the Centers for Disease Control and the National Institutes of Health. In 1999, the Secretary's Advisory Committee on Xenotransplantation was formed to discuss scientific, medical, social, and ethical issues of xenotransplantation.[103]

The guidelines detail requirements for assuring the safety of xenotransplantation to the patient and public. These include certification of the source animals; a current Good Manufacturing Procedures (cGMP) biosecure facility for housing the animals; a cGMP tissue processing laboratory; quality assurance of the animal and transplant tissue; periodic monitoring of recipients and close contacts; archiving of tissues and information; and review by appropriate institutional committees. While the requirements are significant, clinical trials involving xenotransplants are currently underway and have satisfactorily met these requirements.

A greater hurdle will be the need to demonstrate efficacy in a pig-to-nonhuman primate model. The Food and Drug Administration has not issued specific thresholds to be achieved. This will be defined for individual proposals, based on the patients, the proposed procedures, competing and available technologies, and other factors. Some researchers propose a 60% survival rate at 3 months, with at least 10 nonhuman primate recipients surviving to this point.[2] Others point out that primate models are difficult models and that the results with allograft survival underestimated the initial clinical results.

Another proposal is that the initial clinical trial be a small series of transplantations, with perhaps 10 recipients, providing xenografts for candidates with no feasible alternative therapy.[2] These recipients would be followed for a minimum of 3 months before proceeding to more extensive clinical trials.

Xenotransplantation is a very attractive solution to the severe shortage of human heart donors. The transplantation of pig hearts provides significant advantages over human heart transplants. The major deterrent is severe xenograft rejection, which is caused by many antigens and multiple immune reactions. However, the transplantation of pig hearts also provides the opportunity to achieve the goals of transplantation, prolonged graft survival and immune competence within the donor pig before transplantation.

References

1. Annual Report of the US Scientific Registry of Transplant Recipients and the Organ Procurement and Transplantation Network. Transplant data 1989–1998. (February 16, 2001). Rockville, MD, and Richmond, VA: HHS/HRSA/OSP/DOT and UNOS. Available at: http://www.unos.org/frame_Default.asp?Category=anrpt (accessed September 26, 2002).

2. Cooper DK, Keogh AM, Brink J, et al. Report of the Xenotransplantation Advisory Committee of the International Society for Heart and Lung Transplantation: the present status of xenotransplantation and its potential role in the treatment of end-stage cardiac and pulmonary diseases. J Heart Lung Transplant 2000;19:1125–65.

3. Evans RW. Costs and insurance coverage associated with permanent mechanical cardiac assist/replacement devices in the United States. J Card Surg 2001;16:280–93.

4. Transplant Patient DataSource. (February 16, 2000). Richmond, VA: United Network for Organ Sharing. Available at: http://207.239.150.13/tpd/ (accessed August 29,2002).

5. Galili U. Evolution and pathophysiology of the human natural anti-alpha galactosyl IgG (anti-Gal) antibody. Springer Semin Immunopathol 1993;15:155–71.

6. Macchiarini P, Oriol R, Azimzadeh A, et al. Evidence of human non-alpha galactosyl antibodies involved in the hyperacute rejection of pig lungs and their removal by pig organ perfusion. J Thorac Cardiovasc Surg 1998;116:831–43.

7. McKenzie IF, Koulmanda M, Mandel TE, Sandrin MS. Pig islet xenografts are susceptible to "anti-pig" but not Galalpha(1,3)Gal antibody plus complement in Gal o/o mice. J Immunol 1998;161:5116–9.

8. Sato Y, Kimikawa M, Suga H, et al. Prolongation of cardiac xenograft survival by double filtration plasmapheresis and ex vivo immunoadsorption. ASAIO J 1992;38:M673–5.

9. Zhu A. Introduction to porcine red blood cells: implications for xenotransfusion. Semin Hematol 2000;37:143–9.

10. Lau M, Lam T, Morris R. Expression cloning of non-alpha Gal endothelial cell antigens recognized during humoral rejection of pig organ xenografts [abstract]. Transplantation 2002;74:39A.

11. Gambiez L, Salame E, Chereau C, et al. The role of natural IgM in the hyperacute rejection of discordant heart xenografts. Transplantation 1992;54:577–83.

12. Platt JL, Turman MA, Noreen HJ, et al. An ELISA assay for xenoreactive natural antibodies. Transplantation 1990;49:1000–1.

13. Platt JL, Lindman BJ, Chen H, et al. Endothelial cell antigens recognized by xenoreactive human natural antibodies. Transplantation 1990;50:817–22.

14. Platt JL, Vercellotti GM, Dalmasso AP, et al. Transplantation of discordant xenografts: a review of progress. Immunol Today 1990;11:450–6.

15. Dalmasso AP, Vercellotti GM, Fischel RJ, et al. Mechanism of complement activation in the hyperacute rejection of porcine organs transplanted into primate recipients. Am J Pathol 1992;140:1157–66.

16. Platt JL. A perspective on xenograft rejection and accommodation. Immunol Rev 1994;141:127–49.

17. Bach FH, Winkler H, Ferran C, et al. Delayed xenograft rejection. Immunol Today 1996;17:379–84.

18. Saadi S, Platt JL. Immunology of xenotransplantation. Life Sci 1998;62:365–87.

19. Cooke SP, Hederer RA, Pearson JD, Savage COS. Characterization of human IgG-binding xenoantigens expressed by porcine aortic endothelial cells. Transplantation 1995;60:1274–84.

20. Yu PB, Parker W, Everett ML, et al. Immunochemical properties of anti-Gal alpha-1-3-Gal antibodies after sensitization with xenogeneic tissues. J Clin Immunol 1999; 19:116–26.

21. Candinas D, Belliveau S, Koyamada N, et al. T cell independence of macrophage and natural killer cell infiltration, cytokine production, and endothelial activation during delayed xenograft rejection. Transplantation 1996;62: 1920–7.

22. Scheringa M, Schraa EO, Bouwman E, et al. Prolongation of survival of guinea pig heart grafts in cobra venom factor-treated rats by splenectomy. No additional effect of cyclosporine. Transplantation 1995;60:1350–3.

23. Davis EA, Pruitt SK, Greene PS, et al. Inhibition of complement, evoked antibody, and cellular response prevents rejection of pig-to-primate cardiac xenografts. Transplantation 1996;62:1018–23.

24. Hunig T, Bevan MJ. Ability of nude mice to generate alloreactive, xenoreactive and H-2-restricted cytotoxic T-lymphocyte responses. Exp Cell Biol 1984;52:7–11.

25. Vaessen LM, Broekhuizen R, Rozing J, et al. T-cell development during ageing in congenitally athymic (nude) rats. Scand J Immunol 1986;24:223–35.

26. Game DS, Warrens AN, Lechler RI. Rejection mechanisms in transplantation. Wien Klin Wochenschr 2001;113: 832–8.

27. Khalfoun B, Janin P, Machet MC, et al. Discordant xenogeneic cellular interactions when hyperacute rejection is prevented: analysis using an ex vivo model of pig kidney perfused with human lymphocytes. Transplant Proc 1996;28:647.

28. Itescu S, Kwiatkowski P, Wang SF, et al. Circulating human mononuclear cells exhibit augmented lysis of pig endothelium after activation with interleukin 2. Transplantation 1996;62:1927–33.

29. Itescu S, Kwiatkowski PA, Artrip JH, et al. Role of natural killer cells, macrophages, and accessory molecule interactions in the rejection of pig-to-primate xenografts beyond the hyperacute period. Human Immunology 1998;59:275–86.

30. Simeonovic CJ, Ceredig R, Wilson JD. Effect of GK1.5 monoclonal antibody dosage on survival of pig proislet xenografts in CD4+ T cell-depleted mice. Transplantation 1990;49:849–56.

31. Simeonovic CJ, Wilson JD, Ceredig R. Antibody-induced rejection of pig proislet xenografts in CD4+ T cell-depleted diabetic mice. Transplantation 1990;50: 657–62.

32. Wren SM, Wang SC, Thai NL, et al. Evidence for early Th2 T cell predominance in xenoreactivity. Transplantation 1993;56:905–11.

33. Auchincloss H Jr, Moses R, Conti D, et al. Xenograft rejection of class I-expressing transgenic skin is CD4-dependent and CD8-independent. Transplant Proc 1990;22: 2335–6.

34. Friedman T, Shimizu A, Smith RN, et al. Human CD4+ T cells mediate rejection of porcine xenografts. J Immunol 1999;162:5256–62.

35. Desai NM, Bassiri H, Kim J, et al. Islet allograft, islet xenograft, and skin allograft survival in CD8+ T lymphocyte-deficient mice. Transplantation 1993;55:718–22.

36. Bravery CA, Rose ML, Yacoub MH. Proliferative responses of highly purified human CD4+ T cells to porcine endothelial cells. Transplant Proc 1994;26:1157–8.

37. Rollins SA, Kennedy SP, Chodera AJ, et al. Evidence that activation of human T cells by porcine endothelium involves direct recognition of porcine SLA and costimulation by porcine ligands for LFA-1 and CD2. Transplantation 1994;57:1709–16.

38. Fukushima N, Kawauchi M, Bouchart T, et al. Graft atherosclerosis in concordant cardiac transplantation. Transplant Proc 1994;26:1059–60.

39. Scheringa M, Buchner B, Geerling RA, et al. Chronic rejection after concordant xenografting. Transplant Proc 1994;26:1346–7.

40. Lin Y, Vandeputte M, Waer M. Effect of leflunomide and cyclosporine on the occurrence of chronic xenograft lesions. Kidney Int Suppl 1995;52:S23–8.

41. Xiao F, Shen J, Chong A, et al. Control and reversal of chronic xenograft rejection in hamster-to-rat cardiac transplantation. Transplant Proc 1996;28:691–2.

42. Dorling A, Riesbeck K, Warrens A, Lechler R. Clinical xenotransplantation of solid organs. Lancet 1997;349: 867–71.

43. O'Hair DP, McManus RP, Komorowski R. Inhibition of chronic vascular rejection in primate cardiac xenografts using mycophenolate mofetil. Ann Thorac Surg 1994;58: 1311–5.

44. Gammie JS, Kaufman CL, Michaels MG, Ildstad ST. Xenotransplantation: strategies to achieve donor-specific tolerance and immune reconstitution across species barriers through mixed bone marrow chimerism. Mol Diagn 1996;1:219–24.

45. Allan JS. Xenograft transplantation and the infectious disease conundrum. Inst Lab Anim Resources J 1995;37: 37–48.

46. Shalala DE. Draft public health service (PHS) guideline on infectious disease issues in xenotransplantation. Fed Reg 1996;61:49920–32.

47. Martini GA. Marburg agent disease in man. Trans R Soc Trop Med Hyg 1969;63:295–302.

48. Ebola haemorrhagic fever in Zaire, 1976. Bull World Health Organ 1978;56:271–93.

49. Chapman LE, Folks TM, Salomon DR, et al. Xenotransplantation and xenogeneic infections. N Engl J Med 1995;333:1498–501.

50. Deinhardt F. Biology of primate retroviruses. In: Klein G, editor. Viral oncology. New York: Raven Press; 1980. p. 357–98.

51. Michaels MG, Simmons RL. Xenotransplant-associated zoonoses. Strategies for prevention. Transplantation 1994;57:1–7.

52. Morozov I, Sirinarumitr T, Sorden SD, et al. Detection of a novel strain of porcine circovirus in pigs with postweaning multisystemic wasting syndrome. J Clin Microbiol 1998;36:2535–41.

53. Ye Y, Niekrasz M, Kosanke S, et al. The pig as a potential organ donor for man. A study of potentially transferable disease from donor pig to recipient man. Transplantation 1994;57:694–703.

54. Patience C, Takeuchi Y, Weiss RA. Infection of human cells by an endogenous retrovirus of pigs. Nat Med 1997;3:282–6.

55. Martin U, Steinhoff G, Kiessig V, et al. Porcine endogenous retrovirus (PERV) was not transmitted from transplanted porcine endothelial cells to baboons in vivo. Transpl Int 1998;11:247–51.

56. Heneine W, Tibell A, Switzer WM, et al. No evidence of infection with porcine endogenous retrovirus in recipients of porcine islet-cell xenografts. Lancet 1998;352: 695–9.

57. Patience C, Patton GS, Takeuchi Y, et al. No evidence of pig DNA or retroviral infection in patients with short- term extracorporeal connection to pig kidneys. Lancet 1998; 352:699–701.

58. Paradis K, Langford G, Long Z, et al. Search for cross-species transmission of porcine endogenous retrovirus in patients treated with living pig tissue. Science 1999; 285:1236–41.

59. Switzer WM, Shanmugam V, Chapman L, Heneine W. Polymerase chain reaction assays for the diagnosis of infection with the porcine endogenous retrovirus and the detection of pig cells in human and nonhuman recipients of pig xenografts. Transplantation 1999;68:183–8.

60. Oldmixon BA, Wood JC, Ericsson TA, et al. Porcine endogenous retrovirus transmission characteristics of an inbred herd of miniature swine. J Virol 2002;76:3045–48.

61. Elliott RB, Escobar L, Garkavenko O, et al. No evidence of infection with porcine endogenous retrovirus in recipients of encapsulated porcine islet xenografts. Cell Transplant 2000;9:895–901.

62. Guidance for industry. Source animal, product, preclinical, and clinical issues concerning the use of xenotransplantation products in humans. February 7, 2001. http://www.fda.gov/cber/guidelines.htm (accessed September 15, 2002).

63. Draft guidance for industry: precautionary measures to reduce the possible risk of transmission of zoonoses by blood and blood products from xenotransplantation product recipients and their intimate contacts, February 1, 2002. Available at: http://www.fda.gov/cber/guidelines.htm (accessed September 16, 2002).

64. Kirkman RL. Of swine and man: organ physiology in different species. In: Hardy M, editor. Xenograft 25. Amsterdam: Elsevier; 1989. p. 125–31.

65. Hughes HC. Swine in cardiovascular research. Lab Anim Sci 1986;36:348–50.

66. Swindle MM, Horneffer PJ, Gardner TJ, et al. Anatomic and anesthetic considerations in experimental cardiopulmonary surgery in swine. Lab Anim Sci 1986;36:357–61.

67. Vial CM, Ostlie DJ, Bhatti FN, et al. Life-supporting function for over one month of a transgenic porcine heart in a baboon. J Heart Lung Transplant 2000;19(2):224–9.

68. Soin B, Ostlie D, Cozzi E, et al. Growth of porcine kidneys in their native and xenograft environment. Xenotransplantation 2000;7:96–100.

69. Sablinski T, Gianello PR, Bailin M, et al. Pig to monkey bone marrow and kidney xenotransplantation. Surgery 1997;121:381–91.

70. Nair J, Fair JH, Burdick JF, et al. Role of naturally occurring xenoantibodies in hyperacute rejection strengthened by their avid binding to ex vivo pig to human liver xenografts and to isolated pig liver preparations. Transplant Proc 1994;26:1344–5.

71. Cooper DK, Ye Y, Niekrasz M, et al. Specific intravenous carbohydrate therapy. A new concept in inhibiting antibody-mediated rejection—experience with ABO-incompatible cardiac allografting in the baboon. Transplantation 1993;56:769–77.

72. Ghanekar A, Luo Y, Yang H, et al. The alpha-Gal analog GAS914 ameliorates delayed rejection of hDAF transgenic pig-to-baboon renal xenografts. Transplant Proc 2001;33:3853–4.

73. Davis EA, Pruitt SK, Greene PS, et al. Inhibition of complement, evoked antibody, and cellular response prevents rejection of pig-to-primate cardiac xenografts. Transplantation 1996;62:1018–23.

74. Fearon DT. Anti-inflammatory and immunosuppressive effects of recombinant soluble complement receptors. Clin Exp Immunol 1991;86 Suppl 1:43–6.

75. Starzl TE, Murase N, Demetris AJ, et al. Allograft and xenograft acceptance under FK-506 and other immunosuppressant treatment. Ann N Y Acad Sci 1993;685: 46–51.

76. Lin Y, Vandeputte M, Waer M. Effect of leflunomide and cyclosporine on the occurrence of chronic xenograft lesions. Kidney Int Suppl 1995;52:S23–8.

77. Yatscoff RW, Wang S, Keenan R, et al. Efficacy of rapamycin, RS-61443 and cyclophosphamide in the prolongation of survival of discordant pig to rabbit cardiac xenografts. Can J Cardiol 1994;10:711–6.

78. O'Hair DP, McManus RP, Komorowski R. Inhibition of chronic vascular rejection in primate cardiac xenografts using mycophenolate mofetil. Ann Thorac Surg 1994; 58:1311–5.

79. Fujino Y, Kawamura T, Hullett DA, Sollinger HW. Evaluation of cyclosporine, mycophenolate mofetil, and Brequinar sodium combination therapy on hamster-to-rat cardiac xenotransplantation. Transplantation 1994;57:41–6.

80. Goddard MJ, Dunning J, Horsley J, et al. Histopathology of cardiac xenograft rejection in the pig-to-baboon model. J Heart Lung Transplant 2002;21:474–84.

81. Brenner P, Schmoeckel M, Reichenspurner H, et al. Orthotopic heart xenotransplantation (20 days survival) in a hDAF-transgenic pig-to-baboon model [abstract]. Am Soc Transplant. 2000;69:544A.

82. Costa C, Zhao L, Burton WV, et al. Expression of the human alpha1,2-fucosyltransferase in transgenic pigs modifies the cell surface carbohydrate phenotype and confers resistance to human serum-mediated cytolysis. FASEB J 1999;13:1762–73.

83. Costa C, Zhao L, Burton WV, et al. Transgenic pigs designed to express human CD59 and H-transferase to avoid humoral xenograft rejection. Xenotransplantation 2002;9:45–57.

84. Lai L, Kolber-Simonds D, Park KW, et al. Production of alpha-1,3-galactosyltransferase knockout pigs by nuclear transfer cloning. Science 2002;295:1089–92.

85. Dai Y, Vaught TD, Boone J. Targeted disruption of the alpha1,3-galactosyltransferase gene in cloned pigs. Nat Biotechnol 2002;20:251–5.

86. World's first cloned double knock-out pigs lack both copies of gene involved in hyperacute rejection in humans. August 8, 2002. Available at: http://www.ppl-therapeutics.com/welcome/welcome.html (accessed August 22, 2002).

87. Chopek MW, Simmons RL, Platt JL. ABO-incompatible kidney transplantation: initial immunopathologic evaluation. Transplant Proc 1987;19:4553–7.

88. Bach FH, Ferran C, Candinas D, et al. Accommodation of xenografts: expression of "protective genes" in endothelial and smooth muscle cells. Transplant Proc 1997;29: 56–8.

89. Dalmasso AP, Benson BA, Schroeder AA, Abrahamsen MS. Biochemical basis for induction of resistance to human complement in porcine endothelial cells by alphaGAL ligation. Transplant Proc 2000;32:974.

90. Bach FH, Turman MA, Vercellotti GM, et al. Accommodation: a working paradigm for progressing toward clinical discordant xenografting. Transplant Proc 1991;23: 205–7.

91. Fischel RJ, Matas AJ, Platt JL, et al. Cardiac xenografting in the pig-to-rhesus monkey model: manipulation of antiendothelial antibody prolongs survival. J Heart Lung Transplant 1992;11:965–73.

92. Platt JL. A perspective on xenograft rejection and accommodation. Immunol Rev 1994;141:127–49.

93. Sachs DH. Mixed chimerism as an approach to transplantation tolerance. Clin Immunol 2000;95:S63–8.

94. Sykes M, Lee LA, Sachs DH. Xenograft tolerance. Immunol Rev 1994;141:245–76.

95. Rehman A, Tu Y, Arima T, et al. Long-term survival of rat to mouse cardiac xenografts with prolonged blockade of CD28-B7 interaction combined with peritransplant T-cell depletion. Surgery 1996;120:205–12.

96. Buhler L, Awwad M, Basker M, et al. High-dose porcine hematopoietic cell transplantation combined with CD40 ligand blockade in baboons prevents an induced anti-pig humoral response. Transplantation 2000;69: 2296–304.

97. Beschorner WE, Sudan DL, Radio SJ. Heart xenograft survival with chimeric pig donors and modest immune suppression. Ann Surg 2002. [In press]

98. Yang T, Stammers A, Jiang J, et al. Chimeric pig hearts resist hyperacute rejection in ex vivo perfusion model. J Extra Corpor Technol 2001;33:181–4.

99. Sudan DL, Radio SJ, Matamoros A, et al. Effect of surrogate tolerogenesis on the vascular rejection of pig heart xenografts. Transplantation 2000;69:232–5.

100. Beschorner WE, Shearon CC, Yang T, et al. Pretransplant analysis of accommodation in donor pigs. Xenotransplantation 2002. [In press]

101. Yang T, Zhao Y, Beschorner WE, et al. Heart explant from chimeric pig (sheep cells) protected from hyperacute rejection by human blood. Sixth Congress of the International Xenotransplantation Association, Chicago, IL, October 1, 2001.

102. Beschorner WE, Qian Z, Mattei P, et al. Induction of human chimerism and functional suppressor cells in fetal pigs: feasibility of surrogate tolerogenesis for xenotransplantation. Transplant Proc 1996;28:648–9.

103. About the Secretary's Advisory Committee on Xenotransplantation. Available at: http://www4.od.nih.gov/oba/sacx/aboutsacx.htm (accessed September 25, 2002).

CHAPTER 60

ROLE OF GENE THERAPY AND STEM CELLS IN CARDIAC SURGERY

ABDULAZIZ A. AL-KHALDI, MD, PHD, RAY CHU-JENG CHIU, MD, PHD

Since the advent of cardiac surgery in the mid-twentieth century, the focus of surgical therapy has been to repair or substitute abnormal or damaged cardiac anatomic structures in order to palliate or correct functional impairments. Today, we are moving into a new era in which heart diseases may be treated by genetic modification and tissue engineering. Such advances will undoubtedly impact on the cardiac surgery of the future. This chapter reviews the current state of research and clinical trials in gene and cellular therapy of various pathologic conditions relevant to cardiac surgery.

Gene Therapy

The goal of gene therapy is to introduce recombinant genetic material into target cells, in order to change the cellular phenotype or to modify their function such that subsequent local or systemic therapeutic effect is achieved. Theoretical advantages of gene therapy include

1. the potential of long-lasting effect after single local administration, and
2. the potential of changing cellular phenotype or behavior.

The therapeutic genetic materials are introduced into target cells by using various vectors, as listed in Figure 60-1.

Targets for Cardiovascular Gene Therapy

Therapeutic Angiogenesis

This is a novel approach for the treatment of vascular insufficiency. It might be the only hope for patients with advanced disease who are not candidates for standard interventional revascularization techniques. There are three approaches for inducing therapeutic angiogenesis: (1) protein (ligand) therapy; (2) gene therapy; and (3) cell therapy. Angiogenic factors were used in preclinical and clinical studies for the treatment of myocardial or skeletal muscle

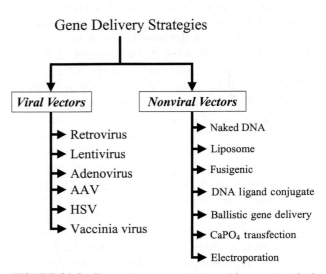

FIGURE 60-1. The most common vectors used for gene transfer in clinical and laboratory studies. AAV = adeno-associated virus; CaPO₄ = calcium phosphate; HSV = herpes simplex virus.

ischemia. Advantages of protein therapy include controlled delivery, established safety, predictable pharmacokinetics and tissue therapeutic levels, and absence of long-term unexpected side effects.[1] Experience with angiogenic factors protein therapy showed several disadvantages such as short tissue half-life, high cost of recombinant molecules, and difficulty in delivering some angiogenic factors as proteins (eg, hypoxia inducible factor [HIF]-1α)

WHICH PATIENT IS A CANDIDATE FOR ANGIOGENIC GENE THERAPY?

Clinical trials of gene therapy for myocardial angiogenesis included patients with advanced coronary artery diseases that are not amenable to interventional therapy. Patients who are considered as ideal candidates for such treatment must have (1) long-standing single- or multivessel disease with evidence of inducible ischemia and myocardial viability and (2) adequate feeder vessels and adequate distal runoff.[2] Therapeutic angiogenesis is not an option for patients with acute coronary syndrome because of the period of delay required for new blood vessel growth. The need for adequate feeder vessel to provide origin and inflow for the new collateral vessels raised the issue of combining angiogenic gene therapy with conventional coronary artery bypass surgery for better results. Patients with a history of cancer (except curable skin cancer), proliferative retinopathy, or angina at rest are not considered candidates for therapeutic angiogenesis.

WHICH ANGIOGENIC FACTOR SHOULD BE USED?

Several angiogenic factors coding genes were used for therapeutic angiogenesis, including vascular endothelial growth factor (VEGF), basic fibroblast growth factor (bFGF), hepatocyte growth factor (HGF), angiopoietin (Ang), and HIF-1α. Initial research experience with these compounds preferred the use of selective factors such as VEGF, which is the most endothelial-specific growth factor, in order to avoid the stimulation of an unwanted overgrowth of fibroblasts and smooth-muscle cells, leading to exacerbation of intimal hyperplasia. Accumulating evidence from laboratory and clinical studies strongly suggests that therapy using a combination of angiogenic growth factors might result in clinically significant better neovascularization from qualitative and quantitative points of view. Normal physiologic angiogenesis is the end result of a synchronized release of several angiogenic factors simultaneously or in sequence. Some of these factors stimulate endothelial cell proliferation and migration (eg, VEGF) and others stabilize the newly formed blood vessels and stimulate the growth of a layer of smooth muscles around them (Ang-1, platelet-derived growth factor-BB). The latter process, called *arteriogenesis*, transforms the new blood vessels into mature arterioles that are less likely to regress and that have more blood flow conductance capacity. The use of VEGF as the only agent in animal models resulted in the formation of only capillaries, and on continuous stimulation, hemangioma formation was noted.[3]

WHICH VECTOR AND DELIVERY TECHNIQUE SHOULD BE USED?

Myocardial angiogenesis requires sustained temporary local delivery of the angiogenic factor, which can be met by using either (1) vectors with transient expression, such as plasmid DNA or adenovirus, or (2) vectors with long-standing expression and a regulatable promoter to allow cessation of gene expression when adequate angiogenesis has been achieved. This can be done by in vivo gene transfer using adeno-associated virus (AAV) or by cell-mediated gene transfer in which cells (eg, myoblasts or endothelium) are cultured in vitro, then transduced (usually using retroviruses) to express the angiogenic factor, and then implanted into the ischemic region. Intramyocar-

dial injection of angiogenic genes directly deliver them into the ischemic regions of the myocardium, which increases the treatment efficiency. The invasiveness needed for this approach encouraged the trial of other delivery methods, including intravenous, intracoronary, and intrapericardial injections. The intravenous and intracoronary injections have the disadvantages of systemic distribution to noncardiac tissues and differential delivery of the therapeutic molecules to areas with better blood flow, as suggested by experience with tracer-labeled growth factor uptake.[4,5] Intramyocardial gene delivery is associated with better efficiency and localization, as compared to intracoronary and intravenous routes. Intrapericardial infusion is limited to patients with a normal pericardial sac; it is not suitable for patients after cardiac surgery and has the disadvantage of indiscriminate delivery of angiogenic factors to the whole myocardium rather than to the ischemic areas only. The superiority of catheter-based versus surgical delivery is not yet determined.

WHAT ARE THE RESULTS OF CLINICAL TRIALS OF THERAPEUTIC ANGIOGENESIS BASED ON GENE THERAPY?

Several phase I clinical trials have been conducted to assess safety, as the main objective, as well as clinical benefits and mechanism of effects (Table 60-1). The two main end points that these trials have considered as clinical benefits are improved survival and improved health-related quality of life. In summary, these phase I clinical trials provided preliminary evidence of safety and efficacy and opened the way for more extensive phase II and III, randomized, double-blind, placebo-controlled trials.

As it stands now, gene transfer for therapeutic angiogenesis is a viable option for patients with advanced ischemic heart disease that is not amenable to standard revascularization techniques. The potential side effects of such therapy include the following:[6]

1. *Accelerated atherosclerosis* is a theoretical risk based on animal studies that showed that the use of angiogenesis inhibitors reduces atherosclerotic plaque growth, which in fact should not be translated necessarily as suggesting that administration of angiogenic factors would enhance atherosclerosis.[7] Several preclinical and clinical studies using VEGF as protein or gene therapy for angiogenesis showed no evidence of increased neointimal thickening and no increased incidence of restenosis.[6]

2. *Development of abnormal hemangioma-like vascular structures* has been described in laboratory experiments where VEGF was overexpressed in skeletal muscle or heart.[3,8] These effects are clearly dose- and duration-related. Hemangiomas have not been reported in preclinical and clinical studies of gene transfer for therapeutic angiogenesis where there is a more physiologic level and duration of gene expression.

3. *Carcinogenesis* as a potential side effect of angiogenic therapy is based on the knowledge that angiogenesis is essential for malignant tumor growth and spread.[9] The

TABLE 60-1. Clinical Trials Published to Date That Used Gene Therapy for Therapeutic Angiogenesis

Investigator (Reference)	Study Protocol	Results
Losordo (103)	Direct intramyocardial injection of phVEGF 165 via mini-left anterior thoracotomy as sole therapy ($n = 5$).	No significant complications. Reduced angina frequency. Reduced area of ischemic myocardium using dobutamine-SPECT sestamibi.
Rosengart (104)	Direct intramyocardial injection of adenovirus carrying the *VEGF 121* gene as adjunct to coronary artery bypass or as sole therapy ($n = 21$).	No systemic or cardiac side effects. Improved angina class. Improved wall motion.
Symes (105)	Direct intramyocardial injection of phVEGF 165 via mini-left anterior thoracotomy as sole therapy ($n = 20$).	One late death (4 months) due to aspiration pneumonia. No significant complications. Reduced angina frequency. Reduced area of ischemic myocardium using dobutamine-SPECT sestamibi.
Laitinen (106)	Randomized, double-blind, placebo-controlled study. Patients received either VEGF plasmid/liposome (P/L), LacZ P/L, or Ringer lactate intracoronary by using a catheter-based technique after percutaneous translumenal coronary angioplasty.	No significant side effects. In control angiography 6 months later, no differences were detected in the degree of coronary stenosis between treatment and control groups.
Vale (107)	Direct intramyocardial injection of phVEGF 165 via mini-left anterior thoracotomy as sole therapy ($n = 13$).	Left ventricular electromechanical mapping showed increased perfusion of ischemic myocardium after gene transfer. SPECT-sestamibi imaging demonstrated significant reduction of ischemic defect size after gene therapy.
Vale (108)	Randomized, single-blind, placebo-controlled pilot study. Patients were randomized to receive either phVEGF-2 ($n = 6$) or placebo ($n = 6$) via catheter-based injection into ischemic myocardium guided by NOGA left ventricular electro-mechanical mapping.	No hemodynamic or electrophysiologic complications. Compared to placebo group, there was significant reduction in angina frequency in patients who received gene transfer up to 360 days of follow-up, reduced ischemia on electromechanical mapping, and improved function by SPECT-sestamibi scanning.
Sylven (109)	Direct intramyocardial injection of phVEGF 165 via thoracotomy as sole therapy ($n = 6$).	Improved angina class. Increased maximal systolic myocardial tissue velocity in all patients about 25%. Improved myocardial perfusion in SPECT scanning in 4 of 6 patients.

VEGF = vascular endothelial growth factor

theoretical concern is that administration of angiogenic factors could stimulate the growth of a latent neoplasm, which so far has not been supported by credible evidence from preclinical or clinical studies. Incidence of cancer in patients who received angiogenic factors (as protein or gene) in published clinical studies were low and inconclusive due to the small number of patients and the short follow-up period.

4. *Retinopathy* is another potential side effect that has not been reported in trials conducted for therapeutic angiogenesis.

5. *Edema* related to VEGF-mediated increase in vascular permeability.

6. *Hypotension* can be caused by VEGF- or bFGF-induced nitric oxide (NO) production. This side effects has been reported in human and animal studies using VEGF or bFGF injection or infusion, but has never been described with angiogenic factor gene transfer studies.

7. *Arrhythmias* are potential side effects resulting from angiogenesis-mediated conduction system instability, altered repolarization and reentry circuits formation.

Prevention of Vein Graft Failure

Either one or more of these four mechanisms can cause vein graft failure: vascular spasm, thrombosis, neointimal hyperplasia, or atherosclerosis. The latter two pathologic processes are the main reasons for the limited intermediate and long-term success of vascular grafts. Neointimal hyperplasia is an adaptive process in response to increased vein wall tension and shear forces that can cause narrowing of the vein lumen in the first year after use as an arterial bypass and predispose to future atherosclerosis. It is a dynamic process that involves intimal smooth-muscle cell proliferation, migration, and production of extracellular matrix proteins. Gene therapy can be used to prevent vascular graft failure by the use of genes that antagonize the four mechanisms. These genes can be introduced (transfected or transduced) into the graft at the time of harvest (intraoperative), just before implantation.

NITRIC OXIDE

NO is a strong vasodilator compound that also exerts antiatherogenic effects by inhibiting platelet aggregation, leukocyte activation, and adhesion, as well as smooth-muscle cell proliferation and migration. With such a profile, NO is an attractive compound to be used in the prevention of vascular conduit failure. NO is synthesized by the NO synthase (NOS) enzyme, which has three isoforms: endothelial NOS (eNOS), which produces NO in blood vessels and plays a major role in vascular function regulation; neuronal NOS (nNOS), which produces NO in the nervous system and is involved in cell–cell signaling and neurotransmission; and inducible NOS (iNOS), which produces NO in leukocytes as part of immunity against pathogens. Previous studies show that vein grafts produce less NO than arteries.[10,11] Such difference may explain the superior long-term patency of left internal mammary artery (LIMA) graft when compared to saphenous vein graft (SVG).[12,13] In vitro studies on SVG showed that adenoviral-mediated gene transfer of NOS resulted in functional transgene expression with increased NO release and significantly inhibited intimal hyperplasia.[14,15] Perivascular delivery of a nitric oxide donor inhibits neointimal hyperplasia in vein grafts implanted in the arterial circulation.[16] Preclinical and clinical studies are being currently conducted to evaluate the effects of NOS gene transfer to SVG before use in arterial bypass.

CELL-CYCLE INHIBITION

Considering neointimal hyperplasia as a vascular proliferative disease makes cell-cycle inhibition a desirable strategy to prevent vein graft stenosis. Several antiproliferative drugs have been used to inhibit neointimal hyperplasia, including heparin, angiotensin-converting enzyme (ACE) inhibitors, platelet-derived growth factor (PDGF) antagonists, angiopeptin (a peptide analog of somatostatin), cytostatic agents such as etoposide or doxorubicin, calcium-calmodulin antagonists, or the microtubule-inhibiting drug colchicine. Clinical trials have failed to show any efficacy of these drugs. Other drugs, such as rapamycin, showed promising results in animal studies, but no clinical data have been published. Gene therapy can be used to inhibit the cell cycle by blocking genes or gene products involved in cell-cycle progression. Such blockade can be achieved by several methods:

1. Antisense oligodeoxynucleotides (ODNs), which are short chains of nucleic acids that are complementary to and bind specific RNA, resulting in blocking of messenger ribonucleic acid (mRNA) translation. Antisense ODNs designed to inhibit the expression of cell-cycle regulatory genes, such as c-myc, c-myb, proliferating cell nuclear antigen (PCNA), and Cdk, have been used successfully in models of vascular lesion formation.[17–19]
2. Ribozymes, which are RNA molecules with enzymatic activity that can be designed to cleave, target mRNA molecules in sequential specific manner. Ribozymes to cell division cycle-2 (CDC-2) kinase and PCNA prevent intimal hyperplasia in rat carotid artery.
3. Decoy ODNs, which are double-stranded nucleic acid chains designed to mimic the chromosomal binding sites of transcription factors (factors that regulate gene expression by binding to chromosomal DNA at specific promoter regions) and to act as "decoys," reducing the availability of transcription factors required for subsequent activation or suppression of target genes.[20] Decoy ODNs that bind transcription factor E2F, which

is responsible for the induction of multiple cell cycle–dependent genes, can inhibit neointimal hyperplasia in balloon-injured arteries and vein grafts.[21] Mann and associates conducted a small prospective randomized double-blind trial of human vein graft treatment with E2F decoy ODN in patients undergoing peripheral bypass surgery.[22] Oligonucleotide was delivered to grafts intraoperatively by ex vivo pressure-mediated transfection. Patients were followed up for 12 months postoperatively with no difference in complication rate between treated and untreated groups. Although this study was not designed to assess efficacy, the enrollment of high-risk grafts led to an overall event rate that allowed comparison of treated and untreated grafts. The investigators found fewer graft failures with the treated grafts compared to controls.

Cell-cycle inhibitory genes can be transduced into vascular cells using a viral vector to prevent neointimal hyperplasia. Examples include p53,[23] a nonphosphorylatable constitutively active form of the retinoblastoma gene product,[24] and Cdk inhibitors p21^{Cip1} and p27^{Kip1}.[25,26]

Prevention of Bioprosthetic Graft Failure

Reduction of bioprosthetic graft thrombogenicity has been the main objective for a large number of preclinical studies. One approach is to seed the luminal surface of these grafts with endothelial cells. Gene therapy has been used to enhance or modulate the function of these endothelial cells before seeding. Retroviral transduction of endothelial cells with the gene for human tissue plasminogen activator before implantation did not show improvement in bioprosthetic graft thrombogenicity.[27] On the other hand, retroviral transduction of the endothelial cells to secrete hirudin and then to seed them onto polytetrafluoroethylene graft resulted in reduced thrombogenicity and neointimal hyperplasia.[28]

Gene Therapy and Cardiac Transplantation

Gene therapy has been extensively used in the field of transplantation, including bone marrow transplantation, solid organ transplantation, and stem cell transplantation. The three main areas where gene therapy might play a major future role in cardiac transplantation are modification of allograft, modification of the host immune response, and prevention of graft arteriopathy.

MODIFICATION OF ALLOGRAFT

Delivery of immunosuppressants directly to allografts by using gene transfer strategies may inhibit immune activation and result in site-specific localized immunosuppression while avoiding the systemic toxicity of conventional immunosuppression. Several animal studies showed that the transfer of immunosuppressing cytokine genes such as transforming growth factor (TGF)-β1 and interleukin (IL)-10 could prolong allograft survival and modulate the immune response. The use of vectors (eg, retroviruses) with stable persistent expression may make this approach clinically applicable and desirable.[29–32] Gene transfer of virally encoded chemokine antagonists vMIP-II and MC148 was found to prolong cardiac allograft survival and inhibits donor-specific immunity.[33] Allograft genetic engineering can also be done to protect the graft against ischemic-reperfusion injury. Genes such as heat shock protein (HSP) 70, when transfected into donor hearts, were found to protect both the mechanical and endothelial function of the graft.[34] Genetic modification of cardiac allograft to overexpress β_2-adrenergic receptor enhanced myocardial function in a rat heterotopic heart transplant model.[35]

The best method for gene delivery to cardiac allograft is not yet established, but it seems that encouraging results are being obtained using intracoronary perfusion techniques. Liposome-mediated gene transfer to cardiac allograft has a much higher efficacy despite that the gene transfer efficiency was lower than that in adenovirus-mediated gene therapy. Also, adenovirus transfection may induce significant negative inotropic and arrhythmogenic adverse effects on transplanted hearts.[36]

MODIFICATION OF THE HOST IMMUNE RESPONSE

Gene transfer technologies have been used to reduce or avoid the use of systemic immunosuppressive therapy by modifying the host immune response to accept the allograft. One approach to achieve this goal is by using suicide genes. These are genes that encode for proteins that can produce toxic substances upon exposure to specific pharmacologic agents, resulting ultimately in the death of cells carrying these genes and possibly of nearby cells, by the "bystander effect." In a well-conducted animal study by Braunberger and colleagues, the suicide gene herpes simplex virus–thymidine kinase (HSV-TK) was used to selectively eliminate the dividing alloreactive T cells upon exposure to ganciclovir (GCV).[37] TK converts GCV into GCV-monophosphate, which is then converted into the toxic metabolite GCV-triphosphate by cellular kinases. By performing heterotopic abdominal heart transplantation in transgenic TK mice, followed by exposure to GCV for 1 week, the authors were able to demonstrate development of a long-lasting tolerance to the cardiac allograft. The developed tolerance was robust as shown by the acceptance of a second cervical allograft of the same haplotype as the first graft. The host mice remained immunocompetent as they were able to reject third-party allograft. Other gene therapy strategies included the transfer of genes that encode for soluble antigens (such as major histocompatibility complex [MHC] class I) that can bind to and neutralize preformed antibodies in sensitized host, thereby protecting the graft from hyperacute rejection.[38] Ex vivo transfection of cardiac allograft with antisense ODN to inhibit the expression of intercellular adhesion molecule (ICAM)-1, an important mediator of T-cell adhesion and co-stimulation, was shown to induce

cardiac allograft tolerance when combined with postoperative systemic administration of monoclonal antibody against leukocyte function antigen-1 (LFA-1), which is the ligand for ICAM-1.[39]

PREVENTION OF GRAFT ARTERIOPATHY

Several studies were conducted for the prevention of cardiac allograft arteriopathy, using principles similar to those mentioned for the prevention of vein graft stenosis, including transfection of eNOS,[40] E2F decoy transfection,[41] human tissue plasminogen activator (htPA) gene transfer,[42] and transfection of antisense CDC-2 kinase ODN.[43]

Gene Therapy for Heart Failure

Genetic engineering of the failed cardiomyocytes to increase expression of proteins that enhance myocardial contractility or prevent further deterioration in function is a novel therapeutic modality. β-Adrenergic receptors are known to be downregulated in heart failure. Overexpression of β_2-adrenergic receptors in cardiomyocytes of animals with induced heart failure resulted in marked increase in contractility and improvement of function in the absence of exogenous β-agonists.[44] Other studies suggested that overexpression of β-adrenergic receptor kinase-1 (betaARK1) inhibitor results in increased contractility without increased injury during ischemia, as compared to overexpression of β_2-adrenergic receptors.[45] Another important molecular target for heart failure gene therapy is the cardiomyocyte calcium transport system. During cardiomyocyte relaxation, 75% of cytosolic Ca^{2+} is removed by sarcoplasmic reticulum Ca^{2+} adensine triphosphatase (ATPase) pump (SERCA2a); the remaining 25% is pumped extracellularly by Na-Ca exchanger. In heart failure, there is reduced activity of SERCA2a resulting in decreased Ca^{2+} uptake with an elevated end-diastolic intracellular Ca^{2+}. In vitro studies show that gene transfer of SERCA2a, to human cardiomyocytes isolated from the left ventricles of patients with end-stage heart failure results in a remarkable increase in contraction and relaxation velocities.[46] Animal studies showed improvement in survival and cardiac metabolism after gene transfer of SERCA2a in a rat model of heart failure.[47] Catheter-based adenovirus-mediated transfer of SERCA2a gene to cardiomyocytes in a rat model of decompensated pressure-overload hypertrophy restored SERCA2a activity to the nonfailing levels, with significant improvement in both systolic and diastolic left ventricular functions.[48] By using a different strategy, inhibiting phospholamban (PLB), another sarcoplasmic reticulum protein that is a potent inhibitor of SERCA2, can result in increased SERCA2a activity and is therefore a potential target to improve the cardiac performance in heart failure. He and associates used adenovirus-mediated gene transfer to express mutants of PLB or antisense RNA of PLB in cultured cardiomyocytes, which resulted in increased SERCA2a activity and myocyte contractility.[49] Several studies have shown that apoptosis (programmed cell death) may contribute to cardiomyocyte loss and cardiac dysfunction in heart failure.[50–53] Attempts to block cardiac apoptosis pathways by using gene therapy techniques included overexpression of Bcl-2 through adenoviral gene transfer, which blocks p53-induced apoptosis in ventricular cardiomyocytes, and adenoviral gene transfer of activated forms of phosphatidy-linositol 3' (PI3)-kinase and Akt (also known as protein kinase B [PKB]), which can block hypoxia-induced cardiomyocyte apoptosis in vitro.[54,55]

Stem Cells

Stem cells are defined as cells that have three important characteristics: (1) unlimited self-renewal, (2) multipotent differentiation potential, and (3) the ability to repopulate tissues upon transplantation (ie, engraftment).[56] There is an exponential increase in the interest to use stem cells in cardiovascular therapy, which emerges from two main potential clinical applications:

1. *Regeneration.* Stem cells can be used to replace and repair the failing heart muscle (cardiomyogenesis or cellular cardiomyoplasty) and to reproduce new blood vessels (therapeutic neovascularization).
2. *Gene therapy vehicle.* Stem cells can be genetically engineered to act as a "platform" for stable local delivery of recombinant therapeutic proteins.

Successful myocardial regeneration using stem cell transplantation requires the fulfillment of four fundamental criteria:

1. Engraftment (survival of the transplanted cells)
2. Differentiation into cardiomyocyte phenotype
3. Normal interaction between host and transplanted cells
4. Mechanical and electrical coupling of transplanted cells

Engraftment largely depends on the absence of immune response against these cells, which makes autologous cells preferable, and the ability of these cells to adapt to the new environment. The differentiation is either induced iatrogenically (using pharmacologic or gene therapy techniques) or by environmental factors (such as adhesion molecules and diffusible factors), which is termed *milieu-dependent differentiation.*

Figure 60-2 illustrates the three sources of stem cells.

Organ-Specific Stem Cells

These cells have extensive proliferation potential and the ability to differentiate into a more mature form of cell to regenerate the organ where they are usually found. Differentiation involves phenotypic change characterized by expression of new cellular markers, receptors, and structural and adhesion molecules that result in histologic and physiologic changes. Examples include hematopoietic stem cells, neural stem cells, hepatic stem cells (oval cells), gastrointestinal stem cells, epidermal stem cells, and skeletal myoblast or satellite cells.[57–61]

The organ-specific stem cells are one step more differentiated than other true pluripotent stem cells. They are

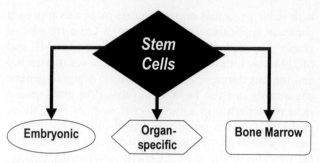

FIGURE 60-2. Sources of stem cells.

already committed to one-cell lineage, a developmental process called *determination.* This can be an advantage because these cells will differentiate "autonomously" into their prespecified lineage without the need for environmental or iatrogenic influences.

Satellite cells (or myoblasts) are committed progenitor cells that are found below the basal lamina in skeletal muscles. Their function is to proliferate in response to injury, with subsequent differentiation into skeletal muscle phenotype and fusion to form myotubes to regenerate the lost muscle fibers. Several animal studies have shown that autologous satellite cells can successfully engraft after transplantation into a myocardial injury model and undergo milieu-dependent in vivo differentiation into myogenic phenotype similar to cardiomyocytes by histologic features (such as longitudinal alignment, centrally located nuclei, and the presence of intercalated discs).[62,63] The transplanted satellite cells differentiate to express markers of fast-twitch skeletal muscle such as fast-twitch skeletal muscle isoforms of myosin heavy chain and SERCA1.[64–66] At the same time, these cells differentiate in vivo to express slow-twitch skeletal muscle markers, including phospholamban and a slow-twitch isoform of myosin heavy chain-β.[65] Expression of cardiac-specific myosin heavy chain-α has never been shown. These data suggest that the myocardial milieu may induce the satellite cells (which are originally programmed to become fast-twitch skeletal muscle) to differentiate into the slow-twitch phenotype of skeletal muscle but not into cardiac phenotype. These slow-twitch fibers were found to contract when stimulated electrically and to be fatigue-resistant, making them suitable for cardiac workload as shown by Taylor and colleagues, who demonstrated improved myocardial function after satellite cell transplantation.[65,67] Transarterial delivery of satellite cells has also successfully shown engraftment and differentiation.[66,68] Electromechanical coupling of the implanted satellite cells to the adjacent myocardium requires the presence of specialized gap junctions that allow exchange of ions and small molecules and represent low-resistance electrical pathways between cardiomyocytes. Gap junctions consist of hexamers of the protein connexin-43. Animal studies have failed to demonstrate the development of gap junctions with connexin-43 between engrafted primary satellite cells and host myocardium, which precludes the electrical coupling between the graft and host muscle cells.[69] In one study, Robinson and associates demonstrated the localization of connexin-43 to some of the interfaces between implanted cells and cardiomyocytes after arterial delivery of myoblast cell line (C2C12) into normal myocardium.[66] The first successful transplantation of autologous myoblast in humans was reported by Philippe Menasché and associates in 2000, and the short-term follow-up showed promising good results (reported in American Heart Association Scientific Sessions 2000/2001).

Embryonal Stem Cells

Embryonal stem (ES) cells are derived from the inner mass of blastocyst or from primordial germ cells.[70–72] ES cells are true stem cells as they have an unlimited self-renewal capacity, can differentiate into all cell lineages in vitro and in vivo, and can repopulate tissues upon transplantation. ES cells potentially represent an unlimited supply of all cell types that can be used in tissue engineering and organ regeneration. Cardiomyocytes derived from ES cells can be differentiated by the appearance of spontaneously and rhythmically contracting myocytes, expression of α- and β-cardiac myosin heavy chain (MHC), α-tropomyosin, myosin light chain 2v (MLC-2v) and atrial natriuretic factor, phospholamban, and type B natriuretic factor, and by exhibiting normal contractile sensitivity to calcium.[73–78] Induction of ES cells to differentiate in vitro can be done by the removal of specific substrate from the ES cell culture system such as the leukemia inhibitory factor (LIF), which is essential for maintaining the undifferentiated phenotype of murine ES cells but not human ES cells.[71,79] Because the differentiation here is nonspecific, in vitro selection by using drug or cell marker is necessary to obtain certain types of cells. Klug and colleagues used drug selection to isolate a pure group of differentiated ES cell–derived cardiomyocytes and were able to show stable engraftment of these cells into the heart for up to 7 weeks.[80] Pharmacologic induction of ES cell differentiation has also been done successfully by using a variety of cytokines, growth factors, and compounds such as vitamin A or retinoic acid (RA), which is known to be a morphogenic and teratogenic compound that can influence gene expression in a complex manner via a family of RA receptors. Wobus and associates showed that RA treatment in vitro accelerated ES cell differentiation into cardiomyocytes with an enhanced development into the ventricular type of cells.[81] Because of their marked multipotency, transplantation of undifferentiated ES cells into adult animals results in the formation of teratomas.[71,82] Consequently, induction, selection, and purification need to be carried out carefully before using these cells for in vivo implantation. The main obstacles facing the introduction of ES cells into clinical practice are the high cost and technical difficulty in isolating, culturing, and handling these cells, as well as the ethical problems related to the source of these cells (ie, human embryos) and the fact that immunosuppression might be necessary to prevent rejection.

Bone Marrow Stromal Cells

When bone marrow is cultured in vitro, it can be divided into two large population of cells: floating hematopoietic stem cells (HSCs) and colonies of adherent fibroblast-like marrow stromal cells (MSCs) that can be easily separated from HSCs by repeated washing. MSCs were first described by Alexander Friedenstein, who called them colony-forming unit fibroblasts (CFU-F).[83] As the name implies, MSCs were believed to provide the physical substrate and anchorage for HSCs because they form both an adventitial coating of the bone marrow sinusoid wall and branching extravascular meshwork. The work of Friedenstein and others showed the ability of these cells to differentiate into bone, cartilage, fibroblast, adipocytes, and muscle tissues, and the name *mesenchymal stem cells* became popular.[84–87] The differentiation capacity of MSCs is not limited to mesodermal tissues; they also differentiate into endodermal (eg, hepatocytes) and ectodermal phenotypes (eg, neurons, astrocytes, and oligodendrocytes).[88–91] A more appropriate name for these cells is *multipotent adult progenitor cells* (MAPCs) as suggested by Verfaillie and colleagues, which reflects their ability to differentiate into various types of cells. They also can differentiate in vitro and in vivo into endothelial cells and cardiomyocytes.[91–94]

MSCs have extensive proliferation capacity. Prockop and associates showed that MSCs can be expanded 100,000-fold in 6 to 8 weeks in an undifferentiated state.[95] Based on these data, MSCs can be considered as stem cells because of their extensive self-renewal, ability to engraft in tissues, and multipotent differentiation capacity. Some investigators do not consider MSCs as true stem cells because it has never been shown that MSCs derived from a single cell colony are capable of differentiating into all cell types. It is well known that MSCs isolated with the current conventional techniques, which depend on using the bone marrow cells that adhere to the culture plates, result in a heterogeneous (or polyclonal) group of cells that are collectively called MSCs. This heterogeneous group of cells might harbor clones with different differentiation capacity, with each clone determined to develop—if exposed to the appropriate stimulus—into specific cell types. This view defines the MSCs as a collection of committed progenitor cells. There are only few markers and antibodies that can be used to identify MSCs, such as the combination of the three monoclonal antibodies SH2, SH3, and SH4, as identified by Caplan, and the antibody STRO-1, expression of which declines as the MSCs start to differentiate and acquire antigens characteristics of more differentiated cell types.[96,97] The use of MSCs in cell therapy has several clinically relevant advantages, including being of autologous origin, abundant and easily available in humans of all age groups, harvestable with minimal morbidity, easy to culture and expand in vitro, and relatively easy to genetically modify to deliver foreign therapeutic genes. Orlic and associates showed that Lin⁻ c-kit^POS bone marrow cells, which were injected in the contracting wall bordering left ventricular infarct in a rat coronary artery ligation model, resulted in newly formed myocardium that occupied 68% of the infarcted portion of the ventricle 9 days after transplanting the bone marrow cells.[98]

The current consensus in the literature is that MSCs constitute a pool of pluripotent cells that acts as a physiologic reserve for continuous body repair and tissue regeneration. The principal factor in recruiting these cells and inducing their transdifferentiation is organ injury. It has been shown that in the presence of acute myocardial infarction, bone marrow cells can be mobilized by cytokines (such as stem cell factor and granulocyte colony-stimulating factor) to migrate to the infarct region and participate in tissue regeneration and repair.[99] Cytokine-induced cardiac repair decreased mortality by 68%, infarct size by 40%, cavitary dilation by 26%, and diastolic stress by 70%, and resulted in increased ejection fraction.

Currently, several studies reported improvement in myocardial function and blood flow after implantation of either whole bone marrow or stromal cell fraction. Hamano and colleagues reported the preliminary result of a clinical trial of therapeutic angiogenesis achieved by the implantation of self bone marrow cells into five patients with ischemic heart disease.[100] They showed that such treatment is generally safe in that small group of patients. Postoperative cardiac scintigraphy showed marked improvement in coronary perfusion in three of five patients. Because of the small size of the treatment groups, significant conclusions cannot be drawn, but the data suggest potential clinical benefits. There are several controversies and questions related to the use of bone marrow cells in cardiac regeneration and therapeutic angiogenesis, including (1) what is the final phenotype of these cells after implantation? (2) what is the nature of the signal that induces myocardial differentiation? (3) what is the proportion of bone marrow cells that are amenable to myocardial or endothelial transdifferentiation? and (4) which part of the bone marrow (whole bone marrow, marrow stromal cells, or hematopoietic cells) should be used for implantation? These questions are still to be answered.

Gene Therapy and Stem Cells

Genetic engineering and modification of stem cells can be used to achieve one or more of the following goals as described by Asahara and colleagues:[101]

1. *Modification of the stem cell potency*, to maintain, enhance, or inhibit their capacity to proliferate or differentiate (ie, the stem cell is the target).

2. *Modification of organ property.* The stem cell progeny that carry the inserted gene can replace genetically disordered organ (ie, progeny is the target).

3. *Acceleration of regeneration* (ie, the regeneration process is the target).

4. *Expressional organization* as the genetically modified stem cells and their derived progeny continuously express therapeutic molecules with local or systemic effects (ie, systemic target).

Conclusion

With the recent advances in the genome project, tissue-engineering technology, and stem cell biology, the gene and cellular therapies reviewed in this chapter will contribute to a paradigm shift in our therapeutic approach to the diseases of the heart, such that the practice of cardiac surgery may be profoundly affected.[102] Further understanding of which signals are presented to the cells and how cells integrate multiple signals to generate a response, coupled with rigorous clinical trials, will usher in the new era of regenerative surgery and medicine, and benefit patients who suffer from cardiac ailments.

References

1. Post MJ, Laham R, Sellke FW, Simons M. Therapeutic angiogenesis in cardiology using protein formulations [review]. Cardiovasc Res 2001;49(3):522–31.

2. Simons M, Bonow RO, Chronos NA, et al. Clinical trial in coronary angiogenesis: issues, problems, consensus. An expert panel summary. Circulation 2000;102:E73–86.

3. Lee RJ, Springer ML, Blanco-Bose WE, et al. VEGF gene delivery to myocardium: deleterious effects of unregulated expression. Circulation 2000;102(8):898–901.

4. Laham RJ, Rezaee M, Post M, et al. Intracoronary and intravenous administration of basic fibroblast growth factor: myocardial and tissue distribution. Drug Metab Dispos 1999;27(7):821–6.

5. Laham RJ. Tissue and myocardial distribution of intracoronary, intravenous, intrapericardial and intramyocardial ¹²⁵I-labeled basic fibroblast growth factor (bFGF) favor intramyocardial delivery [abstract]. J Am Coll Cardiol 2000; 35:10A.

6. Isner JM, Vale PR, Symes JF, Losordo DW. Assessment of risks associated with cardiovascular gene therapy in human subjects. Circ Res 2001;89(5):389–400.

7. Moulton KS, Heller E, Konerding MA, et al. Angiogenesis inhibitors endostatin or TNP-470 reduce intimal neovascularization and plaque growth in apolipoprotein E-deficient mice . Circulation 1999;99(13):1726–32.

8. Springer ML, Chen AS, Kraft PE, et al. VEGF gene delivery to muscle: potential role for vasculogenesis in adults. Mol Cell 1998;2(5):549–58.

9. Folkman J. Tumor angiogenesis: therapeutic implications [review]. N Engl J Med 1971;285(21):1182–6.

10. Jeremy JY, Dashwood MR, Timm M, et al. Nitric oxide synthase and adenylyl and guanylyl cyclase activity in porcine interposition vein grafts. Ann Thorac Surg 1997;63(2):470–6.

11. Luscher TF, Diederich D, Siebenmann R, et al. Difference between endothelium-dependent relaxation in arterial and in venous coronary bypass grafts. N Engl J Med 1988;319(8):462–7.

12. Chello M, Mastroroberto P, Perticone F, et al. Nitric oxide modulation of neutrophil-endothelium interaction: difference between arterial and venous coronary bypass grafts. J Am Coll Cardiol 1998;31(4):823–6.

13. Pearson PJ, Evora PR, Schaff HV. Bioassay of EDRF from internal mammary arteries: implications for early and late bypass graft patency. Ann Thorac Surg 1992;54(6):1078–84.

14. Cable DG, O'Brien T, Schaff HV, Pompili VJ. Recombinant endothelial nitric oxide synthase-transduced human saphenous veins: gene therapy to augment nitric oxide production in bypass conduits. Circulation 1997;96(9 Suppl):II-173–8.

15. Cable DG, Caccitolo JA, Caplice N, et al. The role of gene therapy for intimal hyperplasia of bypass grafts. Circulation 1999;100 Suppl 19:II-392–6.

16. Chaux A, Ruan XM, Fishben MC, et al. Perivascular delivery of a nitric oxide donor inhibits neointimal hyperplasia in vein grafts implanted in the arterial circulation. J Thorac Cardiovasc Surg 1998;115(3):604–12.

17. Morishita R, Gibbons GH, Ellison KE, et al. Intimal hyperplasia after vascular injury is inhibited by antisense cdk-2 kinase oligonucleotides. J Clin Invest 1994;93(4):1458–64.

18. Morishita R, Gibbons GH, Ellison KE, et al. Single intraluminal delivery of antisense cdc2 kinase and proliferating-cell nuclear antigen oligonucleotides results in chronic inhibition of neointimal hyperplasia. Proc Natl Acad Sci U S A 1993;90(18):8474–8.

19. Abe J, Zhou W, Taguchi J, et al. Suppression of neointimal smooth muscle cell accumulation in vivo by antisense cdc2 and cdk2 oligonucleotides in rat carotid artery. Biochem Biophys Res Commun 1994;198(1):16–24.

20. Dzau VJ, Mann MJ, Ehsan A, Griese DP. Gene therapy and genomic strategies for cardiovascular surgery: the emerging field of surgiomics. J Thorac Cardiovasc Surg 2001;121(2):206–16.

21. Morishita R, Gibbons GH, Horiuchi M, et al. A gene therapy strategy using a transcription factor decoy of the E2F binding site inhibits smooth muscle proliferation in vivo. Proc Natl Acad Sci U S A 1995;92(13):5855–9.

22. Mann MJ, Whittemore AD, Donaldson MC, et al. Ex vivo gene therapy of human vascular bypass grafts with E2F decoy: the PREVENT single-centre, randomised, controlled trial. Lancet 1999;354(9189):1493–8.

23. Yonemitsu Y, Kaneda Y, Hata Y, et al. Wild-type p53 gene transfer: a novel therapeutic strategy for neointimal hyperplasia after arterial injury [review]. Ann N Y Acad Sci 1997;811:395–400.

24. Chang MW, Barr E, Seltzer J, et al. Cytostatic gene therapy for vascular proliferative disorders with a constitutively active form of the retinoblastoma gene product. Science 1995;267(5197):518–22.

25. Chang MW, Barr E, Lu MM, et al. Adenovirus-mediated overexpression of the cyclin/cyclin-dependent kinase inhibitor, p21 inhibits vascular smooth muscle cell proliferation and neointima formation in the rat carotid artery model of balloon angioplasty. J Clin Invest 1995;96(5):2260-8.

26. Chen D, Krasinski K, Sylvester A, et al. Downregulation of cyclin-dependent kinase 2 activity and cyclin A promoter activity in vascular smooth muscle cells by p27(KIP1), an inhibitor of neointima formation in the rat carotid artery. J Clin Invest 1997;99(10):2334–41.

27. Dunn PF, Newman KD, Jones M, et al. Seeding of vascular grafts with genetically modified endothelial cells. Secretion of recombinant TPA results in decreased seeded cell retention in vitro and in vivo. Circulation 1996;93(7):1439–46.

28. Lundell A, Kelly AB, Anderson J, et al. Reduction in vascular lesion formation by hirudin secreted from retrovirus-transduced confluent endothelial cells on vascular grafts in baboons. Circulation 1999;100(19):2018–24.

29. Qin L, Chavin KD, Ding Y, et al. Gene transfer for transplantation. Prolongation of allograft survival with transforming growth factor-beta 1. Ann Surg 1994;220(4):508–18.

30. Brauner R, Nonoyama M, Laks H, et al. Intracoronary adenovirus-mediated transfer of immunosuppressive cytokine genes prolongs allograft survival [see comments]. J Thorac Cardiovasc Surg 1997;114(6):923–33.

31. David A, Chetritt J, Guillot C, et al. Interleukin-10 produced by recombinant adenovirus prolongs survival of cardiac allografts in rats. Gene Ther 2000;7(6):505–10.

32. Qin L, Chavin KD, Ding Y, et al. Retrovirus-mediated transfer of viral IL-10 gene prolongs murine cardiac allograft survival. J Immunol 1996;156(6):2316–23.

33. DeBruyne LA, Li K, Bishop DK, Bromberg JS. Gene transfer of virally encoded chemokine antagonists vMIP-II and MC148 prolongs cardiac allograft survival and inhibits donor-specific immunity. Gene Ther 2000;7(7):575–82.

34. Jayakumar J, Suzuki K, Khan M, et al. Gene therapy for myocardial protection: transfection of donor hearts with heat shock protein 70 gene protects cardiac function against ischemia-reperfusion injury. Circulation 2000;102(19 Suppl 3):III302–6.

35. Kypson A, Hendrickson S, Akhter S, et al. Adenovirus-mediated gene transfer of the beta2-adrenergic receptor to donor hearts enhances cardiac function. Gene Ther 1999;6(7):1298–304.

36. Sen L, Hong YS, Luo H, et al. Efficiency, efficacy, and adverse effects of adenovirus vs. liposome-mediated gene therapy in cardiac allografts. Am J Physiol Heart Circ Physiol 2001;281(3):H1433–41.

37. Braunberger E, Cohen JL, Boyer O, et al. T-cell suicide gene therapy for organ transplantation: induction of long-lasting tolerance to allogeneic heart without generalized immunosuppression. Mol Ther 2000;2(6):596–601.

38. Geissler EK, Graeb C, Tange S, et al. Effective use of donor MHC class I gene therapy in organ transplantation: prevention of antibody-mediated hyperacute heart allograft rejection in highly sensitized rat recipients. Hum Gene Ther 2000;11(3):459–69.

39. Poston RS, Mann MJ, Hoyt EG, et al. Antisense oligodeoxynucleotides prevent acute cardiac allograft rejection via a novel, nontoxic, highly efficient transfection method. Transplantation 1999;68(6):825–32.

40. Iwata A, Sai S, Moore M, et al. Gene therapy of transplant arteriopathy by liposome-mediated transfection of endothelial nitric oxide synthase. J Heart Lung Transplant 2000;19(11):1017–28.

41. Kawauchi M, Suzuki J, Morishita R, et al. Gene therapy for attenuating cardiac allograft arteriopathy using ex vivo E2F decoy transfection by HVJ-AVE-liposome method in mice and nonhuman primates. Circ Res 2000;87(11):1063–8.

42. Scholl FG, Sen L, Drinkwater DC, et al. Effects of human tissue plasminogen gene transfer on allograft coronary atherosclerosis. J Heart Lung Transplant 2001;20(3):322–9.

43. Isobe M, Suzuki J, Morishita R, et al. Gene therapy for heart transplantation-associated coronary arteriosclerosis. Ann N Y Acad Sci 2000;902:77–83.

44. Tomiyasu K, Oda Y, Nomura M, et al. Direct intra-cardiomuscular transfer of beta2-adrenergic receptor gene augments cardiac output in cardiomyopathic hamsters. Gene Ther 2000;7(24):2087–93.

45. Cross HR, Steenbergen C, Lefkowitz RJ, et al. Overexpression of the cardiac beta(2)-adrenergic receptor and expression of a beta-adrenergic receptor kinase-1 (betaARK1) inhibitor both increase myocardial contractility but have differential effects on susceptibility to ischemic injury. Circ Res 1999;85(11):1077–84.

46. del Monte F, Harding SE, Schmidt U, et al. Restoration of contractile function in isolated cardiomyocytes from failing human hearts by gene transfer of SERCA2a. Circulation 1999;100(23):2308–11.

47. del Monte F, Williams E, Lebeche D, et al. Improvement in survival and cardiac metabolism after gene transfer of sarcoplasmic reticulum Ca(2+)-ATPase in a rat model of heart failure. Circulation 2001;104(12):1424–29.

48. Miyamoto MI, del Monte F, Schmidt U, et al. Adenoviral gene transfer of SERCA2a improves left-ventricular function in aortic-banded rats in transition to heart failure. Proc Natl Acad Sci U S A 2000;97(2):793–8.

49. He H, Meyer M, Martin JL, et al. Effects of mutant and antisense RNA of phospholamban on SR Ca(2+)-ATPase activity and cardiac myocyte contractility. Circulation 1999;100(9):974–80.

50. Sharov VG, Sabbah HN, Shimoyama H, et al. Evidence of cardiocyte apoptosis in myocardium of dogs with chronic heart failure. Am J Pathol 1996;148(1):141–9.

51. Sharov VG, Sabbah HN, Ali AS, et al. Abnormalities of cardiocytes in regions bordering fibrous scars of dogs with heart failure. Int J Cardiol 1997;60(3):273–9.

52. Li Z, Bing OH, Long X, et al. Increased cardiomyocyte apoptosis during the transition to heart failure in the spontaneously hypertensive rat. Am J Physiol 1997;272(5 Pt 2):H2313–9.

53. Narula J, Haider N, Virmani R, et al. Apoptosis in myocytes in end-stage heart failure. N Engl J Med 1996;335(16):1182–9.

54. Kirshenbaum LA, de Moissac D. The bcl-2 gene product prevents programmed cell death of ventricular myocytes. Circulation 1997;96(5):1580–5.

55. Matsui T, Li L, del Monte F, et al. Adenoviral gene transfer of activated phosphatidylinositol 3'-kinase and Akt inhibits apoptosis of hypoxic cardiomyocytes in vitro. Circulation 1999;100(23):2373–9.

56. Verfaillie CM. Stem cell plasticity. Graft 2000;3(6):296–9.

57. McKay R. Stem cells in the central nervous system [review]. Science 1997;276(5309):66–71.

58. Alison M, Sarraf C. Hepatic stem cells [review]. J Hepatol 1998;29(4):676–82.

59. Potten CS. Stem cells in gastrointestinal epithelium: numbers, characteristics and death [review]. Philos Trans R Soc Lond B Biol Sci 1998;353(1370):821–30.

60. Watt FM. Epidermal stem cells: markers, patterning and the control of stem cell fate [review]. Philos Trans R Soc Lond B Biol Sci 1998;353(1370):831–7.

61. Campion DR. The muscle satellite cell: a review. Int Rev Cytol 1984;87:225–51.

62. Marelli D, Desrosiers C, el Alfy M, et al. Cell transplantation for myocardial repair: an experimental approach. Cell Transplant 1992;1(6):383–90.

63. Chiu RC, Zibaitis A, Kao RL. Cellular cardiomyoplasty: myocardial regeneration with satellite cell implantation. Ann Thorac Surg 1995;60(1):12–8.

64. Koh GY, Klug MG, Soonpaa MH, Field LJ. Differentiation and long-term survival of C2C12 myoblast grafts in heart. J Clin Invest 1993;92(3):1548–54.

65. Murry CE, Wiseman RW, Schwartz SM, Hauschka SD. Skeletal myoblast transplantation for repair of myocardial necrosis. J Clin Invest 1996;98(11):2512–23.

66. Robinson SW, Cho PW, Levitsky HI, et al. Arterial delivery of genetically labelled skeletal myoblasts to the murine heart: long-term survival and phenotypic modification of implanted myoblasts. Cell Transplant 1996;5(1):77–91.

67. Taylor DA, Atkins BZ, Hungspreugs P, et al. Regenerating functional myocardium: improved performance after skeletal myoblast transplantation [published erratum appears in Nat Med 1998;4(10):1200]. Nat Med 1998;4(8):929–33.

68. Taylor DA, Silvestry SC, Bishop SP, et al. Delivery of primary autologous skeletal myoblasts into rabbit heart by coronary infusion: a potential approach to myocardial repair. Proc Assoc Am Physician 1997;109(3):245–53.

69. Reinecke H, Murry CE. Transmural replacement of myocardium after skeletal myoblast grafting into the heart. Too much of a good thing? Cardiovasc Pathol 2000;9(6):337–44.

70. Thomson JA, Kalishman J, Golos TG, et al. Isolation of a primate embryonic stem cell line. Proc Natl Acad Sci U S A 1995;92(17):7844–8.

71. Thomson JA, Itskovitz-Eldor J, Shapiro SS, et al. Embryonic stem cell lines derived from human blastocysts [published erratum appears in Science 1998;282(5395):1827]. Science 1998;282(5391):1145–7.

72. Shamblott MJ, Axelman J, Wang S, et al. Derivation of pluripotent stem cells from cultured human primordial germ cells [published erratum appears in Proc Natl Acad Sci U S A 1999;96(3):1162]. Proc Natl Acad Sci U S A 1998; 95(23):13726–31.

73. Sanchez A, Jones WK, Gulick J, et al. Myosin heavy chain gene expression in mouse embryoid bodies. An in vitro developmental study. J Biol Chem 1991;266(33):22419–26.

74. Muthuchamy M, Pajak L, Howles P, et al. Developmental analysis of tropomyosin gene expression in embryonic stem cells and mouse embryos. Mol Cell Biol 1993;13(6):3311–23.

75. Miller-Hance WC, LaCorbiere M, Fuller SJ, et al. In vitro chamber specification during embryonic stem cell cardiogenesis. Expression of the ventricular myosin light chain-2 gene is independent of heart tube formation. J Biol Chem 1993;268(33):25244–52.

76. Ganim JR, Luo W, Ponniah S, et al. Mouse phospholamban gene expression during development in vivo and in vitro. Circ Res 1992;71(5):1021–30.

77. Boer PH. Activation of the gene for type-b natriuretic factor in mouse stem cell cultures induced for cardiac myogenesis. Biochem Biophys Res Commun 1994;199(2):954–61.

78. Metzger JM, Lin WI, Samuelson LC. Transition in cardiac contractile sensitivity to calcium during the in vitro differentiation of mouse embryonic stem cells. J Cell Biol 1994;126(3):701–11.

79. Williams RL, Hilton DJ, Pease S, et al. Myeloid leukaemia inhibitory factor maintains the developmental potential of embryonic stem cells. Nature 1988;336(6200):684–7.

80. Klug MG, Soonpaa MH, Koh GY, Field LJ. Genetically selected cardiomyocytes from differentiating embryonic stem cells form stable intracardiac grafts. J Clin Invest 1996; 98(1):216–24.

81. Wobus AM, Kaomei G, Shan J, et al. Retinoic acid accelerates embryonic stem cell-derived cardiac differentiation and enhances development of ventricular cardiomyocytes. J Mol Cell Cardiol 1997;29(6):1525–39.

82. Wobus AM, Holzhausen H, Jakel P, Schoneich J. Characterization of a pluripotent stem cell line derived from a mouse embryo. Exp Cell Res 1984;152(1):212–9.

83. Friedenstein AJ, Chailakhjan RK, Lalykina KS. The development of fibroblast colonies in monolayer cultures of guinea-pig bone marrow and spleen cells. Cell Tissue Kinetics 1970;3(4):393–403.

84. Friedenstein AJ, Piatetzky-Shapiro II, Petrakova KV. Osteogenesis in transplants of bone marrow cells. J Embyol Exp Morphol 1966;16(3):381–90.

85. Prockop DJ. Marrow stromal cells as stem cells for nonhematopoietic tissues [review]. Science 1997;276(5309): 71–4.

86. Wakitani S, Saito T, Caplan AI. Myogenic cells derived from rat bone marrow mesenchymal stem cells exposed to 5-azacytidine. Muscle Nerve 1995;18(12):1417–26.

87. Pittenger MF, Mackay AM, Beck SC, et al. Multilineage potential of adult human mesenchymal stem cells. Science 1999;284(5411):143–7.

88. Theise ND, Badve S, Saxena R, et al. Derivation of hepatocytes from bone marrow cells in mice after radiation-induced myeloablation. Hepatology 2000;31(1):235–40.

89. Theise ND, Nimmakayalu M, Gardner R, et al. Liver from bone marrow in humans. Hepatology 2000;32(1):11–6.

90. Kopen GC, Prockop DJ, Phinney DG. Marrow stromal cells migrate throughout forebrain and cerebellum, and they differentiate into astrocytes after injection into neonatal mouse brains. Proc Natl Acad Sci U S A 1999;96(19): 10711–6.

91. Reyes M, Verfaillie CM. Characterization of multipotent adult progenitor cells, a subpopulation of mesenchymal stem cells. Ann N Y Acad Sci 2001;938:231–3.

92. Al-Khaldi A. VEGF-dependent angiogenic response induced by ex vivo cultured marrow stromal cells. Circulation 2001;104(17 Suppl II)II:123.

93. Wang JS, Shum-Tim D, Galipeau J, et al. Marrow stromal cells for cellular cardiomyoplasty: feasibility and potential clinical advantages. J Thorac Cardiovasc Surg 2000;120(5): 999–1005.

94. Makino S, Fukuda K, Miyoshi S, et al. Cardiomyocytes can be generated from marrow stromal cells in vitro. J Clin Invest 1999;103(5):697–705.

95. Colter DC, Class R, DiGirolamo CM, Prockop DJ. Rapid expansion of recycling stem cells in cultures of plastic-adherent cells from human bone marrow. Proc Natl Acad Sci U S A 2000;97(7):3213–8.

96. Haynesworth SE, Baber MA, Caplan AI. Cell surface antigens on human marrow-derived mesenchymal cells are detected by monoclonal antibodies. Bone 1992;13(1): 69–80.

97. Owen M. Stromal stem cells: marrow-derived osteogenic precursor. Ciba Found Symp 1988;136:42–60.

98. Orlic D, Kajstura J, Chimenti S, et al. Bone marrow cells regenerate infarcted myocardium. Nature 2001;410 (6829):701–5.

99. Orlic D, Kajstura J, Chimenti S, et al. Mobilized bone marrow cells repair the infarcted heart, improving function and survival. Proc Natl Acad Sci U S A 2001;98(18):10344–9.

100. Hamano K. Preliminary result of clinical trial of therapeutic angiogenesis achieved by the implantation of self bone marrow cells for ischemic heart disease. Circulation 2001;104(17 Suppl II)II:69.

101. Asahara T. Stem cell therapy and gene transfer for regeneration. Gene Ther 2000;7:451–7.

102. Chiu RCJ. Therapeutic cardiac angiogenesis and myogenesis: the promises and challenges on a new frontier [editorial]. J Thorac Cardiovasc Surg 2001;122:851–6.

103. Losordo DW, Vale PR, Symes JF, et al. Gene therapy for myocardial angiogenesis: initial clinical results with direct myocardial injection of phVEGF165 as sole therapy for myocardial ischemia. Circulation 1998;98(25):2800–4.

104. Rosengart TK, Lee LY, Patel SR, et al. Angiogenesis gene therapy: phase I assessment of direct intramyocardial administration of an adenovirus vector expressing VEGF121 cDNA to individuals with clinically significant severe coronary artery disease. Circulation 1999;100(5):468–74.

105. Symes JF, Losordo DW, Vale PR, et al. Gene therapy with vascular endothelial growth factor for inoperable coronary artery disease. Ann Thorac Surg 1999;68(3):830–6.

106. Laitinen M, Hartikainen J, Hiltunen MO, et al. Catheter-mediated vascular endothelial growth factor gene transfer to human coronary arteries after angioplasty. Hum Gene Ther 2000;11(2):263–70.

107. Vale PR, Losordo DW, Milliken CE, et al. Left ventricular electromechanical mapping to assess efficacy of phVEGF(165) gene transfer for therapeutic angiogenesis in chronic myocardial ischemia. Circulation 2000;102 (9):965–74.

108. Vale PR, Losordo DW, Milliken CE, et al. Randomized, single-blind, placebo-controlled pilot study of catheter-based myocardial gene transfer for therapeutic angiogenesis using left ventricular electromechanical mapping in patients with chronic myocardial ischemia. Circulation 2001;103(17):2138–43.

109. Sylven C, Sarkar N, Ruck A, et al. Myocardial Doppler tissue velocity improves following myocardial gene therapy with VEGF-A(165) plasmid in patients with inoperable angina pectoris. Coron Artery Dis 2001;12(3):239–43.

INDEX

Page numbers followed by f indicate figure; those followed by t indicate table.